Mackie & McCartney
Practical Medical Microbiology

Mackie & McCartney

Practical Medical Microbiology

EDITED BY

J. G. Collee MD(Edin) FRCPath FRCP(Edin)
Robert Irvine Professor of Bacteriology, University of Edinburgh;
Consultant in Bacteriology, Lothian Health Board;
Consultant Adviser in Microbiology, Scottish Home and Health Department

J. P. Duguid CBE MD(Edin) BSc FRCPath
Honorary Member of the Pathological Society of Great Britain and Ireland;
Emeritus Professor of Bacteriology, University of Dundee.
Formerly Reader in Bacteriology, University of Edinburgh;
Consultant in Bacteriology, Tayside Health Board; and
Consultant Adviser in Microbiology, Scottish Home and Health Department

A. G. Fraser MD(Edin) BSc
Senior Lecturer in Bacteriology, University of Edinburgh;
Consultant in Bacteriology, Royal Infirmary, Edinburgh

B. P. Marmion DSc MD(Lond) FRCPath (UK and Aust) FRCP(Edin) FRACP FRS(E)
Visiting Professor, Department of Pathology, University of Adelaide.
Formerly Director, Division of Medical Virology, Institute of Medical and Veterinary Science, Adelaide; and
Robert Irvine Professor of Bacteriology, University of Edinburgh

THIRTEENTH EDITION

Volume 2 of Medical Microbiology

CHURCHILL LIVINGSTONE
EDINBURGH LONDON MELBOURNE AND NEW YORK 1989

CHURCHILL LIVINGSTONE
Medical Division of Longman Group UK Limited

Distributed in the United States of America by Churchill
Livingstone Inc., 1560 Broadway, New York, N.Y. 10036,
and by associated companies, branches and representatives
throughout the world.

First edition (Introduction to Practical Bacteriology) 1925
Second edition 1928
Third edition 1931
Fourth edition 1934
Fifth edition 1938
Sixth edition 1942
Seventh edition 1945
Eighth edition 1948
Ninth edition (Handbook of Practical Bacteriology) 1953
Tenth edition 1960
Eleventh edition 1965
Twelfth edition (The Practice of Medical Microbiology,
Vol 2) 1975
Thirteenth edition (Practical Medical Microbiology) 1989

ISBN 0-443-02332-8

British Library Cataloguing in Publication Data
Mackie, T. J. (Thomas Jones), *1888–1955*
   Mackie & McCartney practical medical
microbiology. – 13th ed.
   1. Medicine. Microbiology
   I. Title. II. McCartney, J. E. (James Elviris), *1891–1969*
III. Collee, J. G. (John Gerald) IV. Mackie, T. J.
(Thomas Jones), *1888–1955*. Medical microbiology.
616'.01

Library of Congress Cataloging-in-Publication Data
(Revised for vol. 2)

Mackie, T. J. (Thomas Jones), 1888–1955.
   Mackie & McCartney medical microbiology.

   Rev. ed. of: Mackie & McCartney's Handbook of
bacteriology. 10th ed. 1960.
   Vol. 2 has title: Mackie & McCartney practical
medical microbiology.
   Contents: v. 1. Microbial infections. – v. 2.
[without special title]
   1. Medical microbiology.   I. McCartney, J. E.
(James Elvins), 1891–   . II. Duguid, J. P.
III. Marmion, B. P. IV. Swain, R. H. A.
(Richard Henry Austin) V. Mackie, T. J. (Thomas Jones),
1888–1955. Handbook of bacteriology. VI. Title.
VII. Title: Medical microbiology.
QR46.M35   1978   616'.01   84-123393

Produced by Longman Group (FE) Ltd
Printed in Hong Kong

Preface

The main purpose of the first edition of the *Introduction to Practical Bacteriology* by Professor T. J. Mackie and Dr J. E. McCartney from the Department of Bacteriology, University of Edinburgh, in 1925, was to give details of methods and the identifying characters of bacteria useful to those engaged in the practice of clinical bacteriology. The original authors carried the book through nine editions, the last being published as the *Handbook of Practical Bacteriology* in 1953.

After the death of Professor Mackie in 1955 and the retirement of Dr McCartney, the editorship was assumed by Mackie's successor in Edinburgh, Professor Robert Cruickshank, who sought to extend the book's value to doctors and students of medicine by increasing its content of clinical, epidemiological and basic microbiological material. This widening of scope and the rise of virology was recognized in the renaming of the eleventh edition as *Medical Microbiology* when it appeared in 1965. With Professor Cruickshank's retirement in 1966 and the appointment of Professor Barrie Marmion to head the Edinburgh Department in 1968, a group of editors and contributors in the Edinburgh and Dundee Departments, with the continuing guidance of Professor Cruickshank, brought on the twelfth edition in two volumes. Volume 1 (1973) contained information of interest to doctors and students and Volume 2 (1975) held technical information useful to the laboratory worker. The editorial contributions of the late Dr R. H. A. Swain to this enterprise are recalled with gratitude.

When the thirteenth edition of Volume 1 was published in 1978 the names of the original editors, Mackie & McCartney, were restored to emphasize continuity with the first nine editions of the book. The present book stands for Volume 2 of the thirteenth edition. But the growth of information and technology has been so great in recent years, and the purposes of the two volumes have so greatly diverged, that this book has been renamed *Practical Medical Microbiology*. It is intended to stand on its own, serving the needs of clinical laboratory workers, as did the first nine editions of Mackie & McCartney.

Advances in technology have provided the microbiologist with such a variety of methods, reagents, equipment and laboratory strategies that we have been forced to be selective. We have described in detail the methods we think likely to be the most useful, with references to alternatives, but it is inevitable that we will have omitted mention of some methods considered valuable by other workers. An important development has been the increased availability from commercial sources of new complex equipment and reagent kits for the rapid performance of biochemical and immunological tests that provide diagnostic information previously unavailable or obtained only by methods too costly in time and labour to be generally applicable. The variety of equipment and kits is too great for us to assess their relative merits from personal experience or to give detailed instructions on their use; the manufacturer's instructions should be consulted. In various chapters and in Appendix 3, we list some sources of supply to assist the laboratory worker. However, a listing does not imply either an endorsement of quality or that the item listed is the only brand available.

Today's wide variety of diagnostic approaches has imposed on clinical microbiologists the major task of selecting the procedures, equipment and strategies most appropriate to the needs of their work. In Chapter 1 we discuss the general problems of organizing a clinical microbiology service. In Chapter 39 we give recommended strategies for the bacteriological examination of the different kinds of clinical specimens and the diagnosis of the different infective syndromes.

With regard to clinical virology, we have not attempted to produce a systematic account of the full range of procedures that would be necessary for a reference virus laboratory. As explained in Chapter 47, we have given details of tests that might be used by the virological section of a general clinical microbiological laboratory. A broad approach has been adopted with advice on effective procedures for direct virus diagnosis (Chapter 48) and serological tests (Chapter 49), as technical advances are widening the scope of the general microbiological laboratory in the prompt and accurate diagnosis of virus infections. We have restricted information on cell and virus culture (Chapter 50) to a few examples that are likely to be relevant in this context.

Some changes of format have been introduced in the present edition. Formerly, the details of technical methods were confined to early chapters, and information about identifying characters was given in later chapters dealing separately with the different groups of microorganisms. In this book, generally applicable methods are still described in the early chapters, 1–15. But more and more, now, different specialized methods are developed for the isolation and identification of particular organisms only, and we have found it convenient to transfer the descriptions of these specialized techniques to a *Methods* section at the end of the chapter on the organisms to which they apply. References in the text of a chapter to the methods given in its *Methods* section are indicated by an asterisk(*).

Abbreviations and conversion factors for measurement units used in microbiology are given in Appendix 1 at the end of the book. Postal regulations relating to pathological specimens and cultures are outlined in Appendix 2. Manufacturers and suppliers of equipment and reagents are identified by key words in the text throughout the book and their addresses are given in Appendix 3. We are very grateful to Mr William Marr for much work in compiling this list.

The official names of antibiotics and other drugs are used throughout the book, for these are the names that should be employed by the laboratory. However, the proprietary names of drugs are often used by staff and patients in clinics and hospital wards, so that it is useful for bacteriologists to have at hand a list showing the equivalence of official and proprietary names. As different proprietary names are current in different countries a national list should be obtained and bacteriologists in Britain are advised to use the British National Formulary.

We have made a change in nomenclature following the example of the seventh edition of Topley & Wilson's *Principles of Bacteriology, Virology and Immunity* by abandoning the double *i* genitive ending in the specific epithets of species binomials, e.g. substituting *Corynebacterium hofmanni* for *C. hofmannii*. The editors have also prevailed upon the authors of the chapters dealing with fungi and protozoa to conform to the convention in this book. The primary aim of nomenclature should be its usefulness to laboratory workers and there is no doubt that the need to remember which epithets require the double, and which the single *i* ending, has been burdensome. The use of nominative epithets, as in *Salmonella london*, has much to recommend it. Our decision to change to the single *i* ending was made at a time when it was understood that the International Committee on Bacterial Nomenclature and Taxonomy was likely to recommend the change, though in the event it did not do so. Readers wishing to use the traditional forms should substitute *ii* for the single *i* ending in all specific epithets derived from proper names except those ending in *r*, e.g. *Proteus rettgeri*.

We regret the frequent changes made by academic taxonomists in the names of bacterial species. Names often have to be changed to reflect changes in classification necessitated by new discoveries, but it seems undesirable that epithets in predominant use should be changed merely to satisfy the niceties of legitimacy or priority. Such changes are upsetting to the practical microbiologist and confusing to the clinician. In this edition, nevertheless, we have had to bow to the trend of usage and substitute *Clostridium perfringens* for *C. welchi* and *Pseudomonas aeruginosa* for *P. pyocyanea*.

The names of the sole or main contributor(s) to each chapter are given under its title, but many chapters contain some material suggested by other members of the team of editors and contributors, so that the designated author of a chapter is not necessarily responsible for all the views expressed in it.

Our thanks are due to many colleagues in many places for information, comments, suggestions and advice. We are particularly indebted to Mrs Joan Collins in Edinburgh and Mrs Julie Maylin in Adelaide, and their colleagues, for so much secretarial help, and to our publishers for their forbearance.

The Editors, 1989

CONVENTIONS FOR TABLES

An attempt has been made to standardize the use of symbols in tables throughout this book; exceptions are detailed in the table footnotes or key. The time of incubation for biochemical tests may be assumed to be 24 h unless otherwise specified in the footnotes or in the text of the appropriate chapter. In general, the following symbols are used:

+ = most strains positive (usually 90% or more)
− = most strains negative (usually 90% or more)
+/− = some strains positive, some negative
± = most strains weak positive
. . . = result not given

Contributors

Robert Brown FIMLS MIBiol
Chief Medical Laboratory Scientific Officer,
Department of Bacteriology, University of
Edinburgh Medical School, UK

Christopher J. Burrell BSc(Med) MB BS PhD
MRCPath FRCPA
Director of Division of Medical Virology,
Institute of Medical and Veterinary Science,
Adelaide; Clinical Professor of Virology,
University of Adelaide, Australia

Joyce D. Coghlan BSc PhD
Formerly Director, Leptospira Reference
Laboratory, PHLS, Colindale, London;
Formerly Lecturer in Bacteriology, University
of Edinburgh Medical School, UK

J. Gerald Collee MD FRCPath FRCP (Edin)
Professor and Head, Department of
Bacteriology, University of Edinburgh Medical
School; Chief Bacteriologist, Royal Infirmary
of Edinburgh; Consultant Adviser in
Microbiology, Scottish Home and Health
Department, Edinburgh, UK

James P. Duguid CBE MD BSc FRCPath
Emeritus Professor of Bacteriology, University
of Dundee, UK; Formerly Reader in
Bacteriology, University of Edinburgh Medical
School, UK

Ronald J. Fallon BSc MD FRCPath FRCP
(Glas)
Consultant in Laboratory Medicine, Ruchill
Hospital; Honorary Clinical Lecturer in
Bacteriology and Immunology, Department of
Infectious Diseases, University of Glasgow, UK

Ian D. Farrell PhD MRCPath
Top Grade Microbiologist, Regional Public
Health Laboratory, East Birmingham Hospital,
UK

Andrew G. Fraser MD BSc
Senior Lecturer, Department of Bacteriology,
University of Edinburgh Medical School;
Honorary Consultant Bacteriologist, Royal
Infirmary of Edinburgh, UK

John R. W. Govan BSc PhD
Senior Lecturer, Department of Bacteriology,
University of Edinburgh Medical School, UK

Doris M. Graham PhD
Senior Lecturer, Department of Microbiology,
University of Melbourne, Australia

David M. Green MD FRCPath
Formerly Senior Lecturer, Department of
Bacteriology, University of Dundee, UK

Norman R. Grist BSc MB ChB FRCP (Edin &
Glas) FRCPath
Emeritus Professor of Infectious Diseases,
University of Glasgow, UK

W. John Herbert MRCVS DTVM (Edin) PhD
Formerly Director of Animal Services,
University of Dundee, UK

Ian Jack MSc
Head, Virus Laboratories, Royal Children's
Hospital, Melbourne, Australia

Matthew Laidlaw MB ChB
Formerly Consultant Bacteriologist, Southern
General Hospital, Glasgow; Consultant
Bacteriologist, Mycobacteria Reference
Laboratory, Glasgow, UK

W. H. Russell Lumsden MD DSc FRCP (Edin)
FRS(E) UK
Senior Research Fellow, Department of
Genitourinary Medicine, University of
Edinburgh, UK

Barbara Magee BA
Department of Biochemistry, University of
Adelaide, Australia

Barrie P. Marmion DSc MD FRCPath (UK
and Aust) FRACP FRCP (Edin) FRS(E)
Visiting Professor, Department of Pathology,
University of Adelaide, Australia; Formerly
Professor of Bacteriology, University of
Edinburgh Medical School, UK

William Marr FIMLS MIBiol
Senior Chief Medical Laboratory Scientific
Officer, Department of Bacteriology,
University of Edinburgh Medical School, UK

Alexander McMillan MD FRCP (Edin)
Consultant Physician and Part-time Senior
Lecturer, Department of Genitourinary
Medicine, University of Edinburgh Medical
School, UK

Rex Stafford Miles MB ChB FRCPath
Senior Lecturer, Department of Bacteriology,
University of Edinburgh Medical School;
Honorary Consultant Bacteriologist, Lothian
Health Board, Edinburgh, UK

Leslie J. R. Milne BSc PhD
Top Grade Mycologist, Mycology Unit, Central
Microbiological Laboratory, Western General
Hospital, Edinburgh, UK

Brian Moore BSc
Formerly Chief Hospital Scientist, Division of
Medical Virology, Institute of Medical and
Veterinary Science, Adelaide, Australia

Richard A. Ormsbee MSc PhD
Formerly Scientific Director, US Public Health
Service, Rocky Mountain Laboratory, NIAID
Hamilton, Montana, USA

David Parratt MD MRCPath
Senior Lecturer, Department of Medical
Microbiology, University of Dundee; Honorary
Consultant, Tayside Health Board, Dundee,
UK

Ian A. Porter MD FRCPath
Former Consultant in Administrative Charge,
Regional Laboratory, City Hospital, Aberdeen;
Honorary Clinical Senior Lecturer, Department
of Bacteriology, University of Aberdeen, UK

Ian R. Poxton BSc PhD
Lecturer, Department of Bacteriology,
University of Edinburgh Medical School, UK

Philip W. Ross TD MD MRCPath MRCP
(Edin) MIBiol
Senior Lecturer, Department of Bacteriology,
University of Edinburgh Medical School;
Honorary Consultant Bacteriologist, Royal
Infirmary of Edinburgh, UK

A. C. Scott MD FRCPath
Consultant Bacteriologist, Central
Microbiological Laboratories, Western General
Hospital, Edinburgh; Formerly Senior Lecturer
in Medical Microbiology, University of
Dundee; Honorary Consultant Bacteriologist,
Tayside Health Board, UK

Sheila S. Scott MB ChB
Lecturer, Department of Medical Microbiology,
University of Dundee, UK

Bernard W. Senior BSc PhD
Lecturer, Department of Medical Microbiology,
University of Dundee, UK

Frank Sheffield MB ChB
Pathologist, The David Bruce Laboratories,
East Everleigh, Wiltshire, UK

A. Simmons MA MB BChir PhD MRCPath
Medical Specialist (Virology), Division of
Medical Virology, Institute of Medical and
Veterinary Science, Adelaide, Australia

J. Douglas Sleigh MB ChB FRCPath FRCP
(Glas)
Reader in Bacteriology, University of Glasgow;
Honorary Consultant Bacteriologist, Royal
Infirmary of Glasgow, UK

Donald M. Weir MD FRCP (Edin)
Personal Professor of Microbial Immunology,
University of Edinburgh Medical School;
Honorary Consultant, Lothian Health Board,
Edinburgh, UK

Allan B. White MB BS FRCPath DipBact
Consultant Microbiologist, Highland Health
Board, Inverness, UK

John F. Wilkinson MA PhD
Professor of Microbiology, School of
Agriculture, University of Edinburgh, UK

David Worswick BSc (Hons)
Principal Hospital Scientist, Division of
Medical Virology, Institute of Medical and
Veterinary Science, Adelaide, Australia

Contents

Organization of the clinical bacteriology laboratory

FUNCTION

The main work of a clinical bacteriology laboratory is to examine specimens from patients for the presence of potentially pathogenic micro-organisms, to detect antibodies to such organisms, to determine the sensitivities of infecting organisms to antimicrobial drugs, and to assess the infective potential of environmental materials. The purpose is quickly and economically to obtain information that will help clinicians to treat their patients or public health officers to prevent the spread of infection in the community. It is to serve the needs of clinical and preventive medicine, rather than the advancement of microbiological science. But subject to these priorities, there is also an obligation to record and investigate new facts encountered in the course of the work.

As most laboratory staff have been trained in microbiology as a science, and many of them also in research, they may tend to regard the examination of a specimen as a research exercise and seek to obtain results with the degrees of precision and certainty required in research, but a patient's interest is generally better served by an early report of the provisional identification of a potential pathogen, and its probable antibiotic sensitivities, than by a delayed report with a precise and confirmed identification. Infections can progress very rapidly, so that speed of reporting is often more important than absolute certainty of the finding. In particular circumstances, however, detailed identification of an infecting organism may be required as a guide to clinical management or as a help in epidemiological tracing.

The principal problems of organizing a bacteriological service are determining the choice and sequence of tests to be applied to each category of specimen, how far the search for pathogens should be pressed, how far isolates should be characterized, the proper balance between economy of labour, speed of reporting and precision of results, what patterns of nomenclature and phrasing should be used in reports, and what new methods should be introduced to exploit advances in medicine and science.

The service should be provided economically and the work should be cost-effective. Labour and resources should not be wasted in gathering information unneeded by the clinician or health officer just because it may be of interest to the microbiologist. Laboratory staff should not be overloaded by the requirement to undertake unnecessary procedures, lest their enforced hurry should cause them to make mistakes in the essential investigations. If there are sufficient resources, some applied research can and should be done on the materials received in a clinical laboratory, but the projects should be carefully planned, with defined objectives, and should generally be done prospectively, and separately from the routine diagnostic work. The quality of the information about patients ordinarily received in the laboratory and the degree of precision of the methods appropriate to clinical needs are likely to be inadequate for the purposes of retrospective research. Thus, a research project loosely based on routine diagnostic work on to which some extra investigations have been grafted is unlikely to yield worthwhile results.

In addition to their main task of providing helpful reports on submitted specimens, the staff of the laboratory have other duties. They should take steps to inform all potential users of the service about the range of investigations available, the supply of specimen containers, the procedures for collecting specimens and the arrangements for transmitting them to the laboratory. They should also be prepared to answer requests for advice on the type of investigations that might be helpful in the diagnosis of particular cases and on the interpretation and significance of findings. They should identify findings that require urgent referral, e.g. by telephone, to the clinician or health officer and they should be prepared to give advice on antibiotic treatment and preventive measures when the recipient of a report may fail to draw the proper conclusions. Other duties of senior staff include the formulation of advice on the investigation of outbreaks of infection, preventive measures to be taken in such outbreaks, procedures for the control of hospital infections and procedures for the sterilization and disinfection of surgical and medical equipment. They should also take part in the in-service education of various categories of health service staff in matters relating to the occurrence, diagnosis and prevention of infection.

STAFFING

The staffing of a clinical bacteriology laboratory will vary with the kind and extent of the clinical and preventive services it supports and the availability of finance and accommodation. In Britain, a microbiology laboratory serving the needs of the hospitals, public health authorities and family doctors of a population of about 250 000 will commonly receive about 150 000 specimens a year. Its staff may ideally include three senior, 'career-grade' graduates, e.g. two trained in medicine and microbiological science (Consultant) and one non-medically-qualified scientist trained in microbiological research (Top-grade or Principal-grade scientist). There should also be one or two medical or science graduates in the training grades that lead to the senior posts. The largest group of staff, e.g. about 20, will be 'technicians' (Medical Labora-

tory Scientific Officers) with either university degrees in science or technical college qualifications. These MLSOs might include a Senior Chief MLSO, in charge of the technical staff, 3–5 Chief or Senior MLSOs, 10 qualified Basic-grade MLSOs and perhaps about 5 Junior MLSOs in training. There will also be a number, e.g. 5–7, of laboratory aides, cleaners, porters and glassware cleaners, and about 4–5 clerical staff who type, issue and file copies of reports.

Medically qualified staff have a special role in organizing the laboratory work in the way best adapted to serve the needs of clinical and preventive medicine, in determining the kinds of examinations to be made on particular specimens and in deciding the content of reports. They are also qualified to give advice on the interpretation of results and on problems of diagnosis, prevention and treatment, and to appreciate the implications of advances in medicine for the kind of investigations the laboratory should be prepared to undertake.

Research-trained scientists have a special role in introducing and evaluating new tests and procedures, and in establishing systems of internal quality control. They are qualified by their training, their familiarity with current literature and their habit of communication with other scientists to appreciate the implications of advances in science for laboratory technology.

Technical staff carry out most of the procedures at the laboratory bench. They become highly proficient in these procedures and experienced in the most efficient way of organizing work at the bench. Senior technical staff have a major responsibility for day-to-day control of the work of technical staff, and for their recruitment, training and discipline. They generally also have a responsibility for the maintenance of equipment, laboratory safety and the ordering and control of supplies.

Whilst the greatest use should be made of the special skills of each category of staff, there should be no unnecessary, rigid demarcation of their duties. As far as practicable, staff in the different categories should work side by side and learn as much as possible of each other's skills and knowledge. Thus, medically qualified staff should not confine themselves to reporting and advisory duties, but should become technically proficient in the common bench procedures so as to gain a full understanding of relevant scientific, training and management issues. Scientific and technical staff should acquire from their medically qualified colleagues as great as possible an understanding of the medical relevance of their work, so that when medically qualified staff are absent, they may undertake reporting and advisory duties within the agreed limits of their competence. Flexibility, cooperation and goodwill among the different categories of staff are essential for the efficient performance of work in a clinical laboratory.

MANAGEMENT

In Britain recently there has been controversy about the form of management of clinical laboratories, whether there should be an appointed director of the laboratory or a consensus management by a laboratory committee representing all categories of staff, and whether, if there is a director, he should be medically, scientifically or technically qualified.

Traditionally, a director of the laboratory has been appointed by the employing health authority and made responsible for all aspects of the running of the laboratory, including standards of performance, expenditure and control of staff. Though formerly such appointments were permanent, employers may now retain the right to transfer the headship from time to time. As the running of a clinical laboratory requires the making of many immediate decisions, management by a committee seems wholly inappropriate. There should be a director who can make decisions without delay. He should, however, determine his policies after wide and frequent consultation with senior members of the different categories of staff, taking advantage of the special skills and experience of each, and those consulted should be assured that their expert views and advice are effectively taken into account. A laboratory committee may usefully serve as a means of consultation, but the director

should have the responsibility for making the final decisions.

The day-to-day management of a clinical laboratory includes much that the director can delegate to other senior staff. Generally, he should delegate to the head of the technical staff most of the managerial work relating to the allocation of duties to technical staff, the recruitment, training and discipline of technical staff, laboratory safety, the maintenance of equipment and buildings, and the ordering of supplies. Similarly, he may delegate responsibility for supervising the quality control of test procedures to a senior member of the scientific staff.

The key area of managerial decisions, to which the director must give the greatest personal attention, concerns the strategy and organization of the service. He has to decide how the work is to be deployed among the different sections of the laboratory, the duties to be undertaken by the different categories of staff, the kinds and sequences of examinations to be done on the different categories of specimens, the arrangements for determining the content and wording of reports, and the arrangements for reporting urgent results and proffering advice to clinicians. He must also decide when new methods are to be introduced and old ones discarded.

As such decisions require a balanced assessment of clinical usefulness, scientific reliability and economy of resources, and an understanding of continuing advances in medicine and science, it is preferable that the person appointed to direct a laboratory should be qualified in both medicine and microbiology, and trained in the methods and practice of scientific research. If no one with this combination of qualifications is available, the person appointed as director must be supported by advice from staff and other colleagues having the special knowledge and experience he lacks.

ELEMENTS OF THE SERVICE

Guidance to users

The laboratory should issue guidance to potential users of the service in a leaflet or booklet distributed to hospital units, medical staff, family doctors and environmental health officers. This leaflet should give the address and telephone number of the laboratory, the times for the normal receipt of specimens and the arrangements for the emergency 'call-out' of staff out of hours and the supply of specimen containers and request forms. It should also outline the range of examinations undertaken in the laboratory and describe the correct procedures for collecting each kind of specimen from the patients and for sending specimens to the laboratory, including the safety precautions to be observed with specimens likely to contain specially dangerous pathogens.

Delivery of specimens

There must be clearly defined arrangements for the collection of specimens from users of the service and their safe delivery to the laboratory. Collection and delivery are usually done by the portering service within the hospital in which the laboratory is located, and by a special van service from other hospitals, clinics and general-practice health centres. Suitable trays or boxes should be provided for safe transport of the specimen containers. If specimens are to be delivered to the laboratory by mail, the postal regulations specifying the types of container and packaging must be observed (see Appendix 2).

Request forms

Request forms should be designed in such a way as to require the clinician to give all the information that may be needed by the laboratory staff to enable them to determine what kind of examinations to make on each specimen and to assist them in interpreting the findings. The form should have indicated spaces for information about the nature and source of the specimen, the type of examination requested, the patient's name, age, sex, address, occupation and recent foreign travel, the hospital unit, and the signature, address and telephone number of the requesting physician.

Clinicians often request examinations in imprecise terms, such as 'culture and sensitivity'

or 'pathogens please'. The microbiologist therefore needs to be given some information about the patient's clinical condition or the clinician's provisional diagnosis to enable him to decide the range of pathogens for which he should search. The request form should ask for this information. Details of any current antibiotic therapy should also be required, for it may help the microbiologist to interpret the results of culture and to select antibiotics for sensitivity tests.

Many laboratories use the request form as a work sheet at the bench, so that the worker can be guided by its information in his choice of tests, interpretation of results and wording of reports. For this purpose, the request form should have a space reserved for the record of the laboratory work and it may be advantageous to have request forms submitted in duplicate so that one copy can be used at the bench and the other kept fair.

Reception of specimens

For safety, the reception of specimens should be undertaken in a room separate from the reporting office and the working laboratories. The work should be done by staff trained in the appropriate safety precautions and the procedure for dealing with leaking specimens. The specimens are unpacked and 'booked in'. The latter process is the recording of information about the patient and specimen. It is generally done by writing in a reception book the patient's name and the kind, place of collection and date of arrival of the specimen. A laboratory serial number is allotted to each specimen and triplicates of it are affixed to the specimen container, the request form and the entry in the reception book. The reception record is required when questions arise about the arrival or non-arrival of specimens, or the stage of their examination when reports are delayed. After being booked-in, the specimens, with their request forms or entries on a work sheet, are distributed to the sections of the laboratory in which they are to be examined. Where records are computerized, the booking-in is done by entry of the patient and specimen information into a computer file and most or all of the information on the request form may be thus recorded. The computer may then be used to prepare work sheets.

Sections of the laboratory

Because the specimens received each day are so numerous, they are normally divided among different groups of staff working in different rooms. Usually one or other of two methods of division, or a combination of the methods, is used. By the first method, all specimens of all kinds received from a particular user group, e.g. a limited number of clinics, hospital wards or general practices, are allocated to a given group or section. The advantages of this method are that staff have the continuous experience of dealing with all kinds of specimens and are helped to correlate the results for different kinds of specimen received from the same patient. Job satisfaction from the varied work and the ability to tailor examinations and interpretations to the needs of individual patients are features of this approach.

By the second method, all specimens of particular kinds are allocated to sections specializing in the examination of these kinds of specimen. Thus, all specimens of urine might be allocated to one section, all specimens of faeces to another, all specimens of pus, exudates and cerebrospinal fluid to a third, all serological specimens to a fourth, and so on. This method of division has great advantages for speed of working, economy of labour and reliability of results. The staff of the section acquire special dexterity in the relevant procedures for their kinds of specimens; they are undistracted by the need to alter procedures from specimen to specimen, have all the required equipment and materials close to hand, and can organize their work on a repetitive, mass-production basis. Because, however, the range of their experience would otherwise be limited, the staff should from time to time be rotated among the different sections so they can learn all branches of the laboratory's work. Special arrangements need to be made to ensure that the results for different kinds of specimens from the same patient are, when significant, considered together. A useful practice to this end is for the staff of all sections

to meet together for a few minutes at the same time each day to report verbally and discuss any important or puzzling findings.

Choice of tests

There is much scope for variation between laboratories in the choice of isolation methods to be applied to each kind of specimen and the choice of identification tests to be applied to each kind of potentially significant microbial isolate. The laboratory should have a carefully considered and clearly formulated policy for the selection of stains, culture media, biochemical tests, serological tests and antibiotics for sensitivity tests to be used in the examination of each kind of specimen, clinical condition and microbial isolate.

A balance must be struck between the extra precision and reliability of results to be gained from the multiplication of isolation methods and identification tests and the need for economy in labour and materials. The greatest effort should be made to diagnose the more serious infections with epidemic potential, but in most infections the use of more than two or three methods of culture is hardly justified by the small improvement gained in the probability of isolating the pathogen.

The degree of precision with which microbial isolates are characterized should be determined by the likely clinical or epidemiological value of a precise identification. When commensal bacteria with potential pathogenicity are isolated from a hospital patient, the clinician generally requires no more detailed information than that a potential pathogen is present and the range of its antibiotic sensitivities. Such an isolate, therefore, may justifiably be identified no further than as, for example, a coliform bacillus, non-haemolytic streptococcus, albus staphylococcus or Gram-negative anaerobic bacillus. In some cases there is a clinical or epidemiological need for full speciation of the isolate, or even for its subspecies typing at a reference laboratory, but these cases are exceptional. They may be recognized by the microbiologist as they arise in the course of his daily work, and then be given special attention. This selective approach avoids the waste of labour and materials incurred in fully characterizing the majority of isolates, for which precise species identification is unnecessary.

Reading of results

The results of bacteriological examinations usually become available in stages on successive days. Microscopical observations on stained films may be obtained on the day of receipt of the specimen and, if significant, be given in a preliminary report to the clinician. Taken in conjunction with the clinical information on the request form, they may help to guide the choice of culture media on which the specimen is to be inoculated. The growths in the primary cultures are usually observed after overnight incubation, i.e. on the second day, when the findings help to determine what further identification tests and what antibiotic sensitivity tests are to be done on subcultures. The results of these later tests are generally available on the third day, when the content of the final report can be decided.

For some types of examination, for example that of urine for significant bacteriuria, diarrhoeal faeces for enteropathogens or sera for specific antibodies, the sequence of test procedures, the criteria for reading the results and the phrasing to be used in reports can be clearly defined in a manual of instructions. It may then be satisfactory to have the results of these examinations read and recorded by technical or scientific staff. For specimens such as those from the respiratory tract, blood cultures and infected exudates, however, where the clinical significance of different organisms needs to be assessed in relation to the clinical information given about the patient, it is preferable that the reading of the primary cultures and the determination of reports should be done by senior, medically qualified staff.

Senior staff, both medical and scientific, should from time to time take part in reading the results for all types of specimens. They should check unexpected or anomalous findings and any finding of serious clinical or epidemiological significance, e.g. that of the presence of tubercle or typhoid bacilli. They should be alert to the possibility of findings being the result of

mistakes, as by the mislabelling of cultures, transfers between the wrong tubes, or the use of faulty reagents or contaminated media, and should decide when tests must be repeated for confirmation of the results. When many examinations have to be made, even skilled and conscientious workers may from time to time make mistakes. Staff should be encouraged to recognize and report any likelihood of their having made a mistake, and should not be made afraid to confess the possibility.

Wording of reports

The aim of the clinical microbiologist is to provide clinicians and health officers with reports that are understandable, instructive and relevant as well as reliable. The laboratory should therefore have a carefully considered policy for the wording of reports and all staff should adhere to that policy. If different members of staff are left free to choose the nomenclature of microorganisms and the pattern of interpretative comment for their reports, a confusing variation is likely to result. The recipients of reports can most quickly learn the significance of particular results if they are reported consistently in the same terms. If the same result is reported in different terms on different occasions, the recipient may be led to imagine that differences of significance are implied.

There are advantages in using the colloquial and clinically indicative names of microorganisms, e.g., typhoid bacillus, Sonne dysentery bacillus, coliform bacillus, commensal-type neisseria and non-cholera vibrio, rather than the formal names, e.g., *Salmonella typhi*, *Shigella sonnei*, *Enterobacter aerogenes*, *Neisseria pharyngis* and *Vibrio cholerae* serotype 23. Where formal names are used, their frequent changing in pursuance of the recommendations of international committees of nomenclature should be avoided. If use is to be made of a formal name thought likely to be unfamiliar to the report's recipient, an interpretative comment should be added, e.g. 'Culture yielded a profuse growth of *Enterobacter aerogenes*, a saprophytic coliform bacillus that may be acting as an opportunistic pathogen in this patient'.

The laboratory's policy for reports should specify not only the wording of interpretative comments, but also the circumstances in which the different comments are to be made. It should, for instance, lay down the circumstances in which the finding of albus staphylococci in a blood culture is to be reported with the comment, 'probably a contaminant from the skin', and without giving its antibiotic sensitivities, and the different circumstances, as in a compromised patient, when the finding is to be reported as 'possibly of clinical significance' and the antibiotic sensitivities given. Similarly, the policy should define the circumstances in which the finding of small or moderate numbers of pneumococci or haemophili in sputum should be reported with their antibiotic sensitivities, so implying a probable clinical significance, and the circumstances in which that finding should be reported as probably due to contamination of the sputum with organisms from the throat, or left unreported.

A policy is also required for reporting the finding of acid-fast bacilli in different specimens. Thus, their finding in sputum might be reported, 'Acid-fast bacilli resembling tubercle bacilli seen in film. Cultures for tubercle bacilli have been set up and will be reported later.' But their finding in urine might be reported more cautiously, 'Acid-fast bacilli seen in film, which, although also alcohol-fast, may be commensal smegma bacilli. Cultures for tubercle bacilli have been set up and will be reported later.'

Particular care must be given to the policy for the wording of negative reports. These should be phrased in such a way as to indicate which pathogens were sought and not found. They should not suggest that tests had been made for a wide range of pathogens when, indeed, methods for detecting only a few types of pathogenic bacteria had been used. The uninformed recipient of a report on a throat swab that 'No pathogens were found' might well imagine that a search had been made for every kind of respiratory-tract pathogen, including viruses, mycoplasmas and chlamydias, when the specimen had been cultured only for pyogenic bacteria.

If a throat swab from acute sore throat has been examined for *Streptococcus pyogenes* the report might properly read, 'Mixed throat organisms present. *Streptococcus pyogenes* not found. Viruses, mycoplasmas and other pathogens not sought.' Similarly, if faeces from simple acute diarrhoea has been examined only for salmonella, shigella and campylobacter, the report should read, 'No salmonella, no shigella, no campylobacter.'

Issue of reports

A variety of arrangements are adopted for the issue of reports. Commonly, the bacteriologist reading the tests writes what is to be reported in an abbreviated form on the worksheet or, if it is used as a worksheet, on a reserved space on the request form. The clerical staff who type the report then translate the abbreviation into the proper, agreed phraseology. To economize in the labour of typists, short-cut methods are often used, particularly in the preparation of 'negative reports', which may comprise up to 80% of the total. Standardized reports may be affixed with an inked stamp or self-adhesive pre-printed label to a reserved space on the request form, or a copy of that form, which is then returned to the physician as the report. This procedure saves the typist the need to copy the patient's identification data as well as the report itself.

All the completed reports should be scrutinized quickly for credibility by senior, preferably medical staff before signature and issue. Anomalous findings may sometimes be detected at this stage, or findings that require urgent consultation with the physician. The signature on the report should be that of the director of the laboratory or a senior staff member to whom the director has delegated the responsibility. It indicates to the recipient whom he should approach for further information or advice about the investigation of the patient or the interpretation of the findings.

Copies of the reports should be filed in the laboratory for later reference and for response to enquiries. A simple system should be adopted, allowing the easy retrieval of recent reports. Reports of long-term interest, e.g. those of findings of tuberculous infection, should be preserved for many years, but negative reports of transient interest may be discarded after a few months. As the responsibility for preserving reports of laboratory findings rests with their recipients, or the hospital records officer, the laboratory needs only to preserve copies of reports to meet its own purposes.

Computerization of reports

There are considerable advantages to be gained from the computerization of laboratory reports and records, and it is likely that when good systems have been well proven their use will become general. The primary aim should be to substitute the rapid, accurate operation of a computer for the slow, laborious and occasionally inaccurate manual work of clerical staff in the booking-in of specimens, the preparation of work sheets and reports, and the filing and retrieval of records.

It is important that the system adopted should not delay or distort the schedule of laboratory work or interfere with changes and developments. It should be sufficiently flexible to enable the bacteriologist to add comments to individual reports and allow changes in the laboratory's policy for the wording of reports to be easily implemented. The request and report forms and other documentation should be designed to permit an immediate reversion to reporting by hand-writing, typing or the affixing of stamps in the event of a computer breakdown.

Request forms may be submitted in duplicate on copying paper and both copies marked on reception with the laboratory's specimen accession number. One copy may then be sent at once with the specimen to the work bench, where its information about the patient may guide the bacteriologist in his choice of tests and interpretation of results; the findings and the result to be reported may be written in a reserved space on it. The other copy may be retained in the reception office, where the clerical staff may copy from it the specimen number and patient data into the computer file. That file serves as a booking-in record and can be obtained as a printed list two or three times a day for reference. The bacteriologist may enter his report directly into a computer terminal or mark it on the request form and pass the form to clerical staff to enter the report into the computer. The computer links the report to the patient data through the specimen's accession number and prepares a final copy for issue through an automatic printer, so obviating typist's work and errors.

Although its primary role is to minimize the need for clerical work in the preparation of reports, computerization confers other advantages in the storage and retrieval of records. It enables the quick retrieval of information about particular patients and the rapid production of cumulative reports on them. It makes easy the derivation of laboratory statistics of various kinds, e.g. the number of specimens of each kind or from each different clinical unit received in a given period, the number of specimens yielding each different species of pathogen, or the antibiotic sensitivities of isolates of particular pathogens. Trends in infection or in the evolution of drug resistance can thus easily be monitored and survey data can be stored and analysed for service or research purposes.

Laboratory manual

A prime responsibility of the director of a laboratory is to compile or supervise the compilation of a laboratory manual of procedures, comprising a collection of instruction sheets for the different sections of the laboratory. The manual should lay down the policy of the laboratory for the kinds and sequence of examinations to be made on each of the different kinds of specimen, the criteria for determining the content of reports, and the standardized wordings of reports.

The adherence of staff to the provisions of the manual should be supervised. Reliance on the verbal communication of policy on procedures from older to newer staff, or from departing to arriving staff in sections of the laboratory subject to staff rotations, is highly unsatisfactory because it often leads to the introduction of unauthorized variations in procedure, and an important drift in technology may escape the notice of senior staff.

As the bench procedures to be laid down in

the manual should be chosen with a view to practicability, reliability and economy of labour at the bench as well as their clinical value and scientific precision, the content of the manual should be determined only after full consultation with the technical and other staff concerned with the work.

The manual should include details or clear references to the methodology of all the tests to be used. Much of the hard work of its preparation may be avoided if sections of a textbook are acceptable. Preferably, copies of relevant sections should be reproduced in the manual for immediate reference at the bench. The manual should also specify the selection and sequence of tests to be applied to each different category of specimen, e.g. pus, sputum, urine and faeces, including the variations to be adopted when the available clinical information indicates the need for special or extra examinations. For example, the manual might specify that throat swabs from persons over 4 years old suffering from acute sore throat, for which the request is only 'pathogens please' or 'culture and sensitivity', should be examined only for *Streptococcus pyogenes* and only by culture on aerobic and anaerobic blood agar plates bearing bacitracin and penicillin disks for identification and sensitivity testing. It might instruct that Vincent's organisms, candida, diphtheria bacilli or other respiratory-tract pathogens should be sought only if specifically requested by the physician or if the patient data on the request form included certain specific indications of the relevant infection.

The manual should further state the types of colonies on primary culture plates that are to be picked for identification and sensitivity tests, the kinds of tests to be applied to these isolates and the criteria for identifying significant pathogens. The criteria for including particular findings in reports and the phraseology of reports should also be laid down.

ACCOMMODATION

The extent and arrangement of laboratory accommodation are constrained by what is available in old buildings and, in new hospitals, usually to a considerable degree by financial and architectural considerations. It is beyond the scope of this book to advise on the design of new laboratories and such advice should be sought from bodies such as central health departments and the Public Health Laboratory Service. Requirements for laboratory safety must be taken into account at an early stage of design.

Some points of importance merit mention here however. The accommodation should be sufficient for the contemporary volume of work with a substantial reserve to provide for a probably progressive yearly increase in demand. It should be capable of flexible use and rearrangement to meet changed patterns of working. Excluding circulation space, corridors, animal rooms, cloakrooms, toilets, etc, about 1000 m^2 of floor space would be required for a bacteriology and virology service meeting the present level of needs of a population of about 250 000.

The groups of staff dealing with the main sections of general bacteriological work may be accommodated in separate bays in a large, open-plan laboratory, or in separate adjacent laboratories. The head technician supervising the technical staff in these laboratories should have a closely adjacent office. At least 10 m^2 of floor space should be available per person. In addition to adequate bench areas for the orderly, uncramped arrangement of specimens, tests and equipment, e.g. 2–3 m of bench per technician, and free wall space for floor-standing equipment, each laboratory should have sufficient office bays, or areas with desks, to enable technical and other staff to perform their paperwork away from the potentially contaminated benches where the bacteriology is done. The director and other senior staff will require separate offices and laboratories. Corridors and passageways should be kept clear and unrestricted by equipment or stored materials.

A special suite of laboratories and offices is required for virology and special laboratories are required for particular functions in bacteriology. A separate room with exhaust ventilated safety cabinets is required for work with dangerous pathogens such as tubercle bacilli and brucellae that may be transmitted by the air. A large room or group of rooms is required for sterilizing discarded specimens and cultures, clean containers and fresh culture media, for washing glassware and for making and dispensing media. Arrangements should be made to minimize exposure of staff to heat, humidity and noise from the autoclaves and glassware washing machines. The staff making and dispensing media should work in a room separate from that used for the sterilizing and washing. There are advantages in having a room reserved for plate pouring, which is kept free from all activities liable to raise dust. It should be provided with laminar flow dust-free cabinets in which the melted agar media can be poured into plates and the plates left open to cool and set.

A large cold room is needed for the storage of culture media, poured plates and labile reagents, and separate store rooms for chemicals, inflammable solvents and general supplies. A small darkroom is required for fluorescence microscopy. A large office with stationery and records stores is required for the clerical staff issuing and filing reports and answering telephoned enquiries, and the provision of an adequate staff common room and library minimizes the waste of time by staff having to visit a distant hospital canteen or library. A special computer room with controlled humidity and temperature may be desirable.

EQUIPMENT

It is convenient and time-saving to have most of the commonly used equipment such as incubators, refrigerators, microscopes and waterbaths located in the laboratories where the main work is done rather than in separate instrument rooms. Exceptions are noisy machines such as centrifuges, rotary incubators and shakers, which are best housed in a separate room. Of all the equipment used in clinical bacteriology, most careful consideration is required in the choice of autoclaves. Different conditions of autoclaving are required for different kinds of materials, e.g. discarded cultures, clean glassware and large volumes of culture media, and it is necessary to have a modern multi-purpose machine that can readily and reliably be switched to different cycles of operation or to have different autoclaves for each different function (Ch. 4).

Expensive, delicate and elaborate equipment is now becoming available to perform rapidly and automatically tests that are slow and sometimes inexact by conventional methods. Any decision to install such equipment should be influenced by considerations of cost effectiveness and clinical value and must take account of the will and ability of staff to maintain the equipment in good working order.

SAFETY PRECAUTIONS

Every clinical bacteriology laboratory must have a defined system for instructing and supervising staff in safety precautions as detailed in Chapter 15. Whilst the head of the laboratory bears the ultimate responsibility for the safety arrangements, another senior member of staff may be appointed to act as Safety Officer to coordinate the arrangements and supervise their implementation. All staff should be offered appropriate immunizations, e.g. that against tuberculosis, and some staff should be trained in first aid and have ready access to basic first aid equipment.

Microscopy

The study of the morphology of very small organisms is of such importance to the microbiologist that he must of necessity be a competent microscopist and, if he is to obtain the best performance from his instrument, he needs to understand the optical principles and construction of the microscope.

In the ordinary optical microscope, the specimen, or *object*, borne on a glass slide is scanned by a focused beam of visible light. Parts of the specimen that are optically dense, having a high refractive index or being coloured with a stain, cast a potential image, like a shadow, in the beam of light, which is magnified in two stages as it passes up the microscope into the eye.

Microscopes designed by different manufacturers differ greatly in the details of their construction and mode of operation, so that the manufacturer's description and instructions for an instrument must be consulted and followed. The descriptions given below are generally applicable for many instruments, but with exceptions in details.

Monocular microscopes have a single eye-piece. They are convenient for use by beginners, who may have difficulty in fusing the images from a binocular microscope, and for demonstrations to a succession of viewers, who would be put to the trouble each time of having to readjust the interocular distance of a binocular head. A monocular microscope is required for photography, but a binocular instrument may be fitted temporarily with an interchangeable monocular head for this purpose.

Binocular microscopes have two eye-pieces. They are to be recommended where much microscopic work has to be done, e.g. in routine examinations, for by the use of both eyes, much eye strain and fatigue is avoided. Such an instrument is illustrated in Figure 2.1. The upright *stand* (5) rests on a heavy *foot* and bears at its upper end an inclined binocular head with two *eye-pieces* (1), above, and a revolving *nose-piece* (3) bearing several *objectives*, below. Attached through a racking mechanism to the middle of the stand is a horizontal platform, or *stage* (6), with a central hole over which the slide with specimen is held by clips. For focusing, the stage is racked upwards or downwards by turning the milled heads of *coarse* and *fine focusing adjustments* (14, 15). For searching different areas of the specimen, the slide can be moved in two directions by turning *mechanical stage adjustments* (11). A built-in *lamp* (16) in the foot of the microscope passes a beam of light upwards through a *field diaphragm* (iris) (13). The beam is focused on to the specimen by a *substage condenser* (8) which is attached beneath the stage, centred by condenser centration adjustments (10) and moved upwards or downwards by the turning of a *condenser focusing adjustment* (7). An *aperture diaphragm* (iris) (9) with a lever for its control is incorporated in the condenser mounting.

In the binocular head (2) the rays of light from the objective are divided equally by a half-silvered surface inclined at 45° which permits half the light to pass through it and reflects the remainder at right angles. Each half of the rays is directed into its appropriate eye-piece by means of prisms. The eye-piece sockets can be moved together or apart to enable the observer to adjust them to his own interpupillary distance,

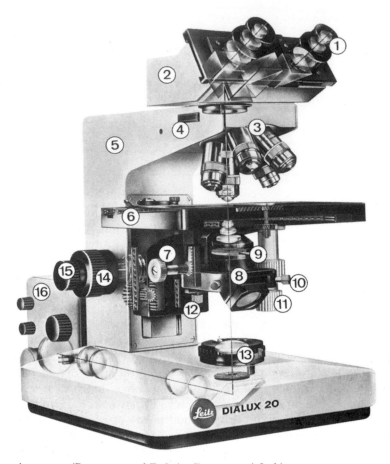

Fig. 2.1 Binocular microscope. (By courtesy of E. Leitz (Instruments) Ltd.)

and the focusing of one of the eye-pieces is adjustable to correct for individual differences between the two eyes.

Inclined binocular microscopes are most suitable for routine use as it is unnecessary to tilt the stand to bring the eye-pieces into a convenient position for the eyes of a seated observer. The stage is kept horizontal, so minimizing the risk of immersion oil or wet preparations running off the slide and soiling it. The inclined body may increase the overall magnification of the microscope by, e.g. 1.5 times, when this factor will be engraved on it. Lower-power eye-pieces, e.g. × 6 or × 8 rather than × 10, should then be used.

Magnification

The purpose of the microscope is to produce an enlarged, well defined image of objects too small to be observed with the naked eye. The degree of enlargement is the *magnification* or *magnifying power* of the instrument and it is expressed as the number of times the length, breadth or diameter, but not area, of the object is multiplied.

It is perfectly possible to design an optical system that will give enormous magnifications, e.g. × 1 000 000, but after a certain degree of magnification the sharpness of the image is lost, the larger images are increasingly blurred and no further detail is revealed. Excessive magnification of this type is known as *empty magnification* and is valueless to the microbiologist. The limit of *useful magnification*, up to which increasing detail is observed, is set by the resolving power, or *limit of resolution* of the microscope lenses, which itself is subject to a limit imposed by the wavelength of the light rays used. With the most powerful lenses, including the 2 mm oil-immersion objective, the limit of resolution is about 0.2 μm and the greatest useful magnification $\times$ 1000 or a little higher.

Magnification is effected in two stages, the first by the objective lenses and the second by the eye-piece lenses. The magnifying powers of the objectives and eye-pieces are engraved on them, and the overall magnification of the microscope can be calculated by multiplying the magnifying power of the objective by that of the eye-piece. If the microscope has an inclined binocular head that increases the magnification by a factor of, e.g. 1.5, the product of the magnifying powers of the objective and eye-piece must be further multiplied by that factor.

The magnifying power of an objective is the optical tube length of the microscope, usually 160 mm, divided by the focal length of the objective. Thus, an objective with a focal length of 2 mm would have a magnifying power of $\times$ 80. Oil-immersion objectives designated as of 2 mm focal length have, in reality, focal lengths a little shorter, so that their magnification is $\times$ 95 or $\times$ 100.

To enable their use at different magnifications, microscopes have a revolving nose-piece bearing several objectives with different focal lengths and thus different magnifying powers. The objective giving the required magnification is revolved into line with the object. The three objectives most commonly used in microbiology are: (1) a low-power 'dry' objective with focal length 16 mm and magnification $\times$ 10, (2) a high-power 'dry' objective with focal length 4 mm and magnification $\times$ 40, and (3) an oil-immersion objective with focal length '2 mm' and magnification $\times$ 100. When these objectives are used with eye-pieces magnifying $\times$ 10, the overall magnifications of the microscope are, respectively, $\times$ 100, $\times$ 400 and $\times$ 1000.

Numerical aperture

Objectives are rated not only by their focal length, but also by their angles of aperture which determine their light gathering powers and abilities to resolve detail. The numerical aperture (NA) may be defined simply as the ratio of the diameter of the lens to its focal length, but is expressed more precisely by the formula:

$$NA = n \, Sin \, U$$

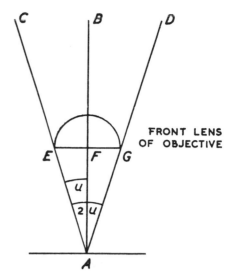

Fig. 2.2 Diagram to illustrate numerical aperture.

when n is the refractive index of the medium between the object and the objective (air, 1; immersion oil, 1.5), and $2U$ is the *angle of aperture*, i.e. the angle formed by the two most divergent rays of light which, starting from the centre of the object, enter the objective and reach the observer's eye (angle CAD, Fig. 2.2).

The theoretical limit of the angle of aperture ($2U$) is 180° and that of U is 90°, i.e. when the objective is in contact with the object. Thus, the greatest possible NA of a dry lens cannot exceed 1.0, for the refractive index (n) of air $= 1$ and Sin 90° $= 1$. Actually, the highest practical NA of a dry lens is 0.95. When immersion oil ($n = 1.5$) is interposed between the object and the objective, the highest theoretical value for n Sin U is 1.5 $\times$ Sin 90°, i.e. 1.5. In practice, the highest NA of an oil-immersion objective, attained in an apochromat, is 1.4, and the NA of an ordinary 2 mm oil-immersion objective is 1.3.

Resolution

The limit of useful magnification of a microscope is set by its resolving power, i.e. its ability to reveal closely adjacent structural details as separate and distinct. This resolving power is expressed quantitatively as the microscope's *limit of resolution* (LR), i.e. the minimum distance between two visible bodies at which they are seen as separate and not in contact with one another. The LR is determined by the wavelength of the light rays (W) and the numerical aperture (NA) of the objective according to the following formula:

$$LR = \frac{0.61 \times W}{NA}$$

Thus, if green light of wavelength 0.55 μm (0.000 55 mm), the best 2 mm oil-immersion apochromatic objective of NA 1.4, and high-power compensating eye-pieces are used,

$$LR = \frac{0.61 \times 0.55}{1.4} = 0.24 \ \mu m$$

This limit of the resolving power of the best light microscope enables even the smallest bacteria to be resolved, but only the very largest of the viruses, e.g. that of smallpox.

For the resolution of smaller bodies, the electron microscope is used. In this, the object is scanned with a beam of electrons having an equivalent wavelength as small as 1/100 000th that of ordinary light. The efficiency of the electromagnetic lenses used to focus the electron beam is, however, much less than that of optical lenses and the resolving power of the electron microscope is therefore only about 250 times better than that of the best light microscope, i.e. LR approximately 0.001 μm, or 1 nm.
Note: 1 nanometre (nm) = 0.001 micrometer (μm) = 0.000 001 millimetre (mm).

Definition

Definition, not to be confused with resolution, is the capacity of an objective to render the outline of the image of an object clear and distinct. It depends on the elimination of optical aberrations inherent in simple glass lenses. *Spherical aberration* is due to the rays passing through the edge of the lens not being brought to the same focus as those passing nearer the centre. *Chromatic aberration* occurs because white light traversing a lens is separated into its component colours of different wavelength which are refracted to different extents and not recombined at the same focus. The result may

be a hazy image fringed with the colours of the spectrum.

Aberrations are corrected by the makers of objectives by combining lenses of different dispersive qualities. *Achromatic objectives* are made by combining convex lenses of crown glass having low dispersive power with concave lenses of flint glass having high dispersive power. This combination, in an assembly of four or more lenses, unites many of the divergent rays of different wavelength to form white light at a common focus. Achromatic objectives are satisfactory for virtually all the microscopical work of clinical microbiology and most research purposes.

Apochromatic objectives represent the highest degree of optical perfection, but are very costly and their expense is justifiable only for critical research work and photomicrography. A good oil-immersion apochromat may have a numerical aperture as high as 1.4 and give almost complete colour correction and maximum resolving power. Its properties depend on its content of the mineral fluorite, which possesses high transparency, a low refractive index and small dispersiveness. Apochromats must always be used with special, *compensating* eye-pieces and a properly centred condenser.

Oil-immersion objectives

Because of the high magnification and resolution required for the study of bodies as small as bacteria, most microbiological work is done with achromatic or apochromatic objectives designed for use with *oil immersion*, which increases the angle of the cone of rays from the object that enters the objective and thus the numerical aperture of the latter. With a 'dry' objective, air is present between the object on the surface of the glass slide and the objective lens (Fig. 2.3, right). An oblique ray of light (ABCD) from the condenser passing through the slide in the direction (BC) of the edge of the objective is refracted outwards (CD) as it leaves the glass (refractive index, n = 1.5) and enters the air (n = 1.0) so that it fails to enter the objective. With an oil-immersion objective, oil (n = 1.5) is present between the slide and the objective and

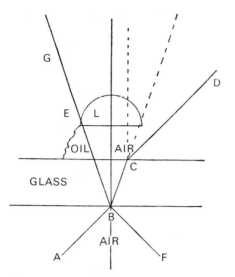

Fig. 2.3 Diagram showing the paths of rays through (1) a dry lens (on right), and (2) an oil immersion lens (on left). Note the refraction of the oblique ray ABCD in passing from the glass slide to air, as compared with the ray FBEG. L is the front lens of the objective.

a similarly oblique ray emerging from the glass into the oil with an equal refractive index is not refracted outwards, but passes straight on into the objective (FBEG). Thus the angle of the cone of rays accepted by an oil-immersion objective is wider than that accepted by a dry lens of similar dimensions.

Because the focal length of the oil-immersion objectives is short and the oil makes it difficult to see the gap separating the lens from the slide, care must be taken when focusing to avoid the lens coming into contact with the slide and so becoming scratched or damaged. Some objectives are constructed with a spring loaded optical train, which reduces the risk of damage from contact with the slide.

Eye-pieces

The functions of the eye-piece are to form a magnified and virtual image of the real image formed by the objective and to carry any micrometer scale or marker to be used with the microscope. *Huygenian eye-pieces* are the most generally useful. They consist of two plano-convex lenses with their plane sides facing upwards and a circular field diaphragm between them to limit the field of view to the central and flattest part of the image. In microbiology, a × 10 eye-piece is generally used with a monocular microscope and a × 6 or × 8 eye-piece with a binocular. *Ramsden eye-pieces* have two plano-convex lenses with the convex sides facing each other and a field diaphragm below the lower lens. They are specially suitable for micrometry, when a scale is placed on the diaphragm. *Compensating eye-pieces* usually contain a triplet system as the lower lens component and are designed to correct the chromatic difference of magnification inherent in particular apochromatic objectives, with which they should always be used. They can be used with advantage with high-power achromats, but should not be used with low-power achromats.

Condensers

The condenser has the function of focusing light on the object. It is mounted below the stage with a rack and pinion mechanism for adjusting its focus and should be fitted with centring screws for critical work with highly corrected objectives. Different types of condenser vary in quality. The simple Abbé condenser, composed of two lenses uncorrected for spherical and chromatic aberrations, is unsuitable for microbiological work. A good quality *achromatic* condenser should be used, corrected for aberrations and having a numerical aperture equal to that of the highest power objective, e.g. NA = 1.37, so that it fills the objective with a solid cone of light. The numerical aperture of such a condenser can be reduced to that of the lower power objectives by adjustment of an iris diaphragm beneath the condenser's bottom lens. As the highest numerical aperture of any dry lens is 1.0, it is necessary for the most critical work with a high power oil-immersion objective to introduce immersion oil between the slide and the top lens of the condenser as well as between the slide and the objective.

Centration of the condenser

After the microscope and illuminant have been set up, close the condenser iris diaphragm to its limit. Rack down the condenser until the image of its iris appears in the field. Adjust the centring screws of the condenser until the image of the iris is in the centre of the field. Open up the iris until its aperture is almost that of the field and make a final adjustment to its centration. Then open the iris fully and rack up the condenser to its normal position.

Focusing of the condenser

The method of focusing the condenser for critical (Köhler) illumination is described below. For less critical work with the high power (2 mm) oil-immersion objective, the condenser should be racked fully or nearly fully upwards to illuminate the field with maximum brightness. With lower power objectives it should be racked downwards, or its top lens swung out of train, to produce even illumination of the field. When an unstained wet film is viewed with a high power objective, the condenser may be similarly de-focused to make bacteria and cells appear more refractile and easily visible, though this procedure leads to some impairment of resolution and definition.

ILLUMINATION

Formerly, light was provided from a lamp separate from the microscope and was reflected upwards into the condenser by a plane mirror mounted on gimbals allowing adjustment of its angle in any direction. Before each use, the position of the lamp and the angle of the mirror had to be adjusted carefully to ensure that the light was properly focused and centred in the microscope field. In most modern instruments, however, the lamp and mirror are built into the foot of the microscope, fixed in their correct positions, so that repeated readjustment is unnecessary.

For simple work with a monocular microscope and Abbé condenser, a 60 watt opal bulb suffices as the illuminant, but with a binocular micro-scope or for critical work a *high-intensity lamp* is required. The latter should have a corrected lamp condenser lens and lamp iris diaphragm to enable the light to be correctly focused and centred into the microscope substage condenser; it should also have a control to enable the intensity of the illumination to be varied according to need.

Light filters. A blue daylight filter is commonly supplied for fitting into a holder beneath the substage condenser when artificial light is used, but a filter is not specially required in ordinary bacteriological work. A pale green filter reduces glare and is restful to the eye; it may also be helpful in making red- or purple-stained objects appear darker and more easily visible.

Köhler illumination. Best results are obtained when illumination with a high-intensity lamp is effected by the Köhler method in which (1) the condenser lens of the lamp focuses an enlarged image of the light source (i.e. lamp filament) on to the iris diaphragm of the substage condenser, and (2) the substage condenser focuses the image of the lamp condenser iris on to the plane of the object (specimen). The following procedures should be performed.

Method of using a high-intensity lamp

1. To prolong the life of the lamp, always move the intensity control to the low, i.e. dim, position before switching either on or off, and avoid running the lamp for long periods at full intensity.

2. Rack up fully the substage condenser of the microscope, i.e. until its top surface is within about 1 mm below the upper surface of the stage.

3. Check that the lamp filament is centred correctly with the lamp condenser lens and open fully the lamp condenser iris ('field iris').

4. If the lamp is separate from the micro-scope, place it 20–25 cm from the mirror of the microscope.

5. Switch on the lamp at low intensity and then increase its intensity to an intermediate level.

6. Adjust the tilt and position of the lamp to direct the beam of light on to the centre of the mirror.

7. Close the substage iris diaphragm and focus the lamp condenser to throw a sharp image of

the filament on to the closed diaphragm. A small hand mirror may be used to assist in the viewing and focusing of the image.

8. Open fully the substage iris diaphragm and move the lamp forwards and backwards until the size of the image of the filament is large enough to fill the lowest lens of the substage condenser.

9. Dim the lamp, place a stained specimen on the stage and focus it with the objective to be used.

10. Close the lamp iris and adjust the mirror, if moveable, so that the image of the lamp iris is in the centre of the field.

11. Open the lamp iris until its image just fills the field.

12. Remove an eye-piece and inspect the back lens of the objective. An image of the filament should appear symmetrically placed and large enough to fill the back lens.

13. For maximum definition, close and focus the lamp iris in the field for each objective just before its use. These adjustments are possible with the 16 mm and 4 mm dry objectives and the 3.5 mm oil-immersion objective, but not with the 2 mm oil-immersion objective.

METHOD OF USE OF LIGHT MICROSCOPE

1. Place the microscope at a convenient position on the bench and adjust the height and position of the observer's chair, so that prolonged viewing may be done in comfort. The eye-pieces of the microscope should be level with, and close to the observer's eyes while he is sitting in a nearly upright position. The forearms or elbows should be rested on the bench in positions that allow the hands convenient access to the focusing and stage adjustments. Observers who wear glasses may be able to dispense with them when using a microscope, but if their defect is of a kind for which the microscope does not compensate, they must take care to prevent their spectacles touching and scratching the lenses of the eye-pieces.

2. Check to ensure that the objectives and eye-pieces are free from dust and immersion oil. If they are not, clean them with a fresh lens tissue. Use only benzol or xylol to remove hardened oil.

3. Rack up fully the substage condenser, i.e. until its top surface is within about 1 mm below the upper surface of the stage (undersurface of the slide). If, when the condenser adjustment is racked to its uppermost position, the top of the condenser is too high, i.e. above the upper surface of the stage, or too low, i.e. not within about 1 mm below the upper surface of the stage, adjust the condenser in its mounting so that it will rack up to the correct position.

4. Check that the filter carrier in the substage is in its correct position and not in an intermediate position where it will obscure the light.

5. Fully open the substage and lamp irises.

6. Switch on the lamp at low intensity and then increase the intensity. For critical work with a high-intensity lamp, make the adjustments described above for obtaining Köhler illumination.

7. Place the slide with the object on the stage, so that it is held by the stage clips and pressed at both ends into close contact with the surface of the stage.

8. First view the specimen with a *low-power* (e.g. 16 mm) dry objective and use the *coarse* focusing adjustment to focus the specimen on the slide. Move an area of the slide with easily visible material into the centre of the field, where it will be available in the smaller field to be focused with the high-power objectives.

Note. Never use the fine focusing adjustment until the specimen has been made visible and brought nearly into focus with the coarse adjustment. Use the fine adjustment only to obtain and maintain exact focus.

9. Adjust the distance between the eye-pieces so that a single field is seen. Focus the microscope on the object to suit the eye using the fixed eye-piece and then focus the other eye-piece to suit the other eye; the specimen object should then be in sharp focus to both eyes simultaneously.

10. If continued examination with the low-power objective is required, diffuse the light uniformly over the field by defocusing the condenser either by racking it down or swinging out its top lens. Reduce the illumination by turning down the intensity control of the lamp,

not by closing the iris diaphragm of the substage or lamp.

11. Before proceeding to use a high-power objective, check that the iris diaphragms are open, the condenser is focused by fully racking up and that the illumination is properly centred.

If it is necessary to re-centre the illumination, close the lamp iris, focus it with the substage condenser. Adjust the substage centring screws until the image of the iris is in the centre of the field. Finally open the lamp iris until the field is *just* completely filled with light.

12. Before using an oil-immersion (e.g. 2 mm) objective, rack down the stage to give adequate clearance between the slide and the objective, and place a moderately large drop of immersion oil on the middle of the specimen central to the light beam focused from the condenser. Take care not to spill oil on the microscope.

13. Rotate the nose-piece until the oil-immersion lens is in position.

14. With the eye at the level of the stage, use the *coarse* focusing adjustment slowly to raise the stage until the oil on the slide makes contact with the objective and the oil 'lights up'. Then, still with the coarse adjustment, raise the stage a little further to bring the surface of the slide as close as possible to the objective lens without actually touching it. Take care to avoid damaging the lens by pressing it against the slide.

15. Apply the eyes to the eye-pieces and, while watching, slowly focus the objective *away* from the slide by lowering the stage with the coarse focusing adjustment. Stop as soon as focus is reached and the specimen is seen. Then, and only then, obtain and maintain exact focus by use of the fine adjustment.

16. If focus is missed, do *not* focus back again while looking into the eye-pieces, for the slide might then accidentally be brought into contact with the objective lens. Failure to find focus is common with the 2 mm oil-immersion objective. It may be due to the slide originally not having been brought close enough to the objective to be within its focal distance or to there not being any visible material on the small area of slide within the field of the objective.

First move the slide so that some visible, e.g. stained, though out-of-focus material is brought into the field. This procedure will ensure that there is visible material to focus. Then, with the eyes level with the stage, use the coarse adjustment to raise the slide until it again comes as close as possible to the objective without touching it. Finally, apply the eyes to the eye-pieces and use the coarse adjustment to focus the objective away from the slide until the specimen is seen in focus. It may be necessary to repeat these manoeuvres several times before focus is found.

17. If the illumination is poor, check that it is properly centred before turning up the intensity control on the lamp.

18. Search the specimen in an orderly way by moving the adjustments of the mechanical stage. Keep a hand on the fine focusing adjustment in order to maintain exact focus during the movements of the slide.

19. After use, wipe the oil from the objective with a clean tissue and clean off any oil that has been spilt on the stage or elsewhere on the microscope. Turn down the light intensity control to low and then switch off the light.

Simple monocular microscope

The foregoing instructions for use apply to a modern binocular microscope with high-intensity illumination. But apart from those relating specifically to the illumination and the binocular eye-pieces, most apply also to the use of a monocular microscope in which the illumination is provided by a low-intensity (e.g. 60 watt) opal bulb, the light from which is reflected into the substage condenser by a moveable mirror beneath it. With this system, great care must be taken to obtain sufficiently intense and properly centred illumination for work with the 2 mm oil-immersion objective. The condenser must be fully racked up to give its proper focus, the substage iris must be kept fully open and the mirror must be kept exactly adjusted to reflect the light centrally into the condenser.

Care of microscope

The microscope is an instrument of precision and care must be taken to preserve its accuracy. It should be kept at a uniform temperature and not exposed to sunlight or any source of heat. It should be moved with care to avoid jarring and mechanical damage, and should be lifted by its fixed upright and foot, not by any moveable part. When not in use it should be protected from dust in its box or under a plastic cover. It should be cleaned at intervals and its working surfaces should be very lightly smeared with soft paraffin. On no account, however, should the component parts of objectives or condensers be unscrewed or dismantled for cleaning.

Spilt or hardened immersion oil is particularly troublesome. Oil dried and hardened on an oil-immersion lens or oil spilt on to a dry lens prevents proper focusing. Oil spilt on to the stage prevents free movement of the slide and oil spilt and dried on moving parts interferes with their movements. *Oil-immersion objectives should be cleaned after use each day* by wiping with a well-washed, fine cotton cloth (handkerchief) or, preferably, with the fine paper tissue known as *lens paper*. A soiled cloth or tissue must not be used, as it may bear grit that will scratch the lens.

Oil left on a lens for a day or more dries, becomes sticky and finally hardens, so that it cannot be removed by simple wiping. It should be removed by repeated wiping with a cloth or tissue soaked in benzol or xylol. Alcohol, acetone, chloroform and other solvents must *not* be used, as they may dissolve the cement holding the lenses and so spoil the objective.

Dry objectives, eye-pieces, condenser lenses and mirror surfaces should be wiped free from dust with a well-washed cotton cloth or a fresh lens paper and any immersion oil spilt on them should be wiped away with a little benzol or xylol. Oil spilt on the stage or elsewhere must similarly be wiped off.

Eye-pieces from time to time may become contaminated internally with dust, so that fuzzy specks are seen in the field. The position of the dirt is readily located in the eye-piece, for the specks move when the eye-piece is rotated in its mount. If the dust is situated on the upper lens, the specks will move if the eye-piece is raised a little with one hand and the upper lens unscrewed with the other. If the dust is on the bottom lens, the specks will move if the mount of that lens is rotated by unscrewing. When the position of the dirt has been located, remove it with a soft camel-hair brush that has been held for a few seconds against a hot electric bulb. If this fails, use a lens paper moistened with *distilled* water.

In binocular microscopes, dust may collect on the prisms in the binocular head. It may be cleaned away with a soft camel-hair brush passed down the eye-piece tubes after removal of the eye-pieces. On no account open the prism case or remove the prisms for cleaning.

Common difficulties in microscopy

A number of troubles may be encountered by those beginning microscopy and the following hints are given to help overcome them.

1. *Inability to find focus or obtain a sharp image with the oil-immersion objective.*

a. See instruction (16) under *Method of use of light microscope* (above).

b. Check that there is no dirt or dried oil adherent to the front lens of the objective. If there is, clean it off.

c. Check that the microscope slide carrying the object has not been put upside down on the stage.

d. Check that the immersion oil has not become so sticky that the slide adheres to the objective and travels up and down with it in the movements of focusing. If so, clean off the old oil and replace with new.

e. Check whether the specimen slide has a film of dried oil and dirt left on it by a previous viewer. If so, clean it off with a lens paper moistened with benzol or xylol.

f. If the specimen is covered with a coverslip, check whether the coverslip is so thick, or whether the layer of mountant is so thick that the objective cannot approach near enough to the specimen to bring it within its focal length.

g. If none of these steps improves matters, consider whether the objective may be faulty. Exchange the objective with one from another microscope and if a sharp image is obtained with the new objective, return the faulty one to the makers.

2. *A dark shadow passes into the field with loss of definition of the image.* This trouble is usually caused by the movement of an air bubble in the immersion oil. With the coarse focusing adjustment, move the slide away from the objective so that contact between the oil and the objective is broken; then remake the contact and re-focus. If this procedure fails, clean the objective and slide with a little benzol to remove the oil, replace with fresh oil and re-focus.

3. *Poor illumination.*

a. Check that the condenser is properly focused, i.e. racked fully upwards. Occasionally it slips downwards in its mounting ring and must be pressed up so that it can be racked up to within 1 mm below the specimen slide. If the condenser is provided with a 'swing out' top lens, check that this lens is in the 'in' position, i.e. in train with the light beam.

b. Check that the substage iris diaphragm is fully open.

c. Check that the illumination is properly centred. If a moveable mirror is used, check that its flat, not concave, surface faces the light and that it is in the correct position to reflect light centrally into the condenser.

EXAMINATION OF UNSTAINED LIVING ORGANISMS: MOTILITY TESTS

Whilst most specimens for microscopy are stained to make them easily visible, the observation of unstained living organisms is required for certain purposes, e.g. to determine whether a culture of bacteria belongs to a species that is motile or to identify erythrocytes, other cells and crystals in infected urine. As unstained organisms may be difficult to focus, special microscopical procedures must be used. With the ordinary light microscope, moreover, it is necessary to defocus the condenser to maximize the contrast between the organism and its background, and this procedure results in some loss of resolution and definition.

The specimen may be a liquid culture, a suspension in broth or saline of agar-grown bacteria, or a body fluid or exudate. It can be examined either in an *unstained wet film* between a slide and a coverslip or in a *hanging-drop preparation*. The former is the simpler method and suffices for most purposes, but the latter provides the organisms with less disturbed and better oxygenated conditions.

Unstained wet film

1. With a glass-marking pen or diamond, draw a line across the middle of a slide. The mark will make it easier to focus the surface of the slide, and thus the film, in the absence of easily visible, stained material.

2. Place beside the line a drop of the liquid specimen or suspension. The drop should be large enough to form a complete film beneath a coverslip, but not so large that much excess fluid exudes at the edges.

3. Apply a coverslip to the drop. Try to avoid trapping large bubbles of air, lest when these are flattened they displace the fluid specimen from a large area of the film.

4. If the film is to be observed over a period of more than a few minutes, it may be sealed against drying by the application of nail varnish or melted soft petroleum jelly to the margins of the coverslip.

5. Observe the film with the low-power 16 mm dry objective. Focus the line and centre it in the field. In the absence of a line, focus and centre the edge of the film or the edge of an air bubble.

6. Turn the high-power 4 mm dry objective into position and focus the line or bubble edge to bring the film into the correct focal plane.

7. Defocus the condenser by racking it downwards, or by swinging out its top lens, to reduce and diffuse the illumination. Unstained cells and bacteria are invisible in intense, focused illumination. Reducing the illumination by defocusing the condenser, rather than by other means, has the additional advantage of rendering the unstained organisms more refractile and easily visible.

8. If necessary, a wet film may be observed

with an oil-immersion objective, but in that case special care must be taken because the viscosity of the oil tends to move the coverslip during the adjustments of focusing and any movements of the slide. Currents so caused in the fluid may give a false appearance of motility in the organisms.

Motility of organisms. When examining living organisms for the property of active locomotion, it is essential to distinguish *true motility*, whereby the organisms move in different directions and change their positions in the field, from either (1) *passive drifting* of the organisms in the same direction in a convectional current in the fluid or (2) *Brownian movement*, which is an oscillatory movement about a nearly fixed point possessed by all small bodies suspended in fluid and due to irregularities in their bombardment by molecules of water.

Hanging drop preparation

1. Use a 'hollow ground' slide, i.e. a glass slide with a shallow, circular concavity in its centre.

2. Encircle the concavity with a line streak of soft petroleum jelly applied with a glass rod to the surface of the slide just outside the concavity.

3. With a glass-marking pen, draw a V-shaped line on the surface of a coverslip and then place a small drop of the liquid culture or suspension on the same side of the coverslip within the angle of the V. As a drop is much thicker than a wet film, make sure that the suspension of culture is not so dense that the crowded organisms obscure one another. If necessary, dilute the suspension.

4. Invert the slide over the coverslip, allowing it to adhere to the jelly. Then quickly turn round the slide so that the coverslip is uppermost. The drop will then be hanging from the coverslip in the centre of the concavity. If too big a drop has been used and it has touched and flowed on to the slide, discard the preparation and prepare another.

5. Proceed to examine first with a low-power objective and then with a high-power one as described above for an unstained wet film.

Warm-stage examinations

The use of a warm stage placed over the main stage of the microscope is very convenient when examining fresh unstained specimens for amoebae and other protozoa, which are more easily observed and identified when moving actively at a temperature of about 37°C. It is also useful for observing the growth or lysis of bacteria in wet films or on blocks of nutrient agar. Several types of warm stage are available, the best types being electrically heated and automatically adjusted to the desired temperature, which is usually 37°C.

MICROMETRY

In bacteriological work the unit of measurement is 0.001 mm, designated a micrometre or μm. The measurement of microscopic objects is accomplished with a *micrometer eye-piece*, the scale in which is calibrated by comparison with a standard *stage micrometer*. The micrometer eye-piece is a special eye-piece of the positive type which bears a graduated scale mounted on its diaphragm and has a movable eye lens for focusing of the scale. The stage micrometer is a microscope slide bearing an engraved scale 1 mm in length and graduated at intervals of 0.01 mm (i.e. 10 μm).

1. Insert the micrometer eye-piece into one eye-piece tube of the microscope. Focus the eye-piece scale with the movable eye-piece lens.

2. Place the stage micrometer on the microscope stage in firm contact with its surface. Centre the scale in the field.

3. With the objective to be used for micrometry, focus the scale of the stage micrometer and move the stage so that the stage and eye-piece scales lie in parallel, side-by-side. With an oil-immersion objective, place oil directly on the stage-micrometer scale.

4. Count the number of divisions on the eye-piece scale that correspond to a definite number, e.g. 10, of divisions in the stage scale. From knowledge that each stage scale division is 0.01 mm, or 10 μm, calculate the length measured by an eye-piece scale division when used with the chosen objective.

5. Remove the stage micrometer and replace it with a slide bearing the specimen to be studied. Focus the specimen with the objective for which the calibration was done and count the number of divisions of the eye-piece scale that just cover the object to be measured. The tube length of the microscope must not be altered between calibration and measurement.

6. Calculate the measurement of the object as in the following example. If with the 2 mm oil-immersion objective 10 stage scale divisions (i.e. $10 \times 10 \ \mu m$) are found equal to 91 eye-piece scale divisions, each eye-piece scale division will correspond to $100/91 \ \mu m$, i.e. $1.1 \ \mu m$, in the field of the 2 mm objective. If, then, the length of a bacterium viewed with the same eye-piece and objective is found to equal 3.5 eye-piece divisions, the length of the bacterium will be $3.5 \times 1.1 \ \mu m$, or $3.85 \ \mu m$.

Photographic micrometry

1. First photograph the organisms or cells with a high-power objective.

2. Without disturbing the microscope or the camera, remove the specimen slide from the microscope stage and replace it with the stage micrometer.

3. After re-adjusting focus on the micrometer scale, photograph the scale. The photographs of the specimen and the scale will then be at exactly the same magnification and enlarged prints of these photographs should be made at exactly the same degree of enlargement.

4. With a pair of fine dividers, take the length (or width) of the organism on its photographic print and then obtain its measurement by applying the dividers to the print of the micro-meter scale, in which one division will represent $10 \ \mu m$.

Electron-microscope micrometry

1. To a suspension of the organisms to be measured, add a suspension of latex particles of known diameter, e.g. 88 or 250 nm.

2. View with the electron microscope and find and photograph a field containing both the organism and some latex particles.

3. Calculate the diameter of the organism by comparison with the known diameter of the latex particles.

It should be remembered that in the electron microscope an organism may be shrunken by drying and heat. This effect may be minimized by suitable fixation.

DARKGROUND MICROSCOPE

Although, as described above, unstained living organisms may be observed in a wet film with the ordinary light microscope, they are seen only faintly, contrasting poorly with their back-ground, and if scanty are difficult to detect. They may be seen much more clearly, and with better resolution, with the darkground microscope or the phase-contrast microscope, which have optical systems that enhance the contrast of unstained bodies. The surfaces and denser internal bodies of bacteria and other cells are shown brightly lit against a dark field in the dark-ground microscope and, usually, in dark contrast against a bright field in the phase-contrast microscope.

The darkground microscope has proved particularly useful for demonstrating the smaller spirochaetes, such as those of syphilis, which are so thin they are practically invisible with the ordinary light microscope, whether in unstained wet films or in fixed films stained by ordinary methods. The bright contrast of the spirochaete in the darkground microscope and the motility it shows in its living, unstained state, make it easy to detect even when in small numbers.

The principle of darkground microscopy is that the specimen is illuminated only by rays of light so oblique that unless they are 'scattered' by objects, e.g. bacteria, of different refractive index from the suspending medium, they fail to enter the objective and reach the eye. Some of the scattered rays from the dense objects enter the objective and reach the eye, so that these objects appear gleaming brightly against a dark background.

There are three requisites for adapting an ordinary microscope for darkground illumi-nation: (1) a darkground condenser, which focuses only oblique rays of light on the specimen, (2) a suitable high-intensity lamp, and (3) a funnel stop which reduces the numerical aperture of the objective to less than 1.0.

Darkground condenser. The special condenser incorporates concentric reflecting mirrors. A central one prevents light rays from passing directly up through the specimen into the objective and reflects them outwards on to a peripheral mirror. The latter reflects the rays inwards on to the specimen at a very oblique angle (Fig. 2.4). The condenser must be furnished with focusing and centring adjustments, for success with darkground illumination depends critically on accurate focusing and centring of the light from the condenser. It is necessary also to use immersion oil between the top lens of the condenser and the bottom of the specimen slide.

Funnel stop. When the objective employed for darkground illumination has a numerical aperture of more than 1, as do ordinary oil-immersion objectives, a special stop must be inserted in it to reduce the numerical aperture to less than 1. This stop consists of a small funnel-shaped piece of metal or plastic that can be fitted into the objective behind its back lens. It can easily be removed later to convert the objective back for bright-field use.

Alternatively, a special objective adaptor with an adjustable iris diaphragm may be used; this enables the numerical aperture to be quickly changed between that for dark-field and that for bright-field microscopy. There are also available special oil-immersion fluorite objectives that can be used without a funnel stop, e.g. a 2 mm objective of numerical aperture 1.15 and a 3.5 mm objective with numerical aperture 0.95.

The slide. The thickness of the slide is critical; it should be only 1.0–1.1 mm. It should be thoroughly clean and free from grease. As the object on the slide must be at the focus of the condenser, which is about 1.2 mm, the use of too thick a slide will prevent proper focusing of the light and result in poor illumination.

The film. The film of fluid containing the specimen should be as thin as possible, so that moving objects are kept in one plane and the background is satisfactorily dark. In a thick film, contrast is diminished and objects frequently move in and out of focus. The thickness of the film is determined by the size of the drop of fluid specimen placed on the slide before the coverslip is laid upon it. If the film is found too thick, it may be thinned by withdrawing fluid with a piece of filter paper or blotting paper applied to its edge. The coverslip itself must be sufficiently thin, e.g. No. 1 grade, not to make contact with the 2 mm objective when that is focused on the specimen. The concentration of bacteria or other material in the fluid specimen must not be too great, for an excessive number of particles will scatter so much light that contrast is lost. If necessary, the specimen should be diluted with saline. When examination is to be prolonged, evaporation from the film should be prevented by sealing its edges with nail varnish or thin smears of petroleum jelly. If either sealant is used, care must be taken when focusing with the 2 mm objective to prevent it coming into contact with the sealant.

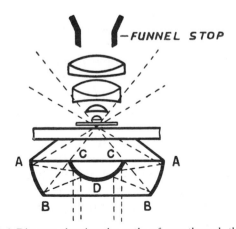

Fig. 2.4 Diagram showing the paths of rays through the darkground condenser and a $\frac{1}{12}$-in-oil-immersion lens fitted with a funnel stop. AB and CDC are reflecting surfaces. The surface at CC is opaque. (After E. Leitz.)

Method of use of the darkground microscope with an oil-immersion objective

1. Turn on the high-intensity lamp at low intensity and then increase the intensity and

centre the illumination. Fully open the lamp iris and substage condenser iris and leave them open. Adjust the mechanical stage so that it will hold a slide with its centre over the substage condenser. Place a funnel stop in the 2 mm oil-immersion objective to reduce its numerical aperture to less than 1.

2. Centre the darkground substage condenser while viewing it with the low-power 16 mm dry objective. Most such condensers have concentric rings engraved on their top lens to show the centre. Rack up the condenser so that its top lens is about 1 mm below the upper surface of the stage. Focus the surface of the lens to bring the engraved rings into view. Any oil left on the condenser will need to be cleaned off, and the illumination may need to be adjusted in order to make the rings easily visible. Then adjust the centring screws of the condenser to bring the engraved rings into a central position concentric with the field.

3. If the condenser does not have engraved centring rings, proceed as in (4) and (5) below and then focus the preparation with the low-power 16 mm dry objective. A bright ring of light should be seen in the field. Focus the condenser slightly up or down, but without breaking oil contact, until the ring of light contracts down to the smallest bright spot obtainable. Move this spot into the centre of the field by adjusting the centring screws of the condenser.

4. Prepare the specimen in a thin wet film between a 1.0–1.1 mm thick slide and a thin coverslip as described above.

5. Lower the condenser so that its top lens is well below the surface of the stage. Place a large drop of immersion oil on its top lens and another drop on the centre of the underside of the slide bearing the wet film. Place the slide on the microscope stage so that the drop of oil on its underside is over the centre of the condenser. Then rack up the condenser until oil contact is made between the whole area of its top lens and the undersurface of the slide. The film should be free from air bubbles. If a complete and bubble-free film is not obtained, remove the slide, add fresh oil and repeat the procedure. Take care during these procedures not to raise the condenser so high that it comes into contact with the slide itself and raises the slide from the stage. Also, avoid putting so much oil between the condenser and slide that it spills down the sides of the condenser.

6. Focus the specimen with the low-power 16 mm dry objective and find a suitable field with material for high-power observation. Turn the high-power 4 mm dry objective into position and focus the specimen with it. If the illumination is not quite central, centre it by adjusting the centring screws of the substage condenser.

7. Place a large drop of oil on the coverslip over the film and turn the 2 mm oil-immersion objective into position so that it just touches this drop. Carefully focus the specimen, taking care to avoid touching the coverslip with the objective by following the procedures (12)–(16) described above under *Method of use of light microscope*.

8. If necessary, slightly adjust the focusing and centration of the substage condenser to obtain an evenly illuminated field in which brilliantly lit objects are seen on a very dark background. In doing so, take care not to break the oil contact between the condenser and the slide. If the dark ground effect is lost, repeat the whole procedure of adjustment with the 16 mm dry objective from step (6) above.

9. After use, turn the light intensity control to low before switching off the lamp and carefully wipe the objective and condenser free from oil.

PHASE-CONTRAST MICROSCOPE

Phase-contrast microscopy provides a second method for observing unstained living organisms with good contrast and high resolution. It does not show up very small or slender objects, such as spirochaetes, as vividly as darkground microscopy, but is more useful than the latter for study of the structure and structural changes in larger microorganisms and tissue cells.

Objects are made to appear in dark-grey contrast against a bright background by causing direct and diffracted rays from them, which differ in their wave phase, to recombine in such a way that they interfere with each other and so reduce the light intensity in the area of the image corresponding to the object. Unstained bacteria and cells consist of alternate strips of material of slightly different refractive indices which act like a diffraction grating and through which diffracted and undiffracted rays of light acquire small phase differences. These differences are maximized by causing the direct and diffracted rays to pass through different thicknesses of glass in a phase plate in the back focal plane of the objective (see Fig. 2.5) which retards the diffracted rays one quarter of a wavelength with respect to the direct rays. As the direct beam is originally more intense than the diffracted beam, its intensity is reduced to the level of the latter by a thin deposit of metal on the part of the phase plate through which it passes. When the two beams are recombined to form an image, the direct and diffracted rays interfere with one another.

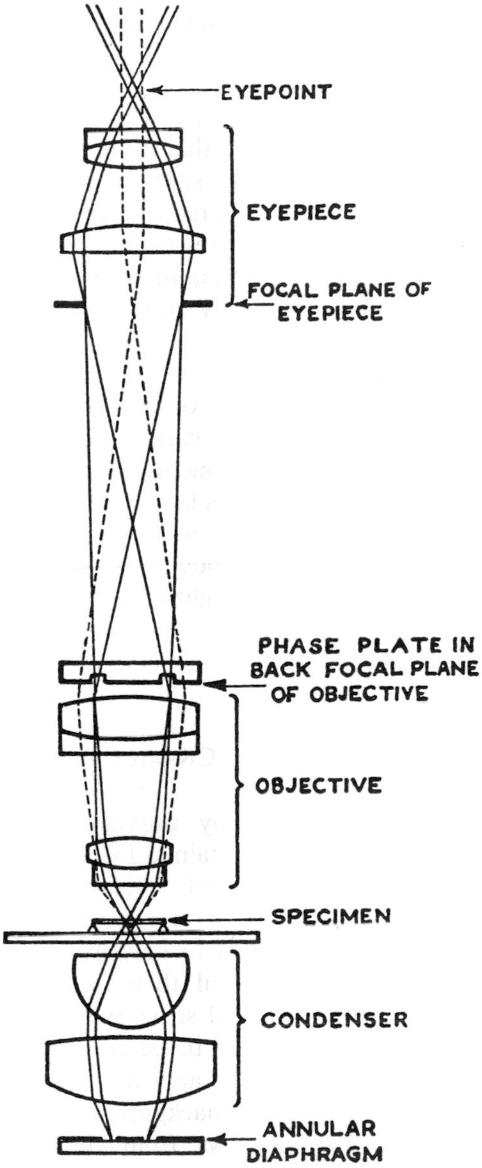

Fig. 2.5 Diagram illustrating the paths of light rays in phase-contrast microscopy. (Reproduced by permission of American Optical Company.)

Requisites

1. The microscope must be provided with a source of high-intensity illumination through an annular diaphragm which transmits a ring of light into the condenser. A different size of annulus is required for use with each objective of different numerical aperture, one of small diameter for the 16 mm objective and one of large diameter for the 2 mm objective. The series of annular diaphragms may be carried on a rotating disk fitted to the bottom of the condenser or be placed interchangeably in a carrier between the lamp condenser and the substage condenser. The size of the annulus is such that the substage condenser forms an image of it in the back focal plane of the objective.

2. The microscope must also be furnished with special phase objectives. These are ordinary objectives with a phase plate fitted in their back focal plane. The phase plate is a disk of glass with a circular trough etched in it. The trough is of such a depth that light passing through it has a phase difference of quarter of a wavelength from that passing through the rest of the plate.

3. An auxiliary telescope is required for observing the image in the back focal plane of the objective. It replaces an eye-piece when being used for this purpose.

Method of use of phase-contrast microscope

Some details of the method of use will differ with the type of microscope and the manufacturer's instructions must be followed. With many microscopes the following instructions will suffice.

1. Turn on the high-intensity lamp at low intensity. Then increase the intensity to half or

three-quarters full and centre the illumination. Fully open the lamp iris and the substage condenser iris and leave them open. Check that the light filter carrier is properly in position. Remove or switch out any annulus from the field of the condenser.

2. Normally begin by using the high-power 4 mm dry objective. Turn the focusing adjustment to give good clearance between the objectives and the stage. Then rotate the 4 mm objective into position.

3. Adjust the substage condenser so that its top lens is about 5 mm below the upper surface of the stage.

4. Place the specimen slide, with the wet film and coverslip uppermost, on the stage in such a position that the film is above the condenser. Press the slide down into uniform contact with the stage.

5. Focus the specimen, looking for the edges of any bubbles (or an indicating line if one has been marked on the slide) for assistance in finding focus. Find a group of organisms or cells to observe while aligning and adjusting the illumination. Focus this group accurately.

6. Replace one eye-piece with the auxiliary telescope. By moving its draw-tube, focus the telescope on the engraved annulus of the phase plate in the objective. Do not alter the focus of the microscope and check that it has remained unchanged by looking down the eye-piece still in place to view the specimen.

7. Place the annular diaphragm appropriate for the objective into position between the lamp and the substage condenser. Focus the substage condenser until the ring of light seen through the telescope is the same size as the engraved annulus on the phase plate. Again check that the microscope is still focused on the specimen by looking down the eye-piece remaining in place.

8. Remove the annular diaphragm again and, while looking down the telescope, adjust the centring screws of the substage condenser until the patch of light (image of the light filament) is centrally placed and lying symmetrically over the engraved annulus on the phase plate.

9. Replace the annular diaphragm and, while looking down the telescope, centre the diaphragm by adjusting the screws on its carrier. The ring of light must be made to fall exactly within the inner and outer margins of the engraved annulus on the phase plate. It should not overlap either margin and should be white, not blue-coloured. Adjust the *size* of the ring of light by adjusting the focus of the substage condenser. Adjust the *position* of the ring of light by adjusting the centring screws on the carrier of the annular diaphragm.

10. Again check that the microscope is still accurately focused on the specimen by looking down the eye-piece in place. Adjust the focus if necessary. After adjustment of the focus, look again down the telescope and re-adjust the ring of light on the engraved annulus.

11. Remove the telescope and replace it with the second eye-piece. Examine the specimen, adjusting the light to a suitable intensity. As searching may require moving of the specimen to areas of different thickness, from time to time use the telescope to check and re-adjust the centration of the ring of light on the annulus.

12. *Examination with 2 mm oil-immersion objective.* Turn the coarse focusing adjustment to give a good clearance between the slide and the objectives. Remove the annular diaphragm from the field of light entering the condenser. Place a drop of immersion oil on the coverslip. Turn the 2 mm objective into position and, with the coarse focusing adjustment, bring the objective into contact with the oil and focus the specimen. Finding focus will be helped if a suitable object has been left in the centre of the field observed with the 4 mm objective.

Then proceed through steps (6) to (11) above, but using the annular diaphragm appropriate to the 2 mm objective.

FLUORESCENCE MICROSCOPE

Fluorescent stains

When certain materials, e.g. oil or fat droplets, or certain dyes are exposed to ultra-violet radiation, they convert this invisible, short-wave radiation into the longer wavelength radiation of visible light, and so become luminous and are said to fluoresce. If, therefore, microorganisms or tissue cells are stained with a fluorescent dye and are examined under the microscope with ultra-violet radiation instead of ordinary visible light, they are seen as bright objects against a dark background.

Some of these fluorescent dyes have a selective affinity for microorganisms or cell components and can be used directly to stain them and so make them easily visible with the ultra-violet, fluorescence microscope. Auramine O, which gives a yellow fluorescence, may be used to stain tubercle bacilli (Ch. 3). Acridine orange R, which has an affinity for nucleic acids, fluorescing orange-red with RNA and yellow-green with DNA, may be used to stain viral nucleic acid in infected cells and tissues (Ch. 3).

Fluorescent antibody: Immunofluorescence

Other fluorescent dyes can be used to label serum antibodies. They are coupled to, or 'conjugated' with, the immunoglobulins and other proteins in an antiserum, so rendering these antibodies and proteins fluorescent. The two dyes most used are fluorescein isothiocyanate, which fluoresces yellow-green, and lissamine rhodamine B (RB200) which gives an orange fluorescence. The fluorescent antiserum is applied like a stain to a film of microorganisms or section of tissue and the fluorescent antibody is allowed to combine firmly with the corresponding antigens in the film. The fluorescent non-antibody proteins are then washed away and the film is examined under the fluorescence microscope. As staining with fluorescent antibody has the high specificity of antigen-antibody reactions, those organisms, cells or cell components seen to fluoresce are specifically identified as containing the antigen corresponding to the fluorescent antibody. Methods for preparing fluorescent antibody and staining films with it are described in Chapter 10 and by Nairn (1976).

Illumination

Many manufacturers supply complete fluorescence microscopes with a suitable, built-in source of ultra-violet (UV) illumination, but an ordinary microscope can be adapted by the provision of a UV lamp and suitable filters.

The best UV source is a high-pressure mercury vapour lamp, such as the Osram HB200, which has a wavelength range of 280–600 nm, so covering the wavelengths of 290–325 nm, required for fluorescein, and 310–350 nm, required for rhodamine. It has a limited life, e.g. about 200 h, and must be enclosed in a protective housing because there is a small risk of explosion that increases as it is used beyond its stated life. Within the housing an aluminium-coated mirror and centring devices are required. The collector lens of the lamp should consist of UV-transmitting crown glass or, better, the more heat-resistant quartz glass.

Two systems of illumination are available, with transmitted UV and with incident UV. The former is the older system and may be applied with an ordinary microscope suitably modified. The latter is the better system and requires the use of a specially designed microscope.

Transmitted UV illumination

The UV radiation is transmitted through a substage condenser on to the specimen film from beneath and the visible light formed by fluorescence in the specimen passes on into the objective and up the microscope. For specimens stained directly with a fluorochrome dye, a bright-ground, three lens, aplanatic condenser is satisfactory, but for specimens stained with fluorescent antibody a darkground condenser gives better results, especially with the higher-power objectives. Auto-fluorescence can be a problem, particularly when a bright-ground condenser is used.

Filters. (1) A primary filter sited close to the lamp ensures the maximum relative emission of radiation of the required wavelengths, e.g. Kodak Wratten 18B or Chance Pilkington OX7 in Britain. (2) A secondary filter is placed in the eye-piece to cut out UV rays which might damage the observer's eye. A Kodak Wratten 2B filter is satisfactory.

Immersion oil. Special non-fluorescent immersion oil is essential and that supplied by Leitz is recommended.

Incident UV illumination

The UV radiation in this system (Ploem 1967) is directed on to the specimen film from above, through the objective, instead of from below, through a substage condenser. It is first directed horizontally from the lamp on to a dichroic mirror set at an angle of 45° in the microscope tube. This interference mirror reflects UV radiation of the required wavelength down the microscope tube and through the objective on to the surface of the specimen. The visible light from the fluorescing specimen then passes back through the objective to the dichroic mirror, which transmits it on through a secondary filter to the eye-piece.

The advantage of the incident UV system is that it gives brighter fluorescence than the transmitted UV system, particularly with the higher-power objectives. Fluorite objectives do not give rise to auto-fluorescence and it is unnecessary to use special immersion oil.

Use of the fluorescence microscope

Procedures for centring and adjusting the illumination should follow the instructions of the manufacturer of the microscope. The work should be done in a dark room lit only by one or two dim 'safe lights' of the kind used in photographic work. A comfortable seating position is necessary, for fluorescence microscopy can be very fatiguing. Before beginning to use the microscope, check that the correct filters are in place, especially that the secondary, 'barrier' filter, which protects the eyes, is present in the eye-piece assembly.

The most difficult part of an examination is to find the plane of focus of the specimen, for out-of-focus fluorescence is often too dim to see. The best method is to use a Teflon-coated slide on which to mount the specimen. A suitable slide is the multispot slide manufactured by Hendley in Britain, which has 6–12 clear circles surrounded by an opaque coating of Teflon. Different specimens are mounted in the clear circles and dried. If they are exudates, secretions or other body materials in which the antigens

may be combined with antibody, the latter is eluted by standing in a glycine-HCl buffer at pH 2.4 for at least 4 h before the film is fixed in methanol or acetone for 10 min, stained and mounted in 10% (v/v) glycerol in phosphate-buffered saline under a coverslip.

The glycine-HCl buffer pH 2.4 is made by adding 32.4 ml of HCl, 0.2 mol/litre, to 50 ml of glycine, 0.2 mol/litre, and making up the mixture to 200 ml with distilled water. A pepsin-HCl buffer consisting of 100 μg pepsin in HCl, 0.1 mol/litre (Ch. 20) is even more effective in removing patient's antibody.

A × 25 or × 40 dry objective is best used for the examination, for even the smallest bacteria such as *Treponema pallidum* are easily observed at these low magnifications when fluorescing. In beginning the examination, find and focus on the edge of the Teflon surrounding each specimen circle. This is easily done and brings the microscope into the focal plane of the specimen, which can then be searched.

If Teflon-coated slides are not available, first scan the film with the low-power 16 mm (× 10) objective to find a large aggregate of fluorescing dust or debris and centre it in the field before changing to the higher-power objective. The aggregate will serve as an easily focused object and facilitate finding the focal plane of the specimen with the latter objective.

Having focused the plane of the specimen, find areas of fluorescence with the colour appropriate to the fluorescent dye being used, e.g. yellow-green for fluorescein. Then confirm that the fluorescence is being emitted from a structure with the morphology of the organism or cell component sought. Unless these two criteria are met, false-positive results will be recorded.

The phenomenon of *quenching* may make it difficult to observe the morphology of fluorescent structures. When a fluorescent structure is moved into the illuminated field, its fluorescence rapidly diminishes, often within a few seconds at the higher magnifications, due to changes produced by the UV radiation in the fluorescent dye. The microscopist must continually move to new, previously unexposed fields in order to see objects with the clearest fluorescence. He will often have to search most of the area of a specimen before he can conclude whether the result is positive or negative.

LOW-POWER MICROSCOPES

Light microscopes with low magnifications, e.g. × 4 to × 50, have special uses in microbiology. The *stereoscopic low-power microscope* is useful for examining the detailed morphology of colonies on culture plates. It has a holder for the culture plate and arrangements for illumination either by transmitted light from below or reflected light from above the level of the plate. Viewing by reflected light is most valuable, for it allows the texture of the surface of the colony to be seen. Illumination by *oblique* transmitted light, giving the effect of darkground illumination, may be arranged with some microscopes; it reveals differences in the texture of the substance of colonies.

The *inverted transmitted-light microscope* is invaluable for examination of virological cell cultures in plates, bottles or tubes, and the cell content of urine samples. The container is placed on the top of the microscope stage with the contained layer of cells nearest to the stage. The lamp and condenser are *above* the stage and focus light down on to the specimen in the container. The objectives, body and eye-pieces of the microscope are *below* the stage, but the eye-pieces are inclined upwards to permit easy viewing.

ELECTRON MICROSCOPE

When it is required to visualize viruses or parts of cells with a diameter less than 0.2 μm (200 nm), which is the limit of resolution of the light microscope, it is necessary to use the electron microscope. The limit of resolution of that instrument may be 0.001 μm (1 nm) or less, making possible the observation of very fine detail.

The object is scanned with a high-speed beam of electrons instead of with visible light, and to allow passage of the electrons, the column, or tube, of the microscope has to be evacuated to make it completely empty of air and gas. The electron beam is focused with electromagnetic 'lenses'. The high resolving power of the instrument is due to the electron beam having a very small equivalent wavelength, about 0.005 nm, or 100 000 times shorter than the wavelength of visible light. If the efficiency of the electromagnetic lenses were as great as that of optical lenses, resolution down to a limit of 0.0025 nm would be possible, but the numerical aperture of an electron microscope lens is very small and, in practice, the best obtainable resolution is in the range of 0.1–0.5 nm.

An object forms an image in the electron microscope because its solid content, particularly its heavy atoms, scatters the electrons and so casts a shadow in the electron beam. If the material in small organisms or particles is not dense enough to show them in sufficient contrast, greater contrast may be provided by outlining them with a layer of heavy metal, e.g. gold or palladium, evaporated on to the dried specimen. This procedure is called 'shadowing' or 'shadow casting', because the dense metal, except where it is absent in shadows cast by the raised parts of the specimen, is relatively opaque to the electron beam and gives the specimen a three-dimensional appearance. Another means of increasing contrast is by applying a solution of heavy metal, e.g. phosphotungstic acid or uranyl acetate, to the specimen during preparation of the film, a procedure called 'negative staining' because the solid parts of the specimen are outlined by the more opaque staining material.

The principal limitation of the electron microscope is that it cannot be used to observe organisms in the wet, living state, for the specimen must be exposed in a vacuum and therefore dried. The shrinking and distorting effects of drying can be minimized by suitable prior fixation of the material to be examined.

Construction of the electron microscope

The electron microscope (see Fig. 2.6) consists of a tubular column (4) at the top of which is

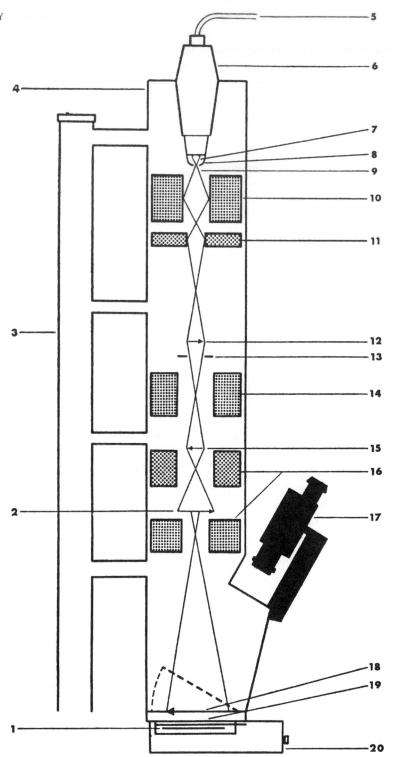

Fig. 2.6 A diagram to show the optical system and component parts of an electron microscope. (1) Photographic plate (2) Primary image (3) Connections from column to vacuum pumps (4) Column (5) 100 000-volt supply (6) Electron gun (7) Hot tungsten-wire filament (8) Cathode shield (9) Electron beam (10) First condenser lens (11) Second condenser lens (12) Object (13) Objective aperture (14) Objective lens (15) Intermediate image (16) First and second projector lenses (17) Focusing binoculars (18) Final image (19) Fluorescent screen (20) Camera.

mounted the source of electrons, the so-called 'electron gun' (6) which emits electrons from a hot tungsten filament serving as a cathode (7). Beneath this filament is placed a 'cathode shield' (8) and an anode with a small hole in its centre. A high voltage, which may be 50 or 100 kV, is applied between the cathode and anode to accelerate the emitted electrons. The life of the cathode filament is limited and it usually requires to be replaced after about 15 h of viewing. A narrow beam of electrons (9) passes at high speed through the hole in the anode and down the column of the microscope. The accelerating voltage must be stabilized with an accuracy better than 1 in 100 000 to ensure that the beam has a uniform velocity. Because the electrons would be scattered by any atoms with which they might collide, the air in the column is completely evacuated and a vacuum of the order of 10^{-6} mm Hg is maintained by the operation of powerful mechanical and oil-diffusion pumps (3).

Focusing and magnification are achieved with a series of 'lenses', which are electromagnets producing accurately controllable magnetic fields. There is a condenser lens system (10 and 11) which focuses a nearly parallel beam of electrons on to the specimen (12) placed beneath it. It is the focusing of the condenser lens that, by diffusing or concentrating the beam, varies the intensity of 'illumination' of the specimen. The different areas of the specimen scatter the impinging electrons to degrees proportional to their thickness and density. The unscattered electrons pass through a small objective aperture (13) and are focused by an objective lens (14) to form a real primary image (2) at a magnification of about × 100. Two projector lenses (16), which have the function of the eye-piece in a light microscope, further magnify part of the primary image to a final magnification of up to × 100 000. The focal length of the electromagnetic lenses can be changed by varying the current flowing through them, so that the degree of magnification can be controlled by the turn of a dial.

The final image (18) is formed on a fluorescent screen (19) at the lower end of the column and is viewed through a glass window. The screen can be withdrawn by the movement of a lever to allow the electrons to impinge and so form an image on a photographic film (1) in a camera beneath it. Owing to the high resolving power of the electron microscope, it is possible to take negatives at magnifications of up to × 100 000 and enlarge them photographically up to × 10. Thus, a useful magnification of up to 1 000 000 diameters can be obtained.

The controls of the microscope are accommodated in panels on its desk. They include dials for the variation of magnification and intensity of illumination, a mechanical control to move the specimen during searching of the field, switches and meters to control and check the voltage, vacuum gauges, and controls for alignment of the electron beam. Switches for the mechanical and diffusion pumps and circuits for stabilizing the voltage form a separate unit.

Specimen holder

The specimen to be examined is mounted on a thin membrane that is relatively transparent to the electron beam. This membrane may be made from collodion or Formvar and stabilized by coating with evaporated carbon. It is supported in a small circular copper grid perforated with holes through which the electrons can pass. After the specimen has been dried, the grid is placed in a special holder and this is introduced into the column between the condenser and objective lenses through an air lock. When the vacuum in the column has been restored, the specimen holder is lowered into position by a lever and the specimen is then focused and examined at the required magnification and a suitable intensity of illumination. Care must be taken to avoid destroying the specimen or its supporting membrane by overlong exposure to a beam of excessive intensity. A × 10 binocular microscope (17) may be used to view the fluorescent screen to facilitate accurate focusing before a photograph is taken.

PREPARATION OF MATERIALS FOR ELECTRON MICROSCOPY

As the penetrating power of the electron beam is slight, only very small objects or very thin sections of tissues can be examined. Specimens are mounted on small copper disks, or 'grids', 2 or 3 mm in diameter, perforated with many apertures in the arrangement of a regular mesh. Grids of 200 mesh size (200 holes per linear inch) provide large holes through which the beam can pass and are often used to mount thin sections. When small objects in suspension, such as bacteria and viruses are to be examined, grids of 400 mesh size are used and these are covered with a thin, electron-transparent film, e.g. of Formvar stabilized with a coating of carbon (see below). The particles are supported on the film which is stretched between the bars of the grid. Grids are manipulated with very fine pointed forceps and are more easily picked up if slightly bent, but sharp bending must be avoided lest it results in damage to the film or section.

Preparation of support film

Formvar cast on glass

The following materials are required:

1. A 2% (w/v) solution of polyvinyl formal (Formvar) in ethylene dichloride, which should not be kept for use more than 4 weeks after its preparation.
2. A small, wide-mouthed flask or jar.
3. A plastic box, about 10 × 10 cm, and a tray.
4. Fresh glass-distilled water.
5. Microscope slides.
6. Lint-free (Velin) tissue.
7. A fine hypodermic or dissecting needle.
8. Fine-pointed forceps.
9. Copper grids of 400 mesh size.
10. Filter paper.

Procedure. 1. Make up a working solution of Formvar by mixing 5 ml of the 2% stock solution with 45 ml ethylene dichloride and pour this working solution into the small flask.

2. Place the plastic box on the tray and fill the box to the brim with glass-distilled water.

3. Clean a glass microscope slide with Velin tissue. Then dip the slide to about half its length in the Formvar solution. After a few seconds, withdraw the slide from the solution and allow it to dry, propped up in a near-vertical position

with its moist end downwards. When dry, the film is transparent.

4. After 5 min, use a sharp needle to cut round the film at one side of the slide, about 1–2 mm from its edge. Then cut the central oblong part of the film into halves.

5. Clean the surface of the distilled water by dragging the edge of a piece of Velin tissue across it.

6. Lower the slide, cut film uppermost, at an angle of 30° into the water. As the slide is slowly pushed under the water the film will float off on to the surface of the water. Observe the floating film by the interference colours it gives in reflected light from a bench lamp. Very thin films, about 20 nm thick, appear dark grey and films about 50–60 nm, which are generally satisfactory, appear an even silver colour.

7. Remove any unwanted scraps of film from the water with a needle.

8. With fine-pointed forceps, place rows of grids, matt side downwards and not quite touching one another, across the surface of one piece of floating film.

9. Take a piece of filter paper about 5 cm square and turn up one corner at right angles to form a handle. Holding this corner, lower the paper so that its flat surface comes to rest on the surface of the water, covering and in contact with the grids.

10. When the whole surface of the filter paper has become moist, lift it from the water and invert it, so that the grids are lifted with it and turned uppermost.

11. Leave the grids on the filter paper to dry overnight, covered against dust. They may be stored on the paper until required for use. When in that position, they have the Formvar film on their upper side.

Formvar-carbon films

Films of Formvar alone, as just described, can be used for the mounting and examination of bacteria and viruses, but when exposed to the electron beam at even moderate intensity, tend to heat up, drift and disintegrate. It is better to use Formvar films stabilized with a coating of evaporated carbon.

Carbon coating is carried out in a vacuum coating apparatus. This consists of a glass bell jar from which the air can be extracted by rotary and diffusion pumps. The base on which the jar stands carries vacuum-tight electrical connections supplying a current at 30 volts between two pointed carbon rods kept in end-to-end contact by a spring.

1. Place the Formvar-coated grids, still on the filter paper, under the bell jar and evacuate the jar to a vacuum of about 10^{-3} Pa.

2. Apply the current to the carbon rods to evaporate carbon on to the paper and grids. Sufficient carbon will have been deposited when the paper becomes a very pale grey, and only several seconds' evaporation should be required to achieve this level.

3. Then switch off the current, close the high vacuum valve and allow the jar to return to atmospheric pressure by the inlet of air.

The Formvar-carbon coated grids need not be removed from the filter paper until required for use. They can be made up in batches and keep well in a dust-free box.

All-carbon films

For work of the highest resolution it is necessary to use grids with all-carbon films that are only about 5 nm thick and show very little background granularity. Unfortunately, such films are also very brittle. They can be made by dissolving the Formvar away from Formvar-carbon coated grids, but unless this is done with great care, the carbon films are liable to become detached from the grids. Alternatively, the vacuum coating apparatus can be used to deposit a film of carbon on a glass slide or a square of clean, freshly cleaved mica. The film is then floated off on to a water surface and collected on grids.

For a detailed discussion of the preparation and properties of specimen supports, see Baumeister & Hahn (1978).

Preparation of suspensions of whole microorganisms

The gross morphology and surface structure of bacteria and viruses, including the fimbriae and flagella of bacteria, can be studied adequately in preparations of whole, intact microorganisms. The preparation of thin sections of the organisms is needed only for studying their internal structure. The organisms should be made up in a clean suspension, freed as far as possible from particulate debris that might obscure them. Their concentration should be sufficiently great, e.g. 10^6–10^8/ml, to ensure that some will be present in most of the small areas of film visible at high magnification.

Bacteria may be fixed by the addition of 0.25% formaldehyde to a suspension or broth culture and then 'washed' by centrifugation and resuspension in distilled water. Extracts of viruses from infected cells, tissues or faeces may require to be concentrated and purified by several cycles of differential centrifugation.

Preparation of the specimen film

With a fine, clean pipette, rinsed free from salts with distilled water, place a small drop of the microbial suspension on the surface of the film coating a grid. The drop must not be so large that fluid spills on to the underside of the grid. If the suspension is free from dissolved substances and the concentration of organisms relatively low, the whole drop may be left to dry on the grid, which should be left in a dust-free atmosphere, e.g. in a desiccator over calcium chloride.

If, however, the suspension is more concentrated and contains a significant amount of dissolved material, it is better to remove most of the drop before it dries. Allow the organisms in the drop to settle on to the film for 0.5–3 min, then remove most of the fluid by touching the drop with the corner of a torn piece of clean filter paper. Finally, leave the film to dry in a desiccator.

Contrast enhancement

The electron-scattering power of the solid content of bacteria and the larger viruses is just sufficient for them to cast a visible image in the microscope, but some means of enhancing the contrast between the organisms and their background is generally used. The methods of shadow casting (metal shadowing), negative staining and positive staining are available. That of negative staining has the greatest use and that of positive staining has its main application in the treatment of ultra-thin sections.

Shadow casting

This is a technique whereby an atomic vapour of electron-dense metal is directed at an angle, e.g. of 15°, and deposited on the specimen (Bradley 1965). The grid is exposed in a vacuum-coating apparatus and a short strip of heavy metal, e.g. gold, palladium or gold-palladium alloy, is placed on a tungsten filament a few inches from the grid and at the correct angle to its surface. The jar is evacuated and an electric current passed through the filament to heat it and evaporate the heavy metal. The metal atoms pass in straight lines in all directions, including that towards the grid. The image given in the microscope is mainly produced by the deposit of metal on the film, as the metal has greater scattering power for electrons than the carbonaceous content of the microorganisms. The increased deposition of metal on the edges of the organism facing towards the filament and the absence of deposition in the shadows behind edges facing away from the filament give the image a clearly outlined, three-dimensional appearance.

Though contrast is excellent, resolution is not as good with shadow casting as with negative staining. Shadow casting has, however, found new applications in enhancing the contrast of free DNA molecules and the contours of surface replicas.

Negative staining

This method was introduced by Brenner & Horne (1959). The mounted specimen is covered with a solution of a compound containing a heavy metal which provides a dark, electron-scattering background. The solid content of the biological structures is less opaque to the electron beam, so that these structures stand out as light areas against the dark background. The stain collects in largest amounts in depressions in the surface of the organisms and in the angle between its edge and the supporting film. The shape of the surface of the organism and its margin are thus clearly shown with dark outlining. The method has been particularly valuable in showing the fine structure of viruses and bacteriophages.

Substances used for negative staining include potassium phosphotungstate, potassium silicotungstate, uranyl acetate and ammonium molybdate. Of these, the phosphotungstate is the most used.

Phosphotungstate (PTA) staining

Prepare a 2% solution of phosphotungstic acid (PTA) in distilled water and adjust it to the required pH (usually 6–7) by the addition of 1 mol/litre potassium hydroxide. If it is found that the stain fails to spread on the specimen film and tends to form dense masses that obscure the specimen, the defect may be corrected by the addition of a trace of serum albumin to the stain to reduce its surface tension, or by reducing the concentration of phosphotungstate. If on the other hand the solution forms too thin a film, the concentration of phosphotungstate may be increased. Attention must be paid to the pH of the stain, for if this is changed the appearance of stained material may be altered.

Two-stage method. 1. Grip the edge of the grid with fine-pointed forceps and hold the grid with its coating film upwards.

2. With a fine pipette, place a drop of specimen suspension on the film on the grid and allow the organisms to settle on the film for 0.5–3 min. The drop must not be so large that fluid spills under the grid.

3. Then remove most of the fluid from the film by touching the drop, but not the surface of the film, with the corner of a torn piece of filter paper.

4. Next, with a fine pipette place a drop of phosphotungstate staining solution on the film and after about half a minute remove most of this fluid with filter paper as in (3).

5. Place the grid, film uppermost, on a piece of clean Velin tissue to dry.

Single-stage method. 1. Mix a drop of specimen suspension and a drop of phosphotungstate stain on a clean glass slide.

2. Place a drop of the mixture on the grid as in (1) and (2) of the two-stage method.

3. After 0.5–3 min, remove most of the fluid with filter paper and allow the film to dry.

When thin all-carbon films are used, the mixture of specimen suspension and stain solution may be applied to the grid with a glass spraying apparatus, but this method should not be used with live pathogenic organisms.

Further information about negative staining methods is given by Glauert (1965), Horne (1965, 1973), Haschemeyer & Myers (1972) and Horne & Wildy (1979).

Preparation of cells and tissues for thin-sectioning

Electron microscopy of thin sections is well established in histopathology, but the method can also be applied in microbiology, e.g. for demonstration of the internal structure of protozoa, the cell walls of bacteria and the intracellular replication of viruses. The procedures are not difficult, but there are many variations of technique that can influence the final microscopic appearance and it is important that changes due to differences in technique are not mistaken for differences among specimens. Some routine methods of preparation are given by Weakley (1981) and the procedures are extensively discussed by Hayat (1970), Glauert (1974), Reid (1974) and Lewis & Knight (1977).

Fixation for sectioning

Tissue fragments, organ cultures or bacterial colonies can be fixed by immersion in baths of fixative. A common procedure is double fixation, in which the tissue is pre-fixed in 2–4% buffered glutaraldehyde, rinsed in three changes of buffer, secondarily fixed in 1% osmium tetroxide, and rinsed again in buffer. Rapid penetration of fixative is needed to prevent autolysis and pieces of specimen should therefore be no larger than about 1 mm^3. Bacteria may be fixed in suspension by the method of Ryter & Kellenberger.

Fixation of microorganisms (Ryter & Kellenberger 1958)

Reagents for fixation

1. Michaelis veronal-acetate buffer

Sodium barbitone	2.94 g
Sodium acetate (hydrated)	1.94 g
Sodium chloride	3.40 g
Distilled water to make	100 ml

2. Kellenberger buffer

Veronal-acetate buffer	5 ml
Distilled water	13 ml
0.1 mol/litre HCl	7 ml
1 mol/l $CaCl_2$	0.25 ml

Adjust to pH 6.0 with the 0.1 mol/l HCl or buffer. Prepare freshly on the day of use.

3. Kellenberger fixative

Osmium tetroxide	0.1 g
Kellenberger buffer	10 ml

4. Tryptone medium

Bacto-Tryptone (Difco)	1 g
Sodium chloride	0.5 g
Distilled water to make	100 ml

5. Sterile agar solution

Agar	2 g
Distilled water to make	100 ml

Sterilize by autoclaving in 5 or 10 ml amounts.

6. Kellenberger washing solution

Uranyl acetate	0.5 g
Kellenberger buffer to make	100 ml

This solution keeps for several weeks at 4°C.

Procedure for fixation

1. Mix 30 ml of a suspension of microorganisms with 3.0 ml of Kellenberger fixative. Centrifuge for 5 min at 1800 *g*.

2. Decant the supernatant fluid and resuspend the microbial deposit in 1.0 ml of Kellenberger fixative to which 0.1 ml tryptone medium has been added.

3. Stand overnight (e.g. 16 h) at ambient temperature (*c*. 18°C).

4. Add 8.0 ml Kellenberger buffer and centrifuge for 5 min at 1800 *g*. Decant the supernatant fluid and resuspend the organisms in the small amount (e.g. 0.1 ml) of residual fluid.

5. Add about 0.03 ml of molten agar at 45°C to the suspension and mix carefully.

6. Pour a drop of the molten agar suspension on to a clean microscope slide and allow it to set firmly.

7. Cut the solidified drop into 1 mm cubes with a razor blade.

8. Place the cubes into the uranyl acetate washing solution and leave for 2 h at ambient temperature. The cubes will then be ready for dehydration and embedding.

The Kellenberger method gives good fixation of nuclear material, but is less satisfactory for preservation of bacterial cell walls. After the introduction of glutaraldehyde for preliminary fixation, Glauert & Thornley (1966) described two modified methods that gave better results with cell walls.

Glauert & Thornley's method A

1. Centrifuge the culture or microbial suspension to form a pellet.

2. Resuspend the pellet in glutaraldehyde solution (2.5% glutaraldehyde in 0.09 mol/litre cacodylate buffer containing 0.01 mol/litre calcium chloride) and leave to fix for 30 min at ambient temperature.

3. Wash the cells three times in cold (1°C) cacodylate buffer.

4. Fix overnight in Kellenberger osmium tetroxide fixative containing 10% (v/v) tryptone medium at ambient temperature.

5. Wash in Kellenberger washing solution (0.5% uranyl acetate in buffer).

6. Embed in agar, dehydrate and embed in Araldite.

7. Stain thin sections with Reynold's (1963) lead citrate.

Glauert & Thornley's method B

1. Suspend bacteria in broth (Difco Heart Infusion Broth containing 0.01% $CaCl_2.6H_2O$).

2. Add an equal volume of cold (1°C) double-strength glutaraldehyde fixative (5% glutaraldehyde in 0.18 mol/litre cacodylate buffer). Fix in a cold room for 1 h, producing a fall of temperature from about 16°C to about 10°C.

3. Centrifuge the suspension and resuspend the deposited organisms in cold single-strength buffer. Leave overnight in cold buffer or wash in three changes of buffer during 3 h.

4. Treat with Kellenberger fixative and uranyl acetate as in method A.

Very small samples of bacteria or cells in suspension may be difficult to process without loss during centrifugation. Some workers therefore prefer to embed small specimens in agar or bovine serum albumin and then fix 1 mm cubes by immersion in fixative.

Embedding and sectioning

Fixed blocks are dehydrated by passage through ethanol and propylene oxide and then embedded in an electron-translucent epoxy resin. Sections 50–90 nm thick are cut with an ultramicrotome. See Glauert (1974) and Weakley (1981) for details.

Positive staining

The positive stains used for electron microscope sections are compounds of heavy metals, some being the same substances that are used at different pH as negative stains. In positive staining, the substance becomes attached to lipids, proteins or carbohydrates in the organism and the stained structures appear as dark (electron opaque) areas or lines in contrast with the lighter background. Osmium tetroxide, uranyl acetate and phosphotungstic acid may act as positive stains at the fixation or dehydration stage. As, however, penetration of these stains into a block may not be adequate, it is usual to restain the thin sections with uranyl acetate followed by Reynold's (1963) lead citrate.

REFERENCES

Barer R 1959 Lecture notes on the use of the microscope, 2nd edn. Blackwell, Oxford

Baumeister W, Hahn M 1979 Specimen supports. In: Hayat M A (ed) Principles and techniques of electron microscopy, vol 8. Van Nostrand Reinhold, New York ch 1

Bradley D E 1965 The preparation of specimen support films. In: Kay D (ed) Techniques for electron microscopy, 2nd edn. Blackwell, Oxford. ch 3

Brenner S, Horne R W 1959 A negative staining method for high resolution electron microscopy of viruses. Biochemica et Biophysica Acta 34: 103–110

Glauert A M 1965 Factors influencing the appearance of biologic specimens in negatively stained preparations. Laboratory Investigation 14: 1069–1079

Glauert A M 1974 Fixation, dehydration and embedding of biological specimens. In: Glauert A M (ed) Practical methods in electron microscopy, vol 3. North Holland, Amsterdam

Glauert A M, Thornley M J 1966 Glutaraldehyde fixation of Gram-negative bacteria. Journal of the Royal Microscopical Society 85: 449–453

Haschemeyer R H, Myers R J 1972 Negative staining. In: Hayat M A (ed) Principles and techniques of electron microscopy, vol 2. Van Nostrand Reinhold, New York ch 3

Hayat M A 1970 Fixation (ch 1). Embedding (ch 2). Sectioning (ch 3). Staining (ch 4). In: Hayat M A (ed) Principles and techniques of electron microscopy, vol 1. Van Nostrand Reinhold, New York

Horne R W 1965 Negative staining methods. In: Kay D (ed) Techniques for electron microscopy, 2nd edn Blackwell, Oxford. ch 11

Horne R W 1973 Contrast and resolution from biological objects examined in the electron microscope with particular reference to negatively stained specimens. Journal of Microscopy 98: 286–298

Horne R W, Wildy P 1979 An historical account of the development and applications of the negative staining technique to the electron microscopy of viruses. Journal of Microscopy 117: 103–122

Lewis P R, Knight D P 1977 Staining methods for sectioned material. In: Glauert A M (ed) Practical methods in electron microscopy, vol 5. North Holland, Amsterdam

Nairn R C 1976 Fluorescent protein tracing, 4th edn. Churchill Livingstone, Edinburgh

Ploem J S 1967 The use of a vertical illuminator with interchangeable dichroic mirrors for fluorescence microscopy with visible light. Zeitschrift Wissenschaft Mikroskopie 68: 129–142

Reid N 1974 Ultramicrotomy. In: Glauert A M (ed) Practical methods in electron microscopy, vol 3. North Holland, Amsterdam

Reynolds E S 1963 The use of lead citrate at high pH as an electron-opaque stain in electron microscopy. Journal of Cell Biology 17: 208–212

Ryter A, Kellenberger E 1958 Etude au microscopie electronique de plasmas contenant de l'acide desoxyribonucleique. Zeitschrift Naturforschung 13b:597

Weakley B S 1981 A beginner's handbook in biological transmission electron microscopy, 2nd edn. Churchill Livingstone, Edinburgh

Wredden J H 1947 The microscope. Churchill, London

Staining methods

As bacteria consist of clear protoplasmic matter, differing but slightly in refractive index from the medium in which they are growing, it is difficult with the ordinary microscope, except when special methods of illumination are used, to see them in the unstained condition. Staining, therefore, is of primary importance for the recognition of bacteria.

The use and general principles of bacterial staining have been discussed in Volume 1, 13th Edition, Chapter 2.

METHODS OF MAKING FILM OR SMEAR PREPARATIONS

Before describing the various staining processes, details of the methods employed in making films must be considered.

Film preparations are made either on coverslips or on 3×1 in glass slides, usually the latter. It is essential that the coverslips or slides should be perfectly clean and free from grease, otherwise films will be uneven. Some manufacturers provide coverslips and slides free from grease and ready for immediate use. If, however, the supply is not sufficiently clean, the slips and slides should be cleaned as follows.

Cleaning slides and coverslips

Slides. A satisfactory method for ordinary use is to wipe the slide with a clean dry cotton cloth and then, holding its end with forceps, roast it free from grease by passing it 6–12 times through a blue Bunsen flame. The heating should be as strong as is possible without cracking the slide. Cracking is rendered less likely by allowing the slide to cool somewhat before laying down, or by laying it on a warmed metal rack. Another method of cleaning is to moisten the finger with water, rub it on the surface of some fine sand soap, and then smear the surface of the slide. After removing the soapy film with a clean cloth the surface is clean and free from grease. For special purposes, slides are cleaned by immersion in concentrated sulphuric acid saturated with potassium dichromate for several days at room temperature. If the slide is perfectly clean a drop of water can be spread over its surface in a thin even film; otherwise the water collects into small drops and a film cannot be made.

After the films have been made and examined the slides should be discarded. *They should not be cleaned and used again, since it is difficult to ensure that all organisms are removed.*

Coverslips. These should be $\frac{3}{4}$ or $\frac{7}{8}$ in^2 and of No. 1 thickness, i.e. 0.1 mm thick. (Thicker coverslips – No. 2 – may prevent the oil-immersion objective from coming near enough for the specimen to be focused.) They are cleaned by the dichromate-sulphuric acid solution as described for slides; they are then well washed, first in tap water and later in distilled water, and stored in a stoppered jar in 50% alcohol. Before use they are dried with a soft clean cloth, such as an old handkerchief. For routine use, the coverslips may be sufficiently clean as supplied by the maker and require only to be wiped free from grit and dust with a clean dry cloth. The newer plastic coverslips should not be used when staining as they melt or buckle during the process. They should be used only for unstained 'wet' preparations.

Making films

In the case of fluid material, e.g. broth cultures, urine, sputum, pus, etc., one loopful (or more) is taken up with the inoculating wire and spread thinly on the slide. A little experience will soon determine the amount required, and in spreading the films it will be found that there are both thick and thin portions, which is not disadvantageous. The slide is then held in the palm of the hand high over a Bunsen flame and dried. The film is fixed by passing the *dried* slide, film downwards, three times slowly through the flame, or by heating through the glass slide. In the latter method the slide is held, film upwards, in the top of the Bunsen flame for a few seconds so that the slide becomes hot. Care must be taken not to char the film, and when the slide is just too hot to be borne on the back of the hand, fixation is complete.

In making films on coverslips and staining them, Cornet's forceps are used to hold the slip in a horizontal position, the forceps resting on the bench.

With solid material, such as cultures on agar, etc., it is necessary to place a loopful of clean water on the slide. The loop is then sterilized and a minute quantity of material, obtained by just touching the growth, is transferred to the drop, thoroughly emulsified, and the mixture is spread evenly on the slide. The resulting film is fixed and dried as above. *Beginners are apt to take more material than necessary from the culture and thus make too thick a film.*

Marking films

Before staining, the end of the slide bearing the film should be marked with numbers or letters to ensure that the identity of the material filmed will be known when the film is later examined microscopically along with films of other materials. A marking diamond or grease pencil may be used to write on the film-bearing side of the slide towards one end of it. A more convenient method involves the use of slides with a ground, matt surface at one end which will take writing with an ordinary graphite pencil. Stick-on paper labels should not be used as they are liable to be soiled or washed off in the staining procedure.

STAINING FILMS AND SECTIONS

Films

The stains are poured directly or filtered on to the slide. The whole area of the film should be covered with a layer of stain thick enough not to dry during the period of staining. Preferably, the area at the end of the slide bearing the identifying mark should not be covered, so that it may be grasped by the fingers or forceps without soiling. When staining is completed, the dye is washed off with water, and the slide is allowed to dry in the vertical position or is placed between two sheets of white fluffless blotting paper or filter paper. The drying of the film is completed over the Bunsen flame. Such stained films may be mounted in Canada balsam under a coverslip, or may be examined unmounted with the oil-immersion lens, a small drop of cedar-wood or synthetic immersion oil being placed directly on the film. If it is desired to mount the preparation later, the oil can be removed with xylol or benzol.

Tissue sections

The sections being embedded in paraffin, it is necessary to remove the paraffin so that a watery stain may penetrate. The paraffin is first removed with xylol (xylene) or benzol (benzene), the xylol or benzol is then removed with alcohol (95% ethanol) and the alcohol is replaced with water. The staining is then done. After staining, the section must be dehydrated with absolute alcohol, cleared in xylol and mounted in Canada balsam under a coverslip. The Canada balsam (which is a resin) is dissolved in xylol in order to render it suitable in consistency.

Alcohol (ethanol) solutions. The reagents most commonly employed in preparation of sections are 'absolute alcohol', which is 100% ethanol, and '95% alcohol', which is a 95% solution of ethanol in water by volume (i.e. 95 ml absolute alcohol plus water to give 100 ml solution).

Industrial methylated spirit (not mineralized) may be used for making up stains, decolourizing stained preparations, dehydrating tissues and treating sections. The type known as 'Toilet spirit, acetone free (66 OP)' is quite satisfactory for use instead of 95% alcohol. Similarly, industrial methylated spirit, absolute (74 OP), can be used instead of absolute alcohol. Not only are these industrial spirits much cheaper than rectified spirit (90% alcohol) and absolute alcohol, but permits for obtaining them duty-free are more readily granted by the customs authorities.

Technique. The slide bearing the paraffin section is placed in a jar of xylol for some minutes to remove the paraffin. The section is then treated with a few drops of absolute alcohol (ethanol), when it immediately becomes opaque. A few drops of 50% alcohol are poured on, and the slide is finally washed gently in water. If the tissue has been fixed in any mercuric chloride preparation, such as Zenker's fluid, the section should be treated with Gram's iodine solution for a few minutes, then with 95% alcohol and finally with water. The sections are now ready to be stained by the appropriate method.

After staining and washing with water, the slide is wiped all round the section with a clean cloth to remove excess of water. The bulk of the water in the section may be removed by pressing between fluffless blotting paper. The section is treated *immediately* with a few drops of 95% alcohol and then with absolute alcohol. The slide is again wiped all round the section, a few more drops of absolute alcohol are poured on and the slide is then immersed in xylol. When cleared, the slide is removed, and excess of xylol round the section is wiped away, a drop of Canada balsam is applied and the section mounted under a No. 1 coverslip. It is essential that the section should not be allowed to dry at any period of the process, and that dehydration with absolute alcohol should be complete in order that the section may be thoroughly cleared.

When the bacteria are readily decolourized with alcohol, aniline-xylol (aniline, 2 parts; xylol, 1 part) should be used for dehydration. After washing, when the slide has been wiped round the section, the preparation is blotted and then treated with the aniline-xylol mixture, which clears as well as dehydrates. The aniline-xylol is then replaced with xylol. This can be done conveniently by holding the slide almost vertically and dropping xylol from a drop bottle on to the slide just above the section. The xylol flows over the section and quickly removes the aniline. The preparation is mounted immediately in Canada balsam.

DPX mounting medium. A mounting medium that replaces Canada balsam has been devised by Kirkpatrick & Lendrum (1939, 1941). It consists of polystyrene (a synthetic resin) dissolved in xylol, with a plasticizer – dibutyl phthalate – to ensure flexibility. There is, however, much shrinkage and the mounting fluid should be applied generously. The mountant termed DPX is made up as follows:

Mix dibutyl phthalate (BDH)	5 ml
with pure xylol	35 ml
and dissolve 'Distrene 80'	10 g

DPX medium is water-clear, inert and does not become acid or cause fading of stained preparations. It is used in the same way as Canada balsam.

If polystyrene of a low molecular weight (about 3000) is used, much less xylol is required and no plasticiser need be added. Moreover, there is practically no shrinkage, which is a great advantage over DPX.

SIMPLE STAINS

These show not only the presence of organisms but also the nature of the cellular content in exudates.

Loeffler's methylene blue

Of the many preparations of this dye, Loeffler's methylene blue is generally the most useful:

Saturated solution of methylene
blue in alcohol   300 ml
KOH, 0.01% in water   1000 ml

Films. Stain for 3 min, then wash with water. This preparation does not readily over-stain.

Sections. Stain for 5 min or longer. The application of the alcohol during dehydration is sufficient for differentiation. Aniline-xylol can also be used for dehydration and clearing.

Polychrome methylene blue

This is made by allowing Loeffler's methylene blue to 'ripen' slowly. The stain is kept in bottles, which are half filled and shaken at intervals to aerate thoroughly the contents. The slow oxidation of the methylene blue forms a violet compound that gives the stain its polychrome properties. The ripening takes 12 months or more to complete, or it may be ripened quickly by the addition of 1.0% potassium carbonate (K_2CO_3) to the stain. The preparation is used in a manner similar to Loeffler's methylene blue. It is also employed in McFadyean's reaction (Ch. 24).

Dilute carbol fuchsin

Made by diluting Ziehl-Neelsen's stain (see below) with 10–15 times its volume of water. Stain for 10–25 s and wash well with water. Over-staining must be avoided, as this is an intense stain, and prolonged application colours the cell protoplasm in addition to nuclei and bacteria.

Negative staining

'Negative staining' is exemplified by *Burri's India ink method*, which was formerly used for the spirochaete of syphilis. A small quantity of India ink is mixed on a slide with the culture or other material containing bacteria, and then by means of another slide or loop a thin film is made; this is allowed to dry before being examined. The bacteria or spirochaetes are seen as clear transparent objects on a dark-brown background. (See below, also India ink methods for capsules.)

Fleming's nigrosin method. A 10% solution of nigrosin (Gurr, BDH) is made in warm distilled water (solution is effected in about an hour) and filtered. Formalin 0.5% (i.e. formaldehyde 0.19%) is added as a preservative. A small drop of the dye is placed on a slide, bacteria are mixed with it and a smear is made with a loop or another slide. A number of preparations can be made on the same slide. Dry and examine.

Nigrosin gives an absolutely homogeneous background, and this is the simplest method of making a preliminary examination of a culture to show shape, size and arrangement of bacteria. Most bacteria stand out as clear objects on a dark field, but some bacilli, such as those of the coliform and haemophilic groups, show in their central portion a slightly dark patch somewhat resembling a nucleus.

GRAM'S STAINING METHOD

This is the most important staining method in bacteriology, and must be employed for the diagnostic identification of various organisms.

Certain bacteria when treated with one of the basic para-rosaniline dyes such as methyl violet, crystal violet or gentian violet (which is a mixture of the two preceding dyes), and then with iodine, 'fix' the stain so that subsequent treatment with a decolourizing agent – e.g. alcohol or acetone – does not remove the colour. Other organisms, however, are decolourized by this process. If a mixture of various organisms are thus stained and subjected to the decolourizing agent, it is found that some species retain the dye, and these are termed 'Gram positive', whereas others are completely decolourized and are termed 'Gram negative'. In order to render the decolourized organisms visible, and to distinguish them from those retaining the colour, a contrast or counterstain is then applied. This counterstain is usually red, in order that the Gram-negative organisms may easily be differentiated from the Gram-positive organisms, which retain the original violet stain.

If Gram's method is properly carried out, Gram-positive organisms and fibrin are stained dark violet in colour. Gram-negative organisms, the nuclei and protoplasm of pus cells and tissue cells are stained pink with the counterstain. To obviate errors from overdecolourizing, a control film of a known Gram-positive organism (e.g. a pure culture of *Staphylococcus aureus*) may be made at one side of the film to be examined. For the recognition of Gram-negative organisms such as gonococci or meningococci in pus, this control must retain the violet stain while the nuclei of the pus cells are stained only with the counterstain.

In the original method of Gram (1884), the smear was stained with aniline-gentian violet, treated with Lugol's iodine (iodine 1 g, KI 2 g, water 300 ml), decolourized with absolute alcohol, and counterstained with Bismarck brown. Later modifications, however, have given better results.

Acetone, as decolourizer appears to give more specific reactions than alcohol, but it acts so quickly that the duration of exposure is difficult to control. The addition of a small concentration of iodine to the acetone was found by Preston & Morrell (1962) to slow the rate of decolouriz-ation without reducing its specificity, so that the period of exposure could be lengthened from about 2–3 s to 30 s, a more controllable time.

Kopeloff & Beerman's (1922) modification

This method, which is a modification of Burke's (1922) method using acetone as decolourizer is recommended for general use.

Solutions

1. Methyl violet stain

Solution A
Methyl violet 6B	10 g
Distilled water	1 litre

Solution B
Sodium bicarbonate ($NaHCO_3$)	50 g
Distilled water	1 litre

Shortly before use, mix 30 volumes of solution A with 8 volumes of solution B. (The mixture is apt to precipitate within a few days and so cannot be kept. Methyl violet solution *without* the addition of bicarbonate acts almost as well in Gram staining and has the advantage of keeping indefinitely. For critical work, however, a freshly made mixture of stain with bicarbonate is to be preferred.)

2. Iodine solution

Iodine	20 g
Sodium hydroxide 1 mol/litre (i.e. 4% NaOH)	100 ml
Distilled water	900 ml

Dissolve the iodine in the NaOH solution and, when it is dissolved, add the distilled water.

3. Basic fuchsin stain

Basic fuchsin	0.5 or 1 g
Distilled water	1 litre

Procedure for films

1. Make a smear on a slide according to the instructions given above under *Making films*. Dry thoroughly in cool air or in warm air *far above* a Bunsen flame. Then, fix by flaming as described above under *Making films*.

2. Cover the whole slide with methyl violet stain and allow this to remain on the slide for about 5 min.

3. Tip off the methyl violet stain, hold the slide at a steep slope and wash off the residual stain with an excess of iodine solution; begin by pouring the iodine on the upper end of the slide and rapidly work downwards. (It is important to use enough iodine solution to wash away all the crystalline deposit that forms when the stain and the iodine mix.)

4. Cover the whole slide with fresh iodine solution and leave it thus for about 2 min.

5. Decolourize with acetone (100%). First tip off the iodine and hold the slide at a steep slope. Then pour acetone over the slide from its upper end, so as to cover its whole surface. Decolour-ization is very rapid, and is usually complete in 2–3 s. After this period of contact the acetone must *at once* be removed by washing thoroughly with water under a running tap. To avoid delay, the tap should be running before the acetone is applied to the slide.

(Kopeloff & Beerman recommended that the acetone should be added to the slide drop by drop until no colour is seen in the washings; they noted that decolourization generally requires less than 10 s and that the time should be reduced to a minimum. We have found that with thin smears, successful results are obtained more consistently if the acetone is flooded over the slide and then washed off with water after only 2 seconds' contact.)

6. Cover the whole slide with basic fuchsin stain and allow this to remain for about 30 s.

7. Wash thoroughly (for about 5 s) in water from the tap, blot and dry in air.

Normally a Gram-stained film is examined under oil-immersion without mounting under a coverslip. The oil can be removed with xylol or benzol if it is desired to preserve the film.

Procedure for sections

1. Remove paraffin with xylol or benzol.

2. Treat the section with absolute alcohol (100% ethanol) and wash in tap water.

3. Cover the slide with methyl violet stain and allow to act for 5 min.

4. Wash off stain with an excess of iodine solution, cover with more iodine and allow to act for 2 min.

5. Decolourize with acetone (see above). The visible violet staining should be removed from the section and this may take one or two seconds longer than is necessary in the decolourization of films.

6. Wash slide in water from tap.

7. Counterstain with basic fuchsin for 30 s.

8. Wipe carefully around the section to remove as much water as possible, dehydrate quickly in absolute alcohol, clear in xylol or benzol and mount in Canada balsam or DPX.

Acetone-alcohol as decolourizer

Kopeloff & Beerman's method is sometimes modified by the substitution of acetone-alcohol in the place of pure acetone as decolourizer. Acetone-alcohol is a mixture of 1 volume of acetone with 1 volume of 95% ethyl alcohol (ethanol). It acts rather more slowly than pure

acetone and decolourization may be prolonged to 10 s or more, and can be more carefully adjusted in duration. It is not, however, considered to be quite as satisfactory as pure acetone in producing specific differential decolourization.

Dilute carbol fuchsin as counterstain

When staining for small Gram-negative bacteria, e.g. haemophilus, campylobacter, these organisms may be more intensely stained and more easily seen if dilute carbol fuchsin is applied for up to 3 min instead of basic fuchsin for 30 s.

Jensen's modification of Gram's method

This modification using alcohol as decolourizer can be recommended for routine bacteriological work. It has been used especially in examination of films of exudates for gonococci and meningococci.

Solutions

1. *Methyl violet stain*

Methyl violet 6B (or crystal violet)	5 g
Distilled water	1 litre

The solution should be made up in bulk and filtered. It keeps indefinitely, and does not precipitate, but should be filtered again before use.

2. *Iodine solution*

Iodine	10 g
Potassium iodide	20 g
Distilled water	1 litre

Dissolve 20 g potassium iodide in 250 ml water, and then add 10 g iodine; when dissolved make up to 1000 ml with water.

3. *Counterstain – neutral red solution*

Neutral red	1 g
1% acetic acid	2 ml
Distilled water	1 litre

Procedure

Films are made, dried and fixed in the usual way.

1. Cover the slide with methyl violet solution and allow to act for about 30 s.

2. Pour off stain and, holding the slide at an angle downwards, pour on the iodine solution so that it washes away the methyl violet. Cover the slide with fresh iodine and allow to act for about 30 s.

3. Wash off the iodine with absolute alcohol (100% ethanol) and treat with fresh alcohol, tilting the slide from side to side until colour ceases to come out of the preparation. This is easily seen by holding the slide against a white background.

4. Wash with water.

5. Apply the counterstain for 1–2 min.

6. Wash with water and dry between blotting paper.

This method is very simple and gives excellent results with freedom from deposit. Safranine, 0.5% in distilled water, may be substituted for neutral red as counterstain. Basic fuchsin, 0.05%, may be used for up to 30 s, but dilute carbol fuchsin should not be used because it tends to stain Gram-negative bacteria so intensely that they may appear Gram-positive.

For the gonococcus and meningococcus in films, *Sandiford's counterstain* is useful, particularly when the organisms are scanty.

Malachite green	0.05 g
Pyronine	0.15 g
Distilled water	to 100 ml

(The stain keeps for about a month only.) Apply the counterstain for 2 min, flood off with water (but do not wash) and blot. Cells and nuclei stain bluish green. Gram-positive organisms are purple-black and gonococci red. It should be noted that not all samples of pyronine are satisfactory for this stain, so that with each new purchase of pyronine the made-up stain should be tested on a film known to contain gonococci or meningococci.

Weigert's modification of Gram's method

This modification which uses aniline-xylol as decolourizer is specially recommended for staining sections of tissue.

Solutions

1. *Carbol gentian violet*

Saturated alcoholic solution of gentian violet	1 part
5% solution of phenol in distilled water	10 parts

(This mixture should be made up each day, as it tends to precipitate.)

2. *Gram's (Lugol's) iodine*

Iodine	1 g
Potassium iodide	2 g
Distilled water	300 ml

3. *Aniline-xylol*

Aniline	2 parts
Xylol	1 part

4. *Carmalum solution*

Carminic acid	1 g
Potassium alum	10 g
Distilled water	200 ml

Dissolve with gentle heat; filter and add 1 ml formalin as preservative.

Procedure for sections

1. Remove the paraffin with xylol or benzol, treat with alcohol, wash with water and counterstain with carmalum for 10 min.

2. Stain with carbol gentian violet for 2–3 min.

3. Pour off stain, replace with Gram's iodine solution and allow to act for 1 min.

4. Dry thoroughly by blotting.

5. Decolourize with aniline-xylol, using several changes until the stain ceases to be removed.

Now examine at this stage under the low power of the microscope; the nuclei of the pus cells should be of a pale-violet colour; if the nuclei are deeply stained, then decolourization is incomplete.

6. Wash with several changes of xylol and dry.

7. Mount in Canada balsam or DPX.

Preston & Morrell's modification of Gram's method

Preston & Morrell's (1962) method uses iodine-acetone as decolourizer. It is recommended for films as giving reliable results without the need for taking great care in adjusting the duration of decolourization.

Solutions

1. *Ammonium oxalate-crystal violet*

Crystal violet	20 g
Methylated spirit (64 OP)	200 ml
Ammonium oxalate, 1% in water	800 ml

2. *Lugol's iodine solution*

Iodine	10 g
Potassium iodide	20 g
Distilled water	1 litre

3. *Liquor iodi fortis* (BP)

Iodine	10 g
Potassium iodide	6 g
Methylated spirit (74 OP)	90 ml
Distilled water	10 ml

4. *Iodine-acetone*

Liquor iodi fortis	35 ml
Acetone	965 ml

5. *Dilute carbol fuchsin*

Ziehl-Neelsen's (strong) carbol fuchsin (see below)	50 ml
Distilled water	950 ml

Procedure

1. Cover slide with ammonium oxalate-crystal violet and allow to act for about 30 s.
2. Pour off and wash freely with Lugol's iodine solution. Cover with fresh iodine solution and allow to act for about 30 s.
3. Pour off iodine solution and wash freely with iodine-acetone. Cover with fresh iodine-acetone and allow to act for about 30 s.
4. Wash thoroughly with water.
5. Counterstain with dilute carbol fuchsin for about 30 s.
6. Wash with water, blot and dry.

It is essential that the whole slide is flooded with each reagent in turn, and that the previous reagent is thoroughly removed at each step.

Modified Preston-Morrell method

A disadvantage of the use of iodine-acetone in the Preston-Morrell method is that an irritant aerosol is produced when the reagent is expelled on to the slide through the jet of a 'squeeze' bottle. The acetone quickly evaporates from the droplets to leave minute, airborne droplet-nuclei of iodine which, when numerous, are highly irritating to the eyes and nose. If many films are being stained in the same room, e.g. in a practical class of students, the atmosphere may become intolerable.

The difficulty may be avoided by reducing the concentration of iodine in the acetone and pouring the reagent carefully to avoid splashing. Good results are obtained by a reduction of the iodine concentration in the acetone to one-tenth that in the standard method and a shortening of the time of decolourization to 10 s.

Solutions

1. *Crystal violet solution*

Crystal violet	10 g
Absolute alcohol (100% ethanol)	100 ml
Distilled water	900 ml

Dissolve the dye in the alcohol, filter and add the water.

2. *Lugol's iodine solution*, as for the Preston-Morrell method.

3. *Liquor iodi fortis*, as for the Preston-Morrell method.

4. *Weak iodine-acetone*

Liquor iodi fortis	3.5 ml
Acetone	1 litre

5. *Dilute carbol fuchsin*, as for the Preston-Morrell method.

Procedure

1. Prepare a dried, heat-fixed smear, mark the end of the slide with an identifying mark and place the slide, smear uppermost, on the staining rack.

2. Cover the slide completely with the crystal violet solution and leave it to act for at least 30 s.

3. Wash off the stain with water from the tap. It is best to do this by lifting the slide with forceps into the stream of water to wash the stain from both sides of it. If this is done, be sure to replace the slide on the rack with the smear side uppermost.

4. Cover the slide completely with Lugol's iodine solution and leave it to act for at least 30 s.

5. Wash off the iodine solution with water from the tap.

6. Cover the slide completely with weak iodine-acetone and leave it to act for about 10 s.

7. Wash off the iodine-acetone with water from the tap.

8. Cover the slide with dilute carbol fuchsin or, if preferred, a weaker counterstain such as basic fuchsin or neutral red (see Kopeloff & Beerman's and Jensen's modifications), and leave it to act for at least 30 s.

9. Wash off the counterstain with water from the tap.

10. Shake off excess water, blot dry by pressing vertically (not rubbing sideways) with clean blotting paper and complete the drying in warm air over a Bunsen flame.

STAINING OF ACID-FAST BACILLI

Ziehl-Neelsen method

This method is a modification of Ehrlich's (1882) original method for the differential staining of tubercle bacilli and other acid-fast bacilli with aniline-gentian violet followed by strong nitric acid. It incorporates improvements suggested, successively, by Ziehl and Neelsen, and is described in a footnote in a paper by Johne (1885).

The ordinary aniline dye solutions do not readily penetrate the substance of the tubercle bacillus and are therefore unsuitable for staining it. However, by the use of a powerful staining solution that contains phenol, and the application of heat, the dye can be made to penetrate the bacillus. Once stained the tubercle bacillus will withstand the action of powerful decolourizing agents for a considerable time and thus still retains the stain when everything else in the microscopic preparation has been decolourized.

The stain used consists of basic fuchsin, with phenol added. The dye is basic and its combination with a mineral acid produces a compound that is yellowish brown in colour and is readily dissolved out of all structures except acid-fast bacteria. Any strong acid can be used as a decolourizing agent, but 20% sulphuric acid (by volume) is usually employed. Acid-alcohol may be used instead and generally gives cleaner films.

In order to show structures and cells, including non-acid-fast bacteria, that have been decolourized, and to form a contrast with the red-stained bacilli, the preparation is counterstained with methylene blue or malachite green.

Solutions

1. *Ziehl-Neelsen's (strong) carbol fuchsin*

Basic fuchsin	10 g
Absolute alcohol (100% ethanol)	100 ml
Solution of phenol, 5% in water	1 litre

Dissolve the dye in the alcohol and add to the phenol solution.

An alternative and quicker preparation is as follows:

Basic fuchsin (powder)	5 g
Phenol (crystalline)	25 g
Alcohol (95% or absolute)	50 ml
Distilled water	500 ml

Dissolve the fuchsin in the phenol by placing them in a 1 litre flask over a boiling waterbath for about 5 min, shaking the contents from time to time. When there is complete solution add the alcohol and mix thoroughly. Then add the distilled water. Filter the mixture before use.

2. *Sulphuric acid*, 20% solution

Place 800 ml water in a large flask. Add 200 ml concentrated sulphuric acid (about 98%; about 1.835 g/ml). The acid should be poured slowly down the side of the flask into the water, about 50 ml at a time. The mixture will become hot. Mix gently; add remainder of acid in same manner.

Note. The acid must be added to the water. It is *dangerous* to add the water to the acid. Great care must be taken to avoid spilling the acid on skin or clothing, or elsewhere. Especial care must be taken to avoid splashing or spurting into the eye. In event of such an accident occurring the eye should at once be washed with an excess of clean water and medical advice sought.

3. *Alcohol 95%*
Ethanol 95 ml plus water to 100 ml

4. *Counterstain*
Loeffler's methylene blue (see above)

Procedure for films

Films are made, dried and fixed by flaming in the usual manner.

1. Cover the slide with filtered carbol fuchsin and heat until steam rises. Allow the preparation to stain for 5 min, heat being applied at intervals to keep the stain hot. The stain must not be allowed to evaporate and dry on the slide; if necessary, pour on more carbol fuchsin to keep the whole slide covered with liquid.

(*Note.* The slide may be heated with a torch prepared by twisting a *small* piece of cotton wool on to the tip of an inoculating wire and soaking it in methylated spirit before lighting. When steam rises from the slide, remove and extinguish the torch. After about 1 min recharge the torch with spirit, relight it, and again heat the slide until the steam rises. Continue in this way for 5 min.)

2. Wash with water.

3. Cover the slide with 20% sulphuric acid. The red colour of the preparation is changed to yellowish brown. After about a minute in the acid, wash the slide with water, and pour on more acid. Repeat this process several times. The object of the washing is to remove the compound of acid with stain and allow fresh acid to gain access to the preparation. The decolourization is finished when, after washing, the film is only very faintly pink.

Decolourization generally requires contact with sulphuric acid for a total time of at least 10 min.

4. Wash the slide well in water.

5. Treat with 95% alcohol for 2 min. This step is optional, and may be omitted; see below.

6. Wash with water.

7. Counterstain with Loeffler's methylene blue or dilute malachite green for 15–20 s.

8. Wash, blot, dry and mount.

Acid-fast bacilli stain bright red, while the tissue cells and other organisms are stained blue or green according to the counterstain used. If tissue cells appear red, the preparation has not been adequately decolourized with sulphuric acid.

Note. The practice of using staining jars in the Ziehl-Neelsen method is to be condemned, as with a positive sputum, stained tubercle bacilli may become detached and float about in the staining fluid or decolourizing agent. After a number of strongly positive films have been passed through the staining jars the number of free stained tubercle bacilli may be considerable. Negative material may, during the staining process, pick up these bacilli and so appear positive when examined microscopically. These false positives can give rise to serious errors of diagnosis. Each slide, therefore, should be stained individually by pouring on the stain from a bottle, the washing done with a stream of tap water and the subsequent decolourizing and staining fluids added to the film from bottles. When drying with blotting paper, a fresh clean piece of paper is used for each slide and then discarded. The practice of using a number of large sheets for drying a succession of slides is also condemned as tubercle bacilli from a positive film may adhere to the blotting paper and subsequently be transferred to a negative film.

Use of alcohol for secondary decolourization. After primary decolourization with sulphuric acid, the film may be treated with 95% alcohol as secondary decolourizer (step 5, above). The basis of this practice is the fact that tubercle bacilli are alcohol-fast as well as acid-fast. One advantage of using alcohol is that decolourization is completed more quickly and the margins and underside of the slide are more completely cleaned and freed from deposits of stain.

Another advantage of using alcohol when the staining is being done for identification of tubercle bacilli, is that certain other acid-fast bacilli, which may be encountered in pathological specimens and may otherwise be confused with tubercle bacilli, are decolourized by alcohol. Thus, specimens of urine often contain the smegma bacillus, an acid-fast bacillus that is a harmless commensal inhabitant in the region of the urethral orifice. Some, though not all strains of smegma bacillus are decolourized with alcohol and the use of alcohol thus lessens, though it does not entirely remove the likelihood of confusion arising in the diagnosis of urinary tract tuberculosis.

Acid-alcohol as decolourizer. Instead of employing 20% sulphuric acid as a decolourizing agent, 3% hydrochloric acid in 95% alcohol (industrial methylated spirit) may be used (i.e. concentrated HC1, 3 ml, and 95% alcohol, 97 ml). The necessity for subsequent treatment with alcohol, as in the original method, is obviated. Acid-alcohol is a more expensive reagent than sulphuric acid, but it is much less corrosive and more convenient to make up and employ, while its use definitely excludes organisms that are acid-fast but not alcohol-fast.

Malachite green as counterstain. Malachite green is also recommended as a counterstain in the Ziehl-Neelsen method. A stock solution of 1% in distilled water is made, and for use a small quantity is diluted with distilled water in a drop-bottle so that 15–20 s application of the weak stain gives the background a pale green tint. Deep counterstaining must be avoided. The pale green background is pleasant for the eyes, and is required for the method in which a deep blue-green filter is used for the easy recognition of tubercle bacilli.

Procedure for sections

Sections are treated with xylol to remove paraffin, then with alcohol, and finally are washed in water.

1. Stain with Ziehl-Neelsen's stain as described for films, but heat gently, otherwise the section may become detached from the slide.
2. Wash with water.
3. Decolourize with 20% sulphuric acid or acid-alcohol as for films. The process takes longer owing to the thickness of the section, and care must be exercised in washing to retain the section on the slide.
4. Wash well with water.
5. Counterstain with methylene blue or malachite green for 0.5–1 min.
6. Wash with water.
7. Wipe the slide dry all round the section, blot with filter paper or fluffless blotting paper, and treat with a few drops of absolute alcohol. Pour on more absolute alcohol, wipe the slide again and clear in xylol.
8. Mount in Canada balsam or DPX.

Modifications of Ziehl-Neelsen method

1. Leprosy bacilli are also acid-fast, but usually to a less degree than the tubercle bacillus. They are stained in films or sections in the same way as the tubercle bacillus, except that 5% sulphuric acid is used for decolourization.
2. Sections of tissues containing 'clubs' caused by *Actinomyces*, *Mycobacterium* and *Nocardia* can be treated with 1% H_2SO_4 to demonstrate the acid-fastness of the clubs.
3. Cultures of some *Nocardia* spp. are acid-fast when decolourized with 0.5% H_2SO_4.
4. Most spores are acid-fast; for methods see *Staining of spores*, below.
5. *Brucella differential stain:* a useful differ-

ential stain for the demonstration of *Brucella abortus* in infected material. Dilute (1 in 10) carbol fuchsin is allowed to act, without heating, for 15 min. The slide is then decolourized with 0.5% acetic acid solution for 15 s, washed thoroughly and counterstained with Loeffler's methylene blue for 1 min. This method may also be used for demonstrating chlamydia in tissue sections.

Fluorochrome staining

Auramine O

This dye can be substituted for carbol fuchsin in the Ziehl-Neelsen method with the effect that the tubercle bacilli fluoresce and become much easier to detect. Heating is unnecessary.

Solutions

1. *Staining solution*

Auramine O	3 g
Phenol	30 g
Distilled water	1 litre

Dissolve the phenol in the water with gentle heat. Add the auramine gradually and shake vigorously until dissolved. Filter and store in a dark stoppered bottle.

2. *Decolourizing solution*: industrial alcohol (ethanol) 75% (v/v) in water containing 0.5% NaCl and 0.5% HCl.

3. *Potassium permanganate solution*

$KMnO_4$	1 g
Distilled water	1 litre

Procedure

1. Stain a thin heat-fixed smear of sputum with the auramine solution for 15 min at room temperature.
2. Wash off the stain with water from the tap.
3. Cover the slide with the acid-alcohol decolourizing solution for 5 min.
4. Wash off the decolourizer with water from the tap; rinse well.
5. Cover the slide with potassium permanganate solution for 30 s.

6. Wash well with water from the tap. Allow to dry in air; do not use blotting paper.
7. Examine the film dry by fluorescence microscopy with a 4 mm objective or, preferably, with an 8 mm objective and high-powered eye-piece. Tubercle bacilli are seen as yellow luminous rods in a dark field. When they have been detected under low power, the morphology of the bacilli is confirmed by observation with an oil-immersion objective.

STAINING OF VOLUTIN-CONTAINING ORGANISMS

Well developed granules of volutin (polyphosphate) may be seen in unstained wet preparations as round refractile bodies within the bacterial cytoplasm. With basic dyes they tend to stain more strongly than the rest of the bacterium, and with toluidine blue or methylene blue they stain metachromatically, a reddish-purple colour. They are demonstrated most clearly by special methods, such as Albert's and Neisser's, which stain them dark purple but the remainder of the bacterium with a contrasting counterstain. The diphtheria bacillus gives its characteristic volutin-staining reactions best in a young culture (18–24 h) on a blood or serum medium.

Albert-Laybourn method

Laybourn's (1924) modification, in which malachite green is substituted for methyl green, is given here instead of the original method of Albert. It is recommended for routine use.

Staining solution

Toluidine blue	1.5 g
Malachite green	2 g
Glacial acetic acid	10 ml
Alcohol (95% ethanol)	20 ml
Distilled water	1 litre

Dissolve the dyes in the alcohol and add to the water and acetic acid. Allow to stand for one day and then filter.

Albert's iodine

Iodine	6 g
Potassium iodide	9 g
Distilled water	900 ml

Note. The iodine solution used in Jensen's modification of Gram's method works equally well.

Procedure

1. Make film, dry in air, and fix by heat.
2. Cover slide with Albert's stain and allow to act for 3–5 min.
3. Wash in water and blot dry.
4. Cover slide with Albert's iodine and allow to act for 1 min.
5. Wash and blot dry.

By this method the granules stain bluish black, the protoplasm green and other organisms mostly light green.

Neisser's method (modified)

The following modification of Neisser's method gives better results than the original:

Neisser's methylene blue stain

Methylene blue	1 g
Ethyl alcohol (95%)	50 ml
Glacial acetic acid	50 ml
Distilled water	1 litre

Procedure

1. Stain with Neisser's methylene blue for 3 min.
2. Wash off with dilute iodine solution (iodine solution of Kopeloff & Beerman's modification of Gram's method, diluted 1 in 10 with water) and leave some of this solution on the slide for 1 min.
3. Wash in water.
4. Counterstain with neutral red solution for 3 min, using the same solution as that employed in Jensen's modification of Gram's method.
5. Wash in water and dry.

By this method the bacilli exhibit deep blue granules and the remainder of the organism assumes a pink colour.

STAINING OF SPORES

If spore-bearing organisms are stained with ordinary dyes, or by Gram's stain, the body of the bacillus is deeply coloured, whereas the spore is unstained and appears as a clear area in the organism. This is the way in which spores are most commonly observed. If desired, however, it is possible by vigorous staining procedures to introduce dye into the substance of the spore. When thus stained, the spore tends to retain the dye after treatment with decolourizing agents, and in this respect behaves similarly to the tubercle bacillus.

Acid-fast stain for spores

Films, which must be thin, are made, dried and fixed in the usual manner with the minimum amount of heating.

1. Stain with Ziehl-Neelsen's carbol fuchsin for 3–5 min, heating the preparation until steam rises.
2. Wash in water.
3. Treat with 0.25% or 0.5% sulphuric acid for one to several minutes, the period being determined by trial for each culture. *Alternatively*, excellent results are obtained by decolourizing in a 2% solution of nitric acid in absolute ethyl alcohol; the slide is dipped once rapidly in the solution and immediately washed in water.
4. Wash with water.
5. Counterstain with 1% aqueous methylene blue for 3 min.
6. Wash in water, blot and dry.

The spores are stained bright red and the protoplasm of the bacilli blue.

It should be noted that the spores of some bacteria are decolourized more readily than those of others and that lipid inclusion granules may stain dark red, appearing like small spherical spores.

Malachite green stain for spores (Method of Schaeffer & Fulton, modified by Ashby (1938))

Films are dried and fixed with minimal flaming.

1. Place the slide over a beaker of boiling water, resting it on the rim with the bacterial film uppermost.

2. When, within several seconds, large droplets have condensed on the underside of the slide, flood it with 5% aqueous solution of malachite green and leave to act for 1 min while the water continues to boil.

3. Wash in cold water.

4. Treat with 0.5% safranine or 0.05% basic fuchsin for 30 s.

5. Wash and dry.

This method colours the spores green and the vegetative bacilli red. Lipid granules are unstained.

STAINING OF CAPSULES

Capsules. The capsules of bacteria present in animal tissues, blood, serous fluids and pus are often clearly stained when these materials are treated by one of the common stains such as basic fuchsin, polychrome methylene blue, Leishman's stain and Gram's stain (which colours them with the red counterstain). Special capsule stains may be of little advantage in such cases. On the other hand, when artificial cultures of bacteria are being examined, the capsules normally are not coloured by ordinary staining methods and special methods must be employed for their demonstration, e.g. 'negative' or 'relief' staining.

The best method for staining capsules on bacteria from cultures in either liquid or solid media is the wet-film India ink method. Dry-film negative staining methods using India ink, nigrosin or eosin are somewhat less reliable since occasionally shrinkage spaces give the appearance of capsules around bacteria that are non-capsulate and occasionally, especially in thick films, capsules may be shrunken or obscured to the point that they are rendered invisible. Dry film methods in which *positive* staining of capsules is attempted are the least reliable and

are not recommended. The advantages and disadvantages of all these different methods are discussed by Duguid (1951).

Loose slime. Many capsulate and some non-capsulate bacteria secrete extracellularly a soluble, viscid material, generally polysaccharide in composition. This may be seen in preparations made by some of the methods used for staining of capsules. The wet-film India ink method is recommended for this purpose. The slime appears as irregular masses of amorphous material lying between the bacteria and outside the capsules of capsulate ones.

Wet India ink films for capsules

If a permanent preparation is required for demonstration of bacterial capsules, it is necessary to use a dry-film method; otherwise capsules are best observed in very thin wet films of India ink. This is the simplest, most informative and most generally applicable method of demonstrating capsules. The capsules do not become shrunken, since they are not dried or fixed, and they are clearly apparent even when narrow.

India ink. A suitable supply of India ink is essential. It must be dense, homogeneous, very finely granular and free from contamination with capsulate or non-capsulate bacteria. A film of the ink alone should be examined on each occasion of use to ensure that it meets these criteria.

Procedure

1. Carefully wipe a microscope slide free from particles of dust or grit.

2. Place a *large* loopful of undiluted India ink on the slide.

3. Emulsify a *very small* portion of solid bacterial culture or a small loopful of liquid culture in the ink. Rub the speck of solid material on the slide surface just beside the ink before mixing it into the ink.

4. Place a clean, grit-free coverslip on the ink drop and press it down through a sheet of blot-

ting paper so that the film becomes very thin and thus pale in colour. The film should be so thin that the bacterial cell with its capsule is 'gripped' between the slide and coverslip, neither being overlaid by ink nor being capable of moving about.

Some practice is required in making satisfactory films of the correct thickness. If the film is left too thick, the capsule is obscured by the overlying ink. If it is pressed too thin, the capsules are crushed or flattened and the ink background becomes too pale to give a good contrast. The commonest errors are to use diluted ink and to make the films too thick.

Appearances. On microscopical examination with the oil-immersion objective the highly refractile outline of the bacterium is seen. Between this refractile surface-membrane and the dark background of ink particles there is a clear space which represents the capsule; the capsular zone may be from a fraction of a micrometre to several micrometres in width. Non-capsulated bacteria do not show this clear zone; the ink particles directly abut the refractile cell wall and, in consequence, these bacteria are not easily seen. When solid bacterial culture is newly mixed with the ink, any *loose slime* in it can be seen as irregular strands and masses, lighter than the ink, which gradually disperse from the bacteria and dissolve in the ink. Loose slime is generally invisible if the preparations are made from cultures in a liquid medium.

Use of phase-contrast microscope. It is recommended that wet India ink films should be examined with a phase-contrast microscope. Since the bodies of the bacteria are not stained in such films their outlines are only faintly visible under the ordinary microscope. With the phase-contrast microscope the bodies of the bacteria appear dark and are seen in clear contrast to the bright capsular zones surrounding them.

Dry India ink films for capsules (method of Butt et al (1936))

1. Place a loopful of 6% glucose in water at one end of a slide. Add a small amount of bacterial culture to this and mix to form an even suspension. Add a loopful of India ink to the drop, and mix.

2. Spread the mixture over the slide in a thin film with the edge of a second glass slide. Dry thoroughly by waving in the air.

3. Fix the film by pouring over it some undiluted Leishman stain or methyl alcohol. Drain off excess at once and dry thoroughly by warming over a flame.

4. Drop on methyl violet solution as used in Gram's stain, and stain for one or two minutes. Wash in water. Blot and dry over a flame.

5. Examine directly with the oil-immersion objective.

The bacteria are stained darkly with the violet dye and any capsule present appears as a clear zone between the stained bacterium and the dark ink background.

DEMONSTRATION OF FLAGELLA

Because of their extreme thinness, flagella are best demonstrated with the electron microscope; metal-shadowed films or films made with phosphotungstic acid (PTA) for 'negative staining' are employed (Ch. 2). Flagella can also be demonstrated by the light microscope, using special staining methods which require most careful attention to details of technique. To make possible their resolution, the flagella must be thickened at least 10-fold by a superficial deposition of stain. In spite of this, their characteristic arrangement and wave form are generally distinguishable.

Staining of flagella by a modification of Leifson's method

The stain, basic fuchsin with tannic acid, is deposited on the bacteria and flagella from an evaporating alcoholic solution. The degree of staining is controlled by an exact determination of the duration of exposure. Good results depend to a large extent on preliminary thorough cleaning and flaming of the glass slides.

1. Clean the glass slides with absolute alcohol, rubbing with a fine cotton cloth. Then immerse

them in concentrated sulphuric acid saturated with potassium dichromate for several days at room temperature or for an hour at 90°C. (In the latter case it is advisable to place the beaker of solution in a strong metal container with sand while heating.) *During all subsequent stages until staining is complete, take care not to finger the slides, even at their edges, and do not let them touch surfaces not properly cleaned and grease-free.* Using forceps, transfer the slides to cleaned Coplin jars in which they will be kept for rinsing, drying and storing; do not overcrowd. Rinse thoroughly with tap water and finally with distilled water. Allow to drain and dry in air with the jar inverted on clean blotting-paper. Store with the jar closed to prevent contamination by air-borne dust. Just before use, flame the slide for a few seconds, passing it with each face downwards about six times through a blue Bunsen flame. Place on a clean warmed metal rack, and allow to cool. Mark or number the slide with a diamond while holding with forceps.

2. Fix the broth culture, or saline suspension of an agar culture, by adding formalin to give a final formaldehyde concentration of 1–2%. Sediment the bacilli by centrifuging at 2000–3000 rev/min, preferably in a horizontal centrifuge. Decant the supernatant liquid and gently resuspend the bacilli in distilled water by rotating the tube alternately in opposite directions, rolling it between the palms of the hand. Centrifuge again and gently resuspend in fresh distilled water so as to obtain a final suspension which is only slightly cloudy, e.g. equal to Brown's opacity standard No. 1. With a flamed platinum loop, place a large loopful of the suspension on the prepared slide and gently spread over an area 1–2 cm in diameter. Allow to dry in air at room temperature or in an incubator at 37°C. Do not fix film.

3. The stain is prepared as follows:

Tannic acid	10 g
Sodium chloride	5 g
Basic fuchsin	4 g

Thoroughly mix the powdered ingredients in these proportions and store dry in a stoppered container. Prepare the solution by adding 1.9 g of the powder mixture to 33 ml of 95% ethyl alcohol and, when mostly dissolved (e.g. in 10 min), adding distilled water to make a final volume of 100 ml. Adjust the pH to 5.0 (at least within 0.2) by addition of NaOH or HCl, using a pH meter. Store the solution in a stoppered bottle in the refrigerator at 3–5°C, where it may remain stable for several weeks.

Alternatively, prepare three stock solutions: (1) tannic acid, 3.0% in water with 0.2% phenol as preservative; (2) sodium chloride, 1.5% in water; and (3) basic fuchsin, 1.2% in 95% ethyl alcohol. (The basic fuchsin must have a pH of 5.0; it may be compounded thus by mixing one part of pararosaniline hydrochloride with three parts of pararosaniline acetate. Allow several hours for solution in the alcohol.) Mix the three solutions in exactly equal proportions to prepare the stain.

4. Place the prepared slide horizontally on a carefully levelled staining rack. Pipette exactly 1 ml stain on to the slide so that it covers the whole surface. Leave at room temperature for exactly the required time, using a stop watch. Several similar preparations should be stained for different times, e.g. for 6, 8, 10 and 12 min, so that the best may be chosen. The optimal duration of staining will vary with the batch of stain, the room temperature and other factors; the apparent thickness of the flagella increases with the duration of staining. Rinse off the stain gently by placing the slide under a slowly running water tap; do not pour off stain before rinsing. Counterstain with methylene blue, e.g. with borax methylene blue for 30 min to colour the bacterial protoplast. Wash with water, rinse with distilled water, drain, dry in air and examine by oil immersion.

STAINING OF INTRACELLULAR LIPID

Burdon's (1946) method

Sudan black stain

| Sudan black B powder | 0.3 g |
| 70% ethyl alcohol | 100 ml |

Shake thoroughly at intervals and stand overnight before use. Keep in a well-stoppered bottle.

Procedure

1. Make a film, dry in air and fix by flaming.
2. Cover the entire slide with Sudan black stain and leave at room temperature for 15 min.
3. Drain off excess stain, blot, and dry in air.
4. Rinse thoroughly with xylol and again blot dry.
5. Counterstain lightly by covering with 0.5% aqueous safranine or dilute carbol fuchsin for 5–10 s; rinse with tap water, blot and dry.

Lipid inclusion granules are stained blue-black or blue-grey, whilst the bacterial cytoplasm is stained light pink.

STAINING OF CELL POLYSACCHARIDES

Periodic acid-Schiff (PAS) method of Hotchkiss (1948)

The polysaccharide constituents of bacteria and fungi are oxidized by periodate to form poly-aldehydes which yield red-coloured compounds with Schiff's fuchsin-sulphite; the proteins and nucleic acids remain uncoloured. The method may be used to reveal fungal elements in sections of infected animal tissue; the fungi stain red, while the tissue material, except glycogen and mucin, fails to take the stain.

Periodate solution. Dissolve 0.8 g periodic acid in 20 ml distilled water; add 10 ml of 0.2 mol/litre sodium acetate and 70 ml ethyl alcohol. The solution may be used for several days if protected from undue exposure to light.

Reducing rinse. Dissolve 10 g potassium iodide and 10 g sodium thiosulphate pentahydrate in 200 ml distilled water. Add, with stirring, 300 ml ethyl alcohol, and then 5 ml of 2 mol/litre hydrochloric acid. The sulphur which slowly precipitates may be allowed to settle out.

Fuchsin-Sulphite solution. Dissolve 2 g basic fuchsin in 400 ml boiling water, cool to 50°C and filter. To the filtrate add 10 ml of 2 mol/litre hydrochloric acid and 4 g potassium meta-bisulphite. Stopper and leave in a dark cool place overnight. Add 1 g decolourizing charcoal, mix and filter promptly. Add up to 10 ml or more 2 mol/litre hydrochloric acid until the mixture

when drying in a thin film on glass does not become pink. Preserved in the dark and well stoppered, the stain remains effective for several weeks.

Sulphite wash. Add 2 g potassium meta-bisulphite and 5 ml concentrated hydrochloric acid to 500 ml distilled water. This should be freshly prepared.

Procedure

1. Dry films in air and fix by flaming. For sections, fix tissue with usual fixatives; bring to 70% ethyl alcohol and wash thoroughly with this.
2. Treat with periodate solution for 5 min at room temperature. Rinse with 70% alcohol.
3. Treat with reducing rinse for 5 min. Rinse with 70% alcohol.
4. Stain with fuchsin-sulphite for 15–45 min.
5. Wash two or three times with sulphite wash solution. Wash with water.
6. Counterstain, if desired, with dilute aqueous malachite green (e.g. 0.002 g/100 ml).
7. Wash with water, dehydrate and mount by the usual methods.

Control sections are prepared similarly, omitting step (2).

Unless easily soluble polysaccharides such as glycogen are to be demonstrated, the method may be simplified by substituting distilled water for the alcohol in the periodate solution and by substituting tap water for rinsing in steps (1)–(3), e.g. see below.

Modified PAS stain for fungi in tissue sections

1. Bring sections to distilled water.
2. Treat for 5 min with a freshly prepared 1% solution of periodic acid in water.
3. Wash in running tap water for 15 min and rinse in distilled water.
4. Stain with fuchsin-sulphite for 15 min.
5. Wash two or three times with sulphite wash solution. Wash with water.
6. Wash in running tap water for 5 min and rinse in distilled water.
7. Counterstain with dilute aqueous malachite

green or with 0.1% light green in 90% alcohol for 1 min.

8. Dehydrate rapidly in absolute alcohol, clear in benzol and mount in Canada balsam.

IMPRESSION PREPARATIONS

This method has been used in the morphological study of mycoplasma cultures and of 'rough' and 'smooth' colonies of various bacteria (Klieneberger 1934; Bisset 1938).

The essential part of the technique is to remove a small slab, about 2 mm thick, of the solid medium (e.g. serum-agar) on which the organism is growing and place it colony downwards on a coverslip. The whole is immersed in fixative, so that the fixing fluid penetrates through the agar to reach the colony. When the bacteria are fixed, the agar is removed carefully from the coverslip which is well washed for two hours in distilled water, suitably stained and mounted. As fixative Bouin's or Flemming's fluid may be used (see below). For staining, methylene blue or dilute carbol fuchsin may be employed, but Giemsa's stain, applied by the slow method, is the most satisfactory for mycoplasmas. The agar slabs, after fixation, may also be embedded, and vertical sections of the colony cut with a microtome.

The 'hot-water transfer' method of Clark et al (1961) is also useful for morphological studies of mycoplasma. The transferred colonies may be stained directly on the slide by Dienes' stain diluted 1 in 10 or by the slow method of Giemsa. In addition, the colonies may be used for immunofluorescence by the direct or indirect methods.

STAINING OF BACTERIAL NUCLEI

Robinow's (1944, 1949) method

The nuclear bodies of bacteria can be differentiated from the cytoplasm if the cells are first treated with 1 mol/litre HC1 at 60°C and then stained wih Giemsa's solution. The following is a modification of Robinow's (1944, 1949) method.

Fixation

Cut a small square block from an agar plate on which the organisms are growing in a thin layer (e.g. as a 4-h old culture) and immerse it, bacteria-carrying side uppermost, in a shallow layer of methyl alcohol for 5 min. Dry the block in air and then place it downwards on a clean coverslip. Remove the agar, dry the film of fixed bacteria deposited on the coverslip and fix in warm alcohol-mercuric-chloride (Schaudinn's fluid) for 5 min. Wash in water and store in 70% alcohol.

Staining

Transfer films from 70% ethyl alcohol to 1 mol/l HC1 at 60°C for 10 min to 'hydrolyse'. Rinse in tap water and twice in distilled water and float on a staining solution made with 2–3 drops of Giemsa stain per ml of phosphate buffer (pH 7.0). Stain for 30 min at 37°C, rinse and mount in water, and examine at once. The nuclei are stained dark purple and the bacterial cytoplasm is only very lightly stained, if at all.

Feulgen staining of deoxyribonucleic acid in the nuclear bodies may be effected by staining with Schiff's fuchsin-sulphite (as for the PAS stain, see above) for 1 h at 15–20°C instead of staining with the Giemsa stain in the above method. The nuclei appear dark pink and the cytoplasm unstained.

To demonstrate the *cell wall*, make impression preparations fixed in Bouin's fluid, as described above. Mordant for 20–30 min with 5–10% tannic acid and stain with 0.02% crystal violet in water for about 1 min. Mount in water.

STAINING WITH ACRIDINE ORANGE

Acridine orange R has a marked affinity for nucleic acids. When cells stained with it are viewed by ultra-violet (UV) radiation, the RNA components fluoresce orange-red and the DNA components yellow-green. The method is of value in studying the growth of viruses in their host cells (Anderson et al 1959, Jamison & Mayor 1965) and for revealing scanty bacteria in wet films, e.g. in the examination of blood cultures in which scanty Gram-negative bacteria may be overlooked in Gram-stained films.

Reagents

1. Acid-alcohol: 3% HCl in 95% ethanol.
2. Acridine orange R, 0.1% in distilled water.
3. Citrate-phosphate buffer pH 3.8. Mix 32.3 ml of 0.1 mol/litre (19.21 g/l) citric acid solution with 17.7 ml of 0.2 mol/litre (28.39 g/l) Na_2HPO_4 solution and make up to 100 ml with distilled water. Check the pH.

Prepare solutions 2 and 3 freshly each week and store them at 4°C, the stain in the dark, covered with foil. On the day of use, dilute the 0.1% acridine orange 1 in 10 with the buffer to obtain 0.01% stain.

Staining cells and exudates

1. Collect living cells, tissue cultures or exudates on coverslips.
2. Without allowing to dry, place the coverslip in the acid-alcohol for 5 min.
3. Rinse for 2 min in two changes of buffer.
4. Stain in 0.01% acridine orange for 4–10 min.
5. Wash in two changes of buffer for 2 min.
6. Mount in buffer under a coverslip and seal the edges.

Staining bacteria in wet films

1. With a 1 μl loop place a drop of 0.01% acridine orange stain on the centre of a slide.
2. With another 1 μl loop add a drop of the specimen, e.g. blood culture fluid, to the stain and mix gently.
3. Ring the drop of mixture with a 'wall' of soft petroleum jelly and apply a coverslip.
4. Examine with a UV fluorescence microscope (Ch. 2) and a ×40 dry objective.

THE ROMANOWSKY STAINS

The original Romanowsky stain was made by dissolving in methyl alcohol the compound formed by the interaction of watery solutions of eosin and zinc-free methylene blue. The original stain has now been replaced by various modifications which are easier to use and give better results; these are Leishman's, Wright's, Jenner's and Giemsa's stains. The peculiar property of the Romanowsky stains is that they impart a reddish-purple colour to the chromatin of malaria and other parasites. This colour is due to a substance which forms when methylene blue is 'ripened', either by age, as in polychrome methylene blue, or by heating with sodium carbonate. The latter method is employed in the manufacture of Leishman's and Wright's stains. The ripened methylene blue is mixed with a solution of water-soluble eosin, when a precipitate, due to the combination of these dyes, is formed. The precipitate is washed with distilled water, dried and dissolved in pure methyl alcohol. (The methyl alcohol, i.e. methanol, must be 'pure, for analysis', and have a pH of 6.5. If too acid, the reaction must be adjusted by the addition of 0.01 mol/l NaOH.) Each modification of the Romanowsky stain varies according to the 'ripening' and the relative proportions of methylene blue and eosin.

The Romanowsky stains are usually diluted for staining purposes with distilled water, when a precipitate is formed which is removed by subsequent washing.

Leishman's stain
(For protozoa in blood films)

This stain may be purchased ready for use or made by dissolving 0.15 g of Leishman's powder in 100 ml pure methyl alcohol (methanol). The powder is ground in a mortar with a little methyl alcohol ('pure for analysis', pH 6.5), the residue of undissolved stain allowed to settle and the fluid decanted into a bottle. The residue in the mortar is treated with more methyl alcohol, and the process is repeated until all the stain goes into solution. The remainder of the methyl alcohol is now added. The stain can be used within an hour or two of making.

Films

Dry unfixed films are used. The stain is first used undiluted, and the methyl alcohol fixes the film. The stain is then diluted with distilled water, and the staining proper carried out.

1. Pour the undiluted stain on the unfixed film and allow it to act for 1 min.

2. By means of a pipette and rubber teat add double the volume of distilled water to the slide, mixing the fluids by alternately sucking them up in the pipette and expelling them. Allow the diluted stain to act for 12 min.

3. Flood the slide gently with distilled water, allowing the preparation to differentiate in the distilled water until the film appears bright pink in colour – usually about 30 s.

4. Remove the excess of water with blotting paper and dry in the air.

It is important that the reaction of the distilled water be neither acid nor alkaline. Any slight variations from neutrality may alter considerably the colour of granules in white blood corpuscles, etc., and give rise to supposed 'pathological' appearances in cells which are really normal. A simple method of ensuring a suitable reaction of the distilled water is to keep large bottles of it – e.g. aspirator bottles – specially for these stains. Add 2 or 3 drops of 1% aqueous neutral red solution. The usual reaction of distilled water is slightly acid, and a few drops of 1% sodium carbonate solution should be added until the solution shows the faintest possible suggestion of pink colour.

Much trouble will be eliminated if a buffer solution is used instead of distilled water for diluting the stain and washing the slide. It is made as follows:

Na_2HPO_4 (anhydrous)	5.447 g
KH_2PO_4	4.752 g

Mix together in a mortar and keep as such. The buffer mixture is quite stable.

Add 1 g of buffer mixture to 2 litres of distilled water and this gives a pH of 7.0, which is suitable for most work.

Some samples of stain may require a slightly more acid solution, of pH 6.8. For this mix

Na_2HPO_4 (anhydrous)	4.539 g
KH_2PO_4	5.940 g

Add 1 g of the mixture to 2 litres of distilled water.

Shute (1950) maintains that 15 s fixation with the undiluted stain is sufficient and that only four drops of stain are necessary. The slide is rocked for 12–15 s and then eight to twelve drops of water are added and thoroughly mixed. Staining proceeds for 15 min and the diluted stain is flooded off in 2–3 s only. If washed for longer, Schüffner's dots will not be seen. Shute advocates a pH of 7.2 for the diluting fluid.

For demonstrating Schüffner's dots in benign tertian malaria the use of Giemsa's stain following Leishman's stain has been recommended by Discombe (1945).

1. Fix thin blood film with Leishman's stain for 15–60 s. Dilute with twice the volume of buffer solution at pH 7.0 and stain for 15 min.

2. Wash off with dilute Giemsa's stain (e.g. Gurr R66, from BDH)–1 drop of stain to 1 ml buffer solution at pH 7.0 – and stain with this for a further 30 min.

3. Wash with buffer solution.

4. Blot and dry.

Sections

1. Treat the section with xylol to remove the paraffin, then with ethyl alcohol and finally distilled water.

2. Drain off the excess of water and stain for 5–10 min with a mixture of 1 part Leishman's stain and 2 parts of distilled water or buffer solution.

3. Wash with distilled water.

4. Differentiate with a weak solution of acetic acid (1 in 1500), controlling the differentiation under the low power of the microscope until the protoplasm of the cells is pink and only the nuclei are blue.

5. Wash with distilled water or buffer solution.

6. Blot, dehydrate with a few drops of absolute alcohol, clear in xylol and mount in Canada balsam or preferably DPX mounting medium.

Giemsa's stain
(For protozoa and spirochaetes)

This consists of a number of compounds made by mixing different proportions of methylene blue and eosin. These have been designated Azur I, Azur II and Azur II-eosin. The preparation can be purchased made up, but batches may vary considerably.

We can recommend the following method of preparation devised by Lillie (1943), which gives consistent and reliable results. It is excellent for staining blood films for malaria parasites, and also mouse or rat blood for trypanosomes.

Stains

1. *Azure B eosinate.* Dissolve 10 g methylene blue in 600 ml distilled water. Add 6.0 ml concentrated sulphuric acid. Bring to the boil and add 2.5 g potassium bichromate dissolved in 25 ml distilled water. Boil for 20 min. Cool to 10°C or lower (place in refrigerator overnight). When cold add 21 g dry sodium bicarbonate slowly with frequent shaking. Then add a 5% solution of eosin (yellowish) and shake constantly until the margin of the fluid appears pale blue or bluish-pink. About 205 ml will be required, and 150 ml of this can be added at once. Filter immediately, preferably on a vacuum funnel with hard paper. When the fluid has been drawn through and the surface begins to crack, add 50 ml distilled water. Allow to drain, and wash again with a second 50 ml distilled water. Now wash with 40 ml ethyl alcohol (95%) and repeat with a second 40 ml alcohol. Dry the precipitate at room temperature or 37°C (not higher). This constitutes Azure B eosinate.

2. *Azure A eosinate.* Proceed exactly as above, but use 5.0 g potassium bichromate (in place of 2.5 g) and dissolve it in 50 ml distilled water.

3. *Methylene blue eosinate.* Dissolve 10 g methylene blue in 600 ml cold distilled water and precipitate as before with 5% eosin solution, filtering and drying as above.

4. *Solvent.* This consists of equal volumes of methyl alcohol (methanol) and glycerol (analytical grades).

5. *Diluting fluid.* This is phosphate buffer solution pH 7.0 (see under Leishman's stain).

Giemsa's solution. To make the finished stain, grind the three eosinates separately into fine powder in separate clean mortars. Then weigh out 500 mg azure B eosinate, 100 mg azure A eosinate, 400 mg methylene blue eosinate, and 200 mg finely ground methylene blue. Decant the mixed powder on to the surface of 200 ml solvent, allowing it to settle in gradually. Then shake frequently for 2 or 3 days, keeping the bottle between 50 and 60°C between shakings. The proportion of stains given above should yield a satisfactory staining picture.

This stain may be used in a manner somewhat similar to Leishman's preparation (the 'rapid method'), or prolonged staining may be carried out, as, for example, in staining spirochaetes (the 'slow method'). In both cases the preparation must be fixed prior to staining, either with methyl alcohol (methanol) for 3 min, or with absolute alcohol (ethanol) for 15 min.

Rapid method

1. Fix films in methyl alcohol for 3 min.
2. Stain in a mixture of 1 part stain and 10 parts buffer solution pH 7.0 for 1 h.
3. Wash with buffer solution, allowing preparation to differentiate for about 30 s.
4. Blot and allow to dry in the air.

This method of staining gives excellent results with thin blood films for malaria parasites, Schüffner's dots being well defined. Trypanosomes are also well demonstrated.

A rapid method with the application of heat is useful for demonstrating spirochaetes.

1. Fix preparations with absolute alcohol (15 min) or by drawing three times through a flame.
2. Prepare a fresh solution of 10 drops of Giemsa's solution with 10 ml of buffer solution

of pH 7.0, shake gently and cover the fixed film with the diluted stain. Warm till steam rises, allow to cool for 15 s, then pour off and replace with fresh stain and heat again.

3. Repeat the procedure four or five times, wash in distilled water, dry and mount.

Slow method

This is a specially valuable method for demonstrating objects difficult to stain in the ordinary way, e.g. certain pathogenic spirochaetes. The principle is to allow the diluted stain to act for a considerable period. As the mixture of stain and water causes a fine precipitate, care has to be taken that this does not deposit on the film.

1. Fix the film in methyl alcohol for 3 min.
2. Mix 1 ml stain with 20 ml buffer solution, pH 7.0, in a Petri dish.
3. Place a piece of thin glass rod in the stain in the dish.
4. Place the fixed slide, film side downwards, in the stain with one end resting on the rod so that there is sufficient stain between the film and the bottom of the dish.
5. Leave to stain for 16–24 h.
6. Wash the slide in a stream of buffer solution.
7. Allow to dry in air, mount and examine.

STAINING OF SPIROCHAETES

Fontana's method for films

Solutions

a. *Fixative*

Acetic acid	1 ml
Formalin (40% H.CHO)	2 ml
Distilled water	100 ml

b. *Mordant*

Phenol	1 g
Tannic acid	5 g
Distilled water	100 ml

c. *Ammoniated silver nitrate*
Add 10% ammonia to 0.5% solution of silver nitrate in distilled water until the precipitate formed just dissolves. Now add more silver nitrate solution drop by drop until the precipitate returns and does not redissolve.

Procedure

1. Treat the film three times, 30 s each time, with the fixative.
2. Wash off the fixative with absolute alcohol and allow the alcohol to act for 3 min.
3. Drain off the excess of alcohol and carefully burn off the remainder until the film is dry.
4. Pour on the mordant, heating till steam rises, and allow it to act for 30 s.
5. Wash well in distilled water and again dry the slide.
6. Treat with ammoniated silver nitrate, heating till steam rises, for 30 s, when the film becomes brown in colour.
7. Wash well in distilled water, dry and mount in Canada balsam.

It is essential that the specimen be mounted in balsam under a coverslip before examination, as some immersion oils cause the film to fade at once.

The spirochaetes are stained brownish-black on a brownish-yellow background.

Becker's method (modified)

The fixative and mordant are as in Fontana's method.

Stain

Basic fuchsin (saturated alcoholic solution)	45 ml
Shunk's mordant B (95% or 100% ethanol 16 ml and aniline oil 4 ml)	18 ml
Distilled water	100 ml

Mix the Shunk's mordant with the alcoholic fuchsin and then add the distilled water. (The glassware should be dry.)

Procedure

1. Filter stain and reagents into jars for use.
2. Make film and dry in air.
3. Place film in fixative for 1–3 min.

4. Wash in water for about 30 s.
5. Treat with mordant for 3–5 min.
6. Wash in water for about 30 s.
7. Place in staining solution for 3–5 min.
8. Wash well in water and drain dry.

Levaditi's method of staining spirochaetes in tissues

This modified method using pyridine is more rapid than the original technique.

1. Fix the tissue, which must be in small pieces 1 mm thick, in 10% formalin (4% formaldehyde) for 24 h.

2. Wash the tissue for 1 h in water and thereafter place it in 96–98% alcohol for 24 h.

3. Place the tissue in a 1% solution of silver nitrate (to which one-tenth of the volume of pure pyridine has been added) for 2 h at room temperature, and thereafter at about 50°C for 4–6 h. Then rapidly wash the tissue in 10% pyridine solution.

4. Transfer to the reducing fluid, which consists of:

Formalin 4% (1.6% H.CHO)   100 parts

to which are added immediately before use:

Acetone (pure)   10 parts
Pyridine (pure)   15 parts

Keep the tissue in this fluid for 2 days at room temperature in the dark.

5. After washing well with water, dehydrate the tissue with increasing strengths of alcohol and embed in paraffin. Thin sections are cut and mounted in the usual way. After removing the paraffin with xylol the sections are immediately mounted in Canada balsam.

FIXATION AND EMBEDDING OF TISSUES

As the ordinary routine bacteriological investigation of tissues is carried out almost exclusively with paraffin sections, this technique only will be described.

The fixed tissue is embedded in paraffin wax to support it during the cutting of the section, and the section is held together by the wax in the process of transferring it to the slide.

The paraffin wax must completely permeate the tissue, but before it can do so, all water must be removed from the material and replaced by a fluid with which melted paraffin will mix.

Water, therefore, is first removed with several changes of alcohol; the alcohol is replaced by some fluid – such as xylol, benzol, acetone, chloroform – which is a solvent of both alcohol and paraffin wax, and the tissue is finally embedded in melted paraffin.

Before removing the water from the tissue preparatory to embedding, the tissue must be suitably fixed and hardened.

The essentials for obtaining good sections are:

1. The tissue must be fresh.

2. It must be properly fixed by using small pieces and employing a large amount of fixing fluid.

3. The appropriate fixing fluid (see below) must be employed for the particular investigation required.

4. The tissue must not remain too long in the embedding bath.

Formalin 10%

Formalin is a 38–40% (w/v) solution of formaldehyde (H.CHO) in water containing 10% methanol to inhibit polymerization (i.e. 38–40 g H.CHO/100 ml solution).

10% commercial formalin (4% formaldehyde) in 0.85% NaCl solution is a good general fixative. It is easily prepared, has good penetrating qualities, does not shrink the tissues, and permits considerable latitude in the time during which specimens may be left in it. Moreover, the subsequent handling of the material is much easier in our experience than in the case of mercuric chloride fixatives, such as Zenker's fluid. Formalin fixation is not as good as other methods where fine detail has to be observed, as, for example, in material containing protozoa. For general routine use, however, it is the most convenient and useful of fixatives. Tissue should be cut into thin slices, about 4 mm thick, and dropped into a large bulk of fixative. The fluid may be changed at the end of 24 h, and fixation is usually complete in 48 h. Specimens are then washed in running water for an hour and transferred to 50% alcohol. In the latter fluid they may be kept for a considerable time without deterioration.

Formalin tends to become acid owing to the formation of formic acid. The strong formalin should be kept neutral by the addition of an excess of magnesium carbonate. The clear supernatant fluid is decanted off when formalin dilutions are required.

Zenker's fluid

Mercuric chloride	50 g
Potassium bichromate	25 g
Sodium sulphate	10 g
Water	1 litre

Immediately before use, add 5 ml of glacial acetic acid per 100 ml of fluid.

The fluid should be warmed to body temperature and only small pieces of tissue must be placed in it. Fixation is complete in 24 h, and thereafter the pieces of tissue are washed in running water for 24 h to remove the potassium bichromate and mercuric chloride. The tissue is then transferred to 50% ethyl alcohol.

It is essential that all the mercuric chloride should be removed, otherwise a deposit will appear in the sections. The bulk of it is removed by washing. The remainder can be removed with iodine during the dehydration stage in alcohol. The material after washing is transferred to 50%, and later to 70% alcohol to which sufficient iodine has been added to make the fluid dark brown in colour. (It is convenient to keep a saturated solution of iodine in 90% alcohol in a drop-bottle, and add a few drops as required.) If the alcohol becomes clear more iodine is added until the fluid remains brown. This indicates that all the mercury salt has been dissolved out by the iodine-alcohol.

Cut sections fixed on slides can also be treated with iodine, e.g. Gram's iodine, for 3–5 min, to remove mercuric chloride.

Animal tissues fixed in Zenker's fluid are more difficult to cut, and sections are apt to float off the slide, particularly if fixation has been unduly prolonged.

Zenker-formol fluid

This is similar to Zenker's fluid except that the acetic acid is omitted and 5 ml of formalin are added per 100 ml immediately before use. It is a useful general fixative for animal tissues.

Mercuric-chloride-formalin

Mercuric chloride, saturated aqueous solution	90 ml
Formalin (40% H.CHO)	10 ml

Small portions of tissue must be used and fixation is complete in 1–12 h. Then transfer to alcohol and iodine as after Zenker's fluid. This fluid fixes with the minimum amount of distortion and the finer cytological details of the cells are retained. It is useful when staining virus inclusion bodies.

'Susa' fixative

Mercuric chloride	45 g
Distilled water	800 ml
Sodium chloride	5 g
Trichloracetic acid	20 g
Acetic acid (glacial)	40 ml
Formalin (40% formaldehyde)	200 ml

This is one of the best fixatives for both normal and pathological tissues. Pieces of tissue not thicker than 1 cm should be fixed for 3–24 h, depending on the thickness. The material should be transferred *direct* to 95% alcohol. Lower grades of alcohol, or water, may cause undue swelling of connective tissue. Add to the alcohol sufficient of a saturated solution of iodine in 95% alcohol to give a brown colour. If the latter fades, more iodine should be added.

The advantages of 'Susa' fixative are rapid and even fixation with little shrinkage of connective tissue. The transference direct to 95% alcohol shortens the time of dehydration, while tissues thus fixed are easy to cut.

Bouin's fluid

This fixative is useful for the investigation of virus inclusion bodies.

Saturated aqueous solution of
  picric acid   75 parts
Formalin   25 parts
Glacial acetic acid   5 parts

This solution keeps well. Use thin pieces of tissue not exceeding 10 mm thick. Fix for 1–12 h according to thickness and density of tissue. Wash in 50% alcohol (not water), then 70% until the picric acid is removed.

Schaudinn's fluid

Absolute ethyl alcohol   100 ml
Saturated aqueous solution of
  mercuric chloride   200 ml

This is an important fixative for protozoa. It may be used cold or warmed to 60°C, when it is more quickly penetrating. It is also a suitable fixative for wet films.

Flemming's fluid

Osmic acid   0.1 g
Chromic acid   0.2 g
Glacial acetic acid   0.1 ml
Water   100 ml

The osmic and chromic acids, when mixed, will keep for only 3–4 weeks. The acetic acid should be added immediately before use.

Embedding and section cutting

After fixation by any of the above-mentioned methods and transference to 50% ethyl alcohol, *small pieces* of tissue are treated as follows:

1. Place in 90% alcohol for 2–5 h.
2. Transfer to absolute alcohol for 2 h.
3. Complete the dehydration in fresh absolute alcohol for 2 h.
4. Transfer to a mixture of absolute alcohol and chloroform (equal parts) till tissue sinks, or overnight.
5. Place in pure chloroform for 6 h.
6. Transfer the tissue for 1 h to a mixture of equal parts of chloroform and paraffin wax, which is kept melted in the paraffin oven.
7. Place in pure melted paraffin in the oven at 55°C for 2 h, preferably in a vacuum embedding oven.

The tissue is embedded in blocks of paraffin. These are cut out, trimmed with a knife, and sections 5 μm thick are cut by means of a microtome. The sections are flattened on warm water, floated on to slides and allowed to dry. Albuminized slides are useful where the staining process involves heating, and where animal tissue is used, especially after fixation with Zenker's fluid. The slides are coated with albumin either by means of a small piece of chamois leather or by the finger tip. The albumin solution is made by adding three parts of distilled water to one part of egg-white and shaking thoroughly. The mixture is filtered through muslin into a bottle, and a crystal of thymol is added as a preservative. It is usual to coat a number of slides and, after drying, these are stored until required. The albuminized side may be identified by breathing gently on the slide; it is not dimmed by the breath, whereas the plain side is.

REFERENCES

Anderson E S, Armstrong J A, Niven J S F 1959 Fluorescence microscopy: observations of virus growth with aminoacridines. Symposium of the Society of General Microbiology, No. IX Cambridge University p 224–255

Ashby G K 1938 Simplified Schaeffer spore stain. Science 87:443

Bisset K A 1938 The structure of 'rough' and 'smooth' colonies. Journal of Pathology and Bacteriology 47: 223–229

Burdon K L 1946 Fatty material in bacteria and fungi revealed by staining dried, fixed slide preparations. Journal of Bacteriology 52: 665–678

Burke V 1922 Notes on the gram stain with description of a new method. Journal of Bacteriology 7: 159–182

Butt E M, Bonynge C W, Joyce R L 1936 The demonstration of capsules about haemolytic streptococci with India ink or azo blue. Journal of Infectious Diseases 58: 5–9

Clark H W, Fowler R C, Brown T McP 1961 Preparation of pleuropneumonia-like organisms for microscopic study. Journal of Bacteriology 81: 500–502

Discombe G 1945 The demonstration of Schüffner's dots in, benign tertian malaria. British Medical Journal 1:298

Duguid J P 1951 The demonstration of bacterial capsules

and slime. Journal of Pathology and Bacteriology 63: 673–685

Ehrlich P 1882 Aus dem Verein für innere Medizin zu Berlin. Deutsche medizinische Wochenschrift 8: 269–270

Geigy 1962 Documenta Geigy Scientific Tables, 6th edn. Geigy Pharmaceuticals, Manchester, p 314

Gram C 1884 Ueber die isolirte Farbung der Schizomyceten in Schnitt und Trockenpräparaten. Fortschritte der Medizin 2: 185–189. See 'The differential staining of Schizomycetes in tissue sections and in dried preparations', In: Brock T D (ed) 1961 Milestones in microbiology. Prentice-Hall, London p 215–218

Hotchkiss R D 1948 A microchemical reaction resulting in the staining of polysaccharide structures in fixed tissue preparations. Archives of Biochemistry 16: 131–141

Jamison R M, Mayor H D 1965 Acridine orange staining of purified rat virus strains X14. Journal of Bacteriology 90: 1486–1488

Johne A 1885 Einzweiffelöser Fall von congenitaler Tuberkulose. Fortschritte der Medizin 3:198 (footnote p. 200).

Kirkpatrick J, Lendrum A C 1939 A mounting medium for microscopical preparations giving good preservation of colour. Journal of Pathology and Bacteriology 49: 592–594

Kirkpatrick J, Lendrum A C 1941 Further observations on the use of synthetic resin as a substitute for Canada balsam. Precipitation of paraffin wax in the medium and an improved plasticizer. Journal of Pathology and Bacteriology 53: 441–443

Kleineberger E 1934 The colonial development of the organisms of pleuropneumonia and agalactia on serum agar and variations in the morphology under different conditions of growth. Journal of Pathology and Bacteriology 39: 409–420

Kopeloff N, Beerman P 1922 Modified Gram stains. Journal of Infectious Diseases 31: 480–482

Laybourn R L 1924 A modification of Albert's stain for the diphtheria bacillus. Journal of the American Medical Association 83:121

Lillie R D 1943 Giemsa stain of quite constant composition and performance, made in the laboratory from eosin and methylene blue. U.S. Public Health Report 58: 449–452

Preston N W, Morrell A 1962 Reproducible results with the Gram stain. Journal of Pathology and Bacteriology 84: 241–243

Robinow C F 1944 Cytological observations on Bact. coli, Proteus vulgaris, and various aerobic spore-forming bacteria with special reference to the nuclear structures. Journal of Hygiene (London) 43: 413–423

Robinow C F 1949 In: Dubos R J (ed) Bacterial cell, Harvard University Press, Cambridge, Mass, Addendum

Shute P G 1950 Thin and thick films showing malarial parasites on the same slide and in the same microscope field. Transactions of the Royal Society of Tropical Medicine and Hygiene 43: 364

Sterilization and disinfection in the laboratory

Sterilization is the freeing of an article from all living organisms, including viable spores. Sterility is a theoretical concept that can never be demonstrated with absolute certainty. There are many difficulties; cultural, technical and statistical (Kelsey 1972). In practice, however, a satisfactory sterilization process is one designed to ensure a high probability of achieving sterility, e.g. a process that kills more than 10^6 organisms (spores) of a defined, exceptionally high degree of resistance.

Disinfection is the freeing of an article from harmful microorganisms. As bacterial endospores capable of causing disease in the intact subject, e.g anthrax spores, are rarely encountered, satisfactory disinfection can usually be achieved by the destruction of all vegetative organisms.

Methods of sterilization and disinfection include the use of heat, chemicals, filtration and radiation, of which heat is the most generally applicable and reliable and should be used wherever possible. *Dry heat* is suitable for glassware, instruments and paper-wrapped articles not spoiled by the very high temperature required, and for water-impermeable oils, waxes and powders, but cannot be used for water-containing culture media. *Moist heat*, which is effective at lower temperatures, is suitable for most culture media and a properly designed autoclave will effectively sterilize media and other water-containing materials in sealed or unsealed bottles, laboratory discards and porous packaged materials.

Gaseous chemical sterilization may be required for heat-sensitive articles, and filtration may be the only means of sterilizing heat-labile fluids.

Radiation, though extensively used in the manufacture of sterile packaged products, e.g. disposable plastic syringes, has few if any applications in the clinical microbiology laboratory. Chemical disinfection is the only convenient procedure for floors, bench tops, wash-basins and other large articles of laboratory furniture.

DRY HEAT

Red heat has its main application in the sterilization of inoculating wires and loops, which should be held almost vertically in a Bunsen flame until red hot along their whole length, almost up to the tip of their metal holder. The points of forceps and the surface of searing spatulae may also be heated to redness. *Flaming* by slow passage through a Bunsen flame may be used to destroy vegetative organisms on the surface of scalpel blades, glass slides, coverslips and the mouths of culture tubes and bottles, but care must be taken not to crack the glass.

Hot air sterilizers

Heating by exposure to hot air is the accepted method for sterilizing loads that cannot be reliably penetrated by steam and can tolerate the high temperatures required, e.g. 160–180°C. It is used particularly for glassware, such as test-tubes, glass Petri dishes, flasks, pipettes and assembled all-glass syringes, and for metal instruments such as forceps, scalpels and scissors. Wrappings of aluminium foil or Kraft paper and stoppers of cotton-wool may be used, though the paper and cotton-wool become slightly charred and some brands of the latter give off volatile antibacterial substances. Hot air is also used to sterilize dry materials in sealed containers, and powders, oils and greases, e.g. petroleum jelly.

Hot air sterilizers should conform to British Standard (BS) 3421. They should be fitted with a fan to provide forced air circulation throughout the oven chamber, a temperature indicator, a control thermostat and timer, open mesh shelving and adequate wall insulation. There should also be a temperature chart recorder and a port for thermocouples. Safety features on new sterilizers should include an overheat cut-out operating at and above 200°C. Door interlocks should be fitted to ensure the heating cycle will not start until the door is shut and that after the cycle it will not open until the temperature has fallen below 60°C (Department of Health and Social Security 1980a Health Technical Memorandum 10).

Preparation of load. 1. Cap glass test-tubes with slip-on aluminium caps and place them vertically in metal racks. The caps will protect the rims of the tubes from airborne contamination during subsequent storage.

2. Stopper the upper ends of pipettes to a depth of about 2 cm with plugs of non-absorbent cotton-wool and place them in metal cannisters or, if for only occasional use, wrap them individually in Kraft paper.

3. Clean all-glass syringes in soap and warm water with a test-tube brush, then rinse and dry them. Lightly smear the piston with silicone grease, insert it into the barrel and work it backwards and forwards several times. Then pack the syringe in an aluminium case with a metal or foil cap or double wrap it in aluminium foil.

4. Wash syringe needles in warm water, clean the channel with a stilette and sharpen the point on an oiled slipstone. Then rinse them with alcohol and pack each separately in a small test-tube with a constriction that will prevent the needle tip touching the bottom.

5. Sterilize screw-capped bottles in hot air only if their caps and liners are made of a material such as metal, Teflon, polypropylene or silicone rubber that will withstand distortion at the sterilizing temperatures.

6. Ensure that all glassware is perfectly dry before placing it in the sterilizing oven. Preliminary exposure in a drying oven at 100°C is recommended.

7. Sterilize powders, fats, oils and greases in sealed glass or metal containers in small amounts not exceeding 10 g in weight or 1 cm in depth.

8. Position the individual articles or packs of the load to allow free circulation of the hot air between and around them. Close the oven door and switch on the source of heat.

Sterilizing cycle. The 'sterilization hold time' does not start until (1) the chamber has reached the chosen sterilizing temperature and (2) a further period has been allowed for all parts of the load to be raised to that temperature. The length of the latter period should be established at the commissioning of the sterilizer by the use of thermocouples distributed throughout a test load of the heaviest and least permeable kind that the machine is expected to process. A master temperature record of this test is produced and details of the 'worst-case' load, such as the size, volume, number, type and distribution of the items, are noted.

Commonly used time–temperature relations for the sterilization hold time are 20 min at 180°C, 40 min at 170°C or 60 min at 160°C (Medical Research Council 1962).

Cooling. This may take up to several hours because of the protective insulation of the oven. It can be hastened by fitting a thermostatically controlled cooling fan, circulating cool outside air drawn in through a HEPA filter, or an external cooling coil.

Do not attempt to open the chamber door until the chamber and load have cooled to below 60°C. Glassware is liable to crack if cold air is admitted suddenly while it is still very hot.

Testing. 1. Compare the temperature record chart produced during each run with the master temperature record to ensure that the performance of the machine has not deteriorated.

2. If the machine is not fitted with a temperature chart recorder, include a Browne's tube No. 3 (Browne) in each load and observe it for

the appropriate colour change (from red to green) at the end of the process.

3. Use biological tests of efficacy only if adequate physical monitoring is not possible, as in the absence of a temperature recorder. Demonstrate that the sterilizing cycle inactivates at least 10^5 spores of *Bacillus subtilis* var *niger* (National Collection of Type Cultures, NCTC10073, American Type Culture Collection, ATCC9372, Collection of Institut Pasteur, CIP77.18). The spores used should have a D value of 5–10 at 160°C (European Pharmacopoeia Commission 1983) and a Z value of about 25. The D value measures the rate of kill at a given temperature and is expressed as the time required, in minutes, to reduce the number of viable organisms by 90%. The Z value is a measure of the thermal resistance of the spore to the process measured as the number of degrees centigrade required to produce a 10-fold change in the thermal death time.

4. Details of additional half yearly and yearly thermocouple tests are given in the Department of Health and Social Security (1980a) Health Technical Memorandum No. 10, and should be complied with wherever possible.

MOIST HEAT

Microorganisms and their spores are killed at lower temperatures by moist heat than by dry heat, but they must be in contact with water, such as that from condensing steam, so that the method is not applicable to waterproof materials such as oils and greases or to dry materials in sealed containers. Moist heat must be used for the sterilization of culture media and other liquids required to retain their content of water.

Pasteurization below 100°C

Heat-labile fluids may be disinfected, though not sterilized, by heating for 1 h at 56°C or for 10 min at 65–75°C. Such treatment is sufficient to kill mesophilic vegetative bacteria. If it is used for serum or other body fluids containing proteins, care must be taken not to allow the temperature to rise above 59°C lest coagulation should occur. The procedure is best carried out

in a waterbath, but a well controlled hot air oven may be used. Its effectiveness should always be checked by subculture on to a range of suitable media.

If the heating is repeated on several successive days, it may be possible to achieve sterility (see Tyndallization, below).

Washing machines

Washing machines using hot water and a detergent may be employed to disinfect eating utensils or items of medical or anaesthetic equipment that would be damaged by autoclaving. They combine a mechanical reduction of the bioburden with a transfer of heat sufficient to kill vegetative organisms. Both parts of the process are important and efficient cleaning at a temperature below 75°C may remove more organisms than less efficient cleaning at a higher temperature (Nyström 1981).

The time required for disinfection is 10 min at 70°C or 1 min at 80°C, though these traditional time-temperature relationships may be excessive. Thus, it is difficult to recover relatively heat-resistant faecal streptococci after exposure for 10 s at 80°C on a clean surface.

The reliability of the process cannot be assumed. Heat must be transferred to all surfaces and the effectiveness of transfer will depend both on the shape of the article and the design of the water jets. Heat penetration also depends on the material of which the article is composed and the degree of its soiling.

Tests of heat disinfection may be done either by attaching thermocouples to the load or by sealing 10^8 streptococci in broth culture in capillary tubes attached to the surface of the articles. In the latter case, bacterial counts are made before and after the processing (Ayliffe et al 1974). Even after adequate biological testing, the performance of a machine may deteriorate dramatically, as for instance by blocking of the water jets, so that regular maintenance is mandatory.

Boiling at 100°C

Heating in water boiling at 100°C for 10 min is sufficient to kill all vegetative bacteria, hepatitis virus and some, though not all, bacterial spores. The method is still occasionally used for medical or surgical equipment when sterility is not essential and better methods are destructive or unavailable.

Metal, glass and rubber items held on a removable tray with a raised edge are immersed in boiling water in a metal bath. The water should be soft, deionized or distilled. First, dismantle and carefully clean the articles to be boiled. Then immerse them completely in the water, avoiding the presence of any trapped air in or between them. Bring back to the boil and do not add fresh articles during the period of boiling. After boiling for 10 min, remove immediately with long-handled sterile forceps. Hold the hot article in the forceps long enough to allow it to dry by evaporation. If a boiled instrument is handled while still wet, skin bacteria may float down from the fingers to contaminate its working end.

Steaming at 100°C

As glass containers are apt to crack if heated directly to boil their contents, it is more convenient to treat bottles, flasks and tubes of fluids and culture media by exposure to steam. Pure steam in equilibrium with water boiling at normal atmospheric pressure (760 mm Hg), i.e. 'free steam', has a temperature of 100°C and exposure to this temperature for 60 min will kill all organisms except slow viruses and the spores of the most resistant mesophilic (e.g. *Clostridium tetani*) and thermophilic bacteria.

When, therefore, an autoclave is not available, a cheap and convenient steamer may be used for the final sterilization of culture media such as broth and nutrient agar. Because, however, steaming at 100°C sometimes fails to sterilize, before the medium is used a portion of it should be incubated to confirm that it is free from viable organisms capable of growing in it under the conditions of its intended use. Being immersed in an atmosphere of steam, little water is lost by evaporation from open containers loosely stoppered with cotton-wool or slip-on metal caps.

As the containers of media are cold when first placed in the steam-filled steamer, they must be left for a period that includes an allowance for heating up to 100°C as well as the required period, e.g. 60 min, for heating at 100°C. The heating-up may be judged to be about 20 min for bottles containing 10–100 ml fluid, 30 min for bottles containing 600 ml and 45 min for a flask containing 2–5 litres. These periods apply only if the water in the steamer is boiling when the containers are introduced. If not, a further period of exposure must be allowed while the water is brought to the boil.

A commoner use of the steamer is to dissolve agar and distribute the ingredients during the initial preparation of most types of culture media. Large unstoppered flasks containing 2–4 litres of medium are steamed and the melted medium is then distributed into smaller containers in which it is sterilized by autoclaving.

Steaming for 30–60 min at 100°C is also used to disinfect some heat-labile culture media such as DCA, TCBS and selenite F, which, because they are selective, are unlikely to support the growth of any heat-resistant bacteria. Selenite F medium dissolved in the cold and distributed in 10 ml amounts in 28 ml Universal containers can be disinfected by steaming for 30 min.

The traditional Koch and Arnold steamers are upright metal tanks with a removable lid incorporating a chimney which allows the free escape of steam while preventing the ingress of air. Water in the bottom of the tank is heated by gas or electricity and the containers of media are laid on a perforated shelf just above the level of the water. Steamers with front-opening doors, as used in commercial catering, are also available.

Tyndallization

Nutrient media may be sterilized by exposure to free steam at 100°C for a period of 20–45 min on three successive days. On each occasion time must be allowed to heat the medium up to 100°C, e.g. 20 min for small containers with up to 100 ml medium and longer for those with larger volumes (see above). Spores that survive the initial heating will germinate in the medium while held at room temperature during the following day and the resulting vegetative bacteria will be killed when the medium is reheated. The process, however, will fail to kill bacteria whose spores cannot germinate in the particular medium or under the conditions of storage between heatings. It is therefore inapplicable to non-nutrient media. Tyndalliz- ation was commonly employed in the past for the sterilization of media containing heat-labile sugars but has now been superseded for this purpose by pressure filtration.

AUTOCLAVES

Autoclaving provides moist heat at temperatures higher than 100°C, the boiling point of water under normal atmospheric pressure. It does so by exposure of the load to steam under increased pressure. This steam is biocidal. As it condenses on the cooler articles of the load it releases both thermal energy (its latent heat) and moisture, which together denature microbial proteins.

Autoclaving is the most reliable method of sterilizing culture media and other laboratory supplies. It should be used for all materials that are water-containing, permeable or wettable, and not liable to be damaged by the process.

Temperature and pressure. Although it is the temperature and not the pressure of the steam that confers the sterilizing effect, the tempera- ture is determined by the pressure. When water boils and is converted into steam at the same temperature, its vapour pressure equals the pressure of the surrounding atmosphere. This occurs at 100°C for normal atmospheric pressure. When water is boiled in a closed vessel under increased pressure, the temperature at which it boils and that of the steam it forms are above 100°C; the greater the pressure the higher the temperature.

Measurements of pressure may be given in a variety of units, in traditional British practice, usually in pounds per square inch (p.s.i. or lb/in^2), but all new autoclaves must be calibrated in bar or m.bar (abs). The following equival- ences may be noted: 1 normal atmosphere = 1 bar = 14.7 p.s.i. = 760 mm Hg = 10^5 N/m^2 = 0.1 mN/m^2 = 100 kPa. It is important to note that the pressures employed in autoclaving may be specified, and shown on the instrument's pressure gauge, either as the degree of pressure above atmospheric or as absolute pressure. Thus a gauge pressure of 2.2 bar (gauge) is equivalent to an absolute pressure of 3.2 bar (abs).

Table 4.1 shows some commonly used press- ures, temperatures and holding times for steril- ization with pure dry saturated steam free from any admixture with air.

Time. The *sterilization hold time* is the time for which the entire load requires to be exposed to pure dry saturated steam at the effective temperature in order to ensure sterilization. It does not allow for the penetration of the load by the steam and heat. It is made up by combining a *holding time* based on the thermal death time of *Bacillus stearothermophilus* (whose thermal resistance exceeds that of the pathogenic clos- tridia) and a small additional *safety time*, orig- inally introduced to compensate for variability within the load.

Before the start of the sterilization hold time, the load requires to be exposed to steam for an additional period long enough to allow the steam to penetrate into it and heat it up to the effective temperature. This is the *heat penetration time*. It varies with the different types of load and

Table 4.1 Time and temperature requirements for sterilization by steam under pressure in the autoclave.

Temperature[a] (°C)	Pressure above atmospheric[b]		Sterilization hold time[c] (min)
	(p.s.i)	(bar)	
115–118	10	0.7	30
121–124	15	1.1	15
134–138	30	2.2	3

[a] Limit given for temperature that must be held throughout load for duration of sterilization hold time to ensure sterilization.

[b] Gauge pressure of pure dry saturated steam required to hold steam at sterilizing temperature given to nearest round figure. Precise relation between pressure and temperature and amounts of energy available as latent heat and sensible heat at each temperature are physical constants, given in tables of thermodynamic properties of fluids.

[c] Time for which sterilizing temperature must be held in all parts of load, shown by thermocouple placed in part of load least accessible to heat and steam penetration. If sterilization period is timed according to temperature of steam in chamber, indicated by thermometer in discharge line, an additional period of *heat penetration time* must be added (see text).

ideally should be determined for each type of load by tests with thermocouples recording the rise of temperature in the least accessible part of the load.

Condensation of steam. When the steam makes contact with the cooler articles in the autoclave it condenses into water on their surfaces and in their interstices. This condensation has three effects of critical importance for the sterilization process. (1) It wets the microorganisms on the articles and so provides this essential condition for their killing by moist heat. (2) It liberates the very large latent heat of steam and so rapidly heats up the articles to the sterilizing temperature. (3) It causes a great contraction in the volume of the steam and so promotes the ingress of fresh steam.

The latent heat liberated by steam as it condenses to water at the same temperature is very great. For example, the amount of the latent heat (h.fg) liberated by dry saturated steam condensing in a closed vessel at 136°C and 3.2 bar (abs) is nearly four times more than the amount of the sensible heat (h.f.) available in the same mass of boiling water at the same temperature and pressure. This latent heat is liberated directly on the surfaces of the articles in the autoclave.

As the steam condenses into water its contraction in volume is very great. Thus, 1670 volumes of steam at 1 bar pressure will contract to form only 1 volume of condensate. The negative pressure created by the contraction draws fresh steam on to the surface and into the interstices of the article. The cycle of condensation, liberation of latent heat and drawing in of fresh steam is then repeated until the article is heated up to the temperature of the steam.

Efficient condensation takes place only if the steam is on the boundary between the vapour and liquid phases. The steam must be both *saturated*, i.e. in free molecular balance with the water from which it is formed, *dry*, i.e. free from suspended droplets of condensed water, and *pure*, i.e. free from admixture with air or other non-condensable gas.

Steam supply. In the simple, pressure-cooker type of autoclave the steam is produced within the chamber by boiling a layer of water at its foot. In larger autoclaves the steam is supplied either from an external boiler attached to the machine or from the main steam supply of the building. In the latter cases, particular care must be taken to prevent the steam becoming either unsaturated due to superheating or wet due to condensation. Mains steam should be supplied to the autoclave at 3.5–4 bar pressure with a dryness fraction of 0.9.

Superheated steam. Steam above the phase boundary, i.e. at a temperature too high for its pressure, behaves as a dry gas. Being unsaturated it fails to condense on the articles of the load, so that the moisturizing and latent heat effects are lost. As, moreover, the temperature and pressure are no longer related, the former cannot be controlled by regulation of the latter. Superheating may be caused by overheating of the jacket of a jacketed autoclave or by too great a reduction of pressure as the steam enters the autoclave or by the processing of too dry a load of textiles, which will absorb an excessive amount of steam.

Wet steam. As latent heat is lost before sensible heat, steam is liable to become wet due to condensation, forming suspended droplets of water, if it is fed to the autoclave through a long, poorly insulated, poorly drained or low velocity supply line. Wet steam delays the removal of air from the autoclave chamber; it may produce wet loads and it provides less latent heat than dry steam. The moisture content of steam is expressed inversely as its *dryness fraction*, which in effect measures the proportion of latent heat still available in it. Steam with a high dryness fraction, over 0.95, may be provided by the use of steam separators or steam traps, or by effecting a large single-step reduction of pressure, as when mains steam at a pressure of about 4 bar is passed through a reducing valve and pressure regulator before entering the autoclave chamber at a pressure of 2.2 bar.

Air removal. Throughout the holding period of sterilization the autoclave must contain only pure steam free from admixture with residual air. Before that period, therefore, all air must be removed from the chamber and the interstices in the load. If an air-steam mixture is left, by Dalton's law the total pressure in the chamber, as shown on the pressure gauge, will consist of the sum of the pressure of the air and the pressure of the steam. Thus the steam's pressure will be less than the gauge pressure and the temperature will therefore be less than that expected from pure steam at gauge pressure. Moreover, bubbles of air trapped in the load will form an insulating layer over solid surfaces, inhibiting condensation and the transfer of heat.

In small simple, pressure-cooker type autoclaves the air is removed by allowing the free escape of steam with entrained air for a sufficient period before sealing the chamber to obtain increased pressure. In downward displacement autoclaves the steam is introduced at the top of the chamber through baffle plates designed to help it scavenge pockets of air in the load; the cooler and denser air-steam mixture and any condensate are discharged by gravity from the foot of the chamber through a near-to-steam trap which opens to let them escape but closes to retain the hotter pure steam. In porous load autoclaves the air may be extracted by an efficient oil-seal high vacuum pump or be diluted out by a succession of steam input pulses alternating with the drawing of a relative vacuum by a water-seal pump capable of handling steam and condensate.

Reasons for the presence of air in the chamber during the holding period include the allowance of insufficient time for steam penetration into and removal of air from the load, the occurrence of a leak in the chamber, and a contamination of the steam supply with air or other non-condensable gas. Leak tests should be made regularly and sophisticated autoclaves may be fitted with air detection devices to cancel any operation when air is present in sufficient quantity to impair sterilization.

Preparation of the load. The materials to be sterilized must be packaged in such a way as to allow the ingress of steam and the removal of air, yet protect them from contamination with bacteria from the environment after their removal from the autoclave. Culture media and liquid reagents are adequately protected in tubes, flasks and bottles closed with cotton-wool stoppers, loose slip-on metal caps or loosely applied screw caps. Instruments and textiles may be autoclaved in permeable wrappings of cloth, plastic or Kraft paper. Articles in *permeable* wrappings must be thoroughly dried before removal from the autoclave, for bacteria can readily pass through moist cloth or paper.

The autoclave should not be packed too fully, space should always be left between the articles or packages of the load to permit the free passage of steam between them. Downward displacement autoclaves must be loaded in such a way that the cooler air can gravitate downwards without encountering any physical barrier; thus packs should be placed vertically rather than horizontally and bowls should be placed on their edge. Wherever possible, avoid autoclaving single small packs in porous load autoclaves. The porous load should occupy more than 10% of the total available chamber space to avoid the possibility of all the residual air being driven into the centre of the single pack.

Fluids in sealed containers. There is one exception to the requirement of complete air discharge from the load. Small hermetically sealed bottles and ampoules of aqueous solutions and culture media can be satisfactorily sterilized in spite of the presence of some air within them. The contained water provides the conditions for moist-heat sterilization, making unnecessary the entry of steam for this purpose, and the contents are heated to the temperature of the chamber steam by the conduction of heat through their walls.

The pressure in the sealed containers is raised above that in the chamber and to avoid the risk of breakages the containers used must not be overfilled and should be strong. Screw-capped cylindrical bottles of from 5–50 ml capacity are relatively safe. Larger volumes (e.g. 500 ml DHSS DIN standard bottles) should be left overnight to cool in a locked chamber or should be left for the time required to cool below 80°C (i.e. about 5–8 h as previously determined by thermocouples placed in the load) or they should be processed in an autoclave fitted with a means of assisted cooling.

Wet loads. Articles in the load may be unduly wetted when the steam supply is wet, i.e. having a dryness fraction of less than 0.95 at the last pressure reducing valve. Even when the steam supply is dry, loads containing a high proportion of metal may become wet, as will loads packed in such a way that condensate can collect inside a metal article or drip from a metal article on to articles below. Drenching of cotton-wool stoppers in tubes or bottles may be minimized by covering them with stout glossy paper.

Drying the load. Even when not drenched with wet steam or excessive condensation, the articles of the load, e.g. packets of textiles, will be moist at the end of their exposure to steam under pressure. They tend to dry by evaporation when, after the holding period, the pressure of the steam is reduced and the autoclave opened. Drying may be promoted by the application of a vacuum before opening the autoclave, as by the use of a steam ejector working on the Venturi principle, a condenser or a vacuum pump.

When a vacuum has been used, air must be reintroduced into the chamber and this air should be passed through a filter which will hold back airborne bacteria that might be driven into and contaminate the load. As a damaged filter would permit airborne contamination, the filter should be inspected regularly and any reduction in the time taken for air re-entry noted.

Cooling aqueous media. The nutritive value of culture media is liable to be impaired if the period of cooling is unduly prolonged. Sugars such as glucose, maltose and lactose may be partially decomposed to form acids, peptones may be broken down, and agar, especially in acid media, may lose its ability to form a firm gel. Even media that are not particularly heat-labile, which can withstand sterilizing at 121°C for 15 min, may be damaged if the period of cooling to under 80°C is prolonged for up to an hour or more. Media should therefore be autoclaved for the minimum period sufficient for ster-

ilization and then be cooled as rapidly as possible. Bottles of media should be small enough for their whole contents to be used on one occasion, so that the need for re-sterilization or re-melting is avoided.

Cooling of small volumes of media in a small, simple unjacketed autoclave is generally rapid enough and does not require assistance, but cooling is liable to be too slow in large bottles of media (e.g. over 500 ml) and in large autoclaves, especially jacketed ones. The latter machines, therefore, should be equipped with a means of hastening the cooling process.

If assisted cooling is not available, it may be necessary to reduce the temperature or the holding period. With care, this may be done without failure to sterilize. Killing of microbes, like impairment of nutrient media, takes place to some degree at all temperatures above about 80°C, though more rapidly, in shorter periods, at the higher temperatures. The overall killing effect of an autoclaving cycle is thus the integration of the effects of the exposures at each temperature for each time interval during the heating-up, holding and cooling periods. When the cooling period is prolonged, therefore, the temperature or time of the holding period may be reduced without detriment. The exact temperature and time to be used for the holding period should be selected after careful trial of reduced values. Uninoculated samples of the media so processed should be incubated to check their sterility before the bulk is issued for routine use.

Simple laboratory autoclave

A small, simple portable autoclave operating like a domestic pressure cooker is convenient for the occasional sterilization of small volumes of aqueous media and small metal or glass instruments. The machine consists of an upright metal tank heated below by electricity or gas and having a lid with a gasket enabling it to be fitted hermetically. The lid bears a manually operated tap for the discharge of air and steam, a pressure gauge and a pressurestat. The last is a pressure-regulated (safety) valve that can be set to open when the pressure of the steam rises above that chosen for sterilization and to close when it falls below it; the pressure and temperature are thus automatically held at the required levels. Before the holding period, air is removed by turbulence and entraining in steam discharged freely through the manually opened valve, a process effective only if the chamber is relatively small. A thermal cut-out device should be fitted to shut off the source of heat in the event of the autoclave boiling dry.

Procedure. 1. Place sufficient water in the foot of the autoclave chamber.

2. Place the articles to be sterilized on a trivet or perforated tray just above the level of the water.

3. Screw down the lid to close the chamber hermetically. Open the manual discharge tap and turn on the source of heat.

4. When the water boils, allow steam and air to escape freely through the discharge tap for a period judged sufficient for the removal of all air; discharge for about 5 min should suffice.

5. Close the discharge tap and allow the pressure to rise until the required level is reached. At that point adjust the pressurestat so that it opens and closes as the pressure rises above and falls below that level. Usually pressure of 1.1 bar (gauge) (15 p.s.i.) and a temperature of 121°C are employed. Heat-labile media, such as malt tellurite agar, may not be able to withstand sterilizing temperatures and may require to be treated at lower temperatures, e.g. 10 min at 115°C. Media processed at lower times and temperatures may not be sterile and should always be tested before use.

6. Allow the autoclaving to continue at the chosen pressure and temperature for the appropriate period. The sterilization hold time (the combined holding and safety times) for sterilization at 121°C is 15 min (Medical Research Council 1959). The additional heat penetration time will vary with the nature of the load. For aqueous media it will be affected by the volume of medium, its viscosity, the size of the vessel, the thickness of its wall and, most importantly, the length of time that the load has taken to reach the sterilizing temperature. In a slowly heating autoclave the temperature of small volumes of fluid follows that of the chamber quite closely. In practice, therefore, a total sterilizing period (the sum of the heat penetration time and the sterilizing hold time) of 15 min is generally adequate for small bottles and tubes containing about 10 ml of medium, and one of 20 min for 500 ml, 25 min for 1000 ml and 30 min for 2000 ml of medium.

7. Turn off the heater and allow the autoclave to cool slowly in the room air until the gauge shows that the chamber is at atmospheric pressure. At exactly this point, open the discharge tap very slowly to allow air to enter the chamber as the cooling and collapse of the steam proceeds. Never open the tap while the chamber is above atmospheric pressure, for the sudden reduction of pressure will cause the medium in loosely stoppered containers to boil over. Do not delay opening the tap until the pressure has fallen much below atmospheric pressure, for an excessive amount of water will then be evaporated and lost from the media.

Even when the cooling period is properly managed and cooling is slow, about 5% of the water in loosely stoppered containers will be lost by evaporation. If the concentration of the medium is critical, 5% of extra water may be added to it before autoclaving. Water is not lost from media autoclaved in small, hermetically sealed containers.

8. When the autoclave is sufficiently cool, open the lid and remove the contents. Tighten the loosely applied screw caps on bottles when these are dry and cool enough to hold.

Larger simple autoclaves. Larger versions of these simple, pressure-cooker type autoclaves may still be found in some laboratories. They are often horizontal and have a door at one end (see Fig. 4.1, upper drawing). They are perfectly adequate for free steaming or medium-pressure autoclaving of aqueous media in loosely stoppered flasks.

The size of the chamber, however, e.g. 15–18 in diameter and 20–30 in long, is too large to permit the effective removal of air, so that working temperatures are not reached at the bottom of the chamber where the cooler air is

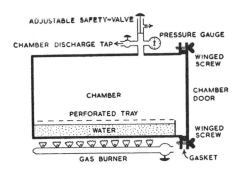

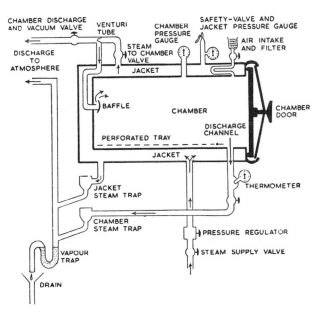

Fig. 4.1 Autoclaves. *Above*: Simple non-jacketed autoclave. *Below*: Steam-jacketed autoclave with automatic gravity discharge of air and condensate, and system for drying by vacuum and intake of filtered air.

Downward displacement laboratory autoclave

This more sophisticated type of autoclave has provision for efficient removal of air from the chamber and load, and may have other useful devices including ones to assist the drying of wrapped and porous loads, to prevent the door being opened while the chamber is under pressure, and for the automatic control of the process. The design of a jacketed machine is shown in the lower drawing in Figure 4.1.

Air removal. For the removal of air, pure steam at the sterilizing temperature, e.g. 121°C, is introduced from an external source into the upper part of the chamber. Percolating downwards through the load, it expels the cooler and therefore denser air and air-steam mixture out through a discharge channel at the foot. A thermostatic steam trap on this channel is set to open on the arrival of air, air-steam mixture or condensate at a temperature of 1°C or more below the sterilizing temperature and to close on the arrival of pure steam at the correct temperature. By repeatedly opening and closing, the trap automatically discharges each lot of air scavenged from the load and completes the removal of free air from the chamber in a heating-up and air displacement period of about 10 min.

A thermometer situated in the discharge line above the steam trap effectively indicates the temperature in the lowest and coolest part of the chamber and when this is shown to be the sterilizing temperature, e.g. 121°C, the free air has been removed from the chamber and the sterilizing period is timed to begin.

Sterilizing. For sterilization at 121°C the total sterilizing period consists of a sterilization hold time of 15 min and a heat penetration time that varies with the nature of the load. During the penetration time, further air is being displaced from the interior of the load and discharged through the steam trap, and the load itself is being heated up to the sterilizing temperature. Ideally the penetration time should be determined by thermocouple tests, but in practice a total sterilizing period of 20 min has been found to be adequate for paper wrapped articles and

layered. This failure goes undetected because the machines are not fitted with a thermometer in a gravity discharge drain. They should not be used for discard loads that must be sterile before disposal.

They are also unsuitable for wrapped articles, as air cannot be extracted from porous loads and there is no means of drying the load and its wrappings. Moreover they are not fitted with a means for assisted cooling and thus are not safe to use for fluids in sealed containers unless the load is left to cool overnight.

30 min for linen packages, and periods from 15–30 min for small to large volumes of aqueous media as described for the simple laboratory autoclave.

At the end of the sterilizing period the steam supply to the chamber is cut off and the chamber, with its load, begins to cool through its door and, if unjacketed, its walls. As the steam collapses by condensation in the chamber, outside air is drawn in to replace it. The incoming air is passed through a filter to exclude dust-borne bacteria and, often, a heating coil to warm it to nearer the chamber temperature.

Cooling of aqueous media. Media in flasks or bottles stoppered with cotton-wool or loosely capped may lose a considerable proportion of their water content either by evaporation, if the cooling period is prolonged, or by boiling, if the pressure is reduced too rapidly. Even when the cooling period is well managed the loss is likely to be about 5% and to compensate for this loss 5% excess water may be added to the media before autoclaving.

Media autoclaved in sealed bottles do not lose water and can be made up at the correct dilution. Sealing, however, increases the chance of breakage and even that of a dangerous explosion if bottles are exposed to thermal shock from a cold draught when the chamber door is opened or mechanical shock on removal from the auto-clave. Slowly cooling bottles may be at a considerable pressure, e.g. a correctly filled bottle at 115°C will have an internal pressure of 3.5 times atmospheric pressure. In the absence of assisted cooling, it may take 5–8 h before the *load* is cooled to 80°C and it is safe to open the autoclave door. If bottles are to be sealed, strong small bottles should be used and they must not be filled to more than 80% of their total capacity. It is important to note that the temperature in the chamber is no guide to the temperature and pressure within the bottle.

Prolonged cooling is a particular problem with this type of autoclave. The heated jacket or insulation necessary to prevent excessive conden-sation within the chamber and to assist in the drying of a porous load inevitably reduces the natural dissipation of heat at the conclusion of the sterilizing period. Cooling times are thus excessively prolonged, taking up to 3 h to cool to 100°C, so frequently having an adverse effect on the nutritive value of the culture medium. Well insulated, downward displacement auto-claves are, therefore, not suitable for processing heat-labile aqueous media unless fitted with a means of assisted cooling.

Drying porous loads. Drying is effected by vaporizing the condensate by means of a vacuum drawn by a Venturi steam injector or a condenser or both these in tandem. The process is assisted by the heated walls of the steam jacketed chamber and in some machines by admitting a continuous bleed of warm, filtered air into the chamber. Drying will probably take 20–30 min depending on the nature of the load.

Air removal from discard loads. Although the downward displacement autoclave will remove air from simple porous loads, it is not the most appropriate machine for sterilizing discarded microbiological materials such as cultures in tubes and Petri dishes, and containers with the residues of clinical specimens. It does not provide for the efficient removal of air trapped at the bottom of pails or bags used to collect the discarded material or from closed dishes, tubes and containers. A Venturi ejector or a condenser does not pull a sufficiently deep vacuum for this purpose. Thus, a survey made by the Public Health Laboratory Service (1978) showed that air removal was inadequate in 22 out of 62 auto-claving cycles tested. Some, but not all of these failures could be attributed to operational errors such as the use of over-large collection containers, sealed plastic bags impervious to steam or occlusion of the container opening.

While it can be argued that a sporicidal effect is not needed for the routine decontamination of discard loads in clinical laboratories (Editorial 1981), the Howie Code (1978) requires that, in Britain, microbiological discards must be placed in containers with solid bottoms and sides, that a temperature of 121°C must be achieved throughout the entire load and that thermo-couples must be used to ascertain the heat penetration time. When this is attempted with a downward displacement autoclave, a cycle of several hours duration may be required. Even in autoclaves of recent design, the mean load lag time, when operating by downward displacement only, was 42 min (Public Health Laboratory Service 1981).

If a multi-purpose laboratory autoclave is not available and a downward displacement autoclave has to be used for the disinfection of discard loads, care must be taken to facilitate the downward displacement of air from the container in which the discards are collected. If a stainless steel pail is used for collection, it should have about six holes 1 cm in diameter cut in a short row in its side about 3 cm from its bottom. To comply with the Howie Code's requirement that a solid-sided container must be used, the pail should be kept in an outer shallow solid box. Most of the air in the pail will be displaced downwards through the holes and any liquid or melted agar escaping from the discards will be retained in the bottom of the pail below the holes and so not escape into the autoclave discharge line.

Multi-purpose laboratory autoclave

Widely different types of load require to be sterilized in the laboratory, e.g. large volumes of aqueous media in hermetically sealed or loosely capped glass containers, heat-labile media that will tolerate only free steaming, clean glassware and other equipment for sterilizing before use, mixed loads of contaminated discard material, and fabrics such as laboratory coats. Different cycles of air removal, holding, cooling and drying are required for the different loads, and autoclaves are now being designed to allow the selection of any one of a number of such cycles, which are controlled automatically.

The essential special features of these autoclaves are the presence of efficient means of assisted air removal and assisted cooling. Safety features should also be included. Door interlocks should be provided to ensure that steam cannot enter the chamber until the door is locked and that the door will not open if the chamber gauge pressure exceeds 0.2 bar or until the chamber temperature has fallen below 80°C. The chamber should be permanently fitted with a temperature-sensitive probe so that the process is controllable by thermocouples reading directly from the load.

Aqueous media. For the sterilization of fluids and agar-containing culture media, the autoclave should be able to meet most of the requirements of British Standard 3970 Part 2. In particular, it should be fitted with a means of accelerated cooling, a control thermocouple and a door interlock that makes it impossible to open the door until the temperature of the *bottled fluid* has fallen below 80°C. Accelerated cooling is required not only to avoid the need to let the autoclave cool naturally overnight to a safe temperature, but also to avoid damage to the nutritive qualities of culture media, even those not particularly heat labile, which may be caused by their prolonged exposure to temperatures above 80°C. Cooling to below 80°C is required to minimize the risk of breakages and explosions when the autoclave is opened.

The bottles must be strong and DIN standard bottles should be used. The volumes of the contents should be kept as small as possible and should not exceed 500 ml for sealed bottles. They should also be small enough to allow the whole contents to be used on a single occasion, so that damage by repeated heating for re-sterilization or the re-melting of agar media can be avoided. The bottles are sealed with tightly applied screw-caps and washers. Larger bottles, closed with loosely applied caps or cotton-wool stoppers can be used, although these will allow some loss of water from the contents and will preclude accelerated cooling by spraying with condensate.

Bottles must not be overfilled, e.g. to over 80% capacity. The pressure inside a hermetically sealed bottle in the autoclave is the sum of the increased pressure of the heated air in the diminished volume above the heat-expanded liquid and the greater saturated vapour pressure of the heated water. At 121°C the air plus vapour pressure inside a bottle filled to 83% capacity is 4 bar absolute, i.e. 2 bar above the steam pressure in the chamber. If the bottle is filled to 90% capacity, the excess pressure will be greater than 11 bar. Serious overfilling, therefore, will result in an explosion.

Before loading into the autoclave, the bottles should be examined and defective ones rejected. The bottles should be placed in the autoclave in a regular and uncrowded pattern, with spaces between them, in conformity with the conditions determined during trials at the commissioning of the autoclave.

Air evacuation and pulsing are not required and the cycle commences with free steaming and downward displacement of air. The duration of the heating-up period should ideally be controlled automatically with a thermocouple placed in one of the largest bottles in the load or a simulator which reproduces the bottles' thermal characteristics. The thermocouple may be put into the drain of the autoclave, in which case it is necessary to allow an additional heat penetration time determined during commissioning with thermocouples placed in the coolest position in the load under the worst conditions of loading, e.g. in a large bottle on a crowded lower level.

After the heating-up period, the sterilizing temperature of 121–124°C is held for the sterilization hold time of 15 min. The steam input to both the chamber and jacket of the autoclave is then cut off and natural cooling commences.

Cooling of the load should be assisted so that the media are cooled to under 80°C within 30 min. The method used may be a spray of condensate continuously passed through a heat exchanger (this is the most effective method but precludes the use of unsealed containers), water cooling in the jacket of the autoclave, water cooling coils in the chamber, or the pumping of filtered air through the chamber. The duration of the cooling period should be controlled with a thermocouple placed in a simulator or a bottle in the slowest cooling part of the load. As the bottle containing the thermocouple may break and therefore show the temperature of the chamber rather than that of the hotter load, the duration of the cooling period should be checked to be about that expected before the door of the autoclave is opened.

If large sealed bottles of media, e.g. over 500 ml capacity, or fluids in plastic bags, are being processed, air ballasting with compressed air is recommended. The air is introduced into the chamber to increase the chamber pressure during the cooling period, thereby reducing the pressure differential between the bottles and the chamber.

However the cooling is managed, the still warm bottles should be handled with care. Gauntlet gloves should be worn and mechanical or thermal shock avoided; thus the bottles should not be laid forcefully on a hard, cold surface.

At the end of each cycle, the temperature record chart should be checked against the master record made on commissioning to ensure that the machine's performance has not deteriorated. Gauge readings should be observed weekly to check they are consistent with previous readings. Additional quarterly, yearly and commissioning tests, with thermocouples are described in the Department of Health and Social Security (1980a) Health Technical Memorandum No. 10, appendix 11, and should be complied with whenever possible.

Free steaming. The multi-purpose autoclave should be capable of giving a free-steaming cycle if a Koch or Arnold steamer is unavailable. A large drain may have to be fitted so that constriction of the profuse flow of steam does not unduly raise the pressure, and hence the temperature in the chamber. As the pressure is still likely to be a little above atmospheric, the temperature may be 1–2°C above 100°C and the period of steaming should be reduced from 90 min to about 60 min to prevent damage to the nutritive value of some media.

Glassware. Some manufacturers produce a special short cycle for the sterilization of clean dry glassware. In practice, clean bottles, lightly capped, can be processed satisfactorily as part of a fluid cycle, though steam penetration into and removal of air from the bottles may not be complete.

Discard loads. The principal difficulty to be overcome is that of removing air from the loosely closed culture plates, bottles and tubes and from the pail or bag in which they are collected. The air may be removed by (1) full-flow free steaming, (2) steam pulsing alternated with the drawing of a partial vacuum by a pump capable of handling both steam and condensate, or (3) the use of a steam lance coupled to a

Hansen valve manifold (Everall et al 1978). Free steaming is the least efficient method and must be prolonged, and steam lances, though effective, make handling problems for the operator. Steam pulsing is recommended. It gives the equivalent of a protracted porous load cycle and a small pre-vacuum may overcome the problem of air entrapment in polystyrene Petri dishes which melt at 60°C early in the process (Oates et al 1983).

Discard loads must not be packed in sealed, impervious plastic bags. Bags must be of pervious nylon or must be opened when placed in the autoclave to allow the replacement of air by steam. High-sided, solid-walled containers such as pails should be avoided because they tend to retain air at the bottom. Perforated, or mesh baskets should not be used, as they allow melted agar to escape into the autoclave's discharge line where it may solidify and cause a blockage. A container with a perforated base or a pail with holes low down in its side may be used, provided it is kept standing in a shallow solid box to catch any spills. It is convenient to use a stainless steel pail with 3–6 holes 1 cm in diameter closely spaced in a short row about 3 cm above its solid base; liquid and melted agar escaping from the discarded cultures is retained in the pail below the level of the holes.

Bottles containing more than 50 ml of fluid must not be processed in the ordinary discard cycle, for the door might be opened when the chamber temperature, but not that of the bottles, is below 80°C. Loose caps are not a safeguard as they may pull up and seal when exposed to the pressure differential between the bottle contents and the chamber. Discarded bottles with more than 50 ml of fluid should be processed separately by the cycle designed for aqueous media.

The time taken for the penetration of the load can be considerably prolonged depending on the nature of the materials and the volume of the discard load. The sterilization hold time is, therefore, set to commence automatically when a controlled thermocouple placed in the coolest part of the load reaches the pre-set temperature. Alternatively, the penetration time for the load can be calculated from extensive thermocouple

readings taken from all parts of the load at not more than monthly intervals (Howie 1978).

A sterilization hold time of $3\frac{1}{2}$ min at 134–138°C is normally employed. At the completion of the sterilizing period partial drying is achieved by evacuating the chamber to 60 m.bar (abs) and then immediately drawing atmospheric air into the chamber through a filter.

The temperature record chart must be checked before each discard load is released to ensure it conforms to the master temperature record. If a recording thermocouple is not fitted, Browne's tubes No. 1 (for 121°C) or No. 2 (for 134°C) should be placed in representative positions in each load, and heat-indicating autoclave indicator tape (3M; DRG) should be put across the mouth of each container. Absolute containment of effluent is unnecessary unless the laboratory is undertaking work with the most dangerous pathogens (Public Health Laboratory Service 1981).

Textile fabrics. The increased availability of disposable laboratory gowns which can be incinerated after use has diminished the need for a sterilizing cycle for such clothing except in laboratories doing much work with category 3 or 4 pathogens. For such textiles as require to be sterilized, a porous load cycle at 134–138°C is used. It may be the same as that used for discard loads except that the time taken for air removal and penetration of the load is not as long. Effective drying, in about 5 min, is achieved by holding the load in a high vacuum (60 m.bar, abs).

Standards. The autoclave should meet the requirements of British Standard 3970 Part 1, although an air detector is seldom fitted. Leak rate tests should be done weekly and the leak should not exceed 1.3 m.bar/min. The temperature recorder chart should be checked on every run to confirm that it conforms with the master temperature record produced on commissioning. Automatic controls should be checked by weekly observation of the gauge readings. Additional quarterly, half yearly and yearly tests with thermocouples are described in the Department of Health and Social Security (1980a) Health Technical Memorandum No. 10, appendix 7.

The advantages of the multi-purpose laboratory autoclave over the simple and downward displacement autoclaves are seen from a comparison of the engineering devices for assisted air removal, drying and cooling generally incorporated in the three types of machine (Table 4.2). Particular models may, however, have devices additional to, or different from those shown.

Table 4.2 Devices in laboratory autoclaves to assist air removal, drying, cooling and safe handling.

Purpose of device	Device present in autoclave of type		
	Simple	Downward displacement	Multi-purpose
Air removal from chamber and porous loads	None	Balanced pressure steam trap	Vacuum pulsing
Drying of wrapped and porous loads	None	Condenser or low vacuum Venturi	High vacuum pump
Air removal from solid-sided containers in discard loads	None	None	Vacuum pulsing
Cooling rapidly to preserve the nutrient quality of culture media	None	None	Condensate spray, or water-cooled jacket
Safe handling, e.g. of bottled fluids	None	Door interlock thermocouple in chamber	Door interlock thermocouple in load

Other autoclaves

High-security autoclave. Pathogenic microbes in the high-risk categories 3 and 4 are not particularly resistant to moist heat. The autoclaving cycles, therefore, are the same as in other laboratory autoclaves. The high-risk organisms, however, are often infective by the airborne route and the autoclaves used for sterilization of material that may contain them are modified in such a way as to contain or sterilize the effluent steam and condensate and the exhaust air.

Discards are placed in Portex nylon bags, which, unlike the usual autoclave bag, allow free penetration of steam and egress of air. The air discharge line leaves the chamber at a high enough level to ensure its freedom from condensate and is fitted with a steam sterilizable filter. The effluent contamination is kept to a minimum by ensuring the chamber is warm before the cycle is begun and that the infected material is contained in solid vessels. The condensate is retained and sterilized within the chamber (Scruton 1983).

Unwrapped instruments and utensils. Bowl and instrument sterilizers are commonly found in the hospital service, but not generally in microbiology laboratories. They operate at 134–138°C and the test criteria are purely physical. They must conform to British Standard 3970 Part 3 and are tested as described in the Department of Health and Social Security (1980a) Health Technical Memorandum No. 10, appendix 12.

Porous load sterilizer. These autoclaves are common in the hospital service, in surgical theatre sterile supply units (TSSU) and central sterile supply departments (CSSD). They are of two main types. The earlier machines have a high pre-vacuum cycle, while the later ones are multi-pulsing. They are unlikely to be found in microbiology laboratories, which are unlikely to be concerned with their routine testing, for the test criteria are purely physical. They operate at 134–138°C and conform to British Standard 3970 Part 1. They are tested as described in the Department of Health and Social Security (1980a) Health Technical Memorandum No. 10, appendix 7.

If biological tests are required, first ensure that the autoclave has passed all its physical checks, including a Bowie-Dick test (Bowie et al 1983), to prove that air removal is effective. Purchase (e.g. from Southern Group Labs) paper disks or strips containing at least 10^6 spores of *B. stearothermophilus* (NCTC10003, ATCC7953, CIP52.81) with a Z factor of 10–14. Place them in the centre of one or more packs in the coolest (lowest) part of the chamber. After autoclaving, transfer them with aseptic precautions into tryptone soy broth pH 7.3 (Oxoid, CM129) and incubate aerobically at 56°C for 5 days. At the same time, incubate a positive, unautoclaved control disk.

Autoclave tape (Bowie et al 1983) on the packs merely provides an indication that the process has been carried out, *not* that the contents are sterile.

Low temperature steam. Exposure to steam at a sub-atmospheric pressure giving a temperature of 73°C for a period of 10–20 min is a reliable and efficient means of disinfection, though not sterilization. The cycle consists of forced air removal by steam and vacuum pulsing followed by the admission of dry saturated steam at an absolute pressure of 263 mm Hg (35.06 kPa). The holding time is 10 min. The load is dried by reducing the chamber pressure to 50 mm Hg absolute (6.67 kPa) to vaporize the residual moisture and then admitting air through a bacterial filter. The machines must comply with British Standard 2970 Part 1 and the test must be carried out as described in the Department of Health and Social Security (1980a) Health Technical Memorandum No. 10. Particular attention should be paid to the air-tightness of the chamber and the steam penetration test.

LOW TEMPERATURE STEAM FORMALDEHYDE

Two processes are used for the sterilization of delicate, heat-labile equipment: (1) exposure to low temperature steam and formaldehyde (LTSF) and (2) exposure to ethylene oxide. Few microbiology laboratories are likely to be responsible for the operation of LTSF machines, but many may be involved in monitoring their efficacy by biological tests, for there are no satisfactory physical ones.

Steam at subatmospheric pressures and therefore at temperatures below 100°C kills the spores of thermophilic bacteria very slowly. Formaldehyde by itself is sporicidal, but only at high concentrations and in the presence of moisture. Together, formaldehyde and steam appear to be synergistic. Very low concentrations of formaldehyde gas in the presence of subatmospheric steam will almost invariably kill spores. The problem lies in bringing the two agents together under optimal conditions.

Saturated steam at an absolute pressure of 263 mm Hg (35.06 kPa) has a temperature of 73°C, which is accepted as standard for the process. The sensible heat of such steam is too low to provide much thermal energy and it is important that the steam be at phase boundary conditions to ensure the liberation of latent heat. The introduction of a large volume of formaldehyde gas wets the steam and causes loss of the latent heat effect (Weymes 1983).

Again, any lowering of the chamber temperature or condensation on cold spots reduces the concentration of monomeric formaldehyde, firstly by conversion to the inactive polymer and then by the formation of dissolved hydrate, which will not penetrate into porous loads or the interior of tubing. Condensation may be minimized by use of a fully jacketed autoclave (including a jacketed door) and heating the jacket slightly above the chamber temperature. Paraformaldehyde is also formed when the concentration of monomer is too high and there is little agreement about the best method of introducing formaldehyde gas into the chamber to minimize the loss. Various pulsing sequences are used and various timings of the delay between the vaporization of formaldehyde and the admission of steam.

Loading. Wash, dry and warm the articles to be sterilized. Do not dry in an oven at a temperature above 60°C. Wrap articles only with materials complying with the specification of the Department of Health and Social Security (1980b). Do not use metal containers. Load articles in the upright position to allow free drainage of condensate.

Sterilization cycle. The cycle varies from one manufacturer to another but generally consists of the following elements. (1) Air removal and steam flush, at an absolute pressure of about 50 mm Hg for about 20 min. (2) Formaldehyde injection, together with steam, in a series of pulses each of 5–10 min duration at an absolute pressure of 50–260 mm Hg. (3) A holding period at 71–75°C for a minimum of 1 h at an absolute pressure of about 263 mm Hg. (4) The formaldehyde is evacuated by a steam flush and an air flush each of about 15 min duration at an absolute pressure of 50–760 mm Hg.

Testing. Proceed to biological testing only if the machine has been commissioned in accordance with Department of Health and Social Security (1980a) Health Technical Memorandum No. 10 and complies with the physical criteria for low temperature disinfection. The test organism is *B. stearothermophilus* (NCTC10003). Paper strips should contain at least 10^6 spores. They must be stored at 4°C for no longer than 6 months before use (Line & Cutts 1982). Spore strips may be purchased from Southern Group Labs.

Place the spore strip in the chamber of a Line & Pickerill (1973) helix. Immediately after the exposure to steam-formaldehyde remove aseptically and immerse the strip in not less than 15 ml tryptone soy broth (Oxoid, CM129) which has been previously incubated to ensure its sterility. The broth should not contain added carbohydrate or a pH indicator dye. Incubate aerobically for 14 days at 56°C, shaking daily. Observe for the development of turbidity, indicating failure of sterilization.

Verify positive cultures by subculture on to nutrient agar plates incubated overnight at 56°C. The colonies should be grey, opaque and about 5 mm in diameter.

When commissioning, five unexposed spore strips and five tubes of media without spore strips are included as positive and negative controls in the test. The test is satisfactory if 10 challenges in a total of not less than 3 processing cycles are all apparently sterile after 14 days (Line & Pickerill 1973). The tests should be done in such a way as to ensure that there is uniformity of the sporicidal effect throughout the chamber; suspend 27 spore strips throughout the chamber in the pattern described in the Department of Health and Social Security (1980b) Health Equipment Information memorandum No. 88, item 95/80.

For routine use, make a single test in a Line & Pickerill helix during each sterilizing cycle, incubate for only 5 days and incorporate a positive control only for each new batch of strips.

Toxicity. Formaldehyde is toxic and irritates the eyes and respiratory tract at concentrations above 2 parts per million, and even at lower concentrations in sensitive individuals. It can also cause allergic dermatitis in man and is carcinogenic at irritant levels in rodents. The permitted peak level of formaldehyde in the environment is 2 p.p.m. (Health and Safety Executive Guidance Note E.H. 15/77, 1977) and there are many machines that fail to contain the environmental air contamination within this value.

Formaldehyde disinfector

Automatic formaldehyde disinfection machines incorporating a heated vaporizing system are rarely used in Britain. They will disinfect, but not sterilize clean exposed surfaces. They should be used only for delicate complex equipment that cannot be protected by filters, cannot stand heating at 73°C and cannot be sufficiently dismantled to allow thorough cleaning with an appropriate disinfectant. They may be unreliable, for in tests on one such device vegetative test bacteria were easily recovered from suction pumps exposed to the process (Babb et al 1982a). Small cabinets in which formaldehyde is generated by heating paraformaldehyde without strict control of temperature and humidity should not be used.

ETHYLENE OXIDE STERILIZER

Although these machines have no place in the diagnostic laboratory, they are used in the hospital service and microbiology staff take part in monitoring the efficacy of the process. Ethylene oxide is used to treat the very small proportion of medical and surgical articles that need to be sterile but cannot withstand even heating at 73°C. The gas is a highly lethal alkyl-ating agent and kills all microorganisms including viruses. Sensitivity to ethylene oxide does not correlate with that to heat, irradiation or other chemical disinfectants and is unaffected by the presence of endospores (Dadd & Daley 1980). Microbes are readily protected by dry proteinaceous material and vegetative bacteria dried in organic material may be more resistant than standard test spores.

Testing. Biological tests are required. The common test organism is *B. subtilis* var *globigii* var *niger* (NCTC10073, ATCC9372). It is easy to grow, its spores survive storage and its col-onies are readily distinguished by their orange pigment from post-sterilization contaminants. Test spores 3M 1222 may be obtained from 3M.

The spores are usually dried on paper or aluminium foil or are injected in aqueous suspension into the lumen of catheters or endo-scopes. Test pieces for determining gas penetration, such as that of Line & Pickerill, are not generally used, but a helix corresponding to a cardiac catheter has been proposed (Gillespie et al 1979). Positive control strips sealed into glass ampoules are included in the test run. Afterwards they are homogenized in broth, diluted and cultured to ensure that the recover-able viable challenge consisted of at least 10^6 spores.

The recovery of test spores is critically influ-enced by the medium, pH and temperature. Glucose tryptone broth or a defined amino acid mixture at pH 6.9 and incubation at 25°C are recommended. Cultures should be examined daily for 14 days for developing turbidity and any turbid cultures should be subcultured to confirm that the growth consists of the test organism. On completion of the test a proportion of the sterile cultures should be challenged by seeding with fresh spores to ensure that the recovery medium has not been made inhibitory by a carry-over of ethylene oxide.

B. stearothermophilus (NCTC10003, ATCC 7953) may also be used, but must be incubated at 56°C. Commercial test packs are available which utilize both types of spores and incor-porate a recovery medium and an indicator.

Hazards. Ethylene oxide is both toxic to man and highly explosive. It should be used only in purpose designed pressure vessels capable of withstanding an explosion; these are fitted with automatic controls and are filled either with 12% ethylene oxide in an inert carrier gas or with pure ethylene oxide supplied from a single-use cartridge; they are operated at subatmospheric pressure in a spark-free environment (Babb et al 1982b). The gas is mutagenic in a variety of animals. Its concentration in the environmental air must not exceed an average of 5 parts per million over an 8 h period, and exposure must be monitored by infra-red spectophotometry at not less than 6-monthly intervals (Department of Health and Social Security 1983). There is no place for 'home made' ethylene oxide cabinets in the laboratory.

STERILIZING FILTERS

Aqueous liquids, including solutions of heat-labile substances, may be sterilized by forced passage through a filter of porosity small enough to retain any microorganisms contained in them. Four main types of filter have been employed for bacteriological purposes, made from earthen-ware, asbestos, sintered glass and membranes of cellulose or other polymer. The first three types are usually adequate for retention of bacteria, but do not retain viruses. They have been almost entirely superseded by membrane filters. Filters not retaining viruses may be unsafe for steril-ization of biological preparations for clinical use.

Earthenware filters. Berkefeld filters are made from kieselguhr, a fossil diatomaceous earth. They can be sterilized by autoclaving and after use should be scrubbed with a stiff brush and boiled in distilled water. Chamberland filters are made of unglazed porcelain and are produced in various grades of porosity. The earthenware filters are made in the form of a hollow 'candle' and the fluid is forced by suction or pressure from the inside to the outside or vice versa. When they become clogged with organic matter they should be heated to redness in a furnace and allowed to cool slowly.

Asbestos filters. Seitz filters consist of a disk of an asbestos composition supported on a perforated metal disk within a metal funnel. The funnel is loosely assembled with the asbestos disk in position and sterilized in the autoclave. Before use, the disk is flushed with sterile saline and the upper part of the funnel is screwed down tightly on to the softened asbestos. After use, the disk is discarded.

Sintered glass filters. These are made from finely ground glass fused sufficiently to make the small particles adhere. They may be supplied in the form of a disk fused into a glass funnel. A special grade for sterilization is manufactured by supporting a specially fine filter on a stronger coarse one. After use they are washed with running water in the reverse direction and cleaned with warm, strong sulphuric acid.

Membrane filters. These membranes are manufactured from a variety of polymeric materials such as cellulose nitrate, cellulose diacetate, polycarbonate and polyester. Being less absorptive than other filters, they have a faster rate of filtration for any given porosity. They are manufactured as disks of from 13–293 mm diameter and with porosities from 0.015–12 μm. A filter is chosen for use that has a porosity fine enough to retain the expected microorganisms and a size and composition suitable for the required type and force of filtration and the volume to be filtered. They are sterilized by autoclaving.

The membranes are made in two main ways. (1) Capillary pore membranes have pores produced by radiation. This process gives a precise pore diameter and density and forms transparent membranes less than 10 μm thick with smooth surfaces and high tensile strength. They are suitable for filtration of viruses, solvents and samples for high pressure liquid chromatography. (2) Labyrinthine pore membranes are thicker, 100–200 μm in depth. They are produced by forced evaporation of solvents from cellulose esters. They are available in pore sizes above 0.1 μm, have a high porosity (about 75%) and give a large liquid throughput before clogging. They are recommended for disinfection of solutions by the removal of

bacteria and yeasts. The 0.22 μm pore size will retain *Pseudomonas diminuta*, the 0.45 μm filter will retain coliform bacilli in water microbiology and the 0.8 μm filter can be used to remove airborne microorganisms in 'sterile' rooms and produce bacteria-free gases.

Procedure. The exact procedure for use varies with the form in which the filter is supplied. Filters may be supplied in plastic holders, pre-sterilized for a single use and then disposal, or they may be mounted in re-usable holders and fitted to the filtration vessel, the whole assembly being autoclaved as a single unit, or the component units may be packed and autoclaved separately for later assembly under aseptic conditions. In the last case, the filter should be handled with flamed or pre-sterilized forceps in a laminar flow clean air cabinet. It is essential that the down-flow side of the filter and the delivery tube of the holder below it should not become contaminated. Generally the delivery tube is inserted through a rubber stopper into a sterile flask or other receptacle for the filtrate. Filtration is assisted by applying a partial vacuum to the receptacle through a side arm fitted with a cotton-wool stopper to prevent any back-flow and ingress of airborne contaminants.

Syringe filters. Membranes of 13 mm and 25 mm diameter are commonly fitted in syringe-like holders of stainless steel or polycarbonate. These can be used for the sterilization of small volumes of fluids, e.g. solutions of heat-labile sugars which are to be added to already sterilized medium held at 56°C. The fluid is forced through the filter by pressing down the piston. Side arms may be fitted to the syringe to enable it to be used in a continuous or serial flow system.

Vacuum and 'in line' filtration. Membranes of 25 and 45 mm diameter are used, either with 'in line' filter holders of Teflon or stainless steel and aluminium, or with vacuum holders of borosilicate glass, polycarbonate or stainless steel. They are suitable for the sterilization or disinfection of large volumes of liquid or air.

Pressure filtration. Large membranes, 100–293 mm in diameter, or filter cartridges housed in pressure filter holders may be used for the production of very pure water for laboratory use. They may be fitted with a Teflon filter so that the assembly is autoclavable with the filter in situ.

Air filters. Large volumes of air may be rapidly freed from infection by passage through HEPA filters (High Efficiency Particle Arresters). A principal use of such filtration in the laboratory is to render safe the air withdrawn from an exhaust-ventilated safety cabinet used for work with dangerous pathogens. Another use is to decontaminate the air input into a laminar flow cabinet used for work, such as plate pouring, that needs to be protected from airborne contamination.

Most safety cabinets are fitted with a disposable pre-filter which reduces the load collected by the main filter and so extends its effective life. The pre-filter should be readily accessible to permit easy changing. It should be tested by the manufacturer in accordance with British Standard 2831 and should be certified as having a gravimetric efficiency of 95% against test dust No. 2.

The main HEPA filter should have an efficiency of 99.997% when tested with hot generated dioctylphthalate chemical smoke or sodium chloride smoke generated in accordance with British Standard 3928 at the filter manufacturer's designed volumetric rate. To measure the penetration of the filter, a sampling point should be provided in the exhaust duct above the filter. The filter must be placed in such a way that contaminated air cannot leak past it; thus, the filter housing should be free standing and not mounted within the wall of the exhaust duct (British Standards Institution 1979).

STERILIZATION BY RADIATION

Ionizing radiation. Gamma radiation emitted from a radioactive element, usually ^{60}Co, provides a reliable means of sterilizing plastic and other materials that would be damaged by heat. It is widely used on a commercial basis for the sterilization of packaged disposable articles such as syringes, but the great cost of the instal-

lation and the need for skilled control makes the method unsuitable for use in the clinical laboratory.

Ultra-violet radiation. Mercury vapour lamps emitting most of their radiation in the region of 250–260 nm are bactericidal and to a lesser extent sporicidal. But the energy levels of the ultra-violet radiation are low and its penetration power poor. These lamps should, therefore, be used only for the disinfection of clean surfaces such as the interior of safety cabinets after cleaning with the appropriate disinfectant. The ultra-violet source must be shielded in such a way as to prevent the radiation falling on the eyes and skin, which it will damage, and must not be left on in a safety cabinet while the cabinet is in use. The lamps have a limited working life and are seriously affected by dirt and dust. The proportion of bactericidal radiation can fall off to insignificant levels without a reduction in the emission of visible light. Although ultra-violet radiation may have value in an ancillary role, by itself it should never be relied on for disinfection.

DISINFECTANTS

The European Committee for the Standardization of Disinfectants defined disinfection as the selective elimination of certain undesirable organisms in order to prevent their transmission, achieved by action on their structure or metabolism, irrespective of their functional state (Reber 1973). Disinfectants kill vegetative bacteria, fungi, viruses and occasionally spores by the destruction of proteins, lipids or nucleic acids in the cell or its cytoplasmic membrane.

General rules for use of disinfectants

1. Unlike chemotherapeutic agents, which selectively attack the microorganisms, disinfectants are more generally toxic and may damage or irritate the skin, conjunctiva and mucosae. Care must be taken to avoid contact with irritant or toxic concentrations and disposable gloves should be worn when handling them (Howie 1978).

2. A disinfectant may have a narrow spectrum of activity against different kinds of micro-organisms. Gram-positive bacteria are most easily killed by many disinfectants, Gram-negative bacteria, especially pseudomonas species, are more resistant, and acid-fast bacteria more resistant still. Activity against viruses and spores may be uncertain or absent. It is necessary, therefore, to choose a disinfectant that is suitable for the purpose required and each laboratory should have a written disinfectant policy specifying the kind and concentration of disinfectant for each type of use.

3. Disinfectants must always be used at the correct concentration. Too little is ineffective and too much may be irritant to the skin. The 'use dilution' may be suggested by the manufacturer on the basis of a Kelsey-Sykes (Kelsey & Sykes 1969) capacity test, but the responsibility for ensuring efficacy rests with the user.

4. The life of a disinfectant varies with its formulation and many disinfectants deteriorate when diluted with water. Disinfectants also deteriorate during use due to their inactivation by the microbes and other organic material to which they are applied. Working solutions should therefore be renewed each day (Department of Health and Social Security 1981).

5. Disinfectants may not kill even susceptible bacteria if these are present in very large numbers or if the disinfectant has been inactivated by excess organic matter or if it is not brought into contact with all the contaminated surfaces. Disinfectant solutions must not be overloaded with bacteria or organic materials such as culture media. All articles to be disinfected must be properly immersed in the disinfectant.

6. Disinfectants take time to act. The time for effective disinfection will vary with the microbial load, the presence of organic material, the temperature, the pH, the nature of the exposed surfaces and the presence of resistant bacteria or spores. Overnight exposure at room temperature, provided fresh contaminated material is not added, is generally considered to be adequate for most purposes.

7. Certain disinfectants are easily inactivated by changes in pH, by the presence of soaps or detergents of opposite polarity, or by the presence of cork, cellulose, cotton, rubber and other discard materials. Disinfectants therefore should not be mixed with other disinfectants or cleaning solutions, and current laboratory procedures should be monitored by regular 'in-use' tests.

Testing disinfectants

Microbiology laboratories may be asked to test the efficacy of disinfectants used in the hospital service, e.g. to determine their Rideal-Walker or Chick-Martin coefficient. These tests compare the disinfectant with phenol for the ability to kill *Salmonella typhi*, but are seldom relevant to the requirements of disinfection in hospitals. The test organism is inappropriate and the test irreproducible. Phenol coefficients are appropriate only for phenolic disinfectants. The Rideal-Walker test, moreover, does not represent a realistic challenge with organic material.

Tests for the minimum inhibitory concentration (MIC) of the disinfectant are equally irrelevant as the number of organisms exposed to the disinfectant is too low and the time of exposure too long. MIC tests are usually done at the unrealistically high temperature of 37°C and without the presence of sufficient organic material.

The choice of a disinfectant should depend on the results of the Kelsey & Sykes (1969) capacity test and the Maurer (1969) stability test. These tests are best carried out in specialist laboratories and, in Britain, advice is available from the Division of Hospital Infection of the Public Health Laboratory Service, Colindale, London. Hospital laboratories should perform only 'in-use' tests to confirm that the chosen disinfectant is effective under the conditions and for the period of its use. This test, for example, should be performed on the diluted disinfectant in a discard jar at the end of the period in which used pipettes, instruments or other material have been added and left overnight.

The in-use test. 1. With a sterile pipette transfer 1 ml of the already used disinfectant into

9 ml nutrient broth in a sterile Universal container.

2. Then at once, with a 0.02 ml pipette place ten 0.02 ml drops of this mixture on to different areas of each of two well-dried nutrient agar plates.

3. Incubate one plate for 3 days at 37°C and the other for 7 days at room temperature.

4. Read the test as showing failure of disinfection if there is growth in more than five drops on either plate.

Any carry-over of a phenolic or hypochlorite disinfectant is neutralized by the dilution in the broth and agar, but an inactivator may have to be used in tests of other kinds of disinfectant. The efficacy of the inactivator must then be checked as described in British Standard 3286 (Maurer 1974).

Disinfection of surfaces

Freshly made up solutions of disinfectant at the appropriate strength should be available on every microbiology work bench, most conveniently in a wash bottle of non-inhibitory plastic. Benches should have an impervious surface that is resistant to damage by disinfectants (well oiled teak is acceptable) and must be cleaned with disinfectant at the end of each working session, even if protected by a disposable covering, e.g. of Benchcote.

Liquid spillages should be immediately treated by the addition of a nearly equal volume of disinfectant. Damaged or broken culture plates should be covered with a cloth soaked in disinfectant for at least 10 min before being swept into an infected waste container with the help of disposable gloves, cloths, paper towels or strong card. If a dust-pan and brush are used for the latter purpose, they must then be autoclaved. If the spillage is very large, a germicidal powder such as Precept Granules (Surgikos) may be used. The eyes, skin and respiratory tract may require to be protected against any excess of liberated chlorine.

Phenolics. Clear soluble phenolic disinfectants such as Clearsol, Hycolin or Stericol are resistant to inactivation by organic matter and are active against a wide range of Gram-positive and Gram-negative bacteria. They are reasonably effective against mycobacteria, but have little activity against endospores, viruses or hepatitis B virus. Their activity is reduced at alkaline pH. Chloroxylenol products are not recommended as they are liable to be inactivated, even by hard water, and when diluted support the growth of pseudomonas. 'White fluids', such as Lysol, are effective but are pungent and irritant to the skin. For use in general bacteriology where organic material is present, and for tuberculous material, the effective concentration for spillage or cleaning is usually 2%.

Hypochlorites. Hypochlorite products, such as Chloros, Domestos, Diversol BX, Sterite and Milton, are readily inactivated by organic material and cationic detergents. They are corrosive to metals and textiles and have poor wetting properties. Buffered solutions at pH 7.5 are said to be less corrosive, but metal surfaces should not be exposed to them for any length of time and hypochlorites should not be used for machinery. They should not be mixed with acids, for they then may give off toxic amounts of chlorine gas.

They are very active against Gram-positive and Gram-negative bacteria and viruses, but somewhat less active against mycobacteria. Buffered hypochlorites are often sporicidal (Death et al 1982). For use in virology and for spilled blood, the effective concentrations are those containing 10 000 parts per million of available chlorine for spillages and 1000 p.p.m. for cleaning.

Glutaraldehyde. Alkaline, acid and non-activated preparations of glutaraldehyde include Asep, Cidex, Clinicide, 3M, Totacide and Triocide. They are usually supplied at the working concentration of 2%. Their ability to penetrate organic material is poor and their use should be restricted to relatively unsoiled surfaces. Glutaraldehyde is less corrosive than hypochlorite and therefore can be used to disinfect centrifuges when virus contamination is likely. Many preparations contain corrosion inhibitors and surfactants and may remain stable for up to 28 days after activation, but the duration of stability should be confirmed in the user's laboratory.

Glutaraldehyde is rapidly bactericidal and virucidal and is effective against mycobacteria and, to a lesser extent, spores, although the killing of spores may require their exposure for at least 3 h. Glutaraldehyde 2% is recommended for defined purposes in virology and immunology, including the decontamination of centrifuges and automated equipment that can resist being damaged by it (Newsom & Matthews 1980).

Ethyl alcohol. Ethanol 70% (v/v) in water is highly active against Gram-positive and Gram-negative bacteria and acid-fast bacilli, but inactive against spores. It is only slightly susceptible to inactivation by organic matter, but has poor powers of penetration and must not be used on heavily soiled surfaces. It can be conveniently removed from disinfected articles by flaming, but the temperature reached on the surface of the article during such flaming is not high enough for sterilization. Ethanol should be used only on perfectly clean surfaces, e.g. glass slides and the tops of culture bottles, for the removal of transient bacteria.

Other disinfectants. Pine fluids, quaternary ammonium compounds, ampholytes and bisguanides are unsuitable for laboratory use as they are inactive against mycobacteria, spores and non-enveloped viruses, and are seriously inactivated by hard water, organic materials and other substances (Maurer 1974; Hoffman 1981).

Discard jars

Large jars containing a suitable disinfectant at the correct concentration should be placed at each work station to receive discarded pipettes, culture tubes and other contaminated materials. The disinfectant should be changed daily and regular in-use testing should be done.

The jars should be filled with a measured volume of water, either tap water or, if the tap water is hard and liable to inactivate the disinfectant, de-ionized water. The jar may be marked with a line on the outside to show the level to which it should be filled. A measured volume of concentrated disinfectant is then added to the jar; this may be done from a small beaker marked at the correct level and kept solely for the purpose. For general bacteriology, where organic matter or tubercle bacilli may be present, a phenolic disinfectant, e.g Hycolin, at a concentration of 2% in water is generally effective. For virology and material soiled with virus-containing blood, a hypochlorite solution containing 2500 parts per million of available chlorine is recommended.

While in use, the discard jars must not be overfilled. All articles must be completely immersed and must not contain bubbles of air. Reusable pipettes must be left overnight without the addition of fresh material to the jar. The jars should be emptied down the discard sink via a sieve. The solid material retained in the sieve should then be placed in an infected waste container for autoclaving or disposal by supervised incineration. The jars should then be thoroughly rinsed and cleaned before refilling with fresh disinfectant.

Disinfection of safety cabinets

Exhaust protective cabinets should be washed down with an appropriate disinfectant after each day's use. Disposable gloves should be worn when doing so. Further decontamination with formaldehyde vapour should be performed once a week. β-propiolactone should not be used, for it is very hazardous, rapidly lethal and probably carcinogenic. Nor should ethylene oxide, which is explosive, acutely toxic and mutagenic.

Formaldehyde disinfection. Place 25 ml of Formaldehyde solution BP (40% formaldehyde) in an electrically heated dish inside the cabinet or in an approved vaporizer built into the cabinet by the manufacturer. Replace the front closure of the cabinet and, if necessary, seal with adhesive tape. Switch on the heater to vaporize the formaldehyde. Leave the closed cabinet filled with the vapour overnight.

Next day switch on the extract fan of the cabinet to remove the formaldehyde vapour and expel it through the HEPA filter into the exhaust duct. After a few minutes open the front closure about 1 cm to increase the airflow. When all the formaldehyde vapour has been extracted, remove the front closure and check the rate of airflow before re-using the cabinet.

If any maintenance work requires to be done on the cabinet, e.g. the cleaning of grids or the changing of filters, it must be done only after formaldehyde disinfection has been carried out and protective gloves and clothing must be worn.

Only in an emergency, if electrical vaporization cannot be used, decontamination can be done by adding 10 g potassium permanganate to 35 ml of 40% formaldehyde solution in a 500 ml beaker placed in the cabinet. This procedure liberates formaldehyde vapour, but it is hazardous. The mixture boils within seconds and there is a risk of explosion if the potassium permanganate is at any time present in excess in relation to the formaldehyde.

Disinfection of rooms

Although only required in exceptional circumstances, the disinfection of a laboratory room may be done with formaldehyde vapour. The efficacy of the process is, however, uncertain, especially at temperatures below 20°C and relative humidities below 70%. Penetration into porous fabrics is slow and every effort must be made to clean and disinfect individually all accessible surfaces. The vapour does not injure wood, rubber, paint, metals or textiles nor damage delicate articles such as cameras, microscopes, electronic controls and SMAC cartridges (Death et al 1982).

Procedure. 1. Before fumigation, seal the room with adhesive tape applied round the edges of doors and windows and over ventilator apertures, etc. to prevent leaks into adjacent rooms, the roof space or out-doors.

2. For each 1000 cubic feet of space (28.3 m³) place 500 ml formaldehyde 40% solution and 1000 ml water in an electric boiler with a safety cut-out when boiling dry and a time switch. Set the latter to open just before the evaporation is completed. Switch on the boiler, leave the room and seal the door.

3. Leave the room filled with formaldehyde and sealed for 24 h.

4. Then open the door and enter the room wearing respiratory protective equipment. Open the windows to allow the vapour to disperse and neutralize any residual formaldehyde with ammonia by exposing 250 ml of SG 880 ammonia per litre of formalin used (Scottish Home and Health Department 1976).

Spraying formaldehyde solution. Spraying a 40% solution is not a satisfactory substitute for vaporization of formaldehyde by boiling as the fine aerosol has poor penetrative power. When decontamination by spraying is attempted, a respirator must be worn and it is necessary to drench all the surfaces of the room and its furniture with a 5% solution of formaldehyde in water.

Disinfection of skin

Laboratory staff must wash their hands thoroughly whenever they become soiled during work or accidentally contaminated with a culture or a leaking specimen. They should also wash their hands at the end of each work period and after removing protective gloves or clothing. They should dry their hands under a hot-air drier or with a disposable paper towel which is discarded into a plastic bag for autoclaving or incineration.

Washing with soap and water removes most of the transient surface contaminants and some of the resident skin commensal bacteria, but because some of the contaminants may remain (Lowbury et al 1981; Pether & Scott 1982), a chlorhexidine or iodine detergent scrub should be used if the hands are likely to have become contaminated with pathogens. These scrubs are 20–30 times more effective than a wash with soap and water (Lowbury & Lilly 1973).

As an alternative or additional precaution the hands may be rubbed with a solution of 0.5%

chlorhexidine and 1% glycerol in 70% isopropyl alcohol (e.g. Phisohex). A small amount, e.g. 5 ml, is rubbed over all parts of the hands and fingers and allowed to dry in (Lowbury & Lilly 1975).

If as result of a laboratory accident the skin is broken, the wound should be cleaned and irrigated with a mild disinfectant such as chlorhexidine with cetrimide (e.g. Savlon). If the unbroken skin is grossly contaminated with bacterial or viral pathogens, it should at once be rinsed with the phenolic or hypochlorite disinfectant available for normal use on the bench, e.g. 2% Hycolin, and then immediately be washed with water.

The commensal bacteria that live in the skin glands and follicles are difficult to reach and kill, and powerful, penetrative disinfectants are required if there is a need to reduce their numbers to a very low level, as in an area through which a specimen of blood is to be collected for culture (see Ch. 7 for methods).

REFERENCES

Ayliffe G A J, Collins B J, Deverill C E A 1974 Tests of disinfection by heat in a bedpan washing machine. Journal of Clinical Pathology 27: 760–763

Babb J R, Bradley C R, Ayliffe G A J 1982a A formaldehyde disinfection unit. Journal of Hospital Infection 3: 193–197

Babb J R, Phelps M, Downes J, Ayliffe G A J 1982b Evaluation of an ethylene oxide steriliser. Journal of Hospital Infection 3: 385–394

Bowie J H, Kelsey J C, Thompson G R 1983 The Bowie and Dick autoclave tape test. Lancet 1: 586–587

British Standards Institution 1979 Methods of test for air filters used in air conditioning and general ventilation, BS 2831. Performance of electrically heated sterilizing ovens, BS 3421. Sterilizers for porous loads, Part 1, BS 3970. Sterilizers for bottled fluids, Part 2, BS 3970. Sterilizers for unwrapped instruments and utensils, Part 3, BS 3970. Method for sodium flame test for air filters, BS 3928. Specification for microbiological safety cabinets, BS 5726,9.1. BSI Publications Manager, 101 Pentonville Road, London Nl 9ND

Dadd A H, Daley G M 1980 Resistance of microorganisms to inactivation by gaseous ethylene oxide. Journal of Applied Bacteriology 49: 89–101

Death J E, Coates D 1979 Effect of pH on sporicidal and microbicidal activity of buffered mixtures of alcohol and sodium hypochlorite. Journal of Clinical Pathology 32: 148–153

Death J E, Hallin B E, Harper G J 1982 Decontamination of automated laboratory equipment. Journal of Clinical Pathology 35: 580–581

Department of Health and Social Security 1980a Health Technical Memorandum No. 10. Sterilizers. Her Majesty's Stationery Office, London

Department of Health and Social Security 1980b Health Equipment Information No. 88. Departmental advice on some aspects of disinfection and sterilization. Her Majesty's Stationery Office, London

Department of Health and Social Security 1981 Interim Advisory Committee on Safety in Clinical Laboratories, Bulletin No. 2. DHSS, London

Department of Health and Social Security 1983 Ethylene oxide sterilizers: risk of environmental contamination. Safety Information Bulletin SIB (8) 2. DHSS, London

Editorial 1981 Sterilization. Journal of Hospital Infection 2: 289–290

European Pharmacopoeia Commission 1983 Biological indicators for the verification of sterilization procedures. 6th Fascicule IX, 1.1. Strasbourg

Everall P H, Morris C A, Yarnall R 1978 Sterilization in the laboratory autoclave using direct air displacement by steam. Journal of Clinical Pathology 31: 144–147

Gillespie E H, Jackson J M, Owen G R 1979 Ethylene oxide sterilization – is it safe? Journal of Clinical Pathology 32: 1184–1187

Health and Safety Executive 1977 Guidance Note EH. 15/77. Threshold limit values for 1977. Her Majesty's Stationery Office, London

Hoffman P N 1981 Disinfectant-impregnated cloths in hospital laboratories. Journal of Hospital Infection 2: 391–392

Howie J H 1978 Code of practice for the prevention of infection in clinical laboratories and post-mortem rooms. Department of Health and Social Security Memorandum. Her Majesty's Stationery Office, London

Kelsey J C 1972 The myth of surgical sterility. Lancet 2: 1301–1303

Kelsey J C, Sykes G 1969 A new test for the assessment of disinfectants with particular reference to their use in hospitals. Pharmaceutical Journal 202: 607–609

Line S J, Cutts D W 1982 Notes on low temperature steam and formaldehyde. Sterile World, June p 3–4

Line S J, Pickerill J K 1973 Testing a steam-formaldehyde sterilizer for gas penetration efficiency. Journal of Clinical Pathology 26: 716–720

Lowbury E J L, Ayliffe G A J, Geddes A M, Williams J D 1981 Control of hospital infection. Chapman and Hall, London. p 72

Lowbury E J L, Lilly H A 1973 Use of 4% chlorhexidine detergent solution (Hibiscrub) and other methods of skin disinfection. British Medical Journal 1: 510–515

Lowbury E J L, Lilly H A 1975 Gloved hand as an applicator of antiseptic to operation sites. Lancet 2: 153–156

Maurer I M 1969 A test for stability and long term effectiveness in disinfectants. Pharmaceutical Journal 203: 529–534

Maurer I M 1974 Hospital hygiene. Arnold, London. p 82–83

Medical Research Council 1959 Sterilization by steam under increased pressure. Lancet 1: 425–435

Medical Research Council 1962 The sterilization, use and

care of syringes. Medical Research Council
Memorandum No. 41. MRC, London
Newsom S W B, Matthews J 1980 A microbiological
survey of automated biochemical machines. Journal of
Clinical Pathology 33: 566–570
Nyström B 1981 Disinfection of surgical instruments.
Journal of Hospital Infection 4: 363–368
Oates K, Deverill C E A, Phelps M, Collins B J 1983
Development of a laboratory autoclave system. Journal
of Hospital Infection 4: 181–190
Pether J V S, Scott R J D 1982 Salmonella carriers; are
they dangerous? Journal of Infection 5: 81–88
Public Health Laboratory Service Subcommittee on
Laboratory Autoclaves 1978 Autoclaving practice in
microbiology laboratories: report of a survey. Journal of
Clinical Pathology 32: 418–422

Public Health Laboratory Service Subcommittee on
Laboratory Autoclaves 1981 Specifications for laboratory
autoclaves. Journal of Hospital Infection 2: 377–384
Reber H 1973 Disinfection: proposal for definition. Second
International Colloquium about the evaluation of
disinfectants in Europe. Zentrablatt für Bakteriologie
157: 7–38
Scottish Home and Health Department 1976 Memorandum
on the control of outbreaks of smallpox, appendix VI.
Her Majesty's Stationery Office, Edinburgh
Scruton M W 1983 Laboratory autoclaves and the safe
handling of microorganisms. Journal of Sterile Services
Management 3: 8–9
Weymes C 1983 Factors influencing the design of LTSF
machines. Sterile World. October p 5–6

pH measurements and buffers, oxidation-reduction potentials, suspension fluids and preparation of glassware

pH IN MICROBIOLOGY

Microorganisms, in common with other living organisms, are very susceptible to changes in the acidity or alkalinity of the surrounding medium. This is important for their growth and for their survival. Whilst many bacteria show vigorous growth within a fairly wide range of acidity or alkalinity, there are others that require this to be adjusted within narrow limits before multiplication takes place. Moreover, all microorganisms have a particular alkaline or acidic or neutral reaction at which growth is optimal.

It is convenient to express acidity and alkalinity in terms of molar hydrogen-ion concentration $[H^+]$. For reasons of practical convenience, $[H^+]$ is usually expressed on a logarithmic or pH scale.

The pH value of a liquid is defined as the logarithm of the reciprocal of the hydrogen ion concentration, i.e.

$$pH = \log \frac{1}{[H^+]}$$

For neutral water, $pH = \log \frac{1}{10^7} = 7$

Two points should be borne in mind about the pH scale.

1. Since it is a *logarithmic* scale, a change of one unit of pH is equivalent to a 10-fold change in hydrogen-ion concentration, that is a 10-fold change in acidity; thus a liquid of pH 5.0 is 10 times more acid than one at pH 6.0, while a liquid of pH 9.0 is 10 times more alkaline than one of pH 8.0. For this reason, the degree of

accuracy required in microbiology makes it necessary always to give values correct to the first decimal place, e.g. 7.0, 7.1 or 7.2.

2. Since it is a *reciprocal* scale, the lower the pH, the greater will be the acidity. A pH value of less than 7.0 indicates an acid solution and greater than 7.0 indicates an alkaline solution. For example, 1 mol/litre HCl has an approximate pH value of 0; 0.1 mol/litre HCl has an approximate pH value of 1; 0.01 mol/litre HCl has an approximate pH value of 2.

Microorganisms are sensitive in varying degrees to the pH of the external environment. Although this is important for survival, it is even more important for growth, where there is an optimum, a maximum and a minimum pH. Media should be adjusted as far as possible to the pH optimal for the growth of the organism concerned. Most pathogenic bacteria have a fairly restricted pH range and grow best around pH 7.3, i.e. at a slightly alkaline reaction. This may be a reflection of the fact that the pH of mammalian blood and tissues is of this order. For example, *Streptococcus pneumoniae* has an optimum pH of 7.8, and a growth range between pH 6.5–8.3. On the other hand, commensal and saprophytic bacteria often have a wider pH growth range. *Escherichia coli* has an optimum pH of 6.5, and a growth range between pH 4.4–7.8. Yeasts and fungi generally have an acid optimum. Not only should growth media be adjusted to the optimum pH, but all suspending fluids should be at a reaction giving the largest survival time (usually of the same order as the optimum pH).

Two types of method are generally employed

for the measurement of pH in the laboratory. These depend either upon the use of electric pH meters or upon pH indicator dyes.

The pH meter

The only accurate method of measuring pH is with a pH meter, and in laboratories where numerous determinations of pH are required, this apparatus is a necessary piece of equipment. It is easy and quick to use although care must be taken in its maintenance.

A pH meter consists of a pair of electrodes or, more commonly now, a single combination electrode which is sensitive to hydrogen-ion concentration and an electrical circuit which measures the e.m.f. developed across the electrode pair. Basic design is similar for most modern combination electrodes. The size and shape varies considerably depending on their intended use. Most have a sheathed glass electrode to prevent breakage. The electrolyte (KCl) in the reference compartment of the electrode is sometimes in a gel, or is sealed to make refilling unnecessary. Flat surface electrodes are useful for measuring the pH of gel surfaces, skin, etc. Detailed descriptions of the theory of pH measurement can be found in appropriate textbooks. Instructions for use of pH meters and electrodes are given in the manuals and pamphlets supplied by the manufacturers.

Methods depending upon the use of pH indicator dyes

Indicator dyes are substances that will change in colour with variations in the pH of the solution in which they are dissolved. For example, phenol sulphone-phthalein (phenol red) is yellow in acid solution and red in alkaline solution. If alkali is gradually added to an acid solution containing phenol red, the change in colour will commence at pH 6.8, the yellow becoming redder until the final red is reached at pH 8.4; thus the 'range' of the indicator is pH 6.8–8.4. Within this range, phenol red has different colours for different pH values and this can be used to determine pH. The range of phenol red is particularly suitable for the adjustment of the pH of bacterial culture media. It must be emphasized that outside the range at which the colour is changing, an indicator can show only whether the solution is more acid or more alkaline than the indicator range. For example, phenol red is yellow at all pH values below 6.8 and is red at all values above 8.4. However, other dyes have their own different ranges in which colour change occurs, and there is now available a series of indicators which will cover the range from pH 1–11. Examples are shown in Table 5.1.

The simplest method of determining the pH of a solution is to use commercially available pH indicator papers. These papers are impregnated with an indicator that gives a change of colour over a specific or general range of pH. The paper can simply be dipped in the solution to be tested or, alternatively, a drop of the solution can be withdrawn by a wire loop or Pasteur pipette and placed on the paper. The resulting colour is compared with the chart supplied with the papers. Sets of wide range and narrow range pH papers are available from several suppliers, e.g. Whatman, BDH. It must be emphasized, however, that these test-papers will give at best

Table 5.1 pH indicators.

Indicator	Range of pH	Colour change
Thymol blue (acid range)	1.2–2.8	Red to yellow
Bromophenol blue	2.8–4.6	Yellow to violet
Bromocresol green	3.6–5.2	Yellow to blue
Methyl red	4.4–6.2	Red to yellow
Litmus	4.5–8.3	Red to blue
Bromocresol purple	5.2–6.8	Yellow to violet
Bromothymol blue	6.0–7.6	Yellow to blue
Neutral red	6.8–8.0	Red to yellow
Phenol red	6.8–8.4	Yellow to purple-pink
Cresol red	7.2–8.8	Yellow to violet-red
Thymol blue (alkaline range)	8.0–9.6	Yellow to blue
Phenolphthalein	8.3–10.0	Colourless to red
Thymolphthalein	9.3–10.5	Colourless to blue
BDH 'Universal'	3.0–11.0	Red-orange-yellow-green-blue-reddish violet

an approximate idea of the pH and the results should always be checked by a more accurate method.

Before pH meters were generally available, two reasonably accurate indicator dye methods were commercially available in kit form and were widely used in laboratories. These methods, the comparator and capillator methods, are now mainly of historic interest and were described in the previous edition of this volume (*Medical Microbiology*, Vol. 2, 12th Edn).

BUFFERS

Not only is it important to have the suspending fluids for microorganisms within a certain pH range, it is also important to keep the pH within the same range. Most microorganisms produce acids or alkalis as a result of their metabolic activities and these must be prevented from altering the pH of the environment too radically. For example, bacteria when grown on a medium containing a sugar generally produce acid intermediates or end-products (e.g. formic, acetic, propionic, butyric or lactic acids). This is particularly true of fermentation under relatively anaerobic conditions. If these acidic products were allowed to accumulate in an unbuffered medium, the organism would soon be killed by the low pH produced.

It is, therefore, preferable and often essential to include buffers in culture media and in suspending fluids. These buffers tend to resist changes in hydrogen-ion concentration. They are usually formed by mixing a weak acid with its salt, although a weak alkali and its salt can also be used. Buffering action is due to the fact that a weak acid is only weakly dissociated while its salt with an alkali metal is strongly dissociated. Thus, whereas 0.1 mol/litre acetic acid is only 1.35% dissociated, 0.1 mol/litre sodium acetate is 97% dissociated. If hydrogen ions are added to such a buffer solution, they will react with the high concentration of salt anions to form non-ionized acids. This weak acid, once formed, does not tend to ionize appreciably and, at the same time, its ionization is opposed by the high concentration of anions present. Therefore hydrogen ions have been added, but have been removed, leaving the pH of the solution only slightly altered.

Generally speaking, the buffering power of a mixture of a weak acid and its salt is greatest when the two are present in equimolar proportions. From such mixtures, buffers can be prepared covering a range of about 1 pH unit on each side of the pH given by an equivalent mixture (the pK of a buffer). Outside this range, the buffering capacity falls off very rapidly. Although the concentration of the buffer determines its ability to resist changes in hydrogen-ion concentration, the actual pH given by a certain mixure is only slightly affected by dilution.

Preparation of some common buffers

1. Citrate buffer

Stock solution A: 0.1 mol/litre solution of citric acid (19.21 g in 1000 ml).

Stock solution B: 0.1 mol/litre solution of sodium citrate (29.41 g $C_6H_5O_7Na_3.2H_2O$ in 1000 ml).

x ml of A + y ml of B, diluted to a total of 100 ml

x	y	pH
46.5	3.5	3.0
43.7	6.3	3.2
40.0	10.0	3.4
37.0	13.0	3.6
35.0	15.0	3.8
33.0	17.0	4.0
31.5	18.5	4.2
28.0	22.0	4.4
25.5	24.5	4.6
23.0	27.0	4.8
20.5	29.5	5.0
18.0	32.0	5.2
16.0	34.0	5.4
13.7	36.3	5.6
11.8	38.2	5.8
9.5	40.5	6.0
7.2	42.8	6.2

2. Acetate buffer

Stock solution A: 0.2 mol/litre solution of acetic acid (11.55 ml in 1000 ml).

Stock solution B: 0.2 mol/litre solution of sodium acetate (16.4 g of $C_2H_3O_2Na$ or 27.2 g of $C_2H_3O_2Na.3H_2O$ in 1000 ml).

x ml of *A* + *y* ml of *B*, diluted to a total of 100 ml

x	y	pH
46.3	3.7	3.6
44.0	6.0	3.8
41.0	9.0	4.0
36.8	13.2	4.2
30.5	19.5	4.4
25.5	24.5	4.6
20.0	30.0	4.8
14.8	35.2	5.0
10.5	39.5	5.2
8.8	41.2	5.4
4.8	45.2	5.6

3. Citrate-phosphate buffer

Stock solution A: 0.1 mol/litre solution of citric acid (19.21 g in 1000 ml).

Stock solution B: 0.2 mol/litre solution of dibasic sodium phosphate (28.39 g of Na_2HPO_4 or 71.7 g of $Na_2HPO_4.12H_2O$ in 1000 ml).

x ml of *A* + *y* ml of *B*, diluted to a total of 100 ml

x	y	pH
44.6	5.4	2.6
42.2	7.8	2.8
39.8	10.2	3.0
37.7	12.3	3.2
35.9	14.1	3.4
33.9	16.1	3.6
32.3	17.7	3.8
30.7	19.3	4.0
29.4	20.6	4.2
27.8	22.2	4.4
26.7	23.3	4.6
25.2	24.8	4.8
24.3	25.7	5.0
23.3	26.7	5.2
22.2	27.8	5.4
21.0	29.0	5.6
19.7	30.3	5.8
17.9	32.1	6.0
16.9	33.1	6.2

15.4	34.6	6.4
13.6	36.4	6.6
9.1	40.9	6.8
6.4	43.6	7.0

4. Phosphate buffer

Stock solution A: 0.2 mol/litre solution of monobasic sodium phosphate (31.2 g $NaH_2PO_4.2H_2O$ in 1000 ml).

Stock solution B: 0.2 mol/litre solution of dibasic sodium phosphate (28.39 g of Na_2HPO_4 or 71.7 g of $Na_2HPO_4.12H_2O$ in 1000 ml).

x ml of *A* + *y* ml of *B*, diluted to a total of 200 ml

x	y	pH
92.0	8.0	5.8
87.7	12.3	6.0
81.5	18.5	6.2
73.5	26.5	6.4
62.5	37.5	6.6
51.0	49.0	6.8
39.0	61.0	7.0
28.0	72.0	7.2
19.0	81.0	7.4
13.0	87.0	7.6
8.5	91.5	7.8
5.3	94.7	8.0

5. Barbitone (Veronal) buffer

Stock solution A: 0.2 mol/litre solution of sodium barbitone (sodium diethyl barbiturate).

Stock solution B: 0.2 mol/litre HCl.

50 ml of *A* + *x* ml of *B*, diluted to a total of 200 ml

x	pH
1.5	9.2
2.5	9.0
4.0	8.8
6.0	8.6
9.0	8.4
12.7	8.2
17.5	8.0
22.5	7.8
27.5	7.6
32.5	7.4

39.0	7.2
43.0	7.0
45.0	6.8

Note: Solutions more concentrated than 0.05 mol/litre may crystallize on standing, especially in the cold.

6. Tris (hydroxymethyl) aminomethane HCl (Tris HCl) buffer

Stock solution A: 0.2 mol/litre solution of tris (hydroxymethyl) aminomethane (24.2 g in 1000 ml).
Stock solution B: 0.2 mol/litre HCl.
50 ml of *A* + *x* ml of *B*, diluted to a total of 200 ml

x	pH
5.0	9.0
8.1	8.8
12.2	8.6
16.5	8.4
21.9	8.2
26.8	8.0
32.5	7.8
38.4	7.6
41.4	7.4
44.2	7.2

7. Boric acid-borax buffer

Stock solution A: 0.2 mol/litre solution of boric acid (12.4 g in 1000 ml).
Stock solution B: 0.05 mol/litre solution of borax (19.05 g in 1000 ml; 0.2 mol/litre in terms of sodium borate).
50 ml of *A* + *x* ml of *B*, diluted to a total of 200 ml

x	pH
2.0	7.6
3.1	7.8
4.9	8.0
7.3	8.2
11.5	8.4
17.5	8.6
30.0	8.8
59.0	9.0
115.0	9.2

8. Bicarbonate-CO_2 buffer

The pH of these buffers is markedly dependent on temperature. The following examples are for a temperature of 37°C.

Concentration of $NaHCO_3$	pH of buffer when concentration of CO_2 in gaseous phase is		
	5%	10%	20%
0.02 mol/litre	7.4	7.1	6.8
0.05 mol/litre	7.8	7.5	7.2

9. Carbonate-bicarbonate buffer

Stock solution A: 0.2 mol/litre solution of anhydrous sodium carbonate (21.2 g in 1000 ml).
Stock solution B: 0.2 mol/litre solution of sodium bicarbonate (16.8 g in 1000 ml).
x ml of *A* + *y* ml of *B*, diluted to a total of 200 ml

x	*y*	pH
4.0	46.0	9.2
9.5	40.5	9.4
16.0	34.0	9.6
22.0	28.0	9.8
27.5	22.5	10.0
33.0	17.0	10.2
38.5	11.5	10.4
42.5	7.5	10.6

'Good' buffers

Before 1966 it was difficult to find a suitable buffer for the biological range of pH 6–8. Those available suffered several drawbacks especially if used in cell-free systems. Phosphate buffer often causes precipitation of polyvalent cations. It is a metabolite or inhibitor of many biological systems and is a poor buffer above pH 7.5. Tris-(hydroxymethyl) aminomethane (Tris) is a poor buffer below pH 7.5 and is often inhibitory. In 1966 Good et al described a series of hydrogen ion buffers which covered the 'biological' range with pKa values of 6–8. Most were zwitterionic N-substituted amino acids. In designing these buffers such properties as maximum solubility in water, inability to form complexes with biological materials, having minimal salt effects and being both stable and chemically inert were considered as important as their buffering capacity. Of these buffers N-hydroxyethylpiperazine-N-ethane-sulphonic acid (HEPES) has proved the most popular. Others are now available and are readily obtained (e.g. from Sigma). The 'Good' buffers as they are commonly referred to are slowly superseding the more traditional buffers listed above. They should be the buffers of choice in any studies involving cell-free systems and tissue culture work. Zwitterionic buffers are usually used at concentrations of between 10 and 100 mmol/litre. Adjustment of the pH is by HCl or NaOH of equal concentration. At the lower concentrations the salt effect of these buffers is negligible. For further details see Ferguson et al (1980).

OXIDATION-REDUCTION (REDOX) POTENTIALS

The oxidation-reduction conditions in a medium are very important in the growth of certain bacteria. Strict aerobes are able to grow only in the presence of dissolved oxygen while strict anaerobes require reducing conditions and hence absence of dissolved oxygen. This may be related to the metabolic character of the organism, a strict aerobe obtaining its energy and intermediates only through oxidation involving oxygen as the ultimate hydrogen acceptor, a strict anaerobe utilizing hydrogen acceptors other than oxygen, while a facultative anaerobe can act in both ways. However, strict anaerobes may actually be poisoned by the presence of oxygen, perhaps due to the production of toxic hydrogen peroxide which cannot be removed by catalase, or superoxide free radicals which cannot be removed by superoxide dismutase, or possibly due to the oxidation of certain essential groupings in the organism, e.g. the sulphydryl groups of proteins.

We may consider oxidizing agents as substances capable of taking up electrons and reducing agents as substances able to part with electrons. It is therefore possible to determine the intensity level of oxidizing or reducing conditions in a system by the net readiness of all the components in that system to take up, or part with, electrons. This ability is usually expressed as the oxidation-reduction (redox) potential of the system.

Redox potentials can be measured best by virtue of the fact that when an 'unattackable' electrode is immersed in a solution, an electrical potential difference is set up between the electrode and the solution, and the magnitude of this potential depends on the state of oxidation or reduction of the solution. This electrode potential (or, more shortly Eh) can be measured in millivolts, and the more oxidized a system, the higher (or more positive) is the potential; in more reduced systems the potential is lower (or more negative). By measuring the electrode potential it is possible to determine and follow the reducing conditions in cultures at different periods and to grade different systems in order according to their state of oxidation or reduction. This measurement can usually be carried out by coupling up a potentiometer with an electrode pair of platinum electrode (the 'unattackable' electrode) and a standard calomel electrode. The redox potential can then be measured by the millivolt scale provided on most commercial pH meters.

Although the redox potential of a bacterial culture may be measured accurately by electrical methods, an approximate idea of the state of reduction may sometimes be obtained by adding various special dyes (oxidation-reduction indicators) and observing by the colour changes how much they are reduced. Table 5.2 lists some redox indicators and the Eh at which they are fully reduced.

It should be noted that in a growing culture

Table 5.2 Redox indicators.

Redox dye	Redox potential at pH 7[a]
Methylene blue	+ 11 mV
Resazurin	− 42 mV
Phenosafranine	− 252 mV
Neutral red	− 325 mV
Standard oxygen electrode	+ 810 mV
Standard hydrogen electrode	− 421 mV

[a] Redox potential below which dye becomes colourless.

of bacteria the Eh of the medium may fall appreciably during the growth phase. It will depend on the starting Eh of the medium, the size of the inoculum, the degree of aeration and the growth rate. Strict anaerobes are unable to grow unless the Eh is low enough. This can be achieved by prereducing the medium by boiling to drive off any dissolved oxygen. Also reducing agents such as thioglycollate or cysteine can be added. (See Chs 7 and 36 for methods of cultivation of anaerobes.)

For fuller discussion on redox potentials in microbiology, see Jacob (1970).

WATER

Tap water contains many impurities and is unsuitable for the preparation of defined culture media, for chemical solutions and for many other uses in the laboratory. These impurities can largely be removed by distillation or deionization.

Distilled water

Distilled water is normally prepared in a commercial metal-lined still which will deliver it at the rate of 1–250 litres/h, depending on size. However, for some purposes this water is insufficiently pure, and it may be necessary to use an all-glass distillation apparatus. It is often advisable to add a knife point of potassium permanganate and a few pellets of sodium hydroxide to the tap water before commencing distillation in order to oxidize steam-volatile organic compounds which might otherwise be carried over into the distillate. For some experimental methods such as tissue culture it may be necessary to repeat the distillation in a glass still to give doubly glass-distilled water.

It is useful to check the purity of distilled water at times by simple conductivity testers. Satisfactory distilled water should have a conductivity no greater than that given by 1.5 p.p.m. of NaCl, and preferably below 1 p.p.m.

Deionized (dermineralized) water

Ion-exchange resins may be used to deionize water. A simple apparatus consists of an anion- and a cation-exchanger in two columns of glass tubing about 2 m tall and 3 cm in diameter. A variety of resins are available for the purpose. Tap water or distilled water is passed over each of the resins in turn. The columns must be periodically regenerated by rinsing with 10% aqueous HCl for the cation-exchanger and 10% aqueous NaOH for the anion-exchanger. After regeneration, the columns are rinsed with distilled water until the final product has a neutral reaction. Commercial deionizers are available, e.g. those supplied by Elga or Permutit, which have the advantage of being transportable and of requiring no external source of heat or electricity. Deionized water should be equivalent to double glass-distilled water and should have a very low conductivity. This should be checked periodically (see above). However, it may carry dissolved organic compounds derived from the resins.

FLUIDS FOR CELL SUSPENSION AND DILUTION

A variety of fluids may be used for the suspension of microorganisms, blood cells or tissue culture cells. These fluids should preserve, as far as possible, the cells in their original condition. The following points should be noted:

1. They should have an osmotic pressure nearly isotonic with the cell to be suspended. This is particularly true of mammalian cells, e.g. red blood cells, where lysis readily occurs in non-isotonic media. Microorganisms are generally more resistant to changes in the external osmotic pressure, but suspension in water or very dilute salt solutions may cause loss of viability.

2. Suspension fluids should preferably contain a buffer to keep the cells at their optimum pH.

3. Certain ions may be necessary for the optimal maintenance of cells, particularly with mammalian cells. Moreover, they may be required for certain in-vitro reactions, e.g. agglutination, complement fixation, etc. In some cases a source of energy such as glucose may be required.

4. Other additions may be made for specific

purposes. The following suspensions and diluent fluids are commonly used. In all cases analytical grade reagents (when available) should be made up in distilled or deionized water.

Physiological saline

A solution of 0.85% NaCl in water. This solution is sometimes called normal saline, a term which should be discarded because of its chemical connotation. It is also often referred to as 'saline'. The solution has an osmotic pressure roughly equivalent to that of mammalian blood serum and can therefore be used for the suspension of blood cells as well as for most micro-organisms. However, the solution contains no buffer and it is recommended that phosphate-buffered saline be used as a general suspension fluid in the laboratory.

Buffered salines

As stated previously, it is preferable to have a buffer present in a suspending fluid or diluent and a variety of solutions containing NaCl but with a buffer added have been proposed. They should all have a final osmotic pressure roughly equivalent to that of physiological saline. A series of solutions can be prepared by diluting standard buffer solutions of the required pH with physiological saline to a strength of 0.01 mol/litre. If a greater buffering power is required, the concentration of buffer must be increased and of saline decreased.

The following types of buffered saline are recommended for various purposes:

Phosphate buffered saline

NaCl	8 g/litre
K_2HPO_4	1.21 g/litre
KH_2PO_4	0.34 g/litre

This solution gives a pH of about 7.3 and also provides potassium and phosphate ions. It is a very useful general diluent and suspending fluid.

Azide saline. Sodium azide at a concentration of 0.08% is added to physiological saline or phosphate buffered saline. The azide acts as a preservative preventing microbial decomposition and is often used for the dilution of serum, etc.

Borate-calcium saline

NaCl	8 g/litre
$CaCl_2$	1 g/litre
H_3BO_3	1.2 g/litre
$Na_2B_4O_7.10H_2O$	0.052 g/litre

This solution, pH *c*. 7.3, is used for haemag-glutination experiments where calcium is required and phosphate should be absent.

Veronal-NaCl diluent

NaCl	8.5 g/litre
Barbitone (diethyl-barbituric acid)	0.575 g/litre
Sodium barbitone	0.2 g/litre
$MgCl_2.6H_2O$	0.168 g/litre
$CaCl_2$	0.028 g/litre

A stock solution ($\times$ 5 conc.) is made by dissolving 5.75 g barbitone in 500 ml hot distilled water. Add 85 g NaCl and make up to *c*. 1400 ml. Dissolve 2 g sodium barbitone in 500 ml distilled water and add it to the NaCl-barbitone solution. Make up to 2000 ml. Add 1.68 g $MgCl_2.6H_2O$ and 0.28 g $CaCl_2$. For use dilute 1 in 5 with distilled water. The pH is 7.1–7.2.

This saline (available as CFT diluent tablets, Oxoid BR16) may be used for complement fixation tests and gives more reproducible results than physiological saline. If glass tubes are used for the reaction mixtures, there may be absorption of complement on to the glass. To reduce this, add 0.1% inactivated rabbit serum, 0.1% gelatin or 0.1% bovine serum albumin.

Complex suspending media

More complex media are required for the suspension and dilution of microorganisms and other cells where optimum viability must be maintained. For example, in viable counts of many bacteria, physiological saline may be to some extent bactericidal and must be replaced by solutions containing other ions as well as a buffer. For these fluids prepare solutions listed

Table 5.3 Complex suspending media.

Reagent at stated concentration in water	Mix solutions in the proportions for				
	Ringer	Locke	Krebs-Ringer		
			Plain	Bicarbonate[b]	Phosphate
NaCl (9.0 g/litre)	100	100	100	100	100
KCl (11.5 g/litre)	4	4	4	4	4
CaCl$_2$ (12.2 g/litre)	3	3	3	3	3
KH$_2$PO$_4$ (21.1 g/litre)	—	—	1	1	—
MgSO$_4$.7H$_2$O (38.2 g/litre)	—	—	1	1	1
NaHCO$_3$ (13.0 g/litre)	—	3	—	21	—
Phosphate buffer pH 7.4 (0.1 mol/litre)[a]	—	—	—	—	20

[a] 17.8 g Na$_2$HPO$_4$.2H$_2$O + 20 ml 1 mol/l HCl diluted to 1 litre.
[b] The solution should be gassed with 5% (v/v) CO$_2$ in O$_2$, air or N$_2$.

in Table 5.3 which are all isotonic with mammalian serum and can be mixed in any proportions. The mixtures, although of different composition, will remain isotonic.

To simplify preparation and handling, the first five solutions can be made up in concentrations five times those listed. They are stable for months when stored in the cold.

The Krebs-Ringer solution seems to be the most generally useful for the suspension of mammalian cells and is also valuable for many bacteria.

It is also possible to use a defined minimal medium for bacterial suspension; if growth is to be avoided, leave out the nitrogen source or the carbon and energy sources.

PREPARATION AND CLEANING OF GLASSWARE

New glassware

New glassware requires special attention because of the resistant spores which may be present in the straw and other packing material and also because it tends to give off free alkali which may be sufficient to interfere with the growth of certain organisms. Consequently it should be placed in 1% HCl overnight, washed in tap water and distilled or deionized water and autoclaved.

Screw-capped bottles are subjected to a special cleansing process by the makers whereby surface alkali is removed, and the above treatment is unnecessary. The bottles may be used without further treatment, as received from the manufacturers.

Cleaning of glassware (including tissue culture glassware) for laboratory use

Ideally all contaminated glassware should be autoclaved before cleaning. If this is not possible glass containers with discarded cultures can be placed in 3% lysol or similar disinfectant after use. Containers contaminated with tubercle bacilli or spore-bearing organisms such as *Bacillus anthracis* or *Clostridium tetani* must be autoclaved. The discarded cultures and their containers are then placed in a hot detergent solution and cleaned with a test-tube brush (or other suitable brush) and placed in a laboratory washing machine and treated as recommended by the manufacturers of the machine and detergent, finally rinsing in deionized water. The glassware is then allowed to drain and is dried in a hot air oven or cabinet. Dry sterilize at 160°C for 3 h.

Cleaning of glassware for biochemical work

For most purposes cleaning in one of the modern detergents (e.g. Decon, Labdet, etc.) according to the manufacturer's instructions is all that is necessary. Some workers, however, still prefer 'chromic acid' cleaning:

1. Remove any grease with petroleum. Wash with warm tap water.

2. Place in dichromate-sulphuric acid cleaning solution for 12–24 h.

3. Remove and wash by rinsing in hot tap water at least four times and in distilled water twice.

4. Dry in oven if the glassware is not used for accurate volumetric purposes.

Dichromate-sulphuric acid cleaning solution ('Chromic acid'). Dissolve 63 g of sodium (or potassium) dichromate by heating with 35 ml water. Cool and add concentrated H_2SO_4 to 1 litre. Technical grade reagents may be used. This fluid should be handled with care; preferably rubber gloves and an apron should be worn. If clothes or skin are splashed with the fluid, they should be immediately washed in water and any residual acid neutralized with sodium carbonate solution. This, in time, is washed off with water.

Cleaning of pipettes

1. If contaminated with infected material, place the used pipette into a 3% (v/v) lysol solution and leave until convenient to wash. (The lysol solution is best contained in a rubber or plastic cylinder about 40 cm high and 10 cm in diameter. The points of the pipettes are not liable to be broken when dropped to the bottom of the cylinder).

2. Rinse in tap water.

3. If necessary, steep overnight in detergent or dichromate-sulphuric acid cleaning fluid (see above).

4. Wash with tap water followed by deionized water in an automatic pipette washer.

5. If required, the top end of the pipette is plugged with cotton wool; this is pressed entirely within the end of the pipette so that there are no protruding strands of cotton to prevent close fitting of a rubber teat or other pipette-filling device which may later be attached to operate the pipette.

6. To sterilize the pipettes, pack them in aluminium or copper cylinders with slip-on lids or in lengths of wide-bore glass tubing stoppered with cotton wool. Place in a hot air oven at 160°C for 3 h.

Note: Accurately calibrated volumetric glassware should never be heated in an oven, since the expansion and contraction of the glass makes the graduations inaccurate. Such glassware should be kept separate from that intended for sterilization.

REFERENCES

Ferguson W J, Braunschweiger K I, Braunschweiger W R, Smith J R, McCormick J J, Wasmann C C, Jarvis N P, Bell D H, Good N E 1980 Hydrogen ion buffers for biological research. Analytical Biochemistry 104: 300–310

Good N E, Winget G D, Winter W, Connolly J N, Izawa S, Singh R M M 1966 Hydrogen ion buffers for biological research. Biochemistry 5: 467–477

Jacob H E 1970 Methods in microbiology, vol 2. London, Academic Press. p 91

Culture containers and culture media

Only in exceptional cases can the identity of a microorganism be established by its morphological characters. It is therefore usually essential to obtain a culture by growing the organism in an artificial culture medium, and if more than one species or type of organism are present, each requires to be carefully separated or isolated in pure culture. In this process there are three distinct operations:

1. The preparation of a suitable culture medium.

2. The initial removal of other organisms from the medium and its containers by sterilization. Bacteria are ubiquitous and are present in the material and on the articles used for making media. These contaminating organisms must be destroyed or removed so that the culture medium is rendered sterile.

3. The cultivation of the organism and its isolation from others present in the material to be examined. Techniques for the separation of mixed cultures are described in the next chapter, and the general subject of bacterial nutrition and conditions for growth has been dealt with in the 13th Edition, Volume 1, Chapter 3.

Liquid and solid media

There are two broad groups of media, liquid and solid. Many liquid media containing different nutrients have been devised and most bacteria will grow in at least one of them. However, liquid media have two disadvantages. Growths usually do not exhibit specially characteristic appearances in them and, except when they are designed for a particular biochemical test, they are of only limited use in identifying species.

Also, organisms cannot be separated with certainty from mixtures by growth in liquid media. If solid media are used, these advantages are overcome. On solid media the appearances exhibited by the colonies of different bacteria are useful in identification; and solid media are almost indispensable for the isolation of pure cultures. It is only occasionally that organisms can be grown directly from the body in pure culture so that solid media are almost always needed for the examination of pathological specimens.

Gelatin was used by the early bacteriologists to make the first solid media; pieces of potato impregnated with nutrient solutions can be used as solid media; serum or egg can be coagulated by heating in an inspissator to make media solid; but agar is most commonly used for this purpose.

Agar-agar or 'agar' for short, is derived from certain seaweeds. In watery solutions it gives a firm gel that remains unmelted at all incubation temperatures and that is generally bacteriologically inert, being decomposed or liquefied only by a few varieties of marine bacteria. In these respects it is more suitable than gelatin; a 15% solution of gelatin melts at 24°C and gelatin is decomposed by many proteolytic bacteria. Agar does not add to the nutritive properties of a medium and a suitable agar should be free from growth-promoting as well as growth-inhibiting substances.

The melting and solidifying points of agar solutions are not the same. At the concentrations normally used, most bacteriological agars melt at about 95°C and solidify only when cooled to about 42°C. The ability of agar to be melted is an advantage compared with the inability of serum or egg to be melted, and the low solidifying point of agar allows heat-sensitive nutrients to be mixed with it in the molten state at temperatures as low as 45°C.

Containers for media and cultures

Flasks stoppered with cotton wool, test tubes stoppered with cotton wool or with slip-on metal caps, and screw-capped bottles of different capacity and shape can be used as containers for media and cultures. Cotton-wool plugs must be discarded after each use. Air passing into the tubes as a result of changes in temperature or pressure, as when cultures are incubated anaerobically, is filtered through the wool; such protection is not provided by metal caps. Screw-capped bottles are made of clear white flint glass, the neck having an external screw thread. The caps are made of aluminium and each has a rubber washer 3 mm thick of special rubber that is not inhibitory to bacterial growth. Screw-capped bottles are air-tight and thus do not allow their contents to dry out during storage. Media in bottles can be kept almost indefinitely. A list of bottles that covers practically all needs is given in Table 6.1.

Glassware must be thoroughly cleaned before use for culture media and new glassware may

Table 6.1 A list of useful bottles.

Bottle	Total capacity (ml)
80 oz round	2400
40 oz round	1190
20 oz round	600
10 oz round	290
5 oz round	140
1 oz round (H 53), McCartney	28
$\frac{1}{2}$ oz round	15
$\frac{1}{4}$ oz round, bijou	6
1 oz universal container	28
8 oz medical flat	236
6 oz medical flat	180
4 oz medical flat	125
3 oz medical flat	85
2 oz medical flat	60
1 oz medical flat	33
2 oz squat (J1/2)	65

require special treatment to remove free alkali. When bottles are cleaned for re-use the old caps and washers may be discarded and replaced with new caps and washers. If undamaged caps are to be re-used they should be thoroughly washed and dried, care being taken to see that there is no moisture between the washer and the cap, since this can interfere with sterilization.

Petri dishes are shallow flat-bottomed circular clear glass or plastic containers with lids; they are normally *c.* 90 mm in diameter, but smaller and larger dishes are available for special purposes. Melted agar medium solidified in a Petri dish provides a large surface area for the culture of bacteria or fungi. It is important to allow access of the desired atmosphere, e.g. anaerobic, CO_2-enriched etc., to the surface of the medium. Accordingly, devices are used to ensure that the lids of glass plates do not become sealed by water of condensation during incubation. Some plastic Petri dishes have ridges on the inner surface of the lid to ensure that the plates are 'vented'.

The use of plastic Petri dishes, e.g. Sterilin, is a substantial saving of labour. They are supplied sterile by the manufacturer and are disposable after one use. Care must be taken to ensure that plastic used for Petri dishes is not inhibitory to microorganisms, especially mycoplasmas, and also to tissue cultures for which specially treated dishes are available. Some plastics are oxidizing and unsuitable for anaerobic media. Vented and non-vented plastic Petri dishes are commercially available.

Copper salts are inimical to the growth of many organisms and copper utensils should not be used for the preparation of media.

Adjustment of pH of culture media

The pH of a culture medium should always be checked and adjusted if necessary as described in Chapter 5. The pH always rises as the temperature falls and allowance for this must be made if the pH is tested when the medium is hot. During autoclaving, solutions that have been adjusted to be a little on the alkaline side of neutrality tend to fall by about 0.1 unit.

Distribution of unsterilized media

In general, media are initially tubed or bottled without sterile precautions. All media are distributed as liquids. Gelatin and agar media are first melted and distributed while hot; for safety it is usual to cool melted agar media to 55°C before distribution. Clean but unsterile glassware is used, and the medium and container together are subsequently sterilized by heat. A simple apparatus is a glass funnel, fixed in a burette stand, with a short length of rubber tubing and a glass delivery nozzle fitted to the stem and controlled by a pinchcock. More sophisticated dispensing machines are commercially available and are recommended for busy laboratories.

Tubing and bottling of media

Liquid media may be distributed in test tubes or bottles. In general, a test tube is half-filled. Small screw-capped bottles in the range 5–30 ml may be almost completely filled (c. 85%), as they can be safely autoclaved with the caps tight (but note the precautions in Ch. 4). Larger bottles (more than 50 ml capacity) should not be filled more than 75–80% full. Solid media are generally prepared by the addition of agar or gelatin in powder form with initial heating and mixing to ensure even dispersal of the ingredients. Distribution of the molten medium may be done at this stage, as for liquid media, without careful sterile precautions. Thereafter, the solid media are sterilized by autoclaving.

Sterilization of prepared media

The choice of method to be used to sterilize a medium depends on whether or not the ingredients are decomposed by heat. If autoclaving will not damage the medium, it is the best method of sterilization, and its application is discussed in Chapter 4.

The sterilization time at a particular temperature is the sum of the heat penetration time, which is variable, and the holding time, which is constant for media prepared under clean conditions for each temperature. The heat penetration time and consequently the sterilization time, varies greatly with the volume of medium and also with the container. For test tubes containing 10 ml of medium, a sterilization time of 15 min at 121°C, or 35 min at 115°C, is required. McCartney bottles containing 10 ml of medium require 20 min at 121°C. Larger amounts of medium require longer sterilization times and so do small amounts of medium in large containers. Recommended sterilization times at 121°C are summarized in Table 6.2. Molten agar requires the same sterilization time as liquid media: but if agar is solid, 5–10 min must be added for melting.

Table 6.2 Sterilization times at 121°C.

Volume of medium	Container	
	Flask	Bottle
10 ml	15 min	20 min
100 ml	20 min	25 min
500 ml	25 min	30 min
1 litre	30 min	40 min

Tubes and bottles of medium must be put in the autoclave so that steam has free access to them. Wire crates are suitable holders, but tins are unsuitable unless holes have been punched in them. Care must be taken that bottles of medium are not packed tightly in a holder, otherwise breakages may occur.

Sometimes lower temperatures, such as 115°C, for times ranging from 10–20 min are recommended for 'sterilization' of media containing ingredients that are not very stable to heat. These conditions are not strictly reliable for sterilization and should be used only for media distributed in small quantities. They are usually satisfactory because it is unlikely that many heat-resistant spores would be present in media prepared under clean conditions.

Steaming at 100°C, either for a long time, e.g. 90 min on one occasion or for shorter times on several occasions, is not a sure way of sterilizing media. Spores are not invariably destroyed at 100°C and will not be destroyed by successive heatings at 100°C unless they are incubated in the intervening periods under conditions in which they will germinate to yield heat-sensitive vegetative organisms. Samples of media steam-treated in this way should be incubated as a routine assurance that they are sterile. Repeated steaming for short periods (tyndallization) is inadequate for the sterilization of *non-nutrient* solutions, e.g. pure sugar solutions, as any spores in them are unlikely to germinate and grow out between steamings.

If any of the ingredients of a medium are liable to be spoiled by autoclaving, the complete medium should not be sterilized by heat. In such cases, it is usual to autoclave the thermostable ingredients of the medium and to add the sterile heat-sensitive ingredients with sterile precautions. Some heat-sensitive ingredients such as blood, serum or egg-yolk can be obtained sterile from natural sources. Others must be sterilized by filtration through a bacterial filter (Ch. 4).

Some selective media that cannot be auto-claved contain ingredients that are inhibitory to the most probable contaminants. These media are sometimes prepared without the sterilization of some ingredients, reliance being placed on the inhibitors to suppress contaminants. The method is usually successful but must always be regarded as less than ideal.

Distribution of sterilized media with sterile precautions

Liquid media

Sterile precautions for tubing and bottling liquid media are necessary if an ingredient of the medium is heat-labile – for example, certain sugars used in fermentation test media. The ingredients that are stable to heat are prepared and sterilized, the unstable ingredient (previously sterilized in a suitable way) is added with sterile precautions and the medium is distributed with sterile precautions into sterile containers.

Alternatively the heat-stable part of the medium may be distributed into clean glassware without sterile precautions and then sterilized. The sterile unstable ingredient can later be added from a sterile graduated pipette or syringe.

Tubing and bottling of solid media

Solid media may be distributed in test tubes or bottles, as for liquid media. This may be done for storage, often prior to supplementation. If the solid medium is to be used for direct culture in a tube or bottle, the shape in which the medium is allowed to solidify depends on the method of inoculation for which it is to be used. The commonest shape is the 'slope' or 'slant', which provides a large surface area of medium for inoculation. For $6 \times \frac{5}{8}$ in (150 × 16 mm) test tubes, 5 ml of medium is sufficient and it is allowed to set at such an angle that there is a thick butt at the bottom (Fig. 6.1). When a large number of tubes of agar have to be sloped, special trays that allow the tubes to be laid at the correct angle are useful. After cooling, fresh agar slopes contain 'water of condensation' at the foot of the tube; this should not be allowed to run over the surface of the medium or wet the plug or cap.

If the medium is to be used for a 'stab' or 'shake' culture the test tube is half filled with the medium, which is allowed to solidify in the upright position.

Screw-capped bottles can be substituted for test tubes. The amounts of medium for slopes in

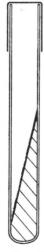

Fig. 6.1 Slope of solid medium in test tube. A cotton-wool plug may be used instead of the slip-on metal cap illustrated here.

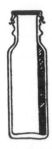

Fig. 6.2 Slope of solid medium in screw-capped bottle.

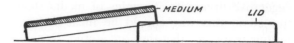

Fig. 6.3 The drying of an agar plate before inoculation.

1 oz and bijou (6 ml) bottles are 5 ml and 2.5 ml respectively. The medium may be allowed to set at an angle to form a butt as in test tubes, but it is easier to inoculate with a loop if it is parallel to the side of the bottle (Fig. 6.2). For stab or shake cultures, 1 oz bottles are half-filled with medium.

Agar media stored in 4, 6 or 8 oz medical flat bottles melt much more quickly than agar in 3, 5 or 10 oz round bottles.

Pouring plates

Solid media in Petri dishes are often called 'plates'. For a dish of 90 mm diameter, 14 ml of medium is usually ample.

Plates are always poured with sterile precautions. Bulk medium is prepared sterile and is poured into sterile Petri dishes. Care must be taken to avoid contamination from the air during pouring. It is desirable to pour plates on a bench in a small room free from draughts and preferably within an inoculation hood or cabinet (see Ch. 7). To reduce condensation of water on the Petri dish lids, the medium should be cooled to 52°C before pouring. The melted medium is poured into the dishes on a flat surface and the dishes are left undisturbed until the medium has set. In separating organisms from mixed cultures by plating, it is essential that the surface of the medium should be dry. When plates have been poured, the steam from the hot liquid condenses on the surface of the medium and this moisture is undesirable. It is removed by drying the poured and set plates in a warming or drying cabinet at 60°C for 15–30 min, depending on the medium (Fig. 6.3). If care is taken to avoid disturbing dust, there is very little risk of contamination of the medium by air organisms.

Machines are commercially available for the automatic distribution of melted medium and for the automatic stacking of the prepared plates.

Inspissation of serum and egg media

The serum in Loeffler's medium and egg in media such as Löwenstein-Jensen medium are usually solidified in an apparatus called an inspissator. It consists of a water-jacketed copper box, the temperature of which can be regulated automatically. The serum or egg medium is tubed and placed in special racks, so that the tubes are at the correct angle for forming slopes. The temperature used is between 75°C and 85°C. At this temperature the protein is completely solidified, but the temperature is not so high as to cause bubbles of steam to disrupt the surface of the medium. As medium in tubes is apt to dry if kept in the inspissator for any time, a small opening should be present in the inner wall communicating with the top of the water-chamber above the level of the water. Water vapour can enter the interior of the inspissator and the medium is kept moist. If an electric inspissator without a water-jacket is to be used, it is better to dispense media in bottles rather than in tubes with cotton-wool stoppers.

CULTURE MEDIA

Some bacterial species are able to grow under a wide range of conditions, but others are very exacting. Artificial culture media generally provide sources of carbon, energy and nitrogen in the form of available carbohydrates and amino acids (see *Medical Microbiology* 13th Edn, Vol. 1, p. 37). Special media provide specific requirements that may include inorganic salts, or particular growth factors.

Defined synthetic media

Chemically defined media are used for various experimental purposes. They are prepared exclusively from pure chemical substances and their exact composition is known. The ingredients should be of analytical reagent quality and are dissolved in distilled or demineralized water.

Simple synthetic media contain a carbon and energy source such as glucose or lactate, an inorganic source of nitrogen, usually in the form of ammonium chloride, phosphate or sulphate, and various inorganic salts in a buffered aqueous solution. They provide the basic essentials for the growth of many non-parasitic heterotrophs, but they will not support growth of most kinds of parasitic bacteria.

Complex synthetic media incorporate, in addition, certain amino acids, purines, pyrimidines and other growth factors. They can therefore be used for the growth of more exacting bacteria.

Routine laboratory media

The majority of organisms to be studied in medical bacteriology are either pathogens or commensals of the human body, and in order to obtain suitable growths the artificial culture medium should provide nutrients and a pH (about 7.2) approximating to those of the tissues and body fluids. For routine purposes many of these nutrients are supplied by aqueous extracts of meat and peptone, which is a product of the digestion of protein.

Basal media such as nutrient broth and peptone water are generally used as simple media and as the basis of supplemented enriched media.

Enriched media are prepared to meet the nutritional requirements of more exacting bacteria by the addition of substances such as blood, serum and egg to a basal medium.

Selective media contain substances that inhibit or poison all but a few types of bacteria. They facilitate the isolation of particular species from a mixed inoculum. If a liquid medium favours the multiplication of a particular species, either by containing enrichments that selectively favour it or inhibitory substances that suppress competitors, cultures from mixed inocula are called *enrichment* cultures. These cultures fail to indicate the proportion of the species present in the inoculum.

Indicator media incorporate some substance that is changed visibly as a result of the metabolic activities of particular organisms. Combinations of enriched media with selective agents and indicator systems are frequently used in the diagnostic laboratory.

Transport media are devised to maintain the viability of a pathogen and to avoid overgrowth of other contaminants during transit from the patient to the laboratory.

Storage media and conditions for the maintenance of bacterial cultures are discussed later in this chapter.

COMMON INGREDIENTS OF CULTURE MEDIA

Water

Tap water is often suitable for culture media, particularly if it has a low mineral content, but if the local supply is found unsuitable, glass-distilled or demineralized water must be used instead. Small amounts of copper are highly inhibitory to bacterial growth so that copper-distilled water cannot be used for media. Suitable demineralizers are commercially available.

Agar

Agar is prepared in several countries from a variety of seaweeds; the product is clarified, dried and finally supplied as the dried strands or as a powder. There are considerable differences in the properties of the agars manufactured in different places, and even between different batches from the same source. Japanese and New Zealand agars are well known and were formerly predominant, but agars are now available from many parts of the world. The exact concentration to be used may require some adjustment according to the batch of agar and also according to the other constituents of the medium. A concentration of 1–2% usually yields a suitable gel, but the manufacturer's instructions should be followed.

The chief component of agar is a long-chain polysaccharide, mainly composed of D-galacto-pyranose units. It also contains a variety of impurities including inorganic salts, a small amount of protein-like material and sometimes traces of long-chain fatty acids which are inhibitory to growth. The minerals present are mainly magnesium and calcium, and agar is thought to exist as the magnesium or calcium sulphate esters of the polysaccharide.

In preparing agar media, the appropriate amount of agar powder or fibre is added to the liquid medium and dissolved by placing the mixture in a steamer at 100°C for 1 h or longer. Most agars dissolve to give a clear solution but sometimes it is necessary to filter off particulate impurities and, possibly, excess phosphates from the nutrient liquid.

Agar can be added to any nutrient liquid medium if the advantages of a solid medium are desired. Nutrients that are not damaged by autoclaving may be added to the medium before dissolving the agar. Such media can be sterilized and allowed to set for storage, being remelted in the steamer before use. However, nutrients that are damaged by autoclaving must be prepared sterile separately from the agar base. The sterilized agar base can be melted in the steamer and cooled to about 45–50°C before adding any heat-labile ingredients, but once these are added the medium must at once be distributed for its final use because it cannot be remelted without damaging the heat-sensitive ingredients.

Agar is hydrolysed to products that do not solidify on cooling if it is heated at a low pH. Agar usually does not alter the pH of the medium to which it is added but if it contains free acid this must be neutralized before it is autoclaved. For media whose pH is about 5, such as those for lactobacilli and fungi, heating should be reduced to a minimum after the agar is in an acid solution. After autoclaving, the medium may be allowed to solidify in bulk but it should be remelted with as little heating as possible and then be wholly distributed for its final use; it

should not be partly used, allowed to solidify and later heated a third time.

Peptone

Peptone consists of water-soluble products obtained from lean meat or other protein material such as heart muscle, casein, fibrin or soya flour, usually by digestion with the proteolytic enzymes, pepsin, trypsin or papain. The important constituents are peptones, proteoses, amino acids, a variety of inorganic salts including phosphates, potassium and magnesium, and certain accessory growth factors such as nicotinic acid and riboflavin. Peptone is supplied as a golden granular powder with a low moisture content, preferably under 5%, and usually a slightly acid reaction, giving a pH between 5 and 7 in a 1% solution. It is hygroscopic and soon becomes sticky when exposed to air; stock bottles should therefore be kept firmly closed. According to the starting materials and mode of preparation, the brands of peptone supplied by different manufacturers show appreciable differences in composition and growth-promoting properties; moreover, variations may occur between different batches of one brand.

The essential requirements of a good peptone include the ability to support the growth of moderately exacting bacteria from small inocula, the absence of fermentable carbohydrates, a low content of contaminating bacteria and a very low content of copper. Apart from the standard grades of bacteriological peptone, some manufacturers supply special grades of peptone recommended for particular purposes, e.g Neopeptone, Proteose peptone, mycological peptone, etc.

Casein hydrolysate

This consists largely of the amino acids obtained by hydrolysis of the milk protein casein. It also contains phosphate and other salts, and certain growth factors. Hydrolysis is effected either with hydrochloric acid, when the product is neutralized with sodium carbonate and so becomes very rich in sodium chloride, or with a proteolytic enzyme (trypsin). The acid hydrolysate is the poorer nutritionally because tryptophane is largely destroyed during the hydrolysis and some other amino acids are reduced in amount; tryptophane must therefore be added to the medium to make it suitable for tryptophane-requiring bacteria. The more expensive enzymic hydrolysate contains abundant tryptophane and the full range of amino acids, and does not require such supplementation. Casein hydrolysate may be substituted for peptone in broth and other media. It is of particular use in experimental work where a nearly defined medium is required, since its composition is more constant and more fully known than that of other peptones. Thus it may be added to a minimal synthetic medium to render it suitable for growth of exacting bacteria.

Meat extract

A commercially prepared meat extract known as Lab-Lemco (Oxoid) is used as a substitute for an infusion of fresh meat. Meat extract is manufactured by Liebig's process in which the products of hot water extraction of lean beef are concentrated by evaporation. The product contains a wide variety of water-soluble compounds, including protein degradation products, e.g. gelatin, albumoses, peptones, proteoses and amino acids and other nitrogen compounds such as creatine, creatinine, carnosine, anserine, purines and glutathione (total N about 10%); it also contains many mineral salts (KH_2PO_4 and NaCl most abundantly), accessory growth factors (e.g. thiamine, nicotinic acid, riboflavin, pyridoxin, pantothenic acid and choline) and some carbohydrates.

Yeast extract

Commercial yeast extract is prepared from washed cells of brewer's or baker's yeast. It contains a wide range of amino acids (amounting to nearly 50% of its mass), growth factors (especially of the vitamin B group) and inorganic salts (particularly potassium and phosphate); over 10% of yeast extract is carbohydrate, including glycogen, trehalose and pentoses. Yeast extract is used mainly as a comprehensive

source of growth factors and may be substituted for meat extract in culture media.

Malt extract

Malt extract is prepared commercially by extracting the soluble materials from sprouted barley in water at about 55°C. The liquor is strained and concentrated by evaporation at a temperature below 55°C to yield a brown viscous material. It consists mainly of maltose (about 50%), starch, dextrins and glucose, and contains about 5% of proteins and protein breakdown products, and a wide range of mineral salts and growth factors, such as thiamin, nicotinic acid, riboflavin, biotin, pantothenic acid, pyridoxin, folic acid and inositol. For use in mycological media it must not contain added sugar or cod-liver oil.

Blood

Blood for use in media must be collected with aseptic precautions adequate to exclude bacterial contamination and preserve the blood in its original sterile condition. Any attempt to sterilize blood by heat would lead to disintegration of the cells, coagulation of cell and serum proteins, and denaturation of the red haemoglobin to brown derivatives. It must be rendered non-coagulating by defibrination or by the addition of citrate or oxalate; defibrination is recommended because it involves no additive that might alter the nutritive properties of the medium.

For defibrination, a bottle containing glass beads is half filled with the blood, stoppered at once and shaken continuously for 5 min. Oxalated blood is prepared by bleeding the animals into bottles containing 10 ml of a 10% solution of neutral potassium oxalate/litre of blood. For citrated blood, which is often preferred to oxalated blood, the blood is collected and gently but thoroughly shaken in a bottle containing sodium citrate 60 mg /10 ml of blood, e.g. 0.3 ml of a 20% solution of sodium citrate.

The sterile blood is immediately distributed in 5 or 10 ml amounts in sterile ½ oz screw-capped bottles and stored in the refrigerator. It will keep for up to 2 months. It must not be allowed to freeze or the cells may be lysed.

Sterile horse blood can be obtained commercially. Alternatively blood may be collected from rabbits and other laboratory animals, sheep, oxen and horses at the abattoir or from man.

Human or animal blood may contain antibiotics. These can be detected by testing with a bacterium sensitive to a wide range of antibiotics. Donor blood sometimes contains glucose and is unsuitable for some purposes. Even screened human blood may contain hepatitis viruses or human retroviruses and strict precautions should be taken when handling it (see Marmion & Tonkin 1972; and Ch. 15 of this book).

Small amounts of blood may be obtained from rabbits, up to 20–30 ml from the ear vein and about 50 ml/kg body weight by cardiac puncture. The procedures for withdrawing blood aseptically in these ways are described in Chapter 14.

Serum

Serum for use in media need not be collected with aseptic precautions because it can be filter-sterilized. Sterile animal sera can be obtained commercially.

Serum may also be prepared from unsterile defibrinated or oxalated blood.

Serum is sterilized by filtration through a suitable membrane filter or Seitz filter. It may be stored at 3–5°C in the refrigerator until required for use.

Serum, like blood, may contain antibiotics or hepatitis viruses.

DEHYDRATED CULTURE MEDIA

Several manufacturers (e.g. Oxoid, Lab M, Difco, BBL) prepare numerous culture media in dehydrated form. Although in general they are not equal in quality to freshly made media they are significantly labour-saving, being easy to reconstitute for use. However, claims that dehydrated media are absolutely constant and reliable cannot be substantiated. Microbiologists who use dehydrated media must be constantly vigilant, rejecting media whose performance falls below standards that have already been achieved and also encouraging improvements. As a minimum a small batch from every bottle of medium should be tested before it is taken into use, noting colony size and germination rate as well as the ability of the medium to perform any special function. More stringent quality control tests such as those recommended by Stokes (1968) or Cowan (1974) are advisable (see also Anderson & Faine 1971).

Dehydrated media tend to deteriorate during storage. Storage conditions should comply with the manufacturer's instructions or, if unspecified, should be cool and dry. There must be adequate mixing and solubilization of dehydrated ingredients. Quality control by the exchange of simulated clinical specimens (Stokes & Ridgway 1980), though aimed primarily at evaluating the standard of laboratory methods, will also tend to sustain the standard of dehydrated media.

It is a false economy to use any but a first-class basal medium. Enrichment with natural products, such as blood, does not compensate for a poor base. The basal medium should be suitable for enrichment for special purposes such as to show haemolysis, particularly by streptococci, and to grow fastidious species. A suggested minimum of four dehydrated culture media for primary cultivation of specimens in a diagnostic laboratory is:

1. *Nutrient broth*. A broth base from which nutrient broth, cooked meat broth, etc., can be made, e.g. Nutrient Broth No. 2 (Oxoid).

2. *Nutrient agar*. Used to make blood agar, heated blood agar, etc., e.g. Columbia Agar (Oxoid).

3. *MacConkey agar*. A medium without added sodium chloride is chosen as this inhibits the spreading of *Proteus* spp., e.g. MacConkey agar without salt (Oxoid). Sodium chloride can be added if especially desired.

4. *Sensitivity test agar*. An 'ordinary' nutrient agar is not suitable for antibiotic sensitivity testing as various inhibitors may be present. Diagnostic Sensitivity Test Agar (Oxoid) is widely used.

The dehydrated media listed are those with which the authors are familiar. Additional special media can be added to suit local conditions.

RECIPES FOR CULTURE MEDIA

The recipes for a range of general bacteriological culture media are given here. Special media, and media for virological, mycological and protozoological use, are discussed in the relevant chapters.

The recipes that follow are for the use of laboratories that still prefer to prepare their own media from fresh ingredients, a practice that one hopes will continue long enough to ensure that dehydrated media are as good as, if not better than, the freshly made media that they replace. Dehydrated cooked meat broth tends to be particularly defective.

Davis and Mingioli minimal medium and its variants

This completely synthetic defined medium is suitable for growth of a wide variety of bacteria for research purposes.

Basal medium

Glucose, sterile 10% solution	20 ml
Dipotassium hydrogen phosphate, K_2HPO_4	7 g
Potassium dihydrogen phosphate, KH_2PO_4	3 g
Sodium citrate, $Na_3C_6H_5O_7.2H_2O$	0.5 g
Magnesium sulphate, $MgSO_4.7H_2O$	0.1 g
Ammonium sulphate, $(NH_4)_2SO_4$	1 g
Agar, if required	20 g
Distilled water to	1 litre

Trace element solution

Ferrous sulphate, $FeSO_4.7H_2O$	0.5 g
Zinc sulphate, $ZnSO_4.7H_2O$	0.5 g
Manganese sulphate, $MnSO_4.3H_2O$	0.5 g
Sulphuric acid, H_2SO_4, 0.1 mol/litre	10 ml
Distilled water	1 litre

Since glucose is partly decomposed when autoclaved in the presence of phosphate, it is added as a sterile solution after the remainder of the medium has been autoclaved.

Essential minerals other than those in the basal medium are likely to be present in sufficient amounts contaminating agar, water and other ingredients. If necessary, 5 ml of the trace element solution and also 1 ml of a 1% calcium chloride solution may be added per litre of medium.

The large phosphate content is required to buffer the acid that is formed by fermentation of glucose, the mixture shown giving a pH of 7.1. If it is required that the phosphate content of the medium should be low, a citrate or bicarbonate buffer may be used. Thus a pH of 7.1 is obtained by incorporation of $NaHCO_3$ 0.3% in the medium and incubation of the culture in an atmosphere containing 20% carbon dioxide.

Other sugars may be substituted for the glucose. The citrate may be omitted. Particular amino acids or growth factors may be added, or a mixture of the essential amino acids in the form of a vitamin-free casein hydrolysate to give a nearly defined medium.

BASAL MEDIA

Nutrient broths form the basis of most media used in the study of the common pathogenic bacteria. They should be of the best quality possible, because enrichment does not fully compensate for a poor basal medium. There are three types of nutrient broth: meat infusion broth consisting of a watery extract of lean meat to which peptone is added; meat extract broth prepared as a mixture of commercial peptone and meat extract; and digest broth consisting of a watery extract of lean meat that has been digested with a proteolytic enzyme so that additional peptone need not be added. Digest broths are economical and are good for obtaining luxuriant growths of exacting organisms. However, cultures tend to die out rapidly in them. The proteolytic enzyme may be trypsin or papain, attention being paid to the optimum temperature and pH for activity of the enzyme.

Meat infusion broth

Lean meat, ox heart or beef	500 g
Water	1 litre
Peptone	10–20 g
Sodium chloride, NaCl	5 g

The type of meat used is an important factor in determining the quality of the broth. It should be fresh, not frozen. Horse flesh is cheap, but is usually not so fresh, and, coming from older animals, is more fibrous than beef. In addition it contains a higher percentage of fermentable sugar which may make the broth unsuitable for many purposes, such as the preparation of toxins.

Carefully remove all fat from the meat and mince it as finely as possible. Add the minced meat to the water and extract for 24 h in the cold, for example in the refrigerator, then strain through muslin and squeeze the meat residue. The extract is bright red and often has a thin surface layer of fat which can be removed by skimming with a piece of filter paper. Boil for 15 min or steam at 100°C for 2 h. The extract becomes brown and turbid because haemoglobin is altered and soluble proteins are coagulated. Filter through a Whatman No. 1 paper. If filtration is done when the medium is hot, it may be necessary to use a hardened filter paper. The extract should be clear and light yellow in colour. Make the volume up to 1 litre with water, add the peptone and salt and dissolve by heating. Filter. The reaction of the broth will be acid because of lactic acid from the meat. Adjust to the desired pH, usually 7.5, which will give a final pH of 7.4 when cold; distribute to tubes or bottles and sterilize by autoclaving at 121°C for 15 min.

Meat extract broth

Peptone	10 g
Meat extract (Lab-Lemco, Oxoid)	10 g
Sodium chloride, NaCl	5 g
Water	1 litre

Mix the ingredients and dissolve them by heating briefly in the steamer. When cool, adjust the pH to 7.5–7.6. A precipitate of phosphates may appear and this may be removed by filtration through filter paper. If clarity of the broth is essential, the mixture should be adjusted to pH 8.0, heated at 100°C for 30 min to precipitate most of the phosphates, cooled, filtered and finally adjusted to pH 7.5. Distribute in tubes or bottles and sterilize by autoclaving at 121°C for 15 min.

The medium should be clear. The presence of a deposit, generally of phosphates, does not interfere with the nutrient value of the medium, but it may hinder the recognition of slight bacterial growth indicated by a developing turbidity.

Hartley's digest broth

Pancreatic extract

Fresh pig pancreas	500 g
Water	1500 ml
Absolute alcohol or methylated spirit	500 ml
Concentrated hydrochloric acid, HCl	c. 2 ml

Remove fat, mince the pancreas and mix it with the water and alcohol. Shake the mixture thoroughly in a large stoppered bottle and allow it to stand for 3 days at room temperature, shaking occasionally. Strain through muslin and filter through paper. Measure the volume of the filtrate and add the concentrated HCl to give a final concentration of 0.1%. This causes a cloudy precipitate which settles in a few days and can be filtered off, although this is not essential.

This extract keeps for about 2 months in stoppered bottles in the cold. If used at once there is no need to add acid, whose action is to retard the slow deterioration of the trypsin.

Preparation of complete medium

Lean meat, ox heart or beef	1500 g
Water	2500 ml
Sodium carbonate, Na$_2$CO$_3$, 0.8% solution	2500 ml
Pancreatic extract	50 ml
Chloroform	50 ml
Concentrated hydrochloric acid, HCl	40 ml

Mix the minced meat and water and heat them in the steam sterilizer until a temperature of

80°C is reached. Add the sodium carbonate, cool to 45°C and add the pancreatic extract and chloroform. Incubate the mixture at 37°C for 6 h or 45°C for 3 h, stirring frequently. When digestion is complete, add the acid, steam at 100°C for 30 min and filter. The broth is stored in an acid condition in 5-litre screw-capped bottles with 0.25% of chloroform. Shake vigorously and frequently in the next 2 or 3 days. Store in a cool, dark place.

For use, adjust to pH 8.0 with sodium hydroxide 1 mol/litre and steam at 100°C for 1 h to precipitate phosphates. Filter while hot and allow to cool. Adjust the reaction to pH 7.6, distribute and autoclave at 115°C for 20 min.

Horse flesh digest broth

This medium is specially suitable for cultivating haemolytic streptococci when an abundant growth is required.

Horse flesh	900 g
Water	3500 ml
Sodium carbonate, Na_2CO_3	12 g
Pancreatin	17.5 g
Concentrated hydrochloric acid, HCl	20 ml
Peptone, high quality	35 g
Calcium chloride, $CaCl_2$	4.4 g
Sodium bicarbonate, $NaHCO_3$	7 g

Mince the meat and mix it with 1500 ml of cold water, raising the temperature to 80°C. Add the remainder of the cold water and the sodium carbonate. Adjust the pH to 8.0, add the pancreatin and keep the mixture at 56°C for 6 h. Add the acid, boil at 100°C for 30 min to arrest digestion and filter. Add the peptone, adjust the pH to 8.0, add the calcium chloride, steam and filter when cold. Add the sodium bicarbonate and filter through a Seitz filter.

Store in bottles. Sterility checks on representative samples are of special importance with filter-sterilized media.

Nutrient agar

Nutrient agar is nutrient broth solidified by the addition of agar. It should be noted that nutrient agar is frequently referred to as 'agar', the context making clear that the agar-broth mixture is meant and not the pure, non-nutritive agar itself. Japanese agar yields a gel of suitable firmness at a concentration of about 2% and New Zealand agar at about 1.2%.

Semi-solid agar

For special purposes agar is added to media in concentrations that are too low to solidify them. At 0.2–0.5% it yields a semi-solid medium through which motile, but not non-motile, bacteria may spread. The actual concentration of the agar used for this purpose must be determined by careful experiment; the choice is influenced by such factors as the quality of the agar and the ingredients and method of preparation of the medium. At 0.05–0.1%, agar prevents convection currents and retards the diffusion of air into media used for anaerobic and micro-aerophilic organisms.

Firm agar

If agar is added to media in concentrations greater than that necessary for solidification, 'spreading' bacteria such as *Proteus vulgaris* and *Clostridium tetani* will grow as discrete colonies. The necessary concentration must be determined by experiment but 6% of Japanese agar and 4% of New Zealand agar are usually satisfactory. Firm agar takes longer to dissolve and to cool and is more difficult to handle than agar at ordinary concentrations.

Peptone water

The medium is used chiefly as the basis for carbohydrate fermentation media (see Ch. 8). Nutrient broths may contain a small amount of sugar derived from meat and it is essential that the basal medium to which various carbohydrates are added for fermentation tests should be free from natural sugars. It is also used to test the formation of indole.

Peptone	10 g
Sodium chloride, NaCl	5 g
Water	1 litre

Dissolve the ingredients in warm water, adjust

the pH to 7.4–7.5 and filter. Distribute as required and autoclave at 121°C for 15 min.

ENRICHED CULTURE MEDIA

Blood agar

Blood agar is widely used in medical bacteriology. In addition to being an enriched medium, it is an indicator medium showing the haemolytic properties of bacteria such as *Streptococcus pyogenes*. It is generally poured as plates.

The medium is prepared by adding sterile blood to sterile nutrient agar that has been melted and cooled to 50°C. The appropriate amount of blood can be poured from a screw-capped bottle. No pipette is necessary as the screw cap keeps the lip of the bottle sterile.

The concentration of blood may be varied from 5–50% for special purposes; 10% is the most usual concentration. Either human or animal blood may be used. Horse blood is the commonest, and safety considerations have excluded the use of human blood for culture work in many laboratories.

A fairly thick layer of medium is required to prevent excessive drying during incubation and if this consists entirely of 10% blood agar, the medium is almost opaque when viewed by transmitted light and haemolysis is difficult to see. Double-layer blood agar overcomes this difficulty. A thin layer of melted nutrient agar, about 7 ml for a 9 cm Petri dish, is poured and allowed to set. Then a similar thin layer of 10% blood agar is poured on top of the first layer. Any bubbles caused by the mixing of the blood and agar can easily be removed by drawing a Bunsen flame quickly across the surface of the medium in the dish.

Blood broth

Nutrient broth to which 5–10% of blood has been added with sterile precautions is occasionally used as an enriched liquid medium.

Heated blood agar ('chocolate agar')

This medium is suitable for *Haemophilus influenzae* and other fastidious organisms such as the neisseriae and the pneumococcus. During heating the red cells are ruptured and nutrients are liberated.

It is prepared by heating 10% of sterile blood in sterile nutrient agar. Melt the agar, cool it in a waterbath at 75°C, add the blood and allow the medium to remain at 75°C, mixing the blood and agar by gentle agitation from time to time until the blood becomes chocolate-brown in colour, within about 10 min. Then pour as slopes or plates.

Lysed blood agar

This medium is suitable for subculture of gonococci and has been used in sulphonamide sensitivity tests.

Lysed blood. Blood can be lysed by heating at 55–56°C for approximately 1 h, or by alternate freezing and thawing, or by treatment with saponin (Ch. 21).

Preparation of complete medium

Nutrient agar	100 ml
Lysed blood	10–20 ml

Melt the nutrient agar, cool to 50°C, add the lysed blood and pour plates.

Serum agar and broth

Serum agar is generally used as slopes.

It is prepared by adding 10% of sterile serum to sterile nutrient agar that has been melted and cooled to 55°C. In an emergency, a useful but less satisfactory serum medium can be made by running a few drops of sterile serum over the surface of a nutrient agar slope or plate.

Serum broth is prepared by adding 10% of sterile serum to sterile nutrient broth.

Egg yolk agar

This medium and other modifications for lecithinase (phospholipase-C) tests are described in Chapters 8 and 37.

Fildes agar and broth

Fildes peptic digest of blood is added to nutrient broth or agar in the proportion of 2–5% after heating at 55°C for 30 min to remove the chloroform. It stimulates the growth of *Haemophilus* and *Clostridium tetani* and the toxin production of *C. perfringens*.

Fildes peptic digest of blood. Peptic digestion of blood liberates nutrients from red cells. Fildes digest is prepared as follows:

Sodium chloride, NaCl, 0.85%	150 ml
Hydrochloric acid, HCl, pure	6 ml
Defibrinated sheep blood	50 ml
Pepsin (B.P. granulated)	1 g
Sodium hydroxide, NaOH, 20% aqueous	*c.* 12 ml
Chloroform	0.5 ml

In a stoppered bottle, mix the saline, acid, blood and pepsin. Heat at 55°C overnight. Then adjust the pH to 7.0 with the NaOH solution. Add the chloroform and shake the mixture vigorously.

This peptic digest of blood keeps well for months.

Glucose agar and broth

Glucose added to nutrient media promotes luxuriant growth of many organisms. It also acts as a reducing agent, and glucose agar is used for deep stab and shake cultures of anaerobes.

If glucose is added before autoclaving the medium, some darkening of it may occur. It is better to prepare a 20% solution of glucose separately, add a drop of phosphoric acid to ensure that the pH is not more than 7.0, and autoclave at 115°C for 20 min; this sterile glucose solution can then be added aseptically to the sterile basal medium.

Concentrations of 0.1, 0.25 and 1% glucose are used; 1% is the commonest.

Glucose blood agar

The incorporation of blood 5–10% (v/v) in glucose agar produces a rich medium for special purposes. Prompt acid production by cultures in this medium may be a disadvantage.

Todd Hewitt meat infusion broth (modified from Todd & Hewitt 1932)

This enriched broth contains glucose 0.2% and is adjusted to pH 7.8. It is of use for the luxuriant growth of organisms such as streptococci.

Meat, minced	450 g
Water	1 litre

Stir the meat in the water and leave at 4°C overnight to give an infusion broth; remove the fat and heat the meat particles and the broth at 85°C for 30 min. Filter out the meat particles and adjust the volume of the filtered broth to 1 litre. Add the following ingredients in the order stated.

Peptone	20 g
NaOH, 10 mol/litre	2.7 ml
NaHCO$_3$	2 g
Glucose	2 g
Na$_2$HPO$_4$.12H$_2$O	1 g
NaCl	2 g

Heat gently to 100°C and boil for 30 min; adjust to pH 7.8, re-filter to remove precipitated phosphates and sterilize at 115°C for 20 min.

Mueller Hinton agar

This medium was originally formulated for the isolation of pathogenic *Neisseria* species (Mueller & Hinton 1941). Nowadays it is more commonly used in conjunction with high potency antibiotic disks, for the determination of antibiotic sensitivity patterns by the Kirby-Bauer technique (Bauer et al 1966, see Ch. 9).

Beef infusion	300 ml
Casein hydrolysate	17.5 g
Starch	1.5 g
Agar	10 g
Distilled water to	1 litre

Emulsify the starch in a small amount of cold water, pour into the beef infusion and add the casein hydrolysate and the agar. Make up the volume to 1 litre with distilled water. Dissolve the constituents by heating gently at 100°C with agitation. Filter if necessary. Adjust the pH to 7.4. Dispense in screw-capped bottles and sterilize by autoclaving at 121°C for 20 min. Pour plates.

Loeffler serum medium

This medium is especially useful for cultivation of the diphtheria bacillus, producing luxuriant growth in 12–18 h with characteristic staining of the organism by Neisser's and Albert's methods (Ch. 3). It is also used to show proteolytic properties, particularly of *Clostridium* species.

Sterile ox, sheep or horse serum	300 ml
Nutrient broth	100 ml
Glucose	1 g

Dissolve the glucose in the broth and autoclave at 115°C for 20 min. Add the glucose broth to the serum with sterile precautions and distribute in sterile test tubes or in 2.5 ml amounts in sterile $\frac{1}{4}$ oz bottles. To inspissate, tubes are laid on a sloped tray but bottles are laid flat with the caps tightly screwed on. The temperature is then slowly raised to 80–85°C and maintained for 2 h, when the serum coagulates to a yellowish-white solid.

If an inspissator is not available, the serum may be coagulated by placing the slanted tubes at the top of a steam sterilizer, where the temperature is a little below 100°C, for 5–7 min. Overheating causes expansion of air bubbles and the formation of steam from the fluid droplets in the partially solidified material, leading to disruption of the medium.

Inspissated medium should be allowed to cool before being handled. Medium in screw-capped bottles can be stored for a long period of time.

Cooked meat broth

The original medium is known as 'Robertson's bullock-heart medium', but the following modification of Lepper & Martin (1929) is recommended. It is suitable for growing anaerobes in air and also for the preservation of stock cultures of aerobic organisms. The inoculum is introduced deep in the medium in contact with the meat.

When cooked meat broth is to be used as a *recovery* medium for spores, following heat resistance tests, or prolonged storage of cultures, the incorporation of a little soluble starch or serum in the medium is an improvement, presumably because the inhibitory effect of fatty acids is thus neutralized.

Fresh bullock heart	500 g
Water	500 ml
Sodium hydroxide, 1 mol/litre	1.5 ml

Mince the heart, place in the alkaline boiling water and simmer for 20 min to neutralize the lactic acid. Drain off the liquid through a muslin filter and, while still hot, press the minced meat in a cloth and dry partially by spreading it on a cloth or filter paper. In this condition it can be introduced into bottles without soiling them.

Peptone infusion broth

Liquid filtered from cooked meat	500 ml
Peptone	2.5 g
Sodium chloride, NaCl	1.25 g

Steam at 100°C for 20 min, add 1 ml pure hydrochloric acid and filter. Bring the reaction of the filtrate to pH 8.2, steam at 100°C for 30 min and adjust reaction to pH 7.8.

Preparation of complete medium. Place meat in 1 oz bottles to a depth of about 2.5 cm and cover with about 15 ml nutrient broth. Autoclave at 121°C for 20 min. After sterilization, the pH of the broth over the meat is about 7.5. If test tubes are used the surface of the medium may be covered with a 1 cm layer of sterile liquid paraffin, but this is not essential.

A tall column of meat is essential because conditions are anaerobic only where there are meat particles. There need be only sufficient broth to extend about 1 cm above the meat.

The use of commercially available dried meat particles is not recommended. However, a good nutrient broth, e.g. Oxoid No. 2, serves well in place of the home-made peptone infusion broth described above.

Thioglycollate broth

In addition to a reducing agent and semi-solid agar, this medium contains methylene blue or resazurin to act as an oxidation-reduction potential indicator which should show that the medium is anaerobic except in the surface layer.

Any nutrient broth can be made anaerobic in this way. The formula given here is that prescribed in the Pharmacopeia of the USA (1970) for sterility tests. It contains only half (0.05%) the usual concentration of sodium thioglycollate (0.1%).

Yeast extract, water soluble	5 g
Casein hydrolysate, pancreatic digest	15 g
Glucose	5.5 g
L-cystine	0.5 g
Agar	0.75 g
Sodium chloride, NaCl	2.5 g
Sodium thioglycollate (mercapto-acetate)	0.5 g
Resazurin sodium solution, 1 in 1000, freshly prepared	1 ml
Water	1 litre

Dissolve the ingredients other than thioglycollate and resazurin by steaming at 100°C. Add the thioglycollate and adjust the pH to 7.3. If there is a precipitate, heat without boiling and filter hot through moistened filter paper. Add the resazurin solution, mix thoroughly, distribute and sterilize at 121°C for 15 min. Cool at once to 25°C and store in the dark, preferably between 20°C and 30°C. Do not use the medium if it has evaporated enough to affect its fluidity. If more than the upper third is pink in colour, anaerobic conditions may be restored once only by steaming at 100°C for a few minutes.

MacConkey agar

This is a useful medium for the cultivation of enterobacteria. It contains a bile salt to inhibit non-intestinal bacteria and lactose with neutral red to distinguish the lactose fermenting coliforms from the lactose-non-fermenting salmonella and dysentery groups. The concentration of sodium taurocholate may be reduced to suit less tolerant organisms. The omission of sodium chloride from the medium prevents the spreading of Proteus colonies.

Peptone	20 g
Sodium taurocholate, commercial	5 g
Water	1 litre
Agar	20 g
Neutral red solution, 2% in 50% ethanol	c. 3.5 ml
Lactose, 10% aqueous solution	100 ml

Dissolve the peptone and taurocholate (bile salt) in the water by heating. Add the agar and dissolve it in the steamer or autoclave. If necessary, clear by filtration. Adjust the pH to 7.5. Add the lactose and the neutral red, which should be well shaken before use, and mix. Heat in the autoclave with 'free steam' (c. 100°C) for 1 h, then at 115°C for 15 min. Pour plates.

The medium should be a distinct reddish-brown colour. When the medium is stored for any length of time the neutral red indicator tends to fade. To overcome this the medium is made up and stored without neutral red, indicator being added and thoroughly mixed before pouring plates.

MEDIA FOR BLOOD CULTURE

There is a wide range of media used for blood culture; factors that govern the choice are discussed in Chapter 7. The media described here represent a range from which selections may be made, but individual variations and permutations are numerous. Many commercially produced media are available in specially designed containers (see Ch. 7).

Brain heart infusion broth with cooked meat particles (BHI/CMP)

This medium allows the growth of nutritionally exacting aerobic and/or anaerobic bacteria. Brain Heart Infusion Broth (BHI, Oxoid) is distributed into bottles containing meat particles prepared from fresh meat as described for cooked meat broth medium (above). A 4 oz medical flat bottle should contain a 2.5 cm layer of cooked meat particles overlaid with 70 ml BHI broth. Each bottle has a perforated metal screw cap with a black rubber liner. A protective foil cap is fitted over the screw cap before autoclaving.

If the filled bottles are autoclaved (121°C, 20 min) with the caps loose and subsequently tightened as soon as they are cool enough to handle so that a partial vacuum is created on further cooling (Collee et al 1977), this makes the medium particularly suitable for the culture of anaerobes; however, small numbers of airborne contaminants may be introduced during the cooling stage and the very low level of contamination may be missed at the quality control stage. We have found it safer to autoclave the bottles with the caps tight. The cooked meat medium is adequately reduced for anaerobic work by this amended procedure, but its shelf-life is less prolonged.

An alternative way to protect the exposed outside surface of the rubber liner in the perforated cap is to apply a plastic Viskap (see *Medical Microbiology*, Vol. 2, 12th Edn, p. 163), but contamination of the liner sometimes occurs with this procedure.

Brain heart infusion broth

This is reconstituted from the dehydrated form according to the manufacturer's instructions (e.g. Oxoid). The medium is not particularly suitable for the isolation of anaerobes. Miniature bottles (1 oz) of this medium have a place in blood culture methodology for young children and neonates from whom small volumes of blood are taken and in whom anaerobic pathogens are not commonly encountered.

Distribute the reconstituted broth in 20 ml amounts into 1 oz medical flat bottles with perforated screw caps and rubber liners. Autoclave with caps tight at 121°C for 20 min. The exposed area of the liner in the perforation should be covered with a foil cap added before autoclaving.

Thioglycollate broth

This medium (see above) supports the growth of anaerobes and aerobes and has been used as described or in modified form by many workers for blood culture purposes. It is more easily prepared but slightly less effective than BHI/CMP medium (Ganguli et al 1982).

Castaneda medium

The original medium provided both solid and liquid phases in one blood culture bottle for the isolation of brucellae from blood. A suitable version for this purpose is given here. It should be noted that the technique is applicable to any blood culture and that there are many other systems that now combine a solid and liquid phase (Ch. 7), including the Roche Septi-Check assembly.

Solid phase. About 30 ml of sterile glucose serum agar (see above) is allowed to set with aseptic precautions on one of the narrow sides of a sterile 4 oz medical flat bottle (Fig. 6.4).

Liquid phase. Sterile glucose serum broth (*c.* 20 ml) is aseptically added to each bottle when the agar has solidified.

The complete medium, in bottles sealed with a rubber liner and a perforated screw cap protected with a foil cap, should be incubated at 37°C for several days as a sterility check before use.

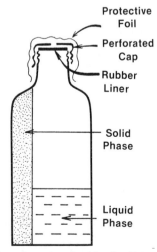

Fig. 6.4 Castaneda system for blood culture.

Saponin broth

This is a special medium for viridans streptococci which may be slightly sensitive to Liquoid. Citrate prevents clotting and saponin causes immediate lysis of the patient's blood.

Sodium citrate, $Na_3C_6H_5O_7.2H_2O$	2 g
Saponin, white (BDH)	1 g
Nutrient broth, sterile	1 litre

This medium cannot be heated above 100°C and care should be taken in making it to reduce contamination to a minimum. Dissolve the ingredients and check that the pH is 7.6. Distribute and heat in steam at 100°C for 20 min on each of three successive days.

Liquoid broth

Liquoid (sodium polyanethol sulphonate) is a good anticoagulant because it is generally not inhibitory and it has the added advantage of annulling the natural bactericidal action of blood. It is obtainable from Sigma, Kodak or Koch Light.

Liquoid solution, 5% in 0.85% NaCl in water	10 ml
Nutrient broth	1 litre

Mix the ingredients and check that the pH is 7.6. Distribute and sterilize at 121°C for 15 min. The final concentration of Liquoid is 0.05%.

Blood culture medium with p-aminobenzoic acid

There may be enough sulphonamide in the bloodstream or other body fluids of patients treated with sulphonamide compounds to prevent the growth of bacteria when culture is carried out. Sulphonamides are antagonized by p-aminobenzoic acid and its addition to the medium will prevent the bacteriostatic action of the sulphonamide. It has also been found valuable in media for the isolation of pathogenic cocci and, even if no sulphonamide has been administered, p-aminobenzoic acid improves the nutritive qualities of the medium.

p-Aminobenzoic acid is stable and withstands autoclaving. It is added in the proportion of 5–10 mg/100 ml of medium.

Blood culture medium with penicillinase

Benzylpenicillin, phenoxymethyl penicillin or ampicillin (amoxycillin) present in specimens from patients on treatment can be destroyed by penicillinase. 1 ml of penicillinase solution (Wellcome) inactivates 100 000 units of penicillin. A suitable dilution containing 0.01 ml of the solution should be added with aseptic precautions to 100 ml of sterile broth for blood culture. Broad spectrum β-lactamases also active against some cephalosporins are available (e.g. from Sigma).

MEDIA FOR PRESERVATION AND STORAGE OF CULTURES

The choice of media used for storage or maintenance of bacteria is dictated by experience and takes account of the special requirements of the species and the strain. For general purposes, cooked meat broth, nutrient agar slopes, semi-solid nutrient agar stabs, blood agar or heated blood agar slopes in small screw-capped bottles often serve well. A few special media are given here.

Egg saline medium

The modification of Dorset's egg medium, in which the broth is replaced by saline and no malachite green is added, is good for preserving cultures of Gram-negative bacilli.

Beaten whole egg	75 ml
Sodium chloride, NaCl, sterile 0.85% solution	25 ml

Prepare the beaten egg, mix and dispense the medium with sterile precautions in 2–3 ml amounts in bijou bottles. Inspissate in a slanted position at 75–80°C for 1 h.

If the medium has been prepared without sterile precautions it can be allowed to cool for a few hours after inspissation and then autoclaved at 121°C for 15 min with the screw caps tightened. If the screw caps are loose, some of the slants may be disrupted by bubbles of steam.

Chalk cooked meat broth

This modification of cooked meat broth is intended for the preservation of stock cultures of clostridia.

Calcium carbonate, $CaCO_3$, 0.1 g and possibly also some minced cooked egg white is added to each bottle of cooked meat broth before the final autoclaving.

Enriched media for maintenance of Haemophilus and Neisseria and other fastidious organisms

A semi-solid medium prepared by adding 2 parts of nutrient broth to 1 part of molten nutrient agar at 50°C is supplemented with serum 10% for fastidious *Neisseria* spp., or Fildes peptic digest broth 10% for *Haemophilus* spp.

The sterile medium is aseptically dispensed in 3 ml amounts into bijou bottles. When seeded with the culture, the medium is overlaid with sterile liquid paraffin (Baker & Breach 1980).

TRANSPORT MEDIA

When the patient is not close to the bacteriological laboratory there is a risk that the pathogen in a bacteriological specimen may not survive or may be overgrown by non-pathogens during the time it takes to transport the specimen to the laboratory. Some media have been devised to protect pathogens during such a delay. Sterile disposable swab kits incorporating Amies transport medium with or without charcoal are commercially available (e.g. Exogen, Medical Wire). We have found them very useful for the submission of specimens by general practitioners.

Stuart's transport medium

This soft agar medium is used to maintain the viability of gonococci on swabs during their transmission through the post to a laboratory.

It is essential that the distilled water used in the medium be free from chlorine. To ensure this, it should be passed through an ion-exchange resin column before use.

Sodium thioglycollate (mercapto-acetate)	1 g
Sodium glycerophosphate	10 g
Calcium chloride, $CaCl_2$	0.1 g
Agar (Oxoid No. 1)	6 g
Methylene blue, 0.1% aqueous	4 ml
Distilled water	1 litre

Dissolve all the solids in the distilled water at 100°C. Adjust the pH to 7.3–7.4. Add the methylene blue solution and distribute in bijou bottles, filling nearly full. Autoclave at 121°C for 15 min and immediately tighten caps. When cool, the medium should be colourless.

Preparation of swabs. Take swabs of absorbent cotton wool on applicator sticks and boil for 5 min in phosphate buffer 0.07 mol/litre at pH 7.4. Shake off excess moisture and immerse in a 1% watery suspension of finely powdered charcoal, such as BDH activated charcoal, twirling until the cotton wool is black. Shake off excess moisture, place in test tubes, plug these with cotton wool, dry in oven and sterilize in oven at 160°C for 90 min.

Alternatively, use charcoal-treated swabs obtained commercially.

Amies transport medium (Amies 1967)

As patients dislike the use of swabs impregnated with charcoal in Stuart's system, Amies incorporated the charcoal into his modified medium, of which several variations are commercially produced.

Sodium thioglycollate (mercapto-acetate)	1 g
Sodium chloride, NaCl	3 g
Potassium chloride, KCl	0.2 g
Calcium chloride, $CaCl_2$	0.1 g
Magnesium chloride, $MgCl_2.6H_2O$	0.1 g
Sodium hydrogen phosphate, Na_2HPO_4	1.15 g
Potassium dihydrogen phosphate, KH_2PO_4	0.2 g

Charcoal (finely powdered)	10 g
Agar (Oxoid No. 1)	4 g
Distilled water	1 litre

Dissolve the chemical salts and the agar in the distilled water at 100°C. Add the charcoal. Check the pH (7.2). Dispense, with regular stirring to keep the charcoal in suspension, into bijou bottles filled nearly full. Autoclave at 121°C for 15 min and cool. Frequent inversion of the bottles during cooling is needed to distribute the charcoal.

Pike's medium

This medium is used to preserve *Streptococcus pyogenes*, pneumococci and *Haemophilus influenzae* in nose and throat swabs. It is blood agar containing crystal violet 1 in 1 000 000 and sodium azide 1 in 16 000 distributed as for stab cultures in tubes or bottles.

Glycerol saline transport medium for typhoid bacilli

If there is likely to be a delay of some hours before specimens of faeces for culture reach the laboratory this transport medium prevents other intestinal organisms from overgrowing the typhoid bacilli.

Glycerol	300 ml
Sodium chloride, NaCl	4.2 g
Disodium hydrogen phosphate, Na_2HPO_4, anhydrous	10 g
Phenol red, 0.02%, aqueous	c. 15 ml
Water	700 ml

Dissolve the sodium chloride in the water and add the glycerol. Add the phosphate and steam to dissolve it. Then add enough phenol red to give a purple-pink colour, judged by pouring a small quantity of the solution into a Universal container. Distribute in 6 ml amounts in Universal containers and autoclave at 115°C for 20 min.

The fluid should not be used if it becomes acid, indicated by a change in colour to yellow.

Identification of culture media

Many methods of identifying and labelling culture media in their containers include the use of marking ink and colour codes etc. For further details, see *Medical Microbiology*, 12th Edition, Volume 2, Chapter 5, p. 146.

STORAGE OF CULTURE MEDIA

Prepared sterilized media in individual screw-capped bottles (e.g. broths and nutrient agars) can be stored at room temperature for weeks, but some deterioration is likely to occur. Poured plates of agar media held on the bench deteriorate quickly and are often contaminated.

It is essential to have some form of cold storage in the laboratory for the preservation of blood, serum and culture media.

For the smaller laboratory, one of the domestic refrigerators of $1-2 m^3$ capacity is suitable; larger laboratories require a correspondingly larger cabinet, or an insulated cold room with the refrigerating plant outside. The temperature should be maintained between 4–5°C (39–41°F); it should never be so low as to cause freezing, as this may be detrimental.

Plates of agar media can be held for short periods not exceeding 7–10 days, but note that changes in hydration with concentration of ingredients may occur, the pH may alter, the Eh changes, and bacterial or fungal contamination can be a problem.

It is also convenient to have 'deep freeze' refrigerators working at low temperatures in the range −10 to −40°C for the preservation of sera and made-up solutions of labile preparations such as antibiotics and amino acids.

QUALITY CONTROL

The quality of microbiological culture media must be assessed as a routine in the laboratory. This applies to media prepared in the laboratory from raw materials and to media reconstituted from commercially available packs or bought in ready-made form. Manufacturers of these dehydrated or ready-to-use media operate their own quality control systems but laboratories should have their own in-house checks. This ensures prompt detection of poor performance that may be attributable to deterioration in storage of the stock, or laboratory errors in weighing and measuring and pH control, or to variations in the quality of the local water or the laboratory's sterilizing procedures. Quality control is advisable before each batch of medium is issued for use – or should be done in parallel with the first issue when fresh media are in regular use.

If the sterility of sterile additives such as blood and serum, and sterile solutions of supplements such as growth factors, is not checked before they are added to a batch of sterile base medium, the sterility of the complete medium cannot be positively assured. In practice, the risk is sometimes taken with products or in-house procedures that have a good record.

Quality control should always be supervised by a senior and experienced member of staff. De-ficiencies or contamination revealed by these checks should be investigated so that the problem is defined and remedied.

For lists of known positive and negative test organisms and advice on methodology, see the following sources:
1. Cowan (1974), Appendices A and E.
2. European Committee for Clinical Laboratory Standards Vol. 4, No. 4. Standard for Quality Assurance, Part 2: Internal Quality Control in Microbiology. Beuth Verlag, Berlin. (In (press.)
3. Stokes & Ridgway (1980), Chapter 10.

These reference cultures have a useful role in this context, but it should be borne in mind that wild strains of demanding species may be more exacting than the stock strains that are used. The reference culture should be inoculated lightly on the medium to be tested, e.g. to give c. 100 colonies per plate. After incubation, the quality and quantity of growth obtained on the test medium should be noted, e.g. number, size and character of colonies, pigment production etc.

REFERENCES

Amies C R 1967 A modified formula for the preparation of Stuart's transport medium. Canadian Journal of Public Health 58: 296–300

Anderson K F, Faine S 1971 Quality control of culture media. College of Pathologists of Australia. Broadsheet No 10

Baker F J, Breach M R 1980 Medical microbiological techniques. Butterworth, London. p. 485

Bauer A W, Kirby W M M, Sherris J C, Turck M 1966 Antibiotic susceptibility testing by a standardized single disc method. American Journal of Clinical Pathology 45: 493–496

Collee J G, Duerden B I, Brown R 1977 Recovery of anaerobic bacteria from small inocula – a model for blood culture studies. Journal of Clinical Pathology 30: 609–614

Cowan S T 1974 Cowan & Steel's Manual for the identification of medical bacteria, 2nd edn. Cambridge University Press

Ganguli L A, Turton L J, Tillotson G S 1982 Evaluation of fastidious anaerobe broth as a culture medium. Journal of Clinical Pathology 35: 458–461

Lepper E, Martin C J 1929 The chemical mechanisms exploited in the use of meat media for the cultivation of anaerobes. British Journal of Experimental Pathology 10: 327–334

Marmion B P, Tonkin R W 1972 Control of hepatitis in dialysis units. British Medical Bulletin 28: 169–179

Mueller J H, Hinton J 1941 A protein-free medium for primary isolation of the gonococcus and meningococcus. Proceedings of the Society of Experimental Biology and Medicine 48: 330–333

Pharmacopeia of the United States of America 1970 18th edn. Sterility tests. p 851

Stokes E J 1968 Quality control in diagnostic bacteriology. Proceedings of the Royal Society of Medicine 61: 457–463

Stokes E J, Ridgway G L 1980 Clinical bacteriology, 5th edn. Arnold, London. p 28–29

Todd E W, Hewitt L F 1932 A new culture medium for the production of antigenic streptococcal haemolysin. Journal of Pathology and Bacteriology 35: 973–974

Cultivation of bacteria

General methods of culture and preservation of microorganisms are described here. Special methods applicable for particular purposes are referred to elsewhere in the appropriate chapters. Personal safety precautions are described in Chapter 15.

INSTRUMENTS USED TO SEED CULTURE MEDIA

The instrument is chosen according to the nature of the medium and inoculum. Inoculating wires are widely used. The original type of inoculating wire was of platinum, No. 23 SWG, 2 in (6.5 cm) long, but 'Nichrome' or 'Eureka' resistance wire, No. 24 SWG, is now generally used. However, nichrome is oxidizing and either stainless steel or platinum-iridium is a better choice for work with anaerobes. One end of the wire is inserted into a special aluminium holder.

The wire is sterilized by holding it vertically in a Bunsen flame so that the whole length becomes red-hot at the same time. A wire charged with particulate growth, such as that of the tubercle bacillus, should be sterilized in a loop incinerator, or a hooded Bunsen burner (Fig. 7.1) to avoid spurting of particles of unsterilized culture from the wire onto the bench.

Wire loop. The free end is bent in the form of a flat, circular and completely closed loop of 2–4 mm internal diameter. This is the most useful of the inoculating wires. It takes up a considerable amount of solid culture or a large drop of liquid. *Note*: Pre-sterilized disposable loops and other applicators made of plastic are

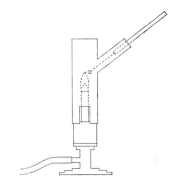

Fig. 7.1 A Bunsen burner hooded with a metal tube to avoid spurting of unsterile particles during flaming of a charged wire loop.

commercially supplied in packs. They are particularly convenient for work in containment cabinets and anaerobic work stations etc., when Bunsen burners cannot be used.

Straight wire. This is used for stab cultures and also for picking off single colonies.

Thick wire (c. No. 60 SWG). Used as a loop, this is more rigid and is very useful for lifting thick viscid sputum; as an L-shaped wire, it is used to handle tenacious growths such as fungal colonies.

Scalpel. A sterile scalpel is used for making inoculations with scrapings from tissues and ulcers.

Sterile pipettes. Graduated 1 ml or 10 ml glass pipettes are used for liquid inocula between 0.1 and 10 ml. These pipettes are stoppered with a cotton-wool plug in their upper end to guard against contamination of their interior, or accidental aspiration of their contents. They are wrapped in paper or placed in a container and sterilized in the hot-air oven. Disposable plastic pipettes are a useful but expensive alternative. Because of the danger of infection, pipettes must not be placed in the mouth, but must be operated by a rubber bulb or an alternative device.

Sterile capillary pipettes. These are made by heating the middle of a piece of glass tubing of 5 mm bore and 20 cm long in a hot Bunsen flame; when the glass has softened, the two ends are pulled out and a thin capillary is produced in the middle. This is nicked with a carborundum disk and broken and two pipettes are obtained. It is important to start with lengths of tubing that have had their ends smoothed by rotation in a hot flame, otherwise injuries frequently occur when teats are being fitted. The capillary ends are cut to a convenient length with a file or carborundum disk and the other smoothed ends are plugged with cotton-wool. They are placed in a container such as a large test tube (e.g. 8 × 1 in, 20.3 × 3.8 cm) which is then stoppered with cotton-wool, or covered with paper or aluminium foil and sterilized by dry heat. An alternative method is to prepare the 20 cm lengths of glass tubing with cotton-wool plugs in each end, wrap them in bundles of 8–10 in Kraft paper, sterilize in the hot-air oven and draw the capillaries in a flame just before they are required for use. These pipettes are useful for the sterile transfer of liquid in volumes that do not need to be measured accurately.

Capillary pipettes delivering measured drops. Small measured volumes are conveniently delivered with sterile capillary pipettes that have been prepared to give drops of a known volume. The pipettes are drawn from glass tubing as described above. When cool, the capillary is inserted into the appropriate hole of a Morse drill gauge and pressed through until it engages. For water drops of 0.020 ml the hole used is Morse 59 (i.e. 0.041 in diameter), for 0.025 ml Morse 55 (0.052 in), for 0.030 ml Morse 52 (0.063 in), for 0.035 ml Morse 47 (0.078 in) and for 0.040 ml Morse 43 (0.089 in). Exactly at its point of impaction in the hole, the capillary is scored with a glass-cutter (e.g. a vulcanite carborundum disk), and broken off squarely. The wide end of each pipette is then plugged with cotton-wool and the pipettes are packed in a large test tube or a small tin and sterilized in the hot-air oven. In use, the liquid is drawn into the pipette by a teat. For accurate work, there should be a good volume of fluid in the pipette which should be held vertically, tip down, and the drops should be expelled at a constant rate of about 40 per minute, i.e. taking about 1 s for the gradual expulsion of one drop. The drop size may differ slightly in the case of liquids with different densities and surface tensions from that of water and the pipette should be calibrated directly for the particular liquid by measuring the volume of 100 drops. For further details consult Miles et al (1938).

Plastic pipettes, pipette tips, constant volume pipettes, repeater pipettes. These and related commercially available devices for the dispensing of a range of small volumes of fluid with accuracy and safety are widely used and for many purposes have replaced glass pipettes.

CULTURE PROCEDURES

The bench should be free from dust and wiped with disinfectant at least before the start of each day's work. Air currents should be reduced to a minimum by closing windows and doors and restricting the movement of people in the room. During inoculation, a culture medium should be uncovered for only a few seconds. The following description applies to operators who are right-handed.

Place the lighted Bunsen burner and inoculating instruments to the right of the bench, and cultures and media to the back and the left. Plate cultures and unseeded plates should be placed with the lid on the bench and the bottom containing the medium uppermost. The caps or plugs of tubes and bottles should be loosened for easy removal.

Media to be seeded should be labelled at this stage, indicating the inoculum and the date, with a glass-marking pen or pencil or self-adhesive label. Labelling should be done on the bottoms of Petri dishes, on tubes and on bottles rather than on lids or caps which can be mistakenly placed on other cultures. Labels should be checked for accuracy while media are being seeded.

During inoculation the right hand holding the inoculating instrument charged with culture material from the specimen should be moved as little as possible and the left hand should bring the media to it.

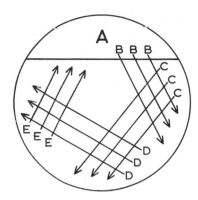

Seeding a plate

It is better to use a loop to seed a plate as a straight wire cuts the agar.

Lift the bottom of the Petri dish containing medium from its lid with the left hand and hold it round the side with thumb and middle finger. In most cases the method of plating-out shown in Figure 7.2 is employed. The inoculum is smeared thoroughly over area A to give a 'well-inoculum' or 'well'. The loop is re-sterilized and then drawn from the well in two or three parallel lines on to the fresh surface of the medium (B, B, B); this process is repeated as shown, care being taken to sterilize the loop, and cool it on unseeded medium, between each sequence. At each step the inoculum is derived from the most distal part of the immediately preceding strokes. Another quicker method of achieving a dilution of the inoculum that is high enough to yield separate colonies is to change to a 4 mm loop after spreading the well, sterilize it and use one side of the loop to spread an area B and the other side as a fresh sterile surface to make a succession of several strokes across the plate as shown in Figure 7.3.

Fig. 7.2 The commonly adopted pattern of plating-out on solid medium. The area A is the well, and successive series of strokes B, C, D and E are made with the loop sterilized between each sequence.

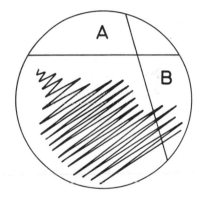

Fig. 7.3 An alternative plating procedure in which one edge of a larger loop is used to make a secondary well B. The other edge is then used to make a succession of strokes across the remaining unseeded area.

When the inoculum is small or the medium is selective it can be more heavily inoculated (Fig. 7.4). Several loopfuls of the specimen are used to spread the well (A); the loop is re-sterilized in a flame, recharged by rubbing it over area A and then used to seed the remainder of the plate by successive parallel strokes, B, C and D, drawn in the directions indicated in the diagram. When this method is used with small inocula or selective media, well separated colonies can be obtained from a heavy inoculation except, of course, in the well of the plate.

Subcultures from liquid media may be distributed with a spreader. This is made by bending a piece of glass rod of 3 mm diameter at a right angle in the blowpipe flame, the short limb used for spreading being 2 cm long. Spreaders may be

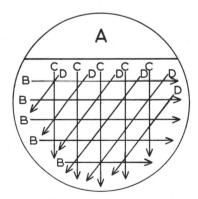

Fig. 7.4 A plating procedure used when the inoculum is scanty or when a highly selective medium is used (see text).

sterilized in the hot-air oven, a number being packed in a metal tin with a 'press-on' lid loosely applied. Alternatively, a sterile capillary pipette or a capillary tube held horizontally may be heated about 1 cm from its tip in the pilot flame of a Bunsen burner. As the glass softens, the end of the pipette bends at right angles and this forms a spreader. The inoculum is placed on the plate with an inoculating loop or capillary pipette and then, with a sterilized spreader, it is evenly distributed over the surface. If a large inoculum is used, incubation will result in a confluent growth called a 'lawn'. Media seeded in this way may be used for disk diffusion tests for assessing sensitivity to antibiotics and other chemothera-peutic agents or for phage typing.

Plating machines are commercially available for the automation of this procedure. The pattern of the rotary seeding procedure may be in spiral form with discrete colonies developing at the central or peripheral end of the track. A variation of this rotary approach is used as a routine for the Stokes' procedure in antimicro-bial sensitivity testing (Ch. 9).

After the plate has been seeded, the bottom of the Petri dish is returned to its lid and the loop is flamed or the capillary pipette is discarded into a jar of disinfectant, care being taken to fill the pipette with the disinfectant. Plates are incubated in the inverted position with the lid underneath.

Seeding a tube fitted with a cotton-wool plug or a metal or plastic cap, or a bottle with a screw cap

It is unwise to attempt to manage more than one tube and its cap at a time. The same applies to bottles with screw caps because of the need for a screwing action to remove them.

In addition, when all tubes had cotton-wool plugs it was the practice to flame the mouths of all tubes before and after any manipulation, because the rims of tubes are not covered by plugs and are probably contaminated; in replacing the plug, organisms could be pushed down from the rim into the tube. The situation is quite different with metal caps and screw caps. Accordingly, flaming of the mouths of tubes and

bottles is not done as a routine, though the prac-tice should be observed after any manipulation with a container that has a cotton-wool plug.

Pick up the tube or bottle with the left hand and remove the cap or plug with the crooked third and fourth fingers of the right hand. Slopes of solid media are seeded by lightly smearing the surface of the agar with the loop or wire in a transverse zig-zag pattern taking care not to cut the agar. Stab cultures in solid media are inoculated by plunging the wire into the centre of the medium and withdrawing it in the same line to avoid splitting the medium. Liquid cultures are usually inoculated from a solid medium by inclining the tube or bottle at an angle of about 45° and depositing the inoculum on its wall above the surface of the liquid at its lower end. When the container is returned to the vertical position, the inoculum is below the surface of the liquid. Capillary pipettes or loops may be used for inoculation from liquid media.

After inoculation withdraw the loop, wire or pipette. Flame the mouth of the tube if it has a cotton-wool plug. Replace the cap or plug and return the tube or bottle to its place, at the same time flaming the loop or wire or discarding the pipette into disinfectant as described above. Check that the cap or plug has been replaced firmly.

Shake cultures

These are made by melting nutrient agar in a test tube, cooling it to 45°C and inoculating it while molten from a liquid medium with a drop from a capillary pipette or a wetted straight wire, depending on the desired size of inoculum. With-draw the pipette or wire and flame the mouth of the tube if it has a cotton-wool plug. Replace the cap or plug and discard the pipette into disinfec-tant or flame the wire. Mix the contents of the tube by rotation between the palms of the hands before the agar solidifies.

Seeding several tubes and bottles of media from a single colony

As in tests for the identification of enterobacteria, it is best to use a wire to pick a single colony.

The media are arranged in order for inoculation, firstly liquid media without carbohydrate, such as peptone water, then liquid media containing carbohydrate, then solid media for stab culture such as motility test medium. The wire charged with inoculum is lightly touched on the moist wall of each tilted liquid medium in turn, then streaked lightly on the solid media and plunged into the deep cultures, and then it is flamed.

Multiple spot inoculation on plates

When large numbers of test strains or reagents are to be spot inoculated on to specially prepared media, as in procedures such as phage typing, bacteriocin testing and sensitivity testing, it is convenient to use a multipoint inoculating device. This may be a hand-held simple array of inoculating loops or points (Brown 1973) or a mechanical multiple inoculator (Denley). The multiple points are charged in wells arranged in a fixed pattern and this is transferred to a plate bearing an orientation mark so that the individual loci can be subsequently identified.

Ørskov's method for studying the morphology of growing bacterial cells

This elegant method allows the maintenance of living cultures under continuous observation so that the development of individual bacteria and also that of colonies can be studied.

Cubes of suitable size not exceeding 3–4 mm in thickness are cut out of an agar plate with a sterilized knife. They are transferred with the knife to a sterilized microscope slide. The agar is now seeded with the organism by a fine stroke. With first a low-power objective the stroke is defined and then with a higher power an area is found where the bacteria lie sufficiently scattered. With a suitable lamp and objective and with the diaphragm closed down, young bacteria appear as strongly refractile and well defined bodies. The area is then registered by means of the vernier scales on the mechanical stage. The slide is removed and placed in a Petri dish with a piece of moist filter paper in the bottom, and the dish is incubated at a suitable temperature. The selected area is then examined at intervals and the changing features observed. In this way the development of individual bacteria can be studied and also that of colonies at each stage. An electrically heated microscope incubator allows a colony to be observed microscopically throughout its period of growth and this is very convenient for these and similar studies.

INOCULATION HOODS OR CABINETS

It is advisable, as far as possible, to carry out some inoculation procedures under a hood, but the operator should clearly understand the operation of the particular system that he employs. Some positively ventilated systems are designed primarily to prevent contamination of the culture and subculture media. For example, Figure 7.5 illustrates a cabinet in which filtered air passes from the back panel to the front. This is useful for the manipulation of sterile media as in dispensing or plate-pouring procedures; it should be noted that this system blows virtually into the face of the operator and must not be used for the

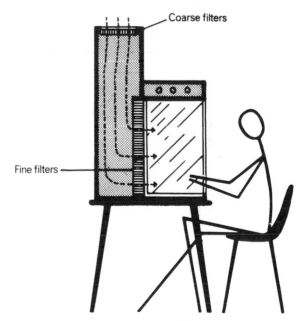

Fig. 7.5 An inoculation cabinet in which a laminar flow of filtered air is delivered at the rear and passes forward over the handling area. Note that this system safeguards the work but must not be used for the manipulation of infective material as the airstream is directed towards the operator.

manipulation of potentially infective material or for cell culture work with tissue cells that may carry infective agents (see Ch. 15).

Whilst there are clear advantages in the use of exhaust protective cabinets for the safety of the operator when special pathogens are handled, the usefulness of a cabinet that does not have positive ventilation, a so-called still air cabinet (Fig. 7.6), merits consideration for general laboratory work that does not involve pathogens assigned to special containment categories. For example, Containment Level 1 work could be done in a still air hood with advantages that include delineation of the area of possible contamination on the bench, and a degree of protection of the media from airborne contaminants. If a gas Bunsen burner is used in

a still-air cabinet, care must be taken to ensure that the burner is not left unattended in the 'on' position or with the pilot light on. The danger is that the flame may blow out and the gas then fills the cabinet; when the operator returns and lights the Bunsen, the cabinet explodes. The solution is to employ a pressure plate device that allows the gas to flow only when the operator's hand rests upon it (e.g. Touchomatic Bunsen, from Horwell or Gibco).

AEROBIC CULTURE

Incubation of cultures at 37°C is standard practice in the culture of bacteria pathogenic to man.

Other temperatures for incubation are 43°C

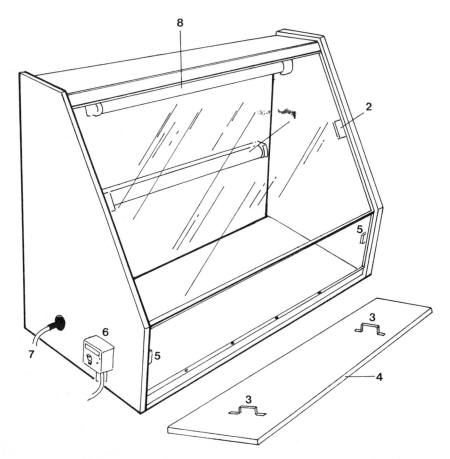

Fig. 7.6 A still air cabinet is useful for general laboratory work. (1) Ultra-violet tube; (2) housing for removable door panel when cabinet is in use; (3) handle; (4) removable door panel held by magnetic catches; (5) magnetic catch; (6) light and/or UV switch; (7) gas inlet; (8) electric light tube.

for campylobacters, 30°C for cultivating leptospires and some bacteria, 25–28°C for many fungi, and 22°C ('cool incubator') for some fungi and for gelatin cultures. Incubators may be heated by electricity, gas or oil, according to the facilities of the laboratory. In some hot countries, a coupled cooling system is needed when the ambient temperature rises above 37°C.

Some laboratories have a warm room kept at 37°C by gas or electricity in which large quantities of material can be incubated. The room has a regulating mechanism similar to that of the ordinary incubator to keep the temperature constant; if electrically heated it should be fitted with a device to cut off the current for the room at the main switch if the temperature rises above 40°C.

In order to prevent drying of the medium when prolonged incubation is necessary, as in the cultivation of the tubercle bacillus, screw-capped bottles should be used instead of test tubes or plates.

Culture in an atmosphere with added carbon dioxide

Capnophilic

Some organisms, such as *Brucella abortus* and capnophilic streptococci require extra CO_2 in the air in which they are grown and others, such as the pneumococcus and gonococcus, grow better in air supplemented with CO_2 5–10%. An anaerobic jar or a similar container can be used for the purpose. Anaerobic jars used in this way should not contain a catalyst and should preferably not serve such a double role as their efficiency is prejudiced. The required amount of air is withdrawn with a vacuum pump and replaced with CO_2 from a cylinder or football bladder as described for anaerobic culture. A simpler method is to generate CO_2 inside the container by lighting a candle in it just before putting on the lid or by adding hydrochloric acid to a marble chip, but the more elegant procedure of adding relatively pure CO_2 gas to a proper container is preferable. An alternative approach for small numbers of cultures is to use a CO_2-generating kit such as those produced by Oxoid or BBL. CO_2 incubators which provide a predetermined and regulated amount of CO_2 in a suitably humid atmosphere are commercially available; they are a preferable approach and should be in general use.

Whichever method is used, screw caps on containers of liquid media must not be tight and should preferably be replaced by a closure that allows entry of CO_2. Petri dishes should be vented.

Culture in a microaerophilic atmosphere

For the culture of truly microaerophilic species such as *Campylobacter jejuni* and *Actinomyces israeli*, an atmosphere of 6–7% O_2 is needed. This can be done by an evacuation replacement method with N_2 as the major replacement gas and 5–10% CO_2. The N_2/CO_2 mixture in this system is preferable to an H_2/CO_2 mixture which is potentially explosive.

When an organism combines a microaerophilic requirement with a CO_2 requirement, as in the case of *C. jejuni*, the candle jar has an apparent advantage; however, the CO_2 concentration in a candle jar is about 17% (see Butzler 1984) and this is not sufficiently low for the growth of pure cultures of a microaerophilic organism. Hence the use of an evacuation procedure is preferred, or convenient commercial alternatives such as the Campy-Pak system (BBL) or the Campylobacter Gas Generating Kit (Oxoid).

ANAEROBIC CULTURE

Obligate anaerobes will not grow from small inocula unless oxygen is absent and the Eh of the medium is low.

Although the routine use of an anaerobic cabinet or gas-flushing system is not essential in clinical bacteriology (see Watt et al 1974), prompt and reliable growth of anaerobes is dependent on care in their handling and incubation. Exposure of the organisms to atmospheric and to dissolved oxygen should be kept to a minimum.

Freshly steamed liquid media are at least temporarily anaerobic. This principle is used when deep nutrient agar with 0.5% glucose is seeded with minimal shaking and solidified rapidly by placing the tube in cold water.

Colonies of anaerobes develop best in the depth of the tube, becoming fewer and smaller towards the surface. Usually there is no growth of strict anaerobes in the top centimetre of medium.

Liquid media soon become aerobic unless a reducing agent is added. Reducing agents include glucose 0.5–1%, ascorbic acid 0.1%, cysteine 0.1%, sodium mercaptoacetate or thioglycollate 0.1%, or the particles of meat in cooked meat broth. Iron strips or ordinary iron nails, sterilized by flaming and dropped while hot into the medium, have been used in the past as an unsophisticated method of providing anaerobic broth, peptone water media, gelatin and milk for immediate use. The associated deposit of iron hydroxide that develops is a disadvantage, and more elegant approaches are preferred.

The effectiveness of reducing agents can be increased by making a liquid medium semi-solid by incorporating agar to 0.05–0.1%. Liquid media should be 'pre-reduced' by holding in a boiling water bath for 10 min to drive off dissolved oxygen, then quickly cooled to 37°C just before use; sterile preparations of heat-labile ingredients should be added after this heat treatment. Cooked meat broth (Ch. 6) has a special place in anaerobic bacteriology, and thioglycollate broth and its modifications are also very useful (Ch. 6, Ch. 36). For the routine surface culture of anaerobes of medical importance, freshly poured blood agar incorporating a good base is recommended (Ch. 36–38) and 10% CO_2 should be present in the anaerobic atmosphere (Watt 1973). After inoculation, both liquid and solid media should be incubated anaerobically with 10% CO_2 at 37°C, either in jars processed by a standard evacuation procedure (Collee et al 1972); or with a proprietary gas generator envelope (Gaskit, Oxoid; or Gaspak, BBL); or in an anaerobic cabinet, as described in detail below.

Care must be taken to achieve pure cultures. For subsequent tests, a single colony is then picked with an inoculating loop to a tube of pre-reduced cooked meat broth (CMB) and incubated anaerobically for 24 h, or until good growth is seen. This starter culture is used to seed all other test media, the inoculum being one drop from a Pasteur pipette (0.02–0.03 ml). Results from most tests can be read after 24 or 48 h incubation, but it may take up to 4 days to obtain reasonable growth of some organisms. Some anaerobes are killed if the plates on which they are beginning to grow are exposed to atmospheric oxygen before visible colonies form. Tests for pigment production should be incubated for up to 7 days, and for gelatin digestion for up to 14 days before being considered negative.

Anaerobic incubation

For cultures on solid media, oxygen must be removed from the atmosphere above the culture either by using it for combustion or by replacing it with an inert gas. It is recommended that all media for growth of anaerobes should be incubated under strictly anaerobic conditions. A technique of repeated evacuation of jars and filling with an inert gas such as nitrogen was popular in the USA. This flushing method tends to dehydrate cultures and it is not suitable for very strict anaerobes.

The removal of oxygen by combustion is nearly always achieved by combining it with hydrogen to form water in the presence of a palladium catalyst. This method was originally used by McIntosh & Fildes (1916) to produce anaerobic conditions for plate cultures in tins or jars by coating asbestos wool with palladium and enclosing it in wire gauze to reduce the risk of explosion by conducting heat away on the Davy lamp principle.

A significant advance was made when Wright (1943) increased the catalytic activity of palladium by presenting to the hydrogen and oxygen in the jar a large surface heavily impregnated with metallic palladium. This was used successfully by Hayward (1945) as a room-temperature catalyst. A full description of the operation of this type of jar is given by Cruickshank (1968).

Heller (1954) advocated the use of Deoxo pellets in which palladium is coated on alumina. This form of the catalyst has now replaced palladiumized asbestos. Deoxo pellets are available from Whitley, and jars incorporating them as a room-temperature catalyst from Baird & Tatlock.

The following procedure is recommended (Collee et al 1971) to provide anaerobiosis with an increased concentration of carbon dioxide in these jars (Fig. 7.7) as CO_2 enhances the growth of many clinically important anaerobes on solid media. The jar (*c*. 20 × 12.5 cm) should be made of metal or robust plastic with a lid that can be clamped down to make it airtight. Glass jars have been used in the past, but, as explosions occasionally occur, their use is not justified. The lid is furnished with two tubes and taps. One or more capsules containing 3–5 g of palladiumized alumina pellets are suspended under the lid.

The most convenient source of hydrogen and carbon dioxide, either individually or as a mixture, is cylinders of the compressed gases supplied commercially. The pressure in these cylinders is too great for them to be connected directly to the anaerobic jar and they should be fitted with reducing valves to deliver the gases at a low pressure (e.g. 2–3 lb/in^2) via football bladders to the jars (see Fig. 7.7). Petri dishes

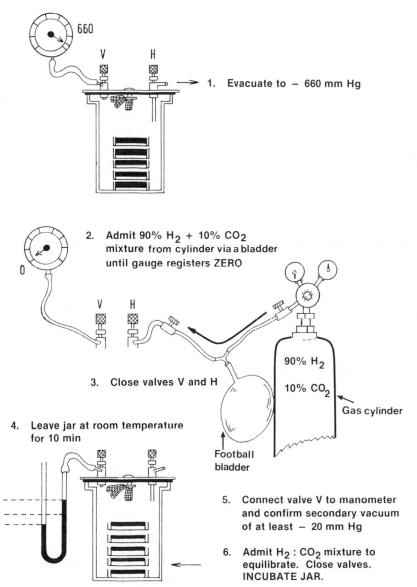

660

V   H

→ 1.   Evacuate to − 660 mm Hg

0

2.   Admit 90% H_2 + 10% CO_2
     mixture from cylinder via a bladder
     until gauge registers ZERO

V   H

90% H_2

10% CO_2

3.   Close valves V and H

Gas cylinder

4.   Leave jar at room temperature
     for 10 min

Football
bladder

5.   Connect valve V to manometer
     and confirm secondary vacuum
     of at least − 20 mm Hg

6.   Admit H_2 : CO_2 mixture to
     equilibrate. Close valves.
     INCUBATE JAR.

Fig. 7.7 A standardized procedure for setting up an anaerobic jar fitted with a 'room-temperature' catalyst.

with the medium uppermost and lid downwards are placed inside the jar. Vented Petri dishes should be used, as sealing of the lid to the bottom of an unvented Petri dish during evacuation of the jar by condensation moisture interferes with removal of oxygen from inside the Petri dish. After putting the plates into the jar the lid is clamped on. Approximately 6/7 of the air is evacuated (pressure reduced to 100 mm Hg, i.e. 660 mm below atmospheric) and this is monitored on a vacuum gauge. The pump is disconnected and the reduced pressure is brought up to 160 mm Hg (600 mm below atmospheric) with CO_2 and then to 760 mm Hg (i.e. atmospheric) with hydrogen from the rubber bladders, monitored on the vacuum gauge. If a 90% H_2 + 10% CO_2 gas mixture is used, the pressure is brought to atmospheric in a single step. The inlet valve is closed and the jar is held on the bench for 10 min. Then the inlet valve is connected to a mercury manometer and opened. If the catalyst is normally active, a decrease in pressure of at least 20 mm Hg occurs within the 10 min period after the admission of hydrogen. More hydrogen or gas mixture is then introduced to equilibrate the pressure and the jar is incubated at 37°C.

The catalytic activity of the palladium may be seriously impaired by moisture and inactive palladium sulphide may be formed from hydrogen sulphide evolved by cultures in the jar. When this happens, heating the sachets at 160°C for a few hours can rejuvenate the catalyst. There is no precise information about the best relationship between the concentrations or amount of palladium on palladiumized alumina pellets and the volume of the jar. An awareness of this problem has always been apparent, from McIntosh & Fildes (1916) who said that a larger jar required more palladium, to Collee et al (1971) who used three capsules (i.e. 3 g) of palladiumized alumina pellets in each jar.

Cultures on solid media for anaerobic incubation should be put in an anaerobic jar as soon as they are seeded. Many non-sporing anaerobes are readily killed by exposure to air and, even with clostridia, spores cannot be relied on to compensate for the toxicity of air to vegetative cells (Watt 1972).

A more expensive but important alternative to this procedure, especially in laboratories where facilities and experience in anaerobic bacteriology are limited, is the 'Gaspak' system (BBL) devised by Brewer & Allgeier (1966). This is marketed by Becton Dickinson. Controlled trials have shown it to be satisfactory for the cultivation of a wide variety of anaerobes of clinical importance when it was used with the Baird & Tatlock anaerobic jar (Collee et al 1972). Water is added to a disposable aluminium foil packet containing pellets of sodium borohydride and cobalt chloride and of citric acid and sodium bicarbonate; the packet is immediately put in the jar and its lid is secured. Reactions then take place to supply hydrogen and carbon dioxide.

The complete Gaspak system comprises a transparent polycarbonate anaerobic jar and a plastic lid fitted with a screened catalyst chamber containing palladiumized alumina pellets. There are no taps in the lid to allow evacuation of the jar, and no vacuum pumps or cylinders of compressed gas are required. An anaerobic indicator, either traditional (Cruickshank 1968) or modified (Brewer et al 1966) is necessary to check the activity of the palladium catalyst.

The Gaskit (Oxoid) is a similar development and is said to yield a more assured volume of carbon dioxide.

The Hungate procedure

More meticulous anaerobic methods to prevent access of air to media during preparation, inoculation and incubation have been developed. One of these methods, the manipulation of all these procedures under oxygen-free gas, was pioneered in 1950 by Hungate (see Hungate 1969), developed by Moore (1966) and has been applied to clinical specimens by McMinn & Crawford (1970). Surface colonies are grown in roll tubes in which a thin layer of agar coats the inside of the tube. The medium must be transparent for surface colonies to be visible, and this precludes the use of blood agar.

Anaerobic cabinets

Anaerobic cabinets are commercially produced for the processing of specimens and the subsequent incubation of cultures and subcultures in an oxygen-free atmosphere enriched with 5–10% CO_2. They have the advantage that all of the processing, including periodic examination of plates and preparation of subcultures, can be done without exposure to oxygen.

These cabinets variably incorporate some, or all, of a number of desirable features including 37°C incubator, bare-handed or fixed-glove operation, electrical outlets, humidity control, atmosphere cleansing, safety controls, and a small sample transfer facility to economize in gas usage. Suppliers of cabinets include Whitley, Raven, Gallenkamp, Horwell, and MDH.

ISOLATION OF PURE CULTURES

Most studies and tests of the physiological, serological and other characters of bacteria are valid only when made on a pure culture, i.e. the growth of a single strain, free from mixture and contamination with other bacteria. For this reason, in the diagnostic examination of mixed infective material, an essential preliminary is the isolation of the pertinent organism in a pure culture. Several techniques are available:

Plating out on a solid culture medium

The solid medium most used is nutrient agar either plain or enriched and usually dispensed as plates. In order to ensure separation, i.e. growth of discrete colonies, the surface of the medium must be dry. The infective material is inoculated on the surface by one of the methods described above so that bacteria are ultimately deposited singly. Where the bacteria are at a sufficient distance from each other (e.g. 1 cm) the whole progeny of each accumulates locally during growth to form a discrete mass, or colony, which is readily visible to the naked eye (e.g. 0.5–5 mm diameter). Each colony is presumed to be a pure culture, consisting exclusively of the descendants of a single cell; it may be picked with a sterile wire to prepare a pure subculture in a fresh medium.

In picking off single colonies, particularly when they are very close to one another, care must be taken that the point of the wire does not touch any of the neighbouring colonies. The culture should first be looked at through the medium held up to the light with the lid removed. To pick off the colony, first sit down with both elbows on the bench. Hold the plate vertically with the left hand, then grasp the holder of the sterilized wire, with the fingers quite close to the wire. Steady the right hand by resting the right little finger on the little finger of the left hand. The selected colony is then easily removed without touching the others. Return the plate to its lid and inoculate the required medium.

Plate culture microscope. Several makers produce low-power binocular magnifiers which are extremely useful for examining plate cultures of organisms; these have a long working distance so that one can pick the colony off the plate while using the instrument. When dealing with bacteria forming small delicate colonies, or where the colonies of the desired organism are few in number, the low-power binocular is invaluable. A magnification of 10 diameters is useful for general work, but with interchangeable eye-pieces and objectives, an instrument with magnifications from 6–30 diameters is available.

Occasionally a mixed colony is formed from two bacteria that have been inoculated close together on the agar or that grow in association, e.g. aerobe and anaerobe. If there is any doubt as to whether a pure colony has been obtained for picking, the colony should be replated immediately on a fresh plate and a single colony picked from this second plating. A culture should not be assumed to be pure unless a subculture from a single colony has been plated, found to be pure and picked again from a single colony on the pure plate. The maintenance of pure cultures necessitates the use of sterilized media, containers and instruments and continuous covering against the deposition of dust-borne bacteria from the air.

Use of selective, enrichment or indicator media

Selective media such as tellurite media for the diphtheria bacillus have been devised so that the majority of organisms likely to be associated with those for which the media are used will not grow, and the isolation of pure cultures is thus facilitated. The risk of contamination of single colonies from selective media is high because bacteria that do not grow may survive under colonies and grow in subcultures.

Enrichment media such as selenite broth for *Salmonella* spp. favour the multiplication of particular species as a step towards their isolation in pure culture.

Indicator media such as Willis and Hobbs medium for *Clostridium* spp. contain ingredients that change in appearance with particular organisms and so assist their isolation.

Use of selective growth conditions

The temperature and atmosphere chosen for a culture automatically preclude the growth of many bacteria. Incubation at 37°C, used for most medically important bacteria, is too warm for some air contaminants which subsequently appear as colonies when plates are kept at room temperature. Some pathogens are selectively favoured by growth at temperatures above 37°C. Strict anaerobes will not grow in air and most facultative anaerobes grow less vigorously under anaerobic than under aerobic conditions.

Selective treatment of the specimen before culture

Heating at 65°C for 30 min or higher temperatures for shorter periods can be used to separate spores from vegetative bacilli but there is no guarantee that spores will germinate under subsequent cultural conditions. Sputum for culture of tubercle bacilli is treated with a chemical, such as NaOH 1 mol/litre or saturated trisodium phosphate, to kill accompanying bacteria.

Animal inoculation

Advantage is taken of the fact that laboratory animals are highly susceptible to certain organisms – for example, the mouse to the pneumococcus. If a mixture of organisms containing the pneumococcus, e.g. in sputum, is inoculated subcutaneously into a mouse, the animal dies of pneumococcal septicaemia in 12–48 h, and from heart blood the organism can be obtained in pure culture. Similarly, the tubercle bacillus can be isolated from contaminating organisms by inoculation of an infected specimen into a guinea-pig. The tubercle bacillus is found in a pure state in the resulting lesions. Advances in the development of culture media now markedly limit the requirement for animal work.

BLOOD CULTURE

The technology of blood culture is reviewed by Gould & Duerden (1983). In most bacterial infections of the blood in man the organisms are not numerous, and it is essential for their demonstration by blood culture that a relatively large amount of blood, e.g. 5–10 ml, should be used as the inoculum. As the blood's natural bactericidal or bacteriostatic action may interfere with the growth of any bacteria present, this effect should be annulled by diluting the blood with medium. There is evidence that up to 10 ml of blood, or probably more, may be added to 100 ml of broth without a detectable antibacterial effect. For practical reasons, it is usual to add 5–7 ml of blood to about 50 ml of medium. The antibacterial effect may be further prevented by some substance incorporated in the medium, such as Liquoid (sodium polyanethol sulphonate); this may have a slightly inhibitory effect on certain species. Saponin broth, in which blood does not clot and is promptly lysed, is sometimes favoured for the isolation of streptococci of the viridans group which may be slightly sensitive to Liquoid. For patients on sulphonamide or penicillin therapy, *p*-aminobenzoic acid or penicillinase respectively may be added.

Castaneda's method of including an agar medium on one of the narrow sides of bottles of broth for blood culture (Ch. 6) is excellent because it allows a subculture to be made without opening the bottle. For use, 5–10 ml of the patient's blood is mixed with the liquid medium and allowed to flow over the agar. The bottle is incubated in the upright position and the agar surface is examined daily for colonies, being seeded every 24–48 h from the blood broth by suitably tilting the bottle.

Broth (*c*. 50 ml) for blood culture is generally dispensed in a special blood culture bottle which may be a 3 oz (90 ml) round bottle or a 4 oz (120 ml) medical flat bottle, with a screw cap. An adequate space above the broth ensures that the blood is not injected under undue pressure and that some air is available for strict aerobes. A smaller bottle is used for neonates and young children and the volumes of blood taken from these patients are appropriately smaller. A hole is punched out of the cap and the rubber washer is re-inserted. In order to protect the surface of the cap and the exposed portion of the rubber washer from contamination before use, the cap and neck of the bottle are covered with a foil cap.

Various commercial devices are available that can be used in place of the conventional blood culture bottle. For example, the Vacutainer Culture Tube System (Becton Dickinson) allows blood to be sampled directly into a partially evacuated 50 ml bottle containing one of a range of supplemented media for the culture of aerobes and anaerobes. The Roche Septi-Check and the Oxoid Signal blood culture systems are more recent developments. The Roche system incorporates a solid and a liquid phase. The Oxoid system exploits the pressure of gas produced by bacterial action to drive liquid medium into an upper chamber and signal growths.

Conventional blood culture procedure

It is essential to avoid contamination, and the following procedures should be undertaken with care:

1. The operator's hands must be clean and dry. Sterile gloves may be worn to protect the operator if there is a possibility of a specific hazard such as hepatitis B or AIDS.

2. Disinfect the venepuncture site on the patient's skin by applying 70% isopropyl alcohol in water with 1% iodine or 1–2% chlorhexidine for at least 1 min and allow to dry.

3. With precautions to avoid touching and re-contaminating the venepuncture site, take the sample of blood.

4. Change the needle with care to avoid touching the shaft or contaminating the operator before inoculating the required volume into each blood culture bottle.

Culture media. It is advisable to seed more than one medium for blood culture. The wide range of available media includes brain heart infusion broth, cooked meat broth, fastidious anaerobe broth, thioglycollate broth and diphasic broth (Castaneda system). All of these perform well and can be used in various combinations; in general, a two-bottle system is most commonly employed, e.g. brain heart infusion (BHI) for aerobes and BHI with cooked meat particles (BHI/CMP) for the anaerobes (Collee et al 1977). As acid formed from glucose fermentation tends to kill bacteria, the addition of glucose to all cultures is not recommended. In suspected cases of enteric fever, the patient's blood may be diluted 1 to 10 in 0.5% sodium taurocholate broth. Special procedures or culture media used for blood culture in the diagnosis of certain infections such as brucellosis and leptospirosis are described in the appropriate chapters.

Incubation. One of each set of bottles should be incubated in an atmosphere of air with 10% CO_2; here it is essential to loosen the caps of bottles during incubation. The routine use of cooked meat broth or fastidious anaerobe broth allows the 'closed' culture of both aerobic and anaerobic bacteria in an aerobic incubator, but the use of an anaerobic cabinet has many advantages.

Subculturing procedures. Growth may produce a generalized turbidity or there may be discrete colonies on the surface of the sedimented red cells. It is most important to make subcultures from all bottles to solid media as a routine; early growth sometimes produces no visible effect in the broth.

Extreme care must be taken to avoid contamination when cultures are opened during subculture to test for growth. Subcultures should be made quickly so that blood cultures do not cool appreciably. Inspection and subculturing of blood cultures should be done at least once during the first day and thereafter at intervals.

Blood cultures received in the laboratory between 9 a.m. and 5 p.m. should have their first subculture done at 10 p.m. that day (see Ganguli et al 1984). If subsequent daily subculturing is thought to be excessive, it is important to ensure that subculture is done at least twice during the first 2–3 days. It is usual to continue incubation and inspection up to 5–7 days with a final subculture then. Prolonged culture is recommended, before the bottles are discarded, in the investigation of some infections such as bacterial endocarditis, brucellosis and some others. Subculture plates should be incubated in air with 10% CO_2 and a parallel series should be incubated anaerobically. Gram-stained smears should be made from any broths that show visible signs of growth as this can allow an early presumptive report. Automated systems for blood culture investigation have been introduced into some laboratories, but there is evidence to show that conventional manual systems still have advantages (Ganguli et al 1985).

The Castaneda system avoids the contamination problem associated with frequent subculturing. A commercially available development (Roche) consists of a clear plastic screw-capped bottle with an internal paddle or dipstick holding sterile medium. At the laboratory, on receipt of the blood culture bottle to which the patient's blood has been added, the screw cap is removed and replaced with this assembly. The blood culture bottle is then transiently inverted so that the contents flow over the medium and the whole assembly is incubated. The inversion can be repeated once or twice daily. As the medium is examined regularly for the development of colonies by direct vision through the clear plastic, the sequential introduction of contaminants into the system is avoided. This is a great advantage over the conventional subculturing procedure.

Quantitative counts of bacteria in blood

These are sometimes useful in differentiating between bacteraemia and septicaemia or for prognostic purposes. A simple procedure is to inoculate 1 ml amounts of blood into several tubes of melted agar and make pour-plates either at the bedside or from unclotted blood in Liquoid in the laboratory.

Clot culture

When blood samples from a patient with suspected enteric fever have been submitted for the Widal test, it is useful as a routine to culture the clot after the serum has been removed.

If it is known that the blood has been withdrawn with strict aseptic precautions, the clot may be placed in a wide tube half-filled with broth, or in a wide-mouth screw-capped bottle containing 80 ml of broth. When there is any doubt as to the presence of contaminating organisms, and this is always a possibility when specimens of blood are sent to the laboratory from a distance, the clot should be transferred directly to a tube of sterile ox bile and disintegrated (with aseptic precautions). After incubation overnight the bile culture is examined for enteric organisms in the usual manner.

A method of clot culture with streptokinase (Calbiochem) has been recommended (Watson 1955). Blood is allowed to clot in 5 ml quantities in sterile screw-capped Universal containers. The separated serum is removed and 15 ml of 0.5% bile-salt broth with streptokinase 100 units/ml is added to each bottle. The streptokinase causes rapid clot lysis with release of bacteria trapped in the clot.

PRESERVATION OF CULTURES

Bacterial species vary greatly in the ability of their cultures to remain alive after the completion of growth (e.g. after 24 h at 37°C). Some species such as *Neisseria gonorrhoeae* and *Streptobacillus moniliformis* are poorly viable and their cultures usually die out within a few days, whether kept at 37°C, at room temperature or at 4–5°C; thus, they must be subcultivated every 2–4 days for maintenance in the laboratory. Other species are much hardier, especially sporing species which may remain viable for many years. There are also many non-sporing species (e.g. Enterobacteriaceae) whose cultures, under suitable conditions, commonly remain viable for many months and often for as much as 10–20 years.

Their prolonged preservation requires the following: (1) that drying of the culture is prevented by hermetic sealing of the tube or bottle with a screw cap and new rubber liner, or with a cotton-wool plug soaked in paraffin wax; (2) that the culture is stored in the dark, and either at room temperature or in a refrigerator at 4–5°C, but not at 37°C; and (3) that the culture be grown in or on a suitable preservation medium or as a nutrient agar stab culture. Organisms of the enterobacteria group may be kept alive on egg saline medium (Ch. 6) for several years without subcultivation; they survive longer than on nutrient agar, and are less liable to vary to the 'rough' state. The culture is grown overnight at 37°C and the screw cap of the bottle is firmly tightened before storing in a dark, cool cupboard. Some organisms other than enterobacteria are better preserved if the bottles are stored at 4°C (but see below). Survival is dependent on the culture not being allowed to dry out.

It is desirable that at least a moderate proportion of the cells in the culture should remain alive; if only a few survive, these may be exclusively resistant mutants, all cells of the original type being lost. Frequent subcultivation also tends to replace the original type by mutants and must therefore be avoided as far as possible. Specific recommendations for the short-term preservation of bacterial cultures have been made by Stokes (1962). Full discussions of media for the maintenance and preservation of bacteria (Lapage et al 1970a) and of culture collections and the preservation of bacteria (Lapage et al 1970b) have been published. Further details of all of the following methods are given by Lapage & Redway (1974).

Regular subculture

Regular subculture of bacterial cultures is not advised as this method can lead, over a period of time, to changes in the original culture that may not immediately be recognized, e.g. contamination by another bacterium especially by spores of *Bacillus* spp.; mutation in which the organism either loses or gains a property not in its original makeup; change in the name or number on the culture due to misinterpretation of writing; or there may be overgrowth of the original strain by a secondary one which was there in small numbers at the original subculture.

Regular subculture may be necessary with certain bacteria that do not readily withstand freezing and/or drying, e.g. some *Neisseria* spp.

Reduced metabolism and periodic transfer

Regular subculture can be reduced by lowering the metabolism of the organism by growing it on a medium containing minimal nutrition, e.g. egg saline slopes or semi-solid nutrient agar stabs, and then sealing the surface of the medium with sterile liquid paraffin to exclude air and reduce dehydration. The culture is then stored at either room temperature or at 4–5°C in a refrigerator. The disadvantages of this method lie mainly in the inconvenience of the liquid paraffin.

Cold storage

This is a common method of preserving strains of bacteria as many can be frozen and remain viable. Damage to bacterial cells at low temperatures can be severe, due, it is believed, to the formation of ice crystals and to the concentration of electrolytes as the water is formed into ice. The damage can be minimized by careful monitoring of the rate of cooling, reducing the amount of electrolytes present to a minimum, adding protective substances such as 'sugars', glycerol or dimethylsulphoxide (DMSO) into the suspending medium and rapid re-warming on reconstitution of the culture.

Temperatures that may be used in this way include:

1. 4–6°C in a domestic refrigerator, although some *Neisseria* spp. and *Haemophilus* spp. do not survive at this temperature.

2. −20 to −40°C in a domestic freezer is a compromise (but see below for preferred methods of long-term storage).

3. −80°C in an ultra-deep freezer, in which the cells are protected by one of the substances

mentioned above or by using a suspension of dried milk.

4. −70°C in solid carbon dioxide, a disadvantage being that cultures will be lost if the solid carbon dioxide is not checked regularly and replenished as it evaporates.

5. In liquid nitrogen at −196°C; this method can be used for a wide range of bacteria as well as for viruses and many other biological cells. Large numbers of strains may be stored in liquid nitrogen storage containers in sterile drinking straws or in special tubes on carriers. Advantages include little loss of viability, rapid resuscitation, ready availability as a living suspension and speed of preparation. A further advantage is that the procedure can be used without delay and the biological character of the stored organism is thus 'fixed' at a very early stage after its isolation. This is the basis of the 'stabilate' concept of Lumsden et al (1973). Disadvantages include the cost of the apparatus and regular supplies of liquid nitrogen, risk of explosion when ampoules are brought into room temperature, loss of large numbers of cultures if careful monitoring of liquid nitrogen levels is not carried out, and possible contamination of the liquid nitrogen in the storage container if an ampoule breaks.

Drying methods

A number of methods for drying suspensions of bacteria for preservation purposes have been developed which are useful in laboratories that cannot afford the expensive equipment used for storing at very low temperatures or for freeze-drying, or in which preservation of cultures is performed infrequently.

1. Paper disks: a thick suspension of bacteria is placed on sterile disks of thick absorbent paper which are then dried over phosphorus pentoxide (P_2O_5) in a desiccator under vacuum.

2. Gelatin disks: again a thick suspension of bacteria is prepared and added to nutrient gelatin. Drops of the bacterial suspension in gelatin are placed on sterile waxed paper or on a plastic Petri dish and then dried off over P_2O_5 under vacuum; this is the method of Stamp (1947).

3. Pre-dried plugs: thick suspensions of bacteria are prepared and drops placed on sterile cellophane (Rayner 1943) or on pre-dried plugs of peptone, starch or dextran (Annear 1956) before drying in a desiccator over P_2O_5 in a vacuum.

4. L-drying: bacteria in small ampoules are dried from the liquid state using a vacuum pump and desiccant and a waterbath to control the temperature. This method is described by Lapage et al (1970b).

Freeze-drying in vacuo (lyophilization)

When bacterial cultures or virus suspensions are dried and kept in the dry state under suitable conditions, they may remain viable for several years; antisera may be preserved similarly without appreciable loss of antibody potency. If such materials are dried from the liquid state, a high salt concentration is produced in the later stages of drying; this causes denaturation of proteins, death of organisms and deterioration of serum. The problem is largely avoided by freeze-drying or lyophilization whereby the culture or serum is dried rapidly in vacuo from the frozen state. The material is frozen by a suitable method and then dried by sublimation of the ice. The sublimation is effected by exposure to an atmosphere of very low pressure (e.g. 0.01 mm Hg or less) which is dried by a chemical desiccant or refrigerated condenser. The dried material is preserved in vacuo or under an inert gas such as nitrogen in hermetically sealed ampoules which are stored in the dark, either at room temperature or preferably in a refrigerator at 4–5°C. This is a convenient means of preserving stock strains of bacteria, guinea-pig complement serum and samples of antisera required for reference or standardization purposes. On a larger scale, it is used for preserving therapeutic antisera, human plasma, antibiotics and vaccines.

Freezing must be very rapid, with the temperature lowered to well below 0°C (e.g. to −20°C), since slow freezing would prolong exposure to the denaturing influence of the suspending salt solution. The liquid should be frozen in a shallow layer with a large surface available for evaporation. Two methods of freezing are available: (1) *prefreezing*, i.e. before the drying process is begun; and (2) *evaporative freezing*, effected during the first stage of the drying process.

Prefreezing is generally employed for large volumes. The liquid is frozen as a layer, or 'shell', lining the walls of the bottle, either by rotating the bottle while immersed nearly horizontally in a bath of ethyl alcohol or acetone and solid carbon dioxide, or of refrigerated coolant, or by spinning the bottle on its vertical axis in a current of refrigerated air.

Evaporative freezing is employed for the smaller quantities that generally suffice for laboratory purposes. The liquid is quickly frozen by the withdrawal of latent heat during its initial rapid evaporation when exposed to the vacuum applied for drying. Precautions must be taken against frothing and spilling during desolution of the atmospheric gases; the 'centrifugal' and 'degassing' methods have been developed for this purpose (see below).

Suspending media for freeze-drying of bacteria

The survival of bacteria during freeze-drying is greatly influenced by the nature of the medium in which they are suspended. Nutrient broth containing peptone 1% and meat extract 1% is a satisfactory medium for the most resistant organisms, e.g. *Streptococcus pyogenes* and *Staphylococcus aureus*, and the moderately resistant, e.g. enterobacteria and brucellae. Broth cultures of these may be dried directly.

Special protective suspending media are necessary for the poorly resistant organisms such as *Neisseria gonorrhoeae*, *Vibrio cholerae* and *Haemophilus influenzae*. Organisms from a fresh stationary phase culture are suspended to a high density equivalent to Brown's opacity standard No. 4 (12th Edn, Ch. 13, p. 308) in the sterile suspending medium just prior to freeze-drying. Various media have been advised, most of which contain sugar, peptone and a colloid (e.g. protein or dextran). Skimmed milk, containing lactose and protein, has been used with success.

The media used at the National Collection of Type Cultures (NCTC) are broth with glucose 7.5% for the enterobacteria, and glucose 7.5% in horse serum sterilized by Seitz filtration for other organisms. Exceptionally fatty batches of serum are avoided.

A suspending medium comprising nutrient broth (Oxoid No. 2) supplemented with rabbit serum or horse serum 10% v/v, inactivated at 56°C for 30 min, and glucose 1% w/v has been used successfully with a wide range of bacteria in the Bacteriology Department, Edinburgh University, for many years. This medium is pre-reduced when it is used for freeze-drying anaerobes.

Greaves' (1944) centrifugal method of freeze-drying

This is a most convenient method for preserving a number of cultures and it is described fully by Lapage et al (1970b). Frothing is prevented by centrifuging the liquid during the first stage of evacuation, and drying until freezing is complete.

Suitable centrifugal freeze-driers are available from several manufacturers. They consist of a drying chamber, usually a polycarbonate bell-jar containing a centrifuge and an attachment for secondary drying manifolds, a trap containing either a freezing coil (condenser) or desiccant trays to remove water vapour, a rotary oil-sealed vacuum pump capable of drawing a negative pressure below 0.04 mm Hg and a Pirani-type vacuum gauge. The liquid cultures or suspensions are dried in special neutral soft glass tubes or ampoules with a stem bore of 6 mm. Plug the ampoules with absorbent cotton wool and sterilize horizontally in the autoclave at 121°C for 20 min or in a dry oven at 160°C for 1 h. The procedure is as follows:

1. Place in each ampoule a small strip of Whatman No. 1 filter paper on which has been typed the number designating the culture to be introduced. The label should be inserted so that the number is easily read when the ampoule is held horizontally with the open end on the right. With a sterile capillary pipette, put 0.25–0.5 ml of liquid culture into the bottom of each small

ampoule (tube type) and up to 2.5 ml into each of the larger ampoules. Discard the original sterility plug into disinfectant and insert a fresh, *loose* plug of sterile, non-absorbent cotton wool, pressing it wholly within the stem of the ampoule, or cap each ampoule with sterile surgical gauze.

2. Prepare the trap for primary drying by cooling the freezing coil to below −40°C or by charging the desiccant trays with fresh phosphorus pentoxide to the extent of at least 3 g of powder/ml of water to be absorbed. *Note*: Phosphorus pentoxide is corrosive and care must be taken to avoid spilling it on the skin, clothing or freeze-dryer. After each use of the dryer, the expended desiccant must be washed from the trays with an excess of water, with care to avoid the corrosive fumes evolved, and the trays are then thoroughly dried. The maker's instructions must be followed for cleaning the apparatus and removing spilt powder.

3. *Primary drying*. Place the ampoules in the nearly vertical holes of the constant speed centrifuge rotor. Cover the centrifuge with the bell-jar and press this firmly into position on the sealing ring of the base plate. (The contact surfaces are previously cleaned with ether and lightly smeared with high-vacuum grease. Edwards supply Apiezon 'M' grease for joints.) While pressing down the jar, switch on first the centrifuge and then the vacuum pump. Observe the fall of the pressure on the gauge. When a low pressure of about 1 mm Hg has been achieved in 5–10 min, it can be assumed that the material is frozen as a thin layer on the inner wall of the ampoule. *Immediately switch off the centrifuge to avoid over-heating*. Leave the vacuum pump running for a period sufficient to complete the primary drying when the pressure should be below 0.1 mm Hg: about 3–6 h for 0.25 ml volumes; 4–8 h for 0.5 ml volumes and 6–12 h for 2.5 ml volumes, depending on the total volume of liquid to be removed. The ampoules should be shielded from sunlight or daylight.

4. Isolate the chamber, open the chamber air-release valve, lift the bell-jar and remove the ampoules. Plug with sterile, non-absorbent wool if previously covered with gauze. Flame the opening and press the loose cotton-wool plug about 6 cm down the stem. While rotating the ampoule, heat the stem in a small glass flame at about 3 cm from its open end, until the glass walls have softened and nearly doubled in thickness. Remove the ampoule from the flame and stretch it to form a capillary neck of about 2 mm external diameter and 1 mm bore. When cool, apply the open end to one of the rubber adaptors on the manifold used for the secondary drying; the manifold is placed so that the ampoules lie horizontally. Any adaptor not in use must be sealed with an empty ampoule.

5. *Secondary drying*. If a chemical desiccant is in use remove the expended material from the trays and replace with fresh phosphorus pentoxide powder. Press the bell-jar into position, close the air-release valve and re-evacuate the chamber. Leave the pump running for a sufficient period to ensure complete drying, e.g. 10 min, until the pressure is 0.05–0.01 mm Hg.

6. Seal the ampoules while they are attached to the manifold with the pump running: heat the capillary neck with a small gas flame, or preferably with a twin-headed sealing attachment; when the glass is melted, pull gently and allow the flame to sever the thin filament so formed. The Pirani gauge will show if a leak develops on the manifold side. When all the ampoules are sealed and set aside, switch off the Pirani guage, open the air-release valve and switch off the pump and discard the desiccant. After 30 min, lay the ampoules on a metal surface and test them for vacuum with a high-frequency vacuum tester; discard any that fail the test.

Recovery of a freeze-dried culture from an ampoule

Check initially that the ampoule is intact; if a high-frequency tester is available, confirm that the contents of the ampoule are still under vacuum. Check the identification label. Mark the ampoule with a file transversely over the cotton-

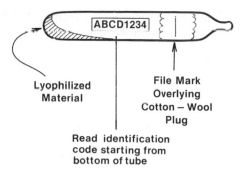

Lyophilized Material

File Mark Overlying Cotton – Wool Plug

Read identification code starting from bottom of tube

Fig. 7.8 An ampoule of lyophilized culture ready for opening.

wool plug. Heat the tip of a glass rod red-hot in a Bunsen flame and apply it firmly to the filed mark on the ampoule which should crack at that point (Fig. 7.8). Allow time for air to enter via the plug; then carefully discard the drawn-out end of the ampoule and the plug into a container of suitable disinfectant, for subsequent autoclaving.

With aseptic precautions, add a small amount of suitably supplemented sterile broth to the ampoule with a sterile Pasteur pipette, expressing and taking up the broth several times to bring the contents of the ampoule into suspension and to soak the paper label. The paper may conveniently adhere to the pipette stem; it should be transferred to the surface of a suitable solid medium for subculture to confirm the absence of contaminants and to obtain prompt colonial growth of the desired strain. The suspended material in the broth should be seeded into one or more suitable fluid media to ensure recovery of the organism after appropriate incubation.

DISPOSAL OF CULTURES

All cultures to be discarded must first be sterilized, even if they are apparently 'negative'. Sterilization is equally important for cultures in reusable containers or in disposable containers such as plastic Petri dishes that may be incinerated, as it is of paramount importance that no living infective material leaves the laboratory.

There are three practical methods by which cultures may be sterilized – incineration, autoclaving and chemical disinfection – but only the first two can guarantee sterility. Chemical disinfection depends on many variables such as adequate access of the disinfectant to the culture, concentration, length of exposure and temperature among others (Ch. 4); these limitations must be borne in mind.

Autoclaving must be used for cultures of *Mycobacterium tuberculosis* and sporing organisms such as *Clostridium tetani* and *Bacillus anthracis*. Note the importance of allowing adequate steam penetration in autoclaving; lids of metal and plastic buckets must be removed and placed in the autoclave and permeable autoclavable bags must be opened at the loading stage. Plastic Petri dishes autoclaved in bins or buckets fuse into a solid lump which may be lifted out when cool for incineration.

Incineration is widely used when the culture containers are disposable, but there may be problems if the incineration procedure is not under the control of the laboratory staff (DHSS 1978; Collins 1983). For example, if material has to be transported some distance, it may be confused with other rubbish and may be dumped without incineration. Another anxiety is that the incinerator may not be functioning properly and may not burn the material completely or may discharge clouds of toxic smoke when plastic materials are burned; in the latter case, an after-burner fitted to the incinerator solves the problem (DHSS 1978). Problems involved in the transport of infected waste from the laboratory are numerous. If there is any uncertainty associated with the use of distant incinerators, the material must be autoclaved before dispatch and it can then be disposed of as harmless rubbish.

Clear written instructions for the disposal of all cultures must be included in the laboratory code. Cultures must be discarded into plastic, colour-coded bags for incineration or into robust bins or buckets (made of stainless steel or autoclavable plastic) or into autoclavable plastic bags. All plastic bags must be supported either in a custom-built frame or in an empty discard bin or bucket. Discard containers must be leak-proof. Containers must never be so full that the lid cannot be placed on top, or the neck of the bag tied off for transport to the sterilization area. Overfull containers cause many problems ranging from bursting open to difficulties in handling and injuries to staff. Disposable containers for discard, such as plastic Petri dishes, must be kept separate from cultures in non-disposable containers such as test tubes and glass bottles.

Further details of the safe disposal of cultures, glassware, sharps and other contaminated materials are dealt with in Chapters 1, 4 and 15.

REFERENCES

Annear D I 1956 The preservation of bacteria by drying in peptone plugs. Journal of Hygiene, Cambridge 54: 487–508

Brewer J H, Allgeier D L 1966 Safe self-contained carbon dioxide-hydrogen anaerobic system. Applied Microbiology 14: 985–988

Brewer J H, Allgeier D L, McLaughlin C B 1966 Improved anaerobic indicator. Applied Microbiology 14: 135–136

Brown D O 1973 Multiple loop inoculator as an aid in bacteriocine typing techniques. Medical Laboratory Technology 30: 351–353

Butzler J-P 1984 Campylobacter infection in man and animals. CRC, Boca Raton, Florida. p 45

Collee J G, Duerden B I, Brown R 1977 Recovery of anaerobic bacteria from small inocula – a model for blood culture studies. Journal of Clinical Pathology 30: 609–614

Collee J G, Rutter J M, Watt B 1971 The significantly viable particle: a study of the subculture of an exacting sporing anaerobe. Journal of Medical Microbiology 4: 271–288

Collee J G, Watt B, Fowler E B, Brown R 1972 An evaluation of the Gaspak system in the culture of anaerobic bacteria. Journal of Applied Bacteriology 35: 71–82

Collins C H 1983 Laboratory-acquired infections. Butterworth, London

Cruickshank R 1968 Medical microbiology 11th edn. (revised reprint). Churchill Livingstone, Edinburgh

DHSS 1978 Department of Health and Social Security, Code of practice for the prevention of infection in clinical laboratories. HMSO, London

Ganguli L A, Keaney M G L, Hyde W A, Fraser S B 1985 More rapid identification of bacteraemia by manual rather than radiometric method. Journal of Clinical Pathology 38: 1146–1149

Ganguli L A, O'Hare W, Hyde W A 1984 Rapid detection of bacteraemia by early subculture. Journal of Medical Microbiology 17: 311–315

Gould J C, Duerden B I 1983 (eds) Symposium report. Blood culture – current state and future prospects. Journal of Clinical Pathology 36: 963–977

Greaves R I N 1944 Centrifugal vacuum freezing; application to the drying of biological material from the frozen state. Nature, London 153: 485–487

Hayward N J 1945 The examination of wounds for clostridia. Proceedings of the Association of Clinical Pathologists 1: 5–17

Heller C L 1954 A simple method for producing anaerobiosis. Journal of Applied Bacteriology 17:202

Hungate R E 1969 A roll tube method for cultivation of strict anaerobes. In: Norris J R, Ribbons D W (eds) Methods in microbiology, vol. 3B. Academic Press, London. p 117

Lapage S P, Redway K F 1974 Preservation of bacteria with notes on other micro-organisms. PHLS Monograph Series No. 7 HMSO, London

Lapage S P, Shelton J E, Mitchell T G 1970a Media for the maintenance and preservation of bacteria. In: Norris J R, Ribbons D W (eds) Methods in microbiology, vol 3A. Academic Press, London, p 1–133

Lapage S P, Shelton J E, Mitchell T G, MacKenzie A R 1970b Culture collections and the preservation of bacteria. In: Norris J R, Ribbons D W (eds) Methods in microbiology, vol 3A. Academic Press, London. p 135–228

Lumsden W H R, Herbert W J, McNeillage, G J G 1973 Techniques with Trypanosomes. Churchill Livingstone, Edinburgh

McIntosh J, Fildes P 1916 A new apparatus for the isolation and cultivation of anaerobic microorganisms. Lancet 1: 768–770

McMinn M T, Crawford J J 1970 Recovery of anaerobic microorganisms from clinical specimens in prereduced media versus recovery by routine clinical laboratory methods. Applied Microbiology 19: 207–213

Miles A A, Misra S S, Irwin J O 1938 The estimation of the bactericidal power of the blood. Journal of Hygiene, Cambridge 38: 732–749

Moore W E C 1966 Techniques for routine culture of fastidious anaerobes. International Journal of Systematic Bacteriology 16: 173–178

Rayner A G 1943 A simple method for the preservation of cultures and sera by drying. Journal of Pathology and Bacteriology 55: 373–375

Stamp Lord 1947 The preservation of bacteria by drying. Journal of General Microbiology 1: 251–265

Stokes E J 1962 Short term preservation of bacterial cultures. Association of Clinical Pathologists, broadsheet No. 40 (new series)

Watson K C 1955 Isolation of Salmonella typhi from the blood stream. Journal of Laboratory and Clinical Medicine 46: 128–134

Watt B 1972 The recovery of clinically important anaerobes on solid media. Journal of Medical Microbiology

Watt B 1973 The influence of carbon dioxide on the growth of obligate and facultative anaerobes on solid media. Journal of Medical Microbiology 6: 307–314

Watt B, Collee J G, Brown R 1974 The isolation of strict anaerobes: the use of an anaerobic cabinet compared with a conventional procedure. Journal of Medical Microbiology 7: 315–324

Wright B M 1943 Improved catalyst for McIntosh and Fildes Anaerobic Jar. Army Pathology Laboratory Service, Current Notes No. 9, p. 8

Tests for identification of bacteria

In this chapter a number of 'biochemical' tests and a few miscellaneous tests, used generally in the identification of microorganisms, are described. Tests used specifically for the identification of a particular organism are described elsewhere in the appropriate section dealing with the organism.

It should be realized that many of the tests described in this chapter are not 'all-or-none' tests; some distinguish between organisms that differ in the rate with which they carry out a particular reaction. It is therefore important to use a method of test that is suitably poised to differentiate the organisms under consideration. For many of the tests given here, a large number of variations have been developed in different laboratories. In these cases, it has been difficult to make a choice of a method and in some instances we have described more than one test for a given reaction. The results obtained with variations on a particular test may not be comparable and it is essential to bear this in mind. Moreover, there may be considerable variation in the commercially available preparations of the reagents used. For example, the tryptophane content of peptone varies according to the mode of preparation and this markedly influences its value as a substrate in the indole test.

Unfortunately many routinely used tests are not yet standardized, but a start has been made by various organizations.

Diagnostic tables showing the biochemical reactions identifying many genera and species of pathogenic and saprophytic bacteria are given by Cowan (1974) and other specialist authors, e.g. Holdeman et al (1977), for strict anaerobes.

Preparation of inoculum for test media

The validity of the identification of an unknown bacterial culture by its reactions in a range of biochemical tests depends absolutely on the use of a *pure* culture of the bacterium for inoculation of the test media. Single, well separated colonies grown on a primary diagnostic plate that has been inoculated with material containing a mixture of bacterial species are usually but not always pure. Some of the colonies are likely to be contaminated with a minor admixture of bacteria of another kind, e.g. an anaerobic or other exacting species that does not grow well under the conditions of culture in the primary plate. If such a colony is accidentally picked and the test media are inoculated either directly from it or from an intermediate slope or broth subculture of it, the contaminating bacteria may grow out selectively in some of the media and give false results.

It is recommended, therefore, that the chosen colony should first be plated out on an unselective culture medium and that an isolated colony on the secondary plate should be used as the inoculum for the tests. This precaution is often omitted in medical diagnostic bacteriology, where speed in obtaining results is important. The results are then not fully reliable and if they are unexpected a freshly purified inoculum culture should be prepared and the tests repeated.

If a larger number of test media have to be inoculated than can conveniently be done from a single colony, the colony should first be subcultured on an agar slope, or in a tube of broth, and this subculture should be used to inoculate the test media. The subculture can then be preserved for making confirmatory or other different tests on subsequent days. It is an unsound practice to use another, apparently similar colony from the primary plate to provide inocula for additional tests.

Controls for tests

The sterility of each batch of test medium should be confirmed by incubating one or two uninoculated tubes of the batch along with the inoculated tests. If the uninoculated tubes show evidence of bacterial growth, the tests and the remainder of that batch of medium should be discarded.

Control tests are also made to confirm that the test media have been made up correctly and that they are used and observed under the proper conditions (see Ch. 6). One tube of each batch of test medium is inoculated with a stock culture of a bacterium known to give a positive reaction and another tube with a stock culture known to give a negative reaction. These positive and negative controls are incubated and examined along with the tests.

TESTS FOR METABOLISM OF CARBOHYDRATES AND RELATED COMPOUNDS

Bacteria differ widely in their ability to metabolize carbohydrates and related compounds. For purposes of identification these differences can be demonstrated by four varieties of test:

1. Test to distinguish between aerobic and anaerobic breakdown of a carbohydrate.
2. Tests to show the range of carbohydrates and related compounds that can be attacked.
3. Tests for specific breakdown products.
4. Tests to show ability to utilize a particular substrate.

Carbohydrates and related compounds may be altered when exposed to normal heat-sterilization temperatures. They may also be altered when heated in the presence of other ingredients of culture media, e.g. peptone, phosphate. For these reasons, it is recommended that the basal ingredients of test media should be heat-sterilized before the carbohydrate or related compound is added. A solution of the compound under test should be sterilized separately and the requisite amount subsequently added with aseptic precautions to the sterile basal medium.

Sterilization of solutions of test compounds by filtration is recommended. However, if heat is to be used, steaming at 100°C is less likely to alter the compound than autoclaving at 121°C. Note that tyndallization (see Ch. 4) is ineffective for pure solutions of sugars etc., as surviving spores will not germinate and grow out in a *non-nutrient* medium. However, tyndallization may be used for sterilization of a sugar solution incorporated in *nutrient* media, e.g. peptone water.

Carbohydrates are particularly susceptible to heat in an alkaline environment and if a carbohydrate solution is to be sterilized by heat, the prior addition of one or two drops of phosphoric acid will ensure that the solution is not alkaline.

Test to distinguish between aerobic and anaerobic breakdown of a carbohydrate

This method (Hugh & Leifson 1953) depends upon the use of a semi-solid tubed medium containing the carbohydrate together with a pH indicator. If acid is produced only at the surface of the medium, where conditions are aerobic, the attack on the sugar is oxidative. If acid is found throughout the tube, including the lower layers where conditions are anaerobic, the breakdown is fermentative.

Medium

Peptone	2.0 g
Sodium chloride, NaCl	5.0 g
Dipotassium hydrogen phosphate, K_2HPO_4	0.3 g
Bromothymol blue (1% aqueous solution)	3 ml
Agar	3 g
Water	1 litre

The pH is adjusted to 7.1 before adding the bromothymol blue and the medium is autoclaved in a flask at 121°C for 15 min. The carbohydrate to be added is sterilized separately and added to give a final concentration of 1%. The medium is then tubed to a depth of about 4 cm.

Method. Duplicate tubes of medium are inoculated by stabbing; one tube is promptly covered with a layer of sterile melted petroleum jelly (yellow soft petroleum) to a depth of 5–10 mm and both are incubated for up to 30 days.

Results. Fermenting organisms (e.g. Enterobacteriaceae, *Aeromonas*, *Vibrio*) produce an acid reaction throughout the medium in the covered (anaerobic) as well as the open (aerobic) tube. Oxidizing organisms (e.g. *Pseudomonas*, *Loefflerella*) produce an acid reaction only in the open tube; this begins at the surface and gradually extends downwards, and may appear only after an alkaline reaction has been present for several days. Organisms that cannot break down the carbohydrate aerobically or anaerobically (e.g. *Alcaligenes faecalis*) produce an alkaline reaction in the open tube and no change in the covered tube.

It should be noted that this medium may also be used for recording gas production and motility.

Tests to show the range of carbohydrates and related compounds that can be attacked.

For practical purposes these tests are of two kinds. The majority are tests simply for the production of acid and gas or acid alone when a pure culture grows in the presence of the test compound. A negative reaction in these tests does not necessarily mean that the culture is unable to utilize the carbon compound. A minority of the tests are more complicated, the principal ones being those for tartrate and citrate fermentation in which breakdown of the substrate is confirmed by showing that it has been removed from the medium or has enhanced growth (see Ch. 29). These tests, in addition to fermentation of mucate, are used in the identification and fermentation typing of salmonellae. They are described in detail by Cruickshank (1968) and will not be repeated here.

Tests for acid and gas or acid alone: 'fermentation tests'

Constituents of fermentation test media

1. A suitable *nutrient medium* as a base to allow the growth of the organism under test, free from substances that might yield acid products. The nature of this medium depends on the nutritional requirements of the organism. Peptone water, serum peptone water and serum agar are commonly used.

2. The *carbohydrate or related compound* under test. A large variety are used and they are often referred to loosely as 'sugars'.
   Monosaccharides
   Pentoses – Arabinose, xylose, rhamnose
   Hexoses – Glucose, fructose, mannose, sorbose, galactose
   Disaccharides
   Sucrose, maltose, lactose, trehalose, cellobiose
   Trisaccharide
   Raffinose
   Polysaccharides
   Starch, inulin, dextrin, glycogen
   Polyhydric alcohols
   Glycerol, erythritol, adonitol, mannitol, dulcitol, sorbitol, inositol
   Glycosides
   Salicin, coniferin, aesculin
   Organic acids
   dextro – tartrate; *laevo* – tartrate; *meso*– tartrate, citrate, mucate, gluconate, malonate.

The test compounds in fermentation test media may be identified by a colour code.

The test compound is usually added in the proportion of 0.5% to peptone water or 1.0% to serum bases. The majority can be prepared as 10% aqueous solutions and sterilized, preferably by filtration. They can be stored in screw-capped bottles in the refrigerator. Rarer compounds may be stored in 15 ml bottles with a perforated cap and rubber washer, similar to the caps of blood culture bottles, and a sterile syringe can be used to withdraw solution from the bottle as required.

It is essential to prepare starch solution immediately before use because it undergoes gradual hydrolysis to glucose which is readily fermented by most medically important bacteria and could give false reactions. Sufficient starch for about 24 bottles can be prepared by adding 5 ml sterile distilled water to 0.15 g soluble starch in a sterile Universal container, screwing on the cap and shaking vigorously. The bottle is placed in a pan of water, brought to the boil and boiled for about 5 min, shaking at intervals to ensure that all the starch is in solution and the contents are homogeneous. The solution is cooled and 0.15 ml is added to 3 ml nutrient medium, usually serum peptone water in bijou bottles (final concentration of starch, 0.15%). The medium should be used within a few weeks after the starch is added.

3. A suitable *indicator* that will change colour only as a result of the formation of acids during the fermentation is required. A variety of indicators with a pK between pH 6 and 8 have been used (see Ch. 5). Some common practical examples are described here:

Andrade's indicator is made by adding NaOH 1 mol/litre to a 0.5% solution of acid fuchsin until the colour just becomes yellow. It is used at a final concentration of 0.005% in the medium and it turns dark reddish pink at about pH 5.5. Andrade's indicator fades fairly rapidly when stored and should not be used unless the media can be utilized within a few months.

Bromocresol purple is made up as a 0.2% solution. For use, 2.5 ml of this solution is added to each 100 ml medium to give a final concentration of 0.005%. Bromocresol purple is yellow at pH 5.2 and violet-purple at pH 6.8. It is recommended instead of Andrade's indicator for media that are likely to be stored for several months.

Phenol red is a solution of phenol sulphonthalein. Add 1.0 g of the reagent to 10 ml NaOH (0.1 mol/litre) and 20 ml distilled water and dissolve by gentle heat. Then add 10 ml HCl (0.1 mol/litre) and make up to 500 ml with distilled water to give a 0.2% solution. For use, 5 ml of this solution is added to each 100 ml of medium giving a final concentration of 0.01%. This indicator does not fade on storage and may be incorporated in bottled media that may not be used for some time. Phenol red is yellow at pH 6.8 and purple-pink at pH 8.4. It is used for serum media because it detects small changes in pH, characteristic of fermentation by nutritionally exacting bacteria.

Bromothymol blue is made up as a 0.2% solution by dissolving 1 g in 25 ml NaOH 0.1 mol/litre mixed with 475 ml distilled water. For use, 1.25 ml of the 0.2% solution is added to each 100 ml medium giving a final concentration of 0.0025%. Bromothymol blue is yellow at pH 6.0 and blue at pH 7.6. It is an alternative to phenol red when the pH change is small and it is used in serum media, broth-based media and in media for organic acid fermentation tests.

4. A small inverted tube (*Durham tube*) completely filled with liquid and containing no air bubbles is usually included in each culture tube or bottle to detect gas (see below).

Preparation of test media

Peptone water fermentation test media

The commonest nutrient medium for fermentation tests is peptone water.

Indicator solution:	
Andrade's	10 ml
or Bromocresol purple	25 ml
Test compound, 10% solution, sterile	50 ml

The nutrient medium (950 ml) is prepared and indicator added. The complete medium cannot be handled in bulk because the process of heat sterilization is used to drive out the air from the Durham tubes which then fill with liquid as the medium cools and fermentation media cannot be heated after adding the test compound. Therefore the base and indicator must be dispensed, sterilized by autoclaving and cooled before the sterile solution of test compound is added aseptically to each individual tube or bottle.

An alternative, easier, but less reliable, method is to add sterile substrate to the sterilized medium in bulk, distribute aseptically into sterile test tubes or bijou bottles, and heat these at 100°C for 20 min only to drive air out of the Durham tubes.

Medium may be dispensed either in 5 ml amounts with 50 × 7 mm Durham tubes, in 125 or 150 × 12.5 mm test tubes with caps or cotton-wool plugs or in 3 ml amounts with 27 × 6 mm Durham tubes in bijou bottles. Medium in bottles can be stored and transported without risk of spilling or of alteration in concentration of ingredients. As a result of shaking during transit, air may enter the Durham tube, but it is easily removed by inverting the bottle, the amount of liquid being such that the open end of the tube is below the surface. When bottles have been seeded the caps should be loosely screwed on to allow access of air.

Broth fermentation media

These may be used instead of peptone water if a more nutritious base is needed.

Meat extract	5 g
Disodium hydrogen phosphate, Na_2HPO_4	2 g
Water	950 ml
Indicator solution (bromothymol blue)	12.5 ml
Test compound, 10% solution, sterile	50 ml

Prepare, sterilize and dispense as for peptone water media.

Bitter medium

This has a special peptone base to distinguish only the reactions of strongly fermenting organisms. It is used with xylose for the 'fermentation typing' of organisms such as *Salmonella typhimurium* and its preparation is described in a previous edition (see Cruickshank 1968).

Serum peptone water fermentation media

These media are suitable for more exacting organisms such as *Corynebacterium diphtheriae*.

Peptone water, pH 7.6	800 ml
Serum	200 ml
Indicator solution: Phenol red	50 ml
or Bromothymol blue	12.5 ml
Test compound, 10%, sterile	10 ml

Some samples of horse serum may contain saccharolytic enzymes and give fallacious results. Batches should be tested before use. Sheep or ox serum is preferable.

Serum media are best sterilized by filtration but if they are not acid they will not coagulate on heating and may be steamed for 20 min on three successive days.

Durham tubes are rarely required for serum media and alternative methods of preparation are therefore practicable. The complete medium can be prepared, sterilized by filtration and dispensed aseptically. Otherwise the nutrient medium and indicator can be prepared, dispensed and steamed for 20 min on 3 successive days, a sterile 10% solution of the carbon compound being added to individual bottles or tubes with sterile precautions.

Hiss's serum water can replace serum peptone water. It consists of 25% serum in distilled water.

Serum agar fermentation media

These are recommended for organisms such as meningococci and gonococci that grow poorly in liquid media.

Basal medium

Peptone	20 g
Sodium chloride, NaCl	5 g
Distilled water	900 ml
Digest broth, pH 7.6	100 ml
Agar	25 g
Phenol red solution, 0.2%	20 ml

Dissolve the peptone and salt in the water by steaming. Adjust to pH 8.4 by making just alkaline to phenolphthalein and steam for 30 min. Filter through a coarse filter paper. Adjust to pH 7.6. Add the broth and agar and steam at 100°C for 45 min or until the agar is dissolved. Filter through a hardened filter paper if necessary, bottle in 100 ml amounts and add 2 ml phenol red to each bottle. Autoclave in 'free steam' for 1 h and then at 110°C for 5 min.

Complete medium

Basal medium	100 ml

Sterile serum (guinea-pig or
   rabbit)   5 ml
Test compound, 10% solution,
   sterile   10 ml

Melt the basal medium, cool to 55°C, add the other ingredients with sterile precautions and dispense as slopes in sterile tubes or bijou bottles.

Solid media in plates for strongly fermenting organisms

Plates of solid media containing carbohydrate may be used to test the fermentation of several pure cultures inoculated as streaks or spots, or to estimate the relative numbers of fermenting and non-fermenting organisms in a mixture plated on the medium. Eosin methylene blue agar or deoxycholate agar (Cruickshank 1968) which gives better differentiation of crowded colonies, is recommended for this purpose with enterobacteria.

Use of test media

Before inoculation, confirm the absence of bubbles of gas from Durham tubes in liquid media. Seed each medium with a speck of solid culture, or a drop or loopful of liquid culture, or a suspension of a solid culture in a sterile liquid. After incubation, examine the media for the presence of a colour change, indicating acid, and for gas formation in the Durham tube. Acid production in liquid serum media may cause coagulation of the serum.

Slopes of solid medium are seeded over the whole surface. The presence of a colour change after incubation indicates acid.

Fermentation reactions are commonly completed within a period of incubation of 24 h, or 48 h for slowly growing species. The identification of many organisms is based on the results recorded at these times. However some quickly growing organisms fail to ferment a given sugar in 24 h but will give 'late' fermentation if incubation is prolonged, up to 40 days. In such cases, tests should be inspected daily and the day on which fermentation first appears should be recorded. 'Late' fermentation is generally due to the emergence of a fermenting mutant.

Tests for specific breakdown products

Methyl red test

The methyl red test is employed to detect the production of sufficient acid during the fermentation of glucose and the maintenance of conditions such that the pH of an old culture is sustained below a value of about 4.5, as shown by a change in the colour of the methyl red indicator which is added at the end of the period of incubation.

Medium (glucose phosphate peptone water)

Peptone	5 g
Dipotassium hydrogen phosphate, K_2HPO_4	5 g
Water	1 litre
Glucose, 10% solution, (sterilized separately)	50 ml

Dissolve the peptone and phosphate, adjust the pH to 7.6, filter, dispense in 5 ml amounts and sterilize at 121°C for 15 min. Sterilize the glucose solution by filtration and add 0.25 ml to each tube (final concentration 0.5%).

Methyl red indicator solution

Methyl red	0.1 g
Ethanol	300 ml
Distilled water	200 ml

Method. Inoculate the liquid medium lightly from a young agar slope culture and incubate at 37°C for 48 h. Add about five drops of the methyl red reagent (see above). Mix and read immediately. Positive tests are bright red and negative are yellow. If the results after 48 h are equivocal, the test should be repeated with cultures that have been incubated for 5 days. For some organisms, incubation at 30°C for 5 days is preferable to incubation at 37°C for 2 or 5 days.

Acetoin production (Voges-Proskauer) test

Many bacteria ferment carbohydrates with the

production of acetyl methyl carbinol ($CH_3.CO.CHOH.CH_3$) or its reduction product 2, 3 butylene glycol ($CH_3.CHOH.CHOH.CH_3$). The substances can be tested for by a colorimetric reaction between diacetyl ($CH_3.CO.CO.CH_3$ – formed during the test by oxidation of acetyl methyl carbinol or 2, 3 butylene glycol) and a guanidino group under alkaline conditions. This test is usually done in conjunction with the methyl red test since the production of acetyl methyl carbinol or butylene glycol usually results in insufficient acid accumulating during fermentation to give a methyl red positive reaction. An organism of the enterobacterial group is usually *either* methyl-red-positve and Voges-Proskauer-negative *or* methyl-red negative and Voges-Proskauer-positive.

Medium. Glucose phosphate peptone water, as for the methyl red test.

Method 1 (O'Meara 1931). Incubate at 37°C or 30°C for 48 h only. Add 0.5 ml of O'Meara reagent (40 g potassium hydroxide and 0.3 g creatine in 100 ml distilled water). Place tubes in a 37°C waterbath for 4 h. Aerate by shaking at intervals. A positive reaction is denoted by the development of an eosin-pink colour, usually in 2–5 min.

Method 2 (Barritt 1936). Incubate at 37°C or 30°C for 48 h. Add 1 ml of 40% potassium hydroxide and 3 ml of a 5% solution of α-naphthol in absolute ethanol. A positive reaction is indicated by the development of a pink colour in 2–5 min, becoming crimson in 30 min. The tube can be shaken at intervals to ensure maximum aeration. α-Naphthol is a carcinogen.

Gluconate test

This is a test for the ability of an organism to oxidize gluconates to the 2 keto-gluconate which subsequently accumulates in the medium. The basis of the test is the change from gluconate, a non-reducing compound when tested with a suitable reagent, to 2 keto-gluconate, which is a reducing compound when so tested.

Medium

Peptone	1.5 g
Yeast extract	1 g
Dipotassium hydrogen phosphate, K_2HPO_4	1 g
Potassium gluconate	40 g
Distilled water	1 litre

The pH, after solution, should be 7.0. Distribute in 10 ml quantities in screw-capped bottles and autoclave at 121°C for 15 min.

Benedict's qualitative reagent. Dissolve sodium citrate 173 g and anhydrous sodium carbonate 100 g by heating in *c.* 800 ml distilled water. Add slowly, with gentle stirring, a solution of $CuSO_4.5H_2O$ (17.4 g in 100 ml of distilled water). When cool, make up to 1 litre with distilled water.

Method. Add 1 ml of the medium aseptically into a clean, sterile tube. Inoculate and incubate at 37°C for 48 h. Then add 1 ml of Benedict's reagent for reducing sugars, place the tube in a boiling water bath for 10 min and observe for the production of a coloured precipitate of cuprous oxide. Alternatively, test with a commercially available system for the detection of reducing sugars. If the Benedict test is used, read as follows:

Positive = green to orange precipitate.
Negative = the blue colour of the reagent is unchanged.

Tests to show ability to utilize a specific substrate

Bacteria that are capable of growing on a simple, chemically defined medium (i.e. *prototrophic* bacteria), can readily be tested for their ability to use a given compound as their sole source of carbon and energy. A defined medium is prepared with the test compound substituted for the normal carbon and energy source. The medium is usually made with agar and poured in plates. The organism is inoculated lightly in a streak or by plating out. After a suitable period of incubation the plate is examined and the appearance of bacterial growth indicates that the bacterium has been able to utilize the test compound.

Growth is often slower on a defined medium than on the ordinary peptone-containing media and observations should be continued for up to 7 days during incubation at 37°C. Usually growth is well developed at 2 days.

The inoculum for these tests should not be heavy and should not be made from a broth culture lest sufficient nutritive organic matter is carried over with the inoculum into the test medium to support a visible amount of growth. Preferably the bacterium is first grown for 18–24 h on an agar slope. A small amount of this growth is suspended in sterile saline solution to give a suspension of about $1–5 \times 10^8$ bacteria/ml and a small loopful of the suspension is used to inoculate the defined medium.

Bacteria that fail to grow on the simple defined medium when glucose and citrate are present as sources of carbon and energy, generally do so because they require as additional nutrients one or more specific amino acids or vitamins; they are described as *auxotrophic*. Growth tests made on further defined media supplemented with single amino acids or vitamins, or different combinations of these, will enable the particular nutritional requirements of an auxotroph to be determined.

Citrate utilization test

This is a test for the ability of an organism to utilize citrate as the sole carbon and energy source for growth and an ammonium salt as the sole source of nitrogen. Koser's liquid citrate medium or Simmons' citrate agar may be used.

Koser's medium (modified)

Sodium chloride, NaCl	5 g
Magnesium sulphate, $MgSO_4$	0.2 g
Ammonium dihydrogen phosphate, $NH_4H_2PO_4$	1 g
Potassium dihydrogen phosphate, KH_2PO_4	1 g
Sodium citrate, $Na_3C_6H_5O_7.2H_2O$	5 g
Distilled water	1 litre

The pH should be 6.8. The medium is dispensed and sterilized by autoclaving at 121°C for 15 min.

Simmons' medium. Simmons' citrate medium is a modification of Koser's medium with agar and an indicator added.

Koser's medium	1 litre
Agar	20 g
Bromothymol blue, 0.2%	40 ml

Dispense, autoclave at 121°C for 15 min and allow to set as slopes.

Method. Inoculate from a saline suspension of the organism to be tested. Incubate for 96 h at 37°C.

The results are read as follows:
1. Koser's citrate medium:
   Positive = Turbidity, i.e. growth.
   Negative= No turbidity.
A positive test should be subcultured into a second tube to eliminate false positives due to an excessive initial inoculum.
2. Simmons' citrate medium:
   Positive = Blue colour and streak of growth.
   Negative= Original green colour and no growth.

Malonate utilization test

Note that ultilization of malonate and deamination of phenylalanine can be combined in one test (see below).

Medium

Yeast extract	1 g
Ammonium sulphate, $(NH_4)_2SO_4$	2 g
Dipotassium hydrogen phosphate, K_2HPO_4	0.6 g
Potassium dihydrogen phosphate, KH_2PO_4	0.4 g
Sodium chloride, NaCl	2 g
Sodium malonate	3 g
Bromothymol blue	0.025 g
Distilled water	1 litre

Adjust the pH to 7.4 if necessary. Sterilize by autoclaving at 121°C for 15 min.

Method. Inoculate from a young agar slope culture and incubate at 37°C for 48 h. Positive results are indicated by a change in colour of the indicator from green to blue due to the rise in pH consequent upon the utilization of sodium malonate.

TESTS FOR METABOLISM OF PROTEINS AND AMINO ACIDS

Proteolytic organisms digest proteins and consequently may liquefy gelatin or coagulated serum. Cultures in meat media cause blackening of the meat, decomposing it and reducing its volume with the formation of foul-smelling products. Some organisms decompose milk proteins. Whereas strongly proteolytic organisms may have all these properties, weakly proteolytic ones may only liquefy gelatin. Liquefaction of gelatin, being the commonest proteolytic property, is used routinely as an index of proteolytic activity but a positive result may take several days to develop.

Gelatin liquefaction

For bacteriological use an edible grade of gelatin is preferred, since this is free from preservatives and inhibitory amounts of heavy metals. Gelatin will not by itself support the growth of many pathogens and it is added to a liquid nutrient medium to produce a firm gel called *nutrient gelatin*. The proportion of gelatin used varies, but 12% is a suitable average.

It is important that the gelatin medium should not be exposed to a high temperature for longer than recommended, otherwise it may be partially hydrolyzed and will not solidify on cooling.

Medium

Nutrient broth	1 litre
Gelatin	120 g

Add the gelatin to the broth and allow it to stand at 4°C overnight. Warm to 45°C to dissolve the gelatin. Adjust to pH 8.4 and steam for 10 min. Cool quickly to 45°C and slowly add the beaten white of two eggs, or 10 g egg albumin dissolved in 50 ml water, or 50 ml serum; this helps to clear colloidal particles from the medium. Steam for 30 min, stirring occasionally. Filter through hardened filter paper. Adjust the pH to 7.6 and bottle in 12 ml amounts. Hold in the autoclave in free steam for 10 min followed by 115°C for 10 min. Remove from the autoclave as quickly as possible and keep at a low temperature.

The resulting medium is perfectly transparent when solid, and should be of firm consistency, yet not so stiff that it is split by the wire when inoculated.

Method. A stab culture is made with an inoculum from an agar slope culture. Pathogenic bacteria are usually grown at 37°C and negative tests may be observed for as long as 30 days. Gelatin at the concentration used melts at about 24°C and is therefore liquid at 37°C. Liquefaction is tested for at intervals by removing the nutrient gelatin cultures from the incubator and holding them at 4°C for 30 min before reading the results.

Gelatin agar

Gelatin breakdown can be demonstrated by incorporating it in a buffered nutrient agar, growing the culture and then flooding the medium with a reagent that differentially precipitates either gelatin or its breakdown products.

Medium

Nutrient agar	1 litre
Potassium dihydrogen phosphate, KH_2PO_4	0.5 g
Dipotassium hydrogen phosphate, K_2HPO_4	1.5 g
Gelatin	4 g
Glucose	0.05 g

Melt the agar and dissolve the phosphates, gelatin and glucose in it, taking care to ensure even distribution of the gelatin. Adjust the pH to 7.0. Sterilize in a flask at 121°C for 30 min. Pour plates.

Mercuric chloride solution

Mercuric chloride, $HgCl_2$	15 g
Hydrochloric acid, concentrated, HCl	20 ml
Water	100 ml

Tannic acid solution. 1% in water.

Method. Seed plates and incubate under appropriate conditions. Flood plates with either mercuric chloride, which causes an opacity in the medium with clear zones around gelatin-liquefying colonies, slow to develop but not fading; or tannic acid, which causes a relative opacity around gelatin-liquefying colonies, quick to develop but fading as the medium also becomes opaque.

Gelatin charcoal disks

The method of Kohn (1953) employing sterile disks or cubes of formaldehyde-denatured gelatin containing finely powdered charcoal is a very rapid and convenient test for proteolysis.

The sterile disk is picked from its bottle with a hot inoculating wire, to which it adheres, and is transferred into a newly inoculated or already grown culture in liquid medium. The culture is incubated with the disk for up to a week at 37°C. (The denatured gelatin does not melt at this temperature.) Liquefaction of the gelatin is shown by the settling of free carbon particles to the bottom of the medium and, later, by the complete disintegration of the disk.

If the disks are added to a culture that is already fully grown or to a dense suspension in peptone water of a young culture grown on agar, liquefaction may be observed after only a few hours' incubation at 37°C.

It is important to include negative and positive controls, even if the disks are commercially produced.

Digestion of milk

Digestion of milk protein may be seen as a zone of clearing around colonies on milk agar. Results can be read in 24–48 h, less than the time usually necessary to see digestion of litmus milk.

Medium

| Nutrient agar, sterile | 87.5 ml |
| Skimmed milk, sterile | 12.5 ml |

Melt the agar, cool to 50°C, add the milk and pour plates.

Method. Inoculate, incubate and examine for zones of clearing.

Hydrogen sulphide production test combined with gelatin liquefaction test

Hydrogen sulphide can be produced at least in small amounts from sulphur-containing amino acids by a large number of bacteria. Methods showing hydrogen sulphide production by suspending strips of paper impregnated with lead acetate above cultures are of variable sensitivity and are of limited value. Precise tests must be poised at a definite level of sensitivity. The method described here is of a sensitivity suitable for group differentiation within the Enterobacteriaceae. Hydrogen sulphide is demonstrated by its ability to form black insoluble ferrous sulphide. The medium is solidified with gelatin and also indicates gelatin liquefaction.

Medium

Meat extract	7.5 g
Peptone	25 g
Sodium chloride, NaCl	5 g
Gelatin	120 g
Distilled water	1 litre
Ferrous chloride, 10% aqueous solution	5 ml

Dissolve all the ingredients except ferrous chloride in water, adjust to pH 7.6, steam and filter. Heat in the autoclave in free steam for 10 min and then at 115°C for 10 min. Remove from the autoclave as quickly as possible and cool to about 55°C. Add the ferrous chloride solution, freshly prepared and sterilized by filtration. Tube the medium in narrow tubes and seal with corks impregnated with paraffin wax.

Method. Inoculate with a straight wire to a depth of 1 cm and incubate at 20°C for at least

7 days. Inspect daily for blackening due to production of hydrogen sulphide and for lique-faction of gelatin.

Indole test

This test demonstrates the ability of certain bacteria to decompose the amino acid trypto-phane to indole which accumulates in the medium. Indole is then tested for by a colori-metric reaction with *p*-dimethyl-amino-benzaldehyde.

Medium

Peptone (brand containing sufficient tryptophane)	20 g
Sodium chloride, NaCl	5 g
Distilled water	1 litre

Adjust the pH to 7.4. Dispense and sterilize by autoclaving at 121°C for 15 min.

Kovac's reagent

Amyl or isoamyl alcohol	150 ml
p-Dimethyl-amino benzaldehyde	10 g
Conc. hydrochloric acid, HCl	50 ml

Dissolve the aldehyde in the alcohol and slowly add the acid. Prepare in small quantities and store in the refrigerator. Shake gently before use.

Method. Inoculate medium and incubate for 48 h at 37°C. Sometimes a period of 96 h at 37°C may be required for optimum accumulation of indole. Add 0.5 ml Kovac's reagent and shake gently. A red colour in the alcohol layer indi-cates a positive reaction.

Amino acid decarboxylase tests

This test (Møller 1955) is based on the ability of some bacteria to decarboxylate an amino acid to the corresponding amine with the liberation of carbon dioxide. The production of these decarboxylases is induced by a low pH and, as a result of their action, the pH rises to neutrality or above.

Medium

Peptone	5 g
Meat extract	5 g
Glucose	0.5 g
Pyridoxal	5 mg
Bromocresol purple (1 in 500 solution)	5 ml
Cresol red (1 in 500 solution)	2.5 ml
Distilled water	1 litre

Dissolve the solids in water and adjust the pH to 6.0 *before* the addition of the indicators. This is the basal medium and to it is added the amino acid whose decarboxylation is to be tested. Divide the basal medium into four portions and treat as follows:

1. Add 1% L-lysine hydrochloride.
2. Add 1% L-ornithine hydrochloride.
3. Add 1% L-arginine hydrochloride.
4. No additions (control).

Readjust the pH to 6.0 if necessary. Distribute 1 ml quantities in small tubes containing sterile liquid paraffin to provide a layer about 5 mm thick above the medium. Autoclave at 121°C for 15 min. *Note*: If the DL components are used, add 2% of the amino acid.

Method. Inoculate lightly through the paraffin layer with a straight wire. Incubate and read daily for 4 days.

The medium first becomes yellow due to acid production during glucose fermentation; later, if decarboxylation occurs, the medium becomes violet. The control should remain yellow.

Phenylalanine deaminase test

This test indicates the ability of an organism to deaminate phenylalanine with the production of phenylpyruvic acid which will react with ferric salts to give a green colour. Deamination of phenylalanine and utilization of malonate can be combined in one test (see below).

Medium

Yeast extract	3 g
DL-phenylalanine	2 g
(or L-phenylalanine	1 g)

Disodium hydrogen phosphate,
Na$_2$HPO$_4$ ... 1 g
Sodium chloride, NaCl ... 5 g
Agar ... 12 g
Distilled water ... 1 litre

Adjust the pH to 7.4, distribute and sterilize by autoclaving at 121°C for 15 min. Allow to solidify in tubes as long slopes.

Method. Inoculate with a fairly heavy inoculum. Incubate for 4 h or, if desired, for up to 24 h at 37°C. Allow a few drops of a 10% solution of ferric chloride to run down over the growth on the slope. If the test is positive, a green colour will develop in the fluid and in the slope.

TEST FOR METABOLISM OF FAT

Hydrolysis of tributyrin

An emulsion of micro-droplets of the fat, tributyrin, in a solid medium makes it opaque. Lipolytic organisms remove the opacity by converting the fat to water-soluble butyric acid.

Medium

Peptone ... 5 g
Yeast extract ... 3 g
Tributyrin (glyceryl tributyrate) ... 10 g
Agar ... 20 g
Water ... 1 litre

The medium is prepared so that the tributyrin forms a stable emulsion in the nutrient agar and the pH is adjusted to 7.5. For exacting organisms the medium may be enriched by addition of 5% of Fildes' extract (Willis 1960).

Method. Inoculate and incubate plates under appropriate conditions. Examine by transmitted light. Colonies of lipolytic organisms are surrounded by wide zones of clearing.

TESTS FOR ENZYMES

Catalase test

This demonstrates the presence of catalase, an enzyme that catalyses the release of oxygen from hydrogen peroxide.

One ml of hydrogen peroxide solution, H$_2$O$_2$ (10 vol), is poured over a 24 h nutrient agar slope culture of the test organism and the tube is held in a slanting position.

Alternatively, a small amount of the culture to be tested is picked from a nutrient agar slope with a clean sterile platinum loop or a clean, thin glass rod (a sealed capillary tube may be used for this purpose), and this is inserted into hydrogen peroxide solution held in a small, clean tube. Enough material may be picked from a single colony to give a reaction by this method.

The production of gas bubbles from the surface of the solid culture material indicates a positive reaction. It occurs almost immediately. A false positive reaction may be obtained if the culture medium contains catalase (e.g. blood agar), or if an iron wire loop is used.

Caution: The possible airborne transmission of a pathogen in the aerosol produced by this test merits careful consideration.

Oxidase test

This test depends on the presence in bacteria of certain oxidases that will catalyse the transport of electrons between electron donors in the bacteria and a redox dye – tetramethyl-*p*-phenylene-diamine. The dye is reduced to a deep purple colour.

The test is used for screening species of *Neisseria*, *Alcaligenes*, *Aeromonas*, *Vibrio*, *Campylobacter* and *Pseudomonas*, which give positive reactions and for excluding the Enterobacteriaceae, all species of which give negative reactions.

Plate method. Cultures are made on a suitable solid growth medium. A freshly prepared 1% solution of tetramethyl-*p*-phenylene-diamine dihydrochloride is poured on to the plate so as to cover the surface, and is then decanted. The colonies of oxidase-positive organisms rapidly develop a purple colour. If subcultures are required from the colonies, they should be made immediately; after 5 min exposure to the reagent it may not be possible to subculture them.

Dry filter paper method. Since the oxidase reagent is unstable and has to be freshly prepared for use, the following method is convenient. Strips of Whatman's No. 1 filter paper are soaked in a freshly prepared 1% solution of tetramethyl-*p*-phenylene-diamine dihydrochloride. After draining for about 30 s the strips are freeze dried and stored in a dark bottle tightly sealed with a screw cap. The papers have a light purple tint and will keep for several months in an airtight container at room temperature. For use, a strip is removed, laid in a Petri dish and moistened with distilled water. The colony to be tested is picked up with a platinum loop and smeared over the moist area. A positive reaction is indicated by an intense deep-purple hue, appearing within 5–10 s, a 'delayed positive' reaction by colouration in 10–60 s, and a negative reaction by absence of colouration or by colouration later than 60 s.

Wet filter paper method. A strip of filter paper is soaked with a little freshly made 1% solution of the reagent and then at once used by rubbing a speck of culture on it with a platinum loop. The result is read as for the dry filter paper method.

Note that the reagent must be freshly made and the bacterial growth must be transferred to the test paper with a clean *platinum* loop or a clean glass rod, since traces of iron will catalyse the reaction and give false positive results. If the colony is small it may be necessary to pick up material from several similar colonies in order to have sufficient to give a strong reaction. When testing colonies from MacConkey medium, a pink-violet colour is due to carry-over from the medium and is not a true oxidase reaction; the true reaction gives an intense purple hue. Dimethyl-*p*-phenylene-diamine oxalate, 1%, may be used in place of the tetramethyl-*p*-phenylene-diamine dihydrochloride in this paper-strip test.

Urease test

Bacteria, particularly those growing naturally in an environment exposed to urine, may decompose urea by means of the enzyme urease:

$$NH_2.CO.NH_2 + H_2O \rightarrow 2NH_3 + CO_2$$

The occurrence of this enzyme can be tested for by growing the organism in the presence of urea and testing for alkali (NH_3) production by

means of a suitable pH indicator. An alternative method is to test for the production of ammonia from urea by means of Nessler's reagent (see below).

Medium 1 (Christensen's medium)

Peptone	1 g
Sodium chloride, NaCl	5 g
Dipotassium hydrogen phosphate, K_2HPO_4	2 g
Phenol red (1 in 500 aqueous solution)	6 ml
Agar	20 g
Distilled water	1 litre
Glucose, 10% solution, sterile	10 ml
Urea, 20% solution, sterile	100 ml

Sterilize the glucose and urea solutions by filtration. Prepare the basal medium without glucose or urea, adjust to pH 6.8–6.9 and sterilize by autoclaving in a flask at 121°C for 30 min. Cool to about 50°C, add the glucose and urea and tube the medium as deep slopes.

The medium may be used as a liquid by omitting the agar.

Method. Inoculate heavily over the entire slope surface and incubate at 37°C. Examine after 4 h and after overnight incubation, no tube being reported negative until after 4 days' incubation. Urease-positive cultures change the colour of the indicator to purple-pink.

Medium 2 (Elek's test)

Urea	4 g
Potassium dihydrogen phosphate, KH_2PO_4, 0.2 mol/litre	50 ml
Sodium hydroxide, NaOH, 0.2 mol/litre	35 ml
Distilled water, ammonia-free	115 ml

This substrate contains 2% urea at pH 7.2. Sterilization of it is unnecessary. It can be stored in the refrigerator in a stoppered bottle with the stopper smeared with petroleum jelly. Freshly prepared substrate should be checked with a known urea-splitting organism, and for the test a negative control and an uninoculated blank must be included. The glassware must be scrupulously clean but not necessarily sterile.

Method. Emulsify sufficient of a 24 h culture of the organism to be tested, in 0.5 ml of the substrate in a small tube. The fluid should be distinctly opalescent. Place the tube in a waterbath at 37°C for 3 h. Remove the tube and add 0.1 ml of Nessler's reagent, and a similar amount to the negative control and blank tubes. Read the result 3 min after adding the Nessler's reagent. Both negative and control tubes must be absolutely colourless. A positive reaction is shown by a colour ranging from a pale but distinct yellow to a dark brown precipitate. The time of incubation is important and should be strictly adhered to.

When isolated colonies are to be examined, the volume of substrate is reduced to 0.3 ml and only one drop of Nessler's reagent used. Readings are taken 4–5 min after nesslerization.

Nessler's reagent. Dissolve 50 g KI in 50 ml water and then add saturated $HgCl_2$ solution until a permanent precipitate just appears. Add 200 ml NaOH solution (5 mol/litre) and make up to 1 litre with water. Take the clear supernate after the precipitate has settled.

ONPG (β-galactosidase) test

Lactose fermentation depends on the production of two enzymes – an induced intracellular enzyme, β-galactosidase, which hydrolyses lactose, and a permease which regulates the uptake of lactose into the cell. Certain bacteria possess the β-galactosidase enzyme but not the permease. These potential lactose fermenters may not produce acid at all in traditional peptone water media or may take several days to do so.

The β-galactosidase (ONPG) test, which determines the presence of the enzyme β-galactosidase by utilizing *o*-nitrophenyl-β-D-galactopyranoside, is used to differentiate late lactose fermenting organisms and is of particular use in the identification of enterobacteria.

Medium

o-Nitrophenyl-β-D-galactopyranoside	0.6 g
Phosphate buffer 0.01 mol/litre, pH 7.5	100 ml

Dissolve without heat and sterilize by filtration.

Add aseptically 1 part of the above to 3 parts of 1% peptone in water at pH 7.5.

Distribute in 2 ml amounts and incubate for 24 h to test sterility. It can then be stored in the refrigerator for up to 1 month.

Method. Inoculate and incubate for 24 h at 37°C. If the test is positive a yellow colour will develop in the fluid. Late lactose fermenters give a positive result more quickly in this medium than in sugar media.

Nitrate reduction test

This is a test for the presence of the enzyme nitrate reductase which causes the reduction of nitrate, in the presence of a suitable electron donor, to nitrite which can be tested for by an appropriate colorimetric reagent. Almost all Enterobacteriaceae reduce nitrate.

Medium

Potassium nitrate, KNO_3 (nitrite-free)	0.2 g
Peptone	5 g
Distilled water	1 litre

Tube in 5 ml amounts and autoclave at 121°C for 15 min.

Test reagent
Solution A. Dissolve 8.0 g of sulphanilic acid in 1 litre of acetic acid 5 mol/litre.

Solution B. Dissolve 5.0 g of α-naphthylamine in 1 litre of acetic acid 5 mol/litre.

Immediately before use, mix equal volumes of solutions A and B to give the test reagent.

Method. Inoculate the medium and incubate for 96 h. Add 0.1 ml of the test reagent to the test culture. A red colour developing within a few min indicates the presence of nitrite and hence the ability of the organism to reduce nitrate.

Note: α-Naphthylamine is potentially carcinogenic.

Lecithinase (phospholipase-C) test

Some bacteria produce enzymes (lecithinases or phospholipases) that split lipoprotein complexes in human serum and hen egg-yolk and produce opalescence or turbidity when grown in media containing these substrates. When the reaction is produced with egg-yolk it is sometimes referred to as the lecithovitellin reaction. The reactions when the substrate is added to a liquid medium and when human serum is added to a solid medium are described here. Note also egg-yolk agar described below.

Tube test (Hayward 1941)

Medium

Nutrient broth, sterile	50 ml
Human serum, sterile	
or Egg-yolk suspension, 10%	50 ml

The egg-yolk suspension is prepared as described for Willis and Hobbs medium in Chapter 37 but is 10% in saline instead of 50%. A sterile egg-yolk broth is obtainable commercially (Oxoid).

Aliquots (0.3 to 1 ml) of medium are dispensed aseptically in sterile tubes. Aliquots of nutrient broth without human serum or egg-yolk are dispensed as controls.

Method. Test and control media are inoculated with a drop of liquid culture or a colony picked from a plate culture. A known lecithinase-producing organism may be inoculated into test and control media as a positive control. In some cases the test can be extended by inoculating an additional test medium and adding antibody to a specific lecithinase, e.g. *Clostridium perfringens* α-antitoxin for the identification of *C. perfringens* (Ch. 37). Some lecithinases are dependent on divalent cations and may be inhibited by sequestering agents or buffers containing calcium-binding salts.

The tubes are incubated under conditions suitable for growth of the species involved and examined for turbidity daily up to five days. A positive reaction usually develops within 24–48 h and is indicated by a pronounced turbidity with a yellowish curd on the surface of the test mixture, easily distinguished from the lesser turbidity caused only by growth in the control and antitoxin tubes. A modification of this method may be used for testing culture filtrates or centrifuged supernates for lecithinase activity with an incubation time of 1–4 h. Tests are more easily read after storage overnight at 4°C or centrifugation to deposit organisms at the bottom and raise the curd to the surface of the mixture in a positive test.

Plate test (Hayward 1943)

Medium

Nutrient agar	100 ml
Human serum, sterile	40 ml

Melt the agar, cool to 50°C, add the serum and pour plates. The medium may be enriched by the addition of 5% Fildes' extract.

Method. Inoculate and incubate under conditions suitable for growth. Lecithinase-producing colonies are surrounded by zones of opalescence. In some cases an additional test can be included by spreading a few drops of antitoxin to a specific lecithinase over half the plate before it is inoculated. Opalescence should be inhibited around colonies on the antitoxin-treated half of the plate (Ch. 37).

Combined tests

Malonate utilization and phenylalanine deaminase test

This combines the two tests already described.

Medium

Ammonium sulphate, $(NH_4)_2SO_4$	2 g
Dipotassium hydrogen phosphate, K_2HPO_4	0.6 g
Potassium dihydrogen phosphate, KH_2PO_4	0.4 g
Sodium chloride, NaCl	2 g
Sodium malonate	3 g
DL-phenylalanine	2 g
Yeast extract	1 g
Distilled water	1 litre

Steam for 5 min and filter through paper. Add 5 ml of a 0.5% solution of bromothymol blue in absolute ethanol. Distribute in 10 ml quantities and autoclave at 121°C for 15 min.

Method. Distribute aseptically in 1 ml volumes in small sterile tubes. Inoculate, incubate overnight, and read results as follows:

1. Malonate utilization test.
Observe colour of medium:
     Blue = positive;
     Green = negative.
2. Phenylalamine deaminase test.

Having recorded the result of the malonate test, acidify with a few drops of HCl 0.1 mol/litre until the colour of the medium becomes yellow. Add a few drops of a 10% aqueous solution of ferric chloride, shake and observe colour:

     Dark green = positive;
     Yellow-buff = negative.

Litmus milk

Milk indicates both saccharolytic and proteolytic properties of bacteria by detecting whether they ferment lactose or digest casein. Lactose fermenters in litmus milk form acid and cause it to become pink. Large amounts of acid will precipitate the casein as a clot and if gas is formed during coagulation the clot will be disrupted by it ('stormy clot'). Proteolytic bacteria may decompose milk proteins to a transparent solution of soluble products. In litmus milk this shows as a change to a clear dark purple solution, usually taking several days and preceded by the formation of a soft, easily disintegrated clot.

Skimmed milk. Steam fresh milk for 20 min and allow it to stand for 24 h in order that the cream may separate. Siphon the milk off from the cream.

Litmus solution

Litmus granules	80 g	
Ethanol, 40% aqueous	*c.* 300 ml	
Hydrochloric acid, HCl 1 mol/l	q.s.	

Grind up the granules, add to a flask containing 150 ml aqueous ethanol and boil for 1 min. Decant the solution, add remainder of the aqueous ethanol and boil for 1 min. Decant and combine the two solutions, making the volume up to 300 ml with 40% aqueous ethanol. Add hydrochloric acid drop by drop, shaking continuously until the solution becomes purple. To test for the correct reaction, boil a tube of tap water and another of distilled water and add a drop of the solution to each. The tap water should be blue and the distilled water mauve.

Preparation of complete medium

Skimmed milk	250 ml
Litmus solution	6.25 ml

Distribute in 5 ml amounts in tubes or screw-capped bottles. Steam for 20 min on three successive days.

The colour fades on storing and it is best to store the skimmed milk, steamed on three successive days, in bulk (e.g. 250 ml) and add the litmus immediately before distribution.

Egg-yolk agar

Egg-yolk indicates both lipase and lecithinase reactions of bacteria. On solid media containing egg-yolk, lipolysis is shown by the formation of a thin, iridescent 'pearly layer' overlying the colonies and a 'confined' opalescence in the medium underlying them, seen best when the colonies are scraped off. Lecithinase is shown by wide zones of opalescence around colonies, more intense and larger than the zones caused by lipolysis (see Willis 1960). Neutralization by antitoxin may be possible (Ch. 37).

Medium

Nutrient agar, sterile	85 ml
Egg-yolk suspension	15 ml

Melt the agar, cool to 55°C and add the egg-yolk. Pour plates.

The medium can be enriched with 5% Fildes' extract. A sterile concentrated egg-yolk emulsion may be obtained from Oxoid.

Method. Inoculate, incubate and examine for wide zones of opalescence indicating lecithinase and for the iridescent layer indicating lipolysis. Flood the plate with a saturated aqueous solution of copper sulphate, stand for 20 min, drain off the excess solution and dry the plate for a short time in the incubator. The greenish-blue colour of copper soaps of fatty acids confirms lipolysis.

MISCELLANEOUS TESTS

Potassium cyanide test

This tests the ability of an organism to grow in the presence of cyanide.

Basal medium

Peptone	3 g
Sodium chloride, NaCl	5 g
Potassium dihydrogen phosphate, KH_2PO_4	0.23 g
Disodium hydrogen phosphate, $Na_2HPO_4.2H_2O$	5.64 g
Distilled water	1 litre

Adjust to pH 7.6 if necessary. Sterilize by autoclaving in flask at 121°C for 30 min. Refrigerate the basal medium until totally chilled.

Cyanide solution

Potassium cyanide, KCN	0.5 g
Distilled water, sterile	100 ml

Preparation of complete medium

Basal medium	1 litre
Cyanide solution	15 ml

Add the cyanide to the cold medium. Distribute in 1 ml amounts in sterile bijou bottles, seal tightly without delay and store at 4°C. The medium will keep for 4 weeks under these conditions.

Method. Inoculate with one loopful from a 24 h nutrient broth culture and incubate at 37°C with the cap tightly screwed down to prevent air exchange. Observe after 24 h and 48 h for turbidity produced by growth.

After use the cyanide in the medium should be destroyed by adding ferrous sulphate and alkali before submitting the cultures for sterilization.

DETECTION OF MOTILITY

In semi-solid agar media, motile bacteria 'swarm' and give a diffuse spreading growth that is easily recognized by the naked eye. Motility may thus be detected more easily than by the microscopical 'hanging drop' method (see Ch. 2).

The exact optimal concentration of agar depends on the particular brand used and must be determined by trial; usually it is about 0.4% of Japanese agar or 0.2% of New Zealand agar. This is dissolved in nutrient broth or peptone water. It is important that the final medium should be quite clear and transparent. Dispense 10 ml amounts in test tubes and leave to set in the vertical position. Inoculate with a straight wire, making a single stab down the centre of the tube to about half the depth of the medium. Incubate under the conditions favouring motility. Examine at intervals, e.g. after 6 h and 1, 2 and 6 days when incubating at 37°C. Freshly prepared medium containing 1% glucose can be used for motility tests on anaerobes.

Non-motile bacteria generally give growths that are confined to the stab-line, have sharply defined margins and leave the surrounding medium clearly transparent (Fig. 8.1a). Motile bacteria typically give diffuse, hazy growths that spread throughout the medium rendering it slightly opaque (Fig. 8.1b). The outgrowth may reach the walls of the tube after a few hours and

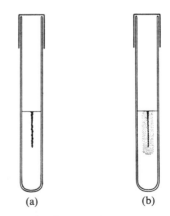

(a)   (b)

Fig. 8.1 Diagram showing growth of a non-motile organism (*a*) restricted to the stab line in semi-solid nutrient agar. The diffuse growth, or 'swarm', of a motile organism (*b*) extends as a zone of turbidity from the stab line.

the foot of the tube after one or two days. It is best observed by contrast while there is still some transparent medium not yet invaded. The incorporation of tetrazolium chloride at a final concentration of 0.005% in the medium is helpful; this is colourless in oxidized form, but the reduced salt is red and indicates where bacterial growth has occurred. With a non-motile strain that yields motile variants, a discrete line of growth is formed along the stab and diffuse outgrowths then fan out from one or two points. Sharply defined finger-like outgrowths may be given by some kinds of poorly motile bacteria, and also by some kinds of non-motile bacteria, apparently by their 'falling' through clefts in the medium; these doubtful cases may be resolved by use of the 'hanging drop' method.

TESTS FOR DIRECT BACTERIAL HAEMAGGLUTININ

Adhesiveness for animal cells is commonly indicated by a tendency of certain bacteria to adhere to and bind together red blood cells and thus cause 'direct bacterial haemagglutination'. The bacterial haemagglutinin may be a fixed part of the bacterial surface (see *fimbriae*, 13th Edn, Vol. 1, Ch. 2) and this type of haemagglutinin is accordingly described as non-diffusible or structural. A few bacterial species produce a soluble amorphous or diffusible haemagglutinin which diffuses into the surrounding medium and, though reacting with red cells, cannot bind the bacteria to these or to other substrates.

Tile test for fimbrial haemagglutinin

Red cells separated from fresh citrated guinea-pig blood are washed twice in physiological saline and made up to a 3% (v/v) suspension in fresh saline. A nutrient broth culture of the test organism is centrifuged to deposit the bacilli. After removal of the culture supernatant, the bacillary deposit is resuspended in the small amount of fluid remaining. A drop of the very dense bacillary deposit is mixed with an equal drop of the red cell suspension in a depression on a white tile at 3–5°C, and the tile is then rocked gently for 5 min while it is warming to room temperature. In the case of most fimbriate organisms, tests made at room temperature (15–20°C) without chilling the tile are entirely satisfactory. A few organisms, however, give haemagglutination at 3–5°C but not at higher temperatures.

The haemagglutination produced by fimbriate organisms is seen with the naked eye and usually develops as a coarse clumping within a few seconds. Weakly active cultures produce a fine granularity within 2–3 min. Very poorly haemagglutinating cultures may show positive reactions only if mixing is continued for up to 30 min. If a very dense bacterial suspension is not used, weak reactions may be missed.

Inhibition of fimbrial haemagglutination with mannose. The incorporation of a small drop of a 2% solution of D-mannose in the haemagglutination mixture (final mannose concentration 0.5%) specifically inhibits type 1 fimbrial haemagglutination (see Duguid & Gillies 1957; Duguid et al 1979).

Tube test for soluble haemagglutinin

To doubling dilutions of the test culture supernate in physiological saline (0.5 ml volumes), 0.5 ml aliquots of a 1% (v/v) red cell suspension in saline are added. The tubes are shaken and allowed to stand at room temperature for 1–2 h. The red cells settle into a characteristic pattern at the foot of each tube and this is conveniently viewed in a mirror. In the absence of haemagglutinin, the red cells form a dense central button. In the presence of soluble haemagglutinin, the red cells fall in a reticulum and this covers the base of the tube. The patterns are very similar to those described for myxovirus haemagglutination.

NEW APPROACHES AND DEVELOPMENTS

In *Medical Microbiology*, 13th Edition, Volume 1, Chapter 4, an account of the biochemical approach to bacterial classification includes considerations of cell-wall composition and DNA composition. In addition to differences in the metabolic products of bacteria that distinguish them and are exploited in our characterization systems, individual differences in chemical constituents of the bacterial cell are of taxonomic significance. Thus, gas chromatography and gas-liquid chromatography can be used in classification and in the detailed identification of bacteria to distinguish genera, species, and sometimes multiple chemotypes; the chromatographic techniques may define end-products of metabolism or may identify specific cell components.

Similarly, in DNA analyses, the DNA base composition as indicated by the G+C ratio (i.e. the percentage amount of guanine and cytosine in the bacterial DNA) is relatively fixed for any one species. Together with DNA homology studies, this provides important information for the characterization and classification of an organism.

These methods, now firmly established in taxonomic work, are forming the basis of some identification procedures that are coming into more general use. The procedures range from determination of the amino-acid composition of cells to complex infra-red spectrometry and mass spectrometry. Considerable advances are also being made in the immunological detection of bacterial antigens of the outer membrane complex by procedures that range from precipitin reactions through counter-current immunoelectrophoresis and polyacrylamide gel electrophoresis to immunoblotting techniques.

There are many possible applications of monoclonal antibodies that hold much promise; some are already exploited, such as the Phade-bact monoclonal GC test (Pharmacia) which is a coagglutination procedure for the rapid identification of gonococci.

Meanwhile, an extension of the traditional approach is to extend the range of identifiable enzymic activities that can be tested by developing a very wide range of special substrates linked with suitable indicator systems. The range of test substrates is matched with the range of organisms to be tested. This is the basis of the commercial systems described below.

Commercial systems

Identification methods are readily available from commercial sources. Some (e.g. Sensititre, Gibco; and API) are essentially a series of miniaturized classical biochemical tests. Dehydrated substances in plastic cups are reconstituted when a suspension of the bacteria under investigation is injected. A biochemical profile of the organisms is obtained after 24–48 h incubation at 37°C. The profile is translated into a numerical code which can be read from a key (Profile Index). Computer-based identification services for unusual organisms are available.

API systems are now widely used by laboratories across the world for the definitive identification of many groups of organisms. The systems include API 20 and API 20NE for enterobacteria and other Gram-negative bacilli, API STAPH for staphylococci and API 20 STREP for streptococci. The RapiD 20E system allows the prompt identification of enterobacteria by detection of pre-formed enzymes in a suspension of the test organism. The rapid system gives a result in 4 h.

Other systems make use of paper disks impregnated with biochemical substrates (e.g. Minitek; BioQuest, from Becton Dickinson). The disks are dispensed into special plates and a suspension of the test organism in broth is added. After incubation a biochemical profile is obtained which is dealt with in a similar way to the API system with numerical codes and computer produced matrices of probabilities.

The Mast ID system uses modified but traditional agar media supplied in sachets sufficient to prepare 200 ml of media. Poured plates will keep for up to 2 weeks. Inoculation with a standardized suspension is by multipoint inoculator which enables the laboratory to test many organisms simultaneously on a series of different media.

REFERENCES

Barritt M M 1936 The intensification of the Voges-Proskauer reaction by the addition of α-naphthol. Journal of Pathology and Bacteriology 42: 441–454

Cowan S T 1974 Cowan & Steel's Manual for the identification of medical bacteria, 2nd edn. University Press, Cambridge

Cruickshank R 1968 Medical microbiology, 11th edn (revised reprint). Churchill Livingstone, Edinburgh

Duguid J P, Clegg S, Wilson M I 1979 The fimbrial and non-fimbrial haemagglutinins of *Escherichia coli*. Journal of Medical Microbiology 12: 213–227

Duguid J P, Gillies R R 1957 Fimbriae and adhesive properties in dysentery bacilli. Journal of Pathology and Bacteriology 74: 397–411

Hayward N J 1941 Rapid identification of *Cl. welchii* by the Nagler reaction. British Medical Journal 1: 811–814

Hayward N J 1943 The rapid identification of *Cl. welchii* by Nagler tests in plate cultures. Journal of Pathology and Bacteriology 55: 285–293

Holdeman L V, Cato E P, Moore W E C 1977 Anaerobe laboratory manual, 4th edn. Virginia Polytechnic and State University, Blacksburg, Virginia

Hugh R, Leifson E 1953 The taxonomic significance of fermentative versus oxidative metabolism of carbohydrates by various Gram negative bacteria. Journal of Bacteriology 66: 24–26

Kohn J 1953 A preliminary report of a new gelatin liquefaction method. Journal of Clinical Pathology 6: 249

Møller V 1955 Simplified tests for some amino acid decarboxylases and for the arginine dihydrolase system. Acta Pathologica et Microbiologica Scandinavica 36: 158–172

O'Meara R A Q 1931 A simple delicate and rapid method of detecting the formation of acetylmethylcarbinol by bacteria fermenting carbohydrate. Journal of Pathology and Bacteriology 34: 401–406

Willis A T 1960 The lipolytic activity of some clostridia. Journal of Pathology and Bacteriology 80: 379–390

Laboratory control of antimicrobial therapy

Much of the work of the clinical microbiology laboratory is done to assist the clinician in the choice of drugs for the treatment of infections. It includes three main components: (1) the identification of relevant pathogens in exudates and body fluids collected from the patient, (2) sensitivity tests done to determine the degree of sensitivity or resistance of the pathogen isolated from the patient to an appropriate range of antimicrobial drugs, and (3) assays of the concentration of an administered drug in the blood or other body fluid of the patient required to control the schedule of dosage.

The clinician's purpose in prescribing an antimicrobial drug is to produce at the site of infection a concentration of it high enough to kill or inhibit the growth of the responsible pathogen, without exerting a significant toxic effect on the patient's tissues. Because nowadays the precise identity of the microorganism causing an infection is seldom implicit in the clinical presentation, the laboratory assists crucially by distinguishing relevant from irrelevant organisms in cultures from the patient and by identifying the species of the former. The different strains of a few pathogenic species are known to have sensitivity characters sufficiently constant to enable the choice of drugs for therapy to be made solely on the basis of the identification of the species, e.g. it may be taken for granted that any strain of *Streptococcus pyogenes* will be highly sensitive to benzylpenicillin, but strains of most pathogenic species differ from one another in their sensitivities, so that it is necessary for the sensitivity pattern of the particular strain isolated from the patient to be determined by sensitivity tests in the laboratory.

Both bacteriologists and clinicians should however bear in mind that the response to therapy in vivo may not always reflect the results of testing the sensitivity of the patient's pathogen in vitro. Thus, therapy for a pathogen found sensitive to a drug in vitro may fail because the drug is not adequately absorbed by the patient, or is unable to penetrate in an effective concentration into the least accessible site of multiplication of the pathogen, or is inactivated by a concomitant drug-resistant bacterium. On the other hand, a pathogen found resistant to a drug in vitro may be eliminated from the body during treatment with that drug either because an exceptionally high dosage is given or as a consequence of the patient's immune response to the infection.

Apart from the value of tests on isolates from individual patients, the accumulated results of sensitivity tests on all isolates of a pathogenic species from patients in a hospital or local community enable informed empirical treatment to be given for serious infections before the results of tests on the individual patients' strains are available. Moreover, by revealing changes in the resistance patterns of local pathogens, these accumulated results often indicate the need for change or control of the local pattern of antibiotic prescribing. Along with pharmacokinetic data, sensitivity tests are also the main means of assessing the potential value of new antimicrobial drugs before they are put to clinical trial.

Assays of the concentration of an antibiotic in the blood serum or other body fluid of a patient under treatment are done mainly when the antibiotic used is one, such as an aminoglycoside, which has toxic effects on the body at concentrations not greatly in excess of that required for its antimicrobial effect. The assays are done on specimens collected at times before and after the administration of a dose that are expected to show the minimum ('trough') and maximum ('peak') concentrations achieved and the results assist the clinician to adjust the dosage schedule so that the drug concentration will mainly be at a non-toxic but effective level, e.g. at about four times the minimum inhibitory or cidal concentration for the infecting organism.

SENSITIVITY TESTS

The results of sensitivity tests are generally reported in the form: 'Organism A isolated, sensitive (or resistant) to antibiotic B'. Such a report implies that the organism is relevant to the patient's clinical condition, that the *minimum inhibitory concentration* (MIC) of the antibiotic for it has been measured in some way, and that, if the organism is reported as 'sensitive', the MIC is less than a half or a quarter the concentration of antibiotic likely to be found in the infected tissues of a patient given the usual schedule of doses, i.e. that the infection is treatable. A larger margin of safety may be required in some infections.

'Resistance' implies that the infection is not treatable with the antibiotic because its MIC exceeds achievable safe tissue or urine levels. Strains described as of 'intermediate sensitivity' may be truly so, especially if the MICs of strains of that species show a unimodal distribution, but they can often be reclassified as sensitive or resistant if retested.

Ideally the bacteriologist might report to the physician the observed MIC of each antibiotic for the patient's infecting organism and leave it to the physician to decide, from his knowledge of the pharmacokinetics of each drug, the likely sites of infection within the patient's body and the concentration of drug likely to be achieved in these sites with the intended dose and route of administration, whether the infection is likely to be sensitive or resistant to therapy. In practice, however, the physician's ability to determine the pharmacokinetic conditions in the individual patient is limited and the bacteriol-

ogist is required to report the MIC findings in terms of 'sensitive' or 'resistant' according to criteria that have gained general acceptance from experience in clinical trials and practice. It must be borne in mind that these evaluations by the bacteriologist are applicable only to cases in which the dosage and method of administration of the drug are those in general use and the absorption and distribution of the drug and the site of infection in the patient's body are not markedly abnormal.

The MIC is measurable in three ways. 1. *Tests with serial discontinuous concentrations*. The organism is exposed to a series of fixed antibiotic concentrations in separate cultures in agar or broth. The different concentrations are produced by dilution, usually serially two-fold, of a solution prepared from antibiotic powder of accurately stated potency supplied for the purpose. They should not be prepared from therapeutic preparations, for the potency of these is not standardized with sufficient precision. The dilution steps should be arranged to give fractions or multiples of a concentration of 1 mg/litre. They may otherwise be prepared by placing commercially available paper disks containing known amounts of antibiotic in the bottom of Petri dishes before adding appropriate volumes of molten agar, or by adding commercially available antibiotic tablets to appropriate volumes of sterile broth, or by adding appropriate volumes of a broth culture of the test organism to the wells of commercially available microtitration plates containing the appropriate amounts of dried antibiotic.

The MIC is generally read as the smallest concentration of antibiotic in the series that prevents the development of visible growth of the test organism. The test can be extended to measure the *minimum bactericidal concentration* (MBC) of the antibiotic by preparing subcultures from each test culture and noting the smallest concentration of antibiotic from which no growth is obtained in the subculture. (Editor's note: Whilst the abbreviation MBC for *minimum bactericidal concentration* is in general use, it is unsatisfactory both because it could stand for *minimum bacteriostatic concentration* and because it is inapplicable to values for non-bacterial pathogens such as fungi and mycoplasmas. MCC, standing for *minimum cidal concentration*, would have been preferable, and it should be used for values for non-bacterial pathogens.)

Tests made thus with a series of concentrations are more expensive and time-consuming than those made by the following methods, which are generally used for routine sensitivity testing, but they are more accurate than the latter and are used to provide reference points for their control. They have a special use in the measurement of the MIC of antibiotics alone or in combination in the management of some serious infections, such as bacterial endocarditis.

2. *Tests with break-point concentrations*. This method is a modification of the foregoing one in which the test organism, along with control strains of known MIC, is exposed to only two or three critical 'break-point' concentrations of the antibiotic in agar or broth. These concentrations are chosen to reflect achievable antibiotic levels in the body fluids, usually blood and urine (Waterworth 1981, 1983). If the organism is inhibited by the lower concentration it is reported as sensitive, if by the higher but not the lower, as of intermediate resistance and if not by the higher concentration as resistant.

3. *Tests with diffusion gradients of concentration*. By this method, the test organism is seeded uniformly over an agar surface and exposed to a continuous concentration gradient of antibiotic diffusing from a paper disk (disk diffusion test). A bacterium sensitive to the antibiotic is inhibited from growing in a circular zone around the paper disk; the lower the MIC of the antibiotic for the organism, the larger the diameter of the zone. A comparison of the zone size with that produced in a parallel test with a control strain gives a measure of the MIC.

None of these in-vitro tests is entirely satisfactory. They provide only an approximation, and sometimes a poor one, to the conditions in the patient's body during treatment. Their accuracy and reproducibility are affected by many variables, e.g. the nature, composition and pH of the test medium, the weight of the bacterial

inoculum, the conditions and time of incubation, the amount of antibiotic present, and the organism's ability to produce an antibiotic-inactivating enzyme. Provided, however, that these limitations are kept in mind, the results are of great value in patient care and in the evaluation of new antibiotics (Phillips 1986). For a full discussion of these methods and their limitations, see Reeves et al (1978).

Novel and as yet largely experimental methods for determining the antibiotic susceptibility of bacteria by, for instance, microcalorimetry, measurement of electrical impedance or conductance of cultures in the presence of antibiotic, radiometric methods, bioluminescence, and the use of DNA probes, have been reviewed by Spencer & Wheat (1986).

Disk diffusion tests

The disk diffusion method is still the most widely used for the routine sensitivity testing of isolates from patients. It is satisfactory for organisms that grow well overnight, i.e. for most of the common pathogenic aerobic and facultatively anaerobic bacteria, rapidly growing anaerobes such as *Clostridium perfringens* and *Bacteroides fragilis*, and rapidly growing fungi such as *Candida albicans*. It is unsuitable for slowly growing organisms, such as the tubercle bacillus, for the antibiotic would have become too diffused before growth had become visible. A method of culture on fixed discontinuous concentrations (method 1, above) should be used for slowly growing organisms, also for measuring accurately the sulphonamide sensitivity of meningococci (Fallon 1978), the penicillin sensitivity of gonococci (Jephcott & Eggleston 1985) and the colistin sensitivity of Gram-negative bacteria (Williams & Leung 1978).

Several forms of disk diffusion test have been advocated, which vary in their methods of standardization, reading and control. 1. *The Kirby-Bauer method* (Bauer et al 1966) is the official method of the USA Food and Drugs Administration. Disks of a single, usually high content of antibiotic are placed on an inoculum of strictly standardized density on Mueller-Hinton agar. Three grades of sensitivity are recognized –

sensitive, intermediate and resistant – by comparing the diameters of the inhibition zones with critical zone diameters in published tables.

2. *The ICS method*, the outcome of a 10 year study by an International Collaborative Study Group (Ericsson & Sherris 1971) is also performed with single, high content disks. The zone diameters are separated into four categories of sensitivity, two of them intermediate, by reference to published regression lines that plot the MIC for many strains of different species against the zone diameter produced by a disk of the strength used in the test. The validity of this method of estimation has been the subject of controversy (Kraseman & Hildenbrand 1980; Arvidson et al 1981).

3. *The comparative method* is widely used in British laboratories. The diameter of the inhibition zone of the test organism is compared with that of a control organism of standard sensitivity tested under identical conditions on a separate plate or, preferably, on the same plate. Disks of low and high antibiotic content may be used, the latter to test organisms from urine, in which many antibiotics become highly concentrated. Three grades of sensitivity are recognized, sensitive, intermediate or indeterminate, and resistant. Testing both the test and control strains on the same plate (Stokes & Ridgeway 1980) eliminates many of the variables likely to affect accuracy, but not those of differences in the weight of the inoculum or speed of growth between the two strains.

There is no British standard for antibiotic sensitivity testing although recommendations for establishing a common method were put forward as long ago as 1971 (Garrod & Waterworth 1971; Stokes & Waterworth 1972). Despite these recommendations, major errors due to variations in technique are commonplace, e.g. the identification of resistant strains as sensitive and vice versa. The frequency of such errors is shown in the publication of analyses of data from the United Kingdom National External Quality Assessment Scheme, which describe common sources of error and the means to avoid them (Snell et al 1982, 1984a). Guidelines for disk diffusion testing for use in EEC member countries are being prepared by the European Committee for Clinical Laboratory Standards, and recommendations for break-point testing by a working party of the British Society for Antimicrobial Chemotherapy (Working Party 1985). Until standard methods are generally agreed, it is recommended that testing should be done by the Stokes same-plate comparative disk diffusion method and particulars for the performance of this method are described below.

Same-plate comparative disk diffusion test

Choice of growth medium. The growth medium must support good overnight growth of the test and control organisms; slow growth can result in the inhibition zones being abnormally large. Supplementation of the medium with whole blood may reduce the activity of antibiotics that are highly protein bound. By contrast, the addition of 5% lysed horse blood is needed to support or enhance the growth of nutritionally exacting species such as the gonococcus and *Haemophilus influenzae*. Lysed horse blood should also be added to certain media for tests with sulphonamides and trimethoprim; its content of thymidine phosphorylase is needed to neutralize the inhibitory effect of thymidine in the medium on the action of these drugs.

Low levels of free Ca^{++} and Mg^{++} ions in the medium increase the action of aminoglycoside antibiotics against *Pseudomonas aeruginosa*, whilst high levels decrease it. Because these ions interact with some constituents of agar, particularly phosphates, during autoclaving, the preparation of a suitable medium is difficult. This problem can be overcome by the use of an appropriate control strain in all tests.

To improve the detection of strains sensitive to mecillinam the medium should be adjusted to an osmolality of less than 400 m.osmol. On the other hand the addition of 5% NaCl to the medium is needed in one of the methods for detecting heteroresistance to methicillin in strains of *Staphylococcus aureus* (Barber 1964, Hewitt et al 1969). Apart from the examples given above, other additions should not be made to the medium unless it is certain that they are necessary and will not interfere with antibiotic activity.

The pH of the medium must be close to 7.3. A more acid reaction decreases the activity of aminoglycoside and macrolide antibiotics, including spectinomycin. Incubation of the test plates in a CO_2-enriched atmosphere or fermentation of sugars in the medium may lower the pH sufficiently to produce this effect. A more alkaline pH favours the action of tetracyclines, novobiocin and fusidic acid, but interferes seriously with the activity of nitrofurantoin.

Consistent and accurate results are most likely to be obtained if one of several suitable commercially available 'sensitivity test' media is used. This medium must be prepared exactly according to the manufacturer's instructions and poured to a depth of 4 mm in flat-bottomed 8.5 cm Petri dishes on a level surface. Once set, the plates may be stored for up to a week at 4°C; their surfaces should be dried with their lids ajar before use.

Preparation of inoculum. The ideal inoculum is one that on overnight incubation gives evenly spread semi-confluent growth. Failure to control the weight and spread of the inoculum is a common source of error. Too heavy an inoculum reduces the size of the inhibition zones produced by many antibiotics and may abolish those produced by some, e.g. sulphonamides. Too light an inoculum not only makes zone diameters difficult to read accurately, but may fail to reveal resistance due to the bacterial production of drug-destroying enzymes.

The inoculum should be prepared from material picked up with a loop from five to ten colonies of the species to be tested. This material should be suspended in saline or broth, or first grown as an overnight culture in broth. The suspension or culture should then be diluted to yield the correct number of colony-forming units in the volume to be inoculated on to the test plate. Precisely how much dilution is needed can be found only by experience, for it depends on the method used to spread the inoculum and the species being tested. Thus, far fewer viable organisms per ml of suspension are needed to produce semi-confluent growth in the case of a rapidly growing, large colonied species, such as *Klebsiella aerogenes* than in that of a slower

growing or small colonied species such as the enterococcus. The density of the suspension to be inoculated should therefore be measured by comparison with an opacity standard, e.g. a barium sulphate suspension, for tests are likely to be less accurate if the required density is judged by eye. Once a satisfactory method of preparing inocula of the proper density has been discovered, it should be written down and strictly followed.

Method of inoculation. The inoculum can be distributed evenly over the test plate by flooding the plate with the bacterial suspension and drying its surface while in a horizontal position before applying the antibiotic disks, but this method is time consuming and potentially hazardous, and so is not recommended. Good results can be obtained by placing a standard loopful of the inoculum suspension on the plate and then spreading it with a dry sterile swab. Alternatively, a swab may be dipped into the suspension, squeezed free from excess fluid against the side of the tube and then rubbed over the plate. A method of preparing swabs impregnated with the control organism and storing them in bulk for up to a week has been described by Felmingham & Stokes (1972). Spreading the inoculum with a wire loop alone is unsatisfactory (Snell et al 1982, 1984a, 1986).

It is often argued that strict control of the density of the inoculum is impracticable in a busy laboratory where many sensitivity tests are done each day, but there is little point in setting up tests without such control if, as is likely, the accuracy of the results will be in doubt, with possible danger to the patient. Any test plates yielding growth indicative of an unsatisfactory inoculum should be discarded unread and the test repeated.

In the original Stokes' method (see Stokes & Ridgeway 1980) the inoculum of the control strain is evenly spread over the upper and lower thirds of a plate and that of the test strain over the central third; uninoculated gaps 2–3 mm wide are left to separate the test from the control areas. Two antibiotic disks are then placed 20–25 mm from the plate rim to straddle each gap; thus four antibiotics can be tested on each plate. A convenient modification of this method (Pearson & Whitehead 1974) facilitates accurate placing of the inoculum and allows up to six disks to be tested on each plate. The plate is placed on a rotating turntable (Denley) and circular areas are seeded by holding the inoculating swab against the plate at appropriate radial positions. The control inoculum is spread over an outer circular area, the test inoculum over the central circular area, and a circular gap 2–3 mm wide is left uninoculated between the two areas, preferably about 13 mm from the plate rim.

When the plate has been seeded by this rotational method, six disks may be placed serially on the gap, and if this is done manually a template should be used to ensure they are placed equidistantly. Alternatively, the six disks can be applied simultaneously in the form of a commercially available paper ring device (e.g. from Mast) or singly, in cartridges held in a spring-loaded six-cartridge dispenser (e.g. from Oxoid). When either of the latter methods is used, the position of the gap between the test and control inocula must be adjusted so that it matches the positions of application of the disks. The application of single disks manually or with a dispenser is to be preferred to the application of a six-disk paper circle, for the results are likely to be more accurate (Snell et al 1982) and changes can be made in the choice of antibiotics to be tested as considered appropriate to the patient's condition.

Whatever the method of applying the disks, it is essential that the full surface of each disk makes firm contact with the seeded agar and that the application be made within a short and standard time of the seeding of the plates.

Prediffusion of antibiotic from the disks may be procured by holding the plates at room temperature for a period before placing them in the incubator to initiate growth of the inoculated bacteria. This practice may improve the reproducibility of results, but is unnecessary except when testing colistin against Gram-negative aerobes (Williams & Leung 1978), when prediffusion for 30 min is recommended. Otherwise, the interval between applying the disks and placing the plates in an incubator should be short and standardized.

Control strains. Four control strains are usually recommended for use with the comparative method: *Escherichia coli* NCTC10418 for tests of coliform bacilli from the urinary tract; *Pseudomonas aeruginosa* NCTC10662 for tests of this species, especially against aminoglycosides; *Clostridium perfringens* NCTC11229 for tests of clostridia against metronidazole and other anticlostridial antibiotics; and *Staphylococcus aureus* NCTC6571, the 'Oxford' staphylococcus, for tests with all other antibiotics except polymyxins.

Because of differences in growth rate, and for other reasons, the use of a control strain of a species different from that of the test strain can reduce the accuracy of the results. Jephcott & Eggleston (1985) have therefore recommended the use of a sensitive strain of *Neisseria gonorrhoeae* rather than the Oxford staphylococcus for tests of gonococcal isolates. And it has been found that a sensitive strain of *Haemophilus influenzae*, NCTC 11931, is a better control than the Oxford staphylococcus for tests of *H. influenzae* against ampicillin, chloramphenicol and tetracycline (Snell et al 1986). A strain of *Bacteroides fragilis*, NCTC 9343, is appropriate when testing rapidly growing Gram-negative anaerobes (Phillips & Warren 1978) and a strain of *E. coli* less sensitive to mecillinam than strain NCTC 10418 when testing coliforms from the urinary tract against this antibiotic (Menday & Tybring 1978). Tests of strains of *S. aureus* that may be heteroresistant to methicillin are more likely to be accurate if a control strain with that resistance is used (Snell 1985). Such a strain is available on request from the Division of Microbiological Reagents and Quality Control, Central Public Health Laboratory, Colindale, London, to laboratories taking part in the United Kingdom National External Quality Assessment Scheme. The use of β-lactamase-producing control strains is recommended when testing the sensitivity of coliforms or *S. aureus* isolates to amoxycillin plus clavulanic acid: *E. coli* NCTC 11560 for the former and *S. aureus* NCTC 11561 for the latter.

Working cultures of control strains should be

grown weekly or monthly from stock cultures that are freeze-dried or frozen at −20°C. They should be maintained on slants of a suitable medium and subcultured as seldom as possible. Inocula are prepared and spread as described for the test strains.

Antibiotic disks. Commercially prepared disks 6 mm in diameter should be used (e.g. Oxoid, Mast). Their content of antibiotic should not vary more than the limits set by the World Health Organization Expert Committee on Biological Standardization (1977) and should be coded as recommended by that committee. The quality of available disks is discussed by Brown et al (1982). Disks and disk dispensers should be stored in sealed containers with a desiccant, bulk stock being kept at −20°C if possible, otherwise at less than 8°C. Working stock, also kept in sealed containers with desiccant, should be stored at less than 8°C. Before they are opened for use, the containers should be allowed to warm up slowly at room temperature to minimize condensation of moisture, which would lead to hydrolysis of the antibiotic. Some workers prefer each day to remove from stock enough disks for the day's work and discard any that are left over on its completion. Stocks of disks should be discarded on their stated expiry date. Metronidazole may deteriorate when exposed to light and disks of it should be kept in the dark as much as possible.

There is little agreement about the correct antibiotic content of disks. Disks with too high a content can produce zones so large that they obliterate most of the growth and make accurate reading impossible. They may also cause to be read as sensitive strains whose MIC is above achievable or safe levels of antibiotic in the tissues. Manufacturers introducing new antibiotics may supply only disks with an unduly high content. It should be remembered, too, that for some time after the disk has been applied to the plate the concentration of antibiotic in the medium near the disk is considerably higher than the disk's content of antibiotic per ml.

Disks of two or more different strengths are produced for about half of the antibiotics used in clinical practice. Organisms from the urinary tract should be tested against the high-content disks to reflect the high concentrations of antibiotic excreted in the urine. Contents tentatively recommended are shown in Tables 9.1 and 9.2.

Particular disk contents shown to improve the accuracy of results (Snell et al 1982) are as follows: for bacteria from the urinary tract, ampicillin 25 μg rather than 10 μg; for staphylo-

Table 9.1 Recommended antibiotic contents of disks for use in diffusion sensitivity tests (in micrograms unless stated otherwise). See Table 9.2 for higher content disks and their uses.

Drug	Content (μg)	Drug	Content (μg)
Amikacin	30	Gentamicin	10
Amoxycillin (20) plus clavulanate (10)	30[a]	Kanamycin	10
		Lincomycin	2
Ampicillin	2	Mecillinam	10
Azlocillin	30	Methicillin	5
Benzylpenicillin[b]	1.2	Metronidazole[c]	5
Carbenicillin	100	Mezlocillin	30
Cefamandole	30	Mupirocin[e]	5
Cefoperazone	30	Nalidixic acid	30
Cefotaxime	30	Neomycin	30
Cefoxitin	30	Netilmicin	10
Cefsulodin	30	Nitrofurantoin	100
Ceftazidime	30	Norfloxacin	10
Ceftriaxone	30	Piperacillin	75
Cefuroxime	30	Rifampicin[f]	2
Cephalothin	30	Sisomicin	10
Cephazolin	30	Spectinomycin	25
Chloramphenicol	2.5 or 5	Streptomycin	25
Cinoxacin	100	Sulphafurazole	100
Ciprofloxacin	5	Sulphamethoxazole	25
Clindamycin	2	Tetracycline	10
Cloxacillin[c]	5	Ticarcillin	75
Colistin	10 units	Tobramycin	10
Cotrimoxazole[d]	25	Trimethoprim	1.25
Erythromycin	5	Vancomycin	25
Fusidate	10		

[a] For *Haemophilus influenzae*, 3 μg.
[b] I.e. 2 units.
[c] For coagulase-negative staphylococci.
[d] Sulphamethoxazole 23.75 μg plus trimethoprim 1.25 μg.
[e] For Gram-positive cocci.
[f] For Gram-positive cocci and *Bacteroides* spp.

Table 9.2 Higher content antibiotic disks for sensitivity of bacteria from the urinary tract, or other purposes as specified. (Contents in micrograms unless stated otherwise.)

Drug	Content (μg)	Other purposes
Ampicillin	25	. . .
Azlocillin	75	. . .
Benzylpenicillin	6	To detect β-lactamase-producing gonococci[a]
Chloramphenicol	25	For clostridia[b] and when topical therapy is intended
Colistin	100 units	For pseudomonads[c]
Mecillinam	25	. . .
Metronidazole	100	For identifying *Gardnerella vaginalis*[d]
Mezlocillin	75	. . .
Neomycin	30	When topical therapy intended
Piperacillin	100	. . .
Rifampicin	100	For Gram-negative species and enterococci[e]
Sulphafurazole	500	For pseudomonads[c]
Tetracycline	30	. . .
Trimethoprim	5	For *Gardnerella vaginalis*[d]

[a] Jephcott & Eggleston (1985)
[b] Phillips et al (1985)
[c] King & Phillips (1985)
[d] Easmon & Ison (1985)
[e] Williams & Leung (1978)

cocci from sites other than the urinary tract, erythromycin 5 μg rather than 10 or 15 μg; for *Pseudomonas aeruginosa* from sites other than the urinary tract, carbenicillin 100 μg rather than 5 μg. Low-content disks are preferable for testing strains of *Haemophilus influenzae* against ampicillin (2 μg rather than 5, 10 or 25 μg), chloramphenicol (2.5, 5 or 10 μg rather than 25 μg) and tetracycline (2, 5 or 10 μg rather than 25 μg). Tests for the sensitivity of strains of *H. influenzae* to amoxycillin plus clavulanic acid should be done with a disk containing 2 μg ampicillin and a disk containing 3 μg amoxycillin plus clavulanic acid, in either case along with a test of the strain's ability to produce β-lactamase (Snell et al 1986); a sensitive strain of the species (e.g. NCTC 11931) should be used as a control. These tests identify strains that are sensitive to ampicillin, strains that do not produce β-lactamase but are resistant to ampicillin (and

therefore to amoxycillin plus clavulanic acid), and strains that are resistant to ampicillin by virtue of the production of β-lactamase. If a disk containing 30 μg amoxycillin plus clavulanic acid is used, many strains in the latter two categories will be wrongly classed as sensitive.

The choice of disks for testing sensitivity to cotrimoxazole is contentious (Edmunds 1978; Lacey & Stokes 1978). A single disk containing a mixture of sulphamethoxazole (23.75 μg) and trimethoprim (1.25 μg) is recommended by the manufacturers. Many workers prefer to test each drug separately, some test with the two drugs separately and also with the combined disk; others seek visible evidence of synergy in the 'pulling out' of contiguous inhibition zones between the sulphonamide and trimethoprim disks placed unusually close together, but the absence of that distortion does not necessarily mean that the two drugs will fail to act synergistically in the body, nor is the opposite necessarily true. Strains resistant to trimethoprim but sensitive to sulphonamides are unlikely to be detected unless the two drugs are tested separately.

Some workers test only with trimethoprim, as cotrimaxazole would not be indicated if the strain were trimethoprim-resistant.

Choice of drugs for tests. The drugs to be tested against each species or category of bacteria should preferably be grouped in sets of six, which is the maximum number to be placed on a single 8.5 cm diameter plate. The members of each set should be those most likely to be used for therapy of infections with a particular species, the preferred method, or infections at a particular body site, or infections with organisms grouped by their Gram reaction.

It is neither possible nor desirable to specify standard sets of drugs because of differences in local prescribing habits, in the resistance patterns of local pathogens, in the relevance of the cost, toxicity, pharmacokinetics and spectrum of activity of the antibiotics to the management of the illnesses of particular patients, and in the extent to which laboratory staff wish to test and report selectively, but the sets chosen should reflect these variables. The standardization of sets does, of course, facilitate the rapid processing of isolates from large numbers of specimens without the need for the choice of drugs to be referred in each case to a senior member of staff.

It is convenient to test routinely those antibiotics that are commonly prescribed by local physicians ('first-line' tests) and to reserve for later ('second-line') tests, should they prove necessary, those antibiotics of which prescription is restricted to special circumstances. First-line tests should include any antibiotic currently being given to the patient, provided its spectrum is relevant to the species being tested.

Isolates of a species need not be tested with drugs that are valueless in the therapy of their infections. Thus, Gram-positive species should not be tested against polymyxins or aztreonam, for neither of these drugs has activity against them. Similarly, Gram-negative species need not be tested against vancomycin, nor enterococci against cephalosporins, nor *Proteus* species against tetracycline, nitrofurantoin or polymyxins. Nalidixic acid and nitrofurantoin should be tested only against isolates from the urinary tract. It is probably unhelpful to test first-generation cephalosporins against *H. influenzae*, and sensible to restrict tests with methicillin and fusidic acid to staphylococci, and tests with chloramphenicol to isolates of *H. influenzae*, salmonellae, Gram-negative anaerobes and anaerobic streptococci from serious infections, and isolates from superficial infections of the ear and eye which may be treated topically.

Only one representative need be tested from any group of closely related drugs amongst which there is cross-resistance. Thus, one tetracycline represents all tetracyclines; the clinical relevance of the sensitivity to minocycline of some tetracycline-resistant strains of *S. aureus* is limited. Colistin can substitute for polymyxin B. Benzylpenicillin represents all the penicillinase-sensitive penicillins when testing staphylococci. Tests with methicillin against *S. aureus* reflect the strain's reaction to all the penicillinase-resistant penicillins, such as flucloxacillin, and the cephalosporins; results are often unreliable if disks of other drugs in this group are tested in the place of one of methicillin. It is not clear whether the

same relations hold true for strains of coagulase-negative staphylococci; the particular penicillin or cephalosporin to be used in treatment should be tested against the isolate. Ampicillin serves for its esters, e.g. bacampicillin and talampicillin, and for amoxycillin. Azlocillin, mezlocillin, piperacillin and ticarcillin should be tested individually. Cephalothin can be used to represent cephalosporins with 'first generation' activity, e.g. cefaclor, cefadroxil, cephalexin, cephapirin and cephradine, but other cephalosporins should be tested individually (except against *S. aureus*), as should also the aminoglycosides and the newer 4-quinolones such as ciprofloxacin, enoxacin, norfloxacin and ofloxacin. Nalidixic acid, however, represents the earlier quinolones such as cinoxacin, oxolinic acid and pipemidic acid against strains from urinary tract infections.

Reading and reporting of results. Discard any plates on which the weight of inoculum is unsatisfactory and repeat the tests.

On satisfactory plates, measure the inhibition zones of the control strain, i.e. the distance in millimetres from the edge of the disk to the zone edge if that is obvious; if it is not, measure to the point of 80% inhibition of growth. The measurement should be made with callipers, a millimetre rule or a ruled template, and on the agar surface, not through the glass or plastic bottom or lid of the dish. The zone sizes of the control strain should fall within limits determined earlier from tests carried out in exactly the same way, and displayed for reference. If they fall outside these limits, repeat the tests after seeking and correcting the cause of the divergence.

It should be noted that some workers measure and describe 'zone size' as the *diameter* of the circular inhibition zone, including the antibiotic disk. In this account, however, it is the *radial width* of the zone *outside* the disk that is described.

If the control strain zones are within the accepted limits, examine the sizes of the inhibition zones of the test strain. If these are as large or larger than those of the control strain, or if growth reaches to the disk's edge, sensitivity or resistance is unequivocal and they do not need to be measured. Otherwise, measure the zone sizes with callipers as described above, for comparing the sizes of the zones of the test and control strains by eye is then insufficiently accurate (Snell et al 1982, 1986).

Some strains of *Proteus* spp. back-swarm into the inhibition zones late during incubation; this growth in the zone should be disregarded and measurements made from the zone edge if it is obvious. Swarming can be prevented by adding to the medium 0.2 mmol/litre (43 mg/100 ml) *p*-nitrophenylglycerol (Sigma) without interfering with the action of a wide range of antibiotics (Senior 1978).

According to the measurements of zone size, three categories of sensitivity can be recognized: (1) *sensitive*, the zone size of the test strain measured as described above is larger than, equal to or not more than 3 mm smaller than that of the control strain; (2) *resistant*, the zone size of the test strain is smaller than 3 mm; (3) *intermediate*, the zone size of the test strain is at least 3 mm, but also 3 mm smaller than that of the control strain.

The validity of the intermediate category has frequently been challenged and many laboratories avoid the phrase in bacteriological reports. Some strains may be truly of intermediate sensitivity, especially if the MICs of the antibiotic for strains in the species are distributed unimodally, but the reporting of their intermediate position is of clinical value only if the antibiotic in question can safely be given in full or increased dosage. The intermediate position of other strains is often questionable; if they are retested, or examined in other ways, e.g. for the production of β-lactamase, they can often be placed in one of the other two categories.

In some circumstances, simply measuring the zone size does not enable the strain to be categorized as sensitive or resistant. The case of β-lactamase-producing strains is discussed in detail below, and in tests of strains of *Proteus* spp. against nitrofurantoin, large inhibition zones may be present but are not a dependable guide to therapeutic sensitivity. The pH of the test plate is considerably less alkaline and therefore less inhibitory to the action of nitrofurantoin than the urine of many patients with proteus infections. For this reason, many workers prefer to record all proteus strains as resistant to nitrofurantoin, irrespective of the size of any zone of inhibition.

The generic (non-proprietary) names of the antibiotics should be used in reporting the results of sensitivity tests. It should be remembered that the laboratory's reports have a considerable influence on the prescribing habits of those to whom they are sent, and that a measure of control over antibiotic prescribing can be exercised by the selective reporting of sensitivity test results (Davies 1982; Cooke et al 1983; Langdale & Miller 1986).

β-lactamase-producing strains. In tests of β-lactamase-producing strains of *S. aureus*, *N. gonorrhoeae* and *H. influenzae* for sensitivity to the penicillinase-destructible penicillins, the zone size is dependent on the growth rate of the test strain relative to that of the control strain and on the amount of the drug-destroying enzyme released by the former during incubation. The zones produced by a disk containing benzylpenicillin in cultures of β-lactamase-producing *S. aureus* are often large, but the growth just outside the edge of the zone is characteristically heaped-up and seen to consist of full-sized colonies. Strains showing this appearance should be reported as resistant regardless of the size of the inhibition zone.

β-lactamase-producing strains of *N. gonorrhoeae* should be recognized by testing chemically for the enzyme. They may be identified provisionally by testing a heavily seeded plate to which is applied a disk containing 6 μg of benzylpenicillin; after incubation the zone of inhibition, if there is one, will measure less than 7 mm (Jephcott & Eggleston 1985).

In tests of β-lactamase-producing strains of *H. influenzae* the inhibition zones around disks containing ampicillin or amoxycillin plus clavulanic acid are often large, especially if disks of too high a content of the antibiotic have been used, e.g. 25 μg of ampicillin or 30 μg of amoxycillin plus clavulanic acid (containing 20 μg of amoxycillin). These strains should also be recognized by testing for β-lactamase and, if positive, be reported as resistant.

Disks of amoxycillin plus clavulanic acid also give rise to problems in the interpretation of zone sizes when other species are being tested. The disk's high content of amoxycillin (20 μg) diffuses further across the plate than its lower content of clavulanic acid (10 μg). If neither the control nor the test strain produces β-lactamase, the difference is of no moment, but if the test strain produces β-lactamase while the control strain does not, the former, because of the restricted diffusion of clavulanic acid and the smaller inhibition zone thereby produced in its growth, is likely to be wrongly classed as resistant to the combined treatment. This problem may be solved in two ways.

1. In tests with a control strain that does not produce β-lactamase, the test strain should be regarded as sensitive if its zone size is greater than or equal to that of the control strain or, in the case of coliform bacteria, not more than 5 mm smaller than that of control strain *E. coli* NCTC 10418; or in the case of strains of *S. aureus*, not more than 10 mm smaller than that of control strain *S. aureus* NCTC6571. The test strain should be regarded as of intermediate sensitivity if its zone size is at least 3 mm but not so great as to fall into the sensitive category as just defined, and as resistant if its zone size is 2 mm or less.

2. The difficulty is better overcome by the use of a suitable β-lactamase-producing strain as the control, e.g. *E. coli* NCTC 11560 or *S. aureus* NCTC 11561. These strains have the advantage of controlling the potency of the clavulanic acid content of the disk, but they have the disadvantage that neither is susceptible to the full range of non-β-lactam antibiotics; both, for instance, are resistant to streptomycin and tetracycline, whilst *E. coli* NCTC 11560 is also resistant to chloramphenicol.

Methicillin resistance in Staphylococcus aureus. In methicillin-resistant cultures of *Staphylococcus aureus* a small and slowly growing proportion of cells can withstand concentrations of the antibiotic that are inhibitory for the remainder. This minority cannot be detected with certainty unless sought under special conditions, i.e. either by carrying out the test on a medium containing 5%

NaCl or by incubating the test plate at 30–34°C (Barber 1964; Annear 1968; Hewitt et al 1969). A disk containing 5 or 10 μg of methicillin should be used and a known methicillin-resistant strain tested simultaneously as a control (Snell 1985).

Tests for β-lactamase

Penicilloic acid is produced when β-lactamases hydrolyse benzylpenicillin. It can be detected (1) by measuring the resulting change in pH, e.g. with an indicator dye, or (2) by its property of reducing iodine and so reversing the blue colour formed when starch complexes with iodine. A third method of detecting β-lactamase depends on the colour change from yellow to red produced on hydrolysis of the β-lactam ring of the chromogenic cephalosporin 87/312, i.e. nitrocefin (Oxoid).

1. *Acid-formation method*. Papers impregnated with penicillin and a pH indicator dye are available commercially. Solid bacterial growth from an overnight culture of a β-lactamase-producing strain applied to the paper lowers the pH and alters the colour of the indicator.

2. *Iodometric method* (Sykes 1978). Prepare in wells in a microtitration plate a heavy suspension (about 10^9 colony forming units/ml) from an overnight culture of the test organism in 0.1 ml of a solution of benzylpenicillin 6 mg/ml in 0.1 mol/litre phosphate buffer pH 7.3. Also set up a control mixture without the organisms. Incubate the plate for up to an hour, or stand it for the same time at room temperature, then mix into the suspension two drops of a freshly prepared 1% solution of soluble starch dissolved by heating at 100°C. Add one drop of iodine reagent, consisting of 2.03 g iodine and 5.32 g potassium iodide in 100 ml distilled water. In a negative test a blue colour persists for at least 10 min; in one positive for β-lactamase the blue colour is rapidly lost.

3. *Nitrocefin test*. Nitrocefin is available impregnated in small rods (Oxoid). If a rod is touched on to a colony of a prolific β-lactamase

producer, a red colour develops within a few seconds. The substance can also be used as a solution. This is prepared at a concentration of 200–500 mg/litre by first dissolving it in dimethyl sulphoxide and then in 0.1 mol/litre phosphate buffer pH 7. The solution will keep its potency for some weeks if stored in a dark bottle. It can be used to detect β-lactamase in one of three ways. (i) Place a drop of the solution on a colony growing on a solid medium. A colour change from yellow to red, denoting a positive test, is often apparent within seconds, but may not become obvious until the plate has been incubated. The red colour is unstable in agar and fades in 2–3 hours. (ii) Add a few drops of solution to an overnight broth culture of the bacterium. A red colour may develop very rapidly, but may not be seen until the culture has been re-incubated for up to 30 min. (iii) Mix equal volumes, e.g. of 50–100 μl, of the solution and a heavy suspension of bacteria from an overnight culture of the test strain in a well in a microtitration plate. In a positive test the red colour develops within 30 min.

Whichever method is used, known positive and negative control strains should be tested in parallel.

Primary sensitivity tests

In these tests the specimen serves as the inoculum. When well mixed a portion of it is spread uniformly over part or whole of one or more primary culture plates and antibiotic disks are applied before the plates are incubated. If the uniformly inoculated part of the plate is less than half its total area, allowing for streaking out to yield separate colonies on the remaining area, only two disks can safely be applied. If the specimen is spread confluently over the whole of a plate, or in a peripheral ring that allows for inoculation of a control strain in the central area, up to six disks may be applied.

Primary sensitivity tests are claimed to have the following advantages. (1) Their results are available the next day, i.e. a day earlier than those of tests on pure subcultures, and the additional labour and cost of performing the subculture tests is avoided. (2) They may help to identify bacteria that have constant patterns of sensitivity to the antibiotics tested. (3) In mixed cultures they may help to separate bacterial species with different sensitivities. (4) They may reveal the presence of small numbers of resistant variants that might not arise rapidly enough to be detected in a pure subculture of the sensitive parent organism.

They have three disadvantages. (1) The weight of the bacterial inoculum cannot be controlled, and because it is often too light the effort of setting up the primary tests may be wasted. (2) It is inconvenient to include a control strain in the primary tests and even when one is included it may in retrospect prove to be of an inappropriate species. (3) Because the identity of any pathogen present is unknown when the test is set up, the choice of drugs to be tested can be made only in terms of the organisms thought most likely to be present.

In practice, it appears that primary sensitivity tests are of most value for specimens of urine, of some value for swabs or pus from patients in accident and emergency clinics, but of little value for specimens from patients already receiving antibiotics or for specimens from sites likely to be heavily contaminated or to yield a heavy mixed flora, e.g. bedsores, varicose ulcers, vaginal swabs and wounds infected with mixed intestinal bacteria.

The value of primary tests on urine samples reflects the fact that the concentration of bacteria in significant bacteriuria is generally close to that needed to produce semi-confluent growth on the culture plate, although it depends on first identifying specimens with significant numbers of organisms, e.g. by microscopical examination, otherwise the labour of setting up the primary tests will often be wasted (Waterworth & del Piano 1976).

It is apparent then that caution must be exercised in reporting sensitivities observed in primary tests. Results should not be reported when the inoculum density is found to have been unsatisfactory. It is perhaps wisest to report the results as only provisional or to confine reporting to species for which the result is almost certainly appropriate, e.g. penicillin sensitivity of an organism identified as *Streptococcus pyogenes* or pneumococcus from the appearance of its colonies and its sensitivity to a diagnostic bacitracin or optochin disk also applied to the primary plate.

Whilst their value as a guide to therapy may be limited, many bacteriologists use primary sensitivity tests to assist in the identification and separation of bacteria in primary cultures. The zone around each antibiotic disk acts in effect as a different kind of selective culture medium and colonies of a resistant species of bacterium may appear in a zone, and be available for picking for identification, while elsewhere on the plate they are masked by those of a more numerous or vigorously growing sensitive species. Thus, colonies of many anaerobic species may be obtained in the zone around a high-content disk of gentamicin or neomycin which inhibits the majority of facultative contaminants and concomitants. Scanty haemophili and enterococci may be observed around penicillin disks. The presence of yeasts may be recognized from the growth of their colonies around all disks of antibacterial antibiotics.

Serial dilution sensitivity tests

These tests are carried out in agar or broth. In the past, because of the labour needed to prepare antibiotic dilutions of known strength, their use was largely restricted to tests of slowly growing organisms for which diffusion tests were unsuitable. Now, however, commercially available tablets and disks containing known amounts of antibiotic (e.g. Adatabs, Mast) have made the accurate preparation of the antibiotic dilutions relatively easy, and prepared series of antibiotic concentrations freeze dried in microtitre trays are also available. As a result, dilution tests are being more widely used, especially tests in agar media containing two or three different 'breakpoint' concentrations (see below). The principal application of dilution tests in broth is to measure the MIC and MBC of suitable antibiotics for bacteria responsible for endocarditis.

Preparation of antibiotic solutions. If this is not to be done by the use of commercially available tablets or disks of known content, solutions should be freshly prepared from powder of known potency supplied by the manufacturer for this purpose. Formulations of antibiotics for use in therapy are unsatisfactory for the tests. Some of these formulations, e.g. esters of chloramphenicol and erythromycin, are inactive in vitro and the potency of therapeutic preparations is seldom stated accurately enough.

Distilled water serves to dissolve most antibiotic powders, but chloramphenicol and erythromycin must first be dissolved in a small amount of ethanol, nitrofurantoin and sulphonamides in a small volume of NaOH solution, and trimethoprim in weak acid (acetic or lactic). For further details, see Reeves et al (1978).

Dilution tests in broth for MIC

Prepare two sets of two-fold dilutions of the antibiotic in sterile broth. The highest concentration should be at least twice as high as that likely to be found in the tissues and the lowest at most half the MIC for the control organism. It is convenient if the final concentrations are multiples or fractions of 1 mg/litre.

Inoculate one set of dilutions with one drop (0.02 ml) of a 1 in 100 dilution in broth of an overnight broth culture of the test strain (i.e. a drop containing about 10^5 to 10^6 colony forming units) and the second set with one drop of a similar suspension of a suitable control strain. The Oxford strain of *Staphylococcus aureus* serves for most antibiotics except the polymyxins. Include in each seeded set a tube of broth without antibiotic to show the suitability of the broth for growth of the oganism and unseeded tubes of broth with and without antibiotic to serve as controls of the sterility and clarity of the broth.

Incubate the tubes for 18–24 h at 37°C and examine them for turbidity due to bacterial growth. Examine the set with the control organism first. Provided the broth sterility control is clear, the tube containing the lowest concentration of antibiotic that prevents visible growth contains the MIC of the antibiotic for the control organism. If this measurement is correct, read and record the MIC for the test organism.

Dilution tests in broth for MBC

The MIC test described above is often extended by subculture to measure the MBC (cidal concentration) as follows. Before incubating the MIC tubes seeded with the test organism, remove a large standard loopful from the tube without antibiotic and spread it over quarter of a plate of nutrient medium free from antibiotic and incubate it. After incubation of the tubes, spread a similar loopful in the same way from each of the tubes not showing visible growth. If possible, incorporate on or in these plates an inhibitor of the antibiotic being tested. After incubation of the subculture plates, examine them for growth. The tube containing the lowest concentration of antibiotic that fails to yield growth on the subculture plate is judged to contain the MBC of antibiotic for the test strain.

By comparing the number of colonies present on the subculture from the antibiotic-free broth before it was incubated, with the numbers on the plate subcultures from the incubated antibiotic-containing tubes, it is possible to identify bacteriostatic action; an incubated tube with a static concentration of antibiotic will yield the same number of colonies as the unincubated antibiotic-free tube. A modest reduction in the number of colonies from an antibiotic-containing tube indicates slow cidal action, and the presence of a few colonies of 'persisters' indicates incomplete killing. Cidal action is indicated by a reduction in the number of colonies by at least 99%.

These interpretations should be made with caution, for the number of colonies appearing when antibiotic-containing tubes are subcultured depends greatly on the weight of the inoculum, a small inoculum favouring the effectiveness of the antibiotic. Great care is needed to avoid splashing some of the inoculum on to the sides of the tubes where live organisms may persist out of contact with the antibiotic during incubation and from where they may be transferred to the subculture plate, grow and wrongly be classed as survivors.

'Break-point' dilution tests in agar

These tests are performed by placing, with a multi-point replica inoculator, a drop of in-oculum of each strain under test on one, two or three agar plates containing different known concentrations of the same antibiotic. A control plate with no antibiotic must be included. An organism tested against two concentrations and inhibited by both is classed as sensitive, one inhibited only by the higher concentration is moderately sensitive, and one not inhibited by either as resistant. Advantages claimed for the method are: up to 30 or more isolates plus the appropriate controls may be tested on a single pair of plates; except in tests with sulphonamides and tests of β-lactamase-producing strains against β-lactam antibiotics, the weight of the inoculum is much less critical than in disk testing; a week's supply of plates may be prepared at one time and stored at 4°C; and automated reading and computer analysis of the results minimizes the labour required and some of the possible errors of the tests.

Disadvantages are: it is difficult to recognize mixed cultures in the test; because patterns of sensitivity are less easily collated than in disk testing their value in identification is much less; and the method as presently practised is no more accurate than disk testing (Snell et al 1984b). There is also controversy about which concentrations of each antibiotic should be used to give results of the greatest clinical relevance. For further details of the method, suggested break-point concentrations of the different antibiotics, and discussions of some of the problems, see Waterworth (1981, 1983), Snell et al (1984b) and Working Party (1985).

Sensitivity tests for mycobacteria

These tests demand considerable technical skill and are potentially hazardous to perform. They are therefore best done in regional reference laboratories furnished with the requisite equipment and expertise. Details of methods of testing in sealed bottles are given by Jenkins et al (1985).

Tests for combined antibiotic action

A physician may treat a patient with more than one antibiotic at a time for one of the following reasons: (1) in serious infections to cover a wide range of possible infecting organisms before the causal one has been identified; (2) to treat mixed infections when one antibiotic alone is insufficient; (3) to prevent the emergence of variants resistant to a single drug; (4) to neutralize antibiotic-destroying enzymes; (5) because the combined drugs act synergistically; (6) to reduce drug-related toxicity.

Two antibiotics acting together in vitro may have one of three effects: (1) *indifference* when the action of each drug in the presence of the other is neither greater nor less than its action when alone; (2) *antagonism*, when the activity of one drug is significantly reduced in the presence of the other; (3) *synergy*, when the antibacterial activity of the mixture, whether static or cidal, greatly exceeds that of either drug alone. It must be appreciated that there has been much debate about these categories. Other workers recognize an *additive* effect; antagonism is then defined as an interaction that is significantly less than additive, and synergy must be shown to be significantly more than a simple additive interaction. See Hamilton-Miller (1985).

Whilst the interaction of one antibiotic with another is often of great theoretical interest, in the diagnostic laboratory tests for synergy are principally made to identify a mixture of two antibiotics that will kill a culture of an organism for which a single bactericidal antibiotic cannot be found, e.g. that of an enterococcal or streptococcal isolate from endocarditis. In such cases synergy is most likely between a β-lactam antibiotic, e.g. a penicillin or cephalosporin, and an aminoglycoside, e.g. gentamicin or netilmicin.

The ways in which two antibiotics may act together to kill a bacterial cell are often complex and can be studied in different ways, e.g. by time-kill experiments, by surface diffusion of antibiotics as in the tambour method described originally by Chabbert and later modified by Anand & Paul (1976; see Garrod et al 1981 for details), or by 'chessboard' titration. Each type of test may give a different answer, and an answer with different clinical relevance (Greenwood 1979). A strong argument can be made for the use of tests with an arithmetic series of drug concentrations rather than the conventional doubling dilutions; this is particularly important when the results are to be plotted as an iso-

bologram (see Hamilton-Miller 1985). The method most often used in clinical laboratories is the 'chessboard' titration described below.

Chessboard titration for combined activity

Prepare by doubling dilution in broth a discontinuous series of concentrations of each antibiotic and mix them together in equal volumes so that each concentration of each drug is present alone and in combination with each concentration of the other in the same final volume of broth.

Into each tube containing antibiotic, and one of broth without antibiotic inoculate one drop of a 1 in 100 broth dilution of an overnight broth culture of the bacterium to be tested. At once remove a standard loopful from the antibiotic-free tube and spread it over quarter of a plate of blood agar. Then incubate the tubes and plate overnight at 37°C.

Next day examine the tubes and record the MICs of the antibiotics acting alone and in combination. The extent of each drug's contribution to any bacteriostatic effect of the mixtures can be expressed as the fractional inhibitory concentration (FIC); this is a fraction in which the denominator is the MIC of the drug acting alone and the numerator is its MIC when acting in combination with the second drug. The combined effect is expressed by adding together the FICs of each drug (Berenbaum 1978). A combined FIC of 1 indicates indifference, one of greater than 1 antagonism, and one of less than 1 synergy. In practice, useful bacteriostatic synergy should not be assumed unless the combined FIC is 0.5 or less (Hallander et al 1982).

If the test is done to identify suitable treatment for streptococcal endocarditis, for which it is valuable (Garrod & Waterworth 1962), it is necessary to extend it to seek a combined *bactericidal* effect capable of sterilizing the culture. A standard loopful from each tube without visible growth after overnight incubation is plated on blood agar and incubated overnight. Next day the presence or absence of growth in the subcultures is read to identify the MBCs of the antibiotics acting alone and in combination.

If a bactericidal combination of concentrations

is not found with the first pair of drugs, further pairs of different drugs must be tested. This can be done by the 'half-chessboard' method. A single concentration of each of six or seven different antibiotics is tested alone and in combination with each of the others in a constant final volume of broth. A control tube of broth free from antibiotic is included.

When the mixtures of antibiotics in broth have been prepared, seed each with a drop of a 1 in 100 dilution in broth of an overnight broth culture of the strain under test. At once remove a standard loopful from the control, antibiotic-free tube and plate it on blood agar. Then incubate both the plate and the tubes of mixtures. Next day subculture from any tubes lacking visible growth on to blood agar.

Such tests against streptococci should be made with (1) penicillins or cephalosporins, (2) aminoglycosides, (3) erythromycin, (4) clindamycin, and (5) rifampicin. Mixtures of (1) with (2), (2) with (3), and (3) or (4) with (5) are those most likely to show synergy. Suitable concentrations (mg/litre) are: benzylpencillin and ampicillin, 2 or 10; cefuroxime, 10; clindamycin, erythromycin, gentamicin, tobramycin and rifampicin, 2; streptomycin, 10.

ANTIBIOTIC ASSAYS

The amount of antibiotic in the blood or other body fluids of patients is measured for four main reasons: (1) to ensure that adequate therapeutic concentrations are being reached, e.g. when oral replaces parenteral administration for a serious infection; (2) to avoid producing toxic concentrations, e.g. when an aminoglycoside, chloramphenicol or vancomycin is being given, or when the patient is very young, elderly or suffering from renal or hepatic failure; (3) to study the pharmacokinetics of the antibiotic; and (4) to correlate the achieved drug level with the clinical outcome. Assays are done for the last two reasons mainly during clinical trials of new antibiotics.

In clinical laboratories, most assays are of blood levels of aminoglycosides, chloramphenicol or vancomycin, done to avoid toxic concen-

trations, or of benzylpenicillin, done to ensure the concentration is therapeutically adequate. For such assays, two samples of blood are needed. The first is taken immediately before the next dose of antibiotic is due to be given; it gives a measure of the lowest, or 'trough' level of antibiotic present, which is the surest indicator of drug accumulation. The second is taken to show the highest, or 'peak' level produced; it should be withdrawn 45–60 min after an intravenous bolus dose, 60 min after an intramuscular dose and 2 h after an oral dose. The exact times at which the samples were withdrawn and the size and route of the dose must be known if the results of the assay are to have any useful meaning.

Until recently, microbiological diffusion methods, particularly the large-plate bioassay, have been the most used for the assay of antibiotics in clinical specimens. Large-plate bioassay is relatively cheap; it is flexible and can be adapted to measure levels of almost any antibiotic; it can be carried out without highly specialized or expensive equipment; and when properly done, is sensitive and precise enough ($\pm15\%$) for most clinical purposes. But it is nonspecific, and the presence of a second, often undeclared antibiotic in the sample usually makes the results meaningless. Moreover, though it can be modified to give a result in 3–5 h for gentamicin (Shanson & Hines 1977) or chloramphenicol (George et al 1981), it is slow, generally needing 18–24 h before results are available, and so can seldom be used to modify, dose by dose, the treatment of a patient whose ability to absorb, conjugate or excrete the antibiotic is deficient or rapidly changing.

Automated assays

It is not surprising, therefore, that other, nonmicrobiological methods of assaying antibiotics have been developed and are increasingly being used. In a rapidly changing field, polarizing fluorescence immunoassay (TDX system, Abbott), fluoro-immunoassay and enzyme immunoassay (EMIT, Syva) are currently the alternative methods most used for the measurement of aminoglycosides and vancomycin. They have the advantages of speed, making results available in

1–2 h, and specificity, their accuracy rarely being affected by the presence of other antibiotics. They are convenient if large numbers of specimens have to be examined each day, but they require the provision of costly, specialized equipment and reagents. Follow the instructions of the equipment's maker.

Large-plate diffusion assay

In this method, the sample to be assayed, e.g. a patient's blood serum, and a series of control standard concentrations of the antibiotic to be measured are applied to agar seeded throughout or on its surface with a sensitive bacterial species. After incubation the diameters of the zones of inhibition are measured. The measurements for the standard solutions are used to construct a dose-response curve from which the concentration of antibiotic in the patient's sample can be read off by interpolation. Diffusion assays, like diffusion sensitivity tests, are affected by many variables. For a detailed discussion of these variables and of how they may be controlled, see Reeves et al (1978), Garrod et al (1981) and De Louvois (1982).

Preparation of plates. Glass-bottomed assay plates, 25 × 25 cm (Mast) accommodate four aliquots of each of 11 samples and 5 standard solutions. Mark one corner of the plate on the outside of the glass. Ensure that the base of the plate is flat and horizontal, so that when agar is poured into it, it will form an even layer. For this purpose, place the plate on a levelling tripod before pouring.

DST agar (Oxoid), adjusted to the appropriate pH, serves for assays of benzylpenicillin (pH 6.8), aminoglycosides (pH 7.8), chloramphenicol (pH 7.4) and vancomycin (pH 7.8). Preferably on the day the assay is to be done, prepare sufficient medium to give a layer from 2–3 mm thick (about 225 ml for a 25 × 25 cm plate) and cool it to 50°C in a waterbath. If the assay organism is to be incorporated in the agar, add it to the agar when the latter has cooled further to about 45°C and mix thoroughly. Quickly warm the glass base of the plate by passing a Bunsen flame across it and pour the seeded molten agar into the plate. Make sure that it

flows evenly over the surface and remove any bubbles by passing a flame rapidly across it before it has set. These last three steps must be carried out quickly. Finally, dry the surface of the plate for 30 min at 37°C and, if it is not to be used at once, store it at 4°C. It is helpful to expose the surface of the agar to ultraviolet radiation for 2–3 min before applying the antibiotic-containing samples, for the elimination of surface growth sharpens the edges of the zones of inhibition and makes easier their accurate measurement.

If the plate is to be seeded on its surface, flood it, after drying, with a diluted culture of the test organism, pipette off the excess and dry it again for 30 min at 37°C. Do not expose such surface-seeded plates to ultraviolet radiation.

Preparation of inocula. A suspension of spores of *Bacillus subtilis* NCTC8236 incorporated in the agar serves for assays of benzylpenicillin, aminoglycosides and vancomycin. Alternatively, *Staphylococcus aureus* NCTC6571 incorporated in the agar can be used for benzylpenicillin or vancomycin; *Klebsiella edwardsi* NCTC10896 in or on the agar for aminoglycosides; and *Sarcina lutea* NCTC8340 or a suitably sensitive strain of *Escherichia coli*, seeded on the agar surface, for chloramphenicol.

Inocula of the non-sporing species should be prepared from stationary-phase (overnight) cultures diluted to the extent that they will produce semi-confluent growth when the assay is read. The exact extent of the dilution must be determined by trial and error; once found, the method should be written down and strictly followed thereafter. Aliquots of the appropriate dilution, sufficient for the seeding of a single plate, can be stored at 4°C for up to 4 weeks or at −70°C or in liquid nitrogen for as long as required.

To prepare a suspension of *B. subtilis* spores, grow the organism on agar slants in bottles of 150–200 ml capacity for 7–10 days at 37°C. When microscopical examination shows that profuse sporulation has taken place, harvest the growth, wash it thrice in changes of distilled water, and finally suspend it in fresh distilled water to a concentration such that only 1–2 ml need be added to the agar to give semi-confluent growth. The suspension can be stored at 4°C for many months.

Standard antibiotic solutions. Prepare these from powders of known potency that have been stored in a desiccator at 4°C. Therapeutic preparations are unsuitable. Prepare concentrations ranging from close to the lower limit of sensitivity of the assay system up to a level slightly higher than the maximum expected in the patient's sample under test, e.g., in mg/litre, benzylpenicillin or gentamicin, 1, 2, 4, 8 and 16; chloramphenicol, 2.5, 5, 10, 20 and 40; vancomycin, 4, 8, 16, 32 and 64.

Weigh out about 100 mg of the antibiotic on an analytical balance and dissolve it in sterile distilled water (chloramphenicol first in 2–3 ml ethanol). If antibiotic in serum is to be assayed, use pooled human serum to produce the dilutions needed for the range of standards. For assays of an aminoglycoside in cerebrospinal fluid, prepare the standards in a solution containing 150 mmol/litre NaCl and 4.5 mmol/litre $CaCl_2$ (Deacon 1976). Concentrated standards, i.e. containing 1 g/litre of aminoglycoside, chloramphenicol or vancomycin in aliquots sufficient for 1 day's work may be stored frozen at $-20°C$ for several weeks, but should not be refrozen after thawing for use. Solutions of benzylpenicillin are best prepared on the day they are to be used.

Patient samples. The samples of blood serum or other body fluid are applied to the plate in wells of 6–9 mm diameter cut with a sterile cork borer; the circular agar plugs must be cut and removed with care not to lift or distort the surrounding agar. Alternatively, the samples may be applied on sterile filter paper disks or in sterile metal, glass or porcelain cylinders placed on the surface of the agar, but the use of wells is preferable. To assist in spacing the wells evenly across the agar, place under the plate a card on which is drawn a square with sides coincident with the visible edge of the base of the plate. Subdivide the square into 64 smaller squares and cut a well over the centre of each of these. The placing of the samples and stan-

11	8	13	3	10	5	16	2
4	12	6	15	7	9	1	14
16	3	10	2	11	8	13	5
7	15	1	14	6	12	4	9
13	5	11	8	16	2	10	3
6	9	4	12	1	14	7	15
10	2	16	5	13	3	11	8
1	14	7	9	4	15	6	12

Fig. 9.1 Randomized number template.

dard solutions should be randomized. To this end, mark each square of the template with a number from 1 to 16 taken in order from a random number table. The finished template will then carry four squares with each of the 16 numbers and no standard or test number should appear twice in the same row or column (e.g. see Fig. 9.1). Several such templates should be prepared and used at random to position the samples in successive assays.

The order in which the standards and test samples are applied should also be randomized. Thus, do not apply all the standards in ascending or descending order first, but intersperse the standards with the test samples and change the order in successive assays. With these arrangements, apply four aliquots of each standard or test sample to the plate, either filling each well to the brim or placing in it a predetermined volume from a fixed volume pipette. Use a fresh pipette for each test sample or standard.

Incubation. Incubate the plate at the temperature and for the time appropriate to the method being used, e.g. for 18 h at 37°C or, for rapid assays of aminoglycosides, for 4 h at 40°C. If a number of assay plates have been set up, place them separately, not stacked on top of one another, in the incubator.

Reading results. Measure the diameter of each zone of inhibition of growth. Do so while it is magnified and centred, either in a zone reader (e.g. as supplied by Leebrook) or as projected from the horizontal position on to a vertical plane surface with an overhead projector. Average the values for the four aliquots of each of the standards and construct the dose-response curve on semi-logarithmic graph paper, plotting the antibiotic concentration on the logarithmic scale and the average zone diameter on the arithmetic.

Then average the zone diameters of the four aliquots of each test sample and calculate the concentration of antibiotic in the test sample by interpolating its average value in the dose-response curve. Do not extrapolate a value for any test sample containing a concentration of antibiotic higher than that in the highest standard; instead, re-assay the sample after diluting it to bring it within the range of the standards.

More complex mathematical treatment of the results by, for instance, the method of Bennett et al (1966) improves the accuracy of the dose-response curve and of the interpolation. If assays are to be done often, it is convenient to arrange for the calculations to be performed by a computer or a programmable calculator (Perkins 1978).

The accuracy of successive assays should be controlled by incorporating in each assay a special standard prepared with the highest possible accuracy and the validity of the laboratory's methods should be checked by the regular assay of externally prepared standards, e.g. those distributed through the UK National External Quality Assessment Scheme (Public Health Laboratory Service, Central Public Health Laboratory, Colindale Avenue, London).

Other antibiotics

Methods of assay of antibiotics other than those mentioned above are not described in this book. For details, see Reeves et al (1978) and De Louvois (1982) or consult the manufacturers of the drug to be assayed.

Assay of one antibiotic in the presence of another

Such assays are best done by an automated method such as the TDX (see above), but may be done by the large-plate diffusion method by the use of an organism resistant to the second antibiotic. Thus, *K. edwardsi* strain NCTC 10896, which is resistant to several other anti-

biotics, may be used for the assay of amino-glycosides. Many interfering β-lactam antibiotics can be inactivated by adding to the assay mixtures a β-lactamase, e.g. Whatman β-lactamase broad spectrum mixture, or a cephalo-sporinase, e.g. that produced by ICN Biomedicals (Selwyn & Bahktiar 1979). Sulphonamides can be neutralized by adding p-aminobenzoic acid, 5–50 mg/litre, to the assay medium, and trimethoprim by adding thymidine, 10 mg/litre. Interfering aminoglycosides can be removed by adsorption on to cellulose phosphate powder (Stevens & Young 1977), of which 50 mg is added to each 0.5 ml of patient's serum. Alternatively, their activity in the assay medium can be neutralized by lowering the pH to 6 if the antibiotic to be assayed is active at that pH.

Serum bactericidal assay

This test measures the cidal activity of the antibiotic-containing blood serum of a patient under treatment against the infecting organism isolated from the patient. It has been widely used to control the treatment of serious infections, especially endocarditis, and is similar in concept to the measurement of minimum bactericidal concentrations (see review by Wolfson & Schwartz 1985).

In tubes of a suitable nutrient broth prepare serial two-fold dilutions of serum from trough or peak blood samples and into each tube inoculate one drop of a 1 in 100 dilution of an overnight broth culture of the patient's infecting organism. Also set up two control tubes of broth, one seeded with the organism, the other not. Before incubating the tubes overnight at 37°C, remove a standard loopful from the seeded control broth and plate it on blood agar to serve as a measure of the weight of inoculum added to the tubes.

The highest dilution of serum that inhibits visible growth of the organism measures the serum's bacteriostatic activity. From each dilution in which growth is not visible, subculture a standard loopful on to blood agar and incubate overnight at 37°C. The highest dilution of serum that kills (or reduces by 99%) the inoculum is a measure of the serum's bactericidal activity.

Among the advantages claimed for the test are that if the patient is receiving two or more antibiotics, it is easier to perform than separate assays of each of the antibiotics. Moreover, a high serum bactericidal activity may indicate synergy between two antibiotics being given to the patient. But despite its extensive use, there is little evidence that the test can predict 'the survival, medical cure or bacteriologic cure' of patients with infective endocarditis (Coleman et al 1982).

REFERENCES

Anand C M, Paul A 1976 A modified technique for the detection of antibiotic synergism. Journal of Clinical Pathology 29: 1130–1131

Annear D T 1968 The effect of temperature on resistance of Staphylococcus aureus to methicillin and some other antibiotics. Medical Journal of Australia 1: 444–446

Arvidson S, Dornbusch K, Ericsson H 1981 Interpretation of the agar diffusion method for bacterial susceptibility testing. Journal of Antimicrobial Chemotherapy 7: 5–14

Barber M 1964 Naturally occurring methicillin-resistant staphylococci. Journal of General Microbiology 35: 183–190

Bauer A W, Kirby W M M, Sherris J C, Turck M 1966 Antibiotic susceptibility testing by a standardized single disk method. American Journal of Clinical Pathology 45: 493–496

Bennett J V, Brodie J L, Benner E J, Kirby W M M 1966 Simplified accurate method for antibiotic assay in clinical specimens. Applied Microbiology 14: 170–177

Berenbaum M C 1978 A method for testing for synergy with any number of agents. Journal of Infectious Diseases 137: 122–130

Brown D F J, Warner M, Bradley J, Taylor C E D 1982 The quality of antimicrobial susceptibility testing disks. Journal of Antimicrobial Chemotherapy 10: 373–382

Coleman D L, Horwitz R I, Andriole V T 1982 Association between serum inhibitory and bactericidal concentrations and therapeutic outcome in bacterial endocarditis. American Journal of Medicine 73: 260–267

Cooke D M, Salter A J, Phillips I 1983 The impact of an antibiotic policy on prescribing in a London teaching hospital. A one-day prevalence survey as an indicator of antibiotic use. Journal of Antimicrobial Chemotherapy 11: 447–454

Davies A J 1982 Testing, reporting and prescribing antibiotics for urinary infections. Journal of Antimicrobial Chemotherapy 10: 7–9

De Louvois J 1982 Factors affecting the assay of antimicrobial drugs in clinical samples by the agar plate diffusion method. Journal of Antimicrobial Chemotherapy 9: 253–266

Deacon S 1976 Assay of gentamicin in cerebrospinal fluid. Journal of Clinical Pathology 29: 54–57

Easmon C S F, Ison C A 1985 Gardnerella vaginalis. In: Collins C H, Grange J M (eds) Isolation and identification of microorganisms of medical and veterinary importance. Academic Press, London, p 120–121

Edmunds P N 1978 Synergy between sulphonamides and trimethoprim in the presence of pus. Journal of Clinical Pathology 31: 162–164

Ericsson H M, Sherris J C 1971 Antibiotic sensitivity testing. Report of an international collaborative study. Acta Pathologica et Microbiologica Scandinavica Section B Supplement 217: 1–90

Fallon R J 1978 Meningococci. In: Reeves D S, Phillips I, Williams J D, Wise R (eds) Laboratory methods in antimicrobial chemotherapy. Churchill Livingstone, Edinburgh. ch 15, p 99–101

Felmingham D, Stokes E J 1972 Sterile swabs as essential equipment for rapid reliable sensitivity tests. Medical Laboratory Technology 29: 198–200

Garrod L P, Waterworth P M 1962 Methods of testing combined antibiotic bactericidal action and the significance of the results. Journal of Clinical Pathology 15: 328–338

Garrod L P, Waterworth P M 1971 A study of antibiotic sensitivity testing with proposals for simple uniform methods. Journal of Clinical Pathology 24: 779–789

Garrod L P, Lambert H P, O'Grady F 1981 Antibiotic and chemotherapy, 5th edn. Churchill Livingstone, Edinburgh. ch 27, p 483–492

George R H, Healing D E, Ould M E 1981 Assay of chloramphenicol in clinical specimens. Journal of Clinical Pathology 34:225

Greenwood D 1979 Laboratory methods for the evaluation of synergy. In: Williams J D (ed) Antibiotic interactions, Academic Press, London. p 53–62

Hallander H O, Dornbusch K, Gezelius L, Jacobson K, Karlsson I 1982 Synergism between aminoglycosides and cephalosporins with antipseudomonal activity: Interaction index and killing curve method. Antimicrobial Agents and Chemotherapy 22: 743–752

Hamilton-Miller J M T 1985 Rationalization of terminology and methodology in the study of antibiotic interaction. Journal of Antimicrobial Chemotherapy 15: 655–658

Hewitt J H, Coe A W, Parker M T 1969 The detection of methicillin resistance in Staphylococcus aureus. Journal of Medical Microbiology 2: 443–456

Jenkins P A, Duddridge L R, Collins C H, Yates M D 1985 Mycobacteria. In: Collins C H, Grange J M (eds) Isolation and identification of microorganisms of medical and veterinary importance. Academic Press, London. p 291–295

Jephcott A E, Eggleston S I 1985 Neisseria gonorrhoeae. In: Collins C H, Grange J M (eds) Isolation and identification of microorganisms of medical and veterinary importance. Academic Press, London. p 150–153

King A, Phillips I 1985 Pseudomonads and related bacteria. In: Collins C H, Grange J M (eds) Isolation and identification of microorganisms of medical and veterinary importance. Academic Press, London. p 3

Krasemann C, Hildenbrand G 1980 Interpretation of agar diffusion tests. Journal of Antimicrobial Chemotherapy 6: 181–188

Lacey R W, Stokes A 1978 Synergy between sulphonamides and trimethoprim in the presence of pus. Journal of Clinical Pathology 31: 165–171

Langdale P, Miller M R 1986 Influence of laboratory sensitivity reporting on antibiotic prescribing preferences of general practitioners in the Leeds area. Journal of Clinical Pathology 39: 233–234

Menday A P, Tybring L 1978 Mecillinam. In: Reeves D S, Phillips I, Williams J D, Wise R (eds) Laboratory methods in antimicrobial chemotherapy. Churchill Livingstone, Edinburgh. ch 10, p 79–81

Pearson C H, Whitehead J E M 1974 Antibiotic sensitivity testing: a modification of the Stokes method using a rotary plater. Journal of Clinical Pathology 27: 430–431

Perkins A 1978 Statistics of plate assays. In: Reeves D S, Phillips I, Williams J D, Wise R (eds) Laboratory methods in antimicrobial chemotherapy. Churchill Livingstone, Edinburgh. ch 25, p 157–163

Phillips I 1986 Resistance as a cause of treatment failure. Journal of Antimicrobial Chemotherapy 18 Suppl C: 255–260

Phillips I, Warren C 1978 Anaerobic bacteria. In: Reeves D S, Phillips I, Williams J D, Wise R (eds) Laboratory methods in antimicrobial chemotherapy. Churchill Livingstone, Edinburgh. ch 14, p 95–98

Phillips K D, Brazier J S, Levett P N, Willis A T 1985 Clostridia. In: Collins C H, Grange J M (eds) Isolation and identification of microorganisms of medical and veterinary importance. Academic Press, London. p 229–230

Reeves D S, Phillips I, Williams J D, Wise R (eds) 1978 Laboratory methods in antimicrobial chemotherapy. Churchill Livingstone, Edinburgh

Selwyn S, Bahktiar M 1979 Inactivation of cephalosporins in blood cultures and mixed assays with a commercially available enterobacter β-lactamase. Journal of Antimicrobial Chemotherapy 5: 318–319

Senior B W 1978 p-Nitrophenylglycerol – a superior antiswarming agent for isolating and identifying pathogens from clinical material. Journal of Medical Microbiology 11: 59–61

Shanson D C, Hines C 1977 Serum gentamicin assays of 100 clinical serum samples by a rapid 40°C Klebsiella method compared with overnight plate diffusion and acetyltransferase assays. Journal of Clinical Pathology 30: 521–525

Snell J J S 1985 Personal communication. (A circular letter to all participants in the UK National External Quality Assessment Scheme)

Snell J J S, Brown D F J, Gardner P S 1982 An antibiotic susceptibility testing trial organised as part of the United Kingdom national external microbiological quality assessment scheme. Journal of Clinical Pathology 35: 1169–1176

Snell J J S, Brown D F J, Gardner P S 1984a Comparison of results from two antibiotic susceptibility testing trials that formed part of the United Kingdom national external quality assessment scheme. Journal of Clinical Pathology 37: 321–328

Snell J J S, Brown D F J, Phua R 1986 Antimicrobial susceptibility testing of Haemophilus influenzae: a trial organised as part of the United Kingdom national external quality assessment scheme for microbiology. Journal of Clinical Pathology 39: 1006–1012

Snell J J S, Danvers M V S, Gardner P S 1984b Comparison of antibiotic susceptibility results obtained with Adatab and disc methods. Journal of Clinical Pathology 37: 1059–1065

Spencer R C, Wheat P F 1986 Novel mechanisms for determining antibiotic susceptibilities. Journal of Antimicrobial Chemotherapy 17: 404–405

Stevens P, Young L S 1977 Simple method for the elimination of aminoglycosides from serum to permit bioassay of other antimicrobial agents. Antimicrobial Agents and Chemotherapy 12: 286–287

Stokes E J, Ridgeway G L 1980 Clinical bacteriology, 5th edn. Reprint. Arnold, London, p 215

Stokes E J, Waterworth P 1972 Antibiotic sensitivity tests by diffusion methods. Association of Clinical Pathologists Broadsheet No. 55: 1–12

Sykes R B 1978 Methods for detecting beta-lactamases. In: Reeves D S, Phillips I, Williams J D, Wise R (eds) Laboratory methods in antimicrobial chemotherapy. Churchill Livingstone, Edinburgh. ch 7, p 64–69

Waterworth P M 1981 Sensitivity testing by the break-point method. Journal of Antimicrobial Chemotherapy 7: 117–126

Waterworth P M 1983 Changes in sensitivity testing. Journal of Antimicrobial Chemotherapy 11: 1–3

Waterworth P M, del Piano M 1976 Dependability of sensitivity tests in primary cultures. Journal of Clinical Pathology 29: 179–184

Williams J D, Leung T 1978 Polymyxins, rifamycins, nalidixic acid and nitrofurantoin. In: Reeves D S, Phillips I, Williams J D, Wise R (eds) Laboratory methods in antimicrobial chemotherapy. Churchill Livingstone, Edinburgh. ch 13, p 88–93

Wolfson J S, Schwartz M N 1985 Serum bactericidal activity as a monitor of antibiotic therapy. New England Journal of Medicine 312: 968–975

Working Party of the British Society for Antimicrobial Chemotherapy 1985 The report of a BSAC working party on breakpoints in in-vitro sensitivity testing

World Health Organization Expert Committee on Biological Standardisation 1977 Requirements for antibiotic susceptibility tests. I. Agar diffusion tests using antibiotic susceptibility discs. Technical Report Series No. 610. WHO, Geneva. p 98–128

Immunological and serological methods in microbial infections

An antibody is an immunoglobulin molecule secreted into the tissue fluids from lymphoid cells which have been exposed to a foreign substance – an antigen. An antigen may be potentially harmful, such as a bacterium or virus, or it may be a harmless bland substance such as foreign serum protein. The antibody can combine only with antigen which is identical or nearly identical with the inducing antigen and not with unrelated antigens. When molecules of antibody and antigen are brought together in solution, they interact with each other by the formation of a link between an antigen-binding site on the immunoglobulin molecule – part of the Fab fragment – and the particular chemical groupings which make up what is termed the antigenic determinant of the antigen molecule. The molecules are held together by non-covalent intermolecular forces which are effective only when the antigen-binding site and the antigenic determinant group are able to make close contact. The better the fit the closer the contact and the stronger the antigen-antibody bond, these factors determining what is often called the affinity of the antibody molecule; antibodies of varying combining quality exist and the overall tendency to combine with antigen is the average ability of the antibodies to combine with antigen or the average intrinsic association constant. This can be calculated experimentally by application of the concepts of chemical equilibria to antigen-antibody interactions. Studies of this type have shown that the affinity of antibodies increases as immunization proceeds and that the dose of antigen can influence the quality of antibody.

The methods used for the detection of antigen-antibody reactions in the laboratory fall into two functional groups: first, procedures designed to elucidate the cytodynamics of antibody formation which involve the study of the behaviour of single cells or small populations of cells; the second group, which is the subject of the present discussion, concerns the detection and quantitation of secreted antibody circulating in the blood or present in the tissue fluids.

The methods used here range in their application from highly specialized studies of the physico-chemical aspects of antigen-antibody interaction to widely used procedures designed to aid in the diagnosis of disease.

In clinical practice serological tests are sometimes supplemented by the results of skin tests carried out on patients, e.g. tuberculin test, Schick test and various intradermal tests for fungal antigens (see Rose & Friedman 1984). For details of specialized techniques in bacterial, viral, fungal and protozoal immunology and tests of immune function see Weir et al (1986).

Table 10.1 at the end of this chapter lists applications of the various types of immunological test in the investigation of microbial and parasitic infections.

Primary interaction and secondary phenomena

In practical terms, the union of antibody with antigen can be detected at two different levels. The first level is that following *primary union* of the two reactants and usually requires that one or other reactant is labelled with a suitable marker such as a fluorescent dye or a radioactive isotope. A simple example of this is the microscopic localization in a tissue of a particular microorganism utilizing an antiserum prepared against the microorganism and labelled with a dye that fluoresces under UV light.

The second level at which antigen-antibody combination can be detected depends on the development, after primary union, of certain changes in the physical state of the complex, resulting in precipitation or agglutination of the components or, alternatively, in the activation of non-antibody components such as serum complement or histamine from mast cells. Reactions of this type occurring subsequent to primary union are termed *secondary phenomena*. This discussion is concerned with the principles of a few of these secondary phenomena which are in common use.

Before considering these reactions individually, it is important to be aware of the difficulties in interpreting results of such tests. The initiation and development of the secondary phenomena constitute a complicated series of events involving many variables such as the type of antibody taking part, the relative proportions of antibody and antigen, characteristics of the antigen molecule, presence of electrolytes, inhibitory substances and unstable components.

Despite these formidable difficulties, the widely and long used secondary phenomena such as precipitation, agglutination and complement fixation have an important role to play as aids in the diagnosis of disease and in the identification of microorganisms.

The secondary phenomena, as already indicated, can bring about several readily observable changes when carried out in vitro and these are used in tests to demonstrate the presence of antibody in the sera of patients suffering from infectious disease, or producing an antibody response to cell antigens as might, for example, occur after incompatible blood transfusion, tissue grafting or in autoimmune states.

Reactions of this type can also be used to identify antigens in the tissue or body fluids and, for example, would be utilized for blood grouping, tissue typing or the identification of microorganisms.

Among the most important of these reactions are *precipitation*, which occurs between antibody and antigen molecules in soluble form; *agglutination*, in which the antibodies directed against surface antigens of particulate materials such as microorganisms or erythrocytes link them together in large clumps or aggregates; and *complement fixation* in which antibody molecules, after reaction with antigen, activate the complex blood components which make up serum complement.

In addition to these widely used serological tests, a number of other effects of antigen-antibody interaction are of medical importance. These include neutralization tests used for example in virus identification, immobilization tests with bacteria and protozoa and skin tests for the reaginic antibody characteristic of anaphylactic states.

The advent of *monoclonal antibodies*, many of which are now available against microbial antigens, is having an increasingly important impact in the detection and identification of these antigens. As these antibodies become more readily available they are likely to replace many of the conventional antisera used in serological diagnosis (see Winstanley & Blackwell 1986).

Quantitative tests: dilutions and titres

In diagnostic serology it is often necessary to determine the amount of a specific antibody in the patient's serum in order to distinguish between the presence of a large amount of antibody produced in response to a current infection and that of a small amount of 'natural' or cross-reacting antibody unrelated to the patient's illness. In routine tests it is impracticable to isolate the specific antibody and measure its mass. Instead, the amount of the antibody is estimated by determining the greatest degree to which the serum may be diluted without losing the power to give an observable effect in a mixture with the specific antigen. Different dilutions of the serum are tested in mixtures with a constant amount of antigen and the greatest reacting dilution is taken as the measure, or *titre*, of the concentration of antibody in the undiluted serum.

Dilutions may be expressed in one of two ways: (1) they may be expressed in terms of the way in which they are made, e.g. a dilution of '1 in 8' is a dilution made by mixing one volume of serum with seven volumes of diluent (usually physiological saline); (2) alternatively, they may be expressed as the factor by which the dilution of the reagent (antibody) is increased, e.g. a dilution of '8' represents an eight-fold increase in dilution.

It is incorrect to express dilutions as fractions, e.g. $\frac{1}{8}$, because the higher dilutions are then represented by the smaller values. In a dilution of 1 in 8, it is the concentration, not the dilution of the reagent that is reduced to $\frac{1}{8}$. It is, moreover, inadvisable to express dilutions in the form '1:8'. as this is the notation generally used to express a ratio; its use for a dilution might be taken to indicate either the ratio between the volume of the serum and that of the diluent or the ratio of the volume of the serum to that of the final mixture of serum with diluent.

Titres should be expressed by the *integers* representing the greatest reacting dilutions, e.g. if the greatest reacting dilution of the serum is 8, the titre is 8. The term 'reciprocal titre' is commonly used in an incorrect sense based on the mistaken use of a fraction to express the endpoint dilution; it should therefore be avoided. Where the endpoint dilution is 1 in 8, it is the titre, not the reciprocal titre, that is 8.

Titres cited by bacteriologists normally indicate the final dilution of the serum in the reaction mixture after all the other reagents have been added, e.g. bacterial suspension and saline diluent. Most titres cited by virologists indicate either the dilution of the serum in the primary reaction mixture with virus or haemagglutinin, or the initial dilution of the serum without adjustment for the further dilution with the added reactants; in the latter case the value is meaningful only in the context of knowledge of the volumes of the reactants added to each mixture.

PRECIPITATION

As a result of the interaction of antibody and antigen molecules in solution, complexes of the two types of molecule will form and precipitation may occur depending on the relative concentration of the two reactants. If a series of tubes

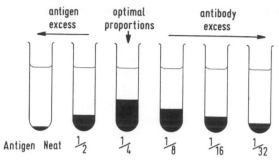

Fig. 10.1 Amount of precipitation observed in a series of tubes with a constant amount of antiserum and a graded dilution of antigen.

is set up (Fig. 10.1), each containing a constant amount of antiserum, and decreasing amounts of antigen are added to the tubes in the row, a haziness will start to appear in the tubes gradually increasing to visible aggregates or precipitates. The amount of precipitation will be seen to increase along the row, reaching a maximum and then falling off with the lower antigen concentration. The tubes where most precipitate appears contain the *optimal proportions* of antigen and antibody for precipitation and the proportions are constant for all dilutions of the same reagents. The composition of the precipitate varies with the original proportions of the antibody and antigen; if antigen is in excess the precipitate will contain relatively more of this component and similarly more antibody if that is present in excess. As can be seen from Figure 10.2, on the antigen excess side of optimal proportions less precipitate appears and this is due to the inability of the antigen-antibody complexes formed to link up to other complexes and so make a large aggregate or lattice which will appear as a visible precipitate (tube 1, Fig. 10.2). Large aggregates of antibody and antigen can form best under conditions of optimal proportions where the antibody and antigen proportions are such that after initial combination of the molecules, free antigen-binding sites and antigen determinant groups remain, enabling the complexes to link up into a large lattice formation (as in tube 2 of Fig. 10.2). In antibody excess all the free determinants of the antigen molecule are soon taken

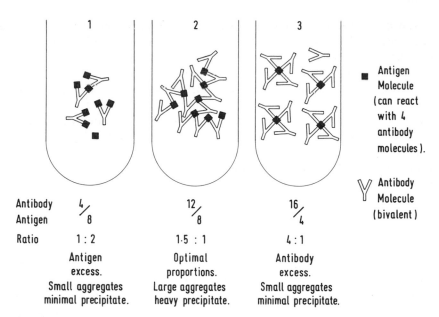

Fig. 10.2 The composition of an antigen-antibody precipitate is determined by the proportions or ratios of the components in the reaction.

up with antibody, so that very little linking can take place between the complexes (as in tube 3 of Fig. 10.2).

The precipitin test can be carried out in a quantitative manner by estimating the protein content of the precipitate at optimal proportions. The qualitative test is much more widely used and is of considerable value in detecting and identifying antigens, having applications in the typing of streptococci or pneumococci. This is done by layering an extract of the organism over antiserum in *tubes*. After a short while, a ring of precipitate forms at the interface (this is called the ring test). The technique is also used in forensic studies and in detecting adulteration of foodstuffs.

A modification of the test in which precipitation is allowed to occur by *double diffusion* in agar gel is very widely used for detecting the presence of antibody in serum or antigen in unknown preparations, and is valuable for showing the identity of different antigen preparations (Fig. 10.3). A concentration gradient forms in the gel, the concentration of a substance decreasing as the molecules diffuse away from the well in which they were placed. Precipitin bands form in the gel in the position where the

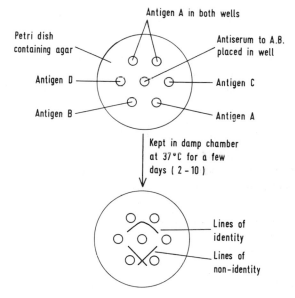

Fig. 10.3 Immunodiffusion or gel diffusion test. Wells are cut in a layer of agar in a Petri dish. Antiserum and antigen solutions are placed opposite each other in the wells and after allowing a few days for diffusion to take place precipitin bands will form where antibody and antigen meet in suitable proportions (optimal proportions). No reactions take place with antigens C and D as the antiserum in the central well contains antibodies only for antigens A and B. Lines of identity as formed between the two A wells enable the technique to be used for identifying unknown antigens.

antigen and antibody molecules reach optimal proportions after diffusion.

When a large number of different antigens are present in a solution, it is difficult to separate the precipitin bands for each of the antigen-antibody reactions by the simple gel-diffusion method just described. In such a situation, a variation of this method can be used to identify the individual components. This modification is particularly valuable in analysing a multicomponent system such as serum. The individual components of serum are first separated by electrophoresis in agar gel and an antiserum, prepared against the serum, is allowed to diffuse towards the separated components, resulting in the formation of precipitin bands. This method, known as *immunoelectrophoresis*, is particularly valuable for showing the presence of abnormal globulin constituents in the serum of patients with myelomatosis and other serum protein abnormalities (see below).

Immunodiffusion in tubes

Double diffusion carried out in tubes 5 cm × 2 cm in which the antigen and antibody diffuse towards each other in a layer of agar is the basis of this technique. The antigen and antibody solutions may be introduced in liquid form, particularly when the concentration of either is low and dilution is not desirable. More conveniently the antigen and antibody can be mixed with agar. The three layers of the system then consist of antigen and antibody mixed with agar separated by a layer of agar. The concentration of the agar used is commonly 0.6%. The precipitin bands form in the middle layer and with strong antisera may be seen within a few hours. Dilution of the antiserum or antigen causes displacement of the band towards the antiserum-agar or antigen-agar interface respectively. This type of immunodiffusion technique in tubes has the distinction of being the most sensitive type of precipitin test available with respect to the quantities of reactants required for formation of visible precipitates. Quantities of reactants too small to form visible precipitates if they were simply mixed together are concentrated in a very narrow zone and can thus form

an observable precipitate. The number of precipitin bands observed in the agar tubes does not necessarily indicate the total number of systems present as some of the bands in complex mixtures may be hidden by others and would only be identified by procedures of high resolving power such as immunoelectrophoresis.

Immunodiffusion has been extensively used in microbiology for the identification of different types and strains of bacteria and viruses (see Table 10.1).

Double diffusion in plates

Sufficient 1% agar in 0.85% NaCl or 0.2 mol/litre phosphate buffer pH 7.2 containing 0.1% sodium azide is poured into a small, flat-bottomed Petri dish to give a perfectly level surface (about 10 ml). When this has solidified, wells are cut in the agar with a cork borer in positions determined by a pattern drawn on a piece of paper which is placed under the Petri dish. More conveniently wells are cut with a gel cutter with, for example, a central well surrounded by six satellite wells. A very large number of different sizes and shapes and arrangements of wells have been used in this technique; the circular central well with equidistant satellite wells is perhaps the most popular. After the wells have been filled, using separate clean Pasteur pipettes, with the antigen and antiserum solutions, e.g. the antiserum in the central well and the antigens in the peripheral wells, the plate is covered and placed in a damp chamber (e.g. a plastic lunch box with a piece of wet filter paper in the base). Diffusion is allowed to occur in the cold (4°C) overnight or longer if necessary. Incubation at 37°C may be used and gives more rapid but less clear cut results; however, certain labile antigens may be denatured at this temperature. The plate is examined by means of incident light using a simple arrangement consisting of a 60 watt electric light bulb with the top covered with a metal light shield, light being reflected into the gel plate from below through an aperture in the light box as shown in the diagram (Fig. 10.4). The types of precipitin bands commonly observed are shown in Figure 10.5. They take the form essen-

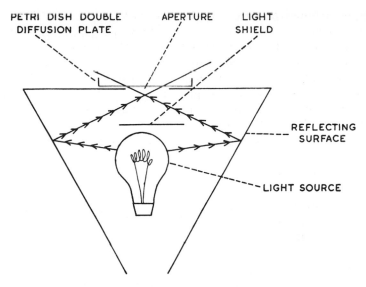

Fig. 10.4 Diagram of viewing box for immunodiffusion.

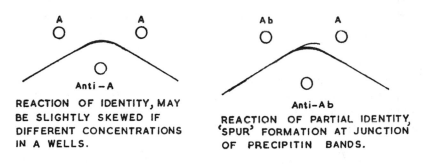

A   A
Anti–A

REACTION OF IDENTITY, MAY
BE SLIGHTLY SKEWED IF
DIFFERENT CONCENTRATIONS
IN A WELLS.

Ab   A
Anti–Ab

REACTION OF PARTIAL IDENTITY,
'SPUR' FORMATION AT JUNCTION
OF PRECIPITIN BANDS.

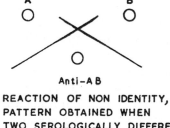

A   B
Anti–A B

REACTION OF NON IDENTITY,
PATTERN OBTAINED WHEN
TWO SEROLOGICALLY DIFFERENT
ANTIGENS ARE USED WITH AN
ANTISERUM CONTAINING
ANTIBODY TO BOTH.

Fig. 10.5 Commonly observed patterns found in double diffusion plates where two antigen solutions are compared using antiserum as the analytic agent.

tially of one of three different patterns: (1) the reaction of identity where the lines are continuous from one well to the next; (2) the reaction of non-identity where the lines cross each other; and (3) the reaction of partial identity which is similar to (1) except for spur formation at the junction of the precipitin bands.

Immunoelectrophoresis

Immunoelectrophoresis can be used for the identification of myeloma proteins, and the changes in globulin levels in such diseases as virus hepatitis, cirrhosis and the reticuloses are distinct enough to suggest the appropriate diagnosis. A glass slide is coated with 1% agar about 1 mm thick made up in either Veronal buffer pH 8.6 (diethylbarbituric acid 1.38 g, sodium barbitone 8.76 g, calcium lactate 0.38 g, distilled water 1 litre) or 0.02 mol/litre potassium phosphate buffer pH 7.2. The former is the buffer commonly used in paper electrophoresis and is available commercially; the latter, however, gives better resolution of the precipitin bands and has a more suitable pH for immunodiffusion. A pattern is made in the agar with a cutter which can be constructed by forcing two large gauge hypodermic needles (1–2 mm internal diameter) with their points sawn off through the centre area of a large cork stopper 4 cm in diameter about 7 mm apart. Between the needles are placed the two halves of a razor blade inserted into the cork so that they are parallel and separated from each other by 1 mm. The cutter is lowered on to the agar on a slide to cut the required pattern and the agar plugs are removed from the wells cut with the needles (a fine Pasteur pipette on a water pump is suitable). The agar between the two parallel cuts made by the razor blades is left in situ until after electrophoresis. The procedure is illustrated in Figure 10.6. The prepared slide is used as a bridge between the two compartments of the electrophoresis apparatus, and is connected to the buffer at each end by means of filter paper wicks. It is important that the wicks are kept damp as they tend to heat up and dry due to the passage of the current. Electrophoresis of the

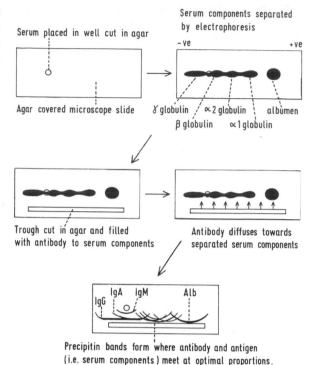

Fig. 10.6 Immunoelectrophoresis. The antigen, e.g. serum, is placed in a small well cut in a layer of agar on a microscope slide. A direct current is applied and differential migration of the serum components takes place. (They are not normally visible in the agar and will show up only if suitably stained.) After electrophoresis for an hour or so, a trough is cut longitudinally in the agar and an antiserum against the electrophoresed antigen is placed in the trough. The two components diffuse towards each other and precipitin bands form. These can be shown up more clearly by staining with a protein stain. This very powerful analytic technique can show up about 30 different components in human serum compared with 4 or 5 by electrophoresis.

antigen (placed in the peripheral wells) is carried out using about 50 volts requiring approximately 2.5 ma per slide for a period (45 min–4 h) sufficient to give adequate separation of the different components of the antigen. Following this the band of agar in the trough between the two razor blade slits is removed and the antiserum run into the trough. The slide is then placed in a humid atmosphere at 4°C or 37°C to allow the development of the precipitin reaction.

The preparation is examined at intervals with the viewing box depicted in Figure 10.4. Any precipitin bands formed can be recorded by drawing the pattern obtained on a piece of paper or the preparation can be photographed. Staining of the bands with a protein stain improves the clarity of the patterns and may even show up precipitin bands which cannot be seen in the unstained preparation. Such stained preparations can conveniently be dried and kept for reference. A suitable procedure for staining and drying is as follows:

1. The unprecipitated protein is washed out of the agar by immersion of the slide for 24 h in the buffer used to make up the agar solution.

2. The slide is then washed for 15 min in 1% acetic acid to remove excess salts.

3. Staining is carried out with a protein stain such as naphthalene black made up to a 1% solution in a solvent containing glacial acetic acid 1 ml, distilled water 49 ml, and methylated spirit 50 ml. Staining should be carried out for about 30 min with this stain.

4. Excess stain is washed out with the solvent to give a preparation with dark blue precipitin bands on a clear background.

5. The preparation is finally soaked in 1% acetic acid containing 1% glycerol for 15 min and dried at 37°C in an incubator.

Crossed immunoelectrophoresis (CIE)

As with immunoelectrophoresis the proteins in the antigen under examination are first separated by agarose gel electrophoresis after which they are electrophoresed at right angles to the original direction into an antibody-containing agarose gel. The precipitates that form show up as sharp peaks (rockets), the height of the peak being determined by the concentration and mobility of the protein. The method also shows up heterogeneity of antigens or identity of various components by fusion or overlapping of patterns. The usual procedure (see Fig. 10.7) is to use 5 × 7.5 cm glass slides coated with a layer of 1% (w/v) agarose (4 ml) in barbitone buffer. The agarose is cut into 5 strips of 5 × 1.2 cm with a razor blade and the strips slightly separated

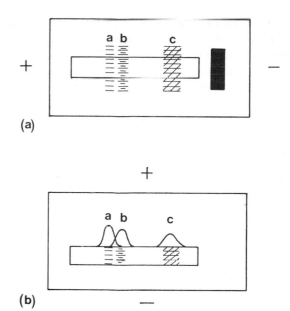

(a)

(b)

Fig. 10.7 Illustration of the principle of crossed immunoelectrophoresis (CIE). (a) Gel layer electrophoresis in agarose gel of mixture containing three constituents with different mobilities. After first run, longitudinal strip removed. (b) Second run; strip laid on antibody-containing gel and a potential gradient applied at 90° to the previous direction. Precipitin bands in the form of arcs develop as illustrated.

from one another. As in immunoelectrophoresis a small well is bored in each strip about 1 cm from one end and in this case close to one of the longitudinal sides of the strip. After placing the sample under test (2–5 μl) into the wells electrophoresis is carried out at 6 V/cm for 1–2 h. Each strip is then transferred to another 5 × 7.5 cm slide, precoated with 0.5% agar (0.2 ml/cm²) and dried overnight at room temperature (or 4–6 h at 40°C). Agarose to which antibody has been added is then poured on to the slide using a level table and adding between 3 and 3.5 ml of the mixture per slide. The preparation is again set up in an electrophoresis tank at 2 V/cm overnight and the precipitin bands examined by staining as described above.

Countercurrent immunoelectrophoresis

In countercurrent immunoelectrophoresis antiserum is placed in one well and the antigen under test in another. In a pH 8.2 gel the immunoglobulins move towards the cathode because of electro-endosmotic flow and if the well containing the antigen is placed on the cathodic side of the antiserum well the antigen which normally will move in the opposite direction towards the anode will meet the antiserum somewhere between the two wells and form a precipitate. This procedure is normally carried out under the same conditions as for immunoelectrophoresis on a precoated microscope slide with two wells (1.5 mm diam) cut in the 1% agarose 1 cm apart on the long axis of the slide. The well closest to the cathode is filled with antigen and the other with antiserum and electrophoresis carried out at 8 V/cm for 30 min. The advantage of this technique over simple immunodiffusion is that a result can be obtained in about 1 h and less antibody and antigen are needed. The two reactants are brought together by the electrophoretic process instead of diffusing in all directions as in simple diffusion. Countercurrent immunoelectrophoresis has been used for the detection of hepatitis B antigen and for bacterial antigen in the CSF of patients with meningitis.

AGGLUTINATION

In this reaction the antigen is part of the surface of some particulate material such as a red cell, bacterium or perhaps an inorganic particle (e.g. polystyrene latex) which has been coated with antigen. Antibody added to a suspension of such particles combines with the surface antigens and links them together to form clearly visible aggregates or agglutinates (Fig. 10.8).

One of the classical applications of the agglutination test in diagnostic bacteriology is the Widal test used for the demonstration of antibodies to salmonellae in serum specimens taken from suspected enteric fever cases (see Ch. 29). Quantitative tube agglutination tests in which the serum is titrated are valuable in determining changes in the immune status of the patient.

Agglutination is the basic technique used in blood grouping, the A, B or O group of the red cells under test being determined by agglutination with a specific antiserum – an anti-A

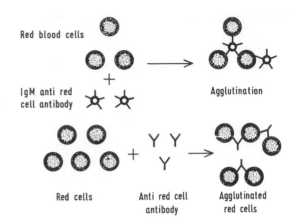

Fig. 10.8 Agglutination reaction. The IgM molecule (*above*) with at least five antigen-binding sites is particularly effective in bringing about agglutination. (cf. IgG *below*).

serum, for example, will agglutinate A cells but not B or O cells. Red cells and inert particles such as polystyrene latex can be coated with various antigens and suitably coated particles are used in a variety of diagnostic tests such as thyroid antibody tests using thyroglobulin-coated cells or latex particles. Hormone-coated red cells or inert particles are used in many hormone assay procedures which are based on the inhibition of the antibody-induced agglutination of the hormone-coated particles by hormone added in the sample under test (Fig. 10.9). Tests of this type are in wide use in pregnancy diagnosis.

Certain viruses, e.g. the orthomyxo- and paramyxo-viruses causing influenza and mumps, have the property of bringing about agglutination of red cells (haemagglutination). Inhibition of haemagglutination by antibody in patient's serum is a widely used diagnostic procedure. The presence of antibody in the patient's serum is thus detected by its ability to link with virus particles and prevent them from bringing about agglutination of the red cells (*haemagglutination inhibition* test; Fig. 10.10).

IgM antibodies capable of agglutinating human red cells (including those of the individual producing the antibody) between 0 and 4°C (*cold agglutinins*) are sometimes found in certain human diseases including primary atypical pneumonia, malaria, trypanosomiasis and acquired haemolytic anaemia.

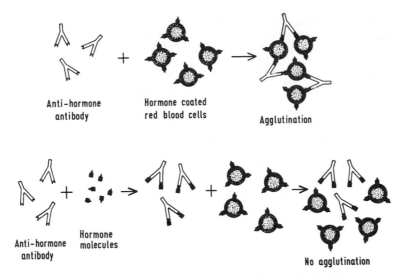

Fig. 10.9 Principle of hormone assay by agglutination inhibition. Red cells coated with hormone are agglutinable by anti-hormone antibody. The addition to the antiserum of a test sample containing free hormone will block the antigen-binding sites and prevent agglutination. The test can be carried out quantitatively by comparing the activity of a known standard hormone preparation with the test sample.

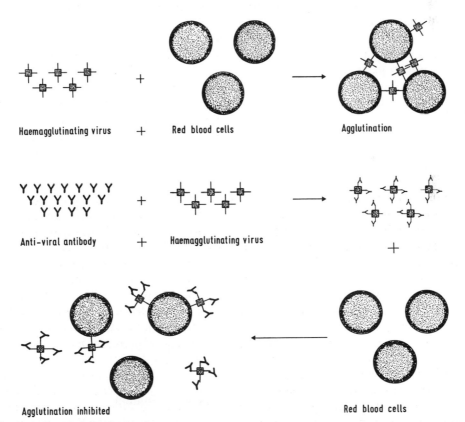

Fig. 10.10 Virus haemagglutination inhibition test. *Above*: cell agglutination is brought about by a variety of viruses (see text). *Below*: this can be inhibited by mixing the virus with anti-viral antibody as shown in the diagram. The test can be quantitated by comparison of serial dilutions of virus alone and virus-antibody mixture.

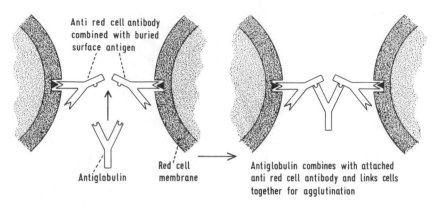

Fig. 10.11 Coombs antiglobulin test. The red cell antibody, probably because it is directed against an antigen situated deep in the cell wall, cannot link two red cells together for agglutination. The addition of an antiglobulin serum brings about agglutination by linking two attached immunoglobulins to one another.

The presence of antibody globulin on a red cell may not result in direct agglutination of the cells, for example in some Rh-negative mothers with Rh-positive infants or in acquired haemolytic anaemia. It is, however, possible to show that the red cells are coated with antibody by using an antiglobulin serum (produced in the rabbit by injecting human globulin) which will bring about agglutination of the cells. This is the basis of the *Coombs test* which is a very widely used serological procedure (Fig. 10.11).

Tube agglutination

In its simplest form an agglutination test is set up in round-bottomed test tubes or perspex plates with round-bottomed wells and a series of doubling dilutions of the antiserum is made up in the tubes; the technical details are important (e.g. see Widal test, Ch. 29). The particulate antigen is then added and after incubation at 37°C agglutination is seen in the bottom of the tubes. The last tube showing clearly visible agglutination is the endpoint of the test. The dilution of the antiserum at the endpoint, e.g. 256, is known as the *titre* of the antiserum and is a measure of the number of antibody units/unit volume of serum, e.g. if the endpoint occurs at a 256 dilution of the antiserum and if the test has been carried out in 1 ml volumes, the titre of the serum is 256 units/ml of serum.

One practical difficulty of importance in agglutination tests is the occasional inhibition of agglutination in the first tubes of an antiserum dilution series, agglutination occurring only in those tubes containing more dilute antiserum. This is known as the *prozone phenomenon* and is probably, in part, due to the stabilizing effects of high protein concentration on the particles, the protein coating the particles increasing their net charge and so bringing about increased electrostatic repulsion between individual particles, thus opposing the efforts of the antibody molecules to link the particles together. However, once the protein concentration is reduced by dilution the antibody molecules can then exert their aggregating effect and bring about agglutination. The agglutination reaction has been shown to require the presence of electrolytes in the suspending medium and is usually performed for this reason at physiological salt concentration.

Blood specimens for agglutination tests are taken by venepuncture, so as to obtain a satisfactory amount of serum for the complete test. At least 5 ml of blood should be obtained, and the blood immediately transferred from the syringe to a dry stoppered sterile tube or screw-capped bottle and allowed to clot. When the serum has separated, it is pipetted off into a sterile tube.

Slide agglutination

This method is useful where only small quantities of culture are available, as in the identification of the whooping-cough bacillus, or where agglutination is carried out with undiluted serum, e.g. in typing pneumococci or typing streptococci by Griffith's method, and it is necessary to use as small a quantity as possible. The method may be applied likewise for identifying organisms of the salmonella and dysentery groups. Slide agglutination is practicable only when the clumping of organisms occurs within a minute or so; it is not suitable where the mixture of organisms and serum has to be incubated.

The procedure can be carried out quite readily on an ordinary slide, but where a number of agglutination tests have to be made it is more convenient to use a piece of 60 mm polished plate glass c. 5 × 15 cm. A long horizontal line is ruled with a grease pencil through the middle of the glass from end to end and then a number of lines are ruled at 1 cm intervals at right angles to this line, thereby dividing the glass into a series of divisions.

A drop of saline is placed in one of the divisions and a small amount of culture from a solid medium emulsified in it by means of an inoculating loop. It is then examined through a hand lens ($\times$ 8 or $\times$ 10), or the low-power microscope, to ascertain that the suspension is even and that the bacteria are well separated and not in visible clumps. With a small loop, 1.5 mm diameter, made from thin platinum wire take up a drop of the serum and place it on the slide just beside the bacterial suspension. Mix the serum and bacterial suspension and examine with the hand lens, or place on the stage of the microscope. Agglutination when it occurs is rapid and the clumps can be seen with the naked eye, but the use of some form of magnification is an advantage. For control purposes, two drops of saline can be placed in adjacent divisions and bacterial culture emulsified in both, one only being mixed with the serum. With streptococci a broth culture is used, and methods for obtaining suitable suspensions for the agglutination test are described in Chapter 17. Two drops of suspension are placed on the slide and a small loopful of the serum mixed with one of them and examined as described above.

While the slide agglutination test is rapid and convenient, its limitations must be realized. In order to obtain rapid agglutination the serum is used undiluted or in low dilutions. In consequence, it may contain normal agglutinins which give non-specific agglutination with organisms other than that against which the serum was prepared. Thus, with regard to the *Salmonella* group particularly, slide agglutination with its high concentration of agglutinins may show low-titre reactions with organisms outside the group which may also have somewhat similar biochemical reactions. It is important therefore to confirm the slide test by quantitative tests in tubes, particularly when any doubt arises or where precise results from agglutination tests are desired. In these tube tests, the demonstration that the organism is agglutinated by the stated maximum effective dilution (titre) of the diagnostic serum confirms the specificity of the reaction and excludes the possibility that low-level cross-reactions are responsible for the positive slide test.

Agglutinin-absorption tests

Agglutinins, like other antibodies, combine firmly with their homologous antigens, and by treating an agglutinating antiserum with the homologous bacteria and then separating the organisms by centrifuging, it is found that the agglutinin has been 'absorbed' or removed by the organisms from the serum.

In certain cases, to prove the serological identity of an unknown strain with a particular species, it may be necessary to show not only that it is agglutinated by a specific antiserum to approximately its titre but also that it can absorb from the serum the agglutinins for the known organism. This becomes necessary owing to the fact that, on immunizing an animal with a particular bacterium, 'group antibodies' for allied organisms are developed, and in some cases these may act in relatively high titre. Absorption with a heterologous strain would remove only the group agglutinins without affecting the specific agglutinin. These effects are exemplified in the *Salmonella* and *Brucella* groups.

The general method of carrying out such absorption tests is to mix a dense suspension of the organism – e.g. 24 h growth on a 9 cm plate of nutrient agar, suspended in 1 ml saline and killed at 60°C (30 min) – with an equal volume of a suitable dilution of the serum, e.g. 64 times the concentration of the known titre. (The bacterial growth must have been thoroughly washed with physiological salt solution, i.e. by mixing with several volumes of saline, centrifuging and repeating the process 2–3 times.) Thus, if the titre is 1600, the dilution used would be 1 in 25. The mixture is incubated for 3–4 h at 37°C and the serum is then separated from the bacteria in a high-speed centrifuge. (In some cases for complete absorption the process may require to be repeated with a similar fresh quantity of bacteria.) The dilution of the serum would now be approximately double the original dilution – in the example taken above, 1 in 50. From the treated serum a series of doubling dilutions is prepared as in direct agglutination tests, so that, when an equal volume of bacterial suspension is added, the series will reach to the known titre of the serum. In the example taken above, the following series of dilutions would be tested: 1 in 50, 1 in 100, 1 in 200, 1 in 400, 1 in 800. After the addition of bacterial suspension these would become: 1 in 100, 1 in 200, 1 in 400, 1 in 800, 1 in 1600.

A control tube is also included, containing suspension but no serum, and the general technique is that employed in direct agglutination tests.

Thus, the identity or non-identity of an unknown culture (X) with a known (A) may be investigated by agglutinin-absorption as follows:

1. Absorb, as above, antiserum to A with a dense suspension of organism X = X-absorbed serum.

2. Test the agglutinating power of X-absorbed serum for A and X.

(A control test would show that the antiserum to A after absorption with A agglutinates neither organism.)

Results:

a. The absorbed serum agglutinates neither A nor X. This indicates that the organisms are identical, because X has absorbed agglutinins for A; to establish this conclusion completely an antiserum to X after absorption with A should agglutinate neither organism.

b. The absorbed serum fails to agglutinate X, but still agglutinates A. This shows that the organisms are not identical, because X has not absorbed the agglutinins for A, though it has removed the heterologous agglutinins.

Coagglutination

The coagglutination (COA) method was first introduced by Kronvall (1973) for the serological typing of pneumococci. COA is based on the principle that staphylococci rich in protein A on their outer surface bind IgG non-specifically through the Fc region leaving specific Fab sites free. The subsequent reaction of Fab with homologous (test) antigen is visualized by clumping of the staphylococci (Fig. 10.12). Most strains of *Staphylococcus aureus* contain protein A but Cowan strain 1 in particular is capable of producing large amounts. Staphylococci are stabilized by treatment with formaldehyde (0.5%) and heat (80°C) prior to coating with antibody (Kronvall 1973). This produces a particle stable for months when stored at 4°C, which is capable of being coated with large amounts of IgG. Antisera used to prepare COA reagents are usually absorbed to remove cross-reacting antibodies before coupling to protein A. In addition to the test reagent comprising non-viable stabilized staphylococci coated with specific IgG, a control reagent is also required which comprises staphylococci coated with IgG from non-immunized rabbits.

The COA test is performed as a simple slide test with a suspension of the presumptive homologous antigen prepared from a bacterial culture or, alternatively, the test can be used directly for detecting the presence of bacterial antigens in serum and urine.

A drop of test and control reagents are added to a slide and each reagent is mixed with a drop of the bacterial suspension or body fluid to be tested. The slide is rocked by tilting at an angle of 45° every few seconds. Reaction normally appears within 2–3 min.

A positive result is denoted by a markedly stronger reaction with the test reagent compared

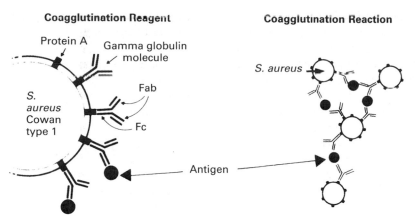

Fig. 10.12 Schematic representation of coagglutination reaction. Presence of antigen demonstrated by cross-linking of specific antibody attached to *Staphylococcus aureus*.

with the control reagent. Absence of reaction with the test reagent indicates a negative result irrespective of any reaction with the control reagent. Occasionally a COA test may be non-interpretable owing to a reaction of similar strength with the test and control reagents. Reagents are stable at 4°C although IgG may slowly leach away from protein A resulting in a loss of sensitivity. Sensitivity may sometimes be restored to a suspension by washing.

Reagents for the identification of *Neisseria gonorrhoeae* (Ch. 21) and serogrouping of *Streptococcus pyogenes* A, B, C, D or G (Ch. 17) are available commercially and are used widely. Reagents are also available commercially for detecting meningococcal, pneumococcal and haemophilus antigen in CSF. COA may be more sensitive than CIE for detecting bacterial antigen in CSF (Jones 1979). However, because protein A staphylococci agglutinate non-specifically with human IgG it is necessary to absorb the CSF with stabilized staphylococci before testing for antigen.

Passive agglutination

In passive agglutination antigens or antibodies are non-specifically absorbed to a carrier such as latex polystyrene beads of uniform diameter (0.8 μm) or erythrocytes. Latex polystyrene beads coated with denatured human IgG were first used to detect rheumatoid factor in serum.

Latex particles coated with globulin from antisera to meningococci, *Haemophilus influenzae* type b or from pneumococcal omni-serum can be used to detect the corresponding antigen in cases of pyogenic meningitis (Fallon 1983). Antigen in the CSF will cause agglutination of the appropriate particles within a few minutes. For the test, two drops of CSF are placed in each of four rings of a glass agglutination plate. One drop of one of the types of coated latex particle is placed in each ring. The slide is gently rocked for up to 3 min when the pattern of agglutination is read. If more than one suspension of latex is agglutinated the result is regarded as a false positive. Reagents are reasonably stable and sensitized latex particles retain their sensitivity for at least 4–6 months if kept at 4°C.

One of the most widely used passive agglutination tests employing erythrocytes is the *Treponema pallidum* haemagglutination (TPHA) test for the serological diagnosis of treponemal infection (Ch. 40). Sheep or avian erythrocytes are first treated with formaldehyde and tannic acid before being sensitized with a sonicate of pathogenic *T. pallidum*. When this reagent (available commercially) is mixed with patient's serum and allowed to stand for a few hours a diffuse carpet of haemagglutination is formed if anti-treponemal antibody is present. In the absence of specific antibody the sensitized erythrocytes settle to form a compact button of cells.

COMPLEMENT FIXATION

The fact that antibody, once it combines with antigen, is able to activate the complement system is used as a way of showing the presence of a particular antibody in a serum, e.g. in the Wassermann test for syphilis or in the identification of viral antigens.

The complement system as currently understood consists of 19 plasma proteins. There are two pathways leading to lysis of cells bearing antibody directed at cell surface antigens – the classical pathway and the alternative pathway. In serology the classical pathway is the one that is used. The complement of most species will react with antibody derived from other species and guinea-pig serum is a common laboratory source of complement – some of the components of complement are heat labile and are destroyed by heating at 56°C for 20–30 min. The individual components of the complement system are taken up by the antigen-antibody complex in a particular order and destruction of the heat-labile components which are taken up early prevents the remaining components from taking part.

For most antigens the reaction of the complement system with the antigen-antibody complex causes in itself no visible effect and it is necessary to use an indicator system consisting of sheep red cells coated with anti-sheep-red-cell antibody. Complement has the ability to lyse the antibody-coated cells, probably by virtue of the esterase activity of one of the components acting on the red cell membrane. In a test the antibody, complement and antigen are first mixed together and after a period of incubation the indicator system, antibody-coated sheep cells, is added. The complement will, however, have been taken up during the incubation stage by the original antibody-antigen complex and will not be available to lyse the red cells. Thus, a positive complement fixation test is indicated by absence of lysis of the red cells whilst a negative test, with unused complement, is shown by lysis of the red cells (Fig. 10.13).

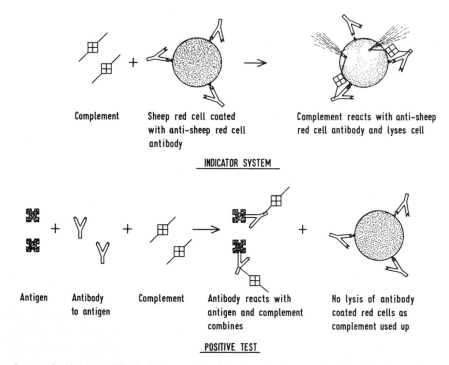

Fig. 10.13 Complement fixation test. The indicator system (sheep red cells coated with antibody to sheep red cells) is normally lysed in the presence of complement (fresh guinea-pig serum) – *above*. If another antibody-antigen system is first mixed with the complement it will no longer be available to lyse the indicator system – *below*.

LABELLED ANTIBODIES

Fluorescence labelled antibody

The precise localization of tissue antigens or the antigens of infecting organisms in the body, of anti-tissue antibody and of antigen-antibody complexes was achieved by the introduction of the use of fluorochrome-labelled proteins. The absorption of UV light between 290 and 495 nm by fluorescein and its emission of longer wavelength green light (525 nm) is used to visualize protein labelled with this dye. The technique is more sensitive than precipitation or complement fixation techniques, and fluorescent protein tracers can be detected at a concentration of the order of 1 μg protein/ml body fluid.

It is advisable to use high avidity antibody from which the immunoglobulin fraction has been purified by salt fractionation (see Johnstone & Thorpe 1982). Antibody (conventional or monoclonal) against individual immunoglobulin classes and subclasses can be obtained commercially conjugated with fluorescein isothiocyanate. If preparing conjugates as described below, conjugates with a satisfactory labelling ratio of dye to protein have an optical density ratio at 495 nm and 280 nm approaching unity. Values below 0.5 indicate low labelling and over 1.5 are likely to result in non-specific staining. A suitable dilution of conjugate to test for obtaining this ratio is usually about 1 in 40. Performance assessment will need to be carried out to establish an optimal working dilution in the test. A useful way to establish specificity of an anti-immunoglobulin is to stain bone marrow cells obtained from patients with a myeloma of known paraprotein type. Conjugates should be freed of non-attached dye by chromatography on Sephadex G-25, and stored in aliquots at −20°C.

It is recommended that prior to examining smears of microorganisms obtained from a patient for attached antibody it is necessary to remove 'blocking' proteins by glycine-HCl buffer, pH 2.4, prior to staining with the fluorescein-conjugated anti-immunoglobulin. When looking for antibody in patient's serum, immunoglobulin of one class can prevent the detection of immunoglobulin of another class by saturating the antigenic sites on a micro-organism. To avoid this, prefractionation of the serum will be required.

Many of the problems of non-specific staining are simply overcome by using diluted conjugates. The appropriate dilution will have been obtained by performance assessment as described above. Recommendations for the testing of fluorochrome-labelled anti-immunoglobulin antibodies are given in the MRC Working Party Report on the use of immunochemical reagents (MRC 1971). For further details of these methods see Johnson & Holborow (1986) and Johnstone & Thorpe (1982).

Some of the uses to which the technique has been put include the localization of the origin of a variety of serum protein components, for example immunoglobulin production by plasma cells and other lymphoid cells. The demonstration and localization in the tissues of antibody globulin in a variety of autoimmune conditions has been shown, including an antinuclear antibody in the serum of patients with systemic lupus erythematosus and thyroid autoantibodies in the serum of patients with Hashimoto's thyroiditis. In the diagnostic field most human pathogens can be demonstrated by immunofluorescence and a tentative diagnosis may be made much sooner than by cultivation; the fluorescent method at present can be used to supplement rather than replace conventional methods.

There are two main procedures in use, the direct and indirect methods (Fig. 10.14). The *direct method* consists of bringing fluorescein-tagged antibodies into contact with antigens fixed on a slide (e.g. in the form of a tissue section or a smear of an organism), allowing them to react, washing off excess antibody and examining under the UV light microscope. The site of union of the labelled antibody with its antigen can be seen by the apple-green fluorescent areas on the slide. The *indirect method* can be used both for detecting specific antibodies in sera or other body fluids and also for identifying antigens. This method differs from the direct method in the use of a non-labelled antiserum which is layered on first, in the same way as described above. Whether or not this antiserum has reacted with the material on the slide is

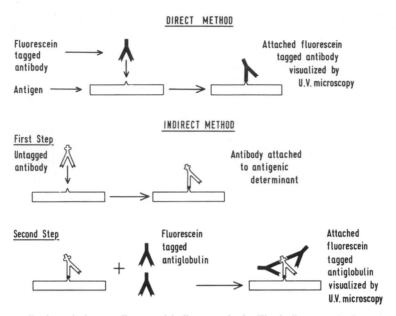

Fig. 10.14 Fluorescent antibody technique – direct and indirect methods. The indirect method can be seen to be more sensitive as two or more fluorescein-tagged antiglobulin molecules can be attached to each immunoglobulin molecule bound to its antigen.

shown by means of a fluorescein-tagged antiglobulin serum specific for the globulin of the serum applied first. Such an antiglobulin serum can be used to detect antibody globulin in sera to a variety of different antigens which gives it a considerable advantage over the direct test; it is also more sensitive. Suitable conjugates are widely available commercially.

Preparation of conjugated antiserum

If using serum from an animal immunized to a given immunoglobulin fraction or to a whole serum it is necessary to separate the globulin fraction from the antiserum prior to conjugation and this is conveniently carried out by 50% saturation with ammonium sulphate as follows:

1. Equal volumes, e.g. 10 ml, of antiserum and saturated ammonium sulphate are chilled separately in universal containers until ice crystals start to form in the antiserum, and then mixed by pouring the ammonium sulphate (all at once) into the antiserum. The mixture is then shaken well and left for 2 h in the cold at 4°C.

2. The precipitated globulin is separated from the supernatant albumin by centrifugation at 3000 *g* in a refrigerated centrifuge at 4°C.

3. The supernatant is removed and the precipitate dissolved in a small volume of distilled water, *just sufficient* to dissolve the globulin completely. The globulin solution is then dialysed overnight against 0.85% NaCl at 4°C to remove the ammonium sulphate.

4. The total protein of the dialysed globulin is then estimated by a convenient method, e.g. the quantitative Biuret method. Provided only a small volume of distilled water was used in the previous step the protein concentration should be 20–30 mg/ml.

Conjugation with fluorescein isothiocyanate. Proteins contain several different chemical groups which can be used for the attachment of fluorochromes. These include the free amino and carboxyl groups at the ends of each protein chain and free amino groups in the lysine side chains. The optimal quantity of fluorescein has been estimated as 0.05 mg/mg of protein. Above this level no further conjugation takes place and progressively larger amounts of protein are denatured.

1. The globulin fraction prepared as indicated above is diluted to 10 mg of protein/ml with 0.5 mol/litre carbonate-bicarbonate buffer pH 9.2

(made up fresh before use) so that the final mixture contains 10% buffer.

2. The solution is chilled to 4°C and 0.05 mg of fluorescein isothiocyanate (BDH) per mg of protein is added. During the addition of the fluorochrome and for the next 18 h the mixture should be stirred continuously, e.g. with a magnetic stirrer, and kept at 4°C.

4. Following conjugation excess fluorescein is dialysed away against phosphate buffered saline (0.01 mol/litre potassium phosphate buffer, pH 7.3; see Ch. 5) in the cold, changing the buffer frequently until the dialysate contains no further dye.

5. The conjugate is finally centrifuged for 45 min at 3000 g at 4°C to remove any precipitated denatured protein.

Conjugation with lissamine rhodamine B (RB200). The fluorochrome is used as the sulphonyl chloride prepared by grinding 0.5 g of RB200 with 1 g of PCl_5 in a mortar (using a fume cupboard). After mixing, 5 ml of acetone is added with stirring for a few minutes and the mixture filtered. This solution should be used within 48 h of preparation. The conjugation process is similar to that for fluorescein isothiocyanate except that 0.2 ml of the solution is used for every 100 mg of protein and after mixing with the globulin stirring need only be continued for 30 min.

Storage of conjugates. Conjugates may be stored at 4°C with the addition of preservative, e.g. merthiolate 1 in 10 000; alternatively they may be stored at −20°C or freeze dried. Prior to use non-specific fluorescence will require to be absorbed from the conjugate.

Enzyme labelled antibody

Similar principles are used as described above except that the antibody is conjugated with an enzyme such as horseradish peroxidase. The technique has the advantage that after addition of the enzyme substrate the stained preparation can be stored. Fluorescein preparations in contrast fade after exposure to UV light. The techniques are fully described in Johnstone & Thorpe (1982) and Weir et al (1986, Ch. 27) and reagents are available commercially (see also *Enzyme immunoassay* below).

Fluorescence polarization

Fluorescein-labelled compounds are also used in fluorescence polarization immunoassay (FIA). FIA is becoming increasingly popular for measuring antibiotic levels in serum. The method, which is extremely rapid, combines competitive protein binding with fluorescence polarization to give a direct measurement without the need for a separation process. The test is based on the principle that antibiotic in the patient sample will compete with fluorescein-labelled antibiotic for a limited number of binding sites on antibodies specific for the antibiotic being measured. The concentration of unlabelled antibiotic from the patient sample will determine how much fluorescein-labelled antibiotic can bind to the specific antibody. A sophisticated optical detection system (Fluorescence Polarization Analyser) is used to measure the increase in the polarization of fluorescent light which results when the fluorescein-labelled antibiotic binds to antibody. The concentration of antibiotic in the patient's serum is determined from an instrument-stored calibration curve of polarization values versus drug concentration. Reagents are available commercially (Abbott) for measuring antibiotics such as gentamicin, amikacin and tobramycin. FIA systems have not yet been used for detection of microbial antigens.

Enzyme immunoassay

Enzyme immunoassays are of two types – the homogeneous type without washing stages (the EMIT system, Syva), and the heterogeneous types known as enzyme-linked immunosorbent assays (ELISA). In the homogeneous assays inactivation of the enzyme label by antibody makes it unnecessary to separate bound from unbound compound as in other immunoassay methods. Homogeneous assays are very rapid but are not very sensitive and are only suitable for the measurement of small molecules.

Competitive protein binding assays such as

EMIT can be used for detecting aminoglycoside antibiotics such as gentamicin, tobramycin, amikacin and kanamycin; easy-to-use reagent kits and convenient processing apparatus are readily available. In these assays the antibiotic, e.g. gentamicin, can be regarded as a hapten. Anti-gentamicin antibody is added to patient's serum containing an unknown concentration of gentamicin; molecules of gentamicin in the serum will immediately bind to antibody sites. Glucose-6-phosphate dehydrogenase-labelled gentamicin is then added to the mixture. Antibody binding sites not already bound with gentamicin from the specimen are immediately occupied by molecules of enzyme-labelled gentamicin. When enzyme-labelled gentamicin binds to the antibody enzymatic activity is reduced. In the case of glucose-6-phosphate dehydrogenase the reaction is followed by monitoring the reduction of the cofactor NAD at 340 nm in the presence of the substrate glucose-6-phosphate.

In contrast to the rapid homogeneous EMIT system the heterogeneous enzyme immunoassays (ELISA) are slow, requiring several incubation and washing stages. However, they are suitable for assaying large molecules and they are very sensitive. Antibodies are conjugated with enzyme by the addition of glutaraldehyde (Engvall & Perlmann 1971) such that the resulting antibody conjugates have both immunological and enzyme activity and can be quantified by their ability to degrade a suitable substrate. Alkaline phosphatase and horseradish peroxidase are the most commonly used enzymes; their respective substrates are p-nitrophenyl phosphate and O-phenylene diamine 2HCl. Enzymatic activity results in a colour change which can be assessed visually or objectively in a simple spectrophotometer.

The test can be done with sensitized carrier surfaces in the form of tubes, beads or plates. Disposable polystyrene or polyvinyl micro-haemagglutination plates are particularly convenient for mass processing. Either antibody or antigen can be detected, in a similar way to that used in radioimmunoassay (RIA). ELISA has not yet become a routine method in most bacteriological laboratories. It is likely that ELISA will find more widespread use in viral serology and in the diagnosis of parasitic diseases (Lancet 1979).

Radioimmunoassay (RIA)

The method is very sensitive and involves the use of either antiserum or more usually antigen labelled with [125]I. The amount of radioactive label bound in antigen-antibody complexes can be measured, and hence the concentration of antigen or antibody in a specimen can be determined.

The underlying principle of the procedure (Fig. 10.15) is to establish a stoichiometric relationship between the antiserum and the antigen and to select the most appropriate conditions as the standard. The equilibrium of this standard is then perturbed by adding the unknown sample (test sample). The extent to which the unknown sample competes in the binding interaction is compared with a standard curve. The concentration of the material in the unknown sample is then read off from the curve. Antibodies for use in these assays should have a high affinity for antigen and the development of monoclonal antibodies has largely overcome earlier difficulties due to inadequately characterized antibodies. For maximum sensitivity, the lowest antibody concentration that will bind a measurable fraction of antigen should be used. It is important to ensure that substances other than those being assayed, that might be present in physiological fluids, do not interfere with the

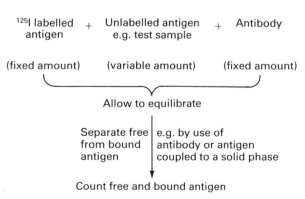

Fig. 10.15 Diagram of principle of competitive binding radioimmunoassay. The amount of labelled antigen bound to antibody is determined by the amount of unlabelled antigen in test sample that competes.

assay. For further details of radioimmunoassay methods see Bolton & Hunter (1986).

MISCELLANEOUS TESTS

The following tests may also find application in some laboratories.

Immobilization. This test depends on the principle that antibody combining with an antigen on a locomotor organ (flagellum, cilium) results in inhibition of motility. The classical application of this reaction is the *Treponema pallidum* immobilization test for the serological diagnosis of syphilis (Ch. 40).

Complement lysis. In the presence of complement antibody combines with a microbial surface antigen causing lysis of bacterium or enveloped virus. Used mainly in research with organisms such as *Vibrio cholerae*, *Escherichia coli* and *Neisseria gonorrhoeae*.

Immune electron microscopy. Antibody combining with viral or surface antigen causes clumping of virus particles visualized by electron microscopy. Used mainly in virus research. The procedures are described in Weir et al (1986, Ch. 35).

'Capsule swelling'. Mixing capsulate bacteria (e.g. pneumococci, *Klebsiella*) with homologous antibody makes possible the direct microscopic visualization of capsules. At one time the antibody was thought to make the capsule visible by increasing the size of the capsule, i.e. the 'Quellung' or swelling reaction; there is some evidence that swelling can occur when the reaction with antibody takes place in the presence of complement, but whether to a visible extent is doubtful (Ch. 18, *Methods*).

Toxin neutralization. Homologous antibody prevents the biological effect of toxin as observed with experimental animals (e.g. intracutaneous or intravenous administration of a mixture of *Clostridium perfringens* toxin and antitoxin to guinea-pigs or mice) or with special culture media (e.g. Nagler reaction, Ch. 37).

Infection with *Streptococcus pyogenes* (Ch. 17) or *Staphylococcus aureus* (Ch. 16) may result in antibody against bacterial haemolysin appearing in the serum. These antibodies are detected by incubating the serum with standard amounts of active haemolysin and noting the degree of inhibition of haemolysis when erythrocytes are added to the mixtures.

Detection of immune complexes. Complexes of antigen and antibody have been demonstrated in many infections and are sometimes responsible for pathological changes, e.g. focal nephritis and endocarditis in streptococcal infections and liver damage and polyarthritis in hepatitis B infections. Many methods are available to detect immune complexes including cryoprecipitation, precipitation by polyethylene glycol and detection of complement components in complexes. A commercial test (Pharmacia) is available for use in diagnosis of bacterial endocarditis. A range of techniques and their limitations are described in Weir et al (1986, Ch. 128).

Table 10.1 Immunological methods used in investigation of microbial and parasitic infections. (For details see appropriate sections in Weir et al, 1986, Vol. 4, Chs 119–123.)

	Precipitation
Bacteriology	Crossed immunoelectrophoresis (CIE) and modifications for identification of antigens of *Neisseria meningitidis*, *N. gonorrhoeae*, *Pseudomonas*, *Clostridium difficile*, *Spiroplasma*, *Salmonella*.
Virology	Double diffusion in agar and CIE for identification and quantitation of many viral antigens, e.g. adenovirus and vaccinia virus. Radioimmunoprecipitation for characterization of antigens of membrane-bound viruses that are difficult to purify, e.g. measles, respiratory syncytial virus. Also in routine use to define antigenic specificity of monoclonal antibodies.
Mycology	Immunodiffusion for detection of precipitins to *Aspergillus*, *Candida*, *Micromonospora*. WHO reference method for antibodies to histoplasmin; serodiagnosis of other systemic mycoses, e.g. coccidioidomycosis. CIE and modifications for detection of immunological responses to many fungi.

Table continued over

Table 10.1 (cont'd)

Protozoology	Immunoelectrophoresis and modifications for characterization of many protozoa, e.g. *Leishmania*.
Helminthology	Immunodiffusion, CIE and modifications for detection of antibodies to many helminths.

Agglutination

Bacteriology	Diagnosis of typhoid fever and brucellosis; serological classification of Gram-negative organisms. Passive haemagglutination for detection of antibody to *Mycoplasma*; diagnosis of syphilis. Coagglutination for identification and typing of *Neisseria gonorrhoeae*, identification and grouping of streptococci. Antistreptolysin 0 titres, influenzal and meningococcal antigens and antibodies.
Virology	Haemagglutination inhibition in influenza, mumps and parainfluenza infections using human or guinea-pig red cells; adenovirus and measles with monkey red cells; reoviruses and many enteroviruses using human red cells; arboviruses using day-old chick or goose red cells.
Mycology	Detection of antibodies to *Candida*, *Cryptococcus*. Classification of *Candida, Torulopsis, Hansenula* and *Debaryomyces*.
Helminthology	Widely used for detection of antibody or antigen, e.g. *Schistosoma mansoni*.

Complement fixation

Bacteriology	Detection of antibodies to *Brucella, Bordetella* and Group A streptococcus.
Virology	Widely used in diagnostic virology, e.g. influenza A and B viruses, adenoviruses.
Mycology	Widely used for diagnosis of histoplasmosis, coccidioidomycosis, blastomycosis and paracoccidioidomycosis.
Helminthology	Widely used for antibody to helminths.

Immunofluorescence

Bacteriology	Detection of pneumococcal antigen in tissues, pathogens in faecal specimens; identification of *Neisseria gonorrhoeae*; serotyping of *Klebsiella* spp.; serodiagnosis of legionellosis; enumeration of bacteria in milk.

Table 10.1 (cont'd)

Virology	Detection of viral antigens in clinical specimens, e.g. rabies, respiratory syncytial and parainfluenza viruses.
Mycology	Systemic mycoses, e.g. histoplasmosis, blastomycosis, coccidioidomycosis, cryptococcosis and sporotrichosis. Detection of organisms in smears or formalin-fixed tissue sections. Detection and quantitation of antibodies to fungal antigens.
Protozoology	Immunocharacterization and tissue localization of populations and subpopulations of parasitic protozoa, e.g. *Leishmania*.
Helminthology	Widely used to detect helminths, e.g. *Schistosoma, Echinococcus, Dirofilaria, Toxocara, Angiostrongylus*.

Enzyme immunoassays (ELISA)

Bacteriology	To identify and quantify bacterial components and to detect antibodies to bacterial antigens, e.g. *Shigella* and *Yersinia*.
Virology	Detection of viral antibodies and antigens, e.g. respiratory syncytial virus in nasopharyngeal aspirates and reovirus-like agents in faeces.
Mycology	Detection of fungal antibodies and antigens, e.g. in aspergillosis, candidosis and extrinsic allergic alveolitis.
Protozoology	Detection of protozoal antibodies and antigens, e.g. *Leishmania, Trypanosoma*.
Helminthology	Widely used, mainly experimentally.

Immunoradiometric assays (RIA)

Bacteriology	Used experimentally for analysis of bacterial antigens.
Virology	Widely used for detection of viral antigens and antibodies, e.g. hepatitis B, HIV.
Mycology	Detection of IgE antibodies in aspergillosis. Assays for antigen in aspergillosis, candidosis and histoplasmosis.
Protozoology	Characterization of antigens of *Trypanosoma*, and sporozoites of *Plasmodium*.
Helminthology	Antibodies to *Schistosoma*.

REFERENCES

Bolton A E, Hunter W M 1986 Radioimmunoassays. In: Weir D M et al (eds) Handbook of experimental immunology, 4th edn. Blackwell Scientific Publications, Oxford. Ch 26

Engvall E, Perlmann P 1971 Enzyme-linked immunosorbent assay (ELISA) Quantitative assay of immunoglobulin G. Immunochemistry 8: 871–874

Fallon R J 1983 Microbiological examination of cerebrospinal fluid. Association of Clinical Pathologists Broadsheet 108

Johnson G D, Holborow E J 1986 Preparation and use of fluorochrome conjugates. In: Weir D M et al (eds) Handbook of experimental immunology, 4th edn. Blackwell Scientific Publications, Oxford. Ch 28

Johnstone A, Thorpe R 1982 Immunochemistry in practice. Blackwell, Oxford

Jones D M 1979 The rapid detection of bacterial antigens. In: Reeves D, Geddes A (eds) Recent advances in infection 1. Churchill Livingstone, Edinburgh. Ch 6, p 91–107

Kronvall G 1973 A rapid slide agglutination method for typing pneumococci by means of a specific antibody absorbed to staphylococcal protein A. Journal of Medical Microbiology 6: 187 190

Lancet 1979 Enzyme immunoassays revisited (Editorial). Lancet 2:780–781

MRC 1971 Working party report on characterization of antisera as reagents. Immunology 20: 3–10

Rose N R, Friedman H (eds) 1984 Manual of clinical immunology. American Society for Microbiology, Washington

Weir D M, Herzenberg L A, Blackwell C C, Herzenberg L A, 1986 Handbook of experimental immunology, 4th edn. Blackwell Scientific Publications Oxford

Winstanley F P, Blackwell C C 1986 Monoclonal antibodies to bacteria and their products. In: Weir D M et al (eds) Handbook of experimental immunology, 4th edn. Blackwell Scientific Publications, Oxford. Ch 113

Examination of water, milk, food and air

EXAMINATION OF WATER

Supplies of drinking water contaminated with sewage or other excreted matter from man and animals may cause diseases like typhoid fever, cholera, campylobacteriosis, amoebiasis and helminthiasis. In the interests of public health, supplies should be tested regularly to confirm their freedom from such contamination. It is impracticable to attempt directly to detect the presence of all the different kinds of water-borne pathogens, any of which may be present only intermittently. Instead, reliance is placed on testing the supply for faecal indicator bacteria. These are the common intestinal commensal bacteria, *Escherichia coli*, *Streptococcus faecalis* and *Clostridium perfringens* (*C. welchi*), which are universally present in, and excreted in large numbers by man and animals. In themselves, they are not dangerous, but their presence indicates that faecal matter has entered the water supply, that the faecal bacteria have not been killed or removed by purification processes and that the supply is therefore liable to contamination with dangerous intestinal pathogens.

It is necessary not only to attempt to detect the presence of the indicator bacteria, but also to enumerate them, for the greater their number, the greater the danger of infection from the supply. The presence of very small numbers of the bacteria in unchlorinated water is usually disregarded, being assumed to have originated from animals and not from the more dangerous excretions of man. Separate counts are made of (1) presumptive coliform bacteria, and (2) confirmed *E. coli* bacteria. If the results of

these tests are difficult to interpret, counts are also made of faecal streptococci and *C. perfringens*.

The methods presented below are generalizations of statutory tests described in the Department of the Environment et al (1982) report 'The bacteriological examination of drinking water supplies 1982', to which reference should be made.

Collection of water samples

1. For collection, use heat-sterilized bottles containing a sufficient volume of sodium thiosulphate to neutralize the bactericidal effect of any chlorine or chloramine in the water. Each bottle of 100 ml capacity should contain 0.1 ml of a fresh 1.8% (w/v) aqueous solution of sodium thiosulphate.

2. When collecting the sample, exercise extreme care to avoid contaminating it with bacteria from the environment. Flame the mouths of taps and hydrants and allow water to run to waste for 3–5 min before running it into the bottle. When sampling from streams or lakes, open the bottle at a depth of about 30 cm with its mouth facing the current and ensure that water entering the bottle has not been in contact with the hand. Sample wells with weighted bottles. Collect at least 100 ml in each bottle.

3. Stopper the bottle, label it with full details of the source of the water and time and date of collection, and deliver it to the laboratory as quickly as possible, at least within 6 h, keeping it in a cool container and protected from light.

Detection and counting of indicator organisms

As the number of indicator bacteria in the water may be small, large volumes of the water have to be cultured. Two methods are available for this purpose, the multiple tube method and the membrane filtration method. Membrane filtration has advantages over the multiple tube test in requiring less labour and materials and in giving results earlier, so that any corrective action required to render the supply safe may be taken sooner. The multiple tube method has the advantages that it can show gas formation by the bacteria and is suitable for the examination of turbid waters containing small numbers of the indicator bacteria, e.g. waters containing numerous saprophytic bacteria that might suppress growth of the coliforms.

Multiple tube test

Measured volumes of water and dilutions of water are added to a series of tubes or bottles containing a liquid indicator growth medium. The media receiving one or more of the indicator bacteria show growth and a characteristic colour change which is absent in those receiving an inoculum of water without indicator bacteria. From the number and distribution of positive and negative reactions, the most probable number (MPN) of indicator organisms in the sample may be estimated by reference to statistical tables.

The indicator medium most used has been MacConkey broth containing bromocresol purple to indicate by its colour change to yellow the formation of acid from the lactose in the broth. The formula is given under *Methods** and a powdered preparation is available commercially (e.g. Oxoid CM5a). An inverted Durham tube is placed in each bottle or tube of the medium. Bacteria capable of growth and the production of acid and gas in MacConkey broth are assumed to be coliform bacilli, i.e. 'presumptive coliforms'.

An alternative selective indicator medium is lauryl tryptose broth* (e.g. Oxoid CM451) in which fermentation of lactose is judged by gas

* Refer to *Methods* section at end of this chapter.

formation and the absence of a pH indicator dye allows indole production to be observed by the addition of rosindole reagent after growth. The medium most strongly recommended is the minerals modified glutamate medium containing lactose and bromocresol purple* (e.g. Oxoid CM607 base, to which sodium glutamate is added). In comparative trials it has given more isolations of *E. coli* than either MacConkey broth or lauryl tryptose broth (e.g. PHLS Standing Committee on the Bacteriological Examination of Water Supplies 1969).

Presumptive coliform count

1. Place 50 ml and 10 ml volumes of indicator broth at double-strength concentration and 5 ml volumes at single strength into suitably sized bottles or tubes containing an inverted Durham tube. Cap and sterilize. After sterilization check that the Durham tubes are free from air bubbles.

2. Invert the bottle containing the sample of water rapidly several times to mix and distribute any deposit. Aseptically discard a little of the water, replace the cap and shake the bottle up and down 25 times.

3. *For waters of good quality*, aseptically pipette one 50 ml volume and five 10 ml volumes of the water into vessels containing corresponding 50 ml and 10 ml volumes of double strength medium.

For waters of doubtful quality, aseptically pipette one 50 ml volume and five 10 ml volumes of the water into vessels containing the corresponding volumes of double strength medium, and five 1 ml volumes into vessels containing 5 ml of single strength medium.

For waters known to be polluted, aseptically pipette five 10 ml volumes into vessels containing 10 ml double strength medium and five 1 ml volumes into vessels containing 5 ml single strength medium. Then prepare a 1 in 10 dilution of the water in quarter-strength Ringer's solution* and, if necessary, to give some negative reactions, higher 10-fold dilutions. Pipette five 1 ml volumes of the 1 in 10 dilution and five 1 ml volumes of any higher dilution into tubes containing 5 ml of single strength medium.

4. Incubate the seeded media aerobically at 37°C.

5. After 24 h and 48 h of incubation, inspect the media and note the number of cultures of each volume of water that show the production of acid (colour change) and gas (a bubble large enough to fill the concavity at the top of the Durham tube). These acid- and gas-producing cultures are considered 'presumptive positive' growths of coliform bacilli, e.g. escherichia, klebsiella or citrobacter. Cultures not showing production of both acid and gas at 48 h are considered negative.

6. By reference to tables of most probable numbers (*Methods*: 2)* in respect of the combination of positive and negative results observed, read off the most probable number (MPN) of presumptive coliform bacilli to be present in 100 ml of the sampled water.

Confirmed Escherichia coli count: Eijkman test

Some spore-bearing bacteria give false-positive reactions in the presumptive coliform test. Their presence is most likely to be misleading in the examination of chlorinated drinking water, for the spores are more resistant to chlorination than coliform bacilli. It is necessary, therefore, to confirm the presence of true coliform bacilli in each vessel showing a presumptive positive reaction and to determine whether these coliform bacilli are *E. coli*. The Eijkman test is used for this purpose, as it gives valid results with inocula of mixed bacteria from the cultures grown in the presumptive coliform test and does not require the preliminary isolation of the bacteria in pure culture.

The test is done by incubating subcultures from the positive presumptive tests at 44 and 37°C in a lactose-containing medium inhibitory to spore-forming bacteria, e.g. lauryl tryptose broth* or brilliant-green lactose bile broth*, and other subcultures at 44°C in tryptone water*. The presence of coliform bacilli is confirmed by the production of gas from lactose at 37°C. That of *E. coli* is confirmed by the production at 44°C of gas from lactose and indole from tryptophan. Two atypical types of *E. coli*, known as irregular

types II and Vl (Wilson et al 1935), are unable to form indole at 44°C, but are rarely found in British water supplies. The formation of indole at 44°C without the formation of gas from lactose at 44°C, even if acid is formed, are the reactions of bacteria other than *E. coli* and are dismissed as negative.

Method. 1. Prepare tubes containing 5–10 ml of either lauryl tryptose (lactose) broth* or brilliant-green lactose bile broth* and an inverted Durham tube, and other tubes containing 5–10 ml tryptone water*. Sterilize and check that afterwards the Durham tubes are free from gas bubbles.

2. Before inoculation, incubate the lactose media in thermostatically controlled waterbaths at 44.0 ± 0.25°C, and at 37°C, and the tryptone waters at 44.0 ± 0.25°C.

3. When the media have reached the incubation temperature, inoculate a loopful or drop of each presumptive positive culture into a tube of the lactose medium at 37°C, another tube of the lactose medium at 44°C and a tube of tryptone water at 44°C. Immediately re-incubate the tubes in the waterbath at their correct temperature.

With each batch of tests, include and treat similarly control cultures known to give the appropriate positive (*E. coli*) and negative (*Klebsiella aerogenes*) results.

4. Remove the tubes incubated at 44°C after 24 h. Add a few drops of Kovac's reagent (Ch. 8), or the essentially similar rosindole reagent of Ehrlich, to the tryptone water cultures, also if desired to the lauryl tryptose cultures. After a few moments check that the reactions of the control organisms are correct. Then examine each culture for gas production and indole formation and record the results.

5. Remove the tubes incubated at 37°C after 48 h, examine them for gas production and record the results.

6. Refer to the tables of most probable numbers*. From the combination of positive and negative results for gas production at 37°C, read off the most probable number of coliform bacilli per 100 ml of water. This value is known as the confirmed coliform count. From the combination

of positive and negative results for gas and indole production at 44°C, read off the most probable number of E. coli per 100 ml of water. This latter value is known as the confirmed E. coli count.

Count of faecal streptococci

If there is difficulty in interpreting the results of the presumptive coliform and confirmed E. coli tests, as when presumptive coliforms are present but E. coli is absent, a demonstration of the presence of faecal streptococci will confirm the faecal origin of the coliform bacilli. The term 'faecal streptococci' refers only to those streptococcal species of Lancefield's group D which normally occur in human and animal faeces. These enterococci can grow in the media used in the presumptive coliform test, where they ferment the lactose with the production of acid but not gas.

Method. 1. Incubate tubes containing 5 ml sterile glucose azide broth* in a waterbath thermostatically controlled at 44–45°C. (Sodium azide is highly toxic and forms explosive compounds with metals. Exercise extreme care in preparing and discarding the medium.)

2. When the tubes have warmed to the incubation temperature, seed them with heavy inocula from all the tubes in the presumptive coliform test that showed the formation of either acid and gas, or acid only. Immediately re-incubate at 44–45°C.

3. After incubation for 48 h, inspect the cultures for acid production shown by a yellow colour change in the bromocresol purple in the medium. Those producing acid contain faecal streptococci.

4. Confirm the presence of faecal streptococci by subculturing each positive glucose azide culture on to a plate of bile aesculin azide agar* incubated at 44–45°C.

5. Examine the plates after a few hours' incubation for a brown-black colouration around the inoculum, which is evidence of hydrolysis of the aesculin and confirms the presence of faecal streptococci.

6. Refer to the tables of most probable numbers* and from the proportion of tubes in the presumptive coliform test from which a confirmed streptococcal result was obtained, determine the most probable number of faecal streptococci in 100 ml of the water sample.

Count of Clostridium perfringens

C. perfringens (C.welchi) is a normal inhabitant of the intestine. Although present in smaller numbers than E. coli, its spores can survive in water for long periods and persist when all other faecal bacteria have died. An examination for their presence in water is valuable in demonstrating remote or intermittent pollution, and in confirming the presence of faecal pollution when only coliforms other than E. coli are cultured from the water.

A count is made of the spores of sulphite-reducing clostridia by first heating the water sample to kill all vegetative bacteria and then doing a multiple tube test by culturing it in differential reinforced clostridial medium (DRCM)*. This medium contains cysteine to permit the growth of anaerobic clostridia and a combination of sodium sulphite and ferric citrate to reveal any growth of sulphite-reducing bacteria by the production of a black precipitate of ferrous sulphide.

Method. 1. Kill vegetative bacteria by heating the water sample in a waterbath for 10 min at 75°C. Control the heating by having beside the sample in the waterbath an equal volume of tap water and a thermometer in the same kind of container as the sample. Start timing the heating period when the thermometer in the tap water reaches 75°C.

2. Aseptically add 50 ml of heated sample to a vessel containing 50 ml double-strength differential reinforced clostridial medium (DRCM)*, five 10 ml volumes of the sample to vessels containing 10 ml double-strength DRCM, and five 1 ml volumes to vessels containing 25 ml single-strength DRCM. If the water may be highly polluted, 1 ml volumes of a 1 in 10 and a 1 in 100 dilution of the sample should be cultured in other vessels containing 25 ml single-strength DRCM. The culture vessels should be

stout screw-capped glass bottles of a size just sufficient to hold the water and the medium. If necessary, aseptically add single-strength DRCM to the bottles until the level reaches the foot of the neck of the bottle; this arrangement minimizes the content of residual air.

3. Screw the caps on the bottles tightly and place the bottles in plastic bags to retain their contents should they explode during incubation. Incubate them for 48 h at 37°C.

4. After incubation, examine the bottles for blackening of the medium, a reaction that can be given by any species of *Clostridium*. Refer to the probability tables* and read from the combination of positive and negative results the most probable number of spores of sulphite-reducing clostridia in 100 ml of water sample.

5. Examine for the presence of *C. perfringens* in the positive, sulphite-reducing cultures by subculturing a loopful from each such culture into a separate tube of litmus milk medium (Chs 8, 37) that has been freshly steamed and cooled and to which a piece of iron wire or nail heated to redness has just been added. The litmus milk should be at least 70 mm deep. Incubate in air for up to 48 h at 37°C.

6. After incubation, and at 48 h, observe the tubes for production of the 'stormy clot' reaction, in which, through fermentation of the lactose, the milk is acidified and coagulated and the clot is disrupted by bubbles of gas and often blown to the top of the tube. This reaction indicates that the inoculated cultures contained *C. perfringens*.

7. Refer to the probability tables* and read from the combination of positive 'stormy clot' results in litmus milk and negative results in both litmus milk and DRCM the most probable number of *C. perfringens* spores in 100 ml of water sample.

Membrane filtration tests

In this method, a measured volume of the water sample is filtered through a membrane with a pore size small enough to retain the indicator bacteria to be counted. The membrane is then placed and incubated on a selective, indicator medium, so that the indicator bacteria grow into colonies on its upper surface. These colonies, which are recognized by their colour, morphology and ability to grow on the selective medium, are counted.

Filtration procedure

1. The filtration apparatus (Baird & Tatlock; Gallenkamp) consists of a base supporting a porous disk under a graduated funnel. Sterilize the apparatus and two extra funnels by autoclaving. Then connect the base to a vacuum source.

2. Procure from a commercial source (e.g. Oxoid) filter membranes of high quality, control grade, 47 mm in diameter and 0.45 μm of pore size. If purchased unsterile, sterilize them by autoclaving for 10 min at 115°C or by boiling in distilled water for 10 min at 100°C. Avoid overheating, which will impair the filtration properties of the membrane. Use each membrane only once.

3. Remove the funnel from the apparatus and with flamed and cooled flat-ended forceps, grasp the edge of a sterile membrane and place it, grid side up, over the porous disk. Replace the sterile funnel securely on the filter base.

4. While the vacuum is still turned off, pour or pipette the requisite volume of the water sample into the funnel. The volume should be chosen so that the colonies to be counted on the membrane will number between 10 and 100. For chlorinated waters, filter a 100 ml volume. For unknown waters, filter a range of different volumes from 10–100 ml. For polluted waters, filter volumes smaller than 10 ml, but add at least 20 ml sterile water to the filter before addition of the sample to ensure dispersion of the bacteria over the membrane.

When filtering different volumes of the same sample, the funnel can be re-used without boiling between uses provided that the smallest volumes are filtered first. When filtering different samples, always sterilize the funnel in boiling water and allow it to cool between its use for each sample. Always filter pure and chlorinated samples before samples known to be polluted.

5. Filter the sample slowly through the membrane by applying a vacuum of about

500 mm of mercury. Stop the evacuation as soon as the sample has been filtered so that as little contaminated air as possible is drawn through the membrane.

6. Remove the funnel and aseptically transfer the membrane, keeping its upper side upwards, on to a sterile paper pad saturated with a selective indicator broth or on to a plate of selective indicator agar medium (see below). Ensure that no air bubbles are trapped between the membrane and the medium.

The absorbent paper pads should be free from toxic substances, approximately 1 mm thick and of at least as great a diameter as the membrane. They can be sterilized in foil-wrapped bundles by autoclaving for 20 min at 121°C. Place the pads in separate sterile Petri dishes before soaking with the special membrane medium. Pour off any excess medium from the saturated pad either before or after the membrane is in position so as to prevent the erroneous formation of confluent growth on the membrane.

7. Incubate the plates holding the membranes under appropriate conditions. Those with absorbent pads must be held in polythene bags or airtight tins containing wads of cotton-wool moistened with water to prevent the pads drying out.

8. After incubation, immediately count the characteristic colonies in a good light and with the aid of a magnifying glass. Express the result as the number of indicator bacteria per 100 ml of water sample.

Presumptive coliform count by filtration

For this test the membranes are cultured on pads soaked with membrane lauryl sulphate broth* (e.g. Oxoid MM615), or an equivalent medium, which is inhibitory to many non-coliform bacteria and on which, because it contains lactose and phenol red, the coliforms grow as yellow-coloured colonies.

1. Filter the water sample as directed above.

2. Incubate the membranes on pads soaked with membrane lauryl sulphate broth first for 4 h at 30°C and then for 14 h at 37°C.

3. Immediately on removal from the incubator, count all the yellow colonies irrespective

of size and, with reference to the volume of water filtered, calculate the number of presumptive coliform bacteria per 100 ml of sample.

Confirmed coliform and Escherichia coli counts by filtration

As some non-coliform bacteria that produce acid but not gas from lactose can form yellow colonies in the presumptive coliform test, the number of yellow colonies that are coliforms must be confirmed by the demonstration of gas formation at 37°C and the number that are *E. coli* by the demonstration that they can form acid and gas from lactose at 44°C and indole from tryptophan at 44°C.

1. Subculture every yellow colony, or a sufficient representative number of them, from the membranes cultured for the presumptive coliform count, each into two tubes of lactose peptone water with phenol red* containing an inverted, medium-filled Durham tube, and a tube of tryptone water*.

2. Incubate one of the tubes of lactose peptone water at 37°C and the other at 44°C. Incubate the tryptone water at 44°C. After about 6 h, subculture growth from the lactose peptone water incubated at 37°C on to a plate of nutrient agar; incubate this plate at 37°C and re-incubate the tube at 37°C.

3. After 24 h incubation; (a) do an oxidase test (Ch. 8) on the colonies on the nutrient agar plate; (b) add a few drops of Kovac's reagent (Ch. 8) to the tryptone water cultures and look for the development of a pink colour denoting indole formation; (c) inspect the lactose peptone water cultures for the formation of acid (yellow colour change) and gas, re-incubating those that are negative for re-examination after a further 24 h at 37°C.

Yellow colonies on membranes are confirmed as being coliform bacteria if they are oxidase negative and form acid and gas in lactose peptone water incubated at 37°C. The oxidase test is required to exclude those *Aeromonas* species that form acid and gas from lactose but are oxidase positive.

Yellow colonies on membranes are confirmed as being *E. coli* if they are oxidase negative, form acid and gas in lactose peptone water incubated at 44°C and form indole in tryptone water incubated at 44°C.

4. From the results, calculate the confirmed coliform count and the confirmed *E. coli* count per 100 ml water sample.

Faecal streptococcus count by filtration

1. Filter the water sample as detailed above.

2. Place the membrane on a surface-dried plate of membrane enterococcus agar* and incubate for 48 h at 37°C.

3. Count all red, maroon and pale pink colonies as being presumptive faecal streptococci.

4. Subculture these presumptive colonies on to slopes of bile aesculin azide agar* and incubate for a few hours in a waterbath at 44–45°C. Inspect the slopes for the development of a brown-black colour, which confirms the presence of a faecal streptococcus.

5. Calculate the number of confirmed faecal streptococci per 100 ml water sample.

Clostridium perfringens count by filtration

1. Kill vegetative bacteria by heating the water sample at 75°C as described for the multiple tube test and, after cooling, filter an appropriate volume through a membrane.

2. Place the membrane face upwards either (a) on a surface-dried plate of membrane clostridial agar* or (b) on the base of a small Petri dish (ensuring no air bubbles are trapped) over which 18 ml molten membrane clostridial agar cooled to 50°C is carefully poured and allowed to set.

3. Incubate the plates in an anaerobic cabinet or jar at 37°C.

4. After 24 h and 48 h of incubation, count all black colonies on the plates as being sulphite-reducing clostridia.

5. Subculture each black colony into a tube of freshly steamed and cooled litmus milk medium containing an iron nail as described for the multiple tube test. Incubate for 48 h at 37°C.

6. Count the colonies that produce a 'stormy clot' as *C. perfringens* and calculate the count of confirmed *C. perfringens* per 100 ml water sample.

Plate count

The plate count expresses the number of all colony-forming bacteria in 1 ml water. It is of limited value by itself, but as a supplementary test it provides information about the amount and type of organic matter in the water which may be useful in indicating the efficiency of the processes used for water treatment or the suitability of the water for large-scale production of food and drink.

Separate plate cultures are incubated at 20–22°C and at 37°C. That at 20–22°C grows mainly the natural saprophytes of soil and water, whilst that at 37°C grows mainly parasitic bacteria derived from human and animal excretions. The true number of viable bacteria and yeasts in the water will be in excess of the counts on these plates, for many of the micro-organisms occur in clumps and many fail to grow under the cultural conditions used.

1. Melt sterile yeast extract agar* and cool it to and maintain it at 50°C until ready to pour plates.

2. Shake the bottle of water sample as described for the multiple tube test. Then aseptically prepare a series of 10-fold dilutions of the water by successively transferring 10 ml volumes through a series of bottles holding 90 ml sterile quarter-strength Ringer's solution* as diluent. According to the count expected, one or two or, rarely, three dilutions will be required.

3. Starting with the highest (most dilute) dilution of the sample and working towards the undiluted sample, aseptically pipette exactly 1 ml of the dilution or sample into each of four sterile Petri dishes.

4. To each plate add 15 ml molten, cool (50°C) yeast extract agar and immediately, and for a brief period, gently rotate the plate clockwise and then anticlockwise to mix the water with the medium. Then leave the agar to set. The interval between preparing the dilutions and mixing them with the agar should not exceed 15 min.

5. Incubate two of the four plates of each dilution for 3 days at 20–22°C and the other two for 24 h ± 3 h at 37°C.

6. Immediately after these periods of incubation, count the colonies on each plate. If there

has to be any delay, meantime refrigerate the plates at 4°C, but count them at least within 24 h. For counting, use an illuminated colony counting apparatus fitted with a magnifying lens and an automatic count recorder. Select for counting the dilution plates that bear between 30 and 300 colonies. Multiply the mean count by the dilution to obtain the plate counts, expressed as the number of colonies per ml water sample after 3 days at 20–22°C or 24 h at 37°C.

If there are less than 30 colonies on the plate from the undiluted sample, report the count as 'approximate only'. If the plates from the highest dilution contain more than 300 colonies either try to count them and report the result as approximate or express the result as 'more than x colonies per ml', calculating x as the dilution factor multiplied by 300.

Interpretation of counts

E. coli is the most numerous coliform in human and animal intestines and is derived almost exclusively from these sources. It does not survive long in water. It is therefore the best indicator of recent human or animal faecal pollution. Its presence in water indicates a potentially dangerous pollution, high counts a heavy or recent pollution and low counts a slight or more remote one.

Other coliform bacilli, e.g. klebsiellas and citrobacters, are much less abundant in faeces than *E. coli* and enter water mainly from soil and vegetation, where they grow as saprophytes. They also survive longer in water than *E. coli*. Their presence in water may therefore indicate either contamination from soil and vegetation or contamination with faecal material at a time remote enough to have allowed the *E. coli* bacteria to die out. The presence of any coliform bacilli in chlorinated water indicates either a failure of the chlorination process or a contamination after chlorination, and the fault should at once be investigated and corrected.

Faecal streptococci are less abundant in faeces than *E. coli* and are often more abundant in animal than human faeces. Speciation of isolates may help to trace the source of pollution, for *Streptococcus bovis* is usually derived from cattle

and sheep, *S. equinus* from horses and *S. avium* from birds; *S. faecium* and *S. durans* are derived from both man and animals, and *S. faecalis* more often from man. Faecal streptococci survive longer in water than *E. coli* and are more resistant to chlorination than the coliforms. Their presence with coliforms, despite the absence of *E. coli*, confirms faecal pollution of the water.

C. perfringens is present in faeces in even smaller numbers than the streptococci and is the least sensitive indicator of faecal pollution. But its spores may survive chlorination and persist in water much longer than the other indicator bacteria, so that its finding in the absence of the latter implies an intermittent or remote pollution, or the result of chlorination in killing the vegetative bacteria, and thus any bacterial pathogens in recently polluted water. In these circumstances the spores themselves do not constitute a hazard to health when the water is used for drinking, but the finding of *C. perfringens* as well as coliform bacilli is suggestive of faecal pollution even in the absence of *E. coli*.

The plate count, as already described, is useful mainly for purposes other than assessing water safety, but a sudden increase in the count at 37°C may be an early sign of pollution and should be investigated. Variation in the count at 22°C usually reflects a change in the season or environment and is of little significance to health.

Bacteriological standards of water quality

The standards applied in Britain are in keeping with those recommended by the World Health Organization (1971) and the European Community (1980). Table 11.1 shows the quality grading as assessed from the *E. coli* and coliform counts.

1. *Water entering a distribution system.* The final treatment of water, usually by chlorination, before it enters the system of pipes distributing it to the public is an effective disinfection. If correctly done, this treatment ensures that no viable coliform bacteria remain in the water. The supply here can be regarded as satisfactory only

Table 11.1 Grades of the quality of drinking water supplies determined by the results of periodic *Escherichia coli* and coliform counts

Quality of supply	Results from routine samples		Tolerance
	Coliform count/100 ml	*E. coli* count/100 ml	
1. Excellent	0	0	In all samples
2. Satisfactory	1–3	0	Provided that coliform organisms do not occur in consecutive samples or in more than 5% of samples
3. Intermediate	4–9	0	
4. Unsatisfactory	10 coliforms *or* 1 or more *E. coli or* any coliform organisms present in consecutive samples, *or* presence of any coliform organisms in more than 5% of routine samples		In any sample

if coliform bacteria are undetectable in all tested samples of 100 ml. Any deviation from this standard, however small, should be reported at once, so that the treatment process can be investigated for faults.

2. *Water drawn from the distribution system.* For various reasons, pure water entering the distribution system may deteriorate in quality before it reaches the consumer's tap, e.g. as a result of unsatisfactory plumbing repairs, use of contaminated materials in construction, and access of coliforms through air valves, hydrants, pumps and leaks in pipes where they are under negative pressure. Thus, although ideally all samples drawn from the distribution system should be free from coliforms, a minimal contamination within the following limits may be tolerated.

E. coli should not be detectable in any 100 ml sample. No more than three coliform bacilli should be found in any 100 ml sample. Coliform bacilli should not be detectable in any two consecutive samples of 100 ml from the same or a closely related sampling point. Coliform bacilli should not be found in more than 5% of routine samples from the system among at least 50 samples examined at regular intervals throughout the year.

When any coliforms are found, the disinfection process should be checked and the water re-sampled from the same and related sites to confirm the original positive finding and locate the possible source of contamination. Even when satisfactory results are obtained on re-testing, the frequency of routine sampling should be increased for a while. The results of the tests should be reviewed annually to obtain an indication of the overall quality of the supply, which may be graded as in Table 11.1 provided that results from at least 50 samplings are available.

3. *Water from unpiped rural supplies.* In the absence of a piped supply, the source of water, e.g. a lake or well, should be protected from obvious sources of excremental pollution. The quality of the water may be considered satisfactory if the coliform count is less than 10/100 ml sample. Water in which this limit is exceeded, or in which more than minimal numbers of *E. coli* are found, should be condemned for drinking.

Examination of water for pathogens

When water is suspected of transmitting a particular infection, an attempt may be made to isolate the causal pathogen from it. Large samples have to be examined by the use of concentration techniques and selective culture media.

Filtration. If the water is clear, concentration may be done by the membrane filtration method previously described, using 500 ml funnels. If it is turbid, a sterile absorbent pad should be substituted for the filter membrane. Before filtering, a sterile suspension of Filter-Aid*, a powdered kieselguhr, is poured over the pad. This retains the bacteria, but is porous enough to enable large volumes of turbid water to be filtered without blockage. After filtration, the pad with the layer of Filter-Aid is transferred to a pre-enrichment medium.

Sewer swab. The method described by Moore (1948) for the isolation of enteric bacteria from sewers may be used. Fold a piece of gauze 1200 cm × 150 cm into eight thicknesses and attach a length of wire or string. Suspend the swab in flowing water or sewage for 48 h so that it may entrap and concentrate a proportion of the passing bacteria, then transfer it into a sterile wide-mouthed, screw-capped jar for delivery to the laboratory.

Resuscitation and selective culture. Resuscitate the bacteria on the swab or filter pad by placing this in a non-selective medium such as buffered peptone water* and incubating for 24 h at 37°C. Then make subcultures in selective and enrichment media appropriate to the species of pathogen being sought.

Legionella. Methods of examining a water supply for the presence of legionella bacteria are discussed in Chapter 35.

Examination of swimming pool water

Swimming pools may be infected with pathogens derived from bathers or from a contaminated water supply. If, however, the pool is chlorinated and free chlorine maintained at an effective level, i.e. 1 part per million, or 2 p.p.m. in heavily used pools, never falling below 0.5 p.p.m., regular bacteriological examination may be unnecessary.

When such examination is required, samples of water should be collected in containers holding sufficient sodium thiosulphate to neutralize the high level of residual chlorine, and coliform and plate counts should be performed. The water may be regarded as satisfactory if coliforms are absent from 100 ml samples and the plate counts at 37°C show no more than 10 colonies/ml in 75% of the samples and no more than 100/ml in the remainder.

EXAMINATION OF MILK

Human infections may be caused by the ingestion of cow's milk which contains either microorganisms derived from the cow, e.g. by contamination with its faeces, or human pathogens derived from milk handlers such as dairy workers. To minimize the risk of such infection from commercial supplies, and also to improve their keeping quality, certain precautions are taken. These include the maintenance of dairy herds free from dangerous infections such as tuberculosis and brucellosis, the maintenance of clean conditions of collection and storage to minimize faecal and other contamination, and the treatment of the milk by heat, e.g. pasteurization, to kill pathogens and spoilage bacteria. According to the conditions of production the milk is marketed as being of certain grades of quality, and bacteriological and chemical tests are routinely done on samples from each bulk supply to ensure that the criteria of the grade advertised have been met.

In Britain the following grades are defined by the Milk (Special Designation) Amendment Regulations 1965 and 1972:

Untreated milk is the unheated milk from tuberculin-tested (and negative) cattle which passes the standard 30 min methylene blue reduction test (see below).

Pasteurized milk is milk that has been heated either (1) at between 63°C and 66°C for 30 min, or (2) at 72°C for at least 15 s, and then immediately cooled to below 10°C. It must pass both the 30 min methylene blue reduction test and the phosphatase test (see below).

Ultra heat treated (UHT) milk is milk that has been heated at 133°C for 1 s and immediately placed in sterile containers. It should grow less than 1000 colonies/ml when incubated for 48 h at between 30°C and 37°C on yeast extract milk agar*.

Sterilized milk is milk that after bottling is heated at 100°C for such a period that it passes the turbidity test (see below).

The designations used in Scotland under the Milk (Special Designations) (Scotland) Order 1965 and 1966 require also that:

Premium milk must contain not more than 15 000 bacteria/ml and not any coliform bacilli in 0.01 ml.

Standard milk must contain not more than 50 000 bacteria/ml and not any coliform bacilli in 0.001 ml.

Pasteurized milk must not contain any coliform bacilli in 0.01 ml.

Statutory tests must be done exactly as described in the Milk (Special Designation) Regulations of England 1963 and Milk (Special Designation) Amendment Regulations 1965 and 1972, and the Milk (Special Designations) (Scotland) Order 1965 and 1966, available from Her Majesty's Stationery Office. They are summarized below.

Samples

If the milk is contained in retail bottles, one unopened bottle constitutes the sample. If in a bulk container, it must be mixed thoroughly with a sterile plunger before a sample is collected from well below the surface with a sterile dipper and poured into a sterile stoppered or screw-capped bottle of about 125 ml capacity. The samples should then be placed in an insulated box, dispatched to the laboratory without delay and examined as soon as possible after arrival, except for samples of untreated milk for the methylene blue test and samples of UHT milk for bacterial counts, which require preliminary holding at particular temperatures (see below).

Methylene blue test

This test is a substitute for a bacterial count. It depends on the dye being reduced and so decolourized by the metabolism of any large number of viable bacteria present in the milk. The rate of reduction is taken as a measure of the degree of bacterial contamination.

1. Because the time of reduction is affected by the temperature at which the milk is held before testing, the samples must be held until the time of testing as follows: (a) from 1 May to 31 October, samples must be held at atmospheric shade temperature, and (b) from 1 November to 30 April, samples must be held at atmospheric shade temperature until 5 pm on the day of sampling, thereafter at 17–20°C. The test should not be done if the atmospheric shade temperature exceeds 21°C.

2. Prepare a 1 in 300 000 solution of methylene blue by dissolving a standard methylene blue tablet from an approved manufacturer (e.g. BDH) in 200 ml cold sterile glass-distilled water

and making up to 800 ml with more of such water. Store the solution in the dark in a refrigerator and use within 2 months.

3. Mix the milk sample thoroughly by inverting the sample bottle about 25 times.

4. Aseptically pipette 10 ml of the sample into a sterile (152 × 16 mm) test tube which has been covered with an aluminium cap during sterilization in a hot air oven.

5. Add 1 ml of methylene blue solution with a 1 ml sterile pipette.

6. Stopper the tube with a rubber stopper that has been sterilized in boiling water. Then invert it once or twice to mix the contents.

7. Place the tube for 30 min at 37°C in a thermostatically controlled waterbath. The water level must be above the top of the milk and the bath covered with a lid to exclude light.

8. With each test incubate as controls (a) 10 ml milk that has been held at 100°C for 3 min, to inactivate its reducing system, plus 1 ml methylene blue, and (b) 10 ml milk plus 1 ml tap water.

9. After incubation, compare the test mixture with control (a) to see whether there is any decolourization in the former, and with control (b) to see whether decolourization is complete.

If the dye is wholly decolourized or decolourized to within 5 mm of the milk surface, the milk fails the test. Record the time for complete decolourization. Untreated milk is considered satisfactory if it fails to decolourize the dye in 30 min.

Phosphatase test

This test determines the inactivation by heat of the enzyme phosphatase which is naturally present in cow's milk. The degree of heating applied in effective pasteurization to kill non-sporing pathogenic microorganisms is sufficient to inactivate the enzyme, and if enzyme activity is still demonstrable in treated milk the pasteurization process has not been properly carried out. The test depends on the ability of the enzyme to liberate p-nitrophenol from disodium p-nitrophenyl phosphate and thereby produce a yellow colour that can be quantified with a colorimeter.

1. Test the milk sample as soon as received or, if that is not possible, after refrigeration overnight.

2. Prepare a buffer solution by dissolving 3.5 g anhydrous sodium carbonate (Na_2CO_3) and 1.5 g sodium bicarbonate ($NaHCO_3$) in 1 litre of distilled water. Store in a refrigerator.

3. Prepare the reagent by dissolving 0.15 g disodium p-nitrophenyl phosphate in 100 ml buffer solution. Store in the dark in a refrigerator and use within 7 days. Never use it if it is yellow.

4. Perform the tests in specially cleaned (152 × 16 mm) test tubes and pipettes kept specially for these tests. When new, they should be cleaned in chromic acid and well rinsed in distilled water, and between tests, washed in hot soda water, rinsed in warm water and then in distilled water, and drained dry.

5. Pipette 5 ml of reagent into each of a number of the specially cleaned test tubes corresponding to the number of the milk samples plus one for a control. Stopper the tubes with rubber bungs that have been sterilized in boiling water. Place the tubes in a waterbath to bring them to 37°C.

6. Thoroughly mix each sample of milk and pipette 1 ml of it into a tube of warmed reagent, re-stopper the tube and shake it to mix the contents. As a control, add 1 ml of milk that has been heated at 100°C for a least 3 min to the remaining tube of reagent, stopper and mix.

7. At once replace the tubes in the waterbath and hold for exactly 2 h at 37°C.

8. After incubation, place the control tube in the left (control) position and a tube of one of the test samples in the right position of a Lovibond comparator fitted with a APTW or APTW7 disk (Baird & Tatlock; Gallenkamp). With the comparator facing a good light, revolve the disk until the control and test samples show the same depth of colour and note the reading. Properly pasteurized milk will have a reading of 10 μg or less p-nitrophenol per ml.

Turbidity test

This is the definitive test for sterilized milk, distinguishing it both from untreated milk and from milk that has merely been pasteurized. The degree of heating necessary for sterilization causes all the heat-coagulable proteins in milk to become precipitable by ammonium sulphate. If the amount of heat applied to milk is insufficient for sterilization, some of its protein will not be precipitated by ammonium sulphate and will be detected by its coagulating and giving turbidity when a filtrate of the ammonium sulphate-treated milk is boiled. Absence of turbidity indicates that the milk has been heated to at least 100°C for at least 5 min. Some bacterial spores may survive this amount of heating, so that the 'sterilized' milk may not keep indefinitely.

1. Add 20 ml of the well-mixed milk sample to a flask containing 4 g ammonium sulphate (analytical grade).

2. Shake the mixture for 1 min to dissolve the ammonium sulphate and allow it to stand for 5 min.

3. Filter the mixture through a folded Whatman No. 12 (12.5 cm diameter) filter paper and collect at least 5 ml of the filtrate in a test tube.

4. Place the test tube in a boiling bath at 100°C for 5 min.

5. Cool the tube in cold water and examine it against a strong light for the presence of any turbidity.

6. Include with each batch of tests a control test of milk that has been heated at 100°C for at least 5 min. This should give no turbidity, nor should properly sterilized milk.

Colony count test

Colony counts assess the number of viable bacteria in the milk and give results easily understood by the dairyman, but the tests are costly in labour and materials, the results are not available for 72 h and errors are great due to the common clumping of bacteria.

1. Thoroughly mix the sample of milk by inverting the bottle about 25 times.

2. Aseptically prepare 1 in 10, 1 in 100 and 1 in 1000 dilutions of the milk in sterile bottles holding 90 ml volumes of quarter-strength Ringer's solution*. Use a sterile, straight-sided 10 ml pipette to transfer 10 ml of the milk into

the first bottle. Mix this dilution by inverting about 25 times, but without vigorous shaking. Then with a separate sterile pipette transfer 10 ml of it into a second bottle. Mix, and with a third pipette transfer 10 ml into a third bottle.

3. Pipette in triplicate 1 ml of the appropriate dilution (1 in 100 for Premium milk, 1 in 1000 for Standard milk) into three sterile Petri dishes and add to each plate 10 ml of yeast extract milk agar* which has been melted and cooled to 45–50°C.

4. Thoroughly mix the contents in each plate by gently moving the plate first in a clockwise and then in an anti-clockwise circular direction. Allow the agar to set. The interval between preparing the dilutions and mixing with the agar should not exceed 15 min.

5. Incubate the plates for 72 h at 30.0 ± 0.5°C.

6. Count the number of colonies, including pin-point ones, in each plate and calculate the mean per plate. Multiply this number by the dilution factor and report the result as 'the number of viable bacteria per ml of milk'.

Ultra heat treated milk. Before making colony counts on UHT milk, incubate the sample in the unopened sample bottle for 24 h at between 30 and 37°C (at 30.0 ± 0.5°C in Scotland). Under Scottish regulations, plate 1 ml of a 1 to 10 dilution mixed with 10 ml yeast extract agar as described above for the standard colony count test. In England, withdraw a standard 0.01 ml loopful of the undiluted milk from below the surface of the sample and mix it with 5 ml molten yeast extract agar at 45–50°C in a 25 ml screw-capped bottle; allow the mixture to solidify as a slope. Incubate the plate or slope for 48 h at 30°C and count the colonies.

Coliform test

This test is usually done in conjunction with a colony count test. It indicates the degree of contamination with coliform bacilli from dust and soiled utensils. The presence of coliforms in milk that passes the phosphatase test indicates that contamination has taken place after pasteurization.

1. Mix the milk and prepare three 10-fold dilutions in quarter-strength Ringer's solution as described for the colony count test.

2. Pipette 1 ml of the appropriate dilution into each of three tubes containing 10 ml single-strength MacConkey broth* and a completely filled Durham tube. Under the Scottish regulations, inoculate from the 1 in 100 dilution for Premium and Pasteurized milks and from the 1 in 1000 dilution for Standard milk.

3. Incubate the tubes for 48 h at 37°C and then look for acid and gas production as evidence of the presence of coliform bacilli.

The absence of acid and gas from at least two of the three tubes is accepted as indicating that the milk has passed the test.

Examination for tubercle bacilli

1. Thoroughly mix the milk sample and centrifuge 100 ml of it, e.g. in two 50 ml lots, under conditions sufficient to deposit any tubercle bacilli e.g. for 30 min at about 1500 *g*.

2. Discard the supernate, make a film from a drop of the sediment and then resuspend the remainder of the sediment(s) in 2.5 ml sterile saline solution.

3. Inject half of the suspension subcutaneously on the inner side of one thigh in each of two guinea-pigs.

4. Stain the film by the Ziehl-Neelsen method and examine it for the presence of acid-fast bacilli which, however, may be only saprophytic mycobacteria.

5. Keep the guinea-pigs under observation for signs of tuberculous lesions. Kill one at 4 weeks, perform a necropsy and examine suspect lesions for tubercle bacilli as described in Chapter 25.

6. If there are no tuberculous lesions, keep the other animal for a further 4 weeks, then kill and examine it.

Examination for brucella infection

Culture for brucella. 1. Charge a swab with cream from the milk sample and inoculate it (a) on to a plate of serum glucose agar made selective for brucella (e.g. Farrell & Robertson's 1972 medium) and (b) into a tube of the brucella enrichment medium of Brodie & Sinton (1975).

2. Incubate the media for up to 2 weeks at 37°C in air with 10% carbon dioxide.

3. At intervals, subculture on two plates each of serum glucose agar* and Farrell & Robertson's medium, incubating for 10 days at 37°C, one plate of each kind in air and the other in air plus 10% CO_2.

4. Identify colonies of brucella by a slide agglutination test with antiserum and other tests described in Chapter 33.

Animal inoculation. 1. Centrifuge 100 ml of milk and mix the sediment with 1 ml of the cream.

2. Inoculate 1 ml of the mixture intramuscularly into each of two guinea-pigs.

3. After 6 weeks kill both animals and with utmost care to avoid accidental dissemination of infected material, collect about 5 ml of blood from the heart and aseptically remove the spleen.

4. Separate serum from the blood and perform an agglutination test with a suspension of *Brucella abortus*.

5. Cut the spleen in two, rub the cut surface over plates of serum glucose agar, incubate the plates and identify brucella colonies as described above.

Milk ring test. This is a very sensitive test for the presence of brucella antibodies in the milk of infected cows, which it may detect even in the bulked supply from a dairy herd.

1. Store the milk overnight at 4°C before testing.

2. Thoroughly mix the milk, put 1 ml into a narrow test-tube, about 75 × 9 mm, and add one drop of stained brucella antigen which is a suspension of *B. abortus* bacilli stained with a blue (haematoxylin) dye. Antigen is obtainable from the Ministry of Agriculture, Fisheries and Food, Central Veterinary Laboratory, New Haw, Weybridge, Surrey, UK.

3. Mix well by shaking, but avoid frothing the milk. Incubate the mixture for 1 h at 37°C in a waterbath.

4. Examine the tube. The presence of a blue cream line above white milk indicates that the milk contains brucella antibodies which have agglutinated the stained bacilli and caused the aggregates to rise with the cream. The presence of a white cream line over blue milk indicates the absence of brucella antibodies. The presence of blue cream over blue milk indicates a low content of brucella antibodies.

The test is unsatisfactory with pasteurized milk and goat's milk. Low fat milk may require the addition of known negative cream. False-positive results may be given by milk collected at the beginning and end of lactation and by milk from cows that have been immunized with the avirulent S19 strain of *B. abortus*.

Whey agglutination test. This is another test for brucella antibodies in milk, which is used only with the milk of an individual cow. Being little influenced by previous vaccination, it is used to confirm a positive milk ring test.

1. Centrifuge the milk and remove the cream.

2. To 10 ml of the skimmed milk add a few drops of rennin (e.g. cheese-making rennet), mix and incubate for 6 h at 37°C.

3. When the milk has coagulated, centrifuge it and collect the clear, colourless whey.

4. Prepare 1 ml volumes of doubling dilutions of the whey from 1 in 10 to 1 in 2560 in narrow (75 × 9 mm) test tubes. Add one drop of a standard suspension of killed *B. abortus* bacilli to each tube.

5. Mix, incubate the tubes for 24 h at 37°C in a waterbath, and read the highest dilution of whey giving agglutination of the bacilli.

Agglutination at a dilution of 40 or higher is evidence of udder infection unless the animal has recently been vaccinated.

Examination of goat's milk

Goat's milk is often consumed by persons allergic to cow's milk and is generally supplied without pasteurization. There is yet no UK legislation about standards or tests for quality. If examination is required, perform colony count tests at 22°C and 37°C, a coliform test, a methylene blue reduction test and a brucella ring test. Satisfactory samples should have a colony count less than 100 000/ml and a coliform count less than 100/ml, pass the methylene blue test, which however is less reliable than with cow's milk, and give a negative brucella ring test, which may be difficult to read on account of the very high fat content. In cases of suspected food-poisoning, examine the sediment from centrifuged milk for *Staphylococcus aureus*, *Salmonella*, *Campylobacter* and *Yersinia enterocolitica*.

Examination of washed milk bottles

These bottles should be examined as recommended by the Ministry of Agriculture and Fisheries (1947) and Davis (1966).

1. Carefully remove the cap from the bottle, aseptically pipette 20 ml quarter-strength Ringer's solution* into the bottle, and replace the cap or insert a sterile rubber bung.
2. Place the bottle on its side and rotate it every 5 min for 30 min so that its inner walls are thoroughly flushed.
3. Inoculate a 5 ml sample of the solution into each of: (a) two plates with 15 ml molten yeast extract agar* at 45–50°C, and (b) two tubes containing 5 ml double-strength MacConkey broth*.
4. Incubate one plate and one tube for 48 h at 37°C and the other plate and tube for 3 days at 22°C.
5. Count the colonies in each plate and multiply the count per plate by four to obtain the count per milk bottle. Examine the tubes for the presence of acid and gas indicating the presence of coliform bacilli.

Satisfactorily washed milk bottles should have a colony count at 37°C less than 200/bottle and should not show the presence of any coliform bacilli. A count of 200–600/bottle is fairly satisfactory and one of more than 600/bottle is unsatisfactory.

EXAMINATION OF CREAM AND ICE CREAM

Sterilized, UHT and pasteurized creams

Examine sterilized and UHT creams by performing colony counts as for UHT milk and coliform tests as for milk (described above). Creams should have a colony count of not more

than 30 000/ml and not show the presence of coliform bacilli in 0.1 ml.

Examine pasteurized cream by performing a coliform test, as for pasteurized milk, and a phosphatase test, as described below.

Phosphatase test for pasteurized cream.
1. Prepare phosphatase reagent as described for the test on pasteurized milk, pipette 15 ml of it into each of two chemically clean tubes and warm these to 37°C.
2. Add 2 g cream to one tube, as the test, and 2 g boiled cream to the other, as a control.
3. Mix well by shaking and incubate the tubes for 2 h at 37°C in a waterbath.
4. Add 0.5 ml of a 30% aqueous solution of zinc sulphate to both tubes, shake them vigorously and then allow them to stand for 3 min.
5. Add 0.5 ml of a 15% aqueous solution of potassium ferrocyanide to each tube and mix well.
6. Filter the contents of each tube through separate Whatman No. 40 filter papers and collect the filtrates in chemically clean tubes.
7. Read the *p*-nitrophenol value of the test sample against the control sample in a Lovibond comparator as described for the phosphatase test on milk. A value greater than 10 μg/ml suggests the sample does not satisfy the regulations. It should be further examined as directed below.

Further phosphatase test. 1. Transfer 10 g cream to each of two chemically clean tubes. To one tube, the test, add an amount of 40% magnesium chloride in distilled water according to the sample's butter fat content: 0.25 ml for 48% fat, 0.35 ml for 35% fat, 0.50 ml for 18% fat, and other volumes by extrapolation. To the other tube, the control, add nothing.
2. Stopper the tubes, mix the contents by inversion, and incubate the tubes for 1 h at 37°C, inverting them from time to time.
3. Transfer 2 g cream from each tube to fresh tubes and repeat the phosphatase test on both, as described above (steps 1–7).

If the intensity of colour in the filtrate of the cream treated with magnesium chloride is greater than that in the control, dilute it 1 in 4 with buffer solution and then compare it again with the control. If the colour in the diluted filtrate is equal to or more intense than that in the control, the original *p*-nitrophenol result is invalid as reactivation has taken place, and the sample is deemed to have passed the test. Otherwise, the original result stands and the sample has failed the test.

Examination of ice cream

Only pasteurized milk should be used in the manufacture of ice cream. Samples should be received in the frozen state and molten ones should be rejected. Allow the frozen sample to melt at 0–2°C immediately before examination.

Methylene blue reduction test. 1. Use this test only for white ice cream.

2. Add 7 ml quarter-strength Ringer's solution and 1 ml standard methylene blue solution 1 in 300 000, prepared as described for the test on milk, to a sterile test tube (152 × 16 mm). Then add 2 ml of the melted ice cream sample.

3. Stopper the tube with a sterile (boiled) rubber bung and mix the contents by inverting it several times.

4. Include with each test a control tube containing boiled instead of unboiled ice cream and a control tube containing Ringer's solution instead of methylene blue.

5. Refrigerate the tubes at 0–4°C until 5 pm, then transfer them to a well insulated waterbath at 20°C in which the water level is above the level of the ice cream.

6. After incubation for 17 h at 20°C, compare the colour in the test and control tubes. Report the tests in which decolourization is complete (or to within 0.5 in of the meniscus) as having decolourized methylene blue in 0 h (i.e. 0 h at 37°C).

7. Mix the contents of the remaining tubes by inversion and place them in a waterbath at 37°C. Remove, examine, invert and replace them at 30 min intervals for up to 4 h, noting the time taken for decolourization of the dye in each.

8. Grade the ice cream according to the decolourization time as follows: Grade 1, no decolourization at 4 h; Grade 2, decolourization in 2.5–4 h; Grade 3, decolourization in 0.5–2 h;

Grade 4, decolourization in 0 h (i.e. after 17 h at 20°C). If ice cream consistently fails to reach Grade 1 or 2, defects in manufacture or handling should be suspected and investigated.

Colony count and coliform tests. These tests are helpful in assessment of coloured ice creams unsuitable for the methylene blue test. Their performance is required in Scotland. They are done in the way described for milk. A colony count of 50 000/g or higher, or the presence of coliform bacilli in 0.01 g is indicative of faults in manufacture or handling.

EXAMINATION OF FOOD

It is frequently necessary to determine the numbers and types of bacteria in food in order to assess and control standards of hygiene and investigate outbreaks of food-poisoning. But as yet there are no generally agreed methods of examination nor any generally agreed standards indicative of safety. The examinations most often done are viable bacterial counts and estimations of the numbers of coliform bacilli, e.g.:

1. Either (a) weigh 10 g food in a sterile container or on sterile grease-proof paper and homogenize it with 90 ml sterile diluent, e.g. Ringer's solution (Ch. 5, Table 5.3), in a blender, or (b) for foods contaminated only on the surface, such as intact vegetables, weigh 100 g food into a sterile jar, add 100 ml sterile diluent, shake well for 20 min, and then assume the diluent contains all the bacteria that were present on the surface of the food.

2. Make serial 10-fold dilutions of the homogenate or diluent and plate them on appropriate media, incubating under appropriate time-temperature combinations. Make coliform counts in MacConkey broth and *Escherichia coli* confirmatory tests by the methods described for water examinations (above).

Frozen foods

Bacterial counts should be done by plating on rich media to enable cold-stressed organisms to multiply. Psychrophiles associated with spoilage require incubation for 5–7 days at 5–7°C. Other bacteria are counted after 2–3 days at 20–30°C.

Ready cooked prawns and shrimps (Mitchell 1970). 1. Chisel 20 g of the food from the frozen block.

2. Place the food in a sterile container in a waterbath for 10–30 min at 44°C to unfreeze.

3. Make colony counts of dilutions of the released juices on blood agar and MacConkey agar plates incubated overnight at 37°C.

Counts of 100 000 colony forming units (cfu)/g are said to be satisfactory, but it is thought unwise to release for consumption samples with counts greater than 1 000 000 cfu/g. Samples with intermediate counts may be released on the condition that they will be used immediately after thawing.

4. Homogenize the food remaining from step (2) and examine it for the presence of food-poisoning bacteria as described later in this chapter.

Frozen vegetables. Coliform bacilli and enterococci are commonly found on vegetables. Make total counts; these are usually low, about 100 000 cfu/g. Examine for and report the presence of any *E. coli*.

Frozen meat pies and complete meals. Frozen pies usually have a low total count, e.g. 5000–30 000 cfu/g, but may contain staphylococci and enterobacteria. Complete meals vary greatly in the kinds and numbers of bacteria present.

Determine the total viable count, the number of coliform bacilli and the number of *Staphylococcus aureus*. For the last, culture on mannitol salt phenol red agar (e.g. Oxoid CM85) for 3 days at 32°C and count the yellow (acid) colonies. It is suggested that the total count after 48 h at 37°C should not exceed 100 000 cfu/g, coliform bacilli should not be present in 0.1 g, and *S.aureus* should not be present in 0.01 g of the food.

Iced lollipops.

1. If the lollipop contains a portion of ice cream, remove that portion and examine it as for ice cream.

2. Allow the iced water part to melt. Remove a small aliquot and determine its pH. If the pH is 4.5 or more acid, a bacteriological examination is not required.

3. If the pH is more alkaline than 4.5, perform plate and coliform counts.

For further information on the microbiology of frozen foods, see Roberts et al (1981).

Canned foods

Food is often preserved in sealed cans which are heated to kill the contained microorganisms, rapidly cooled and finally dried. Spoilage of canned foods is the result of growth of organisms that either have survived the heating process or have been introduced after the heating through a defect in the can.

The amount of heat applied is determined by the kind of food being processed. It should be sufficient to kill vegetative pathogens and the spores of food-poisoning organisms, yet not be so great as to impair the appearance and palatability of the food. Germination of surviving spores and multiplication of microbes entering through a leak are inhibited if the food is acid, e.g. pH 4.5 or lower, contains added salt and nitrate, or is stored at a low temperature.

Accidental under-processing of food may occur through faulty design or careless operation of equipment. Correctly processed food may become contaminated by the entry of bacteria through minute holes or cracks in the can due to faulty construction, rusting or autoclave-induced distortion. Such ingress is especially likely to take place during the cooling process, when a negative pressure develops in the can. The cooling water should therefore be chlorinated and the cans not be handled while still wet.

Examination procedure. 1. In cases of suspected under-processing or spoilage through leakage, examine as many cans as possible from each batch, noting the batch number and code number of each can.

2. With a lens, examine the can for defects, including minute holes, particularly in the seams and any dented or rusted areas.

3. *If the can appears intact and sound*, stimulate multiplication of any organisms present in small numbers by incubating cans for 7 days at 37°C for mesophiles and for 7 days at 55–60°C for thermophiles. Incubate acid foods for 10 days at 25°C.

4. Before opening, scrub the can with soap and water and rinse it with alcohol. Disinfect the area to be opened by flaming, without overheating the contents, or by rubbing with 70% ethanol in water.

5. Puncture the can with a heat-sterilized nail or can opener, then open it sufficiently for a sample to be removed.

6. Note the appearance and smell of the food. Then proceed as in steps 8–10.

7. *If the can has leaks or is swollen*, the contents may be offensive and may be under pressure due to gas formation by spoilage bacteria. Pre-incubation is unnecessary. The area of the surface to be opened should be disinfected with ethanol, not by flaming. Place the can with a sterile nail or can opener in a plastic bag and seal the bag before opening the can, so that anything expelled will be collected within the bag.

8. If the food is liquid, aseptically sample 15–20 ml with a sterile pipette. If solid, sample from both its centre, where organisms are more likely to have survived, and its surface, where leakage contaminants may be present. Take the sample with a sterile cork borer. Expel the core sample with a sterile glass rod into a sterile container and macerate it in a little sterile broth.

9. Make a Gram film of the suspension and inoculate drops of the suspension into appropriate culture media.

Interpret the film with caution, as it may show bacteria that have been killed by the heat processing of the can. The presence of rods resembling *Bacillus* or *Clostridium* bacteria may indicate under-processing, whereas the presence of cocci and Gram-negative rods may indicate contamination through leakage.

Culture on dextrose tryptone bromocresol purple agar (e.g. Oxoid CM75) should be used for the detection of mesophilic and thermophilic species of *Bacillus*, and Robertson's cooked meat medium (Ch. 6) and Crossley's milk medium

(e.g. Oxoid CM213) for the detection and preliminary identification of clostridia. Iron sulphite agar (e.g. Oxoid CM79) should also be seeded if the food smells of bad eggs, and blood agar and MacConkey agar if spoilage through leakage is suspected.

Inoculate the food sample into several plates or tubes of each medium; incubate some aerobically and some anaerobically in the temperature ranges 5–10°C, 22–25°C, 35–37°C and 55–60°C for several days.

10. Identify any organism grown by appropriate tests. *Bacillus stearothermophilus* is a thermophile associated with 'flat sour' spoilage through the formation of acid but not gas; it grows poorly or not at all at 37°C and lower, but forms large acid-producing colonies on dextrose tryptone agar at 60°C. *Clostridium thermosaccharolyticum* and *C. nigrificans* are anaerobic thermophiles which may not grow at 25°C and below. The former produces gas and causes a 'hard swell' of cans, the bulging ends of which cannot be compressed by hand; its colonies have feathery edges. The latter clostridium produces hydrogen sulphide which often blackens the food but, being water soluble, does not bulge the can; it forms black colonies on iron sulphite agar. Food-poisoning bacteria are isolated and identified as described later in this chapter.

Raw, pre-cooked and preserved foods

Poultry. Battery-reared birds are particularly liable to cross-infection with salmonellae and other pathogens, and if under-cooked or cooked after incomplete thawing from the frozen state, may give rise to food-poisoning.

1. Rub a cotton-wool swab over an area of 16 cm^2 of the skin of the bird's breast.

2. Rinse the swab in sterile diluent, e.g. Ringer's solution, and use the suspension to perform colony counts at 22°C on nutrient agar, coliform counts at 30°C on MacConkey agar, and staphylococcal and enterococcal counts at 37°C on blood agar.

3. Examine for salmonella by placing the carcase in a plastic bag along with about 100 ml sterile water. After the carcase has thawed and been thoroughly washed with the water, collect

the liquid from the bag and add it to an equal volume of a double-strength enrichment medium for salmonella. Incubate at 37°C and proceed as for the isolation of salmonella.

Murray (1969) found that in well run establishments for the preparation of poultry carcases, total counts were less than 250 000/16 cm^2 of swabbed skin, coliform counts were less than 1000/16 cm^2, enterococci less than 5000/16 cm^2, and *S. aureus* less than 100/16 cm^2. Low total counts indicate that few spoilage bacteria are present and low counts of coliforms and enterococci suggest that the evisceration technique and handling hygiene are good.

Meat pies and sausage rolls. 1. Open the pie with a sterile knife. Disregard the pastry unless it is obviously spoiled. Examine the internal contents, keeping meat and jelly separate.

2. Homogenize a weighed amount of the meat (or jelly) in sterile diluent and make 1 in 10 and 1 in 100 dilutions of it.

3. Perform total and coliform counts on the two dilutions, incubating the media for 48 h at 30°C.

4. Examine for *Clostridium perfringens* by adding 1 ml volumes of the 1 in 10 dilution to each of five tubes of a diffferential reinforced clostridial medium (DRCM*) (e.g. Reinforced Clostridial Medium, Oxoid CM149) which has been melted and cooled to 50°C. Incubate anaerobically for 48 h at 37°C. Then subculture all tubes showing growth or gas production on to blood agar plates and into litmus milk for identification. Estimate from the probability tables* the most probable number of *C. perfringens*.

Vacuum packed bacon and cooked meats. A low temperature of storage, the absence of oxygen and the presence of salt and nitrate reduce the likelihood of spoilage in such packed foods, but the spores of anaerobes may survive and *Clostridium botulinum* type E may grow in the food at quite a low temperature.

1. Swab the outside of the package with ethanol and open it with sterile scissors.

2. Macerate a weighed amount of food in a small amount of sterile broth and prepare 1 in 10, 1 in 100 and 1 in 1000 dilutions.

3. Perform plate counts of the dilutions on blood agar and MacConkey agar, incubating the plates aerobically for 18 h at 37°C. A total count of 1000/g or less is thought to be satisfactory.

Water cress. This may have been grown in sewage-polluted water. It should be examined for the presence of *E. coli*.

Shellfish. 1. Select 10 shellfish of average size and scrub their shells clean in running tap water with a boiled nail brush.

2. Wash them in sterile water while holding them one by one in sterile forceps.

3. Place them on sterile paper and open each in turn with a sterile knife.

4. Collect the liquor and flesh together in a sterile graduated container and macerate the flesh with sterile scissors.

5. Make the mixture up to a volume of 25 ml with sterile water, add a further 25 ml sterile water, then make 10-fold dilutions.

6. Inoculate 1 ml volumes of each dilution into each of several tubes of MacConkey broth with Durham tubes*, incubate the tubes for 24 h at 37°C and do confirmatory tests for coliform bacilli on the tubes showing acid and gas production.

The shellfish are considered satisfactory if coliform bacilli are absent from at least eight of the ten tested.

Eggs. The shells of hen's eggs may be contaminated with various enterobacteria, pseudomonads, sporing bacteria, yeasts and moulds. The albumen and yolk of newly laid eggs usually contain very few bacteria, but the degree of contamination depends upon the porosity of the shell, the age of the egg, the rate of cooling and the humidity of the environment. Eggs may be contaminated with salmonellae.

Total bacterial counts may be made both on the macerated shell and on the homogenized albumen and yolk of either individual eggs or groups of 10 eggs. The lysozyme content of the homogenate must be diluted sufficiently to allow lysozyme-sensitive contaminants to grow, e.g. by adding one volume of the homogenate to about five volumes of culture medium.

Gelatin. Gelatin is used in the manufacture of ice cream and in the 'topping up' of canned hams and meat pies. It should be examined for coliform bacilli and *Bacillus* spores.

1. Add 5 g gelatin to a bottle containing 100 ml sterile water, mix and allow to stand for 2 h at 0–4°C.

2. Warm the mixture for 15 min in a waterbath at 50°C, mix well and transfer 20 ml of the gelatin solution to a bottle containing 80 ml sterile water.

3. On this 1% gelatin solution (a) perform a total count by inoculating 1 ml and 0.1 ml volumes on to plates holding 15 ml volumes of molten yeast extract agar* at 50°C and, when set, incubating the plates for 48 h at 37°C, and (b) estimate the coliform count by adding 10 ml volumes to 10 ml volumes of double-strength MacConkey broth* and 1 ml and 0.1 ml volumes to 5 ml volumes of single-strength MacConkey broth and incubating for 48 h at 37°C. Refer to tables* for the most probable number (MPN) of coliform bacilli. Do confirmatory tests for *E. coli* on the tubes bearing coliform bacilli.

4. Make a spore count on the remaining 1% gelatin solution by first heating it for 10 min at 80°C to destroy vegetative cells and then adding four 1 ml volumes to four volumes of 14 ml nutrient agar which has been melted and cooled to 50°C, mixing well and pouring in plates. Incubate two plates for 48 h at 37°C and the other two for 48 h at 55°C, and count the colonies.

Gelatin used with canned ham should have a spore count of no more than one colony per plate, i.e. 100 spores/g gelatin, and a total bacterial count not exceeding 10 000/g. Gelatin used in making ice cream should have a total count not exceeding 10 000/g, no coliforms in 0.01 g, and no *E. coli* in 0.1 g.

Cheese. 1. Aseptically take a core sample and grate it with a sterile grater.

2. Homogenize 10 g grated cheese with 90 ml warm sterile diluent.

3. Determine the total count and examine for the presence of *S. aureus*, *E. coli* and salmonellae. Interpret the finding of *S. aureus* with caution as not all types of the species form enterotoxin and, when originally formed in the cheese, enterotoxin may be present long after the staphylococci have died.

Baby foods. Determine the total count of viable bacteria and use both direct plating and enrichment methods to examine for *S. aureus*, coliform bacilli, *E. coli*, *C. perfringens* and salmonellae.

Examination for food-poisoning bacteria

A summary of methods is given below. For further information, see Corry et al (1982).

Salmonellae

Foods especially liable to be infected with salmonellae are poultry, meat, eggs, creams and processed foods made from these ingredients. Methods of isolation of salmonellae are described by Harvey & Price (1975, 1979).

(a) *With food that is uncooked or thought highly contaminated*. 1. Homogenize 50 g of the food in 100 ml 0.1% peptone water.

2. Add 50 ml volumes of the homogenate to two 50 ml volumes of selenite F broth (Ch. 29, *Methods*, with ingredients at double strength). Incubate the cultures for 24 h, the one at 37°C and the other at 43°C.

3. Plate out the cultures on deoxycholate citrate agar (Ch. 29, *Methods*, or Oxoid CM35) and brilliant green MacConkey agar (Ch. 29, *Methods*, or Oxoid CM263) and incubate the plates at 37°C.

4. Examine for salmonella colonies after 24 h and 48 h.

(b) *With food likely to contain few if any salmonellae*. 1. Homogenize 50 g food in 100 ml nutrient broth and incubate the homogenate for 4 h at 37°C.

2. Add 50 ml volumes of the homogenate to selenite F broths and proceed as in steps 2, 3 and 4 above.

Identify suspect colonies as described in Chapter 29.

Staphylococcus aureus

Foods commonly contaminated with *S. aureus* include synthetic creams, custards, trifles and high-salt foods such as hams.

1. Homogenize 10 g food in 100 ml 0.1% peptone water.

2. Plate the homogenate on blood agar or a selective and indicator medium such as mannitol salt agar (Ch. 16, Oxoid CM85), phenol-phthalein phosphate agar (Ch. 16, *Methods*) made selective by the addition of 1250 units polymyxin B per litre, or the mannitol lactose salt gelatin agar, Staphylococcus Medium No. 110 (Oxoid CM145). If counts are required, use the Miles & Misra method (Ch. 12). Incubate the plates for 24–28 h at 37°C.

3. For enrichment of small numbers, add 0.1 ml and 1 ml volumes of the homogenate to 10 ml mannitol salt broth and 10 ml homogenate to 50 ml mannitol salt broth. Incubate overnight at 37°C and plate out on one of the media used in step 2, above, incubating for 24–28 h at 37°C. Growth of *S. aureus* only from the 10 ml inoculum indicates that only very small numbers of the organism were present in the foodstuff.

4. Identify *S. aureus* by the tests described in Chapter 16. Send isolates to a reference laboratory for phage typing, as not all types can cause food-poisoning. For the detection of staphylococcal enterotoxin in food, use the method of Gilbert et al (1972).

Clostridium perfringens

Foods commonly contaminated with *C. perfringens* include meat, meat pies, poultry, stews and gravy.

1. Prepare 10-fold dilutions of a 10% homogenate of the food sample in 0.1% peptone water.

2. Count the viable *C. perfringens* bacilli and spores by the Miles & Misra method (Ch. 12), inoculating drops of the different dilutions on to duplicate plates of blood agar containing 100 mg/litre of neomycin. Incubate the plates for 16–24 h at 37°C, one set aerobically and another anaerobically.

3. Also inoculate 2–3 ml of the food homogenate into each of several tubes of Robertson's cooked-meat broth containing 100 mg/litre of neomycin. Heat some of the tubes for 1 h at 100°C. Incubate both the heated and unheated tubes overnight at 37°C. Then plate from each tube on to two plates of neomycin blood agar; incubate one plate aerobically and the other anaerobically overnight at 37°C.

Heat-sensitive strains of *C. perfringens* produce wide zones of β-haemolysis and do not grow from the heated tubes. Heat-resistant strains also grow from the heated tubes and are usually only slightly haemolytic.

4. Identify isolates by Gram film, colony appearance and the Nagler test (Ch. 37). Then send subcultures to a reference laboratory for typing.

The bacteriological diagnosis of *C. perfringens* food-poisoning depends on the isolation of similar strains from the faeces of patients and from the suspected food. Although heat-resistant strains cause most outbreaks, food-poisoning may also be caused by heat-sensitive strains. The finding of the same strain in large numbers, e.g. 10^5/g or over, in the faeces and food is suggestive of the condition.

Bacillus cereus

Food-poisoning with this organism most often is caused by contaminated rice and rice dishes.

1. Soak 20 g dried rice in 90 ml tryptone water (e.g. Oxoid CM87) for 50 min at room temperature. Then add 90 ml of 0.1% peptone water as diluent. For other foods, prepare a 10% suspension in 0.1% peptone water. Homogenize the suspension.

2. Plate 0.1 ml of dilutions of the homogenate on dextrose tryptone agar (e.g. Oxoid CM75) or the selective medium of Holbrook & Anderson (1980). Incubate the plates for 24 h at 37°C, then leave for a further 24 h at room temperature (*c*. 22°C).

B. cereus forms large, acid-producing 'ground glass' colonies on dextrose tryptone agar and turquoise blue colonies surrounded by a precipitate on Holbrook & Anderson's medium.

3. Confirm the identity of isolates by the tests described in Chapter 24, which gives an alternative method for the isolation and enumeration of *B. cereus* on Baker's phenol-red egg-yolk polymyxin agar. Stain a culture by appropriate methods (Ch. 3), or the combined method of Holbrook & Anderson (1980), to demonstrate the presence of lipid granules and central-to-subterminal oval spores that do not distend the cell.

The causal role of the bacillus is indicated only if large numbers are found in the food, e.g. 10^8/g. Small numbers are often present as harmless contaminants.

Clostridium botulinum

Suspect foods include those that are home canned or bottled, meat, vegetables and fish. Whenever botulism is suspected, reference experts should be consulted immediately (see Ch. 38).

1. Homogenize the food in 0.1% peptone water and inoculate portions of the homogenate into several tubes of freshly steamed and cooled Robertson's cooked-meat broth.

2. Heat half of the tubes at 75–80°C for 30 min and allow them to cool.

3. Incubate all the tubes for 3–5 days at 35°C.

4. Plate out the cultures on to pre-reduced blood agar and egg yolk agar plates and incubate the plates for 3–5 days at 35°C under strictly anaerobic conditions.

5. Identify colonies of *C. botulinum* by fluorescent antibody staining and biochemical tests (Ch. 38). Send subcultures of suspect or confirmed colonies to a reference laboratory.

6. Inoculate a suspension of the food or a suspect pure culture intraperitoneally into guinea-pigs or mice, some of which are protected with *C. botulinum* antitoxin and others with polyvalent gas-gangrene antiserum.

Campylobacter

Suspect foods include raw or inadequately pasteurized milk and processed meats and chickens.

1. Prepare a 10% suspension of the food in 0.1% peptone water and inoculate the suspension on pairs of plates of a selective medium for campylobacter (Ch. 32).

2. Incubate the plates for 48 h, some at 37°C and others at 42°C, all in an atmosphere of approximately 5% O_2, 10% CO_2 and 85% N_2 or H_2.

3. Examine the plates for flat watery colonies and demonstrate their content of oxidase-positive, Gram-negative spirally curved bacilli.

Vibrio parahaemolyticus

Suspect foods include raw fish and shellfish from warm seas, and foods derived from them.

1. Homogenize the food in 0.1% peptone water and plate the homogenate on thiosulphate citrate bile-salt sucrose agar (TCBS)(Ch. 32, *Methods*). Incubate overnight at 37°C.

2. Also add a portion of the homogenate to an equal volume of double-strength alkaline (pH 8.8) peptone water (Ch. 32) and incubate overnight at 25°C. Then subculture on to a TCBS agar plate and incubate the plate overnight at 37°C.

3. Examine the plates for large (2–5 mm) green (i.e. not fermenting sucrose) colonies that are oxidase positive. Identify the colonies by biochemical tests (Ch. 32).

Yersinia enterocolitica

Suspect foods include raw or inadequately pasteurized milk and milk products, and oysters and mussels.

1. Prepare a 10% suspension of the food in phosphate-buffered saline (pH 7.3), inoculate a portion of the suspension into selenite F broth (Ch. 29, *Methods*) and hold the culture for up to 6 weeks at 4°C.

2. Subculture the broth at weekly intervals on to plates of DCA (Ch. 29, *Methods*) or Yersinia selective agar (Oxoid CM653) and incubate for 24 h at 32°C.

3. Examine DCA plates for non-lactose-fermenting colonies and Yersinia selective agar plates for dark red colonies. Test these colonies for urease activity, sucrose fermentation and

motility at 22°C and perform additional biochemical tests to confirm the identity of isolates giving positive reactions in all three tests (Ch. 34).

EXAMINATION OF AIR

Observations of the number of bacteria-carrying particles in air may be required in premises where safe working depends on the air's content of bacteria being kept at a very low level, e.g. surgical theatres and premises where certain foods or pharmaceutical materials are prepared. In hospital wards in which there is an outbreak of cross-infection, it may be required to examine the air for its content of a particular pathogen. The number of bacteria in the air at any time is dependent on a variety of factors, the most important of which are the number of persons present, the amount of their body movements and the amount of disturbance of their clothing. When a room is vacated and left undisturbed, the bacterial content of the air falls to a low level in the course of about 30 min.

Various methods have been devised for measuring the bacterial content of air. A primary distinction must be drawn between those that measure the rate at which bacteria-carrying particles, chiefly the larger particles, are settling by gravity from the air on to exposed surfaces, e.g. the settle plate method, and those that count the number of bacteria-carrying particles contained in a given volume of the air, e.g. the slit sampler method. Each bacteria-carrying dust particle or droplet-nucleus may contain from one to a hundred or more bacteria, though generally only a few. Methods designed to count the total number of bacteria in the air, rather than the number of bacteria-carrying particles, are inconvenient and unnecessary for general use. For further information and references, see Medical Research Council Report (1948), Wolf et al (1959), May (1967) and Noble (1967).

Settle plates

Petri dishes containing an agar medium of known surface area, e.g. 65 cm^2, are left open for a measured period of time. Large bacteria-carrying dust particles settle on to the medium. The plates are incubated and a count of the colonies formed shows the number of settled particles that contained bacteria capable of growth on the medium used and under the conditions of its incubation. Blood agar is suitable for an overall count of the pathogenic, commensal and saprophytic bacteria in the air, an appropriate selective medium may be used to detect a particular pathogen that may be present in only small numbers, and malt extract agar (e.g. Oxoid CM59) may be used for moulds. Incubation is generally aerobic and for 24 h at 37°C, though for saprophytic bacteria it should be for 3 days at 22°C and for moulds, 1–2 weeks at various temperatures from 10–50°C.

The optimal duration of exposure is that which will give a significant and readily countable number of well separated colonies, e.g. 30–100, and will depend on the dustiness of the air. In occupied rooms and hospital wards it is generally between 10 and 60 min (Russell et al 1984).

1. Pour plates and dry off any surface moisture. Mark them with distinctive numbers and prepare a record of the position, time and duration for the exposure of each.

2. Uncover the plate in its chosen position for the measured period of time, then at once replace its lid. It is generally suitable to expose plates on tables and ledges about 1 metre above the ground.

3. Incubate the plates aerobically for 24 h at 37°C or otherwise as described above.

4. Count the colonies, preferably with the use of a plate microscope to detect the smallest ones. Express the result as the number of bacteria-carrying particles settling on a given area in a given period of time.

The method has the advantage of simplicity, but measures only the rate of deposition of large particles from the air, not the total number of large and small bacteria-carrying particles suspended in it. Many plates may have to be used to obtain an overall assessment of conditions in a room, for the count on any one plate is subject to wide variation from the effects of air currents and any temporary dust-raising disturbance in its vicinity.

Slit sampler

The most efficient and convenient of the devices for counting the bacteria-carrying particles suspended in a unit volume of air is the slit sampler introduced by Bourdillon et al (1941). It draws in air from the environment at a fixed rate and causes the suspended particles to impinge on the surface of an agar plate where, on incubation, each forms a colony. The efficiency of collection, even for the smallest bacterial particles, is very high. Thus, about 95% of small bacteria sprayed finely into the air from a suspension of distilled water so that they form droplet-nuclei about 1 μm in diameter are collected. Even respiratory secretion droplet-nuclei down to 0.25 μm in diameter are collected in large numbers (Duguid 1946).

The original and most generally useful form of the device samples the air at the rate of 1 cubic foot (28.3 litres; 0.0283 m³) per minute. Depending on the dustiness of the air, samples of from 1–10 ft³ from occupied rooms generally yield a conveniently countable number of colonies per plate. Later modifications of the sampler (Medical Research Council Report 1948) enable large samples of clean air to be collected at the rate of 20 ft³/min, and minute-to-minute variations in the bacterial content of the air to be recorded. A derivative of the slit sampler separates and enables the counting of particles in four grades of size: >18 μm, 10–18 μm, 4–10 μm and <4 μm (Lidwell 1959). For the measurement of low levels of contamination in ultra-clean air, a sampler that collects 700 litres air/min is recommended by Whyte et al (1983). Instruments may be purchased from C. F. Casella & Co, Ltd, Regent House, Britannia Walk, London N1 7ND.

A Petri dish 9 cm in diameter containing, for example, blood agar is held on a slowly rotating platform in a box closed by an air-tight door. The box is connected to a suction pump which maintains it at a negative pressure of 12 in (305 mm) of water (i.e. 22.6 mm mercury). Air is sucked into the box through a slit 0.33 mm wide and 27.5 mm long with vertical parallel sides about 3 mm deep. At the correct negative pressure, air will enter through a slit of these dimensions at the rate of 1 ft³/min. The slit is positioned above a radius of the plate at a distance of exactly 2 mm from the surface of the agar. As the air-flow is bent laterally at the surface of the medium, the suspended particles are centrifuged forward on to the surface, where they adhere. If the plate remained stationary, the incoming particles would all be deposited in a narrow line beneath the slit, but the rotation of the plate causes them to be spread over a large area.

Method. 1. Pour plates with an even, bubble-free surface exactly level with the underside of the dish. Dry off any free surface moisture. Mark the plates with distinctive numbers and prepare a record of the position, time and size of the sample to be collected on each.

2. Inspect the slit to ensure it is unblocked and free from dust. If necessary, clean it with alcohol and by the insertion of the edge of a piece of stiff paper.

3. Open the door of the box and place the plate centrally and symmetrically on the circular platform. It may be necessary to have the platform covered with some adhesive or gripping material to ensure that the plate rotates with it and does not slip out of position due to vibration transmitted from the suction pump.

4. Raise the platform until the sensing device shows that the surface of the agar is just 2 mm below the slit and fix the platform to its axle at that level.

5. At the correct time, start the motor that rotates the plate and the suction pump that evacuates the sampler. Watching the manometer that records the negative pressure in the sampler, adjust the controllable leak in the suction line so that the pressure is maintained at −12 in water or −22.6 mm mercury.

6. After sampling for the time necessary to collect the required volume of air, switch off the suction pump and the rotor, open the door of the sampler, lower the platform and carefully remove the plate. At once cover the plate with its lid and incubate it for 24 or 48 h at 37°C, or otherwise as required.

7. Count the colonies, preferably with a magnifier or plate microscope to assist the detec-

tion of small ones. It may be found helpful to mark the plate into several parallel strips with the point of a sterile scalpel blade, so that the colonies may be counted in each strip in turn. Express the result as the number of bacteria-carrying particles per given volume of air.

In siting and operating the sampler it should be borne in mind that the major source of bacterial contamination in the air of occupied rooms is the liberation of dust from the skin and clothing by the body movements of the occupants (Duguid & Wallace 1948). The operator should therefore avoid making unnecessary movements in the vicinity of the sampler and stand away from it while the sample is being taken.

Disadvantages of the slit sampler are that it is noisy and relatively cumbersome. Noise can be reduced if the vacuum pump is enclosed with acoustic insulation. The sampler is best separate from the pump and not mounted on its casing lest vibration from the pump interferes with the positioning of the culture plate. Quieter and more portable samplers have been described, but they are less efficient in collecting airborne particles, particularly the smaller ones.

Air centrifuge

The principle of centrifuging particles from the air on to culture medium was exploited by Wells (1933) in his air centrifuge in which the sampled air was passed along a tube lined with nutrient agar which was rotated rapidly on its long axis. A portable, battery-powered instrument of this type is the Reuter centrifugal air sampler supplied by Biotest Folex Ltd, 1649 Pershore Road, Birmingham B30 3DR. It resembles a large cylindrical torch bearing at one end an open-ended drum housing impeller blades. Air is drawn into the drum and subjected to centrifugal acceleration which causes suspended particles to impact on culture medium borne on a plastic strip. After sampling, the strip is removed from the instrument and incubated for 48 h at 37°C, when colonies can be counted.

This sampler is very convenient to transport and use, but it is less efficient than the slit sampler in detecting particles below 5 μm in diameter and the size of the sample may not be accurately controlled (Clark et al 1981; Nakhla & Cummings 1981).

Air contamination standards

The level of bacterial contamination of air is usually expressed as the number of bacteria-carrying particles per m^3 or per ft^3 (= 0.0283 m^3). In studies concerned with airborne infection of man, the particles counted are those that carry bacteria capable of growth on blood agar during aerobic incubation for 24 or 48 h at 37°C. Conventionally ventilated rooms commonly show contamination levels between 150/m^3 and 4000/m^3, and deposition on settle plates at values from 10/m^2 to 1000/m^2 per min. The higher levels are observed when there are many occupants, much bodily movement or other dust-raising activities. Most of the contaminants are harmless saprophytes and commensals, and even when carriers or infected patients are present, usually less than 1%, and commonly only 0.01–0.1% of the airborne bacteria are pathogens.

It was suggested by Bourdillon et al (Medical Research Council 1948) that in surgical theatres providing for most forms of surgery, the bacterial count should not exceed 10/ft^3 (353/m^3), and in theatres for operations on the central nervous system or dressing of burns, it should not exceed 1/ft^3 (35.3/m^3). Stricter standards are now preferred. It is recommended that air entering the theatre from filters should not contain more bacteria-carrying particles than 0.5/m^3, that within 30 cm of the operation site not more than 10/m^3, and that elsewhere in the theatre, not more than 20/m^3. Plastic, Trexler-type isolators should be sampled at the air exhaust point and the air should not contain more bacteria-carrying particles than 1/m^3 (Whyte et al 1983).

Because carriers are commonly present, *S. aureus* is the pathogen most commonly found in air, usually in numbers between 0.1/m^3 and 50/m^3. In rooms occupied by patients with tonsillitis or infected wounds or burns, *Streptococcus pyogenes* may be present in similar numbers. Such levels of contamination may seem small, but it must be remembered that an adult man inhales about 15 m³ of air per 24 h and a baby about 1 m³/24 h. The probability of a person becoming infected will be greatest if he is exposed to a high concentration of airborne pathogens, but no level of contamination, however low, can be regarded as certainly safe. Infection may usually be initiated by the deposition of a single infected particle at a favourable site in the respiratory tract, though the probability of any one such particle initiating infection is likely to be low for the common pathogens, e.g. 10^{-2} to 10^{-5} for the acquisition of *S. aureus* in the nose (Lidwell 1981). It may be high for some, e.g. for the acquisition of *Mycobacterium tuberculosis* in the lungs (Riley 1957).

METHODS: (1) MEDIA AND REAGENTS

MacConkey broth, double strength

Peptone	40 g
Sodium taurocholate	10 g
Lactose	20 g
Sodium chloride	10 g
Bromocresol purple, 1% (w/v) in ethanol	2 ml
Distilled water	1 litre

Dissolve the peptone, taurocholate (bile salt) and sodium chloride in the water by heating and store at 4°C overnight. Filter while still cold, add the lactose and dissolve. Adjust the pH to 7.4 and add the bromocresol purple. Distribute in 10 ml and 50 ml volumes in tubes or bottles each containing an inverted Durham tube and autoclave at 115°C for 10 min.

MacConkey broth, single strength

Dilute the double-strength medium with an equal volume of distilled water. Distribute in 5 ml volumes in tubes or bottles each containing an inverted Durham tube and autoclave at 115°C for 10 min.

Lauryl tryptose broth, double strength

This medium is recommended as an alternative to MacConkey broth by the American Public Health Association (1976). Fermentation of lactose is shown by gas formation and the absence of a pH indicator dye allows the culture to be tested for indole production by the addition of rosindole reagent.

Tryptose	40 g
Lactose	10 g
Sodium chloride	10 g
Di-potassium hydrogen phosphate	5.5 g
Potassium dihydrogen phosphate	5.5 g
Sodium lauryl sulphate, pure (BDH 44244)	0.2 g
Distilled water	1 litre

Add the tryptose, sodium chloride, lactose and phosphates to the water and warm to dissolve. Add the sodium lauryl sulphate, mixing gently to avoid frothing. Adjust to pH 6.8. Prepare single-strength medium by diluting the double-strength medium with an equal volume of distilled water. Distribute the double-strength medium in 10 ml and 50 ml volumes and the single-strength medium in 5 ml volumes in tubes or bottles each containing an inverted Durham tube. Autoclave at 115°C for 10 min.

Minerals modified glutamate medium, double strength

The medium most strongly recommended for the enumeration of coliform bacilli by the multiple tube test is this improved formate lactose glutamate medium modified from Gray (1964; Public Health Laboratory Service Standing Committee on the Bacteriological Examination of Water Supplies 1969).

Lactose	20 g
L(+) Glutamic acid sodium salt	12.7 g
L(+) Arginine monohydrochloride	0.04 g
L(−) Aspartic acid	0.048 g
L(−) Cystine	0.04 g
Sodium formate	0.5 g
Di-potassium hydrogen phosphate	1.8 g
Ammonium chloride	5 g
Magnesium sulphate, $MgSO_4.7H_2O$	0.2 g

Calcium chloride, $CaCl_2.2H_2O$	0.02 g
Ferric ammonium citrate, green scales	0.02 g
Thiamine (aneurin hydrochloride)	0.002 g
Nicotinic acid	0.002 g
Pantothenic acid	0.002 g
Bromocresol purple, 1% (w/v) in ethanol	2 ml
Distilled water	1 litre

Prepare in quantities of 10 litres, but add the lactose and thiamine just before distributing in tubes.

Some of the ingredients are conveniently added to the rest as separate solutions prepared as follows.

Solution 1

L(+) Arginine monohydrochloride	0.4 g
L(−) Aspartic acid	0.48 g
Distilled water	50 ml

Heat to dissolve.

Solution 2

L(−) Cystine	0.4 g
Sodium hydroxide solution, 5 mol/litre	10 ml
Distilled water	90 ml

Heat to dissolve.

Solution 3

Nicotinic acid	0.02 g
Pantothenic acid	0.02 g
Distilled water	5 ml

Dissolve in the cold.

Solution 4

| Ferric ammonium citrate | 0.2 g |
| Distilled water | 10 ml |

Heat to dissolve.

Solution 5

Calcium chloride, $CaCl_2.2H_2O$	5 g
Distilled water	100 ml
Concentrated hydrochloric acid	0.1 ml

Dissolve in the cold, sterilize at 121°C for 20 min and keep as a stock solution.

Solution 6

| Thiamine, best from 100 mg ampoule | 100 mg |
| Distilled water | 100 ml |

Add sterile thiamine to sterile distilled water and store at 4°C for up to 6 weeks.

Prepare 10 litres of double-strength medium. Dissolve the appropriate quantities of glutamic acid sodium salt, sodium formate, di-potassium hydrogen phosphate, ammonium chloride and magnesium sulphate in 9 litres of hot distilled water. Then add the whole volumes of solutions 1, 2, 3 and 4, and 4 ml of solution 5. Adjust the pH to 6.8 or as high as will give pH 6.7 after sterilization. Add 20 ml of 1% bromocresol purple in ethanol. Make up with distilled water (c. 810 ml) to 10 litres. Bottle in 500 ml volumes and autoclave at 115°C for 10 min.

For use, add the necessary amount of lactose and thiamine (solution 6), allow to dissolve and distribute in 10 ml and 50 ml volumes in tubes or bottles containing inverted Durham tubes. Sterilize at 115°C for 10 min.

Single-strength medium. Dilute the double-strength medium with an equal volume of distilled water and distribute in 5 ml volumes in tubes containing inverted Durham tubes, and sterilize at 115°C for 10 min.

Brilliant green lactose bile broth

Peptone	10 g
Lactose	10 g
Ox bile, purified and dehydrated	20 g
Brilliant green, 0.1% (w/v) in water	13 ml
Distilled water	1 litre

Dissolve the peptone in 500 ml distilled water. Dissolve the ox bile in 200 ml distilled water; the pH should be between 7.0 and 7.5. Add the bile solution to the peptone solution, make up with distilled water to about 975 ml, add the lactose and adjust the pH to 7.4. Add the brilliant green and make up the volume to 1 litre. Distribute

5 ml volumes in tubes containing inverted Durham tubes and autoclave at 115°C for 10 min.

Tryptone water

Certain peptones are unsatisfactory for the indole test in cultures grown at 44°C (Burman 1955). Oxoid tryptone has been found satisfactory.

Tryptone, Oxoid L42	20 g
Sodium chloride	5 g
Distilled water	1 litre

Dissolve the ingredients in the water, adjust to pH 7.5, distribute in 5 ml volumes and autoclave at 115°C for 10 min.

Membrane lauryl sulphate broth

This medium is recommended by the Public Health Laboratory Service and Standing Committee of Analysts (1980) for coliform counts by the membrane filtration method.

Peptone	40 g
Yeast extract	6 g
Lactose	30 g
Sodium lauryl sulphate, pure (BDH 44244)	1 g
Phenol red, 0.4% (w/v) in water	50 ml
Distilled water	1 litre

Add the ingredients to the water and mix gently to avoid frothing. Adjust the pH to about 7.6, so the the pH after sterilization becomes 7.4–7.5. Distribute in screw-capped bottles and autoclave at 115°C for 10 min.

Lactose peptone water with phenol red

Peptone	10 g
Sodium chloride	5 g
Lactose	10 g
Phenol red, 0.4% (w/v) in water	2.5 ml
Distilled water	1 litre

Dissolve the ingredients in the water and adjust to pH 7.5. Add the phenol red and distribute in 5 ml volumes in tubes with inverted Durham tubes. Autoclave at 110°C for 10 min. Alternatively, steam at 100°C for 10 min on three

successive days. Test for sterility by incubating at 37°C for 24 h.

Glucose azide broth

This medium is recommended by Hannay & Norton (1947) for the recognition of faecal streptococci from cultures of water samples. Prepare double-strength medium as follows and dilute with an equal volume of distilled water to prepare single-strength medium.

Peptone	20 g
Sodium chloride	10 g
Di-potassium hydrogen phosphate	10 g
Potassium dihydrogen phosphate	4 g
Glucose	10 g
Yeast extract	6 g
Sodium azide	0.5 g
Bromocresol purple, 1.6% (w/v) in ethanol	4 ml
Distilled water	1 litre

Dissolve the ingredients in the water and adjust to pH 6.6–6.8. Distribute in tubes or bottles and autoclave at 115°C for 10 min. *Note*: Sodium azide is highly toxic if ingested or inhaled. Solutions containing it should not be discharged through metal pipework.

Bile aesculin azide agar

Peptone	10 g
Meat extract	10 g
Ox bile, purified and dehydrated	10 g
Sodium chloride	5 g
Aesculin	1 g
Sodium azide	0.15 g
Ferric ammonium citrate, green scales	0.5 g
Agar	10 g
Distilled water	1 litre

Dissolve the ingredients in the water by heating at 100°C. Adjust to pH 7.0 and sterilize at 115°C for 10 min. Pour into plates and store at 4°C in sealed containers to prevent drying.

Membrane enterococcus agar

This medium is recommended by Slanetz &

Bartley (1957) for counting faecal streptococci in water by the membrane filtration method.

Tryptose, Oxoid L47	20 g
Yeast extract	5 g
Glucose	2 g
Di-potassium hydrogen phosphate	4 g
Sodium azide	0.4 g
2,3,5-triphenyltetrazolium chloride (TTC), 1% (w/v) in water	10 ml
Agar	12 g
Distilled water	1 litre

Dissolve the ingredients, except the TTC, in the water, heating at 100°C. The pH should be 7.2. Add the TTC solution, previously sterilized by filtration, mix and at once pour into Petri dishes. Do not store and re-melt. Poured plates may be kept in a sealed container at 4°C for up to 6 months.

Differential reinforced clostridial medium (DRCM)

This medium is recommended by Gibbs & Freame (1965) for the recovery of sulphite-reducing clostridia from food and is useful for the counting of *Clostridium perfringens* in water by the multiple tube test. Make up double-strength medium as follows and dilute with an equal volume of distilled water to prepare single-strength medium.

Basal medium

Peptone	20 g
Meat extract	20 g
Sodium acetate, hydrated	10 g
Yeast extract	3 g
Soluble starch	2 g
Glucose	2 g
L(−) Cysteine hydrochloride	1 g
Distilled water	1 litre

Prepare the basal double-strength medium by adding the peptone, meat extract, sodium acetate and yeast extract to 800 ml of the water. Dissolve the starch in the remaining 200 ml, first making it into a slurry with a little of the water, then boiling the rest of the water and stirring it into the cold slurry. Add the glucose and

cysteine, dissolve and adjust to pH 7.1–7.2.

Distribute 10 ml and 50 ml volumes of the double-strength basal medium into, respectively, 28 ml and 125 ml screw-capped bottles and 25 ml volumes of the single-strength basal medium into 28 ml screw-capped bottles. Autoclave at 121°C for 15 min.

Sodium sulphite and ferric ammonium citrate solutions. Prepare solutions of sodium sulphite (anhydrous) 4% and ferric ammonium citrate (green scales) 7% in distilled water, heating the latter to dissolve. Sterilize by filtration. The solutions may be stored at 4°C for up to 14 days.

Final medium. On the day of use, mix equal volumes of the sodium sulphite and ferric ammonium citrate solutions. Freshly steam and cool the basal media to exclude dissolved oxygen. Aseptically add 0.4 ml and 2.0 ml, respectively, of the sulphite-iron mixture to each 10 ml and 50 ml volume of the double-strength basal medium and 0.5 ml to each 25 ml volume of the single-strength medium.

Membrane clostridial agar

This medium, modified from Burman et al (1969), is used for counting *C. perfringens* in water by the membrane filtration method.

Basal medium

Peptone	10 g
Meat extract	3 g
Glucose	20 g
Sodium chloride	5 g
Agar	15 g
Distilled water	1 litre

Prepare the basal medium by dissolving the ingredients in the water, heating at 100°C. Adjust to pH 7.6 by adding a little 1 mol/litre sodium hydroxide. Distribute in 18 ml volumes in 28 ml screw-capped bottles and sterilize at 121°C for 15 min.

Sodium sulphite solution

Sodium sulphite, anhydrous	10 g
Distilled water	100 ml

Dissolve and sterilize at 121°C for 15 min.

Ferrous sulphate solution

Ferrous sulphate, crystalline	8 g
Distilled water	100 ml

Dissolve at 100°C and sterilize at 121°C for 15 min.

Final medium. Melt 18 ml basal medium, cool to 50°C and add aseptically 1 ml sodium sulphite solution and 0.1 ml ferrous sulphate solution. Mix gently and pour over the membrane in a Petri dish.

Yeast extract agar

This is the medium recommended for making plate counts of the bacteria in drinking water. Dehydrated medium is available from Oxoid (CM19).

Yeast extract	3 g
Peptone	5 g
Agar	15 g
Distilled water	1 litre

Dissolve the yeast extract and peptone in the water. Adjust to pH 7.3. Add the agar and heat at 100°C to dissolve. Distribute in 15 ml volumes in 28 ml universal containers or larger volumes in screw-capped bottles and autoclave at 115°C for 10 min.

Yeast extract milk agar

This medium is recommended for making plate counts of the bacteria in milk supplies and rinse water from dairy and food utensils. It is prepared in the same way as yeast extract agar, but 10 ml fresh or spray-dried, skim or whole milk is added per litre of the broth at the same time as the agar is added. A dehydrated medium is available (Oxoid CM21).

Buffered peptone water

This medium is recommended for the resuscitation of salmonellae and other pathogenic bacteria collected from water on filter pads or sewer swabs (Edel & Kampelmacher 1973).

Peptone	10 g
Sodium chloride	5 g
Di-sodium hydrogen phosphate, anhydrous	3.5 g
Potassium dihydrogen phosphate, anhydrous	1.5 g
Distilled water	1 litre

Dissolve the ingredients in the water, distribute in screw-capped bottles and autoclave at 115°C for 10 min. The pH should be 7.2.

Serum glucose agar

This medium is suitable for the culture of brucella from milk, particularly if made selective by the addition of antibiotics such as bacitracin, cycloheximide and polymyxin B.

Peptone	10 g
Meat extract	5 g
Sodium chloride	5 g
Agar	15 g
Distilled water	900 ml

Dissolve the ingredients in the water with gentle heating, adjust to pH 7.5 and autoclave at 121°C for 15 min. Cool to 52°C and aseptically add:

Sterile horse serum inactivated at 56°C for 30 min	50 ml
Glucose 25% in water, filter sterilized	40 ml

Mix well and pour in plates.

If required, add sterile antibiotic solutions to the melted medium at the same time as the serum and glucose, e.g.

Bacitracin solution, 2000 units/ml	12.5 ml
Cycloheximide solution, 10 mg/ml	10 ml
Polymyxin B solution, 5000 units/ml	1.2 ml

Quarter-strength Ringer's solution

Sodium chloride	2.25 g
Potassium chloride	0.105 g
Calcium chloride, anhydrous	0.12 g
Sodium bicarbonate	0.05 g
Distilled water	1 litre

Dissolve the ingredients in the water, dispense in convenient volumes in screw-capped bottles and autoclave at 121°C for 15 min.

Filter-Aid

This preparation of powdered kieselguhr is used to cover a filter pad for the recovery of pathogenic bacteria from water (Hammarström & Ljutov 1954).

Hyflo-supercel (BDH 33216)	1 g
Distilled water	15 ml

Add the powder to the water in a screw-capped bottle and autoclave at 121°C for 15 min. Shake and pour over the filter pad before filtering the sample of water.

METHODS: (2) TABLES OF MOST PROBABLE NUMBERS

These tables, based on the work of Swaroop (1938, 1951), are used to derive the most probable number (MPN) of bacteria per 100 ml in a sample of water from the numbers of positive and negative reactions in replicate tests of different volumes of the sample examined by the multiple tube method. Adhere to the following rules.

1. Refer only to the results of the replicate tests on three consecutive sample volumes, namely the smallest volume giving some positive reactions and the two immediately larger volumes (examples a and b, Table 11.2). Multiply the MPN value from the table by the preliminary dilution factor, if any, to obtain the MPN/100 ml of the original sample. When volumes of undiluted sample have been tested, read the MPN/100 ml directly from the table.

2. If possible, use results for volumes for which the results are neither all positive nor all negative. If this is not possible, use results for volumes giving positive rather than negative reactions (example c, Table 11.2).

3. If less than three volume sets give positive

Table 11.2 Examples of application of the rules for deriving the most probable number (MPN) of bacteria in a water sample from the numbers of positive reactions in sets of five tubes seeded with different volumes of the sample. The three results to be used to derive the MPN are marked with a dagger (†).

Example (see text)	No. of positive reactions in 5 tubes each seeded from the sample with the volume (ml)					MPN/100 ml
	10	1	0.1	0.01	0.001	
a	5†	3†	2†	0	—	140
b	5	5†	3†	2†	0	1400
c	5†	5†	2†	0	0	540
d	3†	1†	0†	0	—	11
e	0†	1†	0†	0	—	2

reactions start with the largest volume set giving a negative reaction (example d, Table 11.2).

4. If only one volume set gives a positive reaction, refer to this set and the one higher and the one lower (example e, Table 11.2).

Confidence limits. The MPN value may differ considerably from the actual number of bacteria per 100 ml. The 95% confidence limits are shown for the values derived in Table 11.3. Those for the values in Tables 11.4 and 11.5 may be obtained by reference to Swaroop (1951).

Table 11.3 Most probable number (MPN)/100 ml of sample and 95% confidence limits of the value for different results in a set of tests of one 50 ml and five 10 ml volumes.

No. of tubes giving a positive reaction		MPN/100 ml	95% Confidence limits (lower – upper)
1 × 50 ml	5 × 10 ml		
0	0	<1	—
0	1	1	0.5–4
0	2	2	0.5–6
0	3	4	0.5–11
0	4	5	1–13
0	5	7	2–17
1	0	2	0.5–6
1	1	3	0.5–9
1	2	6	1–15
1	3	9	2–21
1	4	16	4–40
1	5	>18	—

Table 11.4 Most probable number (MPN) values/100 ml of sample for a set of tests of one 50 ml, five 10 ml and five 1 ml volumes.

No. of tubes giving a positive reaction			
1×50 ml	5×10 ml	5×1 ml	MPN/100 ml
0	0	0	<1
0	0	1	1
0	0	2	2
0	1	0	1
0	1	1	2
0	1	2	3
0	2	0	2
0	2	1	3
0	2	2	4
0	3	0	3
0	3	1	5
0	4	0	5
1	0	0	1
1	0	1	3
1	0	2	4
1	0	3	6
1	1	0	3
1	1	1	5
1	1	2	7
1	1	3	9
1	2	0	5
1	2	1	7
1	2	2	10
1	2	3	12
1	3	0	8
1	3	1	11
1	3	2	14
1	3	3	18
1	3	4	21
1	4	0	13
1	4	1	17
1	4	2	22
1	4	3	28
1	4	4	35
1	4	5	43
1	5	0	24
1	5	1	35
1	5	2	54
1	5	3	92
1	5	4	161
1	5	5	>180

Table 11.5 Most probable number (MPN) values/100 ml of sample for three sets of tests each of five tubes seeded with a 10 ml, 1 ml or 0.1 ml volume of the sample.

No. of 5 tubes giving a positive reaction			
10 ml	1 ml	0.1 ml	MPN/100 ml
0	0	0	<2
		1	2
		2	4
		3	5
		4	7
		5	9
0	1	0	2
		1	4
		2	6
		3	7
		4	9
		5	11
0	2	0	4
		1	6
		2	7
		3	9
		4	11
		5	13
0	3	0	6
		1	7
		2	9
		3	11
		4	13
		5	15
0	4	0	8
		1	9
		2	11
		3	13
		4	15
		5	17
0	5	0	9
		1	11
		2	13
		3	15
		4	17
		5	19

Table 11.5 (contd) Most probable number (MPN) values/10 ml of sample for three sets of tests each of five tubes seeded with a 10 ml, 1 ml or 0.1 ml volume of the sample.

No. of 5 tubes giving a positive reaction				No. of 5 tubes giving a positive reaction			
10 ml	1 ml	0.1 ml	MPN/100 ml	10 ml	1 ml	0.1 ml	MPN/100 ml
1	0	0	2	2	0	0	5
		1	4			1	7
		2	6			2	9
		3	8			3	12
		4	10			4	14
		5	12			5	16
1	1	0	4	2	1	0	7
		1	6			1	9
		2	8			2	12
		3	10			3	14
		4	12			4	17
		5	14			5	19
1	2	0	6	2	2	0	9
		1	8			1	12
		2	10			2	14
		3	12			3	17
		4	15			4	19
		5	17			5	22
1	3	0	8	2	3	0	12
		1	10			1	14
		2	13			2	17
		3	15			3	20
		4	17			4	22
		5	19			5	25
1	4	0	11	2	4	0	15
		1	13			1	17
		2	15			2	20
		3	17			3	23
		4	19			4	25
		5	22			5	28
1	5	0	13	2	5	0	17
		1	15			1	20
		2	17			2	23
		3	19			3	26
		4	22			4	29
		5	24			5	32

Table 11.5 (contd) Most probable number (MPN) values/100 ml of sample for three sets of tests each of five tubes seeded with a 10 ml, 1 ml or 0.1 ml volume of the sample.

| No. of 5 tubes giving a positive reaction | | | | No. of 5 tubes giving a positive reaction | | | |
10 ml	1 ml	0.1 ml	MPN/100 ml	10 ml	1 ml	0.1 ml	MPN/100 ml
3	0	0	8	4	0	0	13
		1	11			1	17
		2	13			2	21
		3	16			3	25
		4	20			4	30
		5	23			5	36
3	1	0	11	4	1	0	17
		1	14			1	21
		2	17			2	26
		3	20			3	31
		4	23			4	36
		5	27			5	42
3	2	0	14	4	2	0	22
		1	17			1	26
		2	20			2	32
		3	24			3	38
		4	27			4	44
		5	31			5	50
3	3	0	17	4	3	0	27
		1	21			1	33
		2	24			2	39
		3	28			3	45
		4	31			4	52
		5	35			5	59
3	4	0	21	4	4	0	34
		1	24			1	40
		2	28			2	47
		3	32			3	54
		4	36			4	62
		5	40			5	69
3	5	0	25	4	5	0	41
		1	29			1	48
		2	32			2	56
		3	37			3	64
		4	41			4	72
		5	45			5	81

Table 11.5 (contd) Most probable number (MPN) values/100 ml of sample for three sets of tests each of five tubes seeded with a 10 ml, 1 ml or 0.1 ml volume of the sample.

No. of 5 tubes giving a positive reaction			
10 ml	1 ml	0.1 ml	MPN/ 100 ml
5	0	0	23
		1	31
		2	43
		3	58
		4	˙76
		5	95
5	1	0	33
		1	46
		2	63
		3	84
		4	110
		5	130
5	2	0	49
		1	70
		2	94
		3	120
		4	150
		5	180
5	3	0	79
		1	110
		2	140
		3	180
		4	210
		5	250
5	4	0	130
		1	170
		2	220
		3	280
		4	350
		5	430
5	5	0	240
		1	350
		2	540
		3	920
		4	1600
		5	>1800

REFERENCES

American Public Health Association 1976 Standard methods for the examination of water and waste water, 14th edn. American Public Health Association, Washington. p 893

Bourdillon R B, Lidwell O M, Thomas J C 1941 A slit sampler for collecting and counting airborne bacteria. Journal of Hygiene, Cambridge 41: 197–224

Brodie J, Sinton G P 1975 Fluid and solid media for isolation of *Brucella abortus*. Journal of Hygiene, Cambridge 74: 359–367

Burman N P 1955 The standardization and selection of bile salt and peptone for culture media used in the bacteriological examination of water. Proceedings of the Society for Water Treatment and Examination 4:10

Burman N P, Oliver C W, Stevens J K 1969 Membrane filtration techniques for the isolation from water of coli-aerogenes, *Escherichia coli*, faecal streptococci, *Clostridium perfringens*, actinomyces and micro fungi. In: Shapton D A, Gould G W (eds) Isolation methods for microbiologists. Society for Applied Bacteriology Technical Series No. 3. Academic Press, London, p 127

Clark S, Lach V, Lidwell O M 1981 The performance of the Biotest RCS centrifugal air sampler. Journal of Hospital Infection 2: 181–186

Corry J E L, Roberts D, Skinner F A 1982 Isolation and identification methods for food-poisoning organisms. Academic Press, London

Davis J G 1966 A dictionary of dairying. 2nd edn Aberdeen University Press. p. 101–103

Department of the Environment, Department of Health and Social Security, Public Health Laboratory Service 1982 Methods for the examination of water and associated materials. The bacteriological examination of drinking water supplies 1982. Her Majesty's Stationery Office, London

Department of Health and Social Security, Department of the Environment, Welsh Office 1969 The bacteriological examination of water supplies, 4th edn. Her Majesty's Stationery Office, London

Duguid J P 1946 The size and duration of air-carriage of respiratory droplets and droplet-nuclei. Journal of Hygiene, Cambridge 44: 471–479

Duguid J P, Wallace A T 1948 Air infection with dust liberated from clothing. Lancet 2: 845–849

Edel W, Kampelmacher E H 1973 Comparative studies on the isolation of 'sublethally injured' salmonellae in nine European laboratories. Bulletin of the World Health Organization 48: 167–174

European Community 1980 Council Directive No. 80/778/EEC of 15 July 1980 relating to the quality of water intended for human consumption. Official Journal of the European Community L229:11

Farrell I D, Robertson L 1972 A comparison of various selective media including a new selective medium for the isolation of brucellae from milk. Journal of Applied Bacteriology 35: 625–630

Gibbs B M, Freame B 1965 Methods for the recovery of clostridia from foods. Journal of Applied Bacteriology 28: 95–111

Gilbert R J, Wieneke A A, Lanser J, Simkovicova M 1972 Serological detection of enterotoxins in foods implicated in staphylococcal food-poisoning. Journal of Hygiene, Cambridge 70: 755–762

Gray R D 1964 An improved formate lactose glutamate medium for the detection of *E. coli* and other coliform organisms in water. Journal of Hygiene, Cambridge 62: 495–508

Hammarström E, Ljutov V 1954 Concentration technique for demonstrating small amounts of bacteria in tap water. Acta Pathologica et Microbiologica Scandinavica 35: 365–369

Hannay C L, Norton I L 1947 Enumeration, isolation and study of faecal streptococci from river water. Proceedings of the Society for Applied Bacteriology 1:39

Harvey R W S, Price T H 1975 Isolation of salmonellas. Public Health Laboratory Service Monograph No. 8. Her Majesty's Stationery Office, London

Harvey R W S, Price T H 1979 A Review: Principles of salmonella isolation. Journal of Applied Bacteriology 46: 27–56

Holbrook R, Anderson J M 1980 An improved selective and diagnostic medium for the isolation and enumeration of *Bacillus cereus* in foods. Canadian Journal of Microbiology 26: 753–759

Lidwell O M 1959 Impaction sampler for size grading air-borne bacteria-carrying particles. Journal of Scientific Instruments 36: 3–8

Lidwell O M 1981 Some aspects of the transfer and acquisition of *Staphylococcus aureus* in hospitals. In: Macdonald A, Smith G (eds) The staphylococci. Aberdeen University Press, Aberdeen. p 175–202

May K R 1967 Physical aspects of sampling airborne microbes. In: Gregory P H, Monteith J L (eds) Airborne microbes. 17th Symposium of the Society for General Microbiology. Cambridge University Press, Cambridge. p 60–80

Medical Research Council 1948 Studies in air hygiene. Special Report Series No. 262. His Majesty's Stationery Office, London. p 12–53

Ministry of Agriculture and Fisheries 1947 The bacteriological examination of milk bottles. Technique No. B743/TPB. National Milk Testing Advisory Scheme

Mitchell N J 1970 A simplified method for quantitative microbiological examination of deep frozen seafoods. Journal of Applied Bacteriology 33: 523–527

Moore B 1948 The detection of paratyphoid carriers in towns by means of sewage examination. Monthly Bulletin of the Ministry of Health and the Public Health Laboratory Service 7: 241–248

Murray J G 1969 An approach to bacteriological standards. Journal of Applied Bacteriology 32: 123–135

Nakhla L S, Cummings R F 1981 A comparative evaluation of a new centrifugal air sampler (RCS) with a slit air sampler (SAS) in a hospital environment. Journal of Hospital Infection 2: 261–266

Noble W C 1967 Sampling airborne microbes – handling the catch. In: Gregory P H, Monteith J L (eds) Airborne microbes. 17th Symposium of the Society for General Microbiology. Cambridge University Press, Cambridge. p 81–101

Public Health Laboratory Service Standing Committee on the Bacteriological Examination of Water Supplies 1969 A minerals modified glutamate medium for the enumeration of coliform organisms in water. Journal of Hygiene, Cambridge 67: 367–374

Public Health Laboratory Service and the Standing Committee of Analysts 1980 Membrane filtration media for the enumeration of coliform organisms and *Escherichia coli* in water: comparison of Tergitol 7 and lauryl sulphate with Teepol 610. Journal of Hygiene, Cambridge 85: 181–191

Riley R P 1957 Aerial dissemination of pulmonary tuberculosis. American Review of Tuberculosis 76: 931–941

Roberts T A, Hobbs G, Christian J H B, Skovgaard N 1981 Psychrotrophic micro-organisms in spoilage and pathogenicity. Academic Press, London

Russell M P, Goldsmith J A, Phillips I 1984 Some factors affecting the efficiency of settle plates. Journal of Hospital Infection 5: 189–199

Slanetz L W, Bartley C H 1957 Numbers of enterococci in water, sewage and faeces determined by the membrane filter technique with an improved medium. Journal of Bacteriology 74: 591–595

Swaroop S 1938 Numerical estimation of *B. coli* by dilution method. Indian Journal of Medical Research 26: 353–378

Swaroop S 1951 The range of variation of the most probable number of organisms estimated by the dilution method. Indian Journal of Medical Research 39: 107–134

Wells W F 1933 Apparatus for the study of the bacterial behaviour of air. American Journal of Public Health 23: 58–59

Whyte W, Lidwell O M, Lowbury E J L, Blowers R 1983 Suggested bacteriological standards for air in ultraclean operating rooms. Journal of Hospital Infection 4: 133–139

Wilson G S, Twigg R S, Wright R C, Hendry C B, Cowell M P, Maier I 1935 The bacteriological grading of milk. Medical Research Council Special Report Series No. 206. His Majesty's Stationery Office, London

Wolf H W, Skaliy P, Hall L B, Harris M M, Decker H M, Buchanan L M, Dahlgren C M 1959 Sampling microbiological aerosols. US Public Health Monograph No. 60. United States Government Printing Office, Washington DC

World Health Organization 1971 International standards for drinking water, 3rd edn. Palais des Nations, Geneva

Centrifuges, colorimeters and bacterial counts

CENTRIFUGES

One of the best devices for the separation of microorganisms from a suspending fluid is the centrifuge, which achieves the separation of two substances of different density by centrifugal force.

The rate of settling r (cm/s) of spherical particles of density dp and of radius a (cm) in a medium of viscosity η (cgs units) and of density dm is given by Stokes' law:

$$r = \frac{2a^2g(dp - dm)}{9\eta}$$

where g is the acceleration due to gravity (981 cm/s^2).

From this equation, it is evident that the rate of settling of a particle will be increased by the following factors:

1. *An increase in the size of the particle.* Thus, larger microorganisms like yeasts and fungi will sediment faster than bacteria which, in turn, will sediment faster than viruses. Note that the size of the particles is squared in the equation and thus an increase of the radius of the particles by a factor of 2 will increase the rate of settling by a factor of 4.

2. *An increase in the difference between the density of the particles dp and that of the medium dm.* Thus a capsulate bacterium will have a lower average density and be more difficult to sediment than its non-capsulate variant.

3. *A decrease in the viscosity of the medium.* For example, when defibrinated blood is being washed the first sedimentation of the cells from the viscous serum takes much longer than when the cells are suspended in saline.

4. *An increase in the force due to gravity.* This force is increased artificially in the centrifuge. The degree by which this force is increased is measured by the relative centrifugal force (RCF) which can be obtained by the following formula:

$$\text{RCF (in } g) = 1.118 \times 10^{-5} \times R \times N^2,$$

where R = the radius of the centrifuge rotor in cm, being the distance from the centre of the centrifuge shaft to the tip of the centrifuge tube; N = revolutions/min (rev/min).

From this equation, it is evident that the speed of the centrifuge, being squared, is very important in determining the rate of sedimentation. Although an increase in the radius of the machine will increase the rate of sedimentation, it is more efficient and simpler in practice to increase the speed. However, it is most important to express the efficiency of a centrifuge according to the maximum RCF rather than the speed itself, which, without specification of the radius of the centrifuge rotor, is meaningless. The calculation is simple. Thus, a centrifuge rotor with a radius of 10 cm and a speed of 4000 rev/min has an RCF of $1.118 \times 10 \times (4000)^2 \times 10^{-5} = 1788\,g$, say 1800 times the force of gravity. Consequently, particles will sediment in this centrifuge at a rate 1800 times faster than in a tube on the bench.

Types of centrifuge

The choice of a suitable model depends upon the following factors:

1. *The size of the particles to be sedimented.* As shown above, the smaller the particle, the

greater will be the RCF and time required for centrifugation. Machines can be obtained commercially with speeds up to about 75 000 rev/min and RCFs of up to about 500 000 g. To sediment small volumes of micro-organisms in an acceptable time, an RCF of 2000 g is required for yeasts and fungi, 5000 g for bacteria and 150 000 g for viruses. If larger volumes are to be centrifuged, the RCF required would be 5000 g, 20 000 g and 200 000 g respectively.

2. *The volume of material.* Centrifuges can be obtained with capacities of up to at least 15 litres. The fluid to be centrifuged is contained in tubes or buckets, the number and size of which is subject to a wide variation. For very large amounts of material, continuous-flow machines are available. The fluid to be centrifuged is normally continuously passed along the inside of a rotating tube. The particles sediment very quickly in the thin layer of liquid passing along the sides of the tube and the supernate passes out of the machine to be collected. Continuous-flow centrifuges (e.g. Sharples) of this type are common in industry, but are not often used in the laboratory because of aerosol problems.

3. *The temperature required for centrifugation.* In most biological systems it is advantageous and often essential to centrifuge at low temperatures. This prevents metabolism, loss of viability or enzyme activity during centrifugation. Consequently, refrigeration units are built into many centrifuges. This is particularly important in high-speed centrifuges where the temperature may rise due to friction unless refrigeration is used.

For a clinical bacteriology or virology laboratory, a small bench centrifuge taking 10–40 specimen containers of 5–30 ml capacity, with maximum RCF of about 5000 g is essential. These centrifuges and accessories should comply with the Howie safety recommendations (Ch. 15). For more general and research purposes, refrigerated centrifuges with a volume capacity of about 6 litres and a maximum RCF of about 50 000–70 000 g are available. Ultracentrifuges with speeds ranging from 40 000–75 000 rev/min and RCFs of 100 000–500 000 g are available for viruses and rickettsias, and for subcellular frac-

tions. These centrifuges must be refrigerated, and the rotor chamber must be held in vacuo to reduce friction during a run.

Types of rotor

Horizontal swing-out rotors. In these rotors, the sample buckets swing freely from a vertical to a horizontal plane during rotation. Particulate matter moves horizontally through the suspending medium and pellets on the bottom of the container. This type of rotor is recommended in the Howie report for bacteriological work. Special sealed rotors or sealed buckets should be used for pathogens or specimens likely to contain pathogens.

Fixed angle rotors. The sample containers are maintained at a fixed angle of 20–45° during rotation. The advantage of these rotors is that sedimentation is quicker than in a horizontal rotor of similar maximum diameter. This is because the smallest diameter, measured from the centre of the rotor to the top of the sample, is greater than that on the equivalent horizontal rotor. Particulate matter moves horizontally across the container, then slides down the side to pellet at the bottom. Centrifugation should be of sufficient duration to ensure complete pelleting of the material on the bottom of the tube.

The smooth regular outline of fixed angle rotors offers little resistance to air during rotation, so they can attain higher speeds and they are less liable to warm up by friction. A major disadvantage with this type of rotor is the possibility of aerosols, either during a run when there may be leakage between the container and cap, or on removing the cap after a run.

Vertical rotors. A specialized rotor is used for density gradient work (see below). The sample tubes are held in a vertical position during the run, and the rotor must be used on a centrifuge in which acceleration and deceleration is carefully controlled. The major advantage over horizontal swing-out rotors is that lower speeds and shorter run times can be used.

Continuous-flow rotors. The method of separation is similar to that described for continuous-flow centrifuges. This type of rotor is not recommended in medical microbiology because of aerosol problems.

All rotors require regular care and maintenance which should be done according to the manufacturers' instructions.

Types of tubes and bottles

Glass, plastic, cellulose nitrate and stainless steel are the materials of choice. The use of glass culture tubes in centrifuges must be limited to low RCF (about 1000 g) and this is not recommended for bacteriological work. Toughened glass tubes and glass 20 oz bottles can operate at higher RCF (about 4000 g). Plastic containers are made in a variety of materials, e.g. polycarbonate, polypropylene, polyesters, each with their own advantages of clarity, strength and chemical and heat resistance. These containers can withstand very high RCF, but often require to be completely filled and capped. Stainless steel tubes are inert, can be heat sterilized, and can withstand very high RCF.

Method of using the centrifuge

The modern centrifuge has many built-in safety features including out-of-balance detectors, lid interlocks to prevent the lid being opened when the rotor is in motion, overspeed and overheating cut-out devices, and sealed rotor and buckets to cope with potentially dangerous breakages. These features make it difficult to misuse the equipment, but it is still necessary to follow basic instructions:

1. Tubes must be put in the centrifuge in pairs that have been accurately balanced and placed diametrically opposite each other. If there is an odd number of tubes, a balance tube containing water must be prepared. If the buckets are removable from the centrifuge, they should be balanced with the tubes.

2. Before putting tubes into the buckets, make sure that cushions or sleeves are in position at the bottom of the buckets and free from debris, e.g. fragments of glass, otherwise breakages are liable to occur.

3. After the tubes have been placed in position, make sure that the metal buckets in a swing-out head are properly seated and are free to swing, and that all buckets are in place, irrespective of the number actually being used.

4. Close the lid and make sure it is secure. The lid must not be opened when the centrifuge is running. Apart from the danger of an open lid, a decrease in speed due to 'winding' will ensue.

5. Following the manufacturers' instructions, select the speed, time and temperature required. A gradual increase in speed is recommended if this is done manually.

6. When the tubes have been centrifuged sufficiently, switch off the motor. Some centrifuges have an automatic timer switch.

7. Allow the centrifuge to come to a stop. Never slow the rotating head with your hand as brake. This will tend to redisperse the centrifugate by turbulence and may cause serious injuries. Wait until the machine has stopped before attempting to remove the tubes.

8. Periodic maintenance should be done according to the manufacturers' instructions.

Washing of bacteria and other cells

The cell suspension is centrifuged at a suitable speed and preferably at a low temperature. Microorganisms grown on a solid medium are first suspended in liquid by scraping the growth off the surface of the agar with a curved glass rod into a small volume of a suitable suspending fluid. (This suspension may be contaminated with lumps of agar which can be removed by filtration through cheesecloth.) The pellet of cells at the bottom of the centrifuge tube is resuspended and centrifuged. Repeat this washing process one or more times to free the cells from the original suspending medium. The cells are finally made up to the required volume in the required solution.

For metabolic experiments, the cells are washed in a medium similar in composition to the culture medium but with one or more components omitted so that growth does not occur. The 'washed suspension' so obtained is particularly suitable for experiments on catabolism; a substrate and buffer are added so that the breakdown of the substrate can be studied uncomplicated by growth processes or by the metabolism of other substrates. However, it must be realized that some activities 'decay' rapidly after, or during, the preparation of the washed suspension.

Density-gradient centrifugation

In normal centrifugation, the material being centrifuged is forced to migrate though a homogeneous liquid medium. In density-gradient centrifugation, a gradient of a suitable solute, such as sucrose, caesium chloride, Ficoll or Percoll (Pharmacia), is made in the tube in such a way that the density increases with the distance from the axis of rotation. Such a gradient may be formed during the centrifugation process itself (with caesium chloride) or, more commonly, it is prepared by layering or by a gradient maker.

Density-gradient centrifugation can be employed to analyse and separate subcellular particles or viruses. There are three main types of method.

Stabilized moving boundary centrifugation. By the use of a density gradient, the sedimentation constant of a substance can be determined with a preparation centrifuge and a method analogous to classical analytical ultracentrifugation. The gradient is a shallow one and this stabilizes the boundary which might otherwise be destroyed by convection currents. The material to be centrifuged is distributed throughout the tube at the start of the experiment and, after centrifugation, the position of the band or bands formed is found by separating and analysing fractions from the tube.

Zonal centrifugation. In this method, a concentrated preparation is layered on top of a fairly steep gradient in the tube prior to centrifugation. Each component in the preparation will then sediment at its own rate, forming bands or zones in the tube which are separated from each other by distances related to their sedimentation rates. In practice, the separation is mainly related to molecular size. After centrifugation, the components can be removed separately from the tube.

Isopycnic or equilibrium gradient centrifuga-

tion. In this method, a steep gradient is produced to encompass the entire density range of the particles being separated. The preparation is layered on top of the tube as in zonal centrifugation, or is distributed evenly throughout the gradient, and centrifugation is continued until the particles reach positions at which the density of the surrounding liquid is equal to their own. Thus, separation is based solely on density.

PHOTOELECTRIC COLORIMETER AND SPECTROPHOTOMETER

One of the simplest and most accurate methods of measuring the quantity of a microorganism depends upon a turbidity measurement, just as many of the quantitative micro-methods used in biochemistry depend upon the measurement of the depth of colour in a solution. For such measurements, a photoelectric colorimeter or spectrophotometer is more accurate than visual comparison. It is also much quicker and avoids many personal factors such as eye fatigue or colour blindness.

The theory of the instrument as a colorimeter depends upon the application of Beer's law, which states that the extent of diminution in light intensity on passing through an absorbing material depends upon the nature and concentration of the absorbing material and upon the length of the light path. This can be expressed as follows:

$$\log \frac{I_o}{I} = acl$$

where I is the intensity of the beam after passing through the solution, I_o is the incident intensity, a is the extinction coefficient depending upon the particular chromogen, c is the concentration of the chromogen and l is the length of the light path through the solution.

It is possible, therefore, to determine the concentration of a substance by measuring the ratio I_o/I in a vessel of standard dimensions. In photoelectric colorimeters and spectrophotometers, light intensity is measured by photoelectric response which can be made directly proportional to the quantity of light falling on the photoelectric cell.

A range of colorimeters and spectrophotometers is available. There are single and double beam models with visible and/or UV light sources. Different wavelengths of light are produced by coloured filters or, in spectrophotometers, by a diffraction grating.

Automatic scanning is available in some instruments. Most modern instruments utilize standard 10 mm path-length cuvettes, but tubes can be used in some instruments. Directions for the use of a particular machine are supplied by the makers. In all cases a blank solution is used in which the chromogen would be dissolved. A calibration curve should be constructed for the instrument (log I_o/I) against known amounts of chromogen. If Beer's law is obeyed, a straight line is obtained. Readings for test samples are compared with the plot.

The use of such instruments for turbidimetric measurements of bacterial numbers is considered later in this chapter.

COUNTING BACTERIA AND MEASURING BACTERIAL GROWTH

The method used for determining the amount of a microorganism present in a suspension depends upon the kind of information required. In particular, since no constant relation exists between the ratio of increase in protoplasmic mass to rate of multiplication, it is necessary to distinguish clearly between methods which measure multiplication (e.g. total count) and those which measure growth or mass (e.g. total nitrogen content, dry weight, etc.).

Because of variations in average cell size, bacterial counts do not bear a constant relationship to the amount of protoplasmic growth. The amount of protoplasm is better gauged by an opacity measurement, or weighing, or by a total nitrogen estimation. A detailed description of methods to determine viability in cultures is given by Postgate (1969).

An evaluation of the methods that may be used to measure growth by physical and chemical means is given by Malette (1969).

Total count

A total count of the living and dead bacteria in a liquid culture or suspension is made microscopically with a *slide counting chamber*. A suitable chamber (e.g. Hawksley, from Gallenkamp) consists of a thin glass slide with a flat circular platform depressed exactly 0.02 mm below the surface and surrounded by a deeper 'trench'. An area of 1 mm^2 on the platform is marked with a Thoma-type grating of engraved lines into 400 small squares (each 0.0025 mm^2). The chamber is closed with a thick, optically-plane coverslip. When the space between platform and coverslip is filled with a bacterial suspension, the volume over each small square is 0.02 × 0.0025 mm^3, i.e. 0.000 000 05 ml. The average number of bacteria/square is calculated from counts made in sufficient squares (e.g. 100) to yield a significant total number of bacteria (e.g. 100–1000, preferably over 300). Counts are best made in preparations having between 2 and 10 bacteria/square (i.e. 40–200 million/ml). For bacteria occurring in pairs, chains or clusters, an 'individual cell count' may be made of all the cells, or a 'group count' of the groups plus any isolated single cells.

The procedure for a total count is as follows:

1. Fix the bacterial suspension by adding 2–3 drops of 40% formaldehyde/10 ml. Mix thoroughly. If the suspension is too dense, prepare a measured dilution in the range 4–20 × 10^7 bacteria/ml.

2. Wash, rinse, drain and dry the counting chamber and coverslip. Keep them covered until use, free from dust.

3. Place a small drop or loopful of the suspension on the centre of the chamber platform and apply the coverslip. The size of the drop must be such that it will fill the space between platform and coverslip, yet not extend across the 'trench' to float the coverslip from the slide. The coverslip must be applied closely and evenly; it is pressed down until coloured 'Newton's rings' are seen uniformly distributed over the areas of contact.

4. Examine the preparation with a phase-contrast microscope, using the high power dry objective; this shows the unstained bacteria

clearly and allows their distinction from detritus. Alternatively, a darkground microscope may be used, or an ordinary microscope with the iris diaphragm closed or the condenser slightly defocused; it may then be helpful to stain the bacteria by prior addition of freshly filtered methylene blue to a concentration of 0.1%.

5. Count the bacteria in a sufficient number of squares to obtain a total of several hundred bacteria, selecting the squares in a pre-arranged pattern (e.g. all in every fifth row). Focus at different levels for the bacteria that have not settled; most settle on the platform in 5 or 10 min, but some adhere to the coverslip and a few remain in suspension.

6. Calculate the average number of bacteria/square. Multiply this by 2×10^7 and by the dilution factor, if any, to obtain the count/ml in the original suspension. Count two further preparations of the same suspension, and unless they are discordant, take an average of the three results.

If the original suspension contains much less than 4×10^7 bacteria/ml, a haemocytometer with a 0.1 mm chamber depth may be used so as to obtain a significant count in fewer squares. Unstained bacteria are counted with a long-focus phase-contrast microscope, or if an ordinary microscope is used, the bacteria are stained. The preparation is left for 20 min in a moist chamber before counting so that most bacteria may settle on the platform.

Total counts may be done automatically with the Coulter counter (see Kubitschek 1969).

Viable count

Pour-plate method

The number of living bacteria or groups of bacteria in a liquid culture or suspension is counted by a cultural method such as the pour-plate method. A measured amount of the suspension is mixed with molten agar medium in a Petri dish. After setting and incubation, the number of colonies is counted. As a compromise between sampling and overcrowding errors, counts of pure cultures should be made on plates inoculated to yield between 50 and 500 colonies (ideally 200–400).

1. Prepare serial 10-fold dilutions of the bacterial suspension over a range ensuring that one dilution will contain between 50 and 500 viable bacteria/ml. Suitable diluents include buffered saline or balanced salt solution, with or without added material to protect the organisms (e.g. nutrient broth diluted to 20% of normal strength). Pipette 9 ml amounts of diluent into each of several (6–9) sterile test tubes. Mix uniformly the bacterial suspension (vigorous shaking may disrupt cell groups and increase the viable count). With a sterile 1 ml delivering pipette, transfer 1.0 ml suspension into the first tube of diluent; fill and empty the pipette with suspension several times before withdrawing from the original container; remove any excess drop from the outside of the pipette and then slowly deliver its contents into the tube of diluent, touching the wall of the tube but not dipping into the diluent. With a fresh sterile 1 ml pipette, mix the first dilution by filling and emptying several times, and then transfer 1 ml into the next tube of diluent. Make the remaining dilutions in the same way, using a fresh pipette for each.

When counting anaerobic bacteria it is necessary to exclude air. Diluents should be treated to remove dissolved air prior to use; it may be advantageous to use diluents with added non-toxic reducing agents (see Ch. 36). Pipetting should be done carefully to avoid aeration. If possible the whole procedure should be done in an anaerobic chamber.

2. Starting with the greatest dilution, pipette 1 ml amounts of each dilution into each of three 9 cm Petri dishes. Then pour into each dish about 10 ml of clear nutrient agar, melted and cooled to 45–50°C. At once mix by rapidly moving the plate, while flat on the bench, in a combination of side-to-side and circular movements in different directions; continue for about 10 s, taking care not to spill any of the contents. Allow the agar to set and incubate inverted for 2 days at 37°C, or as most suitable for the species examined.

3. Count the colonies in the three plates that were seeded with the dilution giving between 50

and 500 colonies/plate. Multiply the average number/plate by the dilution factor to obtain the viable count/ml in the original suspension.

Surface viable count by spreading method

A surface viable count is made when the bacterium is best grown in surface culture or on an opaque medium. Prior to inoculation, the plate of medium is dried for at least 2 h at 37°C or 10–15 min at 50°C with the lid ajar; it should then be able to absorb all the water of the inoculum within about 15 min, i.e. before the bacteria can multiply. 10-fold dilutions of the bacterial suspension are made as for the pour-plate method. A suitable volume of each dilution, e.g. 0.02–0.1 ml, is pipetted on to the surface of each of three plates and at once spread widely with a sterile glass spreader. The viable count is calculated from the average colony count/plate.

Surface viable count by Miles and Misra method

Alternatively, by the method of Miles et al (1938), the inoculum is deposited as drops from a calibrated dropping pipette. Each drop, 0.02 ml in volume, is allowed to fall from a height of 2.5 cm on to the medium, where it spreads over an area of 1.5–2 cm diameter. Each of five plates receives one drop of each dilution in separate numbered sectors, or separate plates may receive the 5 drops of a dilution. Counts are made in the drop areas showing the largest number of colonies without confluence (up to 20 or more); the total of the five counts gives the viable count/0.1 ml of the dilution.

Methods of measuring growth

Wet weight

Amounts of culture are sometimes measured by wet weight. The moist surface growth on a solid medium is scraped from the medium and weighed at once. However, such estimations are inaccurate because of the difficulty of evaluating the relative contributions of water wetting the bacterial surface and intracellular water. Further, in bacteria forming capsules and slime, the wet weight may greatly overestimate the amount of protoplasm, since it includes the weight of these highly hydrated extracellular substances.

Dry weight

The weight of the dried solid matter of bacteria affords a better measure of their protoplasm. The cells from a known volume of culture are washed free from soluble salts, nutrients and waste products by centrifugation in distilled water. It is assumed that no lysis occurs during this process, and this is not an invariably valid assumption. The whole or a known proportion of the washed cells is placed in a weighed vessel and weighed again after drying to a constant weight by freeze-drying or heating in an oven, e.g. at 120°C for about 3 h. Cool after each heating in a desiccator over P_2O_5 and weigh quickly to prevent adsorption of water.

Total nitrogen

One of the most reliable and constant methods of measuring the amount of bacterial protoplasm for metabolic measurements is by estimation of the nitrogen present in the nitrogenous components of the cells, i.e. mainly proteins and nucleic acids (nitrogen content about 16%). The cells from a known volume of culture are washed by centrifugation to free them from nitrogenous constituents of the medium and from extracellular excretion products. The total nitrogen of the cells is then estimated by the micro-Kjeldahl method. The cells are digested with sulphuric acid using a $CuSO_4$-K_2SO_4-selenium catalyst. The ammonia produced is removed after making the solution alkaline by steam distillation in a suitable still, e.g. a Markham still, trapped in 2% boric acid and estimated either by titration or colorimetrically after the addition of a suitable reagent, e.g. Nessler reagent (see Dawson et al 1969 for fuller details).

Turbidity

The turbidity of a suspension is caused by the

light scattered by particulate matter during its passage through the suspension. Accurate measurements of turbidity, and hence bacterial growth, can be obtained in two ways:

1. By measuring the amount of light scattered directly, a procedure occasionally called nephelometry. This is rarely used in practice.

2. By measuring the light lost from the beam by scattering. Light absorption is assumed to be absent. This loss can be measured accurately in a photoelectric colorimeter or spectrophotometer where a relation similar to Beer's law applies. The expression is the same as that given earlier in this chapter except that the term extinction coefficient is replaced by a constant called the turbidity coefficient. A standard plot can be made of log I_o/I against either the total nitrogen content, the dry weight or total count. The concentration factor applies mainly to protoplasmic mass as the size of the organisms as well as their number determines turbidity.

The following points should be noted:

1. The calibration curve applies only to *a particular organism grown under a particular set of growth conditions*. A new curve must be prepared if a change is made in either of these. It should be noted that the shape of an organism as well as its size will alter turbidity. Further, cells grown in a medium to give a high carbohydrate or fat content generally have a high turbidity/cell.

2. Use a neutral or a blue filter. In a spectrophotometer use a wavelength of 540–600 nm. Light scattering increases very greatly as the wavelength decreases, although it is not advisable to use too low a wavelength since light absorption will become increasingly apparent.

3. For the blank, use the suspending fluid. The growth medium can be used provided the absorption is not altered by growth of the organisms. If it is altered, the cells must be washed and resuspended in fresh solutions.

4. At low concentrations, a linear calibration plot should be obtained, but at higher concentrations a considerable departure from a straight line will normally occur. High cell populations cannot be determined unless they are first diluted to a suitable range.

5. The suspending fluid must be the same as that used for the preparation of the calibration curve.

Turbidity estimations in this way are the easiest and the quickest way of calibrating a bacterial population and they are accurate for comparative studies provided the above points are borne in mind.

An older method of measuring turbidity of bacterial suspensions was by comparing their opacity with that of standard tubes, e.g. Brown's opacity tubes, with the naked eye (see 12th Edn, Vol. 2, Ch. 13 for details). It suffices when greater precision is not required.

REFERENCES

Dawson R M C, Elliot D C, Elliot W H, Jones K M (eds) 1969 Data for biochemical research. Clarendon, Oxford

Kubitschek H E 1969 Counting and sizing micro-organisms with the Coulter counter. In: Norris J R, Ribbons D W (eds) Methods in microbiology, vol 1. Academic Press, London. p 593–610

Miles A A, Misra S S, Irwin J O 1938 The estimation of the bactericidal power of the blood. Journal of Hygiene, Cambridge 38: 732–749

Malette M F 1969 Evaluation of growth by physical and chemical means. In: Norris J R, Ribbons D W (eds) Methods in microbiology, vol 1. Academic Press, London. p 522–566

Postgate J R 1969 Viable counts and viability. In: Norris J R, Ribbons D W (eds) Methods in microbiology, vol 1. Academic Press, London. p 611–628

F. Sheffield

Quantitation in microbiology

Measures and standards

The microbiologist is obliged to make many measurements and comparisons in his routine and experimental work. At the simplest level, he is concerned with relative and absolute sizes of microscopically small objects. In some circumstances, it is quite sufficient to use relative terms and to relate the size of an observed bacterial rod in an exudate, for example, to the relatively 'standard' dimensions of a red blood cell observed in the same field. The fact that a red blood cell is subject to considerable variation in size depending upon osmotic factors, whereas a bacterial cell is rigid, is one of the reasons for regarding the red cell as a very poor standard. When it is necessary to determine cell dimensions accurately, various methods that employ the light microscope, electron microscope or other special equipment are available and these are described in Chapter 2.

In this book, microscopical units of length are used. The micrometre (μm) is one millionth part of a metre or a thousandth part of a millimetre (0.001 mm); the term micron for this measurement is now obsolete. One thousandth of 1 μm was formerly referred to as 1 millimicron (mμ) but is now termed 1 nanometre (nm; 10^{-9} metre). The Angstrom unit (Å; 10^{-10} metre) should not be used now and measurements in this range should be expressed in nanometres (10Å = 1 nm). Thus: metre (m), centimetre (cm), millimetre (mm), micrometre (μm), and nanometre (nm) respectively denote 1, 10^{-2}, 10^{-3}, 10^{-6} and 10^{-9} metre. In general, the dimensions of protozoa, fungi and bacteria fall within the micrometre range and those of viruses are in the nanometre range.

In addition to being concerned with cell dimensions, the microbiologist is greatly concerned with cell numbers. Although a considerable proportion of the observations made in his routine work appear to be essentially qualitative, there are many in which a quantitative element is inferred or actually specified. For example, 'a scanty growth of *Escherichia coli*' isolated from a wound of the perineum may be regarded as less significant than a pure profuse growth of that organism in these circumstances. It must be acknowledged that such measures as 'profuse' and 'scanty' are subject to much observer bias. Much less subjective are the truly quantitative bacteriological procedures for enumeration of bacterial cells in counting chambers and estimation of viable organisms by colony counting, Methods such as these had early application in blood culture work and are now routinely used in the diagnosis of urinary tract infections, examination of sputa and quality control of water supplies, milk and shellfish.

The enumeration of cells in a counting chamber involves direct observation of the bacteria, but the estimation of viable cells defies such direct observation and can be achieved only indirectly by arranging conditions in which each live cell in a preparation grows into a visible colony. Almost all of the measurements that microbiologists are required to make are of attributes that can be measured only indirectly and depend on the interaction of the entity that is to be measured with an *indicator system*. The indicator systems range from the simplest of culture media to the complexity of a whole living animal but in each case the measuring process may be undertaken in a rigorously quantitative manner and so comprise a biological assay, or bioassay.

The use of indicator systems, especially living indicator systems such as laboratory animals, is beset with technical difficulties. The outcome of every interaction between a biologically active substance and an indicator system depends not only on the activity of the substance but also on the responsiveness of the indicator. A resistant indicator reacts only slightly or even not at all; a responsive or susceptible one reacts strongly. Thus, because bacteriological culture media made in different laboratories, and mice challenged on different days, can never be exact replicas and thus react in exactly the same ways, it is never permissible to use such indicators in the way that chemical reagents are used. Reliable quantitation can be achieved only by assays in which the activity of a test substance is compared under exactly comparable conditions with the corresponding activity of an appropriate standard substance.

The standards needed for biological assays of materials of medical importance are held by the World Health Organization which, through its Expert Committee on Biological Standardization, establishes each standard and gives to many an assigned potency stated in International Units (IU). Most standards are freeze-dried materials and thus it is usual for the IU to be defined as the activity present in a stated weight of the dry powder. However, as many standards have been filled into the ampoules very accurately and consistently, it is often more convenient for a worker to dissolve the entire contents of an ampoule in the knowledge that the ampoule contains an accurately defined number of units. WHO standards are held at various International Laboratories for Biological Standards but chiefly at:

Statens Seruminstitut, 80 Amager Boulevard, DK-2300 Copenhagen S, Denmark;

The National Institute for Biological Standards and Control, Blanche Lane, South Mimms, Potters Bar, Hertfordshire, EN6 3QG, UK;

The Central Veterinary Laboratory, New Haw, Weybridge KT15 3NB, UK.

International Standards are available to national laboratories for the purpose of establishing national standards; they are not available for routine use.

International Reference Preparations serve the same purposes as International Standards but have usually been established after less thorough study than that devoted to standards. National Standards are available in many countries and are available in Britain from the National Institute for Biological Standards and Control and from the Central Veterinary Laboratory.

Distribution, mean and error

The repetition of an assay, particularly a biological assay, seldom provides a result that is exactly the same as that obtained in an earlier assay of the same material. However, if the same material is assayed many times the same result is likely to be obtained more than once and histograms can be drawn to show the numbers of results that fall into each of the intervals of an appropriately chosen series. Such histograms may be drawn using either the observed results or a transformation of them, for example, the logarithms of the results. When the observed results approximate to a symmetrical histogram as in Figure 13.1 they are said to be normally distributed; when the logarithms of the results approximate to a symmetrical histogram the results are said to be log normally distributed. When a very large number of results is available the intervals can be very small and their peaks then form the continuous curve shaped like a vertical section through a bell which is superimposed on the histogram in Figure 13.1. Normal distributions have been found for attributes such as height and body weight and log normal distributions for the results of repeated assays of the same biological substance and for attributes such as antitoxin levels in large collections of sera.

An important feature of normal and log normal distributions is that both are wholly defined by only two values, the mean and the

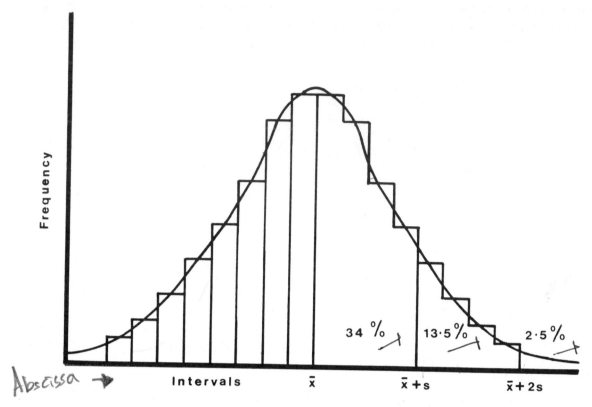

Fig. 13.1 The left side of the diagram shows how a large number of observed values presented as a histogram tends to define the curve of a normal, or log normal, distribution. The right side shows the percentages of observations with values between $\bar{x}$ and $\bar{x} + s$, between $\bar{x} + s$ and $\bar{x} + 2s$ and greater than $\bar{x} + 2s$. Corresponding percentages of observations have values between $\bar{x}$ and $\bar{x} - s$, between $\bar{x} - s$ and $\bar{x} - 2s$ and less than $\bar{x} - 2s$.

standard deviation. The mean is simply the average of all the results and the standard deviation is a measure of the dispersion of the individual results around the mean. In a normal distribution the mean ($\bar{x}$) is the arithmetic mean of the results and the standard deviation (s) is additive; in a log normal distribution the mean is the geometric mean of the results and the standard deviation is multiplicative. In both distributions results that are clustered closely around the mean give rise to small values for the standard deviation and narrow, sharply pointed curves; results that are widely dispersed give rise to large values and widely spread, flattened curves.

The area under the curve of a normal or log normal distribution represents 100% of all the results that may be observed and so the area under any part of the curve defined by two points on the abscissa represents the percentage of results likely to fall in the range between the two points. Regardless of the value of the standard deviation, approximately 34% of values fall between $\bar{x}$ and $\bar{x} + s$ and 13.5% between $\bar{x} + s$ and $\bar{x} + 2s$. Only 2.5% of results, as Figure 13.1 shows, exceed $\bar{x} + 2s$. Thus, since the curve is symmetrical, 5% of results differ from the mean by more than 2s, or the odds against a result that differs from the mean by more than two standard deviations are 19 to 1.

When it is possible to measure an attribute of every member of a defined population, for example the heights of pupils in a particular school, it is possible to calculate both a true mean and a true standard deviation. In biological assays however, it is more usual for data to consist either of results from a sample of a population rather than from an entire population, or from a finite number of assays of a particular substance which could, were there enough of it, be assayed an infinite number of times. Absolute values for the mean and standard deviation are therefore unobtainable, but meaningful estimates can usually be calculated from even very limited data.

Table 13.1 shows in column 1 the estimates in IU/ml of twelve assays of a human tetanus immunoglobulin. Histograms drawn using the observed values and their logarithms do not give a clear indication of whether the values are distributed normally or log normally but, as there is a good deal of external evidence suggesting that such values are log normally distributed, the mean and the standard deviation are calculated on this assumption. Thus, whereas in the case of a normal distribution the observed estimates would be used for the calculations, in the case of a log normal distribution the calculations are a little more complex in that the logarithms of the estimates are used. Column 2 therefore shows the logarithms of the estimates together with their sum, mean and the antilogarithm of the log mean which is the geometric mean titre of the twelve preparations in IU/ml. Column 3 gives the deviations of the logarithm of each value from the logarithm of the mean. Column 4 gives the squares of these deviations, the sum of the squares, the variance (s^2) of the log values which is obtained by dividing the sum of squares by one less than the number of observations (12−1) and the standard deviation (s) which is obtained by taking the square root of the variance. The mean ± twice the standard deviation provides values of 2.439 and 2.335, the antilogarithms of which are 275 and 216 IU/ml. These values which may be expected to encompass 95% of all results comfortably encompass all twelve results given in the first column.

Although the mean derived from the twelve individual estimates is the most reliable estimate of potency that is calculable from the data, it is

Table 13.1 The calculation of the mean, the standard deviation and the standard error of the mean of 12 estimates of the potency of a tetanus immunoglobulin based on the assumption that the estimates are log normally distributed. In this table the calculations are shown in full to illustrate the principles involved but a method that requires much less arithmetic is to be found in textbooks of statistics. Many pocket calculators have programs that provide for the entry of the estimates or the log estimates and give immediate values for the mean and standard deviation.

Observed estimates in IU/ml	Logs of estimates	Deviations of log estimates from log mean	Squares of log deviations
240	2.380	−0.007	.000049
230	2.362	−0.025	.000625
250	2.398	0.011	.000121
240	2.380	−0.007	.000049
220	2.342	−0.045	.002025
240	2.380	−0.007	.000049
240	2.380	−0.007	.000049
260	2.415	0.028	.000784
270	2.431	0.044	.001936
250	2.398	0.011	.000121
260	2.415	0.028	.000784
230	2.362	−0.025	.000625

$\Sigma \log x = 28.643$
mean $= 2.387$
$\equiv 244$ IU/ml

$\Sigma = .007217$
$s^2 = 0.0006561$
$s = 0.026$
log mean $- 2s = 2.335$
$\equiv 216$ IU/ml
log mean $+ 2s = 2.439$
$\equiv 275$ IU/ml

S.E.M. $= \dfrac{0.026}{\sqrt{12}}$
$= 0.0075$
log mean $- 2$ S.E.M.
$= 2.372$
$\equiv 235$ IU/ml
log mean $+ 2$ S.E.M.
$= 2.402$
$\equiv 252$ IU/ml

nonetheless subject to the sampling errors of the estimates from which it is derived. The extent of this error can be found by dividing the standard deviation of the individual estimates by the square root of the number of estimates:

$$\frac{0.026}{\sqrt{12}} = .0075$$

and it is known as the standard error of the mean (S.E.M.)

As the standard error of the mean defines the distribution of means, in this case of means derived from 12 estimates, in much the same way as the standard deviation defines the distribution of estimates, 95% of means can be expected to lie within ±2 standard errors of the mean. Knowing this to be the case it is reasonable to suppose that the true but unknowable potency lies within this range, i.e. between 235 and 252 IU/ml. Although by increasing the number of assays it is possible to narrow the range of two standard errors on either side of the mean, a result such as that given here is sufficiently precise for most purposes.

Useful as the standard error of the mean is as a measure of the range within which a true potency may be expected to lie, its much greater importance is its role in the statistical tests that evaluate the significance of the difference between two means derived from sets of test subjects treated in different ways. The calculations are not difficult and may be found in textbooks of statistics such as that by Bailey (1959), Parker (1973), Finney (1978) and Swinscow (1980).

Estimations of live microorganisms in vitro

The counting of microorganisms is fundamental to quantitative microbiology; the many procedures devised for this purpose attest to the need and to the difficulties.

Bacterial counts

The number of bacteria in a culture or suspension can be estimated either by direct counting of the organisms in a Helber chamber or by means of a Coulter counter or, indirectly, from measurements of opacity or light scattering that have been related to *direct counts*. All such methods provide estimates of the total count but give no indication of the proportion of live organisms, which may be very small. Estimates of the numbers of live bacteria in a preparation, especially if it is a concentrated suspension, may be derived from estimations of oxygen uptake and ATP content, but are obtained more usually by *viable counts* as described in detail in Chapter 12.

Virus infectivity titrations

Estimation of the number of live (infectious) particles in a virus preparation is more complex than the estimation of live bacteria because of the need for a living indicator system. Such a system is provided by cell cultures in which a single infectious virus particle can adsorb to a cell, replicate and cause a readily visible cytopathic effect (CPE). Serial dilutions of the virus preparation are made and each dilution is allocated to a row of wells in a microtitre plate in which cell cultures have been established. Small constant volumes of the dilutions are added to each well in the row to which each dilution is allocated and the trays are incubated for several days. Each well is then examined for cells showing a CPE that indicates virus infection. The dilution of the preparation that would cause a CPE in exactly 50% of the wells is then calculated from the replicates by procedures such as those described by Armitage & Allen (1950). The dilution is the number of 50% cell culture infective doses (CCID50) in the virus preparation used in the assay.

When large numbers of estimates of CCID50 are to be made, automated titration methods are attractive. In such systems the dilutions of the virus preparation are made in small volumes in the wells of the microtitre trays and the indicator cells are added afterwards. In wells in which there is virus, the cells are destroyed by infection, but in wells without virus, the cells fall to the bottom and grow into healthy monolayers. Staining of the trays after incubation makes it possible for the difference to be read automatically by a photometric tray reader that feeds a microprocessor which instantly calculates the titre of the suspension.

An alternative method of estimating infective virus is that of the plaque count. In this method, aliquots of serial dilutions of a test suspension of the virus are placed on relatively large cell culture monolayers, usually in wells in a plastic tray, and time is allowed for the virus to attach to the cells. A thin layer of agar is then poured over the cells and the cultures are incubated. Virus replicates within infected cells, spreads to adjacent cells, and causes small areas of CPE known as plaques. Staining of the monolayer with carbol fuschin or Coomassie blue usually makes the plaques very clear. At one dilution at least the plaques are numerous but sufficiently discrete to be counted; the number multiplied by the dilution factor defines the number of plaque-forming units (pfu) in the test preparation. One CCID50 is roughly equivalent to 0.7 pfu.

Estimations of inactivated preparations in vitro

The inactivation of bacteria, bacterial toxins and viruses by heat or disinfectants is often necessary to make microbial preparations safe for incorporation into reagents and vaccines, but it inevitably precludes the subsequent use of assay procedures dependent on microbial growth or toxicity. Assays based on visible reactions with homologous antibody or antitoxin, however, provide very precise estimates of the concentrations of certain inactivated microbial antigens. Important among such procedures are the precipitin (flocculation) reaction and the single radial diffusion test. (For discussion of the principles of immunological tests, see also Ch. 10.)

The precipitin reaction

Precipitin (flocculation) reactions depend on the union of antigen and antibody in solution to form visible aggregates. Such reactions occur particularly readily with diphtheria and tetanus toxoids and their homologous antitoxins, but only when these substances are mixed at relatively high concentrations. An excellent description of the phenomena is provided by Boyd (1956).

The precipitin reaction is best performed in small narrow tubes held in a rack in a glass sided waterbath maintained at a constant temperature in the range 40–56°C. In the Ramon procedure, serial dilutions of a standard flocculating horse antitoxin calibrated in units known as *Lf equivalents* are made in 5 or 10% steps in the tubes. A constant volume of toxoid, or toxin, is then added to each tube, the total volume being arranged to be about 2 ml. The tubes are placed in the rack and the rack fixed in the waterbath so that only the lowermost quarter of each tube is immersed. Warming of the bottom of each tube and cooling above ensures constant mixing by convection. This speeds the formation of the antigen-antibody floccules which can be observed through the glass and water without removing the tubes from the bath.

The time taken for floccules to appear depends on mixing, temperature, and the concentrations of the reagents, but it always occurs first in the tube that contains antigen and antitoxin in *optimum proportions*. Thereafter, precipitation occurs in the adjacent tubes and slowly extends into the tubes at the extremes of the antitoxin dilution series. In the tube that contains antigen and antitoxin in optimal proportions the number of flocculation equivalents of antitoxin and the amount of antigen expressed in terms of Lf (*Limes flocculationis* = flocculation threshold) are equivalent, and thus the antigen content of the preparation may be expressed in conventional Lf units. Quantitative precipitin reactions are little used today in diagnostic microbiology but are important in the regulation of the amounts of the diphtheria and tetanus toxoids incorporated into vaccines.

Single radial diffusion

Many immunological methods depend on the ability of soluble antigens to diffuse through agar gels. For single radial diffusion a procedure based on the method of Mancini et al (1965) is used. In this method the gels are usually made with 1% agarose but before the liquid gel is poured on to slides a small amount of antibody is added. Wells are punched into the solidified gels and serial dilutions of the antigen to be assayed are pipetted into them. In parallel tests with the same gels, serial dilutions of a standard antigen are similarly processed. The trays are stored in a humid box for 1 or 2 days and then examined for zones of antigen-antibody precipitation around the wells. As the squares of the diameters of the zones are proportional to the concentrations of the antigens in the wells, the potency of the test antigen in terms of the standard can be readily determined. If there is difficulty in identifying the edge of a zone a sharp demarcation can often be obtained by staining with Coomassie blue.

Antibody assays in vitro

The introduction of in-vitro assays of antibodies to bacteria, bacterial toxins and components, and to viruses, not only reduced the cost of such assays but also provided results much more quickly. Of the many methods that are now available the most important are passive haemagglutination (PHA), radioimmunoassay (RIA), enzyme linked immunosorbent assay (ELISA) and virus neutralization tests in cell cultures (see also Ch. 10).

Passive haemagglutination

Passive haemagglutination is a technique that utilizes erythrocytes that have been stabilized with formaldehyde, glutaraldehyde or tannic acid and then coated with an antigen such as tetanus toxoid. When such cells are mixed with a homologous antiserum the antibody binds to the antigen molecules on the cells and thus holds the cells together. The cells are, as the name suggests, passively agglutinated. The test is made quantitative by preparing serial dilutions of a test antiserum and of a standard antiserum in parallel in microtitre trays and by adding antigen-coated cells to both. Agglutination endpoints are read after an hour or two and the titre of the unknown antiserum is calculated by reference to its endpoint dilution and that of the standard. Rigorous controls are always needed for passive haemagglutination assays to exclude the possibility that any agglutination observed is due to non-specific factors in the test serum.

Radioimmunoassay (RIA)

The versatile technique of radioimmunoassay has been impressively deployed in microbiology; an example is the estimation of antibodies in human sera to pneumococcal polysaccharides. Serial dilutions of a reference serum are made and mixed with an excess of a radioactive preparation of the polysaccharide of interest. The antigen-antibody complexes that form are precipitated with $(NH_4)_2SO_4$, washed, counted and assayed for nitrogen, and a curve is drawn relating count to nitrogen content. Test sera appropriately diluted are mixed with quantities of labelled antigen similar to that used to construct the curve and the complexes are similarly precipitated, washed, and counted. The count from each test serum is related to antibody nitrogen by reference to the curve obtained with the reference serum and the antibody content of the test sera expressed in ng of antibody N/ml.

Enzyme linked immunosorbent assay (ELISA)

ELISA of antibodies relies on the ability of many antigens to bind to polystyrene. In this method, described in detail by Voller et al (1977), the wells of a microtitre tray are first filled with a dilute solution of the appropriate antigen and time is allowed for the antigen to bind to the polystyrene before any excess is washed away. Serial dilutions of a standard and of test antisera are then added to the wells and time is allowed for antibody to bind to the fixed antigen. Excess is again washed away. Next a small amount of antibody, usually prepared in a rabbit or goat, and directed against the globulins of the standard and test sera is added. This antibody, prior to use, is linked with an enzyme such as alkaline phosphatase or horseradish peroxidase and so the enzyme also is linked to the standard and test sera fixed in the wells. Excess of this antibody is then washed away and a small amount of a substrate that changes colour under the influence of the enzyme is added. The rate of colour development depends on the amount of enzyme present in a well; this depends on the amount of antibody to which it is linked, which in turn depends on the amounts of standard and test antibody that were available for binding to the antigen. A calibration curve in which the dilutions of the standard antiserum are related to the intensity of colour development is prepared and the potencies of test antisera are determined by comparisons with that curve.

Neutralization tests in cell cultures

The discovery in 1949 that polioviruses would grow in cultured human non-neural cells led very rapidly to the use of tissue cultures, not only for virus assay but also for the assay of antibodies to viruses. The range of cells that can now be cultured in vitro is enormous and, by choosing the appropriate cell type, it is possible to measure antibody to almost any virus. In each assay the principle is to estimate the dilution of serum that neutralizes the infectivity of a convenient, but arbitrary, number of CCID50.

If, for example, the need is to estimate the titre of antibody to poliovirus type 1, it is first necessary to obtain a preparation of the virus and estimate its titre in CCID50 as described in the earlier section. This preparation is then stored under conditions that ensure stability, e.g. frozen, and thereafter appropriately diluted, it can be used in any number of assays. Serial dilutions of the scrum to be assayed are made in tubes and approximately 100 CCID50 of the virus are added to each dilution. The serum-virus mixtures are held, usually overnight, for neutralization to take place and small constant volumes of each mixture are then added to at least five wells in microtitre trays containing established cell monolayers. The trays are incubated for 4 days and the wells then inspected for CPE. The dilution of test serum that protects exactly 50% of the cultures from the cytopathic effects of the virus is calculated from the replicates and this value, the 50% protective dose, is the serum titre. If a standard antiserum to poliovirus type 1 is included in the test, the potency of the test serum can be expressed as a ratio or in units.

Just as assays of virus titre have been automated, so too have assays of antibody. In the case of antibody assays the saving in labour and time can be prodigious when serum samples from a large antibody survey have to be assayed.

Estimations of live microorganisms and toxins in vivo

In the early years of microbiology the most used indicator of biological activity was the laboratory animal. However, during the last quarter of a century the guinea-pig and the mouse have been steadily displaced by in-vitro methods of ever increasing ingenuity. Such methods have been eagerly adopted by microbiologists on the grounds of precision, rapidity, economy and, not least, compassion. Attributes such as these justify the precedence given to in-vitro methods in this chapter.

Although in-vitro assays have greatly reduced the need for assays in vivo there remains a number of assays which must still be performed in animals. Preparations of bacteria, bacterial toxins and viruses can all be assayed for infectivity or toxicity in animals, but the assayist who undertakes such work must ever bear in mind that, even within a single strain of a particular species, the susceptibility of the animals to a particular agent can range remarkably widely. The assayist must take account of this heterogeneity of animal populations.

Although all individuals in a group of apparently similar laboratory animals may be susceptible to a particular pathogen or toxin, some are affected by a dose that is seemingly innocuous to others. This has been extensively investigated by challenging large groups of animals with serial dilutions, usually logarithmic, of a pathogen or toxin. In an experiment with a large number of appropriately chosen dilutions each inoculated into, say, 100 animals, a result such as that shown in Figure 13.2a might well be obtained. The feature of this figure is that as the dilution increases the percentage of survivors increases also. Moreover, whereas at the extremes of the dilution range the change in the death rate between adjacent dilutions is small, in the middle of the range it is quite large.

From the top of the curve in Figure 13.2a it is possible to drop a perpendicular to the abscissa and to read off, albeit a little inaccurately, the dilution of the pathogen that kills virtually all animals. Similarly it is possible to determine from the bottom of the curve, but

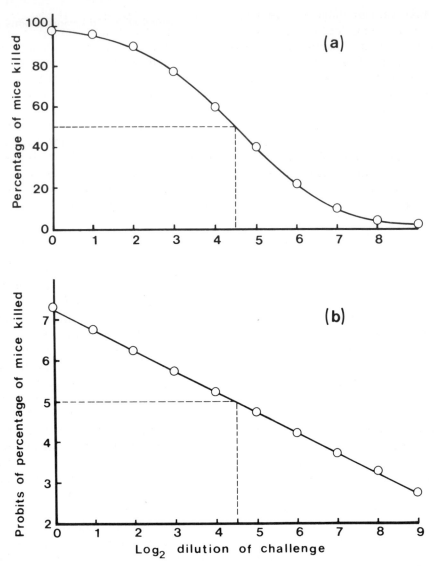

Fig. 13.2 Log dose-response curves showing the mortalities caused by different doses of a pathogen or toxin. Fig. 13.2a shows the typical sigmoid curve obtained by plotting the percentages of mortalities against log doses; Fig. 13.2b the straight line obtained by plotting the probits of the percentages of mortalities against log dose.

equally inaccurately, the dilution that almost all animals withstand. Much more useful, however, is a perpendicular dropped from the intercept of the log dose-response curve and the 50% mortality line. This intercept can be located accurately by reason of the steepness of the slope at this point and so the perpendicular at its intersection with the abscissa provides a correspondingly accurate estimate of the dilution which, had it been one of the dilution series, would have killed exactly 50% of the animals. Each dose of this dilution would contain one 50% lethal dose

or 1 LD50. The methods of Reed & Muench (1938) can be used to calculate the precise dilution that contains 1 LD50 in each dose but it is usually sufficient to plot the curve on semi-logarithmic paper with the dilutions on the logarithmic abscissa and the percentages of survivors on the ordinate and to read off the required value. (See also Ch. 49.)

A difficulty that is often experienced in the drawing of graphs such as that shown in Figure 13.2a, especially when the available points are few, is that the fitting of the curve to the points requires a certain amount of guesswork which leads to uncertainty about the true position of the curve and thus the intersection of the curve with the line representing 50% mortalities. Moreover, the animals towards the extremes of the dilution series are largely wasted as they provide little help with the guessing. These difficulties may be at least partly resolved by transforming the observed percentages of mortalities in each group into values that replace the curve with a straight line. The transformation most often used for this purpose is the *probit* transformation in which the percentages are transformed into corresponding values known as probits by reference to a compendium of statistical tables. The probit corresponding to 50% is 5, lower percentages having probits that diminish towards zero and higher percentages probits that increase towards 10. The conversion of the percentages of mortalities in Figure 13.2a to their probits provides a series of values which, when plotted on the same abscissa, yields the straight line shown on Figure 13.2b. All of the points can be used in the positioning of the line and, if the best possible fit is required, it can be readily calculated by regression analysis. Once the line is fitted the relationship of all probits to doses is established and thus, by reference again to a table of probits, the relationship of all percentages of mortality to dose. In circumstances in which it is possible to use doses that kill or otherwise affect between 10 and 90% of the subjects it is sufficient to use only three serial doses to establish a reliable dose or log dose response curve as long as the doses encompass the dose which would result in a response in 50% of subjects. It must always be remembered, however, that probits are related to the normal distribution and provide straight lines from sigmoid curves only when the observed responses are normally or log normally distributed.

Assays of antibody and antitoxin in vivo

Assays of antibody in vivo measure the true neutralizing potency of an antiserum rather than the combining property that is measured in most in-vitro assays. As these two properties of an antiserum seldom correspond exactly, the in-vivo tests remain necessary for the potency assay of all prophylactic and therapeutic antisera. Very many antitoxins were, in the past, assayed by in-vivo methods but today such procedures are seldom needed in human medicine other than for the potency assay of tetanus antitoxins and immunoglobulins.

In the assay of tetanus antitoxin it is first necessary to determine the correct quantity of toxin to be used. A series of dilutions of tetanus toxin is made in, say, 2-fold steps and the volumes are made up to 4 ml. Next, 1 ml of a solution containing 1 IU/ml of standard antitoxin is mixed with each dilution. After 30–45 min, during which time the toxin and antitoxin interact, 0.5 ml volumes of each mixture are injected into two or more mice. Mixtures containing toxin at low dilution contain some un-neutralized toxin and cause paralysis in the injected animals: mixtures containing toxin at high dilution are without un-neutralized toxin and so are innocuous. Somewhere in the series there is likely to be a mixture that causes paralysis adjacent to a mixture that does not.

In the second stage of the assay a series of dilutions is made in 5 or 10% steps in the range between the adjacent mixtures identified in the first stage. Antitoxin is added as before and more mice are inoculated. Observation of the animals identifies a mixture that causes an obvious but not disabling paralysis on the fourth day. This mixture contains in each 0.5 ml one test dose, the Lp/10 dose, i.e. the dose of toxin which, when mixed with 0.1 IU of antitoxin, is just sufficient to cause paralysis in a mouse 4 days after injection.

In the third stage, serial quantities of the standard antitoxin in the range 0.5–2 IU are placed in a series of tubes and, in so far as a guess allows, similar quantities of test antitoxin are placed in a similar series of tubes. The volumes are made up to 4 ml and then 1 ml of the tetanus toxin diluted to contain 10 Lp/10 doses/ml is added to each tube. After 30–45 min, the mixtures from each tube are injected into mice. Again the mice are observed for paralysis for 4 days.

In the series of mixtures made with the standard, that containing 1 IU of antitoxin is likely to cause paralysis on the fourth day as it contains the Lp/10 dose of toxin and 0.1 IU of antitoxin in each 0.5 ml dose. In the series of mixtures made with the test preparation, any may cause paralysis on the fourth day, but the one that does must clearly contain an amount of antitoxin equivalent to that in the standard series that had the same effect, i.e. 1 IU. Calculations that take account of the dilution of the test preparation rapidly provide the potency of the test antitoxin in IU/ml.

Assays performed as described above give sharp endpoints but are rather insensitive as they estimate antitoxin levels only down to 1 IU/ml. If the small amounts of antitoxin often present in human sera are to be assayed, smaller doses of toxin, e.g. the Lp/100 or Lp/1000 doses, are used but considerable experience is needed in the recognition of the endpoint.

Estimation of protective potency

An antiserum, vaccine or antibiotic may reasonably be expected to protect animals from the ill effects of an inoculum of a pathogen or toxin that would cause disease, even death, in untreated animals. Thus the LD50 of a pathogen or toxin would be greater for the treated animals than for the untreated and the difference would be a measure of the efficacy of the protective preparation. This is indeed so, and assays based on this concept are often used in the early stages of the investigation of a new prophylactic. However, as development proceeds, the need changes to an assessment of activity in terms of a standard and for this purpose comparisons of LD50 are unsatisfactory. Large differences in the dose of the protective agent induce only small differences in LD50 and, furthermore, the results tend to be very imprecise. Worst of all, the method provides only a comparison of the resistance of the two treated groups and that is very different from a comparison of the protective potencies of two products. For this purpose, quantal and quantitative assays of protective potency are needed.

Quantal assay

The principle of the quantal assay is to estimate, under strictly parallel conditions, the dose of a test preparation and the dose of a standard preparation that protect an indicator system in a particular way against an appropriate challenge. In the assay of a vaccine, for example, the doses that are usually estimated are those that protect exactly 50% of the animals from a lethal or other form of challenge and are known as the immunizing doses (ImDs50). As the doses of the standard and the test preparations have the same effects they must, even though they may be of quite different volumes, contain the same amounts of protective activity. Thus the activity of the test preparation can readily be described in terms of the activity of the standard.

Microbiologists who regularly undertake quantal assays know from experience the approximate doses of their standard and test preparations that protect 50% of their animals from the challenge that they use. They therefore make three dilutions, usually in the range 2-fold to 5-fold, of each preparation, ensuring that in each series the mid-dilution dose to be inoculated contains an amount close to the 50% protective dose. The three dilutions of the standard and the three of the test preparation are each allocated to a group of animals, usually at least 16, and one dose is given to each animal.

After about 14 days, during which time the animals that respond to the preparations develop an immune response, all the animals are challenged with the appropriate pathogen. A dose of 50–100 LD50 is usual, but as all the animals receive the same amount the exact dose is not important. At the same time, dilutions of the challenge are inoculated into groups of normal animals to provide an estimate of the size of the challenge and an assurance that it is neither unreasonably small nor large. All the animals are observed for an appropriate time and a record made of those that die in each group.

Table 13.2 shows the results of an assay of this type that was undertaken in mice to estimate the potency of a pertussis vaccine. Clearly the mid-doses of both standard and reference preparation protected about half the animals – the low doses few, and the high doses most. When the percentages of survivors in each group are converted to probits it is possible to depict the result graphically as in Figure 13.3 and, if semi-log graph

Table 13.2 The results obtained in an active mouse protection test for the assay of a pertussis vaccine, their transformation to probits, and the calculation of vaccine potency from the intercepts in the graph in Fig. 13.3.

| | Test vaccine doses | | | Standard vaccine doses | | |
	Low	Mid	High	Low	Mid	High
Survivors out of 32	7	18	29	3	14	25
% of survivors	22	56	91	9	44	78
Probits of %	4.2	5.2	6.3	3.7	4.8	5.8
ImDs50 from graph in Fig. 13.3		7.2μl			0.14 IU	

$$\therefore \text{ Test vaccine contains } \frac{0.14 \times 500}{7.2} = 9.7 \text{ IU/0.5-ml dose}$$

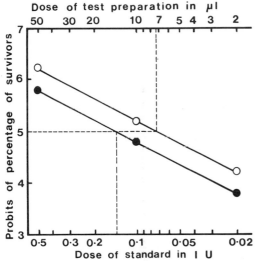

Fig. 13.3 A graphical representation of the results of the 3 + 3 quantal assay given in Table 13.2. The vertical dashed lines show that 50% of animals are protected by 0.14 IU of the standard and by 7.2 μl of the test vaccine. Thus an 0.5 ml dose of vaccine contains $0.14 \times 0.5/0.072 = 9.7$ IU.

paper is used, to read off the amounts of the standard in IU and of the test preparation in ml that protect exactly 50% of the challenged animals. Thereafter a simple calculation provides the potency of the test preparation in IU/ml. However, much better use of the data can be made by probit analysis as described by Finney (1978) as this provides not only a calculated estimate of potency, but also an indication of the precision of that estimate in the form of *fiducial limits*. Moreover the analysis includes tests of validity which warn the assayist if the log dose-response is too shallow or if there are significant

deviations of the log dose-response lines from linearity or parallelism. Many computer programs are now available to make the calculations and save the experimenter a great deal of arithmetical drudgery.

Tests such as those just described are often known as active protection tests, on account of the active immunity evoked by the vaccines, or as 3 + 3 quantal assays, on account of the three doses of each preparation and the all-or-none, quantal, response. Tests with 4 + 4, 3 + 3 + 3 or even larger arrangements are possible and, since the standard preparation need be included only once in any test, tests in which several test preparations are simultaneously compared with a standard are an obvious economy. Such tests have long been used for the potency assay of pertussis vaccines and more recently, in Europe, for the assay of adsorbed diphtheria and tetanus vaccines. Although the description of this type of test has been based on the quantal response of death or survival after challenge, it is perfectly possible to use other quantal indicators such as the first signs of paralysis caused by tetanus toxin or erythema of the skin after the intradermal injection of diphtheria toxin. The advantage of these alternative indicators is that affected animals may be destroyed immediately signs appear and animal suffering is minimized.

Quantitative assays

In a quantitative assay, the activities of a standard preparation and of a test preparation are measured in terms, not of an all-or-none response, but in terms of a response that is, in theory at least, infinitely variable. Examples of the responses used in quantitative assays are the survival times of animals challenged with viruses and treated with antiviral agents, and the serum antibody levels induced by immunization. Clearly a more effective antiviral agent will ensure longer survival and a potent vaccine induce more antibody. The format of quantitative assays may be that of merely two groups, treated and untreated, or more complex with three groups treated with serial dilutions of a test preparation and three groups treated with serial doses of a standard preparation. Relatively simple statistical methods are available for the analysis of the results from both types of test. The disadvantage of many quantitative assays is that they are labour intensive and, despite this, often fail to provide estimates more precise than the less laborious quantal assays.

Microbiological assays

The term microbiological assay is used for assay methods in which microbes, usually bacteria, are used in place of animals as indicators of a biological activity. Two principal forms are used; those in which the assay measures the effect of a growth-inhibiting substance such as an antibiotic, and those in which it measures the activity of a growth-promoting substance such as a vitamin. Both can be performed either in liquid media in a series of tubes containing serial dilutions of the test substance and seeded with appropriate bacteria, or in solid media incorporating the indicator organisms. Though simple in concept, both methods are capable of much sophistication and for details of the procedures readers are referred to Hewitt (1977).

Assays in tubes exploit either the turbidity or acid production caused by bacterial growth to give an index of inhibition or promotion. Serial dilutions of the standard and of the test substance are made in an appropriate medium in tubes and each tube is seeded with the same amount of a suspension of appropriate bacteria. The tubes are incubated for 4–6 h, or longer if necessary, and the bacterial growth is stopped by heat or the addition of a disinfectant. The turbidity or colour change in the medium in each tube is then measured with a nephelometer or densitometer. In assays of the inhibitory effect of antibiotics growth is inhibited at low dilution, and in assays of the growth-promoting effect of vitamins growth is promoted at low dilution. In both cases the activity of the test material can be compared with that of the standard in parallel line assays in which turbidity, colour change or light scattering is plotted against the logarithms of the concentrations.

Assays in agar in plates also depend upon the inhibition or promotion of bacterial growth as an indicator of effect. In this method, however, the measured effect is the diameter of the zone of growth inhibition or promotion surrounding punched wells in the agar into which dilutions of standard and test material have been pipetted. Again, parallel line methods are used to assess the potency of the test material in terms of the standard, but in this case the zone diameter or the square of the zone diameter is plotted against the logarithms of the dilutions.

REFERENCES

Armitage P, Allen I 1950 Methods of estimating the LD50 in quantal response data. Journal of Hygiene (Cambridge) 48: 298–322
Bailey N T J 1959 Statistical methods in biology. English Universities Press, London
Boyd W C 1956 Fundamentals of immunology, 3rd edn. Interscience Publishers, London. p 642–694
Finney D J 1978 Statistical methods in biological assay, 3rd edn. Charles Griffin, London
Hewitt W 1977 Microbiological assay: an introduction to quantitation principles and evaluation. Academic Press, London

Mancini G, Carbonara A O, Heremans J F 1965 Immunochemical quantitation of antigens by single radial immunodiffusion. Immunochemistry 2: 235–254
Parker R E 1973 Introductory statistics for biology. Edward Arnold, London
Reed L J, Muench H 1938 A simple method of estimating 50% endpoints. American Journal of Hygiene 27:493
Swinscow T D V 1980 Statistics at square one, 7th edn. British Medical Association, London
Voller A, Bidwell D E, Bartlett A 1977 The enzyme linked immunosorbent assay. Flowline, Guernsey

Management of experimental animals

INTRODUCTION

Microbiologists have always tried to replace experiments on living animals by in vitro techniques as the latter give more reproducible results. Nevertheless some animal experiments will always be required as many tests depend on physiological interaction of the organs in the intact animal and this cannot be duplicated in vitro. When animals do have to be used, distress to the animal will be minimized if proper attention is given to animal care. The experimenter must try to reduce harmful effects of the intervention and terminate the experiment at any indication of pain or distress.

Legal requirements

Laws intended to safeguard animals from cruelty are on the statute books of most countries. They are usually thought to be sufficient to protect laboratory animals from abuse but, in a few countries, they have been supplemented by separate legislation for the latter purpose. It is essential that all experimenters consult their national legal code before first using any animal for research, for a diagnostic procedure, or for the preparation of an antiserum, however trivial the procedure may seem. Within the European Community a unification of laws relating to animal experimentation is taking place. A *Convention on the Use of Animals in Laboratories* has been accepted by the Council of Ministers and its provisions are in process of being incorporated into the legislation of all the EEC countries.

In the United Kingdom animals are safe-guarded from actions that may be construed as cruel or painful by the *Protection of Animals Act 1911* (*Scotland 1912*). Since 1876, however, it has been possible to obtain a licence that allows bonafide research workers to subject vertebrate animals to experimental procedures 'calculated to cause pain'. The Act under which these licences were issued (the *Cruelty to Animals Act 1876*) was replaced in May 1986 by more stringent legislation, the *Animals (Scientific Procedures) Act 1986*.

Under this Act a two-tier licensing system has been installed. Any person carrying out experiments on animals has to hold a *Personal Licence* signifying their competence to carry out the procedures proposed. Additionally each experiment has to be covered by a *Project Licence*. This is usually issued to the senior experimenter of a group; more rarely to an individual research worker. Applications for the project licence have, inter alia, to show that alternative methods (i.e. those employing non-sentient preparations) cannot be used and to estimate the degree of pain and distress likely to be suffered by the animals. Applications to carry out severe experiments are referred to an advisory committee of experts for advice. Project licences for most types of mild experiment, such as those done by microbiologists, are approved locally.

All procedures that could be viewed as 'experimental' are covered by the new Act including those, such as the preparation of antisera and similar routine procedures, that were outwith the 1876 Act. The breeding and procurement of animals for experimental purposes also comes into the ambit of the new Act and more effective veterinary supervision of animal houses has been instituted. Continuing the provisions of the 1876 Act, all experiments have to be conducted in registered places and these places are visited, unannounced, by Home Office inspectors who hold medical or veterinary qualifications and generally supervise the working of the Act.

Anyone intending to work with experimental animals in the United Kingdom should discuss with the staff of their animal house the licence applications they must make. The staff have detailed knowledge of the procedures to be followed and can also supply the address of the local Home Office inspector. The latter will invariably be found to be helpful and willing to assist. Prospective scientific visitors to the United Kingdom who wish to carry out experiments on animals during their stay are advised to apply for a personal licence well in advance of arrival. Their host should also be informed of the details of the work proposed so that a project licence may be obtained. The Council for International Organizations of Medical Sciences (CIOMS, 1985) has issued *International Guiding Principles for Biomedical Research Involving Animals* which all persons proposing to carry out experiments on animals will find helpful.

Humane experimentation on animals

It is imperative that users of experimental animals give thought to the humanity of the procedures they propose to carry out. In most experiments there are two periods at which distress to the animal may be acute; the time of application of a substance and the time when it produces an effect. In bacteriology, the methods used to introduce materials into an animal's body appear trivial, but they may not always be so. Tests have shown that the method of restraint is a critical factor. Contrary, perhaps, to expectation, close confinement, e.g. in a net or tube, is less disturbing than other techniques and can be recommended. The vehicle in which an inoculum is made up is also important. A balanced salts solution has a measurably less disturbing effect on mice than the more commonly used 0.9% sodium chloride solution.

The consequences of a microbiological experiment may be acutely distressing. Animals may develop inflammation, painful abscesses or illness leading to death. Possible pain and distress must be sympathetically and frequently considered and the animal should be killed immediately the information sought has been obtained. A decision as to the point at which it is to be killed should be agreed before the experiment is started. Until proper information is available, decisions on the degree of pain and distress felt by an animal have to be made by drawing on human experience. It must be realized, however, that this may not always be a good guide. Things that appear innocuous to man may be highly disturbing to another species and vice versa.

So that immediate decisions can be made if an animal is in distress it is essential that contact telephone numbers of the experimenters, both in and out of hours, be available. If the user is away, a deputy, who may be an animal technician, must be informed. Failing all, it should be understood, and so stated in the animal house Code of Practice, that the technician-in-charge has authority to kill or treat with analgesics any animal that appears to be in pain or distress.

The animal user should ensure that attention is not gratuitously drawn to the existence of animal experimentation. In many countries there are groups of persons opposed to the use of animals for any kind of experiment, however innocuous. Their activities may be · violent, including the forcible entry of premises, the release of animals and vandalism of apparatus. Animal houses should be inconspicuous, windows screened from casual observation and exterior labels and direction signs avoided. Doors must be kept locked at all times and access restricted to authorized persons. All inoculations and other manipulations should be carried out within the premises; animals must not be carried to general laboratories for this purpose.

Choice of animal

Species

Most species of animal presently used for experimental purposes were originally chosen because of their ready availability and cheapness rather than because they had been shown physiologically to be the most suitable for the purpose

Table 14.1 Physiological and growth-rate data for experimental animals.

	Rabbit	Guinea-pig	Mouse	Rat	Hamster	Fowl
Rectal temperature (°C)	37–39	37–39	35–39	36–40	36–39	40
Respiratory rate (/min)	35–60	90–150	100–250	70–150	30–140	15–35
Heart rate (/min)	205–235	130–190	500–600	260–450	350	300
Red cell count (10^6/mm^3)	4–7	4–7	7–11	7–10	4–10	2–4
Haematocrit (%)	30–50	35–42	35–45	35–45	39–59	25–45
Blood volume (ml/kg body wt)	70	75	80	50	78	60
Gestation (days)	31	68	19–21	20–22	15–18	21[a]
Litter size(mean)	6	3	8	8	7	—
Litters/year	4	3	9	9	4	—
Weaning age (days)	42–56	2–18	19–21	20–22	20–22	—

Growth-rate: Age	Approximate body weight (g)					
Birth	50	85	1–1.5	4–5	1.5–2.5	—
4 weeks (1 m)	600	240	15	45	35	—
8 weeks (2 m)	1300	450	20–25	200	75	—
12 weeks (3 m)	2100	600	25–30	300	90	—
20 weeks (5 m)	2700	900	25–35	450	120	—
36 weeks (9 m)	5000	1000+	25–35	900	—	—

[a] Period of incubation.

intended. Thus, in the nineteenth century, horses were preferred to cattle and sheep for raising antibodies because worn-out animals were cheap. Research workers out of Europe should not ignore the employment of local species if these are easier to procure, breed, feed and house.

Some species are traditionally associated with particular tests and uses. Legal requirements also exist for named species to be used, e.g. for toxicity testing. Otherwise the species to be used will be decided on grounds such as its known susceptibility to disease, its size in relation to the yield of, e.g. serum, and the ability to afford a statistically significant number of animals. To aid in the choice of animal the weights of the common species at different ages are given in Table 14.1. Once the species has been chosen, consideration should be given to the other distinctions, genetic and microbiological, among laboratory-bred stock.

Genetic status

The traditional laboratory strains of rats and mice are thousands of generations, and possibly thousands of years, removed from their wild relatives. They can be obtained as either outbred or inbred animals.

Outbred animals are, in theory, mated randomly. The degree of heterogeneity of the stock depends on the numbers in the colony. Small groups can easily become inbred unless special steps, i.e. the application of a minimal inbreeding program, are instituted.

Inbred animals are the product of at least 20 sequential brother-sister matings and are effectively genetically identical. Variation in response between individuals is thus enormously reduced so that small numbers can yield a significant result. The ability to transfer tissues and cells between inbred animals has valuable uses in immunology, not least in the production of monoclonal antibodies for the identification of microbial species. Inbred stocks have the disadvantage that the genes in each animal are identical and, therefore, each *stock*, rather than each individual as in an outbred stock, will behave differently in their reactions, e.g. to infection or immunization. It is necessary, therefore, to select by trial the stock that is most suitable for any application. The nomenclature of inbred stocks, which may appear complex, is internationally standardized and regularly updated (Staats 1976).

Hundreds of mutant genes have been identified in mice which have effects on responses to infection, coat colour, presence or absence of enzymes, etc. Many of these may be of value in experimentation; up-to-date lists can be found in the *Mouse News Letter* (see *References*).

Microbiological status

Three types of animals are distinguished according to the type of microbial flora they carry.

1. *Conventional animals* are those bred in normal, open animal rooms without special precautions or microbiological control and so carry an indeterminate flora. Technical advances in isolator design linked with demand has, however, now enabled commercial suppliers to provide laboratory animals of defined microbiological status. These may be specific pathogen free (SPF), or gnotobiotic (germ-free).

2. *Specific pathogen free (SPF) animals* are stocks certified to be free from a published list of possibly pathogenic organisms (Accreditation Microbiological Advisory Committee 1972). They are derived from fetuses obtained from conventional animals by caesarian section and reared and kept in extremely clean, but not sterile, conditions. Monitoring for the presence of viruses, bacteria and other microorganisms and metazoal parasites is carried out (Needham 1979). Even if the construction of the animal house does not permit maintenance of strict SPF status, it is still advisable to purchase such animals. If fresh stock are placed in thoroughly cleaned rooms and steps taken to minimize contamination from old stock, intercurrent infections and the consequent confusion of results will be diminished.

3. *Gnotobiotic animals.* The word gnotobiotic indicates that all the living components of the system are known. Normally there is only one, the animal, and these animals are often called 'germ free', though it is impossible to be sure that all viruses are absent. If such an animal is deliberately infected with several known species of normal gut flora, it is still gnotobiotic. The animals are reared in an entirely sterile environment, usually a large (1.5 × 0.75 × 0.75 m) plastic bag kept inflated with sterile, filtered air. This is the *isolator*. Gloved ports and an airlock enable the inhabitants to be manipulated and supplies and test materials to be inserted. Food is sterilized by cobalt[60] irradiation at 5 Mrad, other materials in an autoclave. The outer surfaces of the packages are sterilized by placing them in the airlock, spraying with 2% peracetic acid and retaining them for 2 h before accepting them into the sterile interior. Gnotobiotic animals are costly to obtain and maintain, but are valuable in some kinds of microbiological experiments. They are, however, abnormal animals; thus gnotobiotic rats and mice, for example, have enormously enlarged caeca.

GENERAL DIRECTIONS FOR CARE OF EXPERIMENTAL ANIMALS

Animal husbandry

This section is written for the information of the scientist who may have to oversee a laboratory animal facility in addition to other duties. It is assumed that trained animal unit staff are available. The notes on animal care that follow are in the nature of comments to provide background information and to highlight points essential to the efficient running of a facility. For detailed information on the construction and maintenance of a facility, and on the care and breeding of common and exotic species recourse should be had to the texts listed in the References. A well qualified senior animal technician will also be found invaluable.

Staff

The well-being of laboratory animals depends entirely on the care, humanity and watchfulness of the staff of the animal house. To keep laboratory animals healthy and contented requires a high degree of technical skill and a full understanding of their ways of life. It must be emphasized that trained animal technicians have to bear much more direct responsibility than many other laboratory staff. Their knowledge and skills are not usually shared with anyone else in a laboratory or hospital. They have to be absolutely certain that supplies are never short, be prepared to take action on their own responsibility in any emergency and to make life and death decisions without hesitation. The standard of those recruited and the quality of the training given should reflect these aspects of the work. Details of training courses for animal technicians in the UK can be obtained from the Institute of Science Technology, the Scottish Technical Education Council and the Institute of Animal Technicians.

Beside duties such as feeding, watering and cleaning, the staff are also responsible for continually observing the animals. A general inspection of every room and every cage should take place first thing each morning, so that remedial action can be taken at once and a report made to the technician in charge. A similar inspection should be made just before leaving the premises in the evening. Though apparently onerous, such inspections can be done rapidly. The eye becomes practised in scanning rows of cages for, e.g., empty water bottles, whilst the nose sniffs out irregularities such as the scent of death, and the ear listens for tell-tale sounds of normal or abnormal behaviour. Beside inspections and routine work, staff should be encouraged to spend time with the animals, getting to know them and gentling them. This is an important aspect of animal care and staff are not wasting time when they play with the stock.

The animal house

This should be self-contained in respect of ventilation, air conditioning, access and staffing whether it be a separate building or part of a general laboratory block. In the latter case a basement site is often convenient as this reduces nuisance to rooms below from leaking floors and pipes. Windows should be omitted except where an uninterrupted supply of electricity cannot be guaranteed. Controlled mechanical ventilation is preferable to open windows. Dark rooms enable the maintenance of lighting cycles appropriate to the various species.

At least 10 changes of air in each hour should be aimed at, but it is essential to avoid draughts. A room temperature between 18 and 21°C is optimal for most species, but rabbits and guinea-pigs show distress above 18°C. Daily records of temperature must be kept for each room, read from a maximum and minimum thermometer or thermograph. The relative humidity should not be allowed to fall below 50%. It is difficult to control but extremely dry conditions must be avoided.

A very high level of cleanliness and hygiene is essential. Rooms should be emptied of all stock in rotation approximately every 4 weeks and the walls, floor and ceiling washed down with disinfectant. Any rooms housing animals on long-term experimentation should be treated as clean from the start. Staff entering them should, on every occasion, wear gowns and overshoes reserved for that room alone so as to minimize spread of infection. All visitors to the animal house should be provided with plastic overshoes as a minimum requirement and preferably also with gowns or disposable coats. Steps should be taken to ensure that persons keeping pets, such as guinea-pigs, never have access to similar experimental animals, as they may carry infection to them.

Allergy to animal products, such as dander from the coat and proteins in the urine of mice, not infrequently occurs in animal house staff. Persons with an atopic history should not be recruited for such positions. Almost complete relief from symptoms can, however, be obtained by wearing a disposable hood and visor supplied with air from a belt-mounted pump and filter (Racal).

Caging

Rats, mice, guinea-pigs and hamsters are best housed in plastic boxes with stainless steel tops. Wire-mesh cages are impossible to clean adequately. Plastic cages are also available for rabbits, the skip-shaped ones being the best. Cages should be tall enough for animals to be able to stand up or stretch to their natural extent. This requirement presents few problems with most species, but the tallest available rat cages should be purchased. Cages are available with wire-mesh floors of various types. These are not recommended for rats or guinea-pigs as they cause sore feet. In some circumstances they may have to be used, e.g. to detect the mating dates of rats by observing 'plugs'. For rabbits the only acceptable perforated floors are those with circular, dished, holes. The excreta falling through are caught in a tray that, for convenience in cleaning, contains a thin layer of horticultural peat or other animal bedding. Fowls can be kept on mesh floors without difficulty. Stock and breeding guinea-pigs can advantageously be kept in large floor pens, which provide an ample exercise area, and do well on this regime.

Bedding

The ideal material for small animals is commercial processed bedding, wood shavings that have been dried, sterilized and dust-extracted. It is highly absorbent, safe and non-irritant. Crude soft-wood shavings or various proprietary forms of absorbent bedding can also be used. If obtained from sawmills or joiner's shops, shavings may have been contaminated by wild rats and mice and must be sterilized by autoclaving before use. Rabbits on perforated floors require no bedding, but if breeding is intended they must be provided with solid floored nest boxes and ample hay.

Cleaning

All species should be transferred to clean cages twice a week or more frequently if daily inspection of the cages shows this to be necessary. The cage tops of small animals are transferred to the new, clean, cages, but water bottles are replaced as necessary. Food hoppers should be cleaned as frequently as the cages. Cages must be handled *one at a time* and great care must be taken to ensure that the correct label is transferred with the animals to the clean cage.

If possible, all cages should be cleaned in an automatic cage washer with a high temperature rinse. Facilities must be provided to autoclave all potentially infective material before it enters the wash-up area; steeping cages in disinfectant is a poor substitute. A separate store should be provided for the clean cages and the routes taken by clean and dirty materials separated as much as possible.

Cage labelling

All cages must be labelled to indicate whether they contain stock animals or animals undergoing experimentation. Labels should be of light card and are best attached to plastic cages by self-adhesive tape (Sellotape). Tape dispensers should be available in each room so that worn-out tape can immediately be replaced. It is essential to institute an invariable routine for moving labels from the old box to the new box when transferring animals so that mistakes do not occur nor unlabelled boxes arrive in the rack. Labels found on the floor of the animal room should *never* be replaced by the finder. The apparently related box should be marked and the owner of the animals informed so that he can check their identity and replace the label if he feels that no error will occur.

Labels for animals under experiment should have space for the name of the experimenter, his department, the nature of experiment, the date the experiment began, and the number, sex, species and description, e.g. strain, of the animal. There should also be a series of pre-printed boxes indicating, for the information of the animal house staff and the Home Office inspector, the main interference that has been carried out on the animals, e.g. i.v., i.p., s.c., BS (blood sampling), and boxes to be ticked if the animals may be a hazard to man or other animals or have been given radio-isotopes. Attachment of a small piece of Biohazard- or Radioactive-symbol tape to the label will draw rapid attention to the latter dangers. The boxes themselves and racks should not bear labels as these tend to be left in place when no danger exists.

Food

Pelleted diets are now available for all species and are preferable in every way to home-made mixtures. Purchase only from manufacturers who provide an analysis. Each bag should bear an expiry date and bags must be used in date order and their residue discarded when they become out of date. Sterile diets for SPF and gnotobiotic use have a very long shelf life. It is especially important that date-expired guinea-pig diets are not used for the vitamin C content must be adequate. Animals fed on pelleted diets require no supplements, except rabbits which should receive ample, preferably daily, supplies of hay if they are not to develop hair balls in the stomach. Hay can also be supplied to guinea-pigs but must always be autoclaved, e.g. in large aluminium boxes or old diet bags (multi-wall paper sacks) tightly tied. A proper vacuum must be drawn at the conclusion of the cycle to ensure a dry product. If autoclaved hay cannot be prepared then it should be omitted from the diet of guinea-pigs as it often carries disease to this species.

Guinea-pigs have an absolute requirement for vitamin C as they cannot synthesize it. Commercial diets contain sufficient if used within their stated expiry date. As an insurance, the diet may be supplemented with cabbage hearts (all outer, contaminated, leaves removed) or vitamin C added to the drinking water, which should be distilled water (Glover & Cotton 1965).

It is essential that food be available to animals at all times but there is no virtue in filling hoppers to overflowing every day if the contents will suffice for a week. Rabbits benefit from strict rationing of their diet, otherwise they may become very fat.

Water

Stock must never lack ready access to drinking water. This is usually supplied from individual bottles for each cage, the bottles having nozzles of various form incorporated into the stopper. Piped water systems can be had but are often unsatisfactory; a leaking nipple can flood a box and drown the inhabitants, whilst a dry nipple is not readily detected. Bottles should be inspected twice a day and any discrepancies investigated. A full bottle may indicate a blocked nozzle or a sick animal (often the first indication

of ill health), an empty one that it has leaked. Wet litter, and hence wet fur, can cause death of the inhabitants from hypothermia. Bottles should be refilled as required; some animals, e.g. rabbits and guinea-pigs, require watering twice or more times a day. Regular cleaning and sterilizing routines for all bottles should be instituted; a laboratory glassware washing machine is useful for this.

Disease in the animal house

Sources

Disease is most frequently introduced into the animal house by the inadvertent purchase of infected stock, though the access of vermin and vermin-contaminated materials play a not insignificant part. It is essential to obtain all animals from breeders (not dealers) who have a reputation to maintain. In the UK the Laboratory Animal Breeders Association (LABA) has instituted an accreditation scheme to take the place of that previously run by the Medical Research Council. The best breeders will supply regular reports on the health and bacteriological status of their stock. Animals should be delivered by the breeder in boxes impervious to dirt, wet and vermin, and with coarse filters over the ventilation holes and properly labelled.

Problems with introduced disease can be eliminated by breeding all stock locally. Except, however, for species and strains not otherwise obtainable, the local breeding of rats and mice is uneconomical. Proper accounting typically shows the real costs to be between 10 and 100 times that of purchase.

Quarantine

Animals may be dispatched by breeders in the early incubation stage of disease, or become contaminated during transit, or a latent infection may be activated by the stress of transport. All animals must, therefore, be quarantined for 2 weeks before being introduced into the main animal house. Quarantine facilities for this purpose should preferably be separate or at least have a door opening from outside the main suite.

All entrances must form an air lock, i.e. have two doors and rodent barriers. Commonsense hygienic precautions should be observed, e.g. inspection of the quarantined stock should be carried out after attending to other animals. Clothing and overshoes dedicated to each quarantine room should be available, and the room cleaned and disinfected after each use.

Signs of health and disease

The earlier symptoms are noticed the easier will it be to control disease. Twice daily inspection of all stock by experienced staff is mandatory. Healthy animals are alert, exhibit the typical posture and movements of their species and strain, have sleek coats, show no discharges at orifices nor perineal staining, and their faeces, smell and vocalization are typical. Any deviation from this pattern, e.g. failure to drink or eat, staring (rough, erected) coat, reluctance to move, noisy breathing, protrusion of the nictitating membrane across the cornea, should be investigated. The affected animals are isolated and necropsy carried out on a selection. Rapid access to bacteriological, virological and histological facilities is essential and these are best associated either with the animal facility itself, a local veterinary centre, or a microbiologist willing to take special interest in these problems. The diverse requirements of the possible pathogens are not routinely catered for in most medical laboratories, nor do the animal house staff always have the influence required to get the examination completed with the rapidity required.

It is occasionally necessary to take an animal's temperature to confirm infection or to monitor its course. This is most easily done with an electronic (thermistor) thermometer, the probe of which is inserted into the rectum. These probes are very small and lubrication is unnecessary. Alternatively, a snub-nosed (rectal) clinical thermometer can be used, lubricated with petroleum jelly. The depth of insertion should be constant from occasion to occasion, say 5 mm in a mouse and 15–20 mm in larger species. Small animals have a considerable temperature gradient

from surface to core. It should also be remembered that animals develop an elevated temperature if they struggle whilst being caught and restrained. The normal ranges to be expected are given in Table 14.1 together with other physiological data.

Disease control

Stock animals that are diseased should be destroyed at once and no attempt made at treatment, except for local injuries. Apart from the danger of spread, recovered or latently infected animals can produce confusion when used for experiments or diagnosis.

Animals under experiment should also be killed when any disease that is likely to spread manifests itself. It is essential to be quite ruthless and act immediately to protect other stock under experiment. Isolate the area, institute special staff hygiene (gowns, overshoes), kill all possibly infected animals, sterilize the cages and clean and disinfect the room. If possible the room should then be left empty for some weeks, or used to house a different species.

Animals infective to man or other animals

When experiments are being carried out with dangerous or highly infective organisms the extent of the precautions required will depend on an assessment of the risks involved. Organisms that may spread to other animals must be considered as well as those dangerous to man. With many pathogens the reservation of a room for a particular experiment with staff wearing protective clothing peculiar to that room, or keeping the animals in a safety cabinet, may suffice.

With some organisms, e.g. *Mycobacterium tuberculosis*, it may be wiser, or mandatory, to keep infected or suspect animals in an isolator. The type of isolator required is opposite in effect to those used to house gnotobiotic animals and its physical integrity need not be so perfect. It consists of a large plastic bag with an air-lock and ports with arm-length gloves, from which air is continually exhausted and filtered to a standard similar to that for safety cabinets. A supporting framework is required to prevent collapse of the structure. If the filtration is adequate and the airflow sufficient, working with such an isolator does not demand the same degree of skill as gnotobiotic technique. It is essential to have an initial supply of caging and other hardware within the isolator sufficient for the expected duration of the experiment. Debris, bedding, and dead animals should be sealed in plastic bags, placed in the air-lock and the exterior of the bags sterilized with peracetic acid before the lock is opened to the outside. The air-lock should have a port to permit this to be done without opening the outer cover.

Code of practice

The working procedures and responsibilities of staff and users of any animal facility should be brought together in a document, the Code of Practice. This Code should be promulgated by the highest authority in the institution of which the facility is a part. Copies must be issued to every member of staff and every user and an acknowledgement signed to the effect that the holder has read and will obey the Code. An outline of a suitable Code of Practice is given by Seamer & Wood (1981). It should cover, inter alia, duties, responsibilities and lines of command between the various grades of staff; access; clothing; movement of animals; control of hazards; action to be taken if animals are found to be in pain; action in the event of fire or other emergencies; control of disease; record keeping by users; first aid arrangements; safety of staff and users.

ORGANIZATION OF EXPERIMENTS

Preparation of animals

Handling

It cannot be too strongly emphasized that laboratory animals handled frequently and sympathetically become tame and easily managed. Users should make daily visits to any animals they intend to manipulate frequently, e.g. for blood sampling. A caress to a rabbit, or a touch of the hand on the bars of a mouse cage will familiarize the inhabitants with the scent of the user. It will not then be a complete stranger who comes to take their blood. Animals should never be handled with gloves or, worse, with forceps except when anaesthetized. Confidence should be attained by manipulating well-tamed individuals before attempting any experimental work. Technicians, also, should be questioned as to the presence of any difficult individuals or strains, before manipulation is begun.

Grouping and randomization

For statistical orthodoxy, animals should be randomly allocated to different treatment groups by prenumbering them and consulting a table of random numbers. This process does not always have the effect intended. It is noticeable that, even within inbred stocks, any box of mice will contain some that are easily caught and others difficult to secure (an example of 'stratification'). With healthy stock this probably derives from the development of a social (pecking) order with resultant physical variation. A random number table may place all the slow mice in one box and the fast ones in another, just as filling the boxes one after another will do. It is preferable to distribute the mice by 'blocking'. Set out all the necessary recipient boxes on a bench and distribute the mice singly to one box after another as they are caught, going round and round until each box contains the required number. The boxes should then be allocated, by random number, to treatments. Similar considerations apply to other species, though the differences are not so marked as they are kept in smaller groups.

When filling boxes, ensure that the sex of the bulk supply is known or an unwanted mixture may result. Do not be surprised if male mice, when distributed, fight violently as they re-establish their social order. Every animal must be permanently marked to identify it and notes on appropriate methods are given for each species. It is usual to number animals in groups within a box, i.e. 1–6, but it is wise also to mark one individual so as to identify the cage from which it comes. An inadvertent interchange of cage labels can then be corrected.

Anaesthesia

For most microbiological purposes only trivial anaesthesia is required. Long-term anaesthetic methods, suitable for major surgery, are detailed in the excellent textbook by Green (1979).

With well gentled animals, many manipulations can be carried out with no anaesthesia and minimal restraint. Where some control is required, ether (diethyl ether) is probably the most useful anaesthetic agent, especially for the inexperienced anaesthetist. Its disadvantages of being irritant (and thus productive of excessive mucous secretions) and flammable being balanced by cheapness and therapeutic safety. Some safety authorities may, however, insist that it only be used within an air extract cabinet (fume cupboard). Methoxyflurane is a recommended substitute with none of the disadvantages and even greater therapeutic safety.

Ether can be used on a cotton-wool pad placed below the metal gauze of a desiccator vessel. A tall, wide-mouthed, lidded jar is preferable as the vapour is better conserved. A 3 litre jar (110 × 140 × 300 mm high) with a layer of gauze at the bottom requires only 10 ml of ether. If used properly, 50 mice can be anaesthetized in this in rapid sequence for intraperitoneal injection. The ether will totally evaporate and the animals will not come into contact with the liquid which is very irritant to the eyes and mucous membranes. Cotton gauze is better than cotton-wool in the jar and a shallow platform of wire gauze helpful.

Animals should be placed in the jar and watched continuously until unconciousness supervenes. Mice must be removed at once or they will die. Remove them with a pair of long forceps, not by tipping them out or reaching in with the hand. These latter manoeuvres will result in loss of vapour and the necessity to add more ether. Second and subsequent ether additions are never as effectively vaporized as the first because the temperature at the bottom of the jar falls further each time. This is the reason for the commonly observed loss of effectiveness of ether jars as work with a large number of animals proceeds.

Anaesthetizing animals in an ether jar exposes the animals to pure ether vapour with no oxygen for respiration nor carbon dioxide to stimulate breathing. On removal to the air they rapidly recover consciousness. If longer term anaesthesia is required an ether vaporizer supplied by an air pump or an oxygen plus 5% CO_2 cylinder should be used. The vapour is piped to an improvized mask or a suitable box. The jar method is, however, simple and to be recommended for rapid control of small animals for injection for infectivity or toxicity testing.

Fentanyl-fluanisone (Hypnorm, Janssen) is an excellent drug combination for the production of neuroleptanalgesia in laboratory animals by intraperitoneal or intramuscular injection. If given with the tranquilizer, muscle relaxant and anticonvulsant drug, diazepam (Valium, Roche), it produces good general anaesthesia. The correct dose rates are given with each species, below. The effect of fentanyl-fluanisone can be reversed by nalorphine 2 mg/kg body weight.

Pentobarbitone sodium (Sagatal, May & Baker) is the traditional injectable anaesthetic agent for laboratory animals but has been surpassed by more recent agents. Analgesia is poor, it produces respiratory depression, hypothermia is a constant danger and recovery is slow. Nevertheless it is still widely used. The general dose rate is 40 mg/kg by the intraperitoneal route. Commercial solution contains 60 mg/ml; this should be diluted 1 in 10 with saline for use in mice. The best results are obtained by placing rather more than the calculated dose in a syringe and then administering half of it as a bolus intravenously. After allowing a few minutes for equilibration, increments of the volume remaining in the syringe are given, also intravenously, until the desired level of anaesthesia is achieved.

Notes on suitable anaesthetics are given later with each species.

Administration by injection

Body fluids

Urine, cerebrospinal fluid, blood and serous fluids should be drawn into the syringe through a needle of the same bore as that to be used for injection. Particles that may cause a blockage are thus rejected. Tenacious material such as pus and sputum may require a wider bore needle than those recommended for each species below.

Cultures

Fluid cultures are easily drawn into the syringe though it may be found advantageous first to pour the culture into a small (50 mm) Petri dish, or wide mouthed bottle. Growths on solid media may be scraped off and suspended in broth or saline, or fluid poured on the culture which is then emulsified with a wire loop.

Tissues

Small fragments of soft tissues such as brain, liver, spleen and kidney are readily homogenized in a glass tissue grinder with a small amount of diluent. If larger volumes of tissue suspension are needed or if firmer tissues such as muscle or lung have to be used, an electrically powered blender is recommended. Tough, fibrous tissues such as skin or chronically inflamed lymph nodes should be cut into small pieces in a sterile porcelain mortar with sterile scissors. Some clean, coarse, acid-washed sand or powdered glass that has been hot-air sterilized is then added. The mixture is well triturated with a pestle, saline being added gradually. On standing for a short time the sand and larger tissue fragments settle and the supernatant fluid can be drawn into a syringe. When intravenous injection of a tissue suspension is intended, care must be taken that no large particles are given. To avoid this, the suspension must be centrifuged at 50–100 g and only the supernatant fluid used.

Syringes

Disposable plastic syringes are convenient and universally used but it should be noted that plasticizers and lubricants can contaminate the inoculum (Inchiosa 1965). The mineral oil used in adjuvants can cause rubber plungers to swell and make the piston difficult to move. All-glass syringes may, therefore, be preferable in some circumstances. They are also recommended for intravenous injections in mice.

Table 14.2 Hypodermic needle sizes: metric and imperial equivalents.

Metric	Imperial	Hub colour
0.5 × 10 mm	25 G × $\frac{3}{8}$ in	Orange
0.5 × 25 mm	25 G × $1\frac{5}{16}$ in	Orange
0.63 × 30 mm	23 G × $1\frac{3}{16}$ in	Blue
0.8 × 40 mm	21 G × $1\frac{1}{2}$ in	Green
1.1 × 50 mm	19 G × 2 in	White

Hypodermic needles are described in the techniques that follow by their metric measurements. Most are labelled in this way but some packs still only show the sizes in inches and Standard Wire Gauge. Equivalents are given in Table 14.2.

Safety precautions

Where possible, to prevent spillage, materials for injection should be transported to the animal house in a closed vial, preferably one sealed with a closure through which a needle may be passed to withdraw the fluid. A small hole can readily be made in the cap of a bijou vial to permit this. When filling syringes it is essential to have available small pads of sterile cotton-wool to receive any material ejected from the needle when purging the syringe of air. Such pads can be prepared from dental rolls or pledgets of cotton-wool wrapped in kraft paper to make a packet about 50 × 50 mm. These are sealed with self-adhesive tape and autoclaved. When required, a corner is cut or torn off and the needle point inserted. Protective pads of this type must always be used when material infective for man or animals is being prepared for injection.

Skin preparation

It is unnecessary to clean or sterilize the skin before making an injection into a normal healthy animal. The same syringe and needle can also be used to inject several individuals in sequence. The needle should be inspected at intervals and replaced if found to be blunted or turned. It is, however, important to realize that, after an injection has been made with a plastic syringe, material from the injected animal will enter the needle as pressure on the plunger is relaxed. This material is passed on to the next animal.

All-glass syringes are less prone to carry over in this way as the barrel and plunger are not compressible.

Collection of plasma and serum

The techniques of withdrawing blood for the preparation of plasma, serum or cells are described for the different species of animals later in this chapter. If *clear* plasma or serum is required, animals should be fasted, with access to water, for about 6 h before bleeding. For most purposes a clear product is unnecessary. Unclotted blood for the preparation of *plasma* or *cells* must be collected through a heparinized needle into a syringe containing heparin solution or other anticoagulant. A final concentration of 5 units of heparin per ml of blood is required. Add 0.1 ml of heparin solution, 5000 units/ml, to 10 ml of saline. Use 0.1 ml of this solution per 1 ml of blood.

For production of *serum*, clotting is best achieved by placing the sample in a 37°C water-bath immediately after collection, not in an incubator. The clot should be separated from the wall of the container after about half an hour. Clotting can also be allowed to take place within the syringe in which the blood is collected. This is particularly effective for fowl blood. Collect about 2 ml of blood into a 2 ml disposable syringe. Remove the needle and draw in a small amount of air to clear the nozzle. Set the syringe vertically in an incubator at 37°C until the blood is firmly clotted. To free the clot draw the plunger down as far as it will go without leaving the barrel. When the clot has retracted, clear serum can be dispensed from the nozzle by working the plunger. The same technique can be used with blood from mammalian species but the serum obtained usually contains some red cells and must be centrifuged before use or storage.

Humane ways of killing animals

The method to be used for killing an animal after experimentation will depend on the purpose to which the cadaver is to be put, what specimens are to be collected before or after death and the skill of the operator. In the UK, standard methods permissible for each species are set out in a Schedule to the 1986 Act. Chemical methods, such as exposure to an overdose of a volatile or parenteral anaesthetic produce no traumatic artefacts but contaminate all specimens with the drug. They are excellent for examination of morbid anatomy and histology. Physical methods leave no adventitious materials in the cadaver but may grossly distort anatomy, promote mixing of materials from different compartments of the body and disseminate materials, possibly infective, into the environment. They can be recommended for the collection of living tissues and cells and are often the most humane for routine use.

Physical methods

These involve breaking the spinal cord in the cervical region, damaging the brain itself or removing the head with a guillotine. Repugnant as the last method is to most operators, it is arguably the most humane. Mice, rats and guinea-pigs may be killed quickly by swinging the animal so that its head suddenly strikes a hard object such as the edge of a bench or sink. This requires confidence and manual dexterity or the result may be quite unacceptable. Practice with recently killed animals should be obtained before attempting it. For most purposes mice are best killed by laying a pencil or similar object across the back of the neck and pressing down whilst the body is pulled sharply backwards. Some internal haemorrhage may result which can interfere with the collection of, e.g., peritoneal macrophages by lavage. Rabbits are killed by allowing them to hang from the left hand by the hind legs and then striking the dorsal surface of the neck sharply with a metal rod or the edge of the right hand to effect dislocation. Birds are held similarly, the neck then being quickly extended and bent back with a sharp jerk.

Chemical methods

Exposure to an overdose of a volatile anaesthetic, usually ether, is the method most easily carried out, but ether, commonly used, is irritant and not particularly humane. It is, also, somewhat unreliable in that animals, unless carefully checked, may appear dead from its effects only to recover later. Chloroform must never be used in, nor be allowed into, the animal house unless confined to a fume cupboard as even small quantities of the vapour are toxic to mice.

Carbon dioxide is both humane and rapid in action. It may be used either piped from a cylinder into a suitable chamber or as dry-ice. The latter is convenient when killing large numbers of mice. A few pieces are placed in a deep container such as a metal waste-paper bin and covered with wood shavings (animal bedding). After a few minutes, filling of the container with CO_2 is tested for with a lighted match. If the container is deep, a cover is not necessary except in draughty areas. The mice are merely dropped in, they behave normally for a few minutes, then collapse, give a single convulsion and are dead.

Where the intravenous route of administration is practicable animals can be killed rapidly with a solution of pentobarbitone sodium (Sagatal or Euthatal, from May & Baker) given quickly at twice the calculated anaesthetic dose (see above). This drug can also be given by other routes but its action is then slow and unreliable and three or four times the anaesthetic dose must be given. Animals can also be killed easily and humanely by the intravenous (or intra-cardiac) injection of a saturated solution of magnesium sulphate, but injection into the bloodstream must be certain.

Disposal of dead animals

The best way to dispose of animal carcases is incineration. Before this is done a careful check must be carried out on each animal to make sure that it is dead. Carcases may be kept in a deep-freeze cabinet or refrigerator before disposal but not if any are contaminated with ether; explosions have occurred due to ignition of ether vapour by a spark from the thermostat or interior light switch.

Post-mortem examinations

All experimental animals should be examined post mortem whatever the apparent cause of death. Where death is expected this can be as cursory or detailed as the experimental protocol demands. Where it is unexpected, or amongst stock animals, a standarized post-mortem report form should be completed. It should be filed in the animal facility for reference. Scrupulous attention to such examinations and reports will often enable an epidemic to be identified at a very early stage. Examinations for this purpose may be as cursory or detailed as time allows; a record of superficial signs and circumstance of death can be enlightening when matched with like reports.

Necropsy

For some purposes a very simple necropsy will suffice, e.g. as part of the post-mortem examination of an animal unexpectedly found dead. The body cavities are opened and the organs viewed superficially for discrepancies from normal.

In most microbiological experiments a primary reason for necropsy will be to recover organisms previously injected into the animal. Such necropsies must be conducted with strict aseptic precautions and, if the organisms present a hazard to man or to other animals, in a safety cabinet. The technique employed is to open each layer of the body with a fresh set of sterile instruments and then to sterilize the surface of organs, by searing with a hot iron, before collecting specimens.

Materials

These are as follows: an animal board, cork can be used but an expanded polystyrene slab or tile is preferable as it can be discarded with the carcase; draftsman's pins, skewers or disposable hypodermic needles with which the body can be fixed to the board; scalpels, 2; scissors, pointed, 4; forceps, rat-toothed, 5; forceps, dissecting, 1; small bone forceps (if it is intended to open the skull), 1; searing iron (spatula, etc), 1; Bunsen burner; Pasteur pipettes; bacteriological loop; specimen containers, media and preservatives as required. The instruments should be of the sterile disposable type or have been sterilized by autoclaving or boiling. A sterile tray or cloth on which they can be laid is also required.

Method

1. Immerse the whole animal in a disinfectant solution or wet the ventral surface with 70% ethanol. This is to prevent loose hairs, dander and dust contaminating exposed organs.

2. Pin the cadaver to the board by its four feet so that it is well stretched.

3. With forceps lift the skin over the abdomen and with scissors snip off a piece of the skin so as to leave a small hole. Lift the edge of the hole, insert the scissor blade and make a median incision through the skin from the lower neck to the perineum. Make subsidiary incisions outwards along the upper parts of the limbs. Hold the skin away from the body as these cuts are made so as not to puncture the body wall. Discard the instruments.

4. Take a fresh pair of forceps and scalpel and dissect away the skin so as to expose abdomen and thorax. Secure the major skin flaps with pins. Discard the second set of instruments.

5. Lift the abdominal wall with forceps and open the peritoneal cavity using scissors. Enlarge the incision along the median line and cut along the costal arch. Pin out the muscle flaps. Discard the instruments.

6. Collect specimens from the abdominal organs. To ensure freedom from contamination, sear surfaces with a hot iron; if care has been taken in opening the body this may not be necessary.

7. Open the thorax by grasping the xyphi-sternum with forceps and then cut through the costal cartilages or ribs on each side of, and well away from, the sternum, using pointed scissors. Reflect the sternum forward. Blood can now be collected from the heart by plunging the tip of a Pasteur pipette through its wall. If the thorax has been cleanly opened there is no need to sear the surface of the heart.

8. If bone marrow is required, remove a femur by cutting the muscles at their attachments with a scalpel and then disarticulating the bone at both ends. Remove the extremities with bone forceps and collect the marrow by lavage or passing a probe (swab-stick) through the cavity.

9. To expose the brain, place the animal on its ventral surface and secure the head with pins through the tip of the nose and the vicinity of the ears. With a scalpel make a midline incision in the skin over the skull, free the skin from the bone and pin the flaps to the board. Depending on the size of the animal, use a scalpel or saw (junior hacksaw) to make a cut across the frontal bones. Again depending on the size of the animal, use dissecting- or bone-forceps to remove the skull piece by piece.

Necropsy of animals infective for man

All necropsies carried out on animals carrying organisms potentially infective for man, or for other animals, should be carried out in a safety cabinet. In some countries the safety precautions will be dictated by legal requirements, with which the operator must familiarize himself. It is essential that the safety cabinet employed has an approved rate of extract air-flow at the working opening. The method employed will essentially be that described above with special arrangements for disposal of the carcase after examination and removal of contaminated materials from the cabinet.

The person carrying out the examination should wear gloves and a disposable apron. The animal board should be placed in an enamel tray and another tray should be available to which organs can be removed for examination and specimen collection. If papier-mâché trays are available these are excellent as they can be discarded. Small plastic bags should be available in the cabinet for disposal of the carcase and all discarded materials. At the end of the examination the filled bags are gently placed in a large plastic sack held open by an assistant outside the cabinet. This sack is sealed and then placed in a multi-walled paper sack for incineration. Non-disposable materials, instruments, etc., are, if small, placed in a metal box for autoclaving. This and any other container is swabbed with disinfectant, e.g. 2% glutaraldehyde, before being removed from the cabinet. Clearing up is conveniently done by an assistant or the operator wearing a fresh pair of gloves and handling contaminated articles with a pair of forceps. The cabinet itself is disinfected or fumigated with formaldehyde as thought fit.

RABBIT

Handling and restraint

To pick up a rabbit approach the animal deliberately but gently. Smooth back its ears and then grasp the loose skin over the shoulders with one hand whilst simultaneously placing the other under the abdomen. Lift gently with both hands and let the animal lie along the arm close to the body whilst carrying it to the bench. Never pick a rabbit up by the ears alone and always keep the hind legs well tucked in to prevent kicking. Place the animal on a non-slippery surface otherwise it may become frightened. A piece of blanket or sacking makes a suitable cover for the bench top, thinner material rucks up too easily.

Well gentled rabbits require little restraint for many manipulations and can be held by an assistant. If an assistant is not available the animal can be rolled up in a towel so that its head protrudes to allow access to the ears. Special boxes are available which fit the animal's body closely; these have a cut out for the neck and an adjustable division to prevent the animal retreating. Such boxes should be used with care; it is easy to break a rabbit's back when holding it in place or by allowing it sufficient room to kick. Many animals will, however, happily sit in such a box which serves to prevent them wandering off whilst preparations and manipulations are carried out. Rabbit restraining boards, to which an anaesthetized rabbit can be fixed on its back for surgery or whilst being terminally bled, are also available commercially or can be improvised.

Identification

As rabbits are usually housed singly problems of identification are less taxing than for other species. Nevertheless the animals should be individually marked as errors can occur and cage labels become interchanged. A note of the coat colour pattern of individuals may be sufficient in particoloured strains. White rabbits can be temporarily marked with stains, picric acid (4% in 70% methanol or detergent solution) or felt pens. More permanent marking is achieved by small metal ear tags or tattooing.

Scarification

The following materials are required for inoculation by scarification; two scalpels, one with a rounded and the other a pointed blade; soap; ethanol, 70%, and swabs.

1. Clip the hair from an area on the flank. Shave the stubble with the rounded scalpel blade after anointing the area with a wetted piece of soap.

2. Clean the skin with ethanol and allow it to evaporate. With the pointed scalpel make a number of parallel scratches with the point. These should be just deep enough to draw blood. Rub the infective material into the scratches with the side of the blade.

Subcutaneous injection

The maximum volume injectable is 1 ml. The materials required are: a syringe and a hypodermic needle, 30×0.63 mm.

1. With the finger and thumb of the left hand pick up a fold of skin over the back or flank. Insert the needle to a depth of about 15 mm through the hollow formed below and between the fingers.

2. Release the skin and move the needle to check that it is placed subcutaneously and not intradermally. Make the injection.

3. Pinch the needle, through the skin, with finger and thumb and squeeze as it is withdrawn so as to close the track. If this is not done leakage may occur.

Intravenous injection

The maximum volume injectable is 5 ml. The materials required are: a syringe; a hypodermic needle, 30×0.63 mm; scissors, curved on flat, and a cotton-wool swab. The injection is made into an ear vein.

1. An assistant secures the animal and grasps an ear tightly at its base to occlude venous return. The veins can usually be seen easily but if the hair is very long it is trimmed with scissors.

2. Choose an engorged vein at the rear margin of the ear. Insert the needle so that it is parallel to the vein and pointed toward the body. Make the injection slowly as the assistant releases the constriction at the base of the ear.

3. Withdraw the needle while pressing a swab on to the point of insertion. Maintain this pressure for a few moments to seal the hole.

Intraperitoneal injection

The maximum volume injectable is 20 ml. The materials required are: a syringe and a hypo-dermic needle, 30 × 0.63 mm.

1. An assistant rolls the rabbit on to its back and grasps its fore and hind feet.

2. Holding the syringe vertically insert the needle 10 mm from the mid line on the left side (operator's right) of the abdomen at the level of the umbilicus to a depth of 15 mm. Do this in a single swift movement with the needle guarded by a finger to control the depth of insertion.

3. Make the injection, withdraw the needle and rub the site of insertion. Immediately allow the rabbit to regain its feet; this will ensure that the muscle and skin layers move in relation to each other and seal the hole.

Intramuscular injection

The maximum volume injectable is 0.5 ml. The materials required are: a syringe and a hypodermic needle, 30 × 0.63 mm. Intra-muscular injections can be made into any suit-ably available muscle mass; the posterior aspect of the thigh is convenient.

1. An assistant holds the rabbit with its left leg stretched out towards the operator.

2. Grasp the animal's left thigh, from the anterior edge, with the left hand so that a pad of muscle forms between forefinger and thumb about half way along the femur.

3. Insert the needle into this pad of muscle, from the rear of the animal, so that it runs between the fingers, to a depth of 10 mm.

4. Gently attempt to withdraw the plunger of the syringe and note whether any blood enters it. If it does, remove the needle and insert it at a slightly different site. If no blood is seen, make the injection and withdraw the needle while pressing with finger and thumb to close the needle track.

Intracerebral injection

The maximum volume injectable is 0.4 ml. The materials required are: anaesthetic apparatus; clippers; swabs; soap; ethanol, 70%; skin disin-fectant; two scalpels; a drill (preferably elec-trical) and 1.5 mm bit; dissecting forceps; a 1 ml syringe; a hypodermic needle, 10 × 0.5 mm; suture material and needle or Michele's clip and applicator, and plasticized, spray-on skin dressing. All instruments must be sterile. A rabbit skull should be examined before the technique is attempted so that the correct site can be located.

1. Remove all hair from the top of the animal's head with the clippers. Swab off as many loose hairs as possible with a damp swab.

2. Anaesthetize the rabbit. Ether or other volatile anaesthetic is preferred for this short procedure (see below).

3. Wet the operation site with a little soap and shave the stubble with a scalpel blade. Clean the area with 70% ethanol and paint it with a skin disinfectant.

4. Make a short incision through the scalp so as to expose a point 2 mm lateral to the sagittal suture and 1.5 mm anterior to the lambdoidal suture. It may be necessary to lift the skin slightly away from the bone with dissecting forceps to ensure that the correct position has been found. Drill a hole through the skull at this point. Swab away any fragments of bone.

5. Insert the needle vertically so that it enters about 6–8 mm into the occipital lobe of the brain. Make the injection and quickly withdraw the needle.

6. Suture or clip the skin over the site and spray the wound with dressing.

Intratesticular injection

The maximum volume injectable is 0.4 ml. The materials required are: anaesthetic apparatus; ethanol, 70%; a syringe, and a hypodermic needle, 30 × 0.63 mm.

1. Anaesthetize the rabbit. A volatile anaesthetic such as ether is suitable for this short procedure.

2. Place the animal on its back and palpate the scrotum. If the testes are not found press steadily on the abdomen until they descend. They are then fixed by an assistant who places a finger over each inguinal ring.

3. Clean the scrotal skin with ethanol. Stretch it tightly over one testis, insert the needle to the centre of the organ and make the injection.

Collection of blood

From marginal vein of ear. Repeated samples of up to 50 ml can be collected at 2–4 week intervals. The materials required are: a scalpel with a curved blade (or razor blade); soap; soft petroleum jelly (Vaseline); cotton-wool swabs; containers for blood (Universal); xylol and ethanol, if required.

1. Restrain the rabbit by rolling it in a blanket or placing it in a rabbit box.

2. Shave the hair from the rear margin of an ear. Smear the skin over the marginal ear vein with petroleum jelly to delay clotting.

3. Grasp the ear near its base so that the venous return is impeded and the vein raised.

4. With a scalpel blade, make a diagonal cut across the vein. The cut should penetrate the skin and vein but not be so deep as to sever the vein. Alternatively, the cut can be made along the vein but this requires more skill if the vessel is not to be missed. The animal will usually jerk violently as the intima of the vein is incised and the operator must be prepared for this.

5. Unless the rabbit is very tame the immediate effect of the cut is to produce vaso-constriction in the ear due to the release of adrenalin. Vasodilation follows after a few minutes; during this time the ear should not be released nor should any sudden movements or noise be made to frighten the animal. Bleeding is best carried out in a quiet room with the door shut. Blood will then start to flow. When the flow begins to slacken, wiping the cut with cotton-wool will usually restart it.

6. When sufficient blood has been collected release pressure on the vein, cover the cut with a small piece of cotton-wool and press firmly. This should stop the flow. If bleeding is persistent, cotton-wool can be held on to the ear with a wire paper clip.

7. Clean all blood from the ear with a damp swab and return the rabbit to its cage. It is important to clean the ear well as dried blood may cause the animal to scratch its ear and reopen the incision.

8. If blood flow is slow vasodilation can be encouraged by wiping the ear with a xylol swab. The resultant flow may, however, be difficult to stop. If xylol is used, the ear must be cleansed with ethanol before the rabbit is returned to its cage.

From central artery of ear. Repeated samples of up to 25 ml can be collected. The materials required are: fentanyl-fluanisone sedative; a 2 ml syringe; a hypodermic needle, 25 × 0.5 mm, for sedation; scalpel or scissors; soap; ethanol, 70%; a hypodermic needle, 40 × 0.8 mm, for bleeding; 50 ml test tube, and a cotton-wool swab.

1. Sedate the animal with fentanyl-fluanisone. This causes vasodilation (see below).

2. Remove the hair over the central artery of the ear with the scalpel or scissors. Clean the skin with 70% ethanol.

3. Place the needle over the artery in line with it and with the point towards the animal's head. Place the test-tube at the needle hub.

4. Insert the needle into the artery. The blood flow will be very rapid and the test tube will fill in a few minutes.

5. Compress the artery with a cotton-wool swab and remove the needle. Press for several minutes to stop blood leakage.

From the heart. Up to 150 ml blood can be collected by terminal bleeding from the heart.

The materials required are: fentanyl-fluanisone sedative; a 2 ml syringe; a hypodermic needle, 25 × 0.5 mm, for sedation; a restraining board with clamps for legs; ethanol, 70%; a transfusion set, two hypodermic needles, 40 × 0.8 mm for bleeding, and a sterile blood bottle.

1. Sedate the rabbit by injecting fentanyl-fluanisone into an ear vein.

2. When sedated transfer the animal to the restraining table and secure it by all four legs. Moisten the chest wall with ethanol.

3. Attach a needle to the transfusion set and the latter to the blood bottle. Insert a second needle in the cap of this to provide an air outlet.

4. With the thumb identify the site on the chest where the heart beat is felt most strongly. Push the bleeding needle through the chest wall at this site to a depth of 20–30 mm. Blood should flow if the needle has been placed correctly. If no blood appears, locate the heart with the tip of the needle and insert it.

5. An assistant now stands on the right side of the animal with a hand on the abdomen to restrain the animal if hypoxaemic convulsions occur.

6. Monitor the heart rate with a thumb at the site of needle insertion. When the heart slows the assistant should release the hind legs and raise the lower part of the animal to maintain blood pressure for as long as possible.

Anaesthesia

Ether is safe but produces considerable excitement on induction. Pentobarbitone at a maximum intravenous dosage of 45 mg/kg body weight will produce light surgical anaesthesia for about 15 min but the recovery time is long. Fentanyl-fluanisone at 0.5 ml/kg intramuscularly produces deep sedation and analgesia for about 30 min. A higher dose, 2 ml/kg should be given by the intravenous route for terminal bleeding.

Antiserum production

The rabbit is widely used for the production of antisera because it responds well to immunization and convenient volumes of blood can readily be collected. Innumerable immunization

protocols have been described in the literature (Herbert 1978); all have their adherents but few are based on comparative experimental data. The following maxims may be found useful:

1. Early antibodies are more specific than those resulting from repeated booster immunizations.

2. Particulate antigens given intravenously stimulate agglutinating IgM type antibodies.

3. Soluble antigens stimulate precipitating IgG type antibodies.

4. Particulate antigens stimulate a rapid response if given intravenously.

5. Soluble antigens should be given subcutaneously or intramuscularly with a depot-forming adjuvant such as alum or in a water-in-oil emulsion.

6. Stable soluble antigens (pure proteins such as ovalbumin) with adjuvant can be given as a single dose.

7. Labile soluble antigens must be given as repeated doses.

8. When depot-forming adjuvants are used patience is an important ingredient of success.

Particulate antigens

Materials such as killed whole bacteria usually stimulate a good antibody response if given intravenously as four to six doses, of gradually increasing amount, at 3 day intervals. Large quantities of antigen are not required for the immunization, 0.5 ml doses containing 10^9 organisms/ml are adequate. A small quantity of blood should be collected just before each injection and tested for agglutinating activity. The main bleed is taken 5 days after the last dose. If the rabbit responds well, anaphylactic shock may occur when the later doses are given. Adrenalin and a syringe must, therefore, be kept at hand.

Stable soluble antigens

Substances that are likely to be stable at 37°C over a reasonable period of time, e.g. serum proteins, toxoids, etc. should be administered in a water-in-oil emulsion or in Freund's complete adjuvant. The latter stimulates the best response but invariably produces an abscess at the injection site. Antibodies to proteins of the tubercle bacillus, as well as against the antigen incorporated into it are also stimulated.

The basis for these two adjuvants is a mineral oil such as pharmaceutical grade light liquid paraffin (or Drakeol 6VR from Pennsylvania Refining, or Bayol F from Esso) combined with an emulsifier, usually Arlacel A (Atlas) in the ratio of 9 parts of oil to 1 part of emulsifier. If Freund's complete adjuvant is required, dried, heat-killed *Mycobacterium tuberculosis*, strain C, or *M. butyricum* is incorporated at the rate of 1 mg/ml of oil. These mixtures can be obtained commercially (Difco).

The easiest way to form the emulsion is to place 2 ml of the oil-emulsifier mixture in a wide-mouthed screw-cap bottle such as a Universal container. An equal volume of antigen solution is then incorporated into the oil in four or five portions. Incorporation is done by taking antigen solution into a syringe and then expelling it rapidly below the surface of the oil through a fine bore (0.5 mm) needle. Between the addition of each portion the bottle is capped and shaken. When all of the antigen solution has been incorporated into the oil, the whole volume of emulsion is taken into the syringe and expelled forcibly through a 0.8 mm bore needle. This is repeated several times to increase the homogenization. For antiserum production a fairly fluid emulsion gives the best results; the homogenization process should not, therefore, be carried too far. The quantity of antigen used will depend on how much is available to the experimenter. It is best to divide it into three and incorporate one part into the emulsion. The other parts are reserved for booster injections. Doses of about 1 mg of serum proteins and 10–100 μg of other materials are sufficient.

Before use, the emulsion is tested for integrity by allowing a drop or two to fall into a beaker of tap water. The drops should either spread over the surface or remain discrete. This indicates a good water-in-oil emulsion. If, on the other hand, the emulsion mixes with the water to form a cloud of particles then it is either an oil-in-water emulsion or, more likely, a mixed or multiple emulsion (Herbert 1965). If this happens do not repeat the emulsifying process but make a note of what is seen and then inject the emulsion as it stands. Mixed emulsions are often more effective for antiserum production than are perfect water-in-oil emulsions. The latter produce very long-lasting but lower responses.

Inject the emulsion, at one site only, subcutaneously or intramuscularly, but never into the foot pad as is often recommended. Placing Freund's complete adjuvant into the foot pad is cruel and unnecessary. An intradermal site will produce an excellent, rapid response but also an unpleasant abscess if Freund's complete adjuvant is used. The site of injection should be examined every few days. If an abscess forms, clip the hair and then treat as an open wound. Healing may be slow.

The antibody response following administration of an antigen in a water-in-oil or Freund's complete emulsion reaches a peak after 8–10 weeks. It then remains at a plateau level for 1 or 2 years, the time depending on the stability of the antigen and the emulsion. A booster dose of antigen, given in saline by the subcutaneous route will produce a maximum secondary response when the plateau has been reached. A secondary response can be elicited from about the fourth week but the peak will not be so high as those produced later nor will it have any influence on the eventual plateau level of antibody response reached. The rabbit is bled for antiserum 5 or 6 days after the booster dose. The site of the booster injection should be observed for abscess formation resulting from an Arthus reaction in highly immune animals.

If the recommended materials are not available, serviceable water-in-oil emulsions can be made by grinding together light liquid paraffin, lanolin and antigen solution in a mortar.

Labile soluble antigens

Labile substances such as tissue homogenates and cell suspensions can be given in water-in-oil emulsions but it is necessary to repeat the dose at weekly intervals for, say, 6 weeks. After a 3 week rest, a booster, not in adjuvant, is given and the antiserum collected 5 days later.

GUINEA-PIG

Handling and restraint

Guinea-pigs are the most easily handled of all experimental animals. Nevertheless they repay gentling and attention by the experimenter with docility and friendliness. They are picked up, or restrained on the bench, with a hand placed over their back so that thumb and forefinger lie on each side of the neck and the fingers round the thorax. If the animal is large it should be supported with a hand under the hindquarters when lifted.

Identification

Coloured animals can be identified by their coat patterns, white strains by marking with stains, picric acid or a felt pen. A similar system to that suggested for mice by Lumsden et al (1973) can be used to indicate individual numbers (see below). More permanent marking is achieved by the use of small metal ear tags.

Subcutaneous injection

The maximum volume injectable is 1 ml. The materials required are: a syringe and a hypo-dermic needle, 30×0.63 mm. The method is as for the rabbit.

Intradermal injection

The maximum volume injectable is 0.1 ml. The materials required are: clippers or scissors, curved on flat; a scalpel with rounded blade, or a razor blade; soap; a 1 ml syringe; a hypo-dermic needle, 15×0.5 mm, and measuring calipers, if required.

1. Clip the hair from a suitable site on the flank or side of the abdomen. Shave the area with a scalpel or razor blade after wetting the coat with a moistened piece of soap. Do not use a safety razor as it will quickly become clogged. It is unnecessary to shave closely; doing so may cause irritation.

2. Partially fill the syringe and then purge it of air. For good intradermal injections it is essential that no air bubbles remain in the syringe or needle. Draw in some air and then, to remove bubbles attached to its walls, shake the syringe vertically as when setting a clinical thermometer. Place a sterile pad on the needle tip and then slowly move the plunger up the barrel, tapping the latter occasionally to dislodge bubbles. This is especially necessary whilst filling the needle hub.

3. If it is intended to make skin-fold measure-ments, mark the proposed site of injection with a felt pen and then measure the skin-fold with calipers.

4. While an assistant secures the guinea-pig, pick up a fold of skin, at the marked site, between the thumb and forefinger of the left hand. Insert the point of the needle, bevel uppermost, near to the surface of the skin so that it will run between thumb and forefinger. Force the needle forward, so that it remains near the skin surface, for about 10 mm.

5. Release the skin-fold and grasp the needle firmly, through the skin, at its point of insertion. Depress the plunger to make the injection. Considerable force will be required if the tip of the needle is within the dermis.

6. Withdraw the needle while compressing the skin along its track between finger and thumb. An intradermal inoculum properly placed will exhibit a persistent, pea-like, swelling on gentle palpation.

Intraperitoneal injection

The maximum volume injectable is 10 ml. The materials required are: a syringe and a hypo-dermic needle, 25×0.5 mm. The method is as for the rabbit. The needle should be inserted to a depth of about 10 mm.

Intramuscular injection

The maximum volume injectable is 0.2 ml. The materials required are: a syringe and a hypo-dermic needle, 25×0.5 mm. The method is as for the rabbit.

Collection of blood

From marginal vein of ear. A sample of up to

0.5 ml can be collected. The materials required are: a hypodermic needle, 25×0.5 mm; a small test-tube; soft petroleum jelly (Vaseline).

1. An assistant holds the guinea-pig. Smear a little petroleum jelly on the ear and then stretch it out to observe the veins.

2. Puncture a vein with the needle. This needs to be done gently; the veins are small and the needle is easily driven through the ear, causing pain and long-lasting vasoconstriction.

3. Hold the ear so that venous return is reduced and collect blood into the test-tube.

From the heart. Volumes of up to 5 ml can be collected at weekly intervals. The materials required are: a 2 ml or 5 ml syringe; a hypodermic needle, 40×0.8 mm, and anaesthetic apparatus.

1. Check that the plunger of the syringe is working freely and then push it fully home. Attach the needle.

2. Anaesthetize the guinea-pig with ether or CO_2. Place it on its back on the bench or hold it in the left hand.

3. Insert the needle in the centre line at the tip of the sternum. Push it forward at an angle of $45°$ to the general body surface until it touches the heart. The beat will be felt.

4. Advance the needle about 6 mm while simultaneously attempting to retract the plunger. Cease forward movement when blood enters the barrel. Collect the blood slowly.

5. Withdraw the needle quickly and allow the animal to recover. It is important that collection be completed and the needle withdrawn before the animal makes any movement on recovering from anaesthesia. Otherwise the heart may be lacerated and fatal cardiac tamponade follow. A mortality of up to 10% may be expected.

Anaesthesia

Injectable anaesthetics are difficult to use in this species. Veins are not easily accessible and if other routes are used, weight-related calculation of the dose is inexact due to the large intestinal contents.

Ether and carbon dioxide can both be used successfully for very short term anaesthesia such as that required for cardiac bleeding. If a guinea-pig is placed in a metal bin containing pieces of solid CO_2 covered with wood shavings it will become unconcious in about 20 s, remain anaesthetized for 60 s and completely recover after another 45 s. Ether is only suitable for short term control because of the excess secretions that it stimulates.

If long term anaesthesia is contemplated in this species the textbook by Green (1979) should be consulted.

MOUSE

Handling and restraint

Most mice are easy to handle with a little practice. It is wise, however, to enquire of the technician in charge of them whether the strain that it is proposed to use is in any way difficult. Some, such as the CBA inbred strain, are very active and likely to jump out of their box as soon as the lid is removed. Young mice of any strain may also do this. Always, therefore, close the door of the room before lifting the lid of their box.

It is customary to pick mice up by the tail, grasping it at the base or mid portion and not by the tip. Docile animals can also be secured by placing the whole hand over them, they will then sit gently exploring between the fingers. To hold a mouse more securely for injection, place it on the bench and then grasp a large fold of skin, at the level of the ears, between thumb and forefinger. It cannot then turn its head to bite. Gentle traction on the tail will stretch the mouse to expose its back and flanks for injection. Rather better initial control will be obtained if the mouse is placed on a cage top and gently pulled backwards by the tail. The animal grasps the metal bars with its forepaws and is effectively immobilized whilst the skin at its neck is grasped.

To expose the abdomen, pick up the mouse at its neck and, holding the hand palm upwards, allow the body to rest in it. The tail is then secured between the last two fingers. The remaining fingers are tucked in below the animal's back so that, when slightly extended, they tense its abdomen for, e.g., intraperitoneal injection.

Identification

The classical way of marking mice is to make small, 1.5 mm diameter, holes in their ears with a punch. Mouse ear punches as received from the maker are not always satisfactory. They should be tested on thin paper and, if necessary, the anvil spread slightly by tapping its tip with a hammer. A complete disk must be cut from the ear otherwise the flap will quickly grow back and the mark be lost. Standard marking schemes will be found in the books listed in the bibliography. The scheme chosen should be widely exhibited in the animal house so that the meaning of the ear punches is known and users do not cause confusion by using a different system.

White mice can be temporarily marked with stains or, more permanently, with picric acid 4% in 70% methanol. A widely used dye marking scheme is given by Lumsden et al (1973). This consists of spots being placed clockwise round the body as viewed from above. The base of the right ear being 1, right forelimb 2, right side of body 3, right hind limb 4, root of tail 5, etc.

Subcutaneous injection

The maximum volume injectable is 0.2 ml. The materials required are: a 1 ml syringe and a hypodermic needle, 15 × 0.5 mm. The method is similar to that for the rabbit.

Intravenous injection

The maximum volume injectable is 0.7 ml of well tolerated, neutral, isotonic solution, but it is wise to limit the volume to 0.1 ml if possible. The materials required are as follows.

Mouse holder. This may be a specially made brass or perforated zinc tube about 35 mm in diameter and 120 mm long, closed at one end and with a rubber bung at the other. The bung has a groove on one edge for the animal's tail. The holder is adjusted to the length of the mouse with cotton-wool swabs. Alternatively a large, 50 ml, disposable syringe may be used. The nozzle end is cut off and replaced by a bung and small holes are made in the side for ventilation. The length is adjusted to suit the mouse by moving the plunger. For use, both types of holder are placed in the clamp of a laboratory stand at a convenient height above the bench.

Other required materials are: a 1 ml syringe, preferably all-glass as there is no lag when the piston is moved; a hypodermic needle, 15 × 0.5 mm; a beaker of hot water at about 40°C, and small pads of cotton-wool.

1. Place the mouse in the holder; it will enter readily. Put in the bung so that the animal's tail lies in the slot, which should be uppermost.

2. Soak a pad of cotton-wool in the hot water and place it on and around the tail to cause vasodilation. Leave in position for 1–2 min.

3. Partly fill the syringe with the material to be injected. Ensure that no large air bubbles are present. Turn the needle so that its bevel lies on the same side as the graduations on the syringe barrel.

4. Hold the tail with the left hand so that it hangs over the forefinger. Observe the dilated veins. Bring the tip of the needle up to one of the veins. Insert it, at a slight vertical angle, just into the skin, then lower it to the horizontal and pass it into the vein.

5. Gently press on the plunger of the syringe, there should be *no* resistance (easily appreciated with an all-glass syringe) and the inoculum should be seen to enter the vein. If any resistance is felt the needle is not in the vein even if the inoculum appears to be entering it. It will, in fact, be in the fascia surrounding the vein and its track will be swollen.

6. When the injection is complete, withdraw the needle; if it was properly placed a drop of blood will follow.

If the first attempt is not successful try again after rewarming the tail. Start near the tip of the tail and work inwards. The technique requires practice. At a first trial the operator may succeed in placing the inoculum intravenously in only 25% of the mice. Preliminary trials should be carried out with an innocuous, but visible, substance such as a suspension of colloidal carbon (Pelikan Indian ink). Mice killed with an overdose of ether usually have dilated tail veins and are suitable for initial attempts at the technique.

Intraperitoneal injection

The maximum volume injectable is 2 ml. The materials required are: a syringe; a hypodermic needle, 10×0.5 mm, and anaesthetic apparatus, e.g. ether jar.

1. Anaesthetize the mouse. Intraperitoneal injection can easily be carried out without anaesthesia but an occasional animal will, on being released, immediately contract its abdomen and eject most of the inoculum through the needle hole. Anaesthesia is also convenient for the rapid injection of groups of mice. The whole group, say six, is dropped into the jar together, removed with long forceps as they become unconscious and rapidly injected. An assistant is essential for this method.

2. Pick up the mouse as described above and inject as for the rabbit. Choose the site so that neither liver nor spleen (on the operator's right) is lacerated and do not insert the needle so deeply that the great vessels are punctured. Release the mouse as the needle is withdrawn.

Prior withdrawal of food overnight, while allowing access to water, considerably reduces the possibility of injection into a viscus (Simmons et al 1963).

Intracerebral injection

The maximum volume injectable is 0.03 ml. The materials required are: ethanol, 70%; a 0.5 or 1 ml syringe; a hypodermic needle, 10×0.5 mm, and anaesthetic apparatus.

1. Anaesthetize the mouse and then clean the top of its head with ethanol.

2. Insert the needle vertically to a depth of 0.5 mm at a point 3 mm from the midline and midway between the outer canthus of the eye and the point of attachment of the ear.

3. Make the injection and withdraw the needle. No dressing is required.

Intranasal instillation

The maximum volume instillable is 0.1 ml. The materials required are: anaesthetic apparatus; a safety cabinet; a Pasteur pipette and a pipette teat. Because of the danger of inhaling an aerosol of infective material it is essential to work in a safety cabinet as used for the necropsy of infective animals.

1. Anaesthetize the mouse and, as soon as its breathing has become even and automatic turn it on its back and introduce the inoculum into the nares on *one side only*.

2. Allow the animal to recover fully while still within the cabinet and preferably allow it to remain there for 30 min after instillation.

Injection of infant mice

Great care and cleanliness is essential when handling the litters if cannibalism by the mother is to be avoided. A 10×0.5 mm needle is used and the following volumes can be given: subcutaneous, 0.03 ml; intraperitoneal, 0.05 ml; intracerebral, 0.03 ml.

Collection of blood

From the tail. The volume obtainable is about 0.3 ml. The materials required are: scissors; a small test tube such as a plastic precipitin tube and a cautery or plastic dressing spray.

1. Cut a small sliver from the tail and milk the tail between two fingers. Sufficient blood will be expressed to make films and counts and even, with persistence, for simple tests. For the latter the blood should be allowed to clot in a 37°C waterbath and, if the clot does not separate from the wall of the test tube, ringed with a bacteriological wire. Serum is taken off with a Pasteur pipette drawn to a fine point.

2. If infective organisms are present in the blood, seal the cut end of the tail by cautery or application of a plastic dressing before the animal is replaced in its box. Otherwise the tail may continue to bleed for some time and contaminate the box.

From the retro-orbital plexus. This is the most efficient way of collecting repeated samples of blood from the mouse. When properly carried out it is entirely humane. In the UK special permission from the Home Office may be required for this technique. The volume obtainable from a 20 g mouse is up to 0.7 ml. The materials required are: a container to receive the blood; a paper towel; a pipette teat and several glass pipettes. Ideally the pipettes should have a tip not exceeding 1.5 mm diameter. A small size of ready-made disposable pipettes can be obtained.

1. It is important that the mouse be held properly so that venous return from the head is reduced.

2. Lift the mouse out of its box and place it on the bench under the left hand.

3. Restrain it by holding the tail with the right hand.

4. Press the animal on to the bench with the backs of the second, third and fourth fingers.

5. Grasp the scruff of the neck by placing the forefinger of the left hand behind the left ear and the thumb over the right ear.

6. Trap a fold of skin from the back of the mouse between the thumb and two distal phalanges of the second finger.

7. Fix the tail with the fifth finger against the palm of the hand and lower the whole hand over the mouse turning its head on to the left side so that the right eye can be approached. Place it on the paper towel. The eyes should now be protruberant due to engorgement of the venous plexus in the orbit.

8. Take a pipette in the right hand and gently insert it into the medial canthus of the right eye so that it is directed below the eyeball. Rotate the pipette on its axis as it is inserted so that it cuts into the wall of the plexus. Puncture of the wall will be felt but blood does not usually flow immediately.

9. Withdraw the pipette slightly (about 1 mm) and blood should enter it.

10. Once blood has entered the pipette the latter should not be moved until the level ceases to rise. Watch the surface of the blood rather than the tip of the pipette. If the flow stops, activate it by moving the pipette in and out of the orbit by increments of about 1 mm rotating it slightly as this is done.

11. When the desired volume of blood has entered the pipette remove it from the eye. Hold it horizontally so that the blood does not run out. Release the mouse at the same moment. Whilst the blood is flowing the pipette need only rest on the fingers.

12. Watch the condition of the mouse carefully while bleeding it, particularly when new to the technique. Properly bled, a mouse should show no ill effects when released. If clotting occurs during the bleeding process change at once to a fresh pipette.

From the heart. The volume of blood obtainable is up to 1.5 ml. The materials required are: a 2 ml syringe; a hypodermic needle, 25 × 0.5 mm; a cork board; adhesive tape; anaesthetic apparatus, and a pencil or rod for killing the mouse. Heart puncture is suitable only for terminal bleeding in this species because cardiac tamponade occurs in a significant number of individuals.

1. Check that the plunger of the syringe is working freely. Lay out two pieces of adhesive tape each about 120 mm long.

2. Deeply anaesthetize the mouse with ether or CO_2 until its breathing stops. The heart will continue to beat.

3. Place the animal on its back on the cork board and quickly secure it with strips of adhesive tape across the fore and hind legs.

4. Follow the cardiac bleeding technique described for the guinea-pig. Be prepared to kill the mouse by cervical dislocation if bleeding fails and the animal shows signs of returning consciousness.

Anaesthesia

Ether is fairly safe for short term anaesthesia but its irritant nature requires that other agents should be used for prolonged unconsciousness. Methoxyflurane (Abbott) appears to be a much more satisfactory anaesthetic. It may be used in a similar manner to ether and it is reputed to be difficult to kill a mouse with it. Carbon dioxide piped into a chamber from a cylinder or prepared in a bucket from dry ice covered with shavings is not suitable for anaesthesia but may be used for terminal bleeding.

Fentanyl-fluanisone provides an excellent sedative for many purposes. Dilute the commercial solution (Hypnorm, Janssen) 1 in 10 with saline and give the diluted drug at the rate of 0.1 ml/30 g body weight by the intraperitoneal route. Maximum effect takes about 5 min to develop. If diazepam at 0.1 mg/30 g is given first by the same route good surgical anaesthesia can be obtained.

RAT

Handling and restraint

No small experimental animal better repays daily handling and gentling with docility and cooperation. Rats can be removed from their cage by picking them up by the tail but it is much better to lift them out with a hand round the thorax. Persons who are nervous of the other animals in a box may find it helpful to lift the animal by the tail on to the right upper arm and then grasp it. An immobilizer made by Scanbur can be strongly recommended. It consists of a metal frame covered with a nylon gauze hammock that extends free on one side. The rat (or mouse or guinea-pig) is placed on the hammock and the free piece of gauze pulled tightly across the animal to immobilize it. The gauze is secured to small projections at the edge of the metal frame leaving the hands free. Injections are made through the gauze. Such an immobilizer produces the least distress and disturbance to the animal of all techniques.

Identification

Ear punches (as for mice) or tattooing may be used. White rats can be marked with dyes or picric acid, again as for mice. Problems of identification are not as great as for mice as fewer animals are kept in each box.

Subcutaneous injection

The maximum volume injectable is 0.4 ml. The materials required are: a syringe and a hypodermic needle, 30 × 0.63 mm. The assistant secures the rat by the neck and tail and presses it to the bench top. Injection is then made in the same manner as for the rabbit.

Intravenous injection

In tail vein. The maximum volume injectable is 0.5 ml. The materials required are: a 1 ml syringe, preferably all glass; a hypodermic needle, 15 × 0.5 mm; a beaker of water at 40°C in an insulated (expanded polystyrene) jacket; cotton-wool swabs, and a V-box. It is convenient to use a polystyrene box about 30 × 30 cm by 20 cm high, such as is used for pathological specimens. This has a V-shaped cut made in one side reaching to the base through which the rat's tail is passed. Its width should be about 15 mm at the top narrowing to 5 mm at the bottom. Alternatively the rat may be rolled up in a piece of towel, secured with safety pins, leaving the tail exposed.

1. Partially fill the syringe and purge it of air.

2. Place the rat in the box with its tail through the slot. Surround the tail with cotton-wool soaked in hot water to dilate the veins or warm it under a table lamp. Rub off any loose skin scales.

3. Hold the tail draped over the forefinger. Insert the needle on top of the tail exactly along the centre line as if to make a subcutaneous injection. It should enter the vein. Blood may be seen to enter a glass syringe if the plunger is relatively loose fitting.

4. Make the injection. Any resistance indicates that the needle is not correctly positioned. A new needle should be used for each injection.

It may help to examine the tail of an albino mouse so that the location of the veins can be seen. They are similarly placed in the rat. The lateral vein may be visible and more easily entered than the dorsal vein. This is a difficult technique to carry out and requires much practice. If males only can be employed, make the injections via the dorsal vein of the penis as described below.

In dorsal vein of the penis. The maximum volume injectable is 0.5 ml. The materials required are: a 1 ml syringe; a hypodermic needle, 25 × 0.5 mm and dissecting forceps.

1. It may be found necessary to use an anaesthetic but, if the assistant is skilled at handling rats, they can be injected without any sedation.

The assistant encourages the rat to climb his left arm so he can grasp it close to its head with his right hand. He then picks it up and turns it over so as to present the underside of its abdomen to the operator.

2. Place the left hand under the animal's back and use the thumb to extrude the penis by pressing at its base. The dorsal vein is now obvious.

3. Grasp the penis gently with the fingers or dissecting forceps to steady the organ and make the injection.

Intraperitoneal injection

The maximum volume injectable is 12 ml. The materials required are: a syringe and a hypodermic needle, 25 × 0.5 mm.

1. An assistant picks up the rat close to the head with the left hand and turns it over so as to present the abdomen to the operator.

2. Grasp both hind legs with the right hand and follow the injection procedure described for the rabbit, taking care to avoid the spleen and great vessels.

Intramuscular injection

The maximum volume injectable is 0.2 ml. The materials required are: a syringe and a hypodermic needle, 25 × 0.5 mm. Anaesthesia may or may not be found necessary depending on the skill of the assistant. The technique is the same as that described for the rabbit.

Collection of blood

From the retro-orbital plexus. The volume obtainable is up to 1 ml. The materials required are: anaesthetic apparatus; a glass pipette of Pasteur type with a tip not exceeding 1.5 mm diameter or a heparinized capillary tube, and a container for the blood.

1. Anaesthetize the animal and then follow the procedure described for the mouse. Collect the blood with a pipette or, more conveniently, through a heparinized capillary tube.

2. For the latter technique, place the animal on an elevated platform or at the edge of the bench. Then insert the tube and allow the blood to flow through it into a test tube placed at a lower level.

From the heart. The volume obtainable from a 250 g rat is 5 ml, which can be collected repeatedly at weekly intervals. The materials required are: a syringe; a hypodermic needle, 40 × 0.8 mm, and anaesthetic apparatus.

1. Follow the method described for the guinea-pig. Collect the blood slowly.

2. When sufficient blood has been obtained, withdraw the needle quickly and allow the animal to recover. It is important that the collection be completed and the needle withdrawn before the animal moves on regaining conciousness otherwise the heart may be lacerated. Mortality may be expected to be up to 10%.

Anaesthesia

Ether is commonly used. It is fairly safe but its irritancy does not make it a good choice for prolonged anaesthesia. Fentanyl-fluanisone (0.1 ml commercial solution for a 250 g rat intraperitoneally) is an excellent sedative and if given with diazepam (0.6 mg intraperitoneally) produces relaxation and analgesia suitable for abdominal surgery.

GOLDEN HAMSTER

Handling and restraint

Golden hamsters (*Mesocricetus auratus*) are often aggressive, particularly older animals and those that have been infrequently handled. If they are to be kept tame they must be repeatedly petted, preferably several times a day. Even so, some remain unpredictable. Hamsters are best picked out of their box between open hands. If then placed on the bench and pressed down with a hand over the back, the scruff of the neck can be grasped and the animal immobilized for various manipulations. The Chinese hamster (*Cricetulus griseus*) is more amenable to handling; techniques are similar to those for the golden hamster.

Identification

Long-lasting identification of the hamster is particularly difficult to achieve by the common methods of staining, ear punching or tagging. If experiments of any length are to be conducted on these animals they must be housed separately and particular care taken that the box labels do not become interchanged.

Injection

The maximum volume injectable subcutaneously is 0.5 ml, that intraperitoneally is 7 ml and that intramuscularly 0.2 ml. The materials required are: a syringe and a hypodermic needle, 25 × 0.5 mm. Follow the methods described for the rabbit.

Collection of blood

Samples can be collected from the retro-orbital plexus, or by cardiac puncture following the techniques described for the rat and guinea-pig.

Anaesthesia

Ether is relatively safe for short periods of anaesthesia. Carbon dioxide can be used to induce rapid narcosis and anaesthesia lasting up to 2 min for cardiac puncture. Fentanyl-fluanisone is an effective sedative at a dose rate of 0.1 ml per 100 g body weight intraperitoneally. Surgical anaesthesia is produced if this is combined with diazepam 0.5 mg/100 g, also given intraperitoneally.

FOWL

Handling and restraint

Domestic fowls (*Gallus domesticus*) are picked up by grasping with both hands round the body so that the wings are secured. They can then be held close to the handler's body with one hand whilst the legs are secured with the other. The bird can now be placed on its back or side on the bench for various manipulations to be carried out. If assistance is not available the bird can be restrained in the following manner:

1. Tie the bird's legs together with string finishing in a bow.
2. Take a second piece of string about 60 cm long. Place its mid point at the front of the neck. Lift the wings and pass the string under them and back to the front. Bend the head back between the wings and close them over it so that it is trapped; the wings are now raised over the birds's back. Tie the string at the front, again with a bow, so as to retain the trapped head between the wings.

This method allows easy access to the wing veins and sites for intramuscular and subcutaneous injection.

Identification

Safety-pin like tags, commercially available with serial numbers imprinted, can be placed in the fore edge of the wing. These give absolute identification of an individual, and can be attached at an early age and left for life.

Leg rings are more easily seen. They are available in a range of colours thus enabling different combinations to be used to identify a large number of individuals. Leg bands are usefully applied in addition to wing tags so that birds can readily be identified and caught. It is important that attention be paid to replacing rings with larger sizes as the bird grows. A spirally wound type can be obtained which expands as the leg increases in diameter.

Subcutaneous injection

The maximum volume injectable is 0.5 ml. The materials required are: a syringe and a hypodermic needle, 25 × 0.5 mm. The injection site is over the breast. The technique is similar to that in the rabbit but the needle should be passed under the skin for its full length and care taken to seal the track by digital pressure or leakage will occur.

Intravenous injection

The maximum volume injectable is 1 ml. The materials required are: a syringe; a hypodermic needle, 25 × 0.5 mm, and cotton-wool swabs.

1. Secure the bird so that the underside of one wing is exposed. Choose one of the veins running over the proximal end of the radius and ulna. If necessary pluck out any down covering it. Occlude the vein by pressure with a finger near the wing root.

2. Tense the skin, and the vein lying below it, with a finger so as to immobilize the vein. The veins are very mobile and it will not be found possible to impale one unless this is done. Insert the needle near the tip of the finger and immediately release the pressure near the root of the wing. This will minimize blood leakage and haematoma formation.

3. Make the injection and as the needle is withdrawn press a swab firmly over the site. Maintain this pressure for at least 1 min. Puncturing a bird's vein almost always leads to haematoma formation. If, therefore, the vein is lacerated but not entered correctly at the first attempt it is best to change to the other wing before trying again.

Intraperitoneal injection

The maximum volume injectable in a 12-week-old bird is 10 ml. The materials required are: a syringe and a hypodermic needle, 30 × 0.63 mm.

Secure the bird so that the abdomen is exposed. Insert the needle midway between the vent and the posterior end of the sternum to a depth of about 10 mm.

Intramuscular injection

The maximum volume injectable in a 12-week-old bird is 0.5 ml. The materials required are: a syringe and a hypodermic needle, 30 × 0.63 mm.

1. An assistant secures the bird on its back so that the breast is exposed. If assistance is not available and the bird has to be tied and laid on its side, the breast is not as accessible.

2. Insert the needle into the breast muscle, from the anterior aspect, parallel to and about 13 mm away from the breast bone, to a depth of 20 mm.

3. Make the injection and then massage the site to distribute the inoculum and close the needle track.

Collection of blood

The volume obtainable is 5 ml from a 12-week-old bird and 10 ml from a full grown cock. The materials required are: a syringe; a hypodermic needle, 40 × 0.8 mm, and cotton-wool swabs.

1. Secure the bird so that the underside of a wing is accessible. Blood is drawn from the veins running over the proximal end of the radius and ulna. Pluck any down obscuring this site.

2. Raise the vein by pressure over the humerus. Working across the body, insert the needle facing away from the bird. Tense the skin so as to immobilize the vein beneath or penetration will be difficult.

3. Draw blood slowly into the syringe so that the thin wall of the vein does not collapse into the bevel of the needle and block it. When sufficient blood has been obtained remove the needle under cover of a cotton-wool swab. Maintain pressure with the swab for several minutes in an attempt to minimize haematoma formation.

Anaesthesia

The anaesthetics commonly available in the animal house are not suitable for birds and there are additional complications in anaesthetizing them due to their air sacs. If anaesthesia is required, the book by Green (1979) should be consulted.

REFERENCES

Accreditation Microbiological Advisory Committee 1972 Microbiological examination of laboratory animals for the purposes of accreditation. MRC Laboratory Animals Centre, London

CIOMS 1985 International guiding principles for biomedical research involving animals. Council for International Organizations of Medical Sciences, Geneva

Glover D J, Cotton D W K 1965 The stability of vitamin C

under various environments. Journal of the Institute of
Animal Technicians 16: 93–96

Green C J 1979 Animal anaesthesia. Laboratory Animals,
London

Herbert W J 1965 Multiple emulsions: a new form of
mineral-oil antigen adjuvant. Lancet 2:771

Herbert W J 1978 Mineral-oil adjuvants and the
immunization of laboratory animals. In: Weir D M (ed)
Handbook of experimental immunology, 3rd edn.
Blackwell Scientific Publications, Oxford

Inchiosa M A 1965 Water-soluble extractives of disposable
syringes. Nature and significance. Journal of
Pharmaceutical Science 54: 1379–1381

Lumsden W H R, Herbert W J, McNeillage G J C 1973
Techniques with Trypanosomes. Churchill Livingstone,
Edinburgh

Needham J R 1979 Handbook of microbiological
investigations for laboratory animal health. Academic
Press, London

Seamer J H, Wood M 1981 Codes of practice. In: Seamer
J H, Wood M (eds) Safety in the animal house, 2nd edn.
Laboratory Animals, London. p 83–94

Simmons V, Cunningham M P, VanHoeve K, Lumsden
W H R 1963 Investigations concerning the destination of
intraperitoneal inocula in mice. Annual Report. East
African Trypanosomiasis Research Organization 1962–63:
25

Staats J 1976 Standardized nomenclature for inbred strains
of mice: 6th listing. Cancer Research 36: 4333–4377

FURTHER READING

Useful books not specifically referred to in the text include
the following:

Festing F W 1980 International index of laboratory
animals, 4th edn. Medical Research Council Laboratory
Animals Centre, London

Hime J M, O'Donoghue P N 1979 Handbook of diseases of
laboratory animals. Heinemann Veterinary Books,
London

Inglis J K 1980 Introduction to laboratory animal science
and technology. Pergamon Press, London

Lepine P, Cadillon J, Chaumont L 1964 Manuel des
inoculations et prélèvements chez les animaux de
laboratoire. Masson et Cie, Paris

Mouse News Letter. Published by The Jackson Laboratory,
Bar Harbour, Maine 04609, USA

UFAW 1987 The UFAW handbook on the care and
management of laboratory animals, 6th edn. Churchill
Livingstone, Edinburgh

Waynforth H B 1980 Experimental and surgical techniques
in the rat. Academic Press, London

Wyatt H V (ed) 1980 Handbook for the animal licence
holder. Institute of Biology, London

Safety in the microbiology laboratory

Those who work in microbiology laboratories are exposed to danger of infection from clinical specimens and laboratory cultures as well as to non-infective dangers such as cuts and other skin injuries, electric shocks, fire and explosion of gases and solvents, burning by corrosive chemicals and acute and chronic poisoning from exposure to toxic substances. In well regulated laboratories such incidents are rare, but constant attention is required to minimize their frequency. The nature of the risks must be well understood and careful precautions taken on a pre-planned and well organized basis. This understanding and the maintenance of good organization and procedures is an essential component of the professional expertise of the laboratory worker – in effect, simply part of good technique. This chapter provides guidance in respect of the infective risks to microbiology workers and their supporting staff. Consideration must extend also to those in the general community who may be endangered by the 'escape' of infection, e.g. by careless disposal without prior disinfection or by the occurrence of infection in a laboratory worker who may transmit it to contacts outside the laboratory.

Immunity from previous natural exposure to infections in the general community or resulting from vaccination gives useful protection against the corresponding pathogens when encountered during laboratory work. This does not justify a casual approach, however, since the immunity may not be complete; unexpected and unusual or exotic pathogens may be encountered in day-to-day work and it is wise to regard all human excretions, secretions, blood serum, tissues and derivatives thereof as potentially infectious. This applies also to similar materials from animals and eggs, whether or not previously inoculated or appearing to be healthy – in fact, all biological materials, even uninoculated cell cultures, should be considered as potentially infectious.

A recent, detailed review of infection hazards, safety regulations, equipment and techniques is available (Collins 1983). The essential information relating to the practice of clinical microbiology is considered below.

OCCURRENCE OF INFECTIONS

It is difficult to assess how often infections are acquired during laboratory work because of the lack of systematic collection and publication of information. However, several surveys and compilations of cases reported in the literature have been published. Sulkin & Pike (1951) sent questionnaires to laboratories in the USA and identified 1342 cases of laboratory-acquired infection, of which 39 were fatal. Sulkin (1961) later described 2348 cases, 107 of them fatal. Pike continued to collect information and published a detailed review in which the following were considered of special concern: typhoid fever, brucellosis, tuberculosis, viral infections, hepatitis and fungal infections (Pike 1979). These data were heavily weighted by infections that were of special interest and study in laboratories in earlier and pre-antibiotic years. Harrington & Shannon (1976) sent questionnaires to 24 000 medical laboratory workers in Britain and made a general survey of safety and health care in British medical laboratories (Harrington & Shannon 1977). They found that in the period 1971–73 the general pattern of sickness absence and accidents resembled that of other working populations, with less sickness absence than other comparable occupational groups, but with excess tuberculosis, diarrhoea, dermatitis, hepatitis and shigellosis in the laboratory group (Harrington 1976).

Most reports concern 'numerators', the numbers of infections recorded on an inevitably selective and incomplete basis. For a valid assessment of the risks and trends one requires the numerators to be associated with corresponding denominators, i.e. the defined populations at risk, normally expressed as person-years of exposure. Such surveys of clinical laboratories in Britain were initiated on a continuing basis by the Association of Clinical Pathologists because of concern about hepatitis. Questionnaires to collect both numerators and denominators were sent out, allowing valid attack rates to be calculated and trends to be assessed even with incomplete data, although the majority of laboratories did in fact cooperate. Crude attack rates of hepatitis fell markedly from 123/100 000 person-years in 1970–74 to 27 in 1975–79 (Grist 1981a). These surveys were extended to cover all types of infection and to additional laboratories identified with the help of the Institute of Medical Laboratory Sciences (Grist 1981b, 1983). The first 5 years of this extended survey (Grist & Emslie 1985) confirm the continued but low incidence of tuberculosis, hepatitis, bacterial bowel infections and various other infections in laboratory workers.

Tuberculosis

This has long been recognized as presenting a serious hazard to laboratory workers. In the recent British surveys 33 cases were reported in the 5 years 1979–83, the incidence rate being 43.8/100 000 person-years. Of these, 12 cases were due to reactivation of pre-existing tuberculosis or other non-occupational factors (Grist & Emslie 1985). The highest incidence was found in mortuary and post-mortem workers,

both medical and other, and in microbiology technicians. This finding is compatible with the main cause being aerosols (see below) generated during the work.

Hepatitis

Hepatitis has also been prominent in reports over the years. In Britain, the incidence in laboratory workers fell markedly after 1974 and during the 5 years 1979–83 the survey revealed 23 cases, the incidence rate being 30.6/100 000 person-years. Of these, the six hepatitis-A infections and one of infectious mononucleosis were attributed to exposure in the general community. There were 11 cases of hepatitis B (plus two not attributed to laboratory work) and three of hepatitis other than type A or B. In these latter 14 cases laboratory infection was known, suspected or at least not excluded (incidence rate 18.6). One of these cases was the only fatality – a mortuary technician who had suffered cuts during his work but had no recognized exposure to hepatitis, and whose infection was diagnosed as 'Non-A Non-B' hepatitis (Grist & Emslie 1985). In most of these cases no accident leading to infection had been recognized, but the highest incidence rates were found in haematology, biochemistry and mortuary post-mortem workers, the high rate of infection being compatible with exposure to blood and infection by overt or inapparent parenteral routes.

Bowel infections

The 1979–83 survey revealed 21 infections, all involving microbiology MLSOs except for one medical virologist who blamed a chicken meal. Infections with shigellae (13 cases) predominated over those with salmonellae (6) and campylobacters (2). Accidental exposure in the laboratory was recorded in seven cases and suspected in several others, emphasizing the need for immaculate technique by microbiology bench workers for their own protection as well as to protect their work from cross-contamination. Ingestion is the likeliest route of infection in this group.

Salmonella typhi was not reported as a laboratory-acquired infection during this survey in Britain, but it is not only the most dangerous, and still potentially lethal, of the intestinal pathogens but has also been an important cause of infection in laboratories in the USA. Blaser & Feldman (1980) reported 24 cases of laboratory-acquired typhoid fever during 33 months in the USA; 21 of these were caused by *S. typhi* deliberately introduced into the laboratories for proficiency testing or research. One of the shigella infections reported in the British survey also arose from quality control testing (Grist & Emslie 1985).

Other infections

Many other laboratory-acquired infections have been reported over the years (Collins 1983). In the 1979–83 survey in Britain they included 12 cases of uncharacterized diarrhoea of uncertain significance. Streptococcal sepsis occurred in persons engaged in morbid anatomy and post-mortem examinations. Malaria was acquired by accidental needle-stick injury during collection of a blood sample. Brucellosis followed work on the open bench with blood cultures from an unsuspected case. Work with *Coxiella burneti*, rickettsiae, *Chlamydia psittaci* and *Francisella tularensis* has long been recognized to entail a high risk of accidental infection, but no such cases were reported in the 1979–83 British survey.

All occupations have their special hazards but although there are risks of infection in laboratory work with microorganisms, they are well recognized and can be contained by good laboratory practice. That this is so is shown by the very small number of infections acquired in recent years in clinical laboratories in relation to the large number of staff employed.

ROUTES OF INFECTION

Inoculation

Literally, inoculation means the introduction of material into an 'eye', as in the horticultural practice of grafting, and by analogy it covers the deliberate or accidental introduction of infection into the body, particularly by a breach of its surface. Thus, it covers the introduction of infection into the eye by splashing or by rubbing with contaminated fingers, injection through the skin by needle-stick injury or the bite of an ectoparasite, incision with a sharp instrument or broken glass, and inunction by the rubbing of material on to the skin or a mucous membrane. There are a few pathogens that can penetrate the skin or mucosa spontaneously, but usually the epithelia have small breaches of continuity that allow a wider range of microbes to reach the tissues.

Ingestion

Infection by the oral route may take place by the licking, sucking or accidental swallowing of infective material. It is specially liable to occur in the mouth-pipetting of cultures or other infected fluids. The cotton-wool plug in the upper end of a pipette does not protect against the risk and the finger placed at the upper end to control the pipette also touches the lips and may itself be contaminated. Infection may also be ingested after touching the mouth with contaminated fingers or writing instruments, or by licking labels contaminated by the fingers, or during eating, drinking or smoking in the laboratory.

Inhalation

Infection may take place by the breathing-in of an infected aerosol or dust. An *aerosol* is a cloud of small droplets of liquid in air. It usually contains many droplets smaller than 0.1 mm in diameter and these droplets dry rapidly to become solid residues, called 'droplet nuclei', so small, e.g. 1–20 μm in diameter, that they may remain air-borne for up to several hours. Invisible aerosols are generated by any action that breaks the continuity of the surface of a liquid: e.g., the withdrawal of a loopful from a broth culture; the bursting of the film of culture in a loop; the vibration of a loop during an inoculation procedure; the sputtering of a charged loop during flaming; the mixing of a suspension with a loop or mixing equipment; the removal of a wet bung, screw-cap or cotton-wool closure from a container; the expulsion of residual fluid from a pipette; allowing liquid to fall in drops into a container instead of pouring it smoothly down the inside surface; the vigorous shaking or high-speed mixing of liquids; the dropping or breaking of culture plates, tubes or bottles; the centrifuging of overfull tubes or tubes with wet rims, or breakages in the centrifuge, especially in angle-head machines.

Infective dusts consisting of particles small enough to remain air-borne for minutes or hours can be produced by spillage of cultures on to the skin, clothing, bench, apparatus or floor. After drying, either in situ or on a cleaning cloth or paper, the residue is readily fragmented by even minor movements into a fine dust and disseminated into the air. Clouds of infective dust or spores can be released by the opening of containers of freeze-dried cultures or the withdrawal of cotton-wool plugs that have dried after being wetted by culture fluid.

Convectional and other air currents can disperse aerosols and dusts widely within a laboratory and also into adjacent rooms. Particles larger than 5 μm in diameter are mainly deposited in the nose and throat, whilst smaller particles can reach the bronchi and lungs.

Hazardous procedures

A number of procedures and situations afford a particular risk of infection. They include the following.

Use of syringe and needle. The operator may puncture his skin with the needle ('needle-stick injury') during use or disassembly of the syringe, or another person may accidentally puncture himself with an improperly disposed, used needle. Aerosol may be liberated from a vibrating needle on withdrawal from a vein or culture. Splashing or spraying may be caused by the forceful ejection of contents, especially if the needle is blown off the syringe. The skin, clothing or bench may be contaminated by leakage from the syringe or back-flow of the inoculum after its injection into an animal.

Pipetting. Infective material may be ingested in mouth-pipetting or be disseminated on to the surroundings in drips or aerosol, especially if the last drop is blown out. Automatic syringes also produce aerosol and splashing. Infective material may be stabbed through the skin on a glass pipette, especially if it is broken or is of the fine-tipped Pasteur type.

Inoculating loop. Vibration of an inoculating wire or 'loop', especially if more than 4–5 cm long, may cause splashing and aerosol production. Flaming of a wet loop or cooling ('sizzling') a hot loop in an agar plate, mixing a slide agglutination test or spreading a film for staining may also liberate infected aerosol.

Petri dishes. Water of condensation on the agar or in the lid may become contaminated and be spilt on to the fingers or the bench.

Mixing, shaking or homogenizing. Shaking produces an aerosol even in a closed container, which can be released on opening the container within a period of several minutes, or through an imperfect seal. Gross contamination of the environment can occur from spillage or breakage during these processes.

Centrifugation. Vibration can generate aerosol within the container and this may be released during the operation or on opening. Careless loading or unloading, breakage of containers during centrifugation or premature opening of the centrifuge to deal with a breakage can lead to gross dissemination of infection.

Freeze drying. Some contamination of air currents from the material being dried is inevitable and the process should be carried out in an otherwise unoccupied room. The opening of the sealed ampoules is also hazardous.

Stoppering tubes. If a tight stopper is applied forcibly or if the tube is faulty, the glass may break and cut the hand, and contents may be spilled.

Safety cabinets. Unless properly installed, maintained and used, these cabinets can disseminate infection into the air of the room or the exhaust duct. Careless use may cause contamination of surfaces within the cabinet, including those of equipment and the hands and arms of the user.

Automated apparatus can become contaminated and also splash samples on surrounding surfaces.

Animal procedures. Work with animals, including inoculation, collection of samples and performance of necropsy, affords many opportunities for injury and infection. Bedding can become contaminated with discharges and excreta and can release infected dust when disturbed. Apparently healthy animals may be carriers of inapparent infections, e.g. salmonellosis, simian herpesvirus B and lymphocytic choriomeningitis.

Transport of specimens. Improperly packaged and inadequately closed samples may leak and contaminate wrappings and attached forms during delivery to the laboratory. The outside of specimen containers may become contaminated during collection of the specimen and should be treated as potentially infected on receipt in the laboratory.

Disposal. Contamination, injury or infection may occur at many points in the procedures for collecting discarded cultures, specimen containers and used equipment, and their decontamination, washing or incineration. Discarded 'sharps' (needles, scalpels, etc.) are a particular danger. The procedures must be carefully planned and supervised as they are often performed by the least-trained staff in the laboratory.

SAFETY ORGANIZATION

Safety codes

Increasing realization of the importance of laboratory infection has led to the establishment of regulatory authorities in a number of countries. The history of official action in Britain has been reviewed by Collins (1983). A further important influence in Britain has been the passing of the Health and Safety at Work Act 1974 which gives legislative grounds on which current codes of practice and their enforcement are based.

Two principal documents provide guidance on the prevention of laboratory infection and containment of pathogens in Britain. These are (1) the Code of Practice for the Prevention of Infection in Clinical Laboratories and Post-mortem Rooms (and subsequent revisions) – the 'Howie Code' (1978) which considers infection risks in all types of clinical laboratory, and (2) the Report of the Advisory Committee on Dangerous Pathogens on the Categorisation of Pathogens according to Hazard and Categories of Containment (ACDP) (Advisory Committee on Dangerous Pathogens 1984). Laboratory workers in Britain must be familiar with both documents. The latter publication supersedes the 'Code of Practice' in terms of classification of pathogens but not, in general terms, in laboratory practice. A new guide to precautions to minimize the risk of infection from specimens known or suspected to be positive for hepatitis B and in the testing of specimens for the presence of hepatitis B antigen or antibodies has been issued (Health Services Advisory Committee 1985). This supersedes the guidance on hepatitis in the Code of Practice. These documents may be used by the Health and Safety Executive to enforce acceptable standards of laboratory practice.

In Britain, pathogens (bacteria, chlamydias, rickettsias, mycoplasmas, viruses, fungi and parasites) are categorized into four hazard groups, based on the inherent hazard of the organism, defined as follows.

Group 1. An organism that is most unlikely to cause human disease.

Group 2. An organism that may cause human disease and which might be a hazard to laboratory workers but is unlikely to spread in the community. Laboratory exposure rarely produces infection and effective prophylaxis or treatment are usually available.

Group 3. An organism that may cause severe human disease and present a serious hazard to laboratory workers. It may present a risk of spread in the community but there is usually effective prophylaxis or treatment available.

Group 4. An organism that causes severe human disease and is a serious hazard to laboratory workers. It may present a high risk of spread in the community and there is usually no effective prophylaxis or treatment.

Only pathogens are listed in the ACDP report. Most fall into group 2, but those falling into groups 3 and 4 are listed in Table 15.1.

An important feature of the ACDP Report is that categorization is the guide to the contain-

Table 15.1 Pathogens in groups 3 and 4 of the ACDP categories.

Bacteria	Group	Bacteria	Group
B. anthracis	3	M. simiae	3
Brucella spp.	3	M. szulgai	3
C. psittaci (avian strains)	3	M. tuberculosis	3
C. burneti	3	Ps. mallei	3
F. tularensis	3	Ps. pseudomallei	3
M. africanum	3	Rickettsia spp.	3
M. bovis (not BCG)	3	S. paratyphi A	3
M. intracellulare	3	S. typhi	3
M. kansasi	3	Sh. dysenteriae (type 1)	3
M. leprae	3	Y. pseudotuberculosis subsp. pestis	3
M. malmoense	3		

Viruses[a]	Group	Viruses[a]	Group
Lymphocytic choriomeningitis	3	Variola	4
Junin, Lassa, Machupo and Mopeia viruses	4	Whitepox	4
Oropouche	3	Monkey pox	3
Rift Valley fever virus	3	Human T-cell leukaemia virus	3
Congo-Crimean haemorrhagic fever virus, Hazara virus	4	Rabies	3
		Eastern equine encephalomyelitis	3
Hantaan, Korean haemorrhagic fever, epidemic nephrosis viruses	3	Venezuelan equine encephalomyelitis	3
		Western equine encephalomyelitis	3
Ebola, Marburg	4	Yellow fever, Japanese B encephalitis, Murray Valley encephalitis (Australia encephalitis), Rocio, St Louis encephalitis viruses	3
Hepatitis B	3		
Herpesvirus simiae (B virus)	3		
Kyasanur forest disease, Omsk haemorrhagic fever, Absettarov, Hanzalova, Hypr, Russian spring-summer encephalitis	4	Kumlinge	3
		Powassan	3

[a] All viruses found in man not listed above are assigned to group 2.

ment necessary when working with an organism. However, in circumstances where the nature of the work or volume of materials used increases the hazard, the categorization may be raised to a higher level. Conversely, if the risk is reduced by working, for example, with a non-virulent organism or a variant that cannot survive except in special cultural conditions, the category may be lowered provided a proper risk assessment has been made and agreed with those working with the organism, and perhaps also with the Health and Safety Inspectorate.

Containment level 1. The categories, or levels, of laboratory containment are numbered to accord with the category of hazard an organism presents. Since organisms falling into hazard category 1 (i.e. group 1) are normally harmless,

the requirements for work with these organisms are only that the laboratory can be cleaned easily and must have washing facilities. As in all laboratories, activities that could lead to infection, such as eating, drinking, smoking, applying cosmetics and mouth-pipetting, must not take place.

Containment level 2. Most pathogens dealt with in clinical laboratories fall into category 2 and will therefore be handled in containment level 2. The laboratory should be easy to clean, access should be limited to laboratory personnel and other specified persons and it should be of adequate size (24 m^3 per worker). Laboratory coats, preferably back or side fastening, must be worn and an autoclave for the sterilization of waste must be readily accessible. Hands and benches must be disinfected after work (see below) and material for disposal must be stored and handled safely. All clinical laboratory suites must contain a class 1 microbiological safety cabinet (see below).

Containment level 3. This category requires in addition that the laboratory should be sited in an area away from general circulation and have a biohazard sign at the entry. A continuous airflow into the laboratory must be maintained during work with pathogens and must be exhausted via a HEPA (high efficiency particle air) filter and procedures must be conducted in a class 1 or 3 (BS 5726:1979) safety cabinet. Gloves must be worn for all work with infective materials. In order to avoid material being taken outside the laboratory, it should have its own equipment such as incubator, centrifuge and refrigerators. Gowns worn by workers must be autoclaved after use and before laundering.

Containment level 4. This is the strictest category of containment. It requires sophisticated air movement control and filtration as well as the use of sealed safety cabinets of class 3, a double-ended autoclave and many other safety features. Very few laboratories should do work with organisms presenting the highest level of risk and so need such expensive facilities.

Table 15.2 Containment requirements for work with microbial pathogens (adapted from ACDP Report 1984). *Key*: +, required; −, not required; ± partial requirement; see text.

Containment requirements	Containment levels			
	1	2	3	4
Laboratory site: isolation from laboratory suite	−	−	±	+
Laboratory: sealable for fumigation	−	−	+	+
Ventilation: inward airflow/negative pressure	−	−	+	+
Airlock: with shower	−	−	−	+
Wash hand basin	+	+	+	+
Effluent treatment	−	−	−	+
Autoclave site: in suite;	−	+	+	+
in lab: double-ended	−	−	−	+
Microbiological safety cabinet	−	+[a]	+	+
Class of cabinet/enclosure	−	1	1,3	3

[a] For clinical microbiology laboratories only.

The requirements for the different containment levels are summarized in Table 15.2, but it is essential that all those responsible for a microbiology laboratory should read the ACDP report to see the requirements set out in full. It is important to note that similar levels of containment are laid down for animal rooms where work with microorganisms is to be conducted. Although the ACDP report supersedes the categorization of pathogens and the classification of laboratory containment in the Howie Code, there is much useful information in the latter Code as well as guidance for containing infection in other clinical laboratories and it too should be read by all those working in such laboratories. Work with certain category 4 pathogens is subject to the Health and Safety (Dangerous Pathogens) Regulations 1981 and in addition a number of pathogens are controlled by the Agriculture and Fisheries Department in the United Kingdom (see Appendix J of ACDP Report 1984).

Other countries have similar codes of practice to those of Britain, for instance, in the United States (US Department of Health and Human Services 1984) where there is an interesting and important difference in the categorization of hepatitis B virus. The World Health Organization has also published a Laboratory Biosafety Manual (WHO 1983).

AIDS

The acquired immunodeficiency syndrome (AIDS) is caused by infection with a retrovirus called a human immunodeficiency virus (HIV) or human T-cell leukaemia virus (HTLV). The serious consequences of the infection have caused concern about the possibility that it may be acquired by laboratory workers from the specimens they examine.

Present information suggests that the risk of infection from accidental exposure to HIV is small, for although large numbers of health care workers have been exposed to percutaneous (e.g. needle-stick) inoculation or splashing of skin and mucosae with blood and other fluids from known HIV-infected patients, very few have become infected (McEvoy et al 1987).

Nevertheless, infection does rarely occur after exposure of apparently intact skin to blood from such patients (Morbidity and Mortality Weekly Report 1987) and laboratory workers must therefore take precautions to avoid not only percutaneous injury and splashing of mucosae, but also any contamination of the skin with blood. Guidelines on the handling of specimens from patients with AIDS have been issued by the Department of Health and Social Security and the Health and Safety Executive (Advisory Committee on Dangerous Pathogens 1986).

AIDS may be caused by retroviruses other than the HIV originally identified as LAV/HTLV III, but infections with these other viruses (HIV 1, HIV 2) are so far uncommon. The human T-cell leukaemia viruses, which include all the HIVs, have been categorized as group 3 pathogens and full containment level 3 precautions must be taken when virus propagation is attempted.

Laboratory organization

Although codes of practice have been drawn up for the prevention of laboratory infection, responsibility rests on the individual worker as well as the laboratory management for the prevention of infection of oneself or other workers and a knowledge and constant practice of the prevention of infection is essential. In the UK, safety at work is subject to statutory control (Health and Safety at Work Act 1974) but this is no substitute for good and careful practice. The director of the laboratory has overall responsibility for safety. He should set up a safety organization and draw up local codes of practice and clear documentation of laboratory procedures which are not only required by law but are an essential part of good laboratory practice.

The appointment of a laboratory safety officer is essential where work at containment level 4 is to be carried out and is valuable in any laboratory. It must not be forgotten that all aspects of safety (e.g. those against fire, mechanical, electrical and chemical hazards) are important as well as those specially associated with microbiology. Microbiological safety is not only confined to the laboratory but also to the handling of infectious material from the time it is taken, from whatever source, until, at the end of the laboratory procedures, infected waste is disposed of safely. There is much helpful guidance on this in the Howie Report, parts of which have now been superseded by guidance issued by the Health Services Advisory Committee (1986) on the labelling, transport and reception of specimens.

Taking of specimens

Take specimens not only without unnecessary contamination of the material but also avoiding self-infection by spillage, creation of an aerosol or gross splashing (especially into eyes) or by injury such as needle stick or contamination of broken skin. Transfer specimens safely to the appropriate robust container; avoid contaminating the outside of the container and tightly close it so as to avoid spillage in transit to the laboratory. Always label containers immediately after the specimen has been placed therein and, if necessary, affix special labels that may be required such as 'HEPATITIS RISK' or 'HIGH RISK' where the specimen may contain for example *Salmonella typhi* or HIV virus. Place the specimen containers in a safe outer container for transport to the laboratory, taking care to ensure that containers remain upright to avoid spillage. If specimens are to travel by external transport, use containers with lids or prepare the specimens as for posting.

Postal regulations

There are special regulations for sending infectious material by post to ensure that the containers do not get broken and their infected contents cannot leak. In the UK, details are available from Postal Headquarters, 33 Grosvenor Place, London SW1X 1PX (see also Appendix 2 and Health Services Advisory Committee 1986). There are also strict special regulations relating to the transport of group 4 pathogens (Health and Safety (Dangerous Pathogens) Regulations 1981).

Reception of specimens

Specimens must be received in a separate area in the laboratory which must not be part of an office or in a public corridor. Where there has been leakage of a specimen either due to a loose container cap or due to breakage of the container, a decision must be taken by a senior member of staff as to whether the specimen is to be discarded or whether the difficulty of obtaining a further specimen, e.g. cerebrospinal fluid, is such that the leaking container should be taken to a safety cabinet for transfer of the specimen to a fresh container. Cover any potentially infected material spilt at the reception area with a cloth or paper towel soaked in disinfectant and leave for at least 10 min before mopping up with cloths, or clearing up with a brush and pan, and placing in an infected-waste container.

Procedures in the laboratory

For most clinical specimens the appropriate containment in the laboratory is at level 2. But where the specimen is known, or likely, to contain a category 3 pathogen, e.g. sputum, faeces from a known case of typhoid, it is at level 3. The basic rules of good laboratory discipline apply at all times so that the worker may avoid infection of himself and others. Any action likely to result in the generation of infective aerosol or the splashing of infective material must be carried out in a safety cabinet (see below).

Mishaps with infective material

Encourage cuts or puncture wounds to bleed and then wash with soap and water. If the eye is splashed rinse at once either with tap water or with irrigating solution held in the laboratory first aid kit. If the skin is soiled with grossly infectious material rinse with 70% alcohol or dilute hypochlorite solution, and then with soap and water. Alcohol will suffice for contamination with vegetative bacteria. Disposable gloves must be worn by persons working with category 3 pathogens and persons with any skin lesions – cuts, abrasions or conditions such as eczema. Deal with small spillages by initial disinfection, then cleaning up and final disinfection. If there

is a gross spillage, or *any* spillage of category 3 organisms outside a safety cabinet, evacuate the room and allow time, at least an hour, for any possible aerosol to be dispersed before entering the area. Then for group 2 organisms proceed as above and for group 3 organisms fumigate the room with formaldehyde. *Report all mishaps* to the Safety Officer or the appropriate member of the laboratory staff, who should record them in an accident book. Deal with spillages in safety cabinets by disinfecting, and if necessary, fumigating the cabinet. Disinfect benches at the end of the day's work with 70% alcohol or hypochlorite (1000 parts per million of available chlorine).

Discard jars

At the start of each day, empty the contents from the previous day, carefully clean the jar, preferably disinfect it by heating to at least 65°C for 10 min, and refill with fresh disinfectant diluted accurately to the correct concentration, e.g. hypochlorite to give 1000 or 10 000 p.p.m. of available chlorine, or phenolic disinfectant, e.g. hycolin, at 1 or 2% concentration. Use hypochlorite for viruses and phenolic disinfectant for tubercle bacilli, the higher concentrations for heavily soiled and the lower for relatively clean equipment. Carefully discard the used pipettes, slides and infective fluids into the disinfectant in such a way as to avoid splashing. Once or twice in the day, test hypochlorite with starch-iodide paper to confirm that it is still active. At regular intervals, e.g. fortnightly, check the adequacy of the disinfectant and concentration used by making an 'in-use' test on the contents of the jar at the end of a day's work (Maurer 1978). Jars must contain enough disinfectant to cover all material placed in them.

Discard material

This must be disposed of safely. Send non-infected material for incineration where appropriate (e.g. paper and plastics). Put broken glass in robust containers to protect workers from injury. Place needles and syringes – infected or not – in robust containers of cardboard or plastic (e.g. Burn bins or Cin bins) to avoid injury of handlers, and incinerate. Autoclave infectious or potentially infectious material before it leaves the laboratory. If material has to be incinerated without prior autoclaving, a member of the laboratory staff should ensure that it is transported safely to, and placed in, the incinerator.

If a gravity displacement autoclave is used, put gloves and gowns (e.g. from category 3 containment) loosely in the autoclave to ensure steam penetration. Put plastic Petri plates into discard boxes or buckets (placing plates on their sides will aid air removal) designed so that air may be discharged during autoclaving and the molten agar collected for disposal. Suitable stainless steel buckets have a wire mesh shelf about 5 cm above the base and several 1 cm holes in one side just below the mesh and 4 cm above the base. The holes permit air discharge, whilst the melted agar or spilt liquids collect in the bottom of the bucket and may later be poured out over the side opposite the holes. Vacuum-assisted autoclaves require no such special containers and autoclave bags or buckets may be used, taking care to avoid molten agar spilling into the chamber drain which would then be blocked when the agar cooled.

Pipetting

Use a rubber teat or automatic suction device, *never the mouth*. Take care neither to draw fluid up as far as the top of the pipette nor to draw bubbles through the liquid. When transferring fluid to another container, first place the tip of the pipette well inside the mouth of the receptacle in contact with its wall and then allow the contents to run gently down the wall. Do not let drops or a jet of fluid fall from the pipette and do not blow out the residual fluid. Do not put the contaminated pipette in a rack or on the bench. At once place it gently into a jar of disinfectant until it is completely submerged.

Hypodermic syringes

Sharp instruments and needles should be avoided as far as possible in microbiology laboratories. Use plastic disposable, not glass syringes. Ensure the needle is firmly attached. When expelling air bubbles, embed the needle in a sterile swab or wad of tissue to soak up any escaping fluid. Empty contents after use *slowly* into disinfectant and discard as above.

Centrifuging

Use only centrifuges with sealable safety buckets. Use the centrifuge strictly according to the operating instructions which should be posted beside it. To avoid breakages by vibration or unseating of buckets, balance the loads accurately and symmetrically and take care to fit the buckets and trunnions properly in place. To balance loads, add water to the tubes, not directly into the buckets. Include a blank set of tubes in each opposing set of carriers to receive the balancing water if it is desired to avoid adding it to the specimens. Use only stout glass or plastic containers that are unlikely to break, preferably screw-capped bottles of the Universal (28 ml), McCartney (28 ml) and bijou (6 ml) series. When filling the bottle, take care not to soil its rim or cap. Do not overfill, e.g. not more than three-quarters full. Cap the tube or bottle firmly, preferably by tight application of a screw-cap over a good rubber washer. Before putting the tube or bottle in the centrifuge bucket, make sure that the supporting rubber pad is correctly in place at the bottom of the bucket and that it is free from fragments of grit or broken glass. When the tube or bottle is in place, make sure that it is supported at its foot, not by the projecting rim of its cap. Avoid rapid acceleration of the centrifuge. After centrifugation, turn the speed controller to zero and allow the centrifuge to come to rest slowly; do not brake it violently or touch the rotor with the hand. Open the lid only after the rotor is at rest. Use the centrifuge only in its proper place, ideally in a separate room.

If a *breakage* occurs during centrifugation, switch off the centrifuge. Remove the buckets with their contents to a safety cabinet, remove the bucket lids and place lids and buckets in a container for autoclaving or into phenolic disinfectant, formaldehyde or glutaraldehyde, but not into hypochlorite because this corrodes metal. If non-sealable buckets have been used leave the centrifuge for at least 10 min after switching off to allow any aerosol to settle before removing buckets and leave a swab soaked in 40% formaldehyde (undiluted formalin) in the closed centrifuge bowl overnight; then swab the bowl with disinfectant and wash with water.

Immunization

Staff of laboratories dealing with infective materials should be immunized against diphtheria, tetanus, poliomyelitis, tuberculosis, typhoid, rubella (for women of child-bearing age) and hepatitis B. Where immunization was not given in childhood, a full course should be given. Recognized prophylactics should also be given where special pathogens, e.g. anthrax, plague, rickettsia, coxiella, *Clostridium botulinum*, are worked with.

SAFETY CABINETS

These cabinets provide a barrier between the worker and infectious material and are designed to prevent infection by splashing or by aerosol. In the United Kingdom, three classes of cabinet are defined by British Standard BS 5726: 1979.

Class 1 cabinets are open-fronted and rely on the walls, glass front and integral tray to contain spillage and splashes. An inward air flow of between 0.7 m/s and 1 m/s provides a protection factor (in general terms a measure of the number of particles which, if liberated in the safety cabinet, will not escape into the room) of at least 1.5×10^5. The air is extracted from the cabinet by a fan situated beyond a HEPA filter which ensures that no infective material is removed from the cabinet by the fan which itself cannot therefore be contaminated as long as the filter is intact.

Class 2 cabinets are also open-fronted but have a flow of filtered air into the cabinet balanced by the extraction of air so that in theory the work in the cabinet is not contaminated by organisms in room air being sucked into the cabinet and the worker is not at risk of infection by organisms liberated from the cabinet. Although in ideal circumstances a class 2 cabinet can provide a protection factor equivalent to a class 1, it is much easier for this protection to be reduced by mechanical or operational factors.

Class 3 cabinets are totally enclosed, gloves for the worker being attached to the sealed front of the cabinet. They are scavenged by air entering and leaving the cabinet through HEPA filters, the circulation being such that the air pressure in the cabinets is below that in the room. Such cabinets provide a high degree of worker protection and are the only ones permissible when dealing with category 4 pathogens. Plastic tents with filtered air inlets and exhausts ('flexible film isolators') are an attractive alternative to rigid class 3 cabinets. They are a development of the tents designed by Trexler & Reynolds (1957) to hold gnotobiotic ('germ free') animals and later adapted for the nursing of patients infected with a category 4 pathogen. Guidance on their use, testing and maintenance has been issued by the Advisory Committee on Dangerous Pathogens (1985). They may well play an increasing role in laboratories where work with dangerous pathogens is carried out.

Use of class 1 and 2 cabinets

These open-fronted cabinets must be sited carefully and should not be used if persons are moving about in the laboratory as draughts from doors, windows or those created by persons walking past a cabinet can draw particles eddying in the front of the cabinet back into the room. Care must be taken that the air from safety cabinets is discharged safely to the outside but never near ventilation intakes or open windows. Because these cabinets protect by virtue of a correct air flow this must be checked daily by viewing the air flow indicator (class 1) and monthly with an anemometer. Good guidance on safety cabinets is presented in Appendices 9 and 14 of the Howie Code as well as detailed information by Collins (1983).

It must be stressed that open-fronted safety cabinets depend on air flow patterns for worker protection, and cannot contain gross splashes or particles ejected from centrifuges, which *must never* be placed in such cabinets. Similarly, air flow patterns can be disturbed by any obstruction, and open-fronted safety cabinets, in particular, must not be cluttered up with equipment. Untidy, overcrowded working conditions are not compatible with safety. Cabinets must be disinfected after working with pathogens and always before any maintenance or change of filter. At the end of a working day, wipe the inside walls and floor with a disinfectant. At the end of a cycle of work and, in any case, at weekly intervals, vaporize formalin inside the cabinet while the aperture of class 1 and 2 cabinets is occluded by a 'night door'. The amount of formalin, 0.05 g/m^3 (approximately 25 ml of formalin BP in a class 1 cabinet) is specified in BS 5726; preferably vaporize it with a thermostatically controlled electric heater. Allow the vapour to act overnight before purging by ventilation through the filter. Ultraviolet lights are not recommended for the disinfection of safety cabinets.

DISINFECTANTS

Disinfectants are needed in the laboratory for the skin, work surfaces, discard jars and spillages. Use as few kinds as possible to avoid confusion and explain their function and limitations to all who use them.

Skin and work surfaces can be decontaminated with 70% ethyl alcohol (industrial methylated spirits with 1% glycerol as an emollient for skin use). This will kill vegetative bacteria and some viruses. If there is any fire hazard and especially if viruses or bacterial spores pose a problem, sodium hypochlorite solution, a cheap disinfec-

tant and rapidly lethal to most bacteria and viruses, may be used. However, it is ineffective against *Mycobacterium tuberculosis*, is neutralized by organic material and is corrosive to metals, but it is free from any marked or persistent irritant or toxic effect. For disinfecting clean surfaces or skin a 1% solution of commercially available hypochlorite solutions such as Chloros or Domestos is adequate. These proprietary disinfectants are 10% solutions of sodium hypochlorite containing 100 000 p.p.m. of available chlorine. Prolonged exposure of skin to hypochlorite should be avoided, the disinfectant being washed off as soon as possible under running water.

Each work place in the laboratory should be provided with one or more deep plastic discard jars filled with disinfectant for the disposal of contaminated pipettes, slides, infective residues, etc. A bottle of disinfectant must be kept for spillages. For discard jars, spillages or any situation where there is organic or tuberculous material a phenolic disinfectant should be used as these disinfectants are more resistant to inactivation than hypochlorite. If work with viruses is being carried out, pipette jars should be filled with hypochlorite solution containing 2500 p.p.m. available chlorine (e.g. 2.5% Chloros) and for blood spillage 10 000 p.p.m. (10% Chloros – 'strong hypochlorite') may be used. If there is much organic matter in a virus spillage or if the corrosive effect of hypochlorite might affect equipment, 2% glutaraldehyde (or similar disinfectant) should be used. Constant exposure to glutaraldehyde can give rise to sensitization. A brief guide to the use of chemical disinfectants in hospitals has been published recently (Ayliffe et al 1984).

REFERENCES

Advisory Committee on Dangerous Pathogens 1984 Categorisation of pathogens according to hazard and categories of containment. HMSO, London

Advisory Committee on Dangerous Pathogens 1985 Guidance on the use, testing and maintenance of laboratory and animal flexible film isolators. HMSO, London

Advisory Committee on Dangerous Pathogens 1986 LAV/HTLV III – the causative agent of AIDS and

related conditions – revised guidelines. HMSO, London

Ayliffe G A J, Coates D, Hoffman P N 1984 Chemical disinfectants in hospitals. Public Health Laboratory Service, London

Blaser M J, Feldman R A 1980 Acquisition of typhoid fever from proficiency-testing specimens. New England Journal of Medicine 303: 1481

Code of Practice for the Prevention of Infection in Clinical

Laboratories and Postmortem rooms 1978 DHSS and others. HMSO, London

Collins C H 1983 Laboratory-acquired infections. Butterworth, London

Grist N R 1981a Hepatitis infection in clinical laboratory staff. Medical Laboratory Sciences 38: 103–109

Grist N R 1981b Hepatitis and other infections in clinical laboratory staff, 1979. Journal of Clinical Pathology 34: 655–658

Grist N R 1983 Infections in British clinical laboratories 1980–81. Journal of Clinical Pathology 36: 121–126

Grist N R, Emslie J A N 1985 Infections in British clinical laboratories 1982–3. Journal of Clinical Pathology 38: 721–725

Harrington J M 1976 The health of medical laboratory workers in Britain. MDThesis, University of London

Harrington J M, Shannon H S 1976 Incidence of tuberculosis, hepatitis, brucellosis and shigellosis in British medical laboratory workers. British Medical Journal 1: 759–762

Harrington J M, Shannon H S 1977 Survey of safety and health in British medical laboratories. British Medical Journal 1: 626–628

Health Services Advisory Committee 1985 Safety in health service laboratories: hepatitis B. HMSO, London

Health Services Advisory Committee 1986 Safety in health service laboratories: the labelling, transport and reception of specimens. HMSO, London

Maurer I M 1978 Hospital hygiene. 2nd edn Arnold, London

McEvoy M, Porter K, Mortimer P, Simmons N, Shanson D 1987 Prospective study of clinical, laboratory, and ancillary staff with accidental exposures to blood or body fluids from patients infected with HIV. British Medical Journal 294: 1595–1597

Morbidity and Mortality Weekly Report 1987 Update: Human immunodeficiency virus infections in health-care workers exposed to blood of infected patients. US Department of Health and Human Services/Public Health Service, Centers for Disease Control. Vol. 36, No. 19.

Pike R M 1979 Laboratory-associated infections: incidence, fatalities, causes and prevention. Annual Reviews of Microbiology 33: 41–46

Sulkin S E 1961 Laboratory-acquired infections. Bacteriological Reviews 25: 203–209

Sulkin S E, Pike R M 1951 Survey of laboratory-acquired infections. American Journal of Public Health 41: 769–781

Trexler P C, Reynolds R J 1957 Flexible film apparatus for rearing and use of germ-free animals. Applied Microbiology 5: 406–412

US Department of Health and Human Services 1984 Biosafety in microbiological and biomedical laboratories. US Government Printing Office, Washington

WHO 1983 Laboratory biosafety manual. World Health Organization, Geneva

Staphylococcus: cluster-forming Gram-positive cocci

The cluster-forming Gram-positive cocci of medical interest belong to the genera *Staphylococcus, Micrococcus, Aerococcus* and *Peptococcus*. Their distinguishing characters are shown in Table 16.1 (Baird-Parker 1974, 1979; Hill 1981). Of these genera, only the staphylococci and peptococci are commonly present as parasites in man and only one species, *Staphylococcus aureus*, is an important primary pathogen. It causes a variety of superficial and deep pyogenic infections.

The other staphylococci, including those listed in Table 16.2, lack primary pathogenicity and are helpfully reported to the physician as 'albus staphylococci' or '*S. albus*'. Of these, *S. epidermidis* and *S. saprophyticus* are commonly, and the other species less commonly present as commensals on the body surfaces. They are thus often found as contaminants in clinical specimens, e.g. in swabs from the skin, nose, throat, wounds, burns and bedsores. Generally their presence is not clinically significant, but they sometimes act as opportunistic pathogens and cause infection in the urinary tract or, in debilitated or immunodeficient subjects, more serious, bacteriaemic infections. Micrococci, aerococci and peptococci may also be found on the body surfaces and occasionally cause opportunistic infections.

Recognition of staphylococci

Staphylococci are initially recognized in a clinical specimen either by their appearance in a film as Gram-positive cocci in clusters or by the appearance of their characteristic colonies in a culture on blood agar, nutrient agar or MacConkey agar.

The colonies, usually 1–3 mm in diameter, are smooth, circular, low convex, glistening and

Table 16.1 Distinguishing characters of four genera of cluster-forming Gram-positive cocci.

Genus	Predominant grouping	Atmospheric requirement	Catalase production	Glucose breakdown	Ecological character
Staphylococcus	Irregular (grape-like) clusters	Facultative[a] (aerobic growth greater than anaerobic)	+	Fermentative[a] (acid formed anaerobically as well as aerobically)	Pathogenic and commensal parasites
Micrococcus	Irregular clusters or tetrads	Strictly aerobic	+	Oxidative (acid formed only aerobically) or inactive	Free-living saprophytes
Aerococcus	Tetrads and small clusters	Facultative (aerobic growth greater than anaerobic)	− or weak	Fermentative	Free-living saprophytes
Peptococcus	Irregular clusters or tetrads	Strictly anaerobic	Weak or variable	Fermentative or inactive	Commensal parasites, opportunistic pathogens

[a] Some staphylococci, e.g. *S. saprophyticus*, grow so poorly under anaerobic conditions that they may be misidentified as micrococci by these criteria; see text.

Table 16.2 Characters distinguishing 10 species of staphylococci (Adapted from Baird-Parker, 1979).
Key: +, > 80% of strains positive; −, > 80% of strains negative; +/−, some strains positive, some negative; ±, weak reaction or rare occurrence in man.

Character	S. aureus	S. intermedius	S. hyicus	S. epidermidis	S. capitis	S. hominis	S. warneri	S. haemolyticus	S. cohni	S. saprophyticus
Occurrence in man	+	−	−	+	±	±	−	+	+	+
Thermostable DNA nuclease	+	+	+/−	−	+/−	+/−	−	−	−	−
Coagulase produced	+	+	+/−	−	−	−	−	−	−	−
Haemolysis on human blood	+	+/−	−	−	−	−	−	+	−	−
Acetoin produced	+	−	−	+	+/−	+/−	+	+	+/−	+
Acid produced aerobically										
from: sucrose	+	+	+	+	+	+	+	+	+	+
trehalose	+	+	+	−	−	+	+	+	+	+
mannitol	+	±	−	−	+	−	+/−	+/−	+	+
Phosphatase produced	+	+	+	+	−	−	−	−	−	−
Growth on medium with 1.6 mg/litre novobiocin	−	−	−	−	−	−	−	−	−	+

Table 16.3 Distinguishing characters of three species of staphylococci.
Key: R, MIC > 2 mg/litre; S, MIC < 0.6 mg/litre.

Character	S. aureus	Albus staphylococci	
		S. epidermidis	S. saprophyticus
Colony colour	Yellow to orange, rarely white	Usually white	Usually white
Coagulase	+	−	−
DNase	+	−	−
Mannitol fermented anaerobically	+	−	−
Novobiocin sensitivity	S	S	R

butyrous. They are distinguished from those of most other bacteria by their golden or white pigmentation and greater opacity for their size. They may form zones of haemolysis on blood agar. They grow on most batches of MacConkey lactose bile-salt agar, on which a pinkish colour is superimposed on their natural pigmentation.

In routine diagnostic work the colony appearance is generally taken as sufficient to identify an isolate as a staphylococcus before proceeding to tests to distinguish whether it is *S. aureus* or an albus staphylococcus. Micrococci and aerococci would give negative results in the tests for *S. aureus* and as they are rarely of clinical significance, little harm will result from their occasional misidentification as an albus staphylococcus.

If, however, a definitive identification of the genus is required, further tests should be done. The colonies should first be filmed to demonstrate the morphology of the cocci and their clusters. They should then be tested for the production of catalase in a subculture grown on 1% glucose agar* to distinguish staphylococci and micrococci (catalase positive) from aerococci and streptococci (catalase negative). The use of a glucose medium for this test avoids false reactions due to pseudocatalase.

Some strains of micrococci are distinguishable from staphylococci because their colonies have either a granular, matt surface or a pink-violet colouration, but most strains form smooth, yellow colonies fairly similar to those of *S. aureus*. The staphylococci are usually distinguished from the micrococci by their ability to grow and ferment glucose under anaerobic conditions in a modified Hugh & Leifson test*, but some, e.g. *S. saprophyticus*, grow so poorly under anaerobic conditions that they are liable to be misidentified as micrococci (Kloos & Schleifer 1975; Baird-Parker 1979). Staphylococci are more reliably distinguished by their ability to grow and ferment glycerol in the presence of 0.4 mg/litre of erythromycin, their sensitivity to 200 mg/l of lysostaphin and their resistance to 25 mg/l of lysozyme in tests by the methods of Schleifer & Kloos (1975).

* Refer to *Methods* at end of this chapter.

Species

Up to 13 species of staphylococci are now recognized (Hill 1981), though not all occur in man and only three, *S. aureus*, *S. epidermidis* and *S. saprophyticus*, do so commonly. The characters distinguishing the 10 more important species are shown in Table 16.2. For most clinical purposes the identification of a species other than *S. aureus* is unnecessary and all the non-aureus staphylococci may be termed albus staphylococci. There is, however, some value in distinguishing between the two commoner albus species, *S. epidermidis* and *S. saprophyticus*, for the latter has a special tendency to infect the urinary tract. A simplified scheme for identifying these three main human species is given in Table 16.3.

STAPHYLOCOCCUS AUREUS

The characters of *S. aureus* absent from most strains of albus staphylococci include a golden colony colour; the production of coagulase, deoxyribonuclease (DNase), α, β, γ, or δ haemolysin, leucocidin, protein A, fibrinolysin and hyaluronidase; the anaerobic fermentation of mannitol; susceptibility to phages of the *S. aureus* typing set; and agglutinability by *S. aureus* typing sera. In routine diagnostic work, reliance is usually placed on the preliminary observation of colony colour followed by a single confirmatory test, preferably that for coagulase or DNase.

Morphology and staining

Spherical cocci, 0.8–1 μm in diameter. In films of pus or from solid medium: grape-like clusters with some single or paired cocci. In broth: small groups, pairs, singles and short chains (less than five cocci in line). Gram-positive, non-sporing, non-motile and, except for rare strains, non-capsulate.

Cultural characters

Facultative anaerobe. Temperature for growth:

range 12–44°C, optimum 37°C. Optimum pH, 7.5.

Nutrient agar. After aerobic incubation for 24 h at 37°C, colonies are 1–3 mm in diameter and have a smooth glistening surface, an entire edge, a soft butyrous consistency and an opaque, pigmented appearance. In most strains the pigmentation is golden, with orange, yellow and cream-buff varieties, but in a few it is white. These white-colonied strains of *S. aureus* are fully virulent. In anaerobic cultures the colonies are smaller and less pigmented.

Blood agar. The colonies have the same appearances as on nutrient agar, but may be surrounded by a zone of β-haemolysis. Haemolysis is more likely to be present if sheep, ox, human or rabbit blood is used instead of horse blood and if incubation is in air with 20% added carbon dioxide.

MacConkey agar. Colonies are pink or pink-orange and small to medium in size, depending on the batch of medium.

Pigmentation. Observation of the golden (orange, yellow or cream-buff) colony colour is useful because it makes possible the provisional identification of *S. aureus* colonies in mixed cultures also containing albus staphylococci. Pigmentation may be poorly developed in 24 h on nutrient agar or blood agar and is then best seen by viewing in daylight the aggregated material scraped up from several colonies on an inoculating wire. It may be enhanced by prolonging incubation at 37°C to 48 h or by the use of special pigment-enhancing media such as milk agar (Christie & Keogh 1940)* or glycerol monoacetate agar (Jacobs et al 1964) or by culture for 5 days at 30°C on a glucose peptone yeast-extract agar (Baird-Parker 1979).

Phenolphthalein phosphate agar. This indicator medium (Barber & Kuper 1951)* assists the identification of *S. aureus* in mixed cultures. All strains of *S. aureus* form phosphatase and their colonies liberate phenolphthalein which, when the plate is exposed to ammonia vapour, gives them a bright pink colour. Most other staphylococci form colonies that remain uncoloured.

Selective salt media. Staphylococci grow so freely on ordinary nutrient media that there is usually no need to use a selective medium for their isolation, but a selective medium may be useful for the isolation and enumeration of staphylococci from materials, such as faeces, food and dust, likely to contain a large predominance of other kinds of bacteria. As staphylococci tolerate higher concentrations of sodium chloride than many other bacteria (Hill & White 1929), useful selective media are cooked meat broth plus 10% NaCl, which may be used for primary enrichment, and milk agar plus 7–10% NaCl, useful for primary plating and for counting the pigmented colonies.*

Mannitol salt agar. This medium, which contains 1% mannitol, 7.5% NaCl and 0.0025% phenol red in nutrient agar, is both a selective and an indicator medium. Most strains of *S. aureus* ferment mannitol and so form colonies surrounded by yellow zones due to acid production, whilst most other staphylococci fail to ferment mannitol and form colonies with red or purple zones.

Coagulase production

The demonstration of coagulase production is the best single test to identify a staphylococcus as belonging to the pathogenic species, *S. aureus.* The only non-aureus staphylococci to produce coagulase are the animal parasites, *S. intermedius* and *S. hyicus*, rarely if ever found in man (Baird-Parker 1979), whilst strains of *S. aureus* failing to produce coagulase are very rare.

The rare coagulase-negative strains of *S. aureus* are, nevertheless, pathogenic and they show most of the biochemical, toxin-producing and other characters of their species. They are probably best distinguished from albus staphylococci by the DNase test (Gramoli & Wilkinson 1978).

Most strains of *S. aureus* form both *free coagulase*, which turns citrated plasma into a firm gel in the tube coagulase test, and *bound coagulase* (clumping factor) which agglutinates the cocci in the slide coagulase test. A few strains form only the one or the other kind.

1. *Tube test.** This is the more reliable of the two tests and should be done in all doubtful

cases. It requires reading at intervals up to 6 h and again after standing overnight, so that its use may delay the reporting of results or a decision as to whether the culture should be tested for antibiotic sensitivities.

2. *Slide test.** This test gives an immediate result, but is less reliable than the tube test. Thus it gives 'false-negative' results with about 5% of coagulase-positive strains. When, therefore, a negative reaction is obtained with a strain thought from its origin or pigmentation to be *S. aureus*, the culture should be retested by the tube method or the DNase test.

3. *Kit tests.* Kits are commercially available which detect bound coagulase in a 'slide' agglutination test on a disposable reaction card. They are convenient to use, give fewer false-negative results than the ordinary slide test and so are more specific for *S. aureus*. As they take only a minute or two to perform, suspect colonies can be identified when the primary culture is read and the delay of about 18 h for the tube coagulase test avoided.

The Staphylase test (Oxoid) demonstrates agglutination of sheep red blood cells sensitized with fibrinogen. The Staphaurex test (Wellcome) detects bound coagulase, protein A or both these substances by the agglutination of latex particles coated with human fibrinogen and immunoglobulin G.

Deoxyribonuclease (DNase) production

Over 99% of coagulase-positive strains of staphylococci produce a heat-stable nuclease that hydrolyses DNA, whilst only a minority, about 20%, of coagulase-negative strains do so (Jeffries 1961; Blair et al 1967). A test for DNase will therefore detect almost all strains of *S. aureus* and screen out the majority of albus strains. The DNase plate test* is very easy to perform, though unlike the less reliable slide coagulase test, it requires overnight incubation. The DNA-containing culture plate is flooded with hydrochloric acid to precipitate unhydrolysed DNA and produce a white cloudiness in the medium.

DNase-positive cultures are surrounded by a clear zone where the DNA has been hydrolysed. The few coagulase-negative staphylococci that are DNase-positive are apt to give only weak reactions, so that cultures showing zones markedly smaller than that of a control coagulase-positive culture should be read as negative, i.e. not as *S. aureus*.

The coagulase-negative staphylococci that produce DNase include not only the rare coagulase-negative, but pathogenic strains of *S. aureus*, but also more numerous strains of various non-pathogenic albus species. If, therefore, the DNase plate test is used as the only identifying test for *S. aureus*, account should also be taken of any golden pigmentation or a predominance of the organism in an infective exudate as indications of its pathogenicity.

The DNase of *S. aureus* is stable on heating for 15 min at 100°C and a test for heat-stable DNase (Lachicha et al 1971; Baird-Parker 1979) is more specific though more laborious than the plate test. But it is still not entirely specific for *S. aureus*, for it gives weak positive results with a few non-pathogenic albus strains (Gramoli & Wilkinson 1978).

Haemolysin production

Nearly every strain of *S. aureus* forms one or more of four haemolytic, membrane-damaging exotoxins, α, β, γ, and δ, which are antigenically distinct and differ from one another in their activity against the red blood cells of different animal species. α-Toxin is most strongly active on rabbit cells, β-toxin on sheep cells, whilst γ- and δ-toxin act about as strongly also on horse and human cells. Strains of albus staphylococci do not form these toxins, but most of them form other haemolysins, one of which, epsilon-haemolysin, acts on rabbit and sheep cells.

Though the effect of the toxins is often seen in the production of zones of haemolysis around colonies on blood agar plates, their specific identification requires tests with different bloods and neutralizing antisera too laborious for use in routine identification of *S. aureus* (Elek & Levy 1950; Elek 1959; McCartney & Arbuthnott 1978).

Enterotoxin production

Between 30 and 50% of strains of *S. aureus* from human sources, particularly those in phage-group III, are able to form an 'enterotoxin'. By growing and forming the toxin in a foodstuff, they can cause the vomiting and diarrhoea of staphylococcal food-poisoning. The toxin produces its effect by an action on the nervous system, not, like other enterotoxins, on the intestinal epithelium. It is relatively heat-stable and may remain active on heating at 100°C for up to 30 min, e.g. in food heated sufficiently to kill the staphylococci; in such a case a diagnosis cannot be made by culture of the food or faeces.

Different strains of *S. aureus* form six anti-genically distinct toxins, A, B, C1, C2, D and E, identified by their precipitation reactions with antisera. Coagulase-negative staphylococci do not form enterotoxin. In man, the ingestion of as little as 1 µg of toxin may cause symptoms within 1–6 h, but no convenient laboratory animal is susceptible. Methods for extracting the toxin from food and identifying it by its reactions with antisera are reviewed by Bergdoll (1970). Casman & Bennett's agar-gel precipitation test as modified by Gilbert et al (1972) detects as little as 0.02 µg toxin/g food.

PV leucocidin, hyaluronidase and fibrinolysin

Methods for demonstrating the production of these substances by *S. aureus* are reviewed by Elek (1959).

Biochemical reactions

By standard methods (Ch. 8), *S. aureus* is shown to form acid but not gas from glucose, maltose, lactose, sucrose and, usually, mannitol. As most strains of albus staphylococci from human sources, but few strains of *S. albus* and micrococci ferment mannitol, this reaction may be observed for the provisional identification of *S. aureus*.

Other reactions of *S. aureus* are: catalase positive on media with 1% glucose; oxidase negative; acetoin produced; nitrate reduced to nitrite; indole negative. Most human strains produce opacity due to lipolysis in egg yolk

(Gillespie & Alder 1952), hydrolyse gelatin and coagulated serum, produce urease and form ammonia from peptone.

Sensitivity to chemical and physical agents

Laboratory cultures survive for months or years. The cocci withstand moist heat at 60°C for 30 min, but are killed in 1 h, are moderately resistant to natural drying and survive in dust and on fomites for several days, weeks or months. They are fairly readily killed by disinfectants used at their proper concentrations, e.g. in a few minutes by 1% Hycolin (clear soluble phenolic) or a hypochlorite solution with 10 000 p.p.m. of available chlorine.

Antibiotic sensitivity

A wide variety of antibiotics have been used for the treatment of *S. aureus* infections and at the time each family of drugs was introduced, most strains were sensitive to them (Table 16.4). Subsequently, however, the selective pressure exerted by the widespread use of penicillin and other popular drugs promoted the proliferation of strains resistant to these drugs. Over 80% of clinical isolates of *S. aureus* in Britain are now

Table 16.4 Minimum inhibitory concentrations (MIC) of different antibiotics for sensitive strains of *S. aureus*.

Antibiotic	MIC (mg/litre)
Benzylpenicillin	0.03
Phenoxymethylpenicillin	0.03
Ampicillin	0.06
Cloxacillin	0.12
Methicillin	2.0
Cephaloridine	0.12
Cephalothin	0.5
Streptomycin	2.0
Neomycin	0.5
Gentamicin	0.06
Chloramphenicol	4.0
Tetracycline	0.12
Erythromycin	0.12
Novobiocin	0.12
Fusidic acid	0.06
Vancomycin	1.0

of the type that forms penicillinase (beta-lactamase) and are resistant to benzylpenicillin, phenoxymethylpenicillin, ampicillin and amoxycillin, and partially resistant to cephaloridine.

Most penicillin-resistant strains are sensitive to the penicillinase-resistant penicillins, e.g. flucloxacillin and methicillin, to cephalothin (MIC 0.5 mg/litre), some other cephalosporins, erythromycin, fusidic acid, vancomycin, cotrimoxazole and Augmentin (amoxycillin plus clavulanic acid). Strains resistant to a variety of drugs, 'multi-resistant' strains, are commonly present in hospitals and may present a difficulty in therapy.

A few of the penicillin-resistant strains are also resistant to methicillin, being able to grow at low therapeutic concentrations of methicillin, flucloxacillin and cephalosporins. The MIC of methicillin for cultures of these strains grown at 37°C is only about 5 mg/litre, but for those grown at 30°C it is about 100 mg/l.

Strains of methicillin-resistant S. aureus (MRSA) have become established as the prevalent strains in a number of hospitals, but it is debated whether they are fully virulent or have epidemic potential (Report 1986; Lacey 1987).

Sensitivity tests

As strains of S. aureus differ in their sensitivity to different antibiotics, the sensitivities of each isolate should be tested. This is most easily done by the disk diffusion method, in which the zone of inhibition of growth of the test organism around an antibiotic disk is compared with that of a standard sensitive organism (Ch. 9). There are, however, some advantages in use of the 'break-point' method, which demonstrates sensitivity or resistance to two critical concentrations of the antibiotic.

In the disk test it is usual to test six antibiotics on each plate and a suitable selection might be benzylpenicillin (0.6 μg, i.e. 1 unit, per disk), methicillin (5 μg), erythromycin (10 μg), cotrimoxazole (25 μg) or trimethoprim (1.25 μg), Augmentin (30 μg) and fusidic acid (10 μg). For staphylococci from urine, novobiocin (5 μg) may be substituted for fusidic acid to distinguish S. saprophyticus (resistant) from S. epidermidis (sensitive). For isolates from sites amenable to topical therapy, e.g. ear or eye, chloramphenicol (25 μg) and neomycin (30 μg) may be substituted for cotrimoxazole and erythromycin. A control test should be done with the fully sensitive 'Oxford' strain of S. aureus (NCTC6571). For tests with Augmentin, a beta-lactamase-producing strain should be used as control.

Beta-lactamase-producing staphylococci may show a fairly large zone of inhibition of growth around a penicillin or ampicillin disk, but are easily recognized by their formation of a heaped-up edge of growth, or a border of large colonies, immediately adjacent to the zone of inhibition. This appearance is quite different from the smoothly tapering edge shown by sensitive cultures. Organisms showing a heaped-up edge should be reported as penicillin- and ampicillin-resistant regardless of the size of the inhibition zone.

Methicillin-resistant staphylococci often appear to be sensitive to methicillin in tests on ordinary medium read after 24 h at 37°C. Resistance is more reliably observed in a separate test made on nutrient agar plus 6% NaCl incubated at 37°C (Hewitt et al 1969). Alternatively, when methicillin is to be tested on a plate of ordinary medium along with other antibiotics, the plate should be incubated at 32–34°C (Drew et al 1972). The result for methicillin may be reported as applying also to cloxacillin, flucloxacillin, oxacillin and most cephalosporins, drugs more commonly used than methicillin itself. The test for sensitivity to methicillin is done primarily to indicate sensitivity to these latter drugs, which need not be tested separately.

Phage-typing

For epidemiological studies and the tracing of sources of infection, strains of S. aureus are generally distinguished from one another by their patterns of susceptibility to lysis by an internationally recognized set of 23 standard typing phages (Oeding 1978). Technical details of the procedure are given by Parker (1972).

Many different phage-types of S. aureus are distinguished on the basis that each shows 'strong' differences from the others in its reactions with at least two of the phages. Lysis

Table 16.5 Staphylococcal phages classified in lytic groups

Lytic group of phages	Designations of phages in lytic group (42D, 187 not in standard set)									
I	29	52	52A	79	80					
II	3A	3C	55	71						
III	6	42E	47	53	54	75	77	83A	84	85
Unclassified	81	94	95	96	(42D)	(187)				

of a culture by one phage is often associated with lysis by one or more other phages and the phages have been classified by such relationships into three *lytic groups*. The organisms lysed only by the phages in one of the lytic groups have been classified in one of three corresponding *phage groups* of staphylococci (Table 16.5).

Drops of the phages at their routine test dilutions (RTD), which give barely confluent lysis of their propagating cultures, are applied to agar plates seeded confluently with the staphylococcus to be typed. After incubation overnight at 30°C the plate is examined for the degree of lysis by each phage and the phage-type of the staphylococcus is reported as the combined designations of the phages that strongly lyse it, e.g. phage-type 52/52A and phage-type 52/52A/80/81 are two common types in phage-group I.

The phage-type of a staphylococcus may occasionally become changed by the loss or gain of a carried, type-determining prophage as the coccus passes from person to person in the community, but it is generally stable enough to serve as a useful epidemiological marker. Thus, in a hospital outbreak of infection lasting a few weeks, the cultures isolated from a carrier and the patients infected by that carrier are likely all to be the same type. Excepting rare, in-vivo variation, differences in phage-type show that the cultures are not epidemiologically related.

Serotyping

Three major serotypes, I, II and III, of *S. aureus* were distinguished by slide agglutination tests with absorbed sera by Cowan (1939) and the method has been developed by Oeding (1978) to distinguish over one hundred serotypes. Serotyping has been used successfully in a few epidemiological studies and can show the relationship between isolates of the same strain that differ in phage-type due to the lysogenization of some of them in vivo. The method, however, has not yet been standardized.

Animal pathogenicity

Strains from human lesions are pathogenic in rabbits; a small quantity of culture produces an abscess when injected subcutaneously and leads to septicaemia, pyaemia and renal abscesses when injected intravenously. Mice and guinea-pigs may be infected, but are less susceptible. Animal tests are not used for diagnosis.

Laboratory diagnosis of staphylococcal infection

Specimens from patients may include pus or wound exudate in a tube or on a swab, blood for culture (e.g. from a patient with pyrexia of uncertain origin), mid-stream urine, sputum from suspected bronchopneumonia, and faeces, vomit and food remains from cases of food-poisoning. Nasal and perineal swabs may be collected from suspected carriers. Staphylococci are relatively hardy, survive well in specimens during transport to the laboratory and are easily recovered on culture.

The main tasks of the bacteriologist are to discover whether *S. aureus* is present and, if present, to what drugs the strain is susceptible. The organism is generally first recognized by the appearance of its pigmented colonies on a blood agar plate and its identity is then confirmed by its reaction in a coagulase or DNase test.

1. Examine a Gram-stained smear of any specimen of pus, wound exudate or sputum, and blood cultures after overnight incubation. The observation of Gram-positive cocci in clusters,

either as sole organism or as the predominant organism among others, may justify the making of a provisional report so that the physician may start treatment with a drug such as flucloxacillin.

2. If the smear of the specimen shows a predominance of staphylococci, or that of a blood culture shows any staphylococci, set up a primary culture test for antibiotic sensitivities (Ch. 9). Inoculate the specimen confluently on a plate of antibiotic sensitivity test agar, apply antibiotic disks and incubate overnight.

3. Also on the first day, plate out the specimen on blood agar to obtain separate colonies. If a coliform infection is possible, plate it also on a MacConkey plate. If the specimen is faeces, vomit or food, plate it also on selective salt milk agar* or salt mannitol agar. Incubate aerobically at 37°C for 24 h.

4. Next day, inspect the plates for golden or white colonies and test any found in a slide coagulase test.* If the organism is coagulase positive, a preliminary report can be issued immediately and antibiotic sensitivities may be given if these have been observed in a primary culture test.

5. Otherwise, suspend one or more of the golden or white colonies in 1–2 ml sterile broth to form a suspension for use as inocula for further tests. A suspension of just visible turbidity (about 10^8 cocci/ml) is required for the antibiotic sensitivity tests and one equivalent to an overnight broth culture (about 10^9 cocci/ml) for the tube coagulase test.

For the tube coagulase test, inoculate 0.1 ml of the dense suspension into 0.5 ml diluted plasma.* For the DNase plate test, spot-inoculate a drop of either suspension on to the DNA plate.* Incubate aerobically at 37°C.

For disk diffusion antibiotic sensitivity tests, confluently inoculate the light suspension on to a plate of antibiotic sensitivity test agar and apply antibiotic disks. Incubate overnight at 37°C or, if methicillin is being tested, at 32°C (Ch. 9).

6. Next day, identify the organism as S. aureus or S. albus from its positive or negative reaction in the coagulase or DNase test. If it is S. aureus, read and report its antibiotic sensitivities.

7. If S. aureus or other pathogen is not isolated, consider the possible clinical significance of any albus staphylococcus isolated. If the clinical data suggest that an albus staphylococcus may have a pathogenic role, e.g. when isolated in significant numbers from urine and identified as S. saprophyticus or when isolated from the blood of an immunodeficient patient (see below), report its presence and antibiotic sensitivities. Otherwise, unless they are specifically requested, withhold the results in case their reporting leads to inappropriate therapy being given.

8. Arrange for phage-typing to be done only if the information is required for epidemiological purposes. Arrange for cultures of S. aureus isolated in outbreaks of food-poisoning, and any remains of implicated food, to be examined for enterotoxin in a reference laboratory.

9. *Serological diagnosis.* Normal human serum frequently agglutinates staphylococci at low titre and many sera contain small amounts of antibodies to staphylococcal toxins, e.g. up to 2 units anti-staphylolysin (anti-α-toxin). In serious staphylococcal infections the titres may be greatly raised, but the absence of antibody does not exclude staphylococcal disease and serological tests are therefore little used. A method for the anti-staphylolysin test is given in the 11th edition of this book.

ALBUS STAPHYLOCOCCI AND MICROCOCCI

These generally non-pathogenic cocci are often present in cultures set up for the isolation of S. aureus and are distinguished from the latter by their negative reaction in the coagulase or DNase test. If required, their species may be identified by the characters shown in Tables 16.1, 16.2 and 16.3, demonstrated by the methods described below*. They may also be identified by tests with a multiple biochemical reaction kit such as API STAPH*.

Being present on the skin, in the mouth and in dust, they are commonly encountered as commensals or contaminants in specimens from skin lesions, wounds, burns, throat, sputum and faeces. Their finding in these specimens is generally of no clinical significance; it is not reported to the physician and the antibiotic sensitivities of the organisms are not tested.

During specimen collection, the commensal cocci of the skin sometimes gain access to blood cultures (in 1–10%) and other specimens such as cerebrospinal fluid, pleural fluid and deep pus that are normally free from commensals. When only small numbers are found in such specimens, even in the absence of other organisms, their presence should be reported as probably being without clinical significance, as, e.g., 'A few albus staphylococci, probably contaminants from the skin', and antibiotic sensitivities not given unless specially requested.

In some circumstances, however, these cocci may have a pathogenic role. They may cause peritonitis in patients on peritoneal dialysis, chronic septicaemia or endocarditis in patients having heart surgery or fitted with an artificial heart valve, meningeal or bacteriaemic infection in patients fitted with a ventriculo-venous cerebrospinal fluid shunt, and septicaemia in immunosuppressed and immunodefective patients. They often cause a bacteriaemic illness in patients treated with an indwelling venous catheter left in place for more than 48 h, but removal of the catheter usually terminates the infection without the need for antibiotic therapy.

Apart from such clinical considerations, the finding of large numbers of cocci in fresh specimens, e.g. more than five colonies per ml patient's blood in a poured-plate blood culture, or their finding in repeated specimens, e.g. in three successive blood cultures, suggests that their presence is due to infection rather than contamination.

When, therefore, the clinical or laboratory data suggest that the cocci may have a pathogenic role, their finding and antibiotic sensitivities should be reported, but with the caution that they may still only be contaminants from the skin.

In most cases it is unnecessary to identify the species of an isolate of an albus staphylococcus, but in cases in which the organism is considered to be the cause of a serious infection, as in a compromised host, and particularly when an attempt is being made to trace the source of the infection, identification of the species may be valuable.

Urinary infection

Albus staphylococci, particularly *S. epidermidis*, derived from the urethral orifice, are commonly present in small or moderate numbers as contaminants in mid-stream specimens of urine, and when their count is less than 10^5/ml, may be disregarded. However, when they number more than 10^5/ml in a fresh specimen of urine, and particularly when identified as *S. saprophyticus* by their resistance to 1.6 mg/litre novobiocin, they are probably the cause of a urinary-tract infection and their presence and antibiotic sensitivities should be reported.

Antibiotic sensitivity

Isolates of albus staphylococci from hospital sources show a greater frequency and a wider spectrum of resistance to different antibiotics than isolates from sources outside hospital. Many strains are resistant to penicillin, ampicillin, methicillin and cloxacillin. The cephalosporins, gentamicin, fusidic acid and vancomycin have been found the most commonly effective drugs.

METHODS

Milk agar

On this medium (Christie & Keogh 1940) large characteristic colonies of staphylococci appear within 24 h. Pigmentation is particularly well developed and easily recognized against the opaque white background.

Fresh or sterilized milk	100 ml
Sterile nutrient agar	200 ml

The nutrient agar must contain 50% more agar than normal, e.g. 2% instead of 1.3%.

Heat fresh milk to 60°C, shake it, then sterilize it by autoclaving at 121°C for 15 min. Avoid repeated sterilization, which causes caramelization and change of colour. Suitable sterilized milk may be obtained commercially.

Melt the agar, cool to 56°C, mix with the milk and pour plates.

Selective salt media

Staphylococci can grow in the presence of 10% or more of sodium chloride, which is inhibitory to many other bacteria, particularly the Gram-negative organisms.

Salt milk agar is a good selective plating medium, with the added advantage of enhancing pigmentation. Prepare it in the same way as milk agar, but add 7–10% sodium chloride to the nutrient agar. The highest concentration of salt makes the medium most selective, but may slightly inhibit the growth of the staphylococci.

Salt cooked meat broth is used as a preliminary enrichment medium to assist the isolation of small numbers of staphylococci from heavily contaminated materials. Prepare it in the same way as cooked meat broth (Ch. 6), but add 10% sodium chloride before sterilizing.

Phenolphthalein phosphate agar

Nutrient agar pH 7.4	98 ml
Sodium phenolphthalein diphosphate, 0.6% solution	2 ml

Take sodium phenolphthalein diphosphate from a fresh batch of the compound, dissolve it in water to 0.6% concentration, sterilize it by filtration and at once add it to melted nutrient agar to the concentration of 0.012% just before pouring into plates. After setting, dry surface moisture from the plates. The complete medium may be stored at 4°C for 1–2 weeks and then be remelted for pouring into plates, but one of the plates should then be tested with ammonia for the presence of free phenolphthalein before the others are used.

Use. Spread the inoculum thinly over the plate and incubate it aerobically for 18 h at 37°C or for 3 days at 30°C. After incubation, place 0.1 ml of ammonia solution SG 0.88 in the lid of the plate and place the dish with the culture over the ammonia for a minute or so. Colonies of *S. aureus* become bright pink.

Coagulase tests

The reagent is human or rabbit plasma. If human plasma is used, for safety it should be from blood known to be free from hepatitis B antigen and HIV antibody. Obtain small volumes of plasma by centrifuging blood to which 0.2–0.3% sodium oxalate or 0.1% ethylenediaminetetraacetic acid (EDTA) has been added.

Collect larger volumes of plasma from outdated, e.g. 3-week-old, human blood containing 0.33% trisodium citrate, discarded from the blood transfusion service. Confirm the suitability of the plasma in slide and tube tests with standard coagulase-positive and coagulase-negative cultures. Then store in 20 ml volumes at −20°C for many months. Store an in-use volume for a week or so in the refrigerator at 4°C. Avoid repeated freezing and thawing.

A disadvantage of the use of citrated plasma is that false-positive reactions are given by some bacteria, e.g. *Streptococcus faecalis*, which may clot the plasma within 8 h by utilization of the citrate.

Slide coagulase test (Williams & Harper 1946).

1. Place a drop of saline (0.85% NaCl) solution or water on a clean microscope slide and, with a minimum of spreading, emulsify in it the material from one or two colonies of the culture under test. If the strain is autoagglutinable and fails to give a smooth, milky suspension, do not proceed with the slide test.

2. In the same way, make a control suspension of a known coagulase-positive culture to confirm the reactivity of the plasma.

3. Dip the tip of a straight inoculating wire into the undiluted plasma warmed to room temperature and stir the adhering traces of plasma (not a loopful) into the drop of bacterial suspension on the slide. Flame the wire and repeat the procedure for the control suspension.

4. Read as a positive reaction the appearance of coarse clumping visible to the naked eye within 5–10 s. Read as negative the absence of clumping or any reaction taking more than 10 s to develop, but re-examine any slow-reacting strains by the tube test.

Tube coagulase test (Gillespie 1943). 1. Prepare

a 1 in 10 dilution of the plasma in saline (0.85% NaCl) solution and place 0.5 ml of the diluted plasma in a small tube.

2. Inoculate into the diluted plasma 0.1 ml of an 18–24 h broth culture (about 10^8 cocci) of the strain under test.

Alternatively, to avoid a day's delay while the broth culture is grown, emulsify a few colonies to give a dense suspension in a small volume of broth and add 0.1 ml of this suspension (about 10^9 cocci) to the diluted plasma.

3. With each batch of tests, set up control tests with known coagulase-positive and coagulase-negative cultures and include a tube of unseeded diluted plasma to confirm that it does not coagulate spontaneously.

4. Incubate the tubes at 37°C, preferably in a waterbath, and examine them for coagulation at 1, 3 and 6 h, and again, if still negative, after standing overnight at room temperature. Examination at each of the prescribed times is necessary as the coagulum may liquefy after it has been formed.

5. Read as positive a test in which the plasma has been converted into a stiff gel, best recognized by its remaining in place when the tube is tilted or inverted (4+ reaction). Read as negative a test in which the plasma remains wholly liquid and free flowing. Read as doubtful a test showing a large (3+) or small (2+) organized clot or several small unorganized clots (1+) surrounded by clear liquid. Re-examine any strain giving a doubtful reaction by another test, such as that for DNase.

Deoxyribonuclease (DNase) plate test

The following method is modified from Jeffries (1961).

1. Prepare DNA agar (e.g. Oxoid DNase Agar) containing per litre: tryptose 20 g, deoxyribonuclease 2 g, sodium chloride 5 g and agar powder 12 g, pH 7.3. Autoclave at 121°C for 15 min, mix well and pour in plates.

2. After setting and drying of the plates, divide each into about six sections by drawing lines on its bottom.

3. Inoculate material from the colony under test by spotting it on to a small area in the middle of one of the marked sections of the DNA plate. Spot-inoculate other cultures to be tested on to other sections, including a control culture of a known DNase-positive strain, e.g. the Oxford strain of *S. aureus*.

4. Incubate the plate aerobically for 18–24 h at 37°C.

5. After incubation, flood the plate with 1 mol/ litre (3.6%) hydrochloric acid to precipitate the unhydrolysed DNA.

6. Let the plate stand for a few minutes until a white cloudiness is seen in the agar and then carefully examine the plate under strong indirect light against a dark background.

7. Read as DNase positive those spot cultures that are surrounded by a clear, uncloudy zone comparable in width to that around the control culture, e.g. 3 mm in radial width from the edge of the colony. Read as negative the cultures with markedly smaller zones and those with no clearing at all.

Biochemical tests

Because some species of albus staphylococci and micrococci grow poorly under the conditions of the standard biochemical tests (Ch. 8), modified methods to demonstrate their distinguishing characters (Tables 16.1 and 16.2) have been recommended by Baird-Parker (1966, 1979).

A kit for easy performance of tests for 19 biochemical reactions distinguishing 22 species and varieties of *Staphylococcus* (API STAPH) is available from API Lab Products.

Modified Hugh & Leifson test

This is a test for the aerobic and anaerobic breakdown of glucose by staphylococci and micrococci (International Subcommittee on Staphylococci and Micrococci 1965; Baird-Parker 1966).

1. Prepare a medium containing per litre: Difco tryptone 10 g, Difco yeast extract 1 g, glucose 10 g, bromocresol purple 0.04 g, Difco agar 2 g, pH 7.2. Distribute in 10 ml amounts in 6 × 0.5 in (15 × 1.3 cm) tubes and autoclave at 115°C for 20 min. If stored, steam briefly at 100°C and cool quickly before use.

2. Inoculate the culture under test into two tubes of the medium by stabbing throughout their length with a long wire loop.

3. Cover one tube of the pair with a layer of sterile liquid paraffin at least 1 in (2.5 cm) deep and incubate both tubes for 5 days at 37°C.

4. Read yellow colouration as acid production from glucose. Staphylococci produce acid by fermentation throughout the depth of the medium both in the anaerobic tube sealed with paraffin and the aerobic, unsealed tube. Micrococci either fail to produce acid in either tube or produce it only by oxidation in the upper part of the aerobic tube.

Sugar fermentations

1. Prepare a medium containing per litre: $NH_4H_2PO_4$ 1 g, KCl 0.2 g, $MgSO_4.7H_2O$ 0.2 g, yeast extract 2 g, bromocresol purple 0.04 g, agar powder 1 g, pH 7.0. Alternatively, use Purple Agar Base (Difco). Autoclave for 15 min at 121°C.

2. While the medium is molten at 46–48°C, add a 10% solution of the sugar sterilized by filtration to give a final concentration of 1% sugar in the medium. Pour 20 ml volumes in Petri dishes and dry off surface moisture.

3. Streak-inoculate up to four broth cultures of strains under test on to each plate and incubate for 5 days at 30°C.

4. Examine the plates daily for an acid (yellow) colour change, which may become reversed on continued incubation.

Acetoin production

1. Prepare a medium containing per litre: tryptone 10 g, Oxoid Lab-Lemco meat extract 3 g, yeast extract 1 g, glucose 20 g, pH 7.2. Distribute in 5 ml amounts into 25 ml screw-capped bottles and autoclave for 20 min at 115°C.

2. Inoculate a drop of broth culture of the strain under test into a bottle of the medium and incubate for 14 days at 30°C.

3. Add 1 ml of 40% potassium hydroxide and 3 ml of a 5% solution of alpha-naphthol in ethanol and shake vigorously for at least 30 s.

4. Read a reddening of the supernatant fluid within 5–10 min as indicating the production of acetoin.

Phosphatase production

1. With carefully rinsed glassware, prepare a 0.005 mol/litre solution of sodium phenolphthalein monophosphate in 0.01 mol/l citric acid-sodium citrate buffer at pH 5.8 and distribute 0.5 ml volumes in 75 × 10 mm tubes.

2. Inoculate a loopful of a well grown culture of the strain under test in heart infusion broth, or a suspension of 10^9/ml agar-grown cocci in broth, into a tube of the solution and incubate for 4 h at 37°C in a waterbath.

3. Add 0.5 ml of 0.5 mol/litre sodium hydroxide and 0.5 ml of 1 mol/l sodium bicarbonate. Then add 0.5 ml of 4-aminoantipyrine (6 g/l) and 0.5 ml of potassium ferricyanide (24 g/l).

4. Read the development of a red colour as indicating the production of phosphatase. This test is more reliable than the phosphatase plate test described above.

Catalase production

1. Prepare a medium containing per litre: Difco Bacto peptone 10 g, Difco yeast extract 1 g, glucose 10 g, sodium chloride 5 g, agar powder 1.5 g, pH 7.1. Autoclave for 15 min at 121°C.

2. Grow the culture under test on this medium overnight at 37°C. Then transfer a small portion of it on a clean platinum wire or glass rod into a tube containing 3% (v/v) hydrogen peroxide and watch for the evolution of bubbles indicative of catalase activity.

Novobiocin sensitivity

1. To molten medium prepared as described above for the catalase test, add a filter-sterilized solution of novobiocin to give a concentration of 1.6 mg/litre and pour plates.

2. Streak-inoculate the cultures under test on to a plate of this medium, incubate aerobically for 24 h at 37°C and examine for the presence (resistant) or absence (sensitive) of growth.

In the routine identification of albus staphylococci isolated from urine it is generally satisfactory to test for novobiocin sensitivity by including a 5 μg novobiocin disk in the usual disk diffusion test for antibiotic sensitivities. *S.* *epidermidis* shows a large zone of inhibition of growth, e.g. over 15 mm in diameter around a 7 mm disk, whilst *S. saprophyticus* shows a much smaller zone or grows right up to the disk.

REFERENCES

Baird-Parker A C 1966 Methods for classifying staphylococci and micrococci. In: Gibbs B M, Skinner F A (eds) Identification methods for microbiologists, part A, the Society for Applied Bacteriology Technical Series No. 1. Academic Press, London. p 59–64

Baird-Parker A C 1974 Micrococcaceae. In: Buchanan R E, Gibbons N E (eds) Bergey's manual of determinative bacteriology, 8th edn. Williams & Wilkins, Baltimore. p 478–489

Baird-Parker A C 1979 Methods for identifying staphylococci and micrococci. In: Skinner F A, Lovelock D W (eds) Identification methods for microbiologists, The Society for Applied Microbiology Technical Series No. 14. Academic Press, London. p 201–210

Barber M, Kuper S W A 1951 Identification of *Staphylococcus pyogenes* by the phosphatase reaction. Journal of Pathology and Bacteriology 63: 65–68

Bergdoll M S 1970 Enterotoxins. In: Montie T C, Kadis S, Ajl S J (eds) Microbial toxins vol III. Academic Press, London. p 265–326

Blair E B, Emerson J S, Tull A H 1967 A new medium, salt mannitol plasma agar, for the isolation of *Staphylococcus aureus*. American Journal of Clinical Pathology 47: 30–39

Christie R, Keogh E V 1940 Physiological and serological characteristics of staphylococci of human origin. Journal of Pathology and Bacteriology 51: 189–197

Cowan S T 1939 The classification of staphylococci by slide agglutination. Journal of Pathology and Bacteriology 48: 169–173

Drew W L, Barry A L, O'Toole R, Sherris J C 1972 Reliability of the Kirby-Bauer disc diffusion method for detecting methicillin-resistant strains of *Staphylococcus aureus*. Applied Microbiology 24: 240–247

Elek S D 1959 *Staphylococcus pyogenes* and its relation to disease. Livingstone, Edinburgh. p 219–312

Elek S D, Levy E 1950 The distribution of haemolysins in pathogenic and non-pathogenic staphylococci. Journal of Pathology and Bacteriology 62: 541–554

Gilbert R J, Wieneke A A, Lanser J, Simkovicova M 1972 Serological detection of enterotoxin in foods implicated in staphylococcal food-poisoning. Journal of Hygiene (Cambridge) 70: 755–762

Gillespie E H 1943 The routine use of the coagulase test for staphylococci. Monthly Bulletin of the Emergency Public Health Laboratory Service 2: 19–22

Gillespie W A, Alder V G 1952 Production of opacity in egg-yolk media by coagulase-positive staphylococci. Journal of Pathology and Bacteriology 64: 187–200

Gramoli J L, Wilkinson B J 1978 Characterization and identification of coagulase-negative, heat-stable deoxyribonuclease positive staphylococci. Journal of General Microbiology 105: 275–285

Hewitt J H, Coe A W, Parker M T 1969 The detection of methicillin resistance in *Staphylococcus aureus*. Journal of Medical Microbiology 2: 443–456

Hill J H, White E C 1929 Sodium chloride media for the separation of certain Gram-positive cocci and Gram-negative bacilli. Journal of Bacteriology 18: 43–57

Hill L R 1981 Taxonomy of the staphylococci. In: Macdonald A, Smith G (eds) The staphylococci. Aberdeen University Press, Aberdeen. p 33–62

International Subcommittee on Staphylococci and Micrococci 1965 Recommendations of the subcommittee. International Bulletin of Bacterial Nomenclature and Taxonomy 15: 109–110

Jacobs S I, Willis A T, Goodburn G M 1964 Pigment production and enzymatic activity of staphylococci; the differentiation of pathogens from commensals. Journal of Pathology and Bacteriology 87: 151–167

Jeffries C D 1961 Comparison of six physiological characteristics of staphylococci from laboratory specimens. American Journal of Clinical Pathology 36: 114–118

Kloos W E, Schleifer K H 1975 Simplified scheme for routine identification of human *Staphylococcus* species. Journal of Clinical Microbiology 1: 82–88

Lacey R W 1987 Multi-resistant *Staphylococcus aureus* – a suitable case for inactivity? Journal of Hospital Infection 9: 103–105

Lachicha R V F, Genigeorgis C, Hoepich P D 1971 Metachromatic agar-diffusion methods for detecting staphylococcal nuclease activity. Applied Microbiology 21: 585–587

McCartney A C, Arbuthnott J P 1978 Mode of action of membrane-damaging toxins produced by staphylococci. In: Jeljaszewicz J, Wadstrom T (eds) Bacterial toxins and cell membranes. Academic Press, London. p 89–127

Oeding P 1978 Genus *Staphylococcus*. In: Bergan T, Norris J R (eds) Methods in microbiology, vol 12. Academic Press, London. p 127–176

Parker M T 1972 Phage-typing of *Staphylococcus aureus*. In: Norris J R, Ribbons D W (eds) Methods in microbiology, vol 7B. Academic Press, London. p 1–28

Report 1986 Guidelines for the control of epidemic methicillin-resistant *Staphylococcus aureus*. Report of a combined Working Party of the Hospital Infection Society and British Society for Antimicrobial Chemotherapy. Journal of Hospital Infection 7: 193–201

Schleifer K H, Kloos W E 1975 A simple test for the separation of staphylococci from micrococci. Journal of Clinical Microbiology 1: 337–338

Williams R E O, Harper G J 1946 Determination of coagulase and alpha-haemolysin production by staphylococci. British Journal of Experimental Pathology 27: 72–81

Streptococcus

The genus *Streptococcus* consists of chain-forming Gram-positive cocci that are facultative anaerobes; related species that are strict anaerobes are discussed in Chapter 36. Pneumococci are separately considered in Chapter 18. Streptococci are catalase negative and this may help to distinguish them from staphylococci and other cluster-forming Gram-positive cocci (see Ch. 16).

The initial classification of streptococci traditionally depends on the type of haemolysis produced on blood agar media. Streptococci usually grow better and often give improved haemolytic reactions when incubated anaerobically. Strains that produce soluble haemolysin (streptolysin O or S) have a definite zone of clearing around colonies on blood agar (β-haemolysis). Some species that do not produce soluble haemolysin cause partial clearing and often green colouration (α-haemolysis). Others are non-haemolytic strains that produce no obvious change around colonies on blood agar; the term 'γ-haemolysis' to denote absence of haemolysis should not be used.

Serological subdivision of the haemolytic streptococci exploits differences in the group-specific polysaccharide antigens in the cell wall. Lancefield thus identified different groups of β-haemolytic streptococci and her scheme now includes 20 serological groups with sequential letters A–H and K–V. Group A β-haemolytic strains, which are responsible for many important human infections, are given the species name *Streptococcus pyogenes*. A variety of other streptococcal species, of various Lancefield groups and haemolytic activities, are also found as pathogens and commensals in man and domestic animals (Table 17.1). It should be appreciated that biochemical and other criteria are also used in defining various species within a single serogroup, e.g. group D streptococci; similarly, some species contain strains of more than one serogroup. A number of species contain strains with different haemolytic reactions, e.g. *S. faecalis, S. agalactiae*. The viridans group of streptococci contains several different species that are α- or non-haemolytic and that may or may not possess Lancefield group antigens; some of these were previously classified as '*S. viridans*' but this is no longer an accepted species name. Reference may be made to Bergey's Manual (Sneath et al 1986) for further details of streptococcal identification; the species of greatest clinical interest are discussed below.

STREPTOCOCCUS PYOGENES (LANCEFIELD GROUP A)

The majority of β-haemolytic streptococci causing infections in man belong to group A and are given the species name *S. pyogenes*. This pathogen is directly responsible for a variety of inflammatory and suppurative conditions such as sore throat, scarlet fever, cellulitis, erysipelas, impetigo, puerperal sepsis, otitis media, septicaemia and wound infections; it is indirectly associated with rheumatic fever, glomerulonephritis and erythema nodosum. It is also found in the throat or nasal cavity in a proportion of apparently healthy people ('carriers').

Morphology and staining

Gram-positive, spherical cocci 0.7–0.9 μm in diameter occurring in chains of varying length, best demonstrated in smears of pus or in liquid

Table 17.1 Classification of streptococci.
Key: NH, non-haemolytic; groups H, K, O, R, S, and T are commonly classified as viridans streptococci.

Serological group	Species	Type of haemolysis	Main habitat
A	*S. pyogenes*	β	Man
B	*S. agalactiae*	α, β or NH	Man, cattle
C	*S. dysgalactiae*	α	Cattle
	S. equi	β	Horses
	S. equisimilis	β	Man, animals
	S. zooepidemicus	β	Animals
D	*S. faecalis*	β or NH	Intestine of
	S. faecium	α, β or NH	man and
	S. durans	α, β or NH	animals
	S. avium	α or NH	Birds
	S. bovis	α or NH	Faeces of animals
	S. equinus	α or NH	Faeces of horses
E, P, U, V	*S. infrequens*	β	Pigs, cattle
F, G	*S. anginosus*	β	Man
H	*S. sanguis*	α	Mouth and
K	*S. salivarius*	α	intestine of man
L	*S. salivarius*	β	Dogs and pigs
M	*S. salivarius*	α or NH	Dogs
N	*S. lactis*	α or NH	Milk and dairy
	S. cremoris	α or NH	products
O	*S. cremoris*	α or β	Man
Q	*S. avium*	α	Birds
R, S, T	*S. suis*	α	Pigs

culture medium. Non-motile, non-sporing, capsulate in very young cultures.

Cultural characters

Facultative anaerobe: optimum temperature for growth 37°C (range 22–42°C). Grows best on blood or serum agar. Colonies are small (0.5–1 mm diameter after 24 h), semi-transparent, low convex, discrete with a matt or glossy surface when freshly isolated (matt colonies contain M antigen). Mucoid colonies may occur when strain is obviously capsulate. Clear, often wide, zone of haemolysis surrounds colonies on horse or sheep blood agar; variable haemolysis with human or rabbit blood agar.

Sensitivity to physical and chemical agents

Killed by 54°C for 30 min. May resist natural drying for weeks if protected from daylight. Laboratory cultures should be stored at 3–5°C in blood broth or cooked meat medium, or freeze-dried. Sensitive to most antiseptics, to benzylpenicillin and to a wide range of anti-microbial drugs; naturally resistant to amino-glycosides; acquired resistance to sulphonamides, tetracyclines, and less commonly to clindamycin and macrolides. *S. pyogenes* is more sensitive to bacitracin than other haemolytic streptococci and this is utilized as a screening test for serogrouping.

Biochemical activities

S. pyogenes is catalase negative and insoluble in bile, but biochemical tests are of little value in laboratory identification.

Exoenzymes and toxins

S. pyogenes produces a number of exoproteins that may play a part in streptococcal patho-genesis; although the products listed below may be virulence factors the evidence linking them with particular aspects of streptococcal infections is still incomplete. Most strains of *S. pyogenes* can produce most of these products under suitable conditions; some are also produced by other groups of β-haemolytic streptococci, e.g. groups C and G. Most of these products are antigenic; tests for antibody to some of them may be of diagnostic value (see below).

Erythrogenic toxins (Dick toxins) are responsible for the rash in scarlet fever. There are three serologically distinct toxins that are antigenic and neutralized by specific antitoxins; the Dick test, in which a test dose of erythrogenic toxin is injected intradermally, detects the presence or absence of such antibodies. Production of these toxins is determined by specific bacteriophages in the lysogenic state.

Haemolysins. Streptococcal haemolysins can also affect many other cells and are better described as cytolysins. *Streptolysin O* is inactivated by oxygen (oxygen-labile); it is produced by the majority of group A streptococci and by some strains of groups C and G. *Streptolysin S* is not inactivated by oxygen (oxygen-stable) and is responsible for the haemolysis produced on the surface of an aerobic blood agar plate; it is not antigenic.

Deoxyribonucleases (DNases) are produced by streptococci of groups A, C and G. There are at least four enzymes, distinguished immunologically and designated A, B, C and D; DNase B is the most common form in *S. pyogenes*.

Streptokinase (fibrinolysin), *hyaluronidase* and *nicotinamide adenine dinucleotidase* (NADase: formerly known as diphosphopyridine nucleotidase – DPNase) are produced by strains of groups A, B, C and G streptococci.

Serum opacity factor (SOF). The ability to produce opacity in horse serum is a characteristic of certain M types of group A streptococci. The SOF is a lipoproteinase closely associated with the M protein and loosely bound to the cell. It is antigenically specific, the specificity corresponding to that of the M antigen.

Cellular antigens

Group-specific carbohydrate. β-haemolytic streptococci are separated into 20 different Lancefield groups on the basis of this major component of the cell wall.

M protein. Group A streptococci can be further subdivided into over 60 Griffith's serotypes on the basis of specific M protein antigens of the cell wall. The M protein, a complex entity, impedes phagocytosis and is responsible for virulence; specific anti-M antibody develops after infection and enhances phagocytosis. Fimbriae on the cell surface that enable the organism to attach to epithelial cells are also M protein.

T protein is another surface antigen complex that may be present in certain group A strains and is used as a marker in epidemiological studies of streptococcal infections. Unlike M proteins, T proteins do not appear to be related to pathogenicity.

R protein. These antigens are present in a few group A serotypes, e.g. Griffith's type 28, but their significance is unknown.

Laboratory diagnosis of β-haemolytic streptococcal infections

This includes identification of β-haemolytic streptococci that have been isolated from the patient and examination of serum for a rising titre of antibody to one or more streptococcal antigens. The bacteriologist's primary aim is to determine whether a β-haemolytic streptococcus is the major pathogen, *S. pyogenes* (group A). The need to identify other groups depends on whether the clinical circumstances suggest that such a less pathogenic streptococcus may be clinically significant.

Culture of streptococci

Organisms are usually cultured from swabs (throat, pus, vaginal, etc.) taken from patients with signs of infection or from suspected carriers; the observation of typical Gram-positive cocci arranged in short chains on microscopic examination of smears of pus may indicate the likelihood of the presence of streptococci. Plate swabs on agar media containing 5–10% blood and incubate for 24 h; haemolysis is often improved in anaerobic cultures. It is good practice to set up both aerobic and anaerobic culture plates for all relevant specimens, e.g. throat swabs, because some group A strains form only O-lysin and fail to show haemolysis on aerobic plates. Although horse or human blood is commonly used, sheep blood is also useful since it inhibits the production of haemolysis by *Haemophilus haemolyticus*, which may easily be mistaken for streptococcal haemolysis. Crystal violet blood agar* and PNF medium* are useful selective media that inhibit many throat commensal organisms; *S. pyogenes* does not grow on MacConkey agar and is always sensitive to benzylpenicillin. Streptococcal colonies that produce β-haemolysis and that are sensitive to benzylpenicillin should be further investigated; a 1 μg disk may be placed on the well of the primary culture plate to give an early indication of penicillin sensitivity.

Bacitracin sensitivity

In some instances, all that the clinician may require to know is whether β-haemolytic strep-tococci have been isolated from a lesion and whether or not they belong to group A; in this case the bacitracin sensitivity of the organism may be tested. Group A streptococci are much more sensitive than other groups but the test is not totally reliable as some non-group-A strep-tococci may also be sensitive to bacitracin. Bacitracin disks* may be added to primary culture plates as part of the initial screen for *S. pyogenes*.

Lancefield grouping

In most cases, full serogrouping should be performed as this will provide epidemiological surveillance of streptococcal infections in the community and hospital and will alert the clin-ician to potentially serious situations, e.g. the isolation of group B streptococci from a neonate. Drug resistance patterns may also be monitored at the same time.

There is now an increasing trend to use commercial kits for streptococcal grouping. These have proved very convenient and reliable

---

* Refer to *Methods* at end of this chapter.

although rather expensive: Streptex (Wellcome) is a latex particle agglutination test; Phadebact (Pharmacia) and Streptosec (Organon) are coag-glutination tests. Although these kits do not require extraction of the carbohydrate antigen from the streptococcal cell this is still essential for the majority of grouping procedures. Two techniques for extraction of the antigen are described below, using hydrochloric acid* or formamide*. Alternative techniques that may be used include: autoclaving (Rantz & Randall 1955); pronase B (Ederer et al 1972); nitrous acid (El Kholy et al 1974); and *Streptomyces albus* enzyme with lysozyme (Watson et al 1975).

After the antigen has been extracted from the cell wall various methods can be used for grouping streptococci. Precipitation tests are detailed below*. Other techniques for strepto-coccal grouping include: slide agglutination (Rosendal 1956; Maxted et al 1976); gel diffusion (Freimer 1963; Rotta et al 1971); counter-current immunoelectrophoresis (Dajani 1973); fluores-cent antibody tests (Moody et al 1958); and enzyme-linked immunosorbent assays (ELISA; Cumming et al 1980).

Typing of group A strains

These tests, which are undertaken only in special-ized laboratories, use specific agglutinating* and precipitating* antisera. Tests for the serum opacity reaction (SOR) may also be used to type group A strains (Maxted et al 1973).

Serological tests

These tests, preferably with paired sera, are used to detect a rise in antibody titre to one or more of the extracellular products of *S. pyogenes*. They may be used to identify or confirm primary infections but are more commonly used for the diagnosis of the non-suppurative sequelae of group A streptococcal infection, such as rheu-matic fever or glomerulonephritis. The anti-streptolysin O (ASO) test (Gooder & Williams 1959) is used most frequently (upper limit of normal 200 Todd units/ml); a commercial latex particle kit is also available (Rapitex ASL, Behring). The anti-DNase B estimation may also be useful (Wannamaker & Ayoub 1960). Other tests, only occasionally used and then only by specialist laboratories, are: anti-streptokinase (ASK), anti-hyaluronidase (ASH) and anti-NADase (WHO Report 1968).

Antibody to M protein on the streptococcal surface can be measured by several tests including the bactericidal and long chain tests but these are complicated and are rarely performed.

STREPTOCOCCUS AGALACTIAE (LANCEFIELD GROUP B)

These organisms have been known since the end of last century as common causes of mastitis in cattle, but it was not until the 1930s that their association with human disease was recognized. Few group B infections were reported in the 1940s and early 1950s, but by the early 1970s group B streptococci had become increasingly common; there appears to be a real change in the incidence and epidemiology of infection. In many ways group B streptococci have now replaced group A, the scourge of the pre-1940s, as the major streptococcal pathogen in sites other than the upper respiratory tract; group B streptococci are particularly associated with septicaemia and meningitis in neonates. The source of infection is usually from the mother (ano-genital commensal carriage is not uncommon) but cross infection may also occur. Infections such as pneumonia, endocarditis, meningitis, cellulitis, arthritis can also occur in adults, particularly in the compromised host.

Accordingly, the isolation of group B streptococci from infections of neonates and puerperal mothers, or from deep infections or infections of compromised patients may be of urgent clinical significance and sensitivity tests should be done. Isolation of these organisms from the respiratory tract, where they may be commensals, is not normally an indication for action.

Culture of group B streptococci

When grown on blood agar plates haemolysis is usually β in nature though not as clear as that produced by group A; sometimes it is closer to the α type, and occasionally no haemolysis is produced at all. Group B streptococci may also grow on MacConkey medium. Colonies may be orange on some media, but pigment is more reliably formed on Islam medium. In epidemiological studies selective media are useful to minimize overgrowth by other organisms, especially if only a few colonies of group B organisms can be cultured from the clinical specimen; nalidixic acid and an aminoglycoside (e.g. gentamicin) are useful selective agents in blood media.* Presumptive tests for identification of group B streptococci include the CAMP reaction,* hydrolysis of sodium hippurate,* and the test for production of orange pigment.*

Typing

Serotyping has been used to study the epidemiology of group B infections (Lancefield 1934). Seven serotypes are identified on the basis of four carbohydrate antigens and the presence or absence of protein antigens; these may be detected by precipitation tests or counter-current immunoelectrophoresis (see Ch. 10). Phage typing has also been developed for group B streptococci (Stringer & Maxted 1979).

GROUP C AND G STREPTOCOCCI

Streptococci of Lancefield groups C and G produce wide zones of β-haemolysis and have been associated with a variety of infections in man, e.g. sore throat, endocarditis, pulmonary infections, skin and wound infections.

GROUP D STREPTOCOCCI

These may cause urinary tract infections, endocarditis, biliary tract infections, suppurative abdominal lesions and ear infections in man. They may participate in mixed infections of wounds but often occur as contaminants in open wounds and bedsores. The commonest species infecting humans is S. faecalis; others include S. faecium and S. durans. These three species are commonly referred to as 'enterococci' or faecal streptococci. *S. faecalis*, usually in the non-haemolytic form, is constantly present as a commensal in the intestine and therefore in the faeces; it is sometimes present in the oral flora.

S. faecalis is characteristically rather larger than *S. pyogenes*, in ovoid pairs or in short chains: non-motile, non-capsulate. Grows readily on ordinary culture media and on MacConkey agar as minute (0.5–1 mm) magenta-coloured colonies; also grows on media with a high salt content. Withstands heat at 60°C for 30 min, a distinguishing feature from other streptococci, and also grows within a wider temperature range (10–45°C). Ferments mannitol with gas production; Voges-Proskauer positive. Strains may be subdivided into specific types according to biochemical and other activities; some strains liquefy gelatin and produce H_2S.

Enterococci are resistant to sulphonamides and benzylpenicillin but relatively sensitive to ampicillin and amoxycillin, which may be used in treatment of urinary tract infection. Resistant to aminoglycosides, but *S. faecalis* endocarditis usually responds to high doses of a combination of a penicillin and an aminoglycoside; vancomycin may be of value for strains that are particularly resistant to other drugs.

Laboratory diagnosis of group D streptococcal infections

Growth on MacConkey medium distinguishes group D enterococci from most other streptococci except those of group B. Identity is most easily confirmed by subculture to bile aesculin azide agar, on which enterococci form black colonies (*Methods*, Ch. 11).

VIRIDANS STREPTOCOCCI

This term presently denotes a group of streptococcal species, some strains of which produce partial haemolysis and green colouration (α-haemolysis) around colonies on blood agar plates although others produce no haemolysis; they are constantly present in large numbers as commensals in the bacterial flora of the mouth and oropharynx. At least six species are recognized: *salivarius, mitior (mitis), milleri, sanguis, mutans* and *pneumoniae*; the latter is dealt with separately in the next chapter of this book in view of its special medical importance. Other species of α-haemolytic streptococci are loosely included in the viridans category by some authors. The medical importance of the viridans group is their association with dental sepsis, caries and bacterial endocarditis. *S. milleri* is associated with deep sepsis, including liver and brain abscesses. *S. mutans, S. mitior* and *S. sanguis* are involved in the production of dental caries, and *S. mitior* and *S. sanguis* are also important causes of endocarditis. The pathogenicity of *S. salivarius* is not clear but this species also may be associated with the production of caries.

'Streptococcus MG' is one of the viridans group with fortuitous serological cross-relationships with *Mycoplasma pneumoniae* (Ch. 45).

Laboratory identification of viridans streptococci

The viridans streptococci resemble *S. pyogenes* morphologically but sometimes may be more ovoid and are usually in short chains: usually grow well on nutrient agar: because of the green colouration, best seen on heated blood agar, they may have to be distinguished from pneumococci (Ch. 18). Table 17.2 summarizes the tests that distinguish the various species that comprise the viridans streptococci. Some viridans streptococci, notably *S. milleri*, are CO_2-dependent or enhanced by CO_2. Since strains may be more resistant to penicillin and other antimicrobial drugs than *S. pyogenes*, isolates from blood culture in bacterial endocarditis should be tested for sensitivity.

The primary recognition of these organisms rests on their α-haemolytic colonies on blood agar, their general failure to grow on MacConkey medium and, in most cases, their sensitivity to penicillin. Remember that some strains of *S. pyogenes* and group B streptococci may give poor haemolytic appearances that may be mistaken for α- or α[1]-haemolysis on aerobic blood agar plates. Note also that some anaerobic cocci may produce α-haemolysis on anaerobic plates.

Table 17.2 Biochemical characterization of viridans streptococci. See *Methods* section for tests used.
Key: +/−, some strains positive, some negative.

Character	S. mutans	S. sanguis	S. salivarius	S. milleri	S. mitior
Acid production from:					
Mannitol	+	−	−	−	−
Trehalose	+	+	+/−	+	+/−
Raffinose	+	+/−	+/−	−	+/−
Salicin	+	+	+	−	+/−
Inositol	+	+	+/−	−	−
Sorbitol	+	−	−	−	−
Hydrolysis of:					
Aesculin	+	+	+	+	−
Arginine	−	+	−	+	−
Starch	−	+	−	+/−	+
Produced from sucrose:					
Levan	−	−	+	−	−
Dextran	+	+	−	−	−

When isolated from the mouth, throat or elsewhere in the respiratory tract, viridans streptococci are generally regarded as harmless commensals. When found in blood, an abscess or a closed lesion, they are more likely to be of pathogenic significance and should be reported, and their antibiotic sensitivities should be determined.

METHODS

Crystal violet blood agar

The addition of a low concentration (1 in 500 000, i.e. 0.0002%) of crystal violet to blood agar inhibits the growth of some bacteria, notably staphylococci, while allowing the growth of streptococci. Crystal violet blood agar is therefore a selective medium for *S. pyogenes*.

Sterile nutrient agar	90 ml
Sterile horse blood	10 ml
Crystal violet, 1 in 1000 aqueous solution	0.2 ml

Melt the agar, cool to 50°C, add the blood and crystal violet and pour plates.

PNF medium (Lowbury et al 1964)

Horse blood agar (5%) with the following addi-

tives is selective for β-haemolytic streptococci, e.g. *S. pyogenes*, but inhibits the growth of staphylococci and coliform species:

Polymyxin B sulphate	17 units/ml
Neomycin sulphate	4.25 μg/ml
Fusidic acid	0.50 μg/ml

Bacitracin sensitivity test (Maxted 1953)

Disks containing 0.04 units of bacitracin may be added to primary culture plates. Streptococci of Lancefield group A are sensitive, i.e. give a large (e.g. >15 mm diameter) zone of inhibition around the disk; most other streptococci are resistant, i.e. give no inhibition or only a small zone. Occasional strains of groups B, C and G may also be sensitive (Coleman et al 1977).

Methods of antigen extraction for Lancefield grouping

Two methods for extraction of the group-specific carbohydrate are described below, using hydrochloric acid or formamide. Since group O polysaccharide is sensitive to formamide such extracts do not react with O antiserum. Acid extracts can also be used in tests for identification of type-specific M antigens (see below).

Hydrochloric acid extract (Lancefield 1933)

Harvest the centrifuged deposit from 50 ml of an overnight Todd Hewitt broth culture in a small tube. Resuspend the deposit thoroughly in 0.4 ml of 0.5 mol/litre HCl. Place the tube in a boiling water bath for 10 min; remove and allow to cool. Add 1 drop of 0.02% phenol red. Neutralize carefully with 0.5 mol/l and then 0.2 mol/l NaOH. The clear supernate after centrifugation is the extract.

Formamide extract (Fuller 1938)

Suspend the deposit from 5 ml glucose broth culture (or scraping of growth from a quarter of a plate) in 0.1 ml formamide and heat in an oil bath at 160°C for 15 min or until almost completely dissolved. Cool, add 0.25 ml acid alcohol (0.5% HCl in 95% ethanol), shake and centrifuge. Add 0.5 ml of acetone to the supernate; shake and spin again. Discard supernate and dissolve precipitate in 0.3–0.4 ml saline; add 1 drop of phenol red and neutralize with 0.5 mol/litre NaOH. (Cross-reactions may occur if the extract is too alkaline.)

Precipitation test for Lancefield grouping

Specific antisera are obtainable from Wellcome. Tests may be performed in the narrowing neck of small Pasteur pipettes. Place a small volume of group A antiserum in the pipette and carefully superimpose the antigen extract. If the extract contains polysaccharide specific for group A, precipitation will be observed at the interface with the serum within 5 min; reactions appearing after this time should not be regarded as positive. Extracts should also be tested with antisera for groups B, C and G routinely, and if necessary with other group sera.

In order to conserve serum, tests may be performed in capillary tubes (Swift et al 1943). Run a 1 cm column of serum into the tube, the exterior of which must be carefully wiped before an equivalent volume of antigen extract is introduced. Allow the contents to run well up the tube and then occlude the upper end with the forefinger until the tube has been placed in a plasticine block. Macroscopic precipitation should be evident within the time limits stated above if the reaction is positive.

Typing of group A streptococci

For the complete epidemiological study of streptococcal infections it is necessary to identify the particular streptococcal serotype. Strains should be identified both by agglutinating (T) and precipitating (M) antisera, since a smaller percentage of strains will thus be regarded as untypable than when either method is employed alone. Antisera may be obtained from the Central Public Health Laboratory, Colindale, London NW9 5HT.

Slide agglutination test

Grow the strain in 5 ml Todd Hewitt broth at 28°C for 18–24 h and thoroughly resuspend the centrifuged deposit in 0.5 ml of supernatant broth. Provided that the suspension is not granular, place 6 loopfuls on a clean glass slide and then mix each with a small (1 mm) loopful of one of the 6 different antiserum pools; rock the slide to and fro for 1 min. If agglutination is noted with one of the pooled antisera, fresh loopfuls of suspension should then be similarly tested with each of the specific sera comprising that particular pool. Strains may react in more than one type-specific serum, but the pattern of such reactions is epidemiologically significant.

Granular suspensions and those that react with many sera should be treated as follows: add 1 drop of Universal Indicator (BDH) and 2 drops of trypsin 1:250 (Difco) to the suspension; adjust the pH to 8.0–8.5 with 0.2 mol/litre NaOH and place in a 37°C water bath for 1 h, shaking every 15 min. On retesting with pooled and specific antisera as above, many such strains will react normally; if results are still unsatisfactory, a further period of 15 min in a 50°C bath may be tried.

Precipitation test

Use acid-extracted antigen prepared for group determination. Test the extract against the relevant antisera by the capillary tube method. Incubate the capillary tubes for 2 h at 37°C and note the results; after overnight refrigeration, examine the tubes again for a white precipitate at the interface. Gel diffusion tests may also be used.

Selective medium for group B streptococci (Baker et al 1973)

Prepare the antibiotic solution, containing 15 μg/ml nalidixic acid and 8 μg/ml gentamicin. Add 0.5 ml of this solution and 0.25 ml of defibrinated sheep blood with aseptic precautions to 4.75 ml of sterile Todd Hewitt broth. This may be used as broth or with the addition of agar as a solid medium.

CAMP test (Christie et al 1944)

Streak a β-lysin-producing *Staphylococcus aureus* strain (NCTC1803) on a blood agar plate; 5% sheep or bovine blood must be used. Then make a single streak of the streptococcal strain perpendicular to the staphylococcal streak; leave about a 1 cm space between the two inoculation lines. Incubate the inoculated plates for 24 h at 37°C in air or in air with 10% CO_2; CAMP (Christie Atkins Munch-Peterson) tests must not be incubated anaerobically because some group A streptococci will then give a positive CAMP reaction. Under aerobic conditions, group B streptococci, but not other streptococci, produce a substance known as CAMP factor that enhances the β-lysin produced by the staphylococcus and an area of increased lysis appears at the junction of the two organisms. This area frequently appears in the shape of an arrowhead.

Sodium hippurate test (Ayers & Rupp 1922)

All group B streptococci hydrolyse hippurate. Some group D and a very few viridans strepto-

cocci do likewise; groups A, C, F and G do not.

The medium consists of 25 g Heart Infusion Broth (Difco) and 10 g sodium hippurate in 1 litre distilled water, dispensed in small screw-capped bottles. Inoculate with two colonies of β-haemolytic streptococci and incubate at 35°C for at least 20 h; centrifuge the medium and pipette 0.8 ml of the clear supernate into a tube. Add 0.2 ml of ferric chloride reagent to the tube and mix well; the reagent contains 12 g $FeCl_3.6H_2O$ in 100 ml 2% aqueous HCl (2% aqueous HCl is made by adding 5.4 ml of concentrated HCl (37%) to 94.6 ml H_2O). The test is positive if a heavy precipitate remains for longer than 10 min. The test is negative if there is immediate clearing of the tube, indicating that the hippurate has not been split. If weak reactions occur, the culture tubes should be reincubated for 24 h and the test repeated. A rapid colorimetric test has also been described (Edberg & Samuels 1976).

Pigment test

On Columbia agar (Oxoid) or a starch/serum agar many group B strains, but not other streptococci, form orange-coloured colonies on anaerobic incubation at 37°C for 18 h (Fallon 1974). The pigmentation is more intense and easily distinguished in cultures on the medium described by Islam (1977).

Tests for identification of viridans streptococci

Methods for performing the tests indicated in Table 17.2 are described by Parker & Ball (1976); commercially available biochemical profile tests, e.g. API 20 Strep, may also be used for the identification of streptococcal species. Alternatively, strains may be submitted to the Streptococcus Reference Laboratory, Central Public Health Laboratories, Colindale, London NW9 5HT, for identification.

REFERENCES

Ayers S H, Rupp P 1922 Differentiation of haemolytic streptococci from human and bovine sources by the hydrolysis of sodium hippurate. Journal of Infectious Diseases 30: 388–399

Baker C J, Clark D J, Barrett F F 1973 Selective broth medium for isolation of group B streptococci. Applied Microbiology 26: 884–885
Christie R, Atkins N E, Munch-Peterson E 1944 A note on

a lytic phenomenon shown by group B streptococci. Australian Journal of Experimental Biology and Medical Sciences 23: 197–200

Coleman D J, McGhie D, Tebbutt G M 1977 Further studies on the reliability of the bacitracin inhibition test for the presumptive identification of Lancefield group A streptococci. Journal of Clinical Pathology 30: 421–426

Cumming C G, Ross P W, Poxton I R, McBride W H 1980 The grouping of β-haemolytic streptococci by enzyme-linked immunosorbent assay. Journal of Medical Microbiology 13: 459–461

Dajani A S 1973 Rapid identification of beta-haemolytic streptococci by counterimmunoelectrophoresis. Journal of Immunology 110: 1702–1705

Edberg S C, Samuels S 1976 Rapid colorimetric test for the determination of hippurate hydrolysis by group B streptococcus. Journal of Clinical Microbiology 3: 49–50

Ederer G M, Hermann M M, Bruce R, Marsen J M, Chapman S S 1972 Rapid extraction method with pronase B for grouping beta-haemolytic streptococci. Applied Microbiology 23: 285–288

El Kholy A, Wannamaker L W, Krause R M 1974 Simplified extraction procedure for serological grouping of beta-haemolytic streptococci. Applied Microbiology 28: 836–839

Fallon R J 1974 The rapid recognition of Lancefield group B haemolytic streptococci. Journal of Clinical Pathology 27: 902–905

Freimer F H 1963 Studies of L forms and protoplasts of group A streptococci. Journal of Experimental Medicine 117: 377–399

Fuller A T 1938 The formamide method for the extraction of polysaccharide from haemolytic streptococci. British Journal of Experimental Pathology 19: 130–139

Gooder H, Williams R E O 1959 Titration of antistreptolysin O. Association of Clinical Pathologists Broadsheet No. 25

Islam A K M S 1977 Rapid recognition of group B streptococci. Lancet 1: 256–257

Lancefield R C 1933 A serological differentiation of human and other groups of haemolytic streptococci. Journal of Experimental Medicine 57: 571–595

Lancefield R C 1934 Serological differentiation of specific types of bovine haemolytic streptococci (group B). Journal of Experimental Medicine 59: 441–458

Lowbury E J, Kidson A, Lilly H A 1964 A new selective blood agar medium for Streptococcus pyogenes and other haemolytic streptococci. Journal of Clinical Pathology 17: 231–235

Maxted W R 1953 The use of bacitracin for identifying group A haemolytic streptococci. Journal of Clinical Pathology 6: 224–226

Maxted W R, Widdowson J P, Fraser C A M, Ball L C, Bassett D C J 1973 The use of the serum opacity reaction in the typing of group A streptococci. Journal of Medical Microbiology 6: 83–90

Maxted W R, Efstration A, Parker M T 1976 Agglutination grouping of streptococci. Lancet 2: 692–693

Moody M D, Ellis E C, Updyke E L 1958 Staining bacterial smears with fluorescent antibody. IV. Grouping streptococci with fluorescent antibody. Journal of Bacteriology 75: 553–560

Parker M T 1976 Streptococci and aerococci associated with systemic infections in man. Journal of Medical Microbiology 9: 275–302

Rantz L A, Randall E 1955 Use of autoclaved extracts of haemolytic streptococci for serological grouping. Stanford Medical Bulletin 13: 290–291

Rosendal K 1956 Grouping of haemolytic streptococci belonging to groups A, C and G: a comparison between the results obtained by precipitation and by slide agglutination. Acta Pathologica Microbiologica Scandinavica 39: 127–136

Rotta J, Krause R M, Lancefield R C, Everly W, Lackland H 1971 New approaches for the laboratory recognition of M types of group A streptococci. Journal of Experimental Medicine 134: 1298–1315

Sneath P H A, Mair N S, Sharpe M E, Holt J G 1986 Bergey's manual of systematic bacteriology, vol 2. Williams & Wilkins, Baltimore

Stringer J, Maxted W R 1979 Phage typing of group B streptococci. Lancet 1:328

Swift H F, Wilson A T, Lancefield R C 1943 Typing group A haemolytic streptococci by M-precipitin reactions in capillary pipettes. Journal of Experimental Medicine 78: 127–133

Wannamaker L W, Ayoub E M 1960 Antibody titres in acute rheumatic fever. Circulation 21: 598–614

Watson B K, Moellering R C, Kunz L J 1975 Identification of streptococci: use of lysozyme and Streptomyces albus filtrate in the preparation of extracts for Lancefield grouping. Journal of Clinical Microbiology 1: 274–278

WHO Report 1968 Streptococcal and staphylococcal infections. WHO Technical Report Series No. 394, Geneva

Streptococcus pneumoniae (pneumococcus)

Pneumococci are involved chiefly in infections of the upper and lower respiratory tracts, often as secondary pathogens after a primary virus infection. They are the commonest bacterial pathogens in lobar and bronchopneumonia and also occur in acute bronchitis, exacerbations of chronic bronchitis, empyema, pharyngitis, sinusitis, otitis media, meningitis, conjunctivitis, peritonitis and arthritis. They cause septicaemia in a proportion of these infections and it is particularly the septicaemic infections that may prove fatal. Before the introduction of antibiotics, pneumococcal infection was one of the commonest causes of death and it still causes many deaths, especially in patients for whom diagnosis and antibacterial therapy is delayed.

The pneumococcus is carried in the nasopharynx by many healthy persons. The carrier rate varies widely between different population groups and between different times in the same group, e.g. from 0 to 70%, but most commonly between 10 and 30% (Straker et al 1939). The pneumococcus generally remains harmless in the carriers, unless it is provoked by a viral infection such as influenza or the common cold to spread to the lower respiratory tract, middle ear, a paranasal sinus or the blood. Such spread is most likely to take place in the first few months after its acquisition in the nasopharynx, as the subject tends to form protective amounts of type-specific antibody on longer carriage.

In its biological characters the pneumococcus resembles the facultatively anaerobic streptococci and is correctly classified in the genus *Streptococcus*. In primary cultures on blood agar its colonies most closely resemble those of the viridans streptococci, from which it must be carefully distinguished (Ch. 17).

Morphology and staining

Gram-positive cocci occurring in pairs (diplococci) or, usually short, chains. The cocci are about 1 μm in diameter; in diplococci they are ovoid or lanceolate in shape, with their distal ends narrowed. They are non-motile and non-sporing and all freshly isolated strains are capsulate.

Cultural characters

Aerobic and facultatively anaerobic. Grows best in air or hydrogen with 5–10% CO_2, for which some strains have a strict requirement. Optimum temperature for growth is 37°C, and range 25–40°C. Grows on ordinary media, but better on media with 5–10% serum, blood or heated blood, which supplies nutrients, pH buffers and catalase. Colonies on blood agar are small, smooth and transparent. Low convex while tiny, they become flattened or depressed centrally, showing the 'draughtsman form', as they grow to a diameter of about 1 mm. Some strains, e.g. of type 3, which form very large capsules, tend to form larger, mucoid colonies, which may remain convex, and some culture media, e.g. Columbia agar, induce other strains to form such large, atypical colonies. A partial clearing of blood and a greenish discolouration (α-haemolysis) is produced underneath and in a narrow zone around the colonies. This resembles the α-haemolytic zone formed by colonies of

Table 18.1 Differential characters of pneumococci and viridans streptococci.

Character	Pneumococcus	Viridans streptococci
Morphology	Ovoid or lanceolate diplococci; some short chains	Short or long chains of rounded cocci
Capsule	Present	Usually absent
Colonies	Become flattened or draughtsman	Convex
Effect on blood agar	Narrow zones of α-haemolysis	Wide or narrow zones of α-haemolysis
Optochin sensitivity	Sensitive	Resistant
Bile solubility	+	−
Inulin fermentation	+	−
Virulence in mice	+	−

viridans streptococci, from which the pneumococci must be distinguished (Table 18.1). In primary cultures on blood agar, the flattened or draughtsman form of their colonies and their generally narrower zones of α-haemolysis helps to identify the pneumococci. Growth may be better anaerobically than aerobically and the haemolysis may then resemble the β-haemolytic type.

The organisms tend to die fairly quickly in cultures, e.g. in the course of a day or two, particularly in aerobic cultures in media without blood. The dead organisms tend to undergo autolysis. Thus an aerobic culture in shallow nutrient broth may be uniformly turbid after 6–12 h and become clear by autolysis within 24 h.

On repeated subculture the capsulate, smooth-colony-forming (S form) pneumococci may give rise to a few non-capsulate, rough-colonied (R form) mutant organisms. The R forms give granular instead of smooth growth in broth and are non-virulent.

Selective culture media

Media have been described which facilitate the isolation of small numbers of pneumococci from sputum heavily contaminated with secondary invaders or throat commensal bacteria, and from throat swabs. They contain antibiotics, particularly an aminoglycoside at a concentration inhibitory to many Gram-negative bacteria but not to pneumococci. One of the most effective appears to be that of Nichols & Freeman (1980)* which contains crystal violet, nalidixic acid and gentamicin, and inhibits the growth of most strains of enterobacteria, diphtheroid bacilli, *Staphylococcus aureus* and *Branhamella catarrhalis*. Unfortunately, like other similar media, it permits the growth of viridans and non-haemolytic streptococci, which are generally the most numerous organisms in sputum and throat secretion and so may still mask the presence of scanty pneumococci. Use of this medium will increase the proportion of sputum specimens from which pneumococci can be isolated, but it is doubtful whether the advantage is great enough to justify seeding it in addition to the plate of non-inhibitory blood agar or heated-blood agar used to grow all the common lung-pathogenic species of bacteria. Moreover, as discussed below under *Laboratory diagnosis*, the clinical significance and value of detecting only small numbers of pneumococci in sputum is doubtful, because their presence may be due to contamination from the throat and mouth.

Biochemical reactions

Catalase negative and oxidase negative. Form acid but not gas from glucose, lactose and sucrose, and many strains also from inulin. A valuable identifying property is the solubility of cultures in bile or bile salt, which brings about autolysis of the cocci.*

Sensitivity to chemical and physical agents

Killed by moist heat at 55°C in 10 min, and readily by most disinfectants. Die fairly quickly in laboratory cultures, which should be freeze-dried rather than subcultured for maintenance of the S form. Differ from other streptococci in being highly sensitive to killing by optochin

* Refer to *Methods* at end of this chapter.

(ethyl hydrocuprein hydrochloride), e.g. at a concentration of 0.001%, nearly a hundred times less than is effective against other streptococci. The optochin sensitivity test* provides the simplest and most reliable means of identifying pneumococci and distinguishing them from viridans streptococci.

Most strains are highly sensitive to benzylpenicillin, other penicillins, cephalosporins, erythromycin, tetracyclines, clindamycin and cotrimoxazole. Their infections are thus amenable to treatment with ampicillin and erythromycin, drugs effective against other common causal agents of pneumonia and often given initially to patients whose infecting organism has not yet been identified. In recent years strains have appeared that show increased resistance to the above named antibiotics, and some strains resistant to all the β-lactam antibiotics and erythromycin have been reported from various parts of the world, notably from South Africa.

Antigenic characters

Some 83 serotypes of pneumococcus are distinguished by differences in the nature of the polysaccharide antigen that composes their capsules and is partly secreted into the culture medium in the form of a loose slime, or 'specific soluble substance' (SSS). The type of a pneumococcus is determined by its reactions with type-specific antisera, tested first in pools and then singly. The tests may be done by agglutination of washed capsulate cocci or precipitation of SSS from culture supernates, but most simply by Neufeld's 'quellung' or 'swelling' reaction,* wherein the homologous specific antiserum coats and outlines with antibody the margin of the hitherto invisible capsule and so makes the cocci appear enlarged. The quellung reaction may be demonstrated directly in tests on a specimen of sputum or pus or with a young broth or blood agar culture. A still quicker method of typing is by slide coagglutination tests with staphylococci coated with type-specific pneumococcal antibody (Kronvall 1973). Pneumococci of some types, e.g. 1, 2, 3, 5, 7, 8, 9, 12, 14, 18, 19 and 23, appear to cause severe infections more commonly than other types, but the frequency of infections with the different types varies from place to place and time to time. Immunity to infection depends mainly on the formation of opsonizing antibody to the capsular antigen and is thus type-specific.

Animal pathogenicity

Most, but not all strains from infective conditions in man are virulent for the mouse, and therein distinguished from viridans streptococci, which are non-virulent. The intraperitoneal injection of a small dose of pneumococci generally causes peritonitis, septicaemia and death of the mouse within 1–3 days. As most respiratory tract commensal bacteria, unlike the pneumococcus, are killed by the mouse's phagocytes, the animal may serve like a selective culture medium and facilitate the isolation of scanty pneumococci from sputum or other specimen heavily contaminated with upper respiratory tract commensals. After inoculation of the specimen, or a young blood broth culture from it, the pneumococcus quickly establishes itself as the predominant organism in the peritoneal cavity and then appears as a pure culture in the mouse's blood. Rabbits also are highly susceptible to the coccus.

Laboratory diagnosis of pneumococcal infections

Diagnosis is generally done by demonstrating the presence of pneumococci in a specimen of sputum, exudate or blood by Gram film and culture, and then identifying the culture in an optochin sensitivity test. This approach is likely to be successful when a heavily infected specimen is collected early in the illness and before the start of antibiotic therapy. If, however, the patient is already on antibiotic therapy, or viable pneumococci are scanty for other reasons, better results may be obtained with tests for the presence of pneumococcal antigen in the specimen by coagglutination (COA), latex agglutination (LA) or countercurrent immunoelectrophoresis (CCIE) with polyvalent or type-specific antisera.* In comparison with one another, COA, LA and CCIE have been found equally sensitive and specific, but COA and LA were easier to perform, more easily read and quicker (1–2 min; Whitby et al 1985). CIE is more useful when large numbers of specimens have to be examined.

There is little difficulty in detecting a pneumococcus by culture and recognizing its pathogenic significance when it is present as sole organism in a specimen of blood, cerebrospinal fluid, or exudate from a site, such as a joint or the middle ear, not normally containing commensal bacteria, but both isolation and the assessment of significance may be difficult if the specimen is one, such as sputum, which is liable to be contaminated heavily with upper respiratory tract secretions and commensal bacteria. Scanty pneumococci may not be detected because they are overgrown in culture by the predominant commensals. If scanty pneumococci are detected, it cannot be assumed that they have a pathogenic role, for they may have entered and contaminated the specimen from a site of harmless carriage in the nasopharynx.

Examination of sputum

Expectorated sputum is the specimen most commonly submitted for examination for pneumococci and it is with sputum that difficulties of isolation and interpretation most commonly arise. Many persons carry pneumococci harmlessly in the throat and some of these cocci, as well as numerous other throat commensal bacteria, are likely to contaminate sputum as it is expelled through the throat and mouth. That such contamination is indeed frequent has been shown by comparison of cultures of bronchial swabs taken by a method excluding contamination from the throat with cultures of throat swabs and expectorated sputum from the same patients (Brumfitt et al 1957; Lees & McNaught 1959). If contaminating pneumococci are found in sputum from a lung infection caused by an undetected agent such as a virus, mycoplasma, legionella or mycobacterium, they may wrongly be thought the causal organism and inappropriate treatment be given to the patient.

Clearly the difficulties of sputum bacteriology could be avoided if all patients could be examined by rigorous swabbing of the bronchi through a bronchoscope by a method like that of Brumfitt et al, but such a procedure is too intrusive and specialized for routine application. The problem of detecting scanty pneumococci in sputum contaminated heavily with other throat commensal bacteria might be overcome if better selective culture media could be developed or if immunological tests for pneumococcal antigen are shown to be sufficiently sensitive and specific with this kind of specimen.

Unfortunately, the available tests for the presence of pneumococcal antigen in sputum may not be sufficiently specific for reliance on the results. Sputum is commonly contaminated with large numbers of *Streptococcus mitis* and other viridans streptococci from the mouth and throat that share antigens with pneumococci. Thus, a polyvalent serum for the capsular antigens of 83 types of pneumococci (Omniserum, from the State Serum Institute of Denmark) was found to cross-react with 68% of strains of viridans streptococci (Holmberg et al 1985).

Quantitative culture has been suggested by Dixon & Miller (1965) as an aid to assessing the significance of pneumococci present in sputum. If the number of pneumococci is large, e.g. 10^6 or more per ml, they will probably have been derived from a pneumococcal infection of the lower respiratory tract; if less than 10^6/ml, they are more likely to have entered the sputum as contaminants from the nasopharynx. It is recommended, therefore, that all specimens of sputum should be cultured quantitatively after homogenization and dilution by a method such as that described in Chapter 19 for examinations for *Haemophilus influenzae*.

Blood culture

Many pneumococcal infections are associated with a bacteriaemia or septicaemia, and whenever such a condition seems possible, a blood culture should be attempted. This procedure is particularly valuable in cases of suspected pneumonia, for it may be possible to isolate pneumococci from the blood in cases in which overgrowth by commensal bacteria prevents their isolation from sputum. Moreover the finding of pneumococci in the blood is much better evidence of their pathogenic role in the lung than is their finding in sputum, where they might be present only as contaminants from the throat.

Cerebrospinal fluid

The bacteriological examination of CSF from cases of suspected meningitis is specially important, for unless promptly treated a pneumococcal meningitis may be fatal. A centrifuged deposit of the CSF should be examined immediately in a Gram film and cultured on plates of blood agar and heated-blood agar incubated in air with 5–10% CO_2. As pneumococci readily undergo autolysis and intact forms may be scanty, the film should be made with both thick and thin areas, and be searched carefully for about 10 min before discarding as negative. A positive finding in the film should be phoned without delay to the physician as it will influence his choice of antibiotic for therapy.

In some cases, particularly if antibiotics have been given before collection of the specimen, the specimen may be devoid of viable cocci and the cultures prove negative. In such cases, pneumococcal antigen is often detectable in the CSF by COA, LA or CCIE tests*. In a comparative study, the COA test for antigen has given positive results in a larger proportion of specimens than either a Gram film or culture. It has, moreover, the advantage over culture in giving a result within a short time after receipt of the specimen. If resources are available, specimens should be examined routinely by a COA test as well as by Gram film and culture.

Identification

The presence of pneumococci is suggested by the finding of Gram-positive diplococci in films and α-haemolytic draughtsman colonies in cultures, and then may at once be reported on a tentative basis to the physician, but some pneumococcal strains form chains and some streptococci, e.g. group B, may form many diplococci. Moreover, some viridans streptococci may form flattened colonies resembling those of pneumococci. An identifying test must therefore be done before a definitive report is made.

The optochin test is recommended as the simplest and most reliable method, though if results are in doubt the bile solubility test should be done as well. The optochin test may be done at the same time as antibiotic sensitivity tests on a plate subculture from colonies on the primary diagnostic plate, but if this is done the definitive report is delayed by a day. Time can be saved by doing these tests on the primary plate, particularly if many Gram-positive diplococci have been seen in a film of the specimen. An optochin disk and a penicillin disk may be placed separately on an area of the plate heavily seeded with diluted sputum, CSF deposit or broth from an incubated blood culture bottle, so that the identification and sensitivity may be known when the pneumococcus-like colonies are first seen.

Instead of an optochin test being made on the primary culture plate, a suspect colony can be identified as pneumococcal by a bile solubility test performed on it in situ, on the plate (Hawn & Beebe 1965) as described under Method 2 below*. The tested colony will then be non-viable and another, similar colony must be subcultured for any further tests.

As antibiotics have replaced type-specific antisera for the treatment of infections, determination of the capsule serotype of a patient's strain is not required for his clinical care. It should be done only if required for the purpose of a well based epidemiological study.

Detection of carriers

The detection of throat carriers of pneumococcus may be required in research studies on carrier rates, but is unnecessary for patient care or the institution of preventive measures. Satisfactory results are obtained with swabs taken conventionally from the oropharynx, but more isolations may be obtained with West's postnasal swabs taken from the nasopharynx (Straker et al 1939). The swabs are usually cultured on plates of blood agar for up to 48 h at 37°C, but the use of a selective medium may help to prevent the masking of small numbers of pneumococci by the throat commensal bacteria. The highest isolation rates are obtained if the swab is finally placed in blood broth for overnight culture and 0.5 ml of the culture inoculated subcutaneously into a mouse; cultures are then seeded from the heart blood and local lesion of mice dying before 5 days or killed after that period.

METHODS

Selective medium

The medium of Nichols & Freeman (1980) is inhibitory to many respiratory-tract bacteria other than the pneumococcus, viridans streptococci and enterococci.

1. Prepare and autoclave Columbia agar as the base medium. Cool to 55°C.

2. Add, with thorough mixing, sterile preparations or solutions of the following, to give the final concentrations as stated:

   defibrinated horse blood to 10%,
   crystal violet to 2 mg/litre (1 in 500 000),
   nalidixic acid to 50 mg/l,
   gentamicin to 2 mg/l.

3. Pour plates, set, dry and seed heavily.

Optochin sensitivity test

This simple and reliable test (Bowers & Jeffries 1955) distinguishes pneumococci from viridans streptococci. Place a paper disk containing 5 μg of optochin (ethyl hydrocuprein) on an area of a blood agar plate that has been spread confluently with material from the specimen or a light broth suspension of pneumococcus-like colonies from the primary diagnostic plate. Incubate at 37°C in air with 5–10% CO_2. A growth of pneumococcus will be inhibited in a zone extending radially for at least 5 mm from the margin of the disk. Viridans streptococci will grow right up to the disk.

Bile solubility test

Pneumococci are soluble in bile; viridans and other streptococci are not. The test may be done by either of the following methods (Cowan 1974).

Method 1. Grow the isolate to be tested for 18 h at 37°C in 5 ml serum, digest broth or infusion broth. While still warm, add 0.5 ml of 10% sodium deoxycholate solution and reincubate at 37°C. Pneumococci are lysed within 15 min and the initially turbid culture becomes clear and transparent. A glucose-containing medium should not be used as the reaction of the culture must not become more acid than pH 6.8.

Method 2. A rapid presumptive test may be made on the primary plate culture. Touch a suspected pneumococcal colony with a loopful of 2% sodium deoxycholate solution at pH 7.0. Incubate the plate for 30 min at 37°C. Colonies of pneumococcus disappear, leaving an area of α-haemolysis on the blood agar.

Control tests should be done with standard cultures of *S. pneumoniae* (positive) and *S. faecalis* (negative).

Swelling test

As there are about 83 capsule serotypes of pneumococci and up to 20 or more may be causing infections in a community at any one time, a wide range of type-specific sera is required for type determination. The sera are laborious to prepare and relatively expensive to purchase, and unless many isolates have to be typed, cultures should be sent for typing to a pneumococcus reference laboratory.

Antipneumococcal rabbit sera may be purchased from the State Serum Institute, Copenhagen, Denmark. Pooled sera ('omnisera') as well as individual type-specific sera may be obtained. A dye such as methylene blue is often added to typing sera so that the bodies of the cocci may be stained and thus made easier to see and distinguishable from the unstained capsules.

The test is done under the microscope in a wet film containing the cocci and antiserum. Pooled sera may be tested first and then in turn the individual type-specific sera until one of them is found to give a positive result. The wet film may be made from a suspension of pneumococcus culture, or directly with the patient's sputum, pus or CSF, or with the peritoneal exudate from an experimentally infected mouse. Ideally the fluid should contain unlysed pneumococci in only moderate numbers; the capsules should be large but there should be little dissolved SSS, which would tend to deviate antibody from them. A suitable suspension of cocci can be prepared from a culture grown in broth for only 5 h or on blood agar or 0.1% glucose blood agar for about 10 h. The cocci should first be suspended in saline (0.85% NaCl), then separated from the saline and dissolved SSS by centrifugation, and finally resuspended to a low density (minimum visible turbidity) in fresh saline.

Place a loopful of the culture suspension or exudate on a microscope slide and mix in a loopful of antiserum. Apply a thin coverslip and examine under oil-immersion either with a phase-contrast microscope or with an ordinary microscope with the condenser slightly defocused to reduce the intensity of illumination. If the serum contains antibodies homologous for the cocci, the margins of the capsules will become refractile and visible, separated from the coccal bodies by the width of the capsules, and agglutination of some of the capsulate cocci may be seen. With heterologous serum the capsules remain invisible and only the coccal bodies can be detected.

Tests for pneumococcal antigen

Coagglutination test (COA). The reagent is a suspension of killed *Staphylococcus aureus* that have been coated with type-specific pneumococcal antibodies bound by their Fc structures to the protein A of the staphylococcal cell wall, so that the FAB combining sites project outwards. When live or dead pneumococci or free pneumococcal antigens (SSS) of the corresponding capsule type are added, they cause coagglutination of the staphylococci which quickly becomes visible to the naked eye in a slide test.

Methods are described by Kronvall (1973) for the preparation of stabilized suspensions of staphylococci by treatment with formaldehyde and heating at 80°C, for coating the cocci with antiserum and for preserving the finished reagent with sodium azide. Type-specific reagents are prepared by coating the cocci with a single type-specific serum. A species-specific 'omni-reagent' is prepared by coating them with a mixture of sera to a wide range of capsule serotypes. Reactions with the type-specific reagents are generally very rapid, seen within seconds, but those with the omni-reagent are weaker and

slower, taking at least a minute to become visible.

Typing by COA. The COA test may be used to type cultures of pneumococci (Kronvall 1973). It gives results in complete agreement with the swelling test, but uses less antiserum and, as not requiring microscopy, is quicker and easier to perform.

1. Place two drops of the typing reagent on the centre of a microscope slide.

2. Emulsify in them one or more colonies of the pneumococcus culture.

3. Observe the slide with the naked eye for up to 2 min while continually mixing. Agglutination, denoting a positive result, usually becomes clearly visible within seconds. Compare the reaction with a parallel test of the same culture in heterologous serum, which should give no, or only minimal granularity.

Diagnosis of infection by COA. The COA test may be used for the rapid diagnosis of infection by the detection of pneumococcal antigen in a clinical specimen. The procedure has been found of especial value in the examination of cerebrospinal fluid for the diagnosis of bacterial meningitis, for it gives results very quickly and may show the presence of pneumococcal antigen even in specimens in which the pneumococci have been lysed by antibiotics or natural antibacterial agents and so become undetectable by film or culture.

Phadebact CSF test kits of species-specific omni-reagents for pneumococcus (83 types), meningococcus (groups A, B, C, Y, W135), and *Streptococcus agalactiae*, and a reagent for *Haemophilus influenzae* type b are available from Pharmacia. The method for their use is as follows.

1. Heat the specimen of CSF at 80°C for 5 min. Remove any contaminating red blood cells by low speed centrifugation.

2. Place one drop of each reagent on their separate sites on a special, marked test slide.

3. Add one drop of the preheated CSF to each drop of reagent.

4. Mix each drop with a separate disposable loop.

5. Continue mixing by tilting the slide to and fro for 1 min.

6. Read the results immediately to avoid misinterpretation of granularity caused by drying of the mixture.

7. Take as a positive result the appearance of agglutination in one of the reagents that is stronger and quicker than any reaction in the other three. Absence of agglutination usually denotes absence of infection with the corresponding organism, but in a few cases where COA is negative, the organism may be grown in culture.

Latex agglutination test (LA). Test kits for LA are available as Wellcogen *Streptococcus pneumoniae* kit from Wellcome. Latex particles coated with an appropriate antibody are used and the test is similar to COA. It gives favourable results in the detection of pneumococcal antigens in CSF, urine and serum.

Counter-current immunoelectrophoresis (CCIE). This method, described by Dulake (1979), is a specially sensitive means of detecting capsular antigen and may give a positive result when the COA test is negative.

REFERENCES

Bowers E F, Jeffries L R 1955 Optochin in the identification of *Str. pneumoniae*. Journal of Clinical Pathology 8: 58–60.

Brumfitt W, Willoughby M L N, Bromley L L 1957 An evaluation of sputum examination in chronic bronchitis. Lancet 2: 1306–1309

Cowan S T 1974 Cowan and Steel's Manual for the identification of medical bacteria, 2nd edn. Cambridge University Press

Dixon J M S, Miller D C 1965 Value of dilute inocula in cultural examination of sputum. Lancet 2: 1046–1048

Dulake C 1979 Counter-current immunoelectrophoresis for the diagnosis of pneumococcal chest infection. Journal of Infection 1: Suppl 2, 45–51

Hawn C V Z, Beebe E 1965 Rapid method for demonstrating bile solubility of *Diplococcus pneumoniae*. Journal of Bacteriology 90:549

Holmberg H, Danielsson D, Hardie J, Krook A, Whiley R 1985 Cross-reactions between α-streptococci and omniserum, a polyvalent pneumococcal serum, demonstrated by direct immunofluorescence, immunoelectrophoresis, and latex agglutination. Journal of Clinical Microbiology 21: 745–748

Kronvall G 1973 A rapid slide-agglutination method for typing pneumococci by means of specific antibody adsorbed to protein-A-containing staphylococci. Journal of Medical Microbiology 6: 187–190

Lees A W, McNaught W 1959 Bacteriology of lower-respiratory-tract secretions, sputum, and upper-respiratory-tract secretions in 'normals' and chronic bronchitis. Lancet 2: 1112–1115

Nichols T, Freeman R 1980 A new selective medium for *Streptococcus pneumoniae*. Journal of Clinical Pathology 33: 770–773

Straker E, Hill A B, Lovell R 1939 A study of the nasopharyngeal bacterial flora of different groups of persons observed in London and South-East England during the years 1930 to 1937. Reports on Public Health and Medical Subjects No. 90, Ministry of Health. His Majesty's Stationery Office, London

Whitby M, Kristinsson K G, Brown M 1985 Assessment of rapid methods for the detection of pneumococcal antigen – detection in routine sputum bacteriology. Journal of Clinical Pathology 38: 341–344

Haemophilus, Gardnerella and other bacilli

Members of the genus *Haemophilus* are obligatory parasites that colonize human and animal mucosae. Three species are pathogenic in man: *Haemophilus influenzae*, which is common in respiratory infections and sometimes the cause of meningitis, conjunctivitis or otitis media; *H. aegyptius* (the Koch-Weeks bacillus), the cause of acute contagious conjunctivitis; and *H. ducreyi*, the cause of the venereal infection, chancroid or 'soft sore'. Other species are commonly commensal in the human mouth and throat, and rarely cause opportunistic infections such as dental abscess, jaw infections, infective endocarditis, and brain abscess; these species include *H. parainfluenzae, H. haemolyticus, H. parahaemolyticus, H. aphrophilus, H. paraphrophilus* and *H. segnis*.

The haemophili are small non-motile nonsporing Gram-negative rods that are facultative anaerobes, but grow poorly in the absence of oxygen, and are exacting in nutritional requirements. Their haemophilic character reflects a requirement for either or both of two substances generally supplied by the addition of blood to a nutrient agar medium. These required nutrients are (1) heat-stable X factor, which is protoporphyrin IX, haemin or some other iron-containing porphyrin, and (2) heat-labile (at 121°C for 30 min) V factor, which is either nicotinamide adenine dinucleotide (NAD), otherwise called diphosphopyridine nucleotide (DPN), or NAD phosphate (NADP), otherwise called triphosphopyridine nucleotide (TPN).

The closest relatives of the haemophili are members of the genera *Pasteurella* and *Actinobacillus*, which are also small non-motile parasitic Gram-negative bacilli, but differ from the haemophili in not requiring X or V factor. In this chapter we deal with the only *Actinobacillus* species parasitic in man, namely *Actinobacillus actinomycetemcomitans*, and also some other Gram-negative bacilli of uncertain affiliation, of which one, *Gardnerella vaginalis*, is commonly present in human vaginosis; the others are present in rarer human infections.

HAEMOPHILUS INFLUENZAE

This bacillus acquired its specific epithet because it was originally thought to be the cause of influenza, which is now known to be a viral infection. It is commonly present as a harmless commensal in the throat and nasopharynx, e.g. in 25–75% of healthy persons, though rarely demonstrable in the mouth. It often acts opportunistically as a secondary pathogen in the upper or lower respiratory tract following a viral infection or some non-infective disease process, e.g. in secondary bronchopneumonia and acute exacerbations in chronic bronchitis, cystic fibrosis or bronchiectasis, and it is sometimes the primary bacterial invader in conjunctivitis, otitis media and paranasal sinusitis.

A minority of strains are capsulate and more virulent than the common non-capsulate strains. They are carried in the nasopharynx in 1–5% of healthy persons and act as primary pathogens, particularly in children under 4 years old, causing severe infections such as acute laryngo-epiglottitis (croup), bronchopneumonia, otitis media, septicaemia, meningitis, and bone and joint infections.

H. influenzae is distinguished from most other

Table 19.1 Distinguishing characters of *Haemophilus* species found in man.
Key: (+), weak positive; $-^+$, a few strains require extra CO_2; +/−, some strains positive, some negative; −/(+), some strains negative, some weakly positive; +L, positive only after incubation for more than 1 day.

Character	H. influenzae	H. aegyptius	H. haemolyticus	H. parainfluenzae	H. parahaemolyticus	H. aphrophilus	H. paraphrophilus	H. segnis	H. ducreyi
X requirement	+	+	+	−	−	(+)	−	−	+
V requirement	+	+	+	+	+	−	+	+	−
CO_2 (5%) requirement	$-^+$	−	−	−	−	+	+	−	−/(+)
β-haemolysis[a]	−	−	+	−	+	−	−	−	−
Haemagglutination[b]	−/(+)	+	−	−	−	−	−	−	−
Acid from glucose	+	+L	+	+	+	+	+	(+)	−/+L
Gas from glucose	−	−	−/+L	−/+L	−/+L	+	+	−	−
Acid from sucrose	−	−	−	+	+	+	+	(+)	−
Acid from D-xylose	+	−	+/−	−	−	−	−	−	−
Indole produced	+/−	−	+/−	−	−	−	−	−	−
Urease activity	+/−	+	+	+/−	+	−	−	−	−
Ornithine decarboxylase	+/−	−	−	+/−	+/−	−	−	−	−

[a] Haemolysis best on ox or sheep blood.
[b] Reaction with human or guinea-pig cells at 4°C.

species of *Haemophilus* by its requirement for both X and V factors (Table 19.1). The only other species requiring both factors are *H. aegyptius* and *H. haemolyticus*, which are sometimes regarded as varieties of *H. influenzae* rather than as distinct species. *H. aegyptius* is distinguished from *H. influenzae* by its stronger haemagglutinating activity and greater infectivity for the conjunctiva, and *H. haemolyticus* by its production of β-haemolysis on blood agar and apparent lack of any pathogenic role.

For a further account of the clinical significance of *H. influenzae* and its laboratory diagnosis, see Turk (1982).

Morphology and staining

Small Gram-negative bacilli, 0.3–0.5 × 1–2 μm, often pleomorphic and showing filamentous and swollen forms in old cultures. Non-motile and non-sporing. Capsules are absent from most strains, but present in a few, more virulent strains: they are demonstrable in thin, India ink wet films (Ch. 3) and by their 'swelling' reaction with type-specific antiserum. Under suitable cultural conditions, some strains form fimbriae, which enable them to cause haemagglutination in a tile test at 4°C with human, guinea-pig, fowl or other animal red cells (Scott & Old 1981).*

Cultural characters

Grows aerobically, and only poorly anaerobically. A few strains require extra CO_2 (5–10%). Temperature range for growth, 20–42°C, optimum 35–37°C. Requires both X factor and V factor, thus grows on blood agar, which contains these factors, but not on nutrient agar which lacks sufficient amounts of them. The amount of V factor in ordinary blood agar is usually suboptimal, so that colonies are very small. Colonies are larger (1) where they are within 1–3 mm of the colony of an organism such as *Staphylococcus aureus* which excretes an excess of V factor ('satellitism'), (2) on blood agar supplemented with 10–20 mg/litre of crystalline NAD while at 55°C just before pouring in plates,

(3) on heated-blood agar ('chocolate agar') made from horse blood, wherein extra V factor is released from the blood cells and serum NADase is inactivated by heating for a few minutes at 75–100°C (Ch. 6), and (4) on a transparent medium containing an extract or digest of blood, e.g. Fildes (1920) agar*, which is a nutrient agar containing a peptic digest of blood, or Levinthal's agar prepared from heated blood (Alexander 1965).*

After 24 h at 37°C on medium with sufficient NAD, the colonies of non-capsulate strains are usually 0.5–1 mm in diameter, circular, low convex, smooth, pale grey and transparent. On Fildes agar they are transparent and have a slightly blue iridescence. In growths on most media they have a fishy, seminal smell which alerts the non-smoking bacteriologist to their possible presence in a mixed culture. The colonies of capsulate strains are larger, e.g. 1–3 mm in diameter, high convex in shape, mucoid and iridescent. The strong iridescence indicative of capsulation consists of red, orange, green and blue shades which alter with the angle of observation. It is best seen by looking obliquely at colonies on a transparent medium illuminated brightly from beneath.

H. influenzae, strictly defined, is non-haemolytic on blood agar, but non-pathogenic β-haemolytic strains, now classified as *H. haemolyticus*, are sometimes present as commensals in the throat and their colonies, unless filmed or serogrouped, may be mistaken for those of *Streptococcus pyogenes*.

Testing X and V requirements

H. influenzae is formally identified by demonstrating the dependence of its growth on a supply of both X factor and V factor (Table 19.1). This is usually done in a disk test* wherein the presence or absence of growth is observed around paper disks impregnated with X factor alone, V factor alone, or X plus V factor placed on a nutrient agar deficient in both X and V. Kilian & Biberstein (1984) point out that the disk test is unreliable as a means of demonstrating the X requirement, for which it gives about 20% of misleading results. They recommend that the X

---

* Refer to *Methods* at end of this chapter.

requirement should be determined by the porphyrin synthesis test of Kilian (1974).*

Selective media

H. influenzae has often to be isolated from specimens, such as throat swabs and sputa, that yield also a mixture of throat commensal bacteria liable to overgrow and mask the haemophili. Media selective for *H. influenzae* are helpful in such cases. Growth of viridans streptococci, neisseriae, diphtheroid bacilli and albus staphylococci may be largely suppressed on blood agar or heated-blood agar containing 0.2–0.5 units/ml of penicillin (Fleming 1929), 5–19 units/ml (80–300 mg/litre) of bacitracin (Hovig & Aandahl 1969; Ederer & Schurr 1971) or 80 mg/l of bacitracin plus 5 mg/l of cloxacillin (Sims 1970). Some pharyngeal neisseriae, actinobacilli and *Eikenella corrodens* can grow on the 300 mg/l bacitracin medium. Fildes (1920) agar, even without additives, is moderately selective for haemophilus because the large content of haemin provided by the blood digest is inhibitory to viridans streptococci, pneumococci and some neisseriae, though not to enterococci and coliforms.

The differential selective medium of Roberts et al (1987)* contains bacitracin as selective agent and sucrose and phenol red to distinguish *H. parainfluenzae*, which ferments the sucrose and forms yellow colonies, from *H. influenzae* which forms smaller, colourless, non-fermenting colonies.

Biochemical reactions

Catalase positive and oxidase positive. Ferments glucose and galactose, and some strains also fructose, maltose or xylose, producing acid but not gas. Does not ferment lactose, sucrose or mannitol. The medium* to be used in the fermentation tests must support good growth to ensure that enough acid can be produced to change the colour of the pH indicator dye. The production of gas from glucose, which distinguishes *H. aphrophilus* and *H. paraphrophilus* from *H. influenzae* (Table 19.1), is demonstrated in the usual way by the inclusion

of an inverted Durham tube in the glucose broth. Methods for a wide range of biochemical tests are described by Kilian (1976) and Broom & Sneath (1981).

Biovars (biotypes)

Kilian (1976) has divided strains of *H. influenzae* into six biovars by their indole, urease and ornithine decarboxylase reactions (Table 19.2). The tests should be done by micro-methods not requiring growth of the inoculated culture (Kilian & Biberstein 1984). The biovar of any strain appears to be stable enough for use as a clone marker in epidemiological studies. Strongly haemagglutinating strains of biovar 3 correspond to *H. aegyptius*. The indole, urease and ornithine reactions are also of some value in identifying other species of *Haemophilus* (Table 19.1).

Table 19.2 Characters of six biovars of *Haemophilus influenzae*.

Character	Biovar (biotype)					
	1	2	3	4	5	6
Indole production	+	+	−	−	+	−
Urease activity	+	+	+	+	−	−
Ornithine decarboxylase	+	−	−	+	+	+

Sensitivity to chemical and physical agents

H. influenzae is killed by moist heat at 55°C in 30 min. It dies within a few days in cultures and exudates held at room temperature, and even sooner at 4°C in the refrigerator. It also dies quickly, e.g. in 1–48 h, in dried secretion and airborne droplet-nuclei.

Most strains are sensitive to a wide range of drugs, including sulphonamides, trimethoprim, benzylpenicillin (though only at a concentration of at least 1 mg/litre, i.e. 1.7 units/ml), ampicillin and amoxycillin (0.25 mg/l), streptomycin, tetracycline, chloramphenicol, erythromycin and gentamicin. Ampicillin or amoxycillin is generally used for severe respiratory infections, cotrimoxazole often for the less severe infections, and chloramphenicol, because of its high diffusibility, for haemophilus meningitis. Some strains, now becoming commoner, are resistant to ampicillin and amoxycillin by virtue of the production of a plasmid-determined β-lactamase, and some strains are resistant to sulphonamides and tetracycline.

Antigenic characters

Non-capsulate strains are antigenically very heterogeneous. They appear to possess a thermostable species-specific somatic antigen, a thermolabile (at 56°C in 24 h) somatic antigen, and antigens that cross-react with those of other *Haemophilus* species. Capsulate strains are divisible into six serovars (serotypes) labelled a–f, identified by agglutination, 'swelling' (Alexander et al 1946) or precipitation tests (Zinnemann 1960) with type-specific antisera. Type b strains, mostly in biovar 1, are responsible for most cases of haemophilus meningitis and laryngo-epiglottitis. Type a is common in sinusitis and types e and f cause occasional respiratory infections.

Animal pathogenicity

Inoculation into animals has no place in the laboratory diagnosis of haemophilus infections. Large doses of non-capsulate cultures inoculated intraperitoneally kill mice in 24–48 h by virtue of their content of endotoxin, not their infectivity. Capsulate strains are more virulent and the intraperitoneal injection of a small dose suspended in mucin may cause a fatal septicaemia.

Laboratory diagnosis

Specimens

Specific diagnosis and therapy are urgently required in the bacteriaemic, life-threatening infections caused by type b capsulate strains in young children, but it is often difficult, e.g. in epiglottitis, otitis media and pneumonia, to obtain a specimen from the local site of infection from which *H. influenzae* can be isolated. In suspected cases of such infections, blood cultures should always be done and an attempt made to demonstrate the presence of type b capsular antigen in body fluids.

In the less acute, e.g. bronchial, infections in adults caused by non-capsulate strains, it is sufficient to attempt to isolate *H. influenzae* from an exudate, e.g. sputum, from the affected site. As haemophili are poorly viable, such specimens should be cultured as soon as possible after their collection. The rate of isolation of *H. influenzae* from sputa may be halved by one day's delay in delivery to the laboratory (May & Delves 1964).

Demonstration of type b antigen in body fluids

Indications of a serious haemophilus infection may be obtained most quickly, within minutes, by the demonstration of type b capsular antigen in the patient's serum, urine or cerebrospinal fluid. Kits are available commercially to demonstrate the antigen by the agglutination of latex particles coated with rabbit antibody to type b antigen (e.g. Wellcogen H. influenzae b test, Wellcome) or by coagglutination with *Staphylococcus aureus* coated with anti-type b antibody (e.g. Phadebact CSF test, Pharmacia). As a false-positive result may be obtained due to the presence of type b antigen absorbed by a throat carrier or a cross-reacting antigen from another organism, a positive finding should, if possible, be confirmed by subsequent isolation of the haemophilus in culture.

Blood culture

Any good blood culture medium may be used, for it will be enriched with X and V factors from the blood sample. To obtain the quickest indication of growth, the culture should be examined after 4–5 h for bacilli showing 'capsule swelling' in a wet film with type b antiserum, as in the swelling test for pneumococci (see *Methods*, Ch. 18). A Gram film should also be examined and subcultures made on heated-blood agar.

Isolation from other specimens

Specimens suspected of containing *H. influenzae* should be examined in a Gram-stained film for the presence of numerous small Gram-negative bacilli. They should then be inoculated on to plates of blood agar supplemented with NAD, heated-blood agar or Fildes digest agar and incubated at 35–37°C in air with 10% CO_2 overnight. When the specimen is from the respiratory tract and likely to contain a mixture of throat commensal bacteria, the media used should include Fildes agar or a heated-blood agar made selective for haemophilus by the addition of penicillin or bacitracin (see *Selective media*, above). Colonies may be recognized by their appearance and smell (see *Cultural characters*, above); their bluish iridescence on Fildes agar is particularly helpful. They should be identified by the demonstration of their X and V requirements, and tested for sensitivity to amoxycillin and cotrimoxazole among other antibiotics.

The isolation of *H. influenzae* and the recognition of its pathogenic role are relatively easy when the organism is present by itself in a specimen from a part of the body that is normally sterile, e.g. in cerebrospinal fluid from meningitis, blood from septicaemia or pus from otitis media, but they are difficult when the specimen is a throat swab or sputum, almost certainly contaminated with a mixture of throat commensal bacteria which often include *H. influenzae* itself. The haemophilus may then be overgrown and masked by the other, more robust commensal bacteria, or it may be found, but only because it was being carried as a commensal in a patient who became infected with a virus or other undetected pathogen. Moreover, when *H. influenzae* is found in a condition that is primarily either viral or non-infective, it has still to be considered whether it is present only as a harmless contaminating commensal or as a significant secondary invader requiring eradication with antibiotics. A guide to its significance in such cases is its number in the specimen; if a colony count suggests that more than about 10^6 bacilli/ml are present, it is wisest to assume they have a pathogenic role.

Throat swabs

Swabs from pharyngitis in older children and adults are not normally examined for *H. influenzae* as this organism is present as a commensal in the throat in 25–75% of healthy persons and, though it may sometimes act as a secondary, and possibly even as a primary invader in the throat, there is no evidence that its eradication with antibiotics is beneficial. In children under 4 years old, however, a capsulate strain may cause severe infection, with spread to the larynx, lung, middle ear or meninges, and it is wise in these cases to examine for *H. influenzae* with view to prescription of the appropriate antibiotic. The number of the colonies should be noted, and whether they are mucoid and capsulate.

Unfortunately, it is almost impossible to obtain a satisfactory specimen from the epiglottis and no attempt should be made to take a throat swab from a child with acute epiglottitis as the interference may precipitate respiratory obstruction. Laboratory diagnosis of haemophilus epiglottitis should therefore be done by blood culture or the demonstration of type b antigen in the serum or urine.

Sputum

Sputa from chest infections should always be examined for the presence of *H. influenzae* in addition to that of other respiratory pathogens such as pneumococcus and *Staphylococcus aureus*. Account must be taken of non-capsulate as well as capsulate strains as these former are common secondary pathogens in the bronchi and lungs. Unless it is collected by aspiration from a bronchus, the sputum is liable to be contaminated with throat secretion and saliva on its passage through the throat and mouth. It is thus liable to become contaminated with small or moderate numbers of *H. influenzae* when, as is commonly the case, these organisms are being carried as harmless commensals in the throat. For this reason, the finding of the organism in a culture of sputum does not necessarily indicate that it is present in the lower respiratory tract (Brumfitt et al 1957; Lees & McNaught 1959).

Some indication of whether or not the haemophilus is infecting the lower respiratory tract may be obtained from observation of its number in the expectorated sputum. If it is present in large numbers, e.g. greater than 10^6/ml, in purulent sputum, or if it is the predominant organism present, it is probably derived from an infection of the bronchi or lungs. No such conclusion should be drawn from its finding in small numbers in a mixed flora of throat commensal bacteria. Observation of the haemophilus colonies on a culture plate that has been seeded with sputum in the conventional way suffices to show whether the organism is a predominant member of the flora present, but does not permit a standardized assessment to be made of its numbers. It is preferable, therefore, to make a quantitative culture of the sputum after it has been homogenized and suitably diluted (Dixon & Miller 1965). A recommended procedure is as follows.

1. Examine the sputum with the naked eye to ensure that it is purulent, i.e. thick, opaque and yellow or green. If it consists of clear, watery saliva, it is unsuitable for examination and a further specimen should be requested.

2. Homogenize the sputum by adding to it an equal volume of a freshly made up solution of a mucolytic agent, e.g. dithiothreitol (e.g. Sputolysin, Calbiochem) or buffered pancreatin (Oxoid) and mix thoroughly. Mixture with dithiothreitol may be carried out continuously on a rocking machine for 30 min at room temperature, alternatively for 15 s on a rapid vortex mixer followed by standing for 15 min at room temperature. Mixture with pancreatin should be done with continuous or occasional shaking for 30 min at 37°C. For safety, the mixing of sputum should be done in a sealed container in a safety cabinet.

3. Examine a Gram-stained smear of the homogenized mixture. The finding of very large numbers of small Gram-negative bacilli, putatively *H. influenzae*, or that of putative pneumococci or *S. aureus*, should be the subject of a provisional report to the physician. If there is a mixed bacterial flora and less than ten polymorphs per squamous epithelial cell, the specimen probably consists largely of saliva.

4. Dilute the homogenized sputum 1 in 100 in sterile nutrient broth; 0.005 ml of the dilution will then correspond to 0.000 025 ml of the original unhomogenized specimen. Plate a 0.005 ml loopful of the dilution on each culture plate, spreading it evenly over half of the plate and streaking out for separate colonies on the other half. After incubation, the presence of 25 or more colonies of the same potential pathogen

indicates that 10^6 or more of these bacteria were present per ml sputum and suggests that they had a pathogenic role. The finding of smaller numbers of any throat-carried species may generally be regarded as insignificant.

The plates seeded should include one of blood agar and one of a medium selective for *H. influenzae*, such as Fildes agar. Up to two antibiotic disks may be placed on the evenly seeded part of each plate to assist species identification and enable the early reporting of findings on the day after receipt of the specimen. Thus, an optochin disk might be placed on the blood agar plate to identify pneumococcus and an amoxycillin disk placed on the Fildes plate to enable immediate reporting of the sensitivity of *H. influenzae*.

5. The identity of *H. influenzae* may be confirmed by tests of its X and V requirements, and its sensitivity to further antibiotics may also be tested, but the patient's interests will probably be better served by reporting the provisional results after 1 day than by waiting a further day until the confirmed results are available.

Cerebrospinal fluid

The examination of CSF for acute suppurative meningitis is detailed in Chapter 39. When *H. influenzae* is present it is commonly seen as small Gram-negative bacilli in the centrifuged deposit of the CSF and an immediate report of the finding will help the physician in his choice of antibiotic. Chloramphenicol is generally the preferred drug for haemophilus meningitis, though not for meningococcal or pneumococcal infection. Among the media seeded with the deposit, V-supplemented blood agar or heated-blood agar should be included to ensure the growth of any viable haemophili. Colonies should be identified by demonstration of the X and V requirements, tested for sensitivity to antibiotics including chloramphenicol and tested for 'swelling' with type b capsular serum.

The CSF may also be tested directly for the presence of type b capsular antigen by a latex agglutination or *S. aureus* coagglutination test (see above). A positive result is sometimes obtained when both the Gram film and the culture are negative, and it enables a definitive diagnosis to be made on the day of receipt of the specimen (Wasilavskas & Hampton 1982).

Antibiotic sensitivity tests

Haemophili fail to grow on the sensitivity test media generally used for other organisms. Tests with antibiotics should be done on heated-blood agar and those with sulphonamides and trimethoprim on Fildes or Levinthal agar. Accurate control of inoculum density (Ch. 9) is essential.

In serious, bacteriaemic infections sensitivity results are required urgently. If, therefore, bacilli are seen on filming a blood culture or cerebrospinal fluid, the specimen should at once be inoculated over a heated-blood agar plate and disks of ampicillin and chloramphenicol applied, so that the sensitivities may be read on primary culture.

Disk-diffusion tests with β-lactam antibiotics may fail to detect resistance in a haemophilus producing β-lactamase. Isolates from serious infections should therefore be tested for β-lactamase. The acidometric paper strip method of Slack et al (1977) gives results within a few minutes. A paper strip impregnated with penicillin and bromocresol purple (e.g. Intralactam strip, Mast) is moistened with distilled water and then rubbed with material from several colonies; if the organisms have produced β-lactamase, the penicillin will be hydrolysed to penicilloic acid and the colour of the strip changed from purple to yellow.

Haemophilus aegyptius

The Koch-Weeks bacillus is sometimes regarded as a variety of *H. influenzae*, but differs from it in having a greater infectivity for the conjunctiva, causing an acute contagious conjunctivitis whilst *H. influenzae* causes only sporadic conjunctivitis, and in not occurring as a commensal in the nasopharynx of healthy subjects. It is also distinguished by being more exacting nutritionally and growing more slowly than *H. influenzae*. Thus, its colonies on heated-blood agar reach only about 0.5 mm diameter in 48 h. Better growth and higher rates of isolation

are obtained on heated-blood agar enriched with 1% IsoVitaleX (BBL) (Vastine et al 1974). *H. aegyptius* differs further from *H. influenzae* in failing to ferment D-xylose, being sensitive to troleandomycin and showing stronger haemagglutinating activity with human or guinea-pig red blood cells in a tile test at 4°C (Davis et al 1950; Scott & Old 1981).

Haemophilus haemolyticus

This haemophilus has also been regarded as a variety of *H. influenzae*, from which it differs in forming zones of β-haemolysis around its colonies on blood agar. The haemolysis is strongest on sheep or ox blood, but is also seen on horse or human blood. The organism is found as a commensal in the throat, but not mouth, in a minority of healthy persons and, unlike *H. influenzae*, appears to be devoid of any pathogenic activity. Its colonies in throat swab cultures grown aerobically on blood agar may be mistaken for those of *Streptococcus pyogenes*, but on anaerobically incubated plates its haemolysis is much weaker, whereas that of *S. pyogenes* is stronger in anaerobic than in aerobic cultures.

Haemophilus parainfluenzae

This organism is distinguished from *H. influenzae* by its non-requirement for X factor, ability to ferment sucrose but not D-xylose, and low pathogenicity. It is normally present as a commensal in the mouth and throat, and also often present in the vagina. It occasionally exercises an opportunistically pathogenic role in endocarditis, conjunctivitis and bronchopulmonary infections in patients with cystic fibrosis. In its general characters it resembles *H. influenzae* (Table 19.1), but it forms larger, more opaque yellowish white colonies on heated-blood agar (e.g. 1–2 mm at 24 h), which are usually smooth but sometimes wrinkled or rough.

Haemophilus parahaemolyticus

This organism resembles *H. parainfluenzae* in most characters but differs in forming β-haemolytic colonies. It is commonly present as a commensal in the mouth and throat, and is occasionally found in cases of oral sepsis and endocarditis.

Haemophilus aphrophilus

This haemophilus is a common commensal in the mouth and dental plaque and an occasional cause of jaw infections, endocarditis and brain abscess. Its distinguishing characters are its production of gas in the fermentation of glucose and its dependence on the addition of 10% CO_2 to air for growth on heated-blood agar. Its colonies are high convex, yellow opaque, and 1–1.5 mm in diameter at 24 h. It has no requirement for V factor but on primary isolation has an apparent requirement for X factor.

Haemophilus paraphrophilus

This resembles *H. aphrophilus* in its occurrence as a commensal and occasional opportunistic pathogen, and in the production of gas from glucose and requirement for extra CO_2. It differs in requiring V factor and not X factor (Table 19.1).

Haemophilus segnis

This is commonly present as a commensal in the mouth, dental plaque and throat, and appears to be almost entirely non-pathogenic. It requires only V factor and grows very slowly, forming opaque whitish colonies up to 0.5 mm in diameter after 48 h.

Haemophilus ducreyi

This haemophilus is the cause of the uncommon venereal disease called chancroid, or 'soft sore', being found in the ulcer, its exudate and the associated buboes. It is not found as a commensal in healthy persons. The organism grows poorly on most media, requires X factor but not V factor, and is inactive in most biochemical tests (Table 19.1). Colonies on heated-blood agar are less than 0.5 mm in diameter after 72 h and growth on ordinary blood agar is even poorer, though some strains show faint β-haemolysis. Better growth is obtained on heated-blood agar enriched with 1% IsoVitaleX (Hammond et al 1978).

Laboratory diagnosis. 1. Aspirate material from a bubo and scrape material from the surface of a sore cleansed with gauze and saline.

2. Attempt to grow primary cultures on moist slopes of coagulated rabbit blood. Prepare these slopes by distributing 1–2 ml amounts of fresh sterile rabbit blood in small test tubes and heating the tubes in the sloped position for 5 min at 55°C. Inoculate the specimen into the serum that separates from the clot.

Alternatively, inoculate the specimen on to moist plates or slopes of 1% IsoVitaleX (BBL) heated-blood agar.

3. Incubate the cultures for 2–3 days at 35–37°C in a humid atmosphere, e.g. in a plastic bag or jar containing wet blotting paper.

4. Subculture any visible growth by plating on heated-blood agar and identify the organism by agglutination with a specific antiserum.

GARDNERELLA VAGINALIS

This organism is a small Gram-negative or Gram-variable bacillus, facultatively anaerobic and nutritionally exacting. It was originally named *Haemophilus vaginalis* and later, because it showed a Gram-positive diphtheroid morphology and the production of volutin granules on Loeffler's serum, *Corynebacterium vaginale*. But its cell-wall structure and composition resemble those of Gram-negative rather than Gram-positive bacteria and it differs from diphtheroid bacilli in lacking catalase activity. It also differs from *Haemophilus* in not requiring either X or V factor, and has therefore been classified in a separate genus of uncertain family affiliation.

It is present in small or moderate numbers as a commensal in the vagina in up to 50% of healthy women, and is present in large numbers, along with anaerobic bacteria, in the vaginal secretion in all or nearly all women with anaerobic vaginosis, a condition of which the main complaint is the occurrence of a foul-smelling discharge. It is also found in the urethra of most male partners of women patients and probably is often transmitted by sexual contact.

Anaerobic vaginosis is characterized by a grey, green or yellow, often frothy discharge with a putrid fishy odour that may be strongest after coitus. The odour is due to the presence of amines such as cadaverine and putrescine, and can be intensified by mixing a drop of 10% KOH with a drop of secretion on a slide held under the nose (amine test). Whereas the secretion of the healthy adult vagina is highly acid, with a pH under 4.5, and has a predominant flora of lactobacilli forming lactic acid as end-product, the secretion in anaerobic vaginosis is less acid, with a pH 5.0 or higher and has a predominant flora of *G. vaginalis*, bacteroides and peptococcus which produce as main products, respectively, acetate and pyruvate, succinate, and butyrate (Spiegel at al 1980). Succinate-forming, anaerobic motile curved Gram-negative rods (*Mobiluncus*) are also present in many cases (Spiegel et al 1983). There is usually little or no inflammation of the vaginal epithelium (vaginitis) and few polymorphs are present in the secretion.

The initial cause of anaerobic vaginosis, which allows the normally scanty gardnerellas and anaerobes to multiply and replace the commensal lactobacilli, is still unknown, as is the exact role of *G. vaginalis*. Almost all cases respond well to treatment with oral metronidazole, e.g. in doses of 500 mg twice daily for 5 days, which produce peak serum levels of about 10 mg/litre. As anaerobes are more sensitive than *G. vaginalis* to metronidazole they are possibly the main target of its action and their synergy with gardnerella may be required both for the pathogenic effect and the development and maintenance of the abnormal flora. Whatever the role of gardnerella, the demonstration of its presence in large numbers in the vaginal secretion is generally considered to be useful confirmatory evidence of the presence of anaerobic vaginosis.

Morphology and staining

A small non-motile rod-shaped Gram-negative bacterium, *c.* 0.5 × 1–2 μm. Under some cultural conditions, e.g. on Loeffler's serum, the bacteria form volutin granules and appear Gram-positive or Gram-variable. Even in vivo their appearance is often Gram-variable and diphtheroid.

Cultural characters

Facultatively anaerobic, slowly growing and exacting in nutritional requirements. It fails to grow on simple nutrient agar, but requires a medium enriched with blood, serum or starch, and a humid aerobic or anaerobic atmosphere preferably enriched with 5% CO_2. Growth is slightly better under anaerobic than aerobic conditions. The optimum temperature for growth is 35–37°C and the optimum pH 6.0–6.5. Incubation should be continued for at least 48 h, as growth may be imperceptible at 24 h.

Colonies on blood agar after 48 h are small, e.g. less than 0.4 mm in diameter, round and dome-shaped. They exhibit β-haemolysis on human or rabbit blood, but not on horse or sheep blood. Growth is slightly better on heated-blood agar and the peptone-starch-dextrose agar of Dunkelberg et al (1970)*. After 48 h on the latter medium, colonies are 0.5–2 mm in diameter, circular, domed, and white-opaque with dark centres.

Various selective media have been described: that of Mickelsen et al (1977)* contains colistin and nalidixic acid, that of Totten et al (1980)* amphotericin, and that of Ison et al (1982)* nalidixic acid, gentamicin and amphotericin.

Biochemical characters

The gardnerella ferments glucose, maltose, dextrin, glycogen and starch with the production of acid but not gas. Its ability to hydrolyse starch may be seen in the production of zones of clearing around colonies on the opaque peptone-starch-dextrose agar of Mickelsen et al (1977). It is catalase negative, oxidase negative and urease negative, and it has the ability to hydrolyse sodium hippurate, an identifying reaction of some value. Its characters are compared with those of *Haemophilus* and other Gram-negative bacilli in Table 19.3. The catalase and oxidase tests may be performed by the usual methods on

Table 19.3 Distinguishing characters of *Haemophilus* species, *Gardnerella vaginalis* and some unclassified facultatively anaerobic Gram-negative bacilli occasionally infecting man.
Key: + T, twitching, fimbriae-dependent motility, no swimming or flagella; +A, X factor required only for aerobic growth; +/− or −/+, some strains positive, some negative; +B, haemolysis best on sheep or ox blood, fair on horse blood; +C, haemolysis on human or rabbit, but not sheep or horse blood; +D, haemolysis on horse blood; (+), weak positive reaction; . . ., result not given.

Character	*Haemophilus spp*	*Gardnerella vaginalis*	*Actinobacillus actinomycetem-comitans*	*Eikenella corrodens*	*Strepto-bacillus moniliformis*	*Cardio-bacterium hominis*	*Chromo-bacterium violaceum*[a]
Motility	−	−	−	+T	−	−	+
X requirement	+/−	−	−	+A	−	−	−
V requirement	+/−	−	−	−	−	−	−
Growth on MacConkey agar	−	−	−	−	−	−	+
β-haemolysis	−/+B	+C	−	−	−	−	+D
Catalase	+/−	−	+	−	−	−	+
Oxidase	+	−	I	+	−	+	+
Acid from glucose	+	+	+	−	+	+	+
Indole	+/−	−	−	−	−	(+)	−
Urease	+/−	−	. . .	−	. . .	−	−

[a] Violet coloured colonies.

growths on heated-blood agar. A technique for fermentation tests is described by Greenwood & Pickett (1984). Hippurate hydrolysis may be tested by the method of Hwang & Ederer (1975).*

Sensitivity to physical and chemical agents

Gardnerella is not salt-tolerant and will not grow on medium with 2% NaCl. It dies out fairly rapidly in culture and working cultures should be transferred every 48 h. It is resistant to colistin, gentamicin and nalidixic acid, which are used in selective media, and to the sulphonamides. It is sensitive to ampicillin, penicillin and trimethoprim, which drugs however are much less effective than metronidazole in the treatment of anaerobic vaginosis. Most strains are sensitive in vitro to high concentrations of metronidazole, e.g. 128 mg/litre, and although strains have been described as sensitive to 2–16 mg/l (Pheifer et al 1978) they are still less sensitive than anaerobes.

Laboratory diagnosis

Anaerobic vaginosis can readily be diagnosed in the clinic by history, physical examination and simple tests on the vaginal secretion (Blackwell & Barlow 1982), but the isolation of gardnerella in the laboratory provides a helpful confirmation.

1. In the clinic the pH of the vaginal secretion may be tested by placing indicator paper for the range pH 4–6 on the vaginal wall. A pH of 5 or higher suggests anaerobic vaginosis or trichomonas vaginitis. A drop of secretion may be subjected to the amine test (see above) and another drop in a wet film may be examined microscopically with the × 40 dry objective for the presence of 'clue cells' (see below), candida and trichomonas.

2. Specimens sent to the laboratory may be high vaginal or endocervical swabs soaked in exudate. If there is to be any delay in delivery they should be placed in tubes of a suitable transport medium, e.g. Stuart's (Ch. 6). Preferably, the physician should take a second swab in the clinic and use it to prepare a smear on a microscope slide, allow this to dry and submit it to the laboratory along with the first swab.

3. In the laboratory, fix the smear with heat and stain it by Gram's method. If a separate smear is not provided, use the swab to make a smear on a sterile slide for Gram staining. Examine particularly for 'clue cells' and large numbers of small Gram-negative or Gram-variable bacilli of diphtheroid morphology.

Clue cells are squamous epithelial cells coated with large numbers of the gardnerella bacilli, a characteristic finding generally present in anaerobic vaginosis. Lactobacilli and polymorphs will be few in number in that condition.

As the pH and microscopic appearances of the secretion in trichomonas vaginitis may resemble those in anaerobic vaginosis, a wet film from the swab in transport medium should be examined microscopically to exclude the presence of trichomonads (Ch. 43).

4. Plate the swab on media including a rich, unselective blood agar or heated-blood agar and a selective agar medium such as that of Mickelsen et al (1977)* or that of Ison et al (1982)*. Incubate anaerobically for 48 h. Look for the presence of small colonies of appropriate morphology, e.g. surrounded by zones of clearing on the starch-containing medium or β-haemolysis on human blood agar.

5. Identify the colonies as *G. vaginalis* by examining their morphology in a Gram film, demonstrating their catalase-negative character to differentiate them from diphtheroids, demonstrating their ability to grow aerobically in 48 h in a humid atmosphere with about 5% CO_2, e.g. in a candle jar containing wet blotting paper, and demonstrating their sensitivity to high concentrations of metronidazole, e.g. by culturing anaerobically on heated-blood agar with a 50 μg disk of metronidazole placed on a confluently seeded area of the plate. Confirmatory tests may also be done for the hydrolysis of hippurate* and haemolysis of human or rabbit blood.

ACTINOBACILLUS ACTINOMYCETEMCOMITANS

This small non-motile Gram-negative bacillus (0.3–0.5 × 0.5–1.5 μm) is an atypical member of the genus *Actinobacillus*, of which it is the only species found in man. Apart from its lack of X and V requirements, it more closely resembles *Haemophilus* (see Table 19.3). It is present in the lesions of about 30% of cases of actinomycosis, usually as a concomitant of a primary pathogen such as *Actinomyces israeli*, but also occurs as a commensal in the healthy mouth and rarely as sole pathogen in jaw infection and endocarditis. It is a facultative organism that grows on plain nutrient agar, best under microaerophilic conditions with added CO_2, when it forms small firm adherent star-shaped colonies. It is sensitive to chloramphenicol, erythromycin, streptomycin and tetracycline.

EIKENELLA CORRODENS

This small Gram-negative bacillus (0.3–0.4 × 1.5–4 μm) shows the unusual character of 'jerking' or 'twitching' motility dependent on its possession of contractile, fimbria-like filamentous appendages. It lacks flagella and the capacity for swimming-type motility. It is a commensal in the human mouth and intestine, but occasionally causes opportunistic infections such as endocarditis and mixed infections with other facultative or anaerobic bacteria, e.g. in periodontal disease and infections related to the mouth. It has also been found in wound infection, brain or liver abscess, meningitis and osteomyelitis, in some cases as sole pathogen.

Culture and identification

It is facultatively anaerobic, but requires haemin for aerobic growth. Specimens should be cultured for up to 5 days at 35–37°C on blood agar plates incubated, in parallel, in highly humid aerobic and anaerobic atmospheres with 10% added CO_2, e.g. in plastic bags or jars containing wet blotting paper. The colonies may be 0.5–1 mm in diameter after 48 h, when they are seen at the bottom of small pits in the medium, and later may develop a spreading edge. The 'corroding' appearance is due to the twitching motility of the bacilli which causes them to disturb and embed themselves into the surface of the agar. Non-fimbriate, and thus non-twitching variant strains form non-corroding, non-spreading colonies.

For isolation from mixed infections, Slee & Tanzer (1976) have described a selective medium containing clindamycin 0.5 mg/litre, KNO_3 2 g/l and haemin 5 mg/l in a nutrient agar made from Todd-Hewitt broth. The organism is catalase negative and oxidase positive, and does not produce acid from glucose or indole from peptone (Table 19.3). It is usually sensitive to ampicillin, benzylpenicillin, cefoxitin, chloramphenicol and tetracycline, and always resistant to clindamycin and metronidazole.

STREPTOBACILLUS MONILIFORMIS

This organism is a normal inhabitant of the nasopharynx of wild and laboratory rats, in which it sometimes causes respiratory, ear or conjunctival infection. It also causes a disease in mice characterized by multiple arthritis and swellings of the feet and legs. In man, it is the cause of one type of rat-bite fever, which may be accompanied by a rash, arthritis, endocarditis, pneumonia or brain abscess. The human infection appears sometimes to be contracted by the ingestion of food or milk contaminated by rats. Another type of rat-bite fever is caused by *Spirillum minus* (Ch. 32) and may be clinically indistinguishable from that caused by the streptobacillus.

Morphology and staining

The organism is a highly pleomorphic, non-motile Gram-negative bacillus. It may appear as short rods, 0.3–0.4 × 1–3 mm, or as elongated filaments which sometimes bear axial fusiform swellings or lateral spherical protrusions.

Cultural characters

It is a nutritionally exacting facultative anaerobe which requires a culture medium with a high proportion of blood or serum. It grows well on moist slopes of Loeffler's serum, on moist plates of nutrient agar containing 20% horse serum, and in 20% serum broth. Plates should be incubated in a humid aerobic atmosphere for 3 days, when the colonies will be raised, smooth, grey, granular and 1–3 mm in diameter. Viability is poor and the cultures die off in 2–4 days.

L-form variants

Variants defective in cell-wall formation are very liable to appear in artificial culture. They are seen alongside the larger streptobacillus colonies as minute (0.1–0.3 mm) colonies with a 'fried egg' appearance representing a denser central portion penetrating the agar surrounded by a thin skirt of bacilli spilling out on to its surface. They consist mainly of small coccoid bodies and can be transferred to slides for staining by excising a square of the agar and fixing it while pressed colony-side downwards on a slide (Ch. 3). The variant can be subcultured by rubbing an agar block with colonies on a fresh plate and then leaving it, colony-side down, during incubation. It breeds true in the L-form.

Laboratory diagnosis

In human infections the streptobacillus can sometimes be isolated from the blood or joint fluid. Collect about 10 ml of the patient's blood or joint fluid into a tube containing 20 mg sodium citrate as anticoagulant and centrifuge it to deposit the bacilli and cells. Inoculate the deposit into 20% serum broth and on to plates of 20% serum nutrient agar and incubate at 37°C in a humid aerobic atmosphere for 3 days. Colonies like 'fluff balls' may be seen on the surface of the sedimented blood cells in the serum broth and both streptobacillary and L-form colonies on the plates.

The organism is catalase negative and oxidase negative (Table 19.3). When inoculated into mice it causes a rapidly fatal generalized infection or a slowly progressive disease with swelling of the feet and joints. It is highly sensitive to penicillin and streptomycin, which may be used successfully for treatment. The L-form variant is resistant to penicillin, but probably incapable of survival and growth in the body.

CALYMMATOBACTERIUM GRANULOMATIS

This organism, found only in man, is the cause of a chronic granulomatous disease called granuloma venereum, granuloma inguinale or Donovanosis, and found mainly in warm humid tropical and subtropical countries. The initial lesion is commonly on the genitals, indicating transmission by sexual contact, but is sometimes elsewhere on the skin and then probably the result of intimate non-sexual contact. There is often an associated bubo. Treatment is with ampicillin or tetracycline.

Morphology and staining

C. granulomatis is a small plump capsulate Gram-negative bacillus, 0.5–1.5 × 1–2 μm, often showing polar staining. In smears from lesions it is seen mainly within the cytoplasm of large mononuclear phagocytes and, when stained with Leishman's or Giemsa's stain, shows a pinkish capsule.

Cultural characters

It is difficult to grow in vitro and is most readily cultured in the yolk sac of a developing chick embryo. Artificial media containing fresh egg yolk have been used successfully by Dienst et al (1948) and Dulaney et al (1948).

Laboratory diagnosis

1. Aspirate material from any bubo present. Also, cleanse the surface of a skin or genital lesion with gauze soaked in saline and scrape and macerate tissue from its base.

2. Make smears of the aspirate and scrapings, stain with Leishman's or Giemsa's stain (Ch. 3) and examine for the presence of intracellular capsulate bacilli. Their finding is diagnostic.

3. If facilities are present, inoculate the aspirate and scrapings into the yolk sac of a 5-day-old embryonated hen's egg, incubate for 3 days and examine Leishman- and Gram-stained smears of the yolk fluid for the typical bacilli.

4. If a suitable antigen, e.g. sterilized culture, is available, inject the recommended dose intradermally into the patient to demonstrate a specific allergic reaction (Chen et al 1949).

CARDIOBACTERIUM HOMINIS

This organism is a small non-motile pleomorphic Gram-negative bacillus. It is a common commensal in the nose and throat of man and a rare cause of endocarditis, diagnosed by its isolation in blood culture. It is a facultative anaerobe, but growth on nutrient, yeast extract or blood agar is poor unless plates are incubated in a humid atmosphere of air with 3–5% CO_2 or in an anaerobic jar. Colonies on blood agar after 48 h are smooth, circular and opaque, 1–2 mm in diameter. *C. hominis* is sensitive to penicillin, chloramphenicol, gentamicin and tetracycline. Its distinguishing characters are shown in Table 19.3.

CHROMOBACTERIUM VIOLACEUM

This organism is a robust, easily grown saprophyte found in soil and water, which rarely causes opportunistic suppurative or septicaemic infections in man. It is a large motile Gram-negative bacillus, 0.6–0.9 × 1.5–4 μm, having a single polar flagellum and usually also one or two lateral flagella, and sometimes showing barred or bipolar staining.

It is a facultative anaerobe and grows readily on simple nutrient media at 35–37°C including MacConkey agar. It is recognized by its production of violet-coloured colonies among other characters (Table 19.3). It is resistant to benzylpenicillin and sensitive to tetracycline.

METHODS

Fildes (1920) blood-digest agar

1. *Peptic digest of blood*

Sodium chloride, NaCl, 0.85% aqueous solution	150 ml
Hydrochloric acid, HCl, pure 35–40% aqueous solution	6 ml
Defibrinated sheep blood	50 ml
Pepsin (BP, granulated)	1 g
Sodium hydroxide, NaOH, 20% aqueous	12 ml
Chloroform, CHCl$_3$	0.5 ml

In a stoppered bottle mix the saline, HCl, blood and pepsin. Heat at 55°C for 2–14 h. Then add NaOH until a sample of the mixture diluted with water gives a deep violet-red colour with cresol red indicator (i.e. at pH about 9). Add further pure HCl drop by drop until a sample of the mixture shows almost no red colour with cresol red, but a definite red tint with phenol red indicator (i.e. at pH 7.2–7.3). Add the chloroform and shake vigorously. The digest will keep at room temperature for several months. Fildes peptic digest of blood is also available commercially, e.g. from Oxoid.

2. *Blood-digest agar.* Just before preparing the medium, heat sufficient of the digest at 55°C for 30 min to remove the chloroform. Melt some nutrient agar and cool it to 50–55°C, then add the digest to it in the proportion of 5 ml to 100 ml, mix well and pour in plates.

The resulting medium, Fildes agar, is a clear yellow medium containing abundant haemin (X factor), NAD (V factor) and other nutrients liberated from the red blood cells. It supports good growth of *H. influenzae* and some other exacting pathogens such as *Clostridium tetani*, while its high content of haemin makes it inhibitory to many bacteria such as throat commensal streptococci.

Levinthal agar

The modified preparation recommended by Alexander (1965) is as follows.

Levinthal stock. 1. Prepare brain heart infusion broth (Difco) according to the maker's instructions.

2. Heat the broth to vigorous boiling and, while boiling, add sterile defibrinated horse blood to a concentration of 10%.

3. Filter the mixture through Whatman filter paper No. 12 and sterilize the clear filtrate by Seitz filtration.

Levinthal agar. 1. Prepare a nutrient agar from 45 g Proteose agar No. 3 (Difco) and 15 g Bacto agar per litre of water. Autoclave.

2. Add one volume of sterile Levinthal stock to one volume of the melted, cooling agar. Mix thoroughly and pour in plates.

Haemophilus differential selective medium

This plating medium of Roberts et al (1987) contains bacitracin to make it selective for haemophilus, and sucrose and phenol red to distinguish *H. parainfluenzae*, which ferments the sucrose and forms large yellow colonies, from *H. influenzae*, which does not ferment sucrose and so forms small colourless colonies. It also contains haemin (X factor), and after the plate has been seeded, a V factor disk is placed on it so that the haemophilus colonies may be identified by their satellite growth around the disk.

Blood agar base (Oxoid No. 2)	40 g
Sucrose	10 g
Phenol red	25 mg
Water	1 litre

Autoclave at 121°C for 15 min, cool to 50°C and, in sterile solutions, add:

Haemin	3 mg
Bacitracin	100 mg

Pour in plates, inoculate the clinical specimen, apply a V factor disk and incubate aerobically.

Note: Depending on the preparation and method of sterilization, a larger quantity of haemin, up to 20 mg, may be required. If incubation is done in atmosphere with added CO_2, the acidic gas may cause a yellow colour change independently of fermentation of the sucrose, which persists until the gas disperses in normal air.

Peptone-starch-dextrose-agar

This medium of Dunkelberg et al (1970) supports the growth of *G. vaginalis* whose colonies after 48 h are recognized by their high-domed shape and whitish opacity with dark centres. If the medium is made opaque by the substitution of insoluble maize starch for the soluble starch in the original formula, the formation of clear zones due to hydrolysis of the starch around the colonies is seen as another identifying feature (Mickelsen et al 1977).

Proteose peptone No. 3 (Difco)	20 g
Soluble (or insoluble maize) starch	10 g
Dextrose (glucose)	2 g
Na_2HPO_4	1 g

NaH₂PO₄.2H₂O	1 g
Agar	15 g
Distilled water	1 litre

$NaH_2PO_4.2H_2O$ 1 g; Agar 15 g; Distilled water 1 litre

Adjust the pH to 6.8 before melting. Autoclave at 121°C for 15 min. Pour in plates.

Selective media for Gardnerella vaginalis

Medium of Mickelsen et al (1977). This medium contains colistin and nalidixic acid to minimize the growth of enteric bacteria and insoluble maize starch to permit the recognition of starch-hydrolysing colonies.

GC agar base (BBL)	36 g
Insoluble maize starch	10 g
Colistin solution 5 g/litre	2 ml
Nalidixic acid solution 7.5 g/litre	2 ml
IsoVitaleX (BBL)	10 ml
Distilled water	1 litre

Dissolve the GC agar base and maize starch in the water, boil for 1–2 min and then add the colistin and nalidixic acid. Autoclave at 121°C for 15 min. Allow to cool to about 55°C and add the IsoVitaleX. Pour 15–18 ml volumes in 90 mm Petri dishes.

Medium of Totten et al (1980). This medium contains amphotericin to inhibit the growth of yeasts and human blood to permit the recognition of *G. vaginalis* colonies producing β-haemolysis on incubation in 5% CO_2 in air for 3 days. Plates are poured with a basal layer of 7 ml of Columbia CNA agar base (BBL) plus 2 mg/litre of amphotericin B and a covering layer of 14 ml of the same medium enriched with 5% citrated human blood.

Medium of Ison et al (1982). This medium is a nutrient agar containing 5% of citrated human blood, amphotericin 2 mg/litre, nalidixic acid 30 mg/l and gentamicin 4 mg/l.

Disk test of X and V requirements

1. Pour a plate of autoclaved nutrient agar deficient in X and V factors. Paper disks impregnated with suitable amounts of X and V factors are available commercially (Oxoid).

2. Inoculate a small portion of the colonial growth under test as a broad streak from side to side across the plate in one of its halves. Inoculate a control culture of *H. influenzae* in a streak across the other half.

3. On to each streak at well spaced intervals apply a paper disk containing X factor, a second disk containing X and V factors, and a third disk containing only V factor.

4. Incubate the plate at 37°C for 24 h in air with 10% CO_2.

5. Read the results as follows. (a) Growth along the whole length of the streak indicates absence of either X or V requirement. (b) Growth only around the X plus V disk indicates requirements of both X factor and V factor. (c) Growth around the X plus V disk and one of the other two disks (e.g. V disk) indicates a requirement only of the factor in that disk.

This test gives false results for X factor requirement in a proportion of cases and for certain identification of the X requirement it is recommended that the porphyrin synthesis test should be done as described below.

Disk test for V requirement. When the X requirement is to be tested separately, the preferred method of testing the V requirement, on a blood-containing medium, may be used.

1. Melt some nutrient agar, add 5% of defibrinated horse blood to it, mix, and *then* autoclave at 121°C to sterilize it and destroy all the V factor in the blood and nutrient agar. Pour in plates. This medium contains abundant X factor.

2. Streak the culture under test across half of a plate and a control culture of *H. influenzae* across the other half. Apply a V factor disk to the middle of each streak and incubate overnight. Growth confined to a zone immediately around the disk indicates a requirement of V factor.

Porphyrin synthesis test

This test (Kilian 1974) demonstrates the ability of a bacterium supplied with δ-aminolaevulinic acid to synthesize and excrete porphobilinogen and other porphyrins, indicating the absence of a requirement for X factor.

Substrate. Prepare a solution of δ-aminolaevulinic acid HCl (Sigma) 2 mmol/litre, $MgSO_4$ 0.8 mmol/l, sodium phosphate buffer pH 6.9, 0.1 mol/l.

Method. 1. Distribute 0.5 ml volumes of the substrate in small glass tubes.

2. Add a large loopful of bacteria from the colonies on a plate culture to a tube of substrate. Incubate for 4 h at 37°C.

3. Observe the tube under a Wood's lamp (i.e. in ultraviolet radiation at 360 nm wavelength) in a dark room. A red fluorescence from either the bacterial deposit or the supernatant fluid in the tube indicates porphyrin synthesis and thus the *absence* of a requirement for X factor. Absence of fluorescence indicates that the bacterium requires X factor for growth.

4. Control the procedure by doing parallel tests on an X-requiring, e.g. *H. influenzae*, and a non-X-requiring haemophilus, e.g. *H. parainfluenzae*.

Haemagglutination tests

Most strains of *H. aegyptius* and many of *H. influenzae* agglutinate red blood cells, but strains differ in the species of cells with which they will react and cultures should therefore be tested in parallel with the red cells of man (group O), guinea-pig, fowl, pig and sheep (Scott & Old 1981). Tests should be done at 4°C as the reactions commonly disappear ('elute') on warming to 20°C, though strong reactions with human cells, as given by most strains of *H. aegyptius*, do not elute till warmed to about 45°C and can therefore be detected in tests done at room temperature, as in the tube tests of Davis et al (1950). The reactions are mannose-resistant.

1. Centrifuge red cells from the blood, wash thrice in saline (0.85% NaCl) and resuspend to 3%(v/v) in saline.

2. Grow the culture under test for 24 h at 37°C on a heated-blood ('chocolate') agar buffered at pH 7.0 with 3.6 g KH_2PO_4 and 6.4 g K_2HPO_4/litre. Harvest the culture in saline to a

high density, about 10^{11} bacteria/ml. It is essential to test the bacteria in high concentration.

3. Mix a large drop of the dense bacterial suspension with a large drop of the 3% suspension of erythrocytes in a depression on a white tile chilled to about 4°C. Rock the tile to and fro for 15 min while keeping it at 4°C. Then look for the presence of fine or coarse clumping of the red cells.

4. Test each strain in parallel with each species of erythrocyte and observe also a control mixture of the erythrocytes in saline to exclude the possibility of their being autoagglutinating.

Fermentation tests on haemophili

Kilian & Biberstein (1984) recommend culture in phenol red broth (Difco) containing 1% of the test carbohydrate and enriched with crystalline nicotinamide adenine dinucleotide 10 mg/litre and crystalline haemin 10 mg/l added from filter-sterilized solutions (Kilian 1976).

Hippurate hydrolysis test

A rapid test developed by Hwang & Ederer (1975) to detect the hydrolysis of sodium hippurate by haemolytic streptococci may be used to demonstrate hippurate hydrolysis by *G. vaginalis*.

1. Prepare a 1% solution of sodium hippurate and dispense it in 0.4 ml volumes in capped or corked tubes, which may be stored at −20°C until required for use.

2. Thaw the tubes and inoculate into each a large loopful of solid colonial growth from a rich blood-containing medium. Emulsify thoroughly.

3. Incubate the tubes for 2 h at 37°C.

4. Then add to each 0.2 ml of ninhydrin solution (3.5 g of ninhydrin in 100 ml of a mixture of equal parts of acetone and butanol).

5. Incubate for a further 10 min at 37°C.

6. Observe the tubes for a purple colour indicating that glycine has been produced on the hydrolysis of hippurate.

REFERENCES

Alexander H E 1965 The haemophilus group. In: Dubos R J, Hirsch J G (eds) Bacterial and mycotic infections of man, 4th edn. Pitman Medical, London. p 724–741

Alexander H E, Leidy G, MacPherson C 1946 Production of types A, B, C, D, E and F *H. influenzae* antibody for diagnostic and therapeutic purposes. Journal of Immunology 54: 207–211

Blackwell A, Barlow D 1982 Clinic diagnosis of anaerobic vaginosis (non-specific vaginitis). A practical guide. British Journal of Venereal Diseases 58: 387–393

Broom A K, Sneath P H A 1981 Numerical taxonomy of *Haemophilus*. Journal of General Microbiology 126: 123–149

Brumfitt W, Willoughby M L N, Bromley L L 1957 An evaluation of sputum examination in chronic bronchitis. Lancet 2: 1306–1309

Chen C H, Dienst R B, Greenblatt R B 1949 Skin reaction of patients to *Donovania granulomatis*. American Journal of Syphilis, Gonorrhea and Venereal Diseases 33: 60–64

Davis D J, Pittman M, Griffitts J J 1950 Hemagglutination by the Koch-Weeks bacillus (*Hemophilus aegyptius*). Journal of Bacteriology 59: 427–431

Dienst R B, Greenblatt R B, Chen C H 1948 Laboratory diagnosis of Granuloma Inguinale and studies on the cultivation of the Donovan body. American Journal of Syphilis, Gonorrhea and Venereal Diseases 32: 301–306

Dixon J M S, Miller D C 1965 Value of dilute inocula in cultural examination of sputum. Lancet 2: 1046–1048

Dulaney A D, Guto K, Packer H 1948 *Donovania granulomatis*: cultivation, antigenic preparation and immunological tests. Journal of Immunology 59: 335–340

Dunkelberg W E Jr, Skaggs R, Kellogg D S Jr 1970 Method for isolation and identification of *Corynebacterium vaginale* (*Haemophilus vaginalis*). Applied Microbiology 19: 47–52

Ederer G M, Schurr M L 1971 Optimal bacitracin concentration for selective isolation medium for haemophilus. American Journal of Medical Technology 37: 304–305

Fildes P 1920 Peptic-blood-agar for culture of *B. influenzae* and general purposes. British Journal of Experimental Pathology 1:129

Fleming A 1929 On the antibacterial action of cultures of a penicillium with special reference to their use in the isolation of *B. influenzae*. British Journal of Experimental Pathology 10: 226–236

Greenwood J R, Pickett M J 1984 Genus *Gardnerella*. In: Krieg N R, Holt J G (eds) Bergey's manual of systematic bacteriology, vol 1. Williams & Wilkins, Baltimore p 587–591

Hammond G W, Lian C J, Wilt W, Albritton W, Ronald A R 1978 Determination of the hemin requirement of *Haemophilus ducreyi*: evaluation of the porphyrin test and media used in the satellite growth test. Journal of Clinical Microbiology 7: 243–246

Hovig B, Aandahl E H 1969 A selective medium for the isolation of *Haemophilus* in material from the respiratory tract. Acta Pathologica Microbiologica Scandinavica 77: 676–684

Hwang M N, Ederer G M 1975 Rapid hippurate hydrolysis method for presumptive identification of Group B streptococci. Journal of Clinical Microbiology 1: 114–115

Ison C A, Dawson S G, Hilton J, Csonka G, Easmon C S F 1982 Comparison of culture and microscopy in the diagnosis of *Gardnerella vaginalis* infection. Journal of Clinical Pathology 35: 550–554

Kilian M 1974 A rapid method for the differentiation of *Haemophilus* strains. The porphyrin test. Acta Pathologica Microbiologica Scandinavica, Section B, 82: 835–842

Kilian M 1976 A taxonomic study of the genus *Haemophilus* with the proposal of a new species. Journal of General Microbiology 93: 9–62

Kilian M, Biberstein E L 1984 Genus II. *Haemophilus*. In: Krieg N R, Holt J G (eds) Bergey's manual of systematic bacteriology, vol 1. Williams & Wilkins, Baltimore. p 558–569

Lees A W, McNaught W 1959 Bacteriology of lower-respiratory-tract secretions, sputum and upper-respiratory-tract secretions in 'normals' and chronic bronchitics. Lancet 2: 1112–1115

May J R, Delves D M 1964 The survival of *H. influenzae* and pneumococci in specimens of sputum sent to the laboratory by post. Journal of Clinical Pathology 17: 254

Mickelsen P A, McCarthy L R, Mangum M E 1977 New differential medium for the isolation of *Corynebacterium vaginale*. Journal of Clinical Microbiology 5: 488–489

Pheifer T A, Forsyth P S, Durfee M A, Pollock H M, Holmes K K 1978 Non-specific vaginitis: role of *Haemophilus vaginalis* and treatment with metronidazole. New England Journal of Medicine 298: 1429–1434

Roberts D E, Higgs E, Cole P J 1987 Selective medium that distinguishes *Haemophilus influenzae* from *Haemophilus parainfluenzae* in clinical specimens: its value in investigating respiratory sepsis. Journal of Clinical Pathology 40: 75–76

Scott S, Old D C 1981 Mannose-resistant and eluting (MRE) haemagglutinins, fimbriae and surface structures in strains of *Haemophilus*. FEMS Microbiology Letters 10: 235–240

Sims W 1970 Oral haemophili. Journal of Medical Microbiology 3: 615–625

Slack M P E, Wheldon D B, Turk D C 1977 A rapid test for beta-lactamase production by *H. influenzae*. Lancet 2: 906

Slee A M, Tanzer J M 1976 Selective medium for isolation of *Eikenella corrodens* from periodontal lesions. Journal of Clinical Microbiology 8: 459–462

Spiegel C A, Amsel R, Eschenbach D, Schoenknicht F, Holmes K K 1980 Anaerobic bacteria in non-specific vaginitis. New England Journal of Medicine 303: 601–607

Spiegel C A, Eschenbach D A, Amsel R, Holmes K K 1983 Curved anaerobic bacteria in bacterial (nonspecific) vaginosis and their response to antimicrobial therapy. Journal of Infectious Diseases 148: 817–822

Totten P A, Amsel R, Holmes K K 1980 Selective differential medium for isolation of *G. vaginalis*. In: Abstracts of the 80th Annual Meeting of the American Society for Microbiology, Miami Beach, May 1980, Washington D C, American Society for Microbiology 1980: 310 abstract

Turk D C 1982 *Haemophilus influenzae*. Public Health Laboratory Service Monograph Series No. 17. HMSO, London

Vastine D W, Dawson C R, Hoshiwara I, Yoneda C, Daghfous T, Messadi M 1974 Comparison of media for the isolation of *Haemophilus* species from cases of seasonal conjunctivitis associated with severe endemic trachoma. Applied Microbiology 28: 688–691

Wasilavskas B L, Hampton K D 1982 Determination of bacterial meningitis: a retrospective study of 80 cerebrospinal fluid specimens evaluated by four in-vitro methods. Journal of Clinical Microbiology 16: 531–535

Zinnemann K 1960 *Haemophilus influenzae* and its pathogenicity. Ergebnisse der Mikrobiologie, Immunologie und Experimentellen Therapie 33: 307–368

Bordetella

The genus *Bordetella* comprises three recognized species of Gram-negative bacilli. *B. pertussis* is a human pathogen incriminated in the majority of cases of whooping cough, a common childhood infection. *B. parapertussis* is also occasionally found in whooping cough. It has been suggested that there may be conversion of *B. pertussis* to *B. parapertussis*, although the evidence is not conclusive (Kumazawa & Yoshikawa 1978). *B. bronchiseptica* is an animal pathogen that occurs only rarely in man as a secondary invader after viral respiratory infections.

Culture of bordetellas requires special media. The traditional medium, Bordet-Gengou, should now be replaced by charcoal-containing blood agar which gives better growth. In diagnostic work, any colony with a typical appearance on appropriate media should be regarded as *Bordetella*; however, microscopy to establish that the organism is a Gram-negative bacillus, and serological identification to confirm the species, are essential.

BORDETELLA PERTUSSIS

Morphology and staining

Small ovoid Gram-negative cocco-bacilli with slight pleomorphism; non-motile and non-sporing. Capsules may be demonstrable in young, freshly isolated cultures.

Cultural characters

The organisms are aerobes with an optimum growth temperature of 35°C. Primary isolation is not possible on conventional media such as blood agar or nutrient agar and requires an enriched medium. Even so, growth of *B. pertussis* on charcoal blood agar is slow and incubation should be continued for at least 5 days. Usually a growth will be recognizable after 72 h as greyish-white colonies with a shiny surface and high convex shape, the typical 'bisected pearl' or 'mercury drop' appearance.

Subsequent cultures may be obtained on less exacting media, e.g. nutrient agar to which charcoal or starch has been added. For long term maintenance it is recommended that charcoal blood agar slopes be used if freeze-drying is unavailable.

Biochemical characters

Biochemical testing has limited value as the organisms have few significant fermentative activities. *B. pertussis* is weakly oxidase positive whereas *B. parapertussis* is oxidase negative.

Sensitivity to physical and chemical agents

B. pertussis is a fragile organism, dying within a few days on culture or on drying. It is killed by heat at 55°C for 30 min and is adequately contained by standard disinfection procedures. The organism is usually sensitive to ampicillin and erythromycin and these drugs have a reasonable therapeutic record in whooping cough. Disk diffusion tests should be carried out by a Stokes procedure with a control organism of known sensitivity (see Ch. 9).

Serological characters

B. pertussis has three major antigens, designated

1, 2 and 3, which can be detected by slide agglutination tests. In recent years the commonest serotype in Britain has been type 1,3 in well immunized and type 1,2 in poorly immunized communities (Preston 1985).

Animal pathogenicity

Intranasal inhalation of *B. pertussis* by mice results in a severe interstitial pneumonia. Mice are also highly susceptible to small intracerebral inoculations with virulent strains and this procedure has been used as a test to monitor the effectiveness of *B. pertussis* vaccines (but see Preston 1966).

B. pertussis produces a number of toxic and enzymic factors, e.g. the heat-labile endotoxin, the histamine sensitivity factor, the lymphocytosis factor, fimbrial and non-fimbrial haemagglutinins, and an adjuvant substance. Any or all of these substances may be important in the pathogenesis of infections caused by *B. pertussis*. For diagnosis, however, they should at present be ignored because they offer no simple route towards identification of the organisms.

BORDETELLA PARAPERTUSSIS

This organism is occasionally found in patients with whooping cough. It can be differentiated from *B. pertussis* by a few simple characters. *B. pertussis* is weakly oxidase positive, grows slowly on bordetella media and does not grow on nutrient agar. *B. parapertussis*, in contrast, is oxidase negative, grows rapidly on bordetella media and will grow on and produce brown discolouration of nutrient agar. Further, an antiserum can be obtained commercially which is specific for *B. parapertussis* and can be used in agglutination tests as described for *B. pertussis*.

BORDETELLA BRONCHISEPTICA

This organism is related antigenically and in toxin production to *B. pertussis*. It is motile, with peritrichous flagella, and grows on ordinary media without the addition of blood. It causes secondary respiratory infections in canine distemper and in rodents and may be a cause of snuffles in rabbits. Human infections occur rarely (Ghosh & Tranter 1979).

LABORATORY DIAGNOSIS OF WHOOPING COUGH

Three methods are available: (1) Isolation of *B. pertussis* by culture from a pernasal swab (2) Identification of the organism in a smear from a pernasal swab by immunofluorescence microscopy (3) The serological demonstration of specific antibodies in the patient's serum. As any one or two of these methods may give negative results while another is positive, two or preferably all three methods should be employed in parallel.

Collection of specimens

The pernasal swab has generally replaced the cough plates or post-nasal swabs which were used in the past. A detailed description of the type of pernasal swab required and its use is given by Abbott et al (1982). Briefly, a sterile cotton-wool swab on a flexible wire is passed gently along the floor of the nose until it meets resistance; the swab, which will collect mucopus, is withdrawn and either plated immediately on charcoal blood agar, or placed in transport medium. If delay in transport is more than 4 h, Amies (1967) transport medium should be used (Hunter 1986). These transport media will support the viability of the organism for only a few hours, and the aim should be to inoculate an appropriate medium as soon as possible. An alternative to the use of pernasal swabs is to use suction catheters (i.e. Auger catheters) to obtain the post-nasal secretions (Regan 1980).

Single swabs taken from infected patients may not always yield bordetellas and it is recommended that up to six swabs taken at intervals of 1–2 days be examined before *B. pertussis* is considered to be absent. Because of the difficulties of isolation even in typical cases of the infection where the appropriate methods of investigation are undertaken, the use of immunofluorescence is recommended for direct identification of the organism in secretions in addition to cultural techniques. Where isolation is repeatedly negative, particularly in adults, serological examination may be appropriate.

Culture of B. pertussis

The preferred medium is charcoal blood agar* to which cephalexin has been added; the antibiotic inhibits other organisms commonly found in specimens but does not restrict the growth of *Bordetella* species. This medium is superior to Bordet-Gengou medium in that it will support a heavier growth of the organism on primary isolation, and the size of the colonies will be larger.

It should be noted that the best medium described to date is the diamidine-penicillin-fluoride medium of Lacey (1954). Although isolation rates of *B. pertussis* on this medium are much better than on the media noted above, the recipe for the medium is complicated and it is unreliable except in the most experienced hands.

Because incubation must be continued for at least 5 days it is necessary to use double-thickness plates and to maintain adequate humidity. If a humidified incubator is not available, a bowl of water should be placed on the floor of the incubator to provide humidity by evaporation. Alternatively, plates can be sealed in plastic bags containing dampened paper towels and incubated in the normal way. If drying of the plates occurs, *B. pertussis* will not grow.

Typical 'bisected pearl' colonies appearing after 3–5 days incubation at 37°C must be investigated further. In practice, any colony growing on charcoal blood medium should be investigated as the colonial morphology is insufficient for diagnosis. Suspect colonies should first be shown to be Gram-negative bacilli and thereafter serologically identified by slide agglutination with specific antisera. A positive agglutination test (see below), together with the growth characteristics and colony appearances, is suf-

* Refer to *Methods* at end of this chapter.

ficient for diagnosis of *B. pertussis* infection (Preston 1970).

Slide agglutination test

Antisera can be obtained commercially from various sources (e.g. Wellcome) but it is important to make sure that *B. pertussis* sera have been absorbed to remove cross-reacting antibody to *B. parapertussis*. For identification of *B. pertussis* it is essential to use a polyvalent agglutinating antiserum which will react with all three major antigens.

The normal method of slide agglutination, with a colony of bacteria emulsified in a drop of saline on a microscope slide, should not be used because the organism harvested from solid medium does not emulsify satisfactorily. The preferred method is to disperse several single colonies in a small volume of saline (e.g. 0.25 ml) by mechanical agitation with a Pasteur pipette or a syringe fitted with a small (21) gauge needle. When a smooth suspension has been obtained in this way, and no clumps are observed, the suspension is transferred as drops to microscope slides. Thereafter, a drop or loopful of antiserum is added to the suspension and the slide is gently rocked for approximately 1 min before the result is observed (see Preston 1970 for details).

The serotyping of *B. pertussis* and *B. parapertussis* is difficult and there are many traps for the unwary. Where typing is thought necessary for epidemiological reasons, cultures of isolated organisms should be sent to a reference laboratory; in the UK the recommended laboratory is the Department of Bacteriology, University of Manchester Medical School, Manchester, MI3 9PT. Cultures are preferably despatched as 2–3 day old specimens on charcoal agar slopes.

Diagnosis by immunofluorescence

B. pertussis cannot be recognized by microscopy in nasopharyngeal secretions unless specific fluorescent antiserum is used. In some studies the technique has proved very valuable and sensitive (Chalvardijan 1966; Linneman et al 1968) whilst in others the method has performed badly (Kendrick et al 1961; Field & Parker 1977; Rossier & Chan 1977). There is little evidence of uniformity of technique in these communications. It is well established that two factors are of importance for the identification of micro-organisms in tissue secretions or exudates by immunofluorescence. The first of these is that the antiserum used must have a high titre of IgG antibody to the organism. To obtain this type of antiserum careful attention must be paid to the immunizing procedure; an example of the appropriate regime is given later in this chapter*. (It is important to recognize that commercial antisera for identification of *B. pertussis* have been developed for agglutination tests and are usually unsatisfactory for the immunofluorescence method.) The second factor is that it must be anticipated that organisms in secretions from an infected patient will have adsorbed antibody which the host has produced. These adsorbed antibodies will block access to the organism by the fluorescent reagents and negative results will be obtained. It is therefore essential to treat the specimens prior to staining in order to remove any host antibody*.

With these modifications the immunofluorescence method can be expected to have a positivity rate of 70–75% in suspected cases of whooping cough, as against 50–55% positivity for repeated culture. The advantages of the immunofluorescence method are that it is sensitive, accurate and rapid (a diagnosis is possible within 12 h), and can produce a result in patients who have been partially treated with antibiotics where the organisms present in the secretions are not viable.

Serological tests

Several serological methods have been used in an attempt to diagnose pertussis infection in culture negative cases for serological tests often give positive results when culture fails to do so. But serological tests are not a substitute for attempted culture, because sometimes the reverse holds. Macaulay (1979, 1981) described direct agglutination, indirect haemagglutination (IHA) and complement fixation tests (CFT). The IHA was considered more sensitive than the

direct agglutination and detected IgM antibody. The CFT detected only IgG antibody. Paired sera must be examined for accurate results. Serum antibody is slow to appear; the first sample should be taken within 2–3 weeks of the onset of symptoms, and the second sample 2–4 weeks later. Single samples are almost impossible to interpret because of previous immunization or clinical whooping cough. A further problem is antibody to *Haemophilus* and *Moraxella* species which cross-reacts with *B. pertussis* (Abbott et al 1982).

Goodman et al (1981) looked for IgA antibody to *B. pertussis* in nasopharyngeal secretions but found this was unusual in acute infections and suggested that its appearance was late, often after disappearance of the organisms. However, Viljanen et al (1982), using the ELISA method for serum antibody to *B. pertussis*, showed that measurement of IgM and IgA antibody was diagnostic in 44–64% of patients after the age of 2 years, whereas culture was positive in only 9%. ELISA results were poor for patients under the age of 3 months but the use of paired sera, looking for a rising titre, increased the accuracy in this group of patients. IgG antibody measurements did not assist diagnosis in any age group.

METHODS

Charcoal blood agar

The traditional Bordet-Gengou medium has been largely replaced by charcoal blood agar, the recipe for which is given below. (We have not included the recipe for Bordet-Gengou medium, but this was given in the 12th Edn, Vol. 2, p. 131.)

Charcoal agar base is prepared as follows:

Beef extract ('Lab- Lemco', Oxoid)	10 g
Starch	10 g
Peptone	10 g
NaCl	5 g
Charcoal, bacteriological grade	4 g
Nicotinic acid	1 mg
Agar	12 g
Water	1 litre

Dissolve the ingredients, except the charcoal, in the water by heating gently. Adjust to pH 7.5–7.6 and add the charcoal. Dispense into suitable containers, shaking the medium occasionally to keep the charcoal in suspension. Autoclave at 121°C for 30 min.

For preparation of *complete medium*, add 10 ml sterile defibrinated horse blood to 100 ml charcoal agar base. Cool the molten agar to 45–50°C. Add the blood, previously warmed to 37°C. For a selective medium for primary culture, add cephalexin to a final concentration of 40 mg/l. Pour 4–5 plates from this volume. Do not dry the poured plates unless they are for immediate use.

The medium may also be dispensed in 5–10 ml amounts in screw-capped bottles and 'sloped'. In this form the medium is useful for the maintenance of stock cultures of *B. pertussis*, with weekly subcultures.

Raising of antiserum to B. pertussis for use in immunofluorescence

The NCTC10911 strain of *B. pertussis* is suitable for raising antibody because it contains antigens 1, 2 and 3. Prepare a suspension of 10^8 orgs/ml in saline and kill by heating at 56°C for 30 min. Emulsify 1 ml of this in 1.1 ml of Freund's complete adjuvant and, after appropriate mixing, inject 1 ml of suspension intramuscularly into a rabbit (0.5 ml into each thigh muscle). The animal must not be further injected for 6 weeks at least, after which time a booster injection is given intravenously; this should contain 10^7 organisms of the same strain in 1 ml saline.

After 7 days, bleed the animal and test the serum for activity in the fluorescence test. A titre of 50 or greater is acceptable. If this is not achieved, the animal should be given weekly booster injections for a minimum of 4 further weeks, using the same dose in saline. If the animal fails to produce a reasonable titre of antibody activity at the end of this time it is advisable to immunize another animal.

To save time, and where facilities allow, immunize at least 4 animals. If several of these produce good diagnostic antisera the sera can be pooled; where only one animal produces a satisfactory response the antiserum can be obtained by repeated booster injections and re-bleeding.

The antiserum obtained will probably have cross-reactivity against staphylococci, yeasts and *Haemophilus* species and this must be absorbed before the reagent is used. Ideally, after absorption the antiserum should produce strong fluorescence with *B. pertussis* at a dilution of 1 in 20, with no reaction at this dilution to other organisms.

Fluorescein labelling of the antiserum is by standard methods (Nairn 1976) or the antiserum can be used in a two-stage procedure with fluorescein-labelled anti-rabbit globulin as the second reagent. The latter is preferable as the labelled second reagent is commercially available, and the introduction of the second step increases sensitivity.

Immunofluorescence staining of smears for identification of B. pertussis

Prepare thin smears from pernasal swabs and allow to dry in air at room temperature. Immerse them in a solution containing 100 μg pepsin in 0.1 mol/litre HCl in a Coplin jar for 4–6 h to remove patient's antibody from the specimen. Remove, fix in methanol or acetone for 10 min and stain by standard procedures (Nairn 1976). Briefly, in the two-stage method, a drop of 1 in 20 rabbit antiserum is added to the specimen which is incubated at room temperature for 30 min in a damp chamber. The slides are washed with 0.1 mol/litre phosphate buffered saline (PBS, pH 7.2, Ch. 8) and a drop of fluorescein-labelled anti-rabbit IgG is added. The slide is incubated for 30 min, washed as before, mounted with glycerol (10%) in PBS and examined using a UV microscope. An incident-light microscope is particularly valuable because examination with a high power lens is necessary.

Include as controls: (1) positive smear of an NCTC strain; (2) labelled antiserum only, to control non-specific attachment of the label to the specimen; and (3) a second smear for each specimen, which is treated with the rabbit anti-pertussis serum previously absorbed with the standard strain used for its production. A convenient way of carrying out these tests is to use microscope slides which have 12 spots/slide, each separated by Teflon. Smear each patient specimen on to a pair of spots, one each on the upper and lower sequences. The upper sequence is treated with the rabbit anti-pertussis serum and the lower sequence with the absorbed control serum. During examination it is then easy to determine that fluorescing organisms in

specimens in the upper sequence do not fluoresce with the absorbed serum. Specificity of the reaction is therefore controlled.

B. pertussis are seen as short bacilli, with vigorous cell wall staining. They are often attached to squamous cell debris in the specimen. It is advisable to test at least three pernasal swabs by this method unless the first is unequivocally positive.

REFERENCES

Abbott J D, Macaulay M E, Preston N W 1982 Bacteriological diagnosis of whooping cough. Association of Clinical Pathologists: Broadsheet 105

Amies C R 1967 A modified formula for the preparation of Stuart's transport medium. Canadian Journal of Public Health 58: 296–300

Chalvardijan N 1966 The laboratory diagnosis of whooping cough by fluorescent antibody and cultural methods. Canadian Medical Association Journal 95: 263–266

Field L H, Parker C D 1977 Pertussis outbreak in Austin and Travis County, Texas, 1975. Journal of Clinical Microbiology 6: 154–160

Ghosh H K, Tranter J 1979 *Bordetella bronchiseptica* infection in man: review and a case report. Journal of Clinical Pathology 32: 546–548

Goodman Y E, Wort A J, Jackson F L 1981 ELISA IgA in nasopharyngeal secretions as an indicator of recent infection. Journal of Clinical Microbiology 13: 286–292

Hunter P R 1986 Survival of *Bordetella pertussis* in transport media. Journal of Clinical Pathology 39: 119–120

Kendrick P L, Elderling G, Eveland W C 1961 Fluorescent antibody techniques: methods for the identification of *Bordetella pertussis*. American Journal of Diseases of Children 101: 149–154

Kumazawa N H, Yoshikawa M 1978 Conversion of *Bordetella pertussis* to *Bordetella parapertussis*. Journal of Hygiene, Cambridge 81: 15–23

Lacey B W 1954 A new selective medium for *Haemophilus pertussis* containing a diamidine, sodium fluoride and penicillin. Journal of Hygiene, Cambridge 52: 273–303

Linneman C C, Bass J W, Smith M H D 1968 The carrier state in pertussis. American Journal of Epidemiology 88: 422–427

Macaulay M E 1979 The serological diagnosis of whooping cough. Journal of Hygiene, Cambridge 83: 95–102

Macaulay M E 1981 The IgM and IgG response to *Bordetella pertussis* in vaccination and infection. Journal of Medical Microbiology 14: 1–7

Nairn R C 1976 Fluorescent protein tracing, 4th edn. Churchill Livingstone, Edinburgh

Preston N W 1966 Potency tests for pertussis vaccine: doubtful value of intracerebral challenge test in mice. Journal of Pathology and Bacteriology 91: 173–179

Preston N W 1970 Technical problems in the laboratory diagnosis and prevention of whooping cough. Laboratory Practice 19: 482–486

Preston N W 1985 Change in the serotype of pertussis infection in Britain. Lancet 1: 510 Letter

Regan J 1980 The laboratory diagnosis of whooping cough. Clinical Microbiology Newsletter 2: 1–3

Rossier E, Chan F 1977 *Bordetella pertussis* in the National Capital Region: prevalent serotype and immunization status of patients. Canadian Medical Association Journal 117: 1169–1171

Viljanen M K, Ruuskanen O, Granberg C, Saluri T T 1982 Serological diagnosis of pertussis: IgM, IgA and IgG antibodies against *Bordetella pertussis* measured by enzyme-linked immunosorbent assay (ELISA). Scandinavian Journal of Infectious Diseases 14: 117–122

Neisseria: Acinetobacter: Branhamella

There are two genera of medically important aerobic Gram-negative diplococci, *Neisseria* and *Branhamella*. The distinguishing features of these are shown in Table 21.1. The meningococcus *N. meningitidis* and the gonococcus *N. gonorrhoeae* are the important pathogens in the genus *Neisseria*; other *Neisseria* species are commonly found as commensals in the upper respiratory tract. *N. meningitidis* gives rise to septicaemia and meningitis with or without septicaemia; it is normally carried in the throat but may be found in other sites such as the genital tract, where its presence is not usually of pathological significance. *N. gonorrhoeae* causes gonorrhoea, a sexually transmitted infection of the genitourinary tract, but may occasionally be found in the throat. Sometimes systemic spread gives rise to disseminated gonococcal infection, characterized by arthritis with or without skin lesions.

Branhamella catarrhalis is the only important member of the genus *Branhamella*, which may now be considered as a subgroup of *Moraxella* (Bøvre, 1984). This organism is normally an upper respiratory tract commensal but occasionally gives rise to respiratory infection, usually as an opportunist pathogen. *B. catarrhalis* was formerly classified in the genus *Neisseria* but differs from *Neisseria* in DNA base content, fatty acid composition, and inability to produce acid from carbohydrates (Catlin 1970).

Neisseria and *Branhamella* are recognized in a clinical specimen by the appearance of oval Gram-negative diplococci with flattened or concave opposing edges and long axes parallel, either lying free in the specimen or, in the case of *N. meningitidis* and *N. gonorrhoeae*, often inside polymorphonuclear leucocytes. The colonies of neisseriae differ according to the species, but all are oxidase positive. Those of the pathogenic *N. meningitidis* and *N. gonorrhoeae* species are small and mucoid, whereas those of other species tend to be larger, may be smooth or rough and tend to be sticky so that colonies adhere to a wire loop. In general, gonococci and meningococci may be distinguished from other neisseriae by their ability to grow on appropriate selective media. However *N. lactamica*, which is

Table 21.1 Distinguishing characters of *Neisseria* and *Branhamella* species.
Key: ±/−, some strains weak positive, some negative.

Species	Pigment	Growth at 22°C	Requirement for blood or serum	Growth on selective media (e.g. MNYC)	Oxidation of carbohydrate(s)
N. gonorrhoeae	−	−	+	+	+
N. meningitidis	−	−	+[a]	+	+
N. lactamica	±/−	−	−	+	+
N. pharyngis	+	+	−	−	+
N. polysacchareae	−	−	−	+	+
B. catarrhalis	−̣	+	−	−	−

[a] However, *N. meningitidis* will grow on Mueller Hinton medium without the addition of blood or serum.

Table 21.2 Sugar utilization reactions of *Neisseria* and *Branhamella* species. For *Methods* see text.

Species	Glucose	Maltose	Fructose	Sucrose	Lactose
N. gonorrhoeae	I	−	−	−	−
N. meningitidis	+	I	−	−	−
N. lactamica	+	+	−	−	+
N. pharyngis					
N. subflava	+	+	−	−	−
N. flava	+	+	+	−	−
N. perflava	+	+	+	+	−
N. sicca	+	+	+	+	−
N. polysacchareae	+	+	−	−	−
B. catarrhalis	−	−	−	−	−

commonly found in the throat and resembles *N. meningitidis* closely on culture, grows well on the selective media, as does *N. polysacchareae*; some strains of *B. catarrhalis* may also grow on the selective media.

N. meningitidis and *N. gonorrhoeae* must be identified accurately both for general medical and for medico-legal purposes; the sugar utilization reactions that distinguish the species of *Neisseria* from each other are shown in Table 21.2. Odugbemi et al (1978) described a simple and inexpensive manganous chloride and Congo red disk method which could increase the efficiency of distinguishing between pathogenic *Neisseria* in laboratories with limited facilities: *N. meningitidis* is resistant to manganous chloride and Congo red whereas *N. gonorrhoeae* is sensitive.

NEISSERIA MENINGITIDIS

N. meningitidis may be differentiated from commensal *Neisseria* and *Branhamella* by its requirement for enriched culture media, the beneficial effect of (if not absolute requirement for) added CO_2 in the atmosphere used for primary isolation, and growth within a narrow temperature range (Table 21.1). It is further differentiated from other species by its utilization of both glucose and maltose and, in capsulated strains, by agglutination with group-specific antiserum; these are the features of principal importance in diagnostic work.

Morphology and staining

Oval Gram-negative diplococci, with flattened or concave opposing edges and the long axes parallel; about 0.8 μm in diameter; typically seen in large numbers inside polymorphonuclear leucocytes. Films from cultures show more rounded cocci and some pleomorphism with irregular staining. Capsules are not ordinarily evident; non-sporing; non-motile.

Cultural characters

Aerobe, but primary cultures grow better in an atmosphere containing 5–10% CO_2. Temperature range 25–42°C, optimum 35–36°C. Optimum pH 7.0–7.4. Strains will grow on Mueller Hinton medium without the addition of blood or serum but grow poorly if at all on most unenriched media. After incubation in 5–10% CO_2 in air for 24 h at 37°C colonies on blood agar are 1–2 mm in diameter, convex, grey and translucent. After 48 h colonies are larger with an opaque raised centre and thin transparent margins which may be crenated. No haemolysis on blood agar. Colonies are slightly larger on heated blood (chocolate) agar than on ordinary blood agar.

Biochemical reactions

Oxidase reaction; quickly positive when the reagent is flooded on to agar cultures. Utilize glucose and maltose but not lactose or sucrose. Occasional strains are found that utilize only glucose or maltose on primary isolation;

repeated subculture of these strains may be necessary before they utilize both sugars. Non-maltose-utilizing strains of *N. meningitidis* may be mistaken for gonococci. This could be of medico-legal importance; if there is any doubt about the identity of the *Neisseria* in this situation it should be forwarded to a reference laboratory for further examination. Recently an organism with the growth and biochemical characteristics of *N. meningitidis* and the serological characteristics of *N. gonorrhoeae* has been isolated from a vaginal swab (Hodge et al 1987). This underlines the importance of seeking expert advice with atypical neisseriae.

Sensitivity to physical and chemical agents

Dies within a few days at room temperature but cultures may be maintained on Dorset's egg medium or heated blood agar slopes in screw-capped bijou bottles for several weeks. Colonies emulsified in peptone water will survive at $-70°C$ or in liquid nitrogen for months, but freeze-drying is preferable for long-term storage. Killed at 55°C in 5 min. Readily killed by disinfectants at their correct use-dilution.

Antibiotic sensitivity

N. meningitidis is sensitive to a wide variety of antibiotics, of which benzylpenicillin, chloramphenicol and rifampicin are the most important; it is also sensitive to the more recent cephalosporins, e.g. cefuroxime and cefotaxime. 10–20% of strains are resistant to sulphonamides.

Serogrouping

The serogroups of meningococci of pathological importance whose polysaccharide antigen structure has been determined are: A, B, C, X, Y, Z, Z^1 (29E) and W135. Further serogroups H, I, K and L have also been described but their pathological significance is not yet clear. A group D was described by Branham (1958) but no capsular polysaccharide specific for this group has yet been demonstrated. Meningococci of groups A and C are those principally associated with epidemics; group B meningococci are the common inter-epidemic strains but recently epidemics due to these organisms have been described in Scandinavia. Non-serogroupable strains are commonly found in carriers, but rarely in disease.

Outer membrane protein and lipoprotein serotypes occur within groups B, C, Y and W135 and may be identified by reference laboratories for epidemiological purposes. A detailed identification of a meningococcus by group, type and subtype antigens, e.g. a Group B meningococcus of type 15 with the protein subtype antigen P1.16 would be shown as B:15:P1.16 (Frasch et al 1985). Types 2, 15, and recently 4, have been particularly associated with Group B meningococcal disease.

Animal pathogenicity

Intravenous inoculation of viable meningococci into rabbits may be fatal within 24 h but animal tests are not used for diagnosis.

Laboratory diagnosis of meningococcal infection

Specimens may include cerebrospinal fluid (CSF), blood for culture (which may come from a patient with meningitis, a haemorrhagic rash or pyrexia of uncertain origin), aspirate from skin lesions or pus from an infected joint. Throat, nasopharyngeal and, in certain circumstances, genital swabs may be collected from suspected carriers. Swabs are plunged into transport medium (e.g. Stuart's) for forwarding to the laboratory; all specimens where meningococcal infection is suspected must be submitted to the laboratory immediately.

Cerebrospinal fluid

1. Perform a cell count (see Ch. 39); the exudate in meningococcal meningitis is typically polymorphonuclear.

2. Centrifuge the remaining CSF. Make a smear of the centrifuged deposit and stain with Gram stain. Stain a second film with methylene blue to determine the cell type; occasionally, diplococci may be seen more easily with this stain. CSF from a typical case of meningococcal meningitis will show Gram-negative diplococci

inside a limited proportion of the pus cells; many are extracellular. If fluorescein isothiocyanate-coupled antiserum is available, a smear of the deposit may be examined for the direct identification of the meningococcal serogroup responsible for infection (Fallon 1983).

3. Divide the supernatant CSF into two aliquots – one to be kept if necessary for biochemical examination, the other to be examined for the presence of meningococcal polysaccharide antigen by counter-immunoelectrophoresis, latex agglutination* or coagglutination.

4. Plate out the specimen on both blood and heated blood agar and incubate at 37°C in 5–10% CO_2 for 24 h. Add Robertson's cooked meat broth to the deposit, incubate overnight and subculture in the same way. Examine colonies appearing after incubation by Gram stain and oxidase reaction.

5. Set up the rapid carbohydrate utilization test (RCUT)* or inoculate a set of Flynn & Waitkins sugar media* for utilization reactions. In addition to glucose, maltose, lactose and sucrose, inoculate an ONPG tube; the ONPG medium base used is Mueller Hinton broth. This latter test will identify strains of *N. lactamica* where lactose utilization on solid media may be slow.

Forward cultures of organisms identified as meningococci by sugar utilization reactions to an appropriate reference laboratory for determination of sulphonamide sensitivity, serogrouping and, where appropriate for epidemiological purposes, serotyping (Dr D. M. Jones, Public Health Laboratory, Withington Hospital, Manchester M20 8LR; Dr R. J. Fallon, Department of Laboratory Medicine, Ruchill Hospital, Bilsland Drive, Glasgow G20 9NB).

6. Set up antibiotic sensitivity tests. Strains resistant to penicillin have not yet been described although for a small proportion of strains the MIC is as high as 0.25 mg/litre; this antibiotic should be tested along with chloramphenicol and rifampicin. Appropriate concentrations are benzylpenicillin 1.2 μg (2 units)/disk, chloramphenicol 10 μg, rifampicin 10 μg. Disk

* Refer to *Methods* at end of this chapter.

testing for sulphonamide sensitivity is satisfactory provided a 25 μg sulphadiazine disk is used in a Stokes technique with a control sensitive meningococcus. Preferably, test by the agar dilution method using Mueller Hinton agar as described by Fallon (1978). The inoculum should be a 1 in 50 dilution of a shaken overnight broth culture and a suitable range of concentrations of sulphadiazine is 0.1, 1, 10, 50 and 100 mg/litre. Strains resistant to 10 mg/l are resistant to sulphonamide therapy; strains resistant to 1 mg/l may not be eradicated from the nasopharynx if sulphonamides are used for chemoprophylaxis.

7. Serogrouping is performed by slide agglutination with hyperimmune sera (Wellcome). Care must be taken to test a strain against antiserum to each serogroup as fine non-specific agglutination may occur which may be thought to be specific unless the reaction with all antisera has been checked. If difficulty is experienced in serogrouping, the culture may be plated on Mueller Hinton agar containing about 5% (depending on the strength of the serum) group-specific antiserum. A halo of precipitate appearing in the medium round the colonies after 24–48 h incubation is a positive reaction (Craven & Frasch 1979).

Blood cultures

Subculture to blood agar and heated blood agar. Incubate cultures in 5–10% CO_2 for 24 h and examine oxidase positive colonies of Gram-negative diplococci as above.

Pus, aspirates and swabs

Examine Gram stained films and inoculate pus, aspirates and swabs on to selective heated blood agar* or Modified New York City (MNYC) medium* in addition to media normally used for the examination of pus from any source.

Serological diagnosis

Paired sera may be tested for the presence of complement-fixing antibodies (Ross & Stevenson 1962). This test is helpful in cases where no organisms have been isolated or in obscure pyrexias, which may be due to chronic meningococcal septicaemia. Specific antibodies to capsular polysaccharide may be demonstrated by a haemagglutination test (Edwards & Driscoll 1967).

NEISSERIA GONORRHOEAE

Morphology and staining of *N. gonorrhoeae* are identical to those of *N. meningitidis* (see above). The main character that distinguishes the gonococcus from the meningococcus is the ability to produce acid from glucose but not maltose.

Cultural characters

A delicate organism with exacting nutritional and environmental requirements. Aerobe, but most strains have an absolute requirement for CO_2. Optimum pH 7.0–7.4. Recommended culture media contain a rich nutrient base supplemented with blood, either partially lysed by heat (chocolate agar) or completely lysed by saponin; unlysed blood agar is not recommended for diagnostic cultures. Selective media are valuable in isolating gonococci from heavily contaminated sites such as the rectum or pharynx.

After incubation for 24 h in a moist aerobic environment enriched with 5–10% CO_2 colonies on Modified New York City (MNYC) medium are small (*c*. 1 mm), grey and convex; after 48 h the colonies are larger (1.5–2.5 mm), sometimes with a crenated margin and an opaque raised centre. Considerable variation in size occurs with gonococcal colonies and on most culture media the colony outline is irregular, unlike the circular colonies of *N. meningitidis*. On Thayer Martin medium growth is slower; although colonies are similar to those on MNYC medium they are usually smaller.

Naturally occurring variants with specific requirements for particular amino acids, bases or vitamins may be detected; this technique (auxotyping) has been applied for epidemiological typing (Catlin 1973).

Biochemical reactions

The gonococcus is oxidase positive and utilizes glucose but not maltose, sucrose, lactose or fructose. The rapid carbohydrate utilization test (RCUT; Young 1978a) measures preformed enzymes and provides a quicker and more reliable identification than conventional growth-dependent sugar tests using solid or semi-solid media (Tapsall & Cheng 1981).

Sensitivity to physical and chemical agents

Readily killed by drying, soap and water, and many other cleansing or antiseptic agents at their correct use-dilution. Organisms may remain viable for a day or so in pus contaminating linen or other fabrics. Cultured gonococci die in a few days at room temperature. Survival can be ensured for several months by harvesting an overnight plate culture into 1 ml of tryptone soya broth containing 6% lactose and freezing at −20 or −70°C. Freeze-drying is the most reliable method for long-term storage of gonococci but storage at −70°C or in liquid nitrogen may be more convenient for intermediate storage.

Antibiotic sensitivity

The gonococcus is usually sensitive to many antibiotics including penicillin, cefuroxime, cefotaxime, spectinomycin, cotrimoxazole, tetracycline, erythromycin and streptomycin. However, sensitivity of isolates may vary geographically making it important to base antibiotic policies on the sensitivity of local isolates.

A definite progression towards decreased sensitivity to various antibiotics has occurred over the past three or four decades. Because of its central role in the treatment of gonorrhoea, sensitivity to penicillin has been studied most widely. By convention, strains with an MIC of 0.125 mg/litre or more are defined as less sensitive or relatively resistant; around 20% of strains in the UK fall into this category. The majority of strains isolated in the UK are fully sensitive to penicillin (MIC <0.125 mg/l). Multiple antibiotic resistance sometimes occurs and may be due to a mutation giving reduced permeability of the outer membrane (Maness & Sparling 1973). The most significant development in recent years has been the emergence of penicillinase-producing *N. gonorrhoeae* (PPNG) giving resistance to high levels of penicillin; tests for β-lactamase production should always be performed.

Mutations also exist which increase the permeability of the membrane, making isolates hypersensitive to certain antibiotics; hypersensitivity may include vancomycin (Exner et al 1982) and therefore influence choice of selective media.

Serogrouping

Antigenic heterogeneity has been demonstrated in purified surface components of *N. gonorrhoeae*, including pilus (fimbrial) protein, lipopolysaccharide and outer membrane proteins, and this has made it difficult to devise a standard scheme for dividing the species into serogroups as in the case of the meningococcus. The coagglutination serogrouping system of Sandström & Danielsson (1980) which is based on differences in the principal outer membrane protein (PrI) is gaining widespread acceptance: using specifically absorbed polyclonal antisera the gonococcus can be divided into two major groups termed WI and WII/WIII. More recently, serogroups WI and WII/WIII have been subdivided into serovars on the basis of their reaction patterns with panels of monoclonal antibodies reactive with epitopes on PrIA and PrIB respectively. The biological and epidemiological significance of gonococcal serogroups and serovars is reviewed in detail by Bygdeman (1988).

Neisseria gonorrhoeae ssp. *kochi*. Mazloum et al (1986) suggested that an unusual neisseria isolated from conjunctival cultures in rural Egypt and originally described by Robert Koch as an atypical gonococcus merits subspecies status. These isolates do not react with the monoclonal antibodies currently used in the serological classification of gonococci.

Laboratory diagnosis of gonorrhoea

The main task of the bacteriologist is to determine whether or not *N. gonorrhoeae* is present in a specimen and, if present, whether or not the strain produces β-lactamase. Since the management of gonorrhoea includes the tracing of infected contacts, laboratory diagnosis is best carried out in association with a special department of genitourinary medicine.

The greater the number of sites examined the better will be the chance of detecting gonococcal infection. Details of specimens required for bacteriological diagnosis are given by Robertson et al (1988). In men urethral samples usually suffice (with rectal cultures in homosexual males) but in women urethral, cervical and rectal specimens should always be examined. Although repeated sampling of multiple sites is ideal, a single well taken endocervical swab will detect approximately 90% of gonococcal infections in women. A high vaginal swab is not suitable and, if this is the only specimen taken, 1 in 3 infected women is likely to be missed.

Throat infection also occurs and should be sought where appropriate. In suspected disseminated gonococcal infection (DGI), specimens may include blood, swabs of skin lesions, or pus aspirated from a joint. Occasionally conjunctival material is examined, particularly in neonatal ophthalmia. Any urine specimen showing Gram-negative diplococci in a Gram stain should be cultured on an appropriate selective medium.

The gonococcus is very fastidious and care is needed in the collection of specimens and their transport to the laboratory. Best results are achieved by the direct inoculation of culture plates with patients' secretions, followed by immediate incubation at 36–37°C in a moist atmosphere containing 5–10% CO_2. When direct plating and immediate incubation is impracticable several transport and culture systems are available. These consist of a selective medium, usually present in a small chamber containing CO_2 or a CO_2-generating system, e.g. Transgrow or Jembec (Martin & Jackson 1975). The media can be inoculated directly from the patient and transported to the laboratory either before or after incubation. Such systems are expensive and it is more usual to send a charcoal-coated swab in Stuart's medium, or preferably Amies's modification of Stuart's medium (see Ch. 6) in which case a plain swab is adequate. Dry swabs should not be sent as the gonococcus is very susceptible to drying.

1. Examine Gram stained smears of urethral discharge from men, and urethral and cervical secretions from women. The observation of characteristic kidney-shaped Gram-negative diplococci lying within polymorphonuclear leucocytes with a few extracellular organisms is typical of gonococcal infection and the smear is reported as positive. If Gram-negative diplococci are seen only extracellularly, the result of the smear examination is equivocal; a diagnosis should not be made on this basis. If no Gram-negative diplococci are seen, report the smear as negative.

Approximately 95% of infected men and 55–60% of infected women will yield a positive smear; if the smear is examined while the patient is at the clinic immediate treatment can be given.

2. Plate out the specimen on selective culture media and, in the case of specimens from normally sterile sites, on the same medium lacking antibiotics; incubate immediately in a moist CO_2-enriched aerobic atmosphere at 37°C.

The original selective medium of Thayer & Martin (TM medium) contains the antibiotics vancomycin, colistin and nystatin. Although widely used in many laboratories TM medium has been criticized because 3–10% of gonococcal strains are inhibited by vancomycin (Mirret et al 1981). A modified TM medium (Martin et al 1974) gives superior results; however, MNYC medium* is preferred because it gives better growth and the use of lincomycin as selective agent avoids the problem of vancomycin sensitivity.

3. Examine plates after 24 h incubation and test suspect colonies by touching with a cotton bud soaked in oxidase reagent: oxidase positive bacteria turn the contact area of the bud purple within 5–15 s. If oxidase positive, Gram stain an identical colony. Incubation of primary isolation plates is continued for 48 h and cultures are re-examined by the above procedures before any specimen can be reported negative.

A presumptive diagnosis of gonorrhoea made on the basis of oxidase positive Gram-negative diplococci growing on selective medium is approximately 99% accurate for specimens taken from the male urethra and female urethra, cervix or rectum. A presumptive diagnosis of gonor-

rhoea is much less reliable in the case of rectal cultures from homosexual males. Particular attention must be paid to throat cultures where gonococcal and meningococcal colonies may coexist; Gram-negative diplococci isolated from the throat are most likely to be meningococci.

4. If there is sufficient growth on the primary isolation plate set up the rapid carbohydrate utilization test (RCUT)*, including a tube to detect β-lactamase production. Otherwise subculture on antibiotic-free medium and incubate overnight to obtain sufficient material for the test.

5. Recently a coagglutination test* using monoclonal antibodies reactive with epitopes on PrI has become available and this test may be used in place of the RCUT (Young & Reid, 1988) for identification of an isolate. These reagents, which are 100% specific, do not cross-react with N. lactamica or meningococci and, provided that the test is properly controlled, a positive reaction is a reliable indicator of gonococcal infection at any site. Although the sensitivity is very high (99.7%) it is prudent to confirm the identity of any non-reactive genital isolate by RCUT. Biochemical confirmation is also recommended whenever medico-legal proceedings may be involved.

6. Inoculate a suitable non-selective medium (e.g. the isolation medium lacking antibiotics) with the growth from several colonies and place a 6 μg penicillin disk on the well. If the zone of inhibition is less than 20 mm after overnight incubation test for β-lactamase by the filter-paper acidometric method* or by the chromogenic cephalosporin method (Ch. 9).

Since the majority of patients with gonococcal infection will have been treated on the basis of a positive smear, antibiotic tests other than those to detect β-lactamase are of little help in the initial management of the patient. However, they are important in planning rational therapy for use in the geographical area concerned; it is sufficient to test only a proportion of isolates in a laboratory with a high number of positive cultures. The sensitivity of all gonococci isolated from complicated and disseminated infections or after treatment failure should be tested.

If antibiotic sensitivity tests are indicated

prepare a turbid suspension of organisms in peptone water for use as inoculum in the agar dilution or disk diffusion sensitivity test. Diffusion tests using disks of several strengths can be made to give acceptable results but an agar dilution method is preferable (Jephcott 1981). The Adatab system available commercially (Mast), provides tablets containing suitable quantities of a wide variety of antibiotics. This system, suitably controlled, makes accurate agar dilution testing a practical proposition for most laboratories.

7. In suspected disseminated gonococcal infection, set up blood cultures with a biphasic medium (Jephcott 1981) and incubate in a CO_2 incubator with standard closures replaced by cotton-wool plugs. Immunofluorescence staining may be of value in examining exudate from skin lesions (Tronca et al 1974). Culture on non-selective media may be advisable.

Quality control

Reliable diagnosis or exclusion of gonococcal infection depends upon high microbiological standards. Procedures must be subjected to proper quality control and the efficiency of culture carefully monitored. The percentage of microscopy-positive specimens that fail to yield gonococci on selective medium (possibly because of antibiotic sensitivity) should be determined by correlating the results of microscopy and culture; a figure of 1–2% is acceptable.

Serological diagnosis

The low sensitivity and specificity of existing serological tests, and the persistence of antibody due to past infection, limit their value in clinical practice. Serological tests are not suitable for screening for gonococcal infection and should not be used in this way to diagnose or exclude gonorrhoea. The gonococcal complement fixation test (GCFT) is the only serological test for gonococcal infection that has been much used in clinical practice. This test may occasionally be useful in conjunction with culture in suspected disseminated gonococcal infection but the GCFT should not be performed as a routine.

COMMENSAL NEISSERIAE

These organisms occur on various mucous surfaces of the body; they are regularly found in the throat, nose and mouth and, less frequently, on the genital mucosae. When inflammatory or other pathological conditions affect these mucous membranes, Gram-negative diplococci may constitute a prominent feature of the bacterial flora and may possibly act as secondary infecting agents in such conditions. The commensal neisseriae are much less well characterized than the important human pathogens described above.

Neisseria lactamica. Carriage of this organism occurs more frequently in infants and young children than in adults. Morphology and staining is similar to *N. meningitidis* but it differs in its relative lack of virulence and ability to utilize lactose. It grows readily on selective media and some strains cross-react with antisera raised against gonococci and meningococci. Whenever Gram-negative diplococci are isolated from the throat, biochemical tests are required to provide accurate differentiation between *N. lactamica* and the meningococcus and gonococcus.

Neisseria pharyngis. The classical nasopharyngeal commensals *N. subflava*, *N. flava*, *N. perflava* and *N. sicca* are included in the umbrella species *N. pharyngis*; their main characters are given in Tables 21.1 and 21.2. Most of these nasopharyngeal commensals produce moist pigmented colonies and utilize glucose, maltose, fructose and sucrose when tested by the RCUT. Although *N. sicca* utilizes the same sugars, colonies are dry, tough, adherent to the medium and opaque.

Neisseria polysacchareae (which resembles the meningococcus in appearance) grows on selective media, utilizes glucose and maltose (Riou et al 1983), and is found in the nasopharynx of healthy carriers (Boquete et al 1986). Unlike *N. meningitidis* it produces polysaccharide when grown on medium containing 5% sucrose and lacks gamma-glutamyl aminopeptidase activity.

Neisseria cinerea has been isolated as a commensal, frequently from the oropharynx and less commonly from genital sites (Knapp et al 1984). Occasionally it is isolated on selective medium, when it resembles *N. gonorrhoeae*. Although considered to be asaccharolytic it may utilize glucose in certain biochemical test systems (Dossett et al 1985). *N. cinerea* is non-reactive in the coagglutination test for the gonococcus. Lack of DNase helps to differentiate it from *B. catarrhalis*.

Neisseria flavescens. This organism was described in 1930 as the causative pathogen in a group of cases of meningitis in America but has not with certainty been isolated since. It resembled the meningococcus in morphology but on blood agar produced golden-yellow colonies. Initially the isolates did not utilize carbohydrates but later developed the ability to produce acid from glucose, maltose and sucrose. It may be biologically related to *N. pharyngis*.

Neisseria mucosa differs from other members of the group in being definitely capsulate and producing mucoid colonies. It has been isolated only sporadically from cases of meningitis, endocarditis and also opportunistic infections (Gini 1987). Its carbohydrate utilization reactions are similar to *N. sicca* but it reduces nitrates and, like *N. polysacchareae*, it synthesises polysaccharide. There is much variation in the characters of the organisms described under this name (Brodie et al 1971; Johnson 1983).

BRANHAMELLA CATARRHALIS

The characters of *B. catarrhalis* that are useful in identification include oxidase positivity, inability to produce acid from sugars and ability to grow on medium lacking blood. *B. catarrhalis* is antigenically distinct from commensal neisseriae; there are no recognized serogroups.

Morphology and staining

Oval Gram-negative cocci about 0.8 μm in diameter. Sometimes organisms are single, but more often in pairs with adjacent sides flattened; occasionally found in groups of four as a result of characteristic division in two successive planes at right angles to one another. On occasion they may be found inside polymorphonuclear leucocytes.

Cultural characters

Aerobe with optimum temperature about 36°C but growth of many strains occurs at 22°C. Although CO_2 may enhance growth there is no absolute requirement. Most strains grow on nutrient agar. After incubation for 24 h colonies on blood or heated blood agar are 1–2 mm in diameter, non-haemolytic, often friable, white or greyish, convex with an entire margin later becoming irregular. After 48 h colonies are larger, more elevated with a raised opaque centre. Most strains do not grow on media selective for pathogenic neisseriae.

Biochemical reactions

Oxidase positive; does not produce acid from glucose, maltose, sucrose, lactose or fructose; reduces nitrate to nitrite.

Sensitivity to physical and chemical agents

Appears to be more resistant than the meningococcus or gonococcus. Cultures may remain viable for several months at 20°C if prevented from drying. May survive in sputum for 3–4 weeks.

Susceptible to a wide range of antibiotics but many strains produce β-lactamase and are resistant to penicillin and ampicillin. Sensitivity tests can be carried out by disk or agar dilution methods as for meningococci and gonococci.

Laboratory diagnosis

B. catarrhalis is normally considered to be a harmless commensal of the upper respiratory tract and is most often encountered when examining throat swabs and specimens of sputum. The finding of a few colonies of *B. catarrhalis* in a mixed culture containing other upper respiratory tract commensal organisms is probably of little or no significance. However, in patients with compromised lung function, *B. catarrhalis* may be a pathogen of the lower respiratory tract. In these patients a relatively pure growth of *B. catarrhalis* is often obtained from sputum and other specimens such as transtracheal aspirates.

Specimens should be cultured on blood agar and a selective medium. After overnight incubation in 5–10% CO_2 in air cultures are examined by the oxidase test and, if positive, Gram stained. Oxidase positive Gram-negative diplococci are then tested by the RCUT for their ability to utilize sugars and to produce β-lactamase. If the isolate grows well on selective medium it should also be shown to be immunologically distinct from *N. gonorrhoeae* and *N. meningitidis* by the tests described previously. Recent reports (Doern & Morse 1980) suggest that clinically significant isolates of *B. catarrhalis* grow well on modified TM medium, produce β-lactamase and do not grow on nutrient agar at 22°C. The extent of the correlation between pathogenicity, β-lactamase production and ability to grow on selective media remains to be elucidated.

MORAXELLA, KINGELLA AND ACINETOBACTER

Organisms classified in the family Neisseriaceae include *Moraxella*, *Kingella* and *Acinetobacter* spp.

Moraxella. The genus *Moraxella* includes *Moraxella lacunata* which causes a form of purulent conjunctivitis classically presenting as an angular blepharo-conjunctivitis. The moraxellas occur as components of the normal flora of the upper respiratory tract, the conjunctiva, the skin and the genital tract. Moraxellas may be involved in opportunist infections in compromised patients.

The moraxellas are stout Gram-negative cocci or short stout rods; they typically occur in pairs and may simulate gonococci. They are strict aerobes, non-capsulate, non-motile. *M. lacunata* and *M. atlantae* require serum for growth but some other species are less demanding. Loeffler medium is pitted by colonies of *M. lacunata* and the variant *M. liquefaciens*. *M. lacunata* cannot grow on MacConkey agar but some other species can. The moraxellas are relatively inactive in

biochemical tests. Moraxellas are oxidase positive and usually catalase positive. They do not ferment sugars and do not produce indole or H_2S. *M. lacunata* produces a gelatinase. Sensitivity to penicillin has been regarded by some workers as a feature of the moraxellas that distinguishes them from acinetobacters.

Kingella. These are Gram-negative rods and the genus contains three species that differ from *Moraxella* in being saccharolytic and catalase negative. They are of low pathogenicity but, as they grow on Thayer Martin medium and are oxidase positive, they could be mistaken for pathogenic neisseriae.

Acinetobacter. This genus contains strictly aerobic short, stout, often capsulate, non-motile Gram-negative (or Gram variable) bacilli or coccobacilli (often diplococco-bacilli) that grow well on simple media. They are usually free-living saprophytes in soil and water. The genus contains only one species, *Acinetobacter calcoaceticus*, which embraces two variants; *A. calcoaceticus* var. *anitratus* produces acid oxidatively from dextrose whereas *A. calcoaceticus* var. *lwoffi* does not. This terminology supersedes earlier terms such as *Herellea vaginicola* and *A. anitratum* which correspond to the *anitratus* variant, and *Mima polymorpha* and *Moraxella lwoffi* which correspond to the *lwoffi* variant. In the past, *Achromobacter* species names were also assigned to these variants.

Acinetobacter organisms occur frequently as components of the commensal flora of man and animals and are therefore regular contaminants of the hospital environment. They are increasingly recognized as opportunist pathogens associated with infections that range from bronchopneumonia to septicaemia in compromised patients. Predisposing factors include the presence of a prosthesis, endotracheal intubation, intravenous catheters, and prior antibiotic therapy in a seriously ill patient in hospital.

A. calcoaceticus is oxidase negative, catalase positive, and indole negative. Some strains produce urease. Acinetobacter organisms do not reduce nitrates and do not ferment sugars. The *anitratus* variant produces acid from dextrose and other sugars oxidatively but the *lwoffi* variant does not. Colonies are white or cream coloured, smooth, circular with an entire edge, sometimes raised and opaque, and may show surface spreading. Some strains are haemolytic on blood agar. Some strains liquefy gelatin slowly. All strains are penicillin resistant. Hospital strains of *Acinetobacter* are often resistant to many other antibiotics. Most strains are resistant to sulphonamides, penicillins including ampicillin, the cephalosporins, erythromycin, the tetracyclines and chloramphenicol. They are often resistant to gentamicin and other aminoglycosides (see Bergogne-Berezin & Joly-Guillou 1985). It is essential to guide antimicrobial management by antimicrobial sensitivity tests.

Hospital strains can be traced by a combination of biotyping, antibiograms, serotyping, bacteriocin typing and immunofluorescence tests, but these approaches to tracing have limitations at present (see Stone & Das 1986).

METHODS

Modified New York City (MNYC) medium
(Young 1978b)

Preparation of yeast dialysate. Mix 908 g baker's yeast to a smooth paste with 2.5 litres distilled water. Autoclave at 110°C for 10 min and dialyse against 2 litres distilled water for 48 h at 4°C. Dispense the dialysate (material outside sac) into 25 ml amounts and autoclave at 121°C for 15 min. Store at −20°C.

Ingredients

GC Medium Base (Difco)	36 g
Yeast dialysate	25 ml
Human or horse blood (100 ml), lysed with 5 ml of 10% saponin	105 ml
Glucose (10%) sterilized at 115°C for 10 min	10 ml
Colistin (6 mg/litre)	1 ml
Lincomycin (1 mg/l)	1 ml
Trimethoprim (5 mg/l)	1 ml
Amphotericin B (1 mg/l)	1 ml

Method. Dissolve the GC agar base in 856 ml distilled water and autoclave at 121°C for

15 min. Allow to cool and hold at 50°C. Add lysed blood, glucose, yeast dialysate and the antibiotics. Mix and pour plates.

Set up quality control cultures by inoculating plates from each batch of medium with the following cultures: *N. gonorrhoeae* (a recent clinical isolate); *N. meningitidis*; *N. pharyngis*; *Staphylococcus aureus*; *Escherichia coli*; *Proteus mirabilis*; *Candida albicans*. Incubate plates in a CO_2 incubator as for gonococcal cultures. Release a batch of plates for routine use only if the medium supports good growth of the pathogenic neisseriae while inhibiting completely the growth of *N. pharyngis* and the other test organisms.

Products for the preparation of MNYC medium are available commercially (GC Agar Base, CM367; Yeast Autolysate Supplement, SR105; LCAT Antibiotic Supplement, SR95: Oxoid).

Selective heated blood agar

Heated blood (chocolate) agar may be made selective for the pathogenic neisseriae by the addition of vancomycin 3 mg/litre, colistin 7.5 mg/l and nystatin 12 500 units/l (or use Oxoid VCN Antibiotic Supplement, SRlOl). This medium facilitates the isolation of pathogenic neisseriae in mixed cultures; appearances are the same as on non-selective heated blood agar.

Rapid carbohydrate utilization test (RCUT) and penicillinase test (Young 1978a)

In the RCUT, preformed enzyme is measured by adding a suspension of the overnight growth of the test organism to a buffered (non-nutrient) solution containing the sugar to be tested and a pH indicator. β-lactamase can be detected by substituting ampicillin for sugar. Acid production resulting from sugar utilization or from the splitting of ampicillin to penicilloic acid is detected by a colour change of the pH indicator from red to yellow.

Buffer-salt solution (BSS). Prepare by mixing the following solutions: 40 ml 0.1 mol/litre

K_2HPO_4; 12 ml 0.1 mol/l KH_2PO_4; 100 ml 8% (w/v) KCl; 10 ml 1% (w/v) aqueous phenol red; and 838 ml sterile distilled water. Check pH and if necessary adjust to 7.10–7.15. Dispense in 20 ml amounts in screw-cap bottles and store at −20°C.

Sugar solutions. Prepare 100 ml of 10% (w/v) solutions in distilled water of glucose, maltose, sucrose, fructose and lactose; filter sterilize, dispense in 4 ml amounts and store at −20°C.

Note: some batches of maltose contain excessive amounts of glucose and give false positive results; Extra Pure Maltose (BDH) gives satisfactory results. Commercial carbohydrate disks are available for preparation of RCUT substrates (*Neisseria* Identification Disks, Oxoid DD7).

Ampicillin solution. Dissolve the contents of a 500 mg vial of sodium ampicillin (Beecham) in 2 ml BSS to give a concentration of 250 mg/ml. Dispense in 200 μl amounts and store at −20°C.

Method. 1. Each week (or more often if required) thaw one bottle of BSS, one of each sugar, and one of ampicillin and store at 4°C for daily use.

2. Set out 5 tubes (70 × 10 mm) for each suspect gonococcal isolate from a genital site, and 7 tubes for each non-genital or atypical isolate. Add 20 μl of glucose, maltose, sucrose and ampicillin respectively to 4 individual tubes for the genital isolates; also add 20 μl of fructose and lactose respectively to the extra 2 tubes for non-genital isolates.

3. Add 100 μl of BSS to each of the tubes containing sugar or ampicillin and 300 μl BSS to the remaining tube.

4. Harvest growth from a 16–24 h culture with a cotton-tipped swab and make a thick suspension in the 300 μl of BSS. Transfer 30 μl of the suspension to each sugar-containing tube and to the ampicillin tube. Shake tubes and incubate at 37°C in a waterbath.

5. Examine tubes after 30–60 min and make a definitive reading after 3 h. A yellow colour (occasionally yellow-orange) is positive; red is negative.

Each day set up a β-lactamase-producing *N.*

gonorrhoeae and a strain of *N. meningitidis* as controls.

The RCUT can also be conveniently performed in microtitre plates. The appropriate reagents are dispensed in wells and the plates stored at −20°C until required.

Serum-free agar sugars (Flynn & Waitkins 1972)

Supplement. Solution A: dissolve 1 g of L-glutamine in 90 ml distilled water. Solution B: dissolve ferric nitrate 0.05 g in 10 ml distilled water. Prepare the supplement by adding 90 ml of solution A to 10 ml of solution B.

Sugars. 10% solutions of glucose, sucrose or maltose, sterilized by filtration.

Method. Boil 36 g of GC Medium Base (Difco) in 970 ml distilled water and when clear add 20 ml of the supplement and 10 ml of phenol red (0.2% stock solution). Adjust to pH 7.6 with NaOH (1 mol/litre), and distribute in 90 ml volumes in screw-cap bottles. Autoclave at 121°C for 10 min. Cool to 50°C. Add 10 ml of the appropriate sugar solution (aseptically) to 90 ml of medium to give a final concentration of 1% sugar. Dispense 3 ml amounts into sterile 5 ml screw-cap bottles and allow to set as slopes.

For use, slopes should be inoculated heavily and incubated at 37°C in an atmosphere containing 5–10% CO_2, the screw caps of the containers being loosened. A positive result (colour change to yellow) should be obtained after overnight incubation, although cultures should routinely be kept for 48 h. With very small inocula a longer period of incubation may be necessary.

Filter-paper acidometric test for β-lactamase production (Sng et al 1981)

Penicillin solution. Prepare 0.05 mol/litre phosphate buffer, pH 8.0, by dissolving 37.5 mg KH_2PO_4 and 842 mg $Na_2HPO_4.2H_2O$ in 100 ml distilled water. Dissolve 5% crystalline benzylpenicillin (buffer-free) and 0.2% bromocresol purple in this buffer. Divide into small aliquots and store at $-20°C$. When an aliquot is in use keep at 4°C.

Method. Place a piece of Whatman No. 1 filter paper (5 × 6 cm) in a Petri dish. Add penicillin solution dropwise to saturate the paper. With a bacteriological loop transfer several colonies from the test culture and spread over an area of *c.* 5 mm diameter. Several different strains may be tested on the same paper, separated from each other by about 1 cm.

Incubate paper at 37°C for 30 min with the Petri dish cover on. Examine paper and note yellow zones formed by β-lactamase-producing strains. Each day set up a β-lactamase-producing and a penicillin-sensitive strain of *N. gonorrhoeae* as controls.

Coagglutination test

This is a rapid (10 min) coagglutination slide test which uses protein-A-containing staphylococci with murine monoclonal antibodies bound by the Fc portion to the protein A. The test uses two reagents, WI and WII/III, composed of separate pools of monoclonal antibodies reactive with PrIA and PrIB respectively. When a test sample containing gonococci, usually a primary culture of an isolate, is mixed with the reagents, the specific monoclonal antibodies react with the appropriate PrI antigen. A coagglutination lattice is formed which is visible to the naked eye. Kits are available from Pharmacia. The test should be performed, according to the manufacturer's instructions, with a light suspension of the organism boiled in 0.9% saline. The unit volume of reagents may be reduced to 15 μl for economy.

Polysaccharide antigen of *N. meningitidis* Groups A, B, C, Y and W135 can be detected in CSF (treated to remove non-specific reactions) by coagglutination with a kit available from Pharmacia.

Latex agglutination

The polysaccharide antigens of meningococci can be detected in CSF, urine (concentrated if necessary) or serum, by agglutination of antibody-coated latex particles. Body fluids must be heated or centrifuged to remove non-specific reactions. The group B reagent will cross-react with *Escherichia coli* K1 antigen which may be found in neonatal meningitis. Kits are available from Wellcome.

REFERENCES

Bergogne-Berezin E, Joly-Guillou M L 1985 An underestimated nosocomial pathogen, *Acinetobacter calcoaceticus*. Journal of Antimicrobial Chemotherapy 16: 535–538

Boquete M T, Marcos C, Sáez-Nieto J 1986 Characterisation of *Neisseria polysacchareae* sp. nov. (Riou, 1983) in previously identified noncapsular strains of *Neisseria meningitidis*. Journal of Clinical Microbiology 23: 973–975

Bøvre K 1984 Family VIII. Neisseriaceae. In: Krieg N R, Holt J G (eds), Bergey's manual of systematic bacteriology. Williams and Wilkins, Baltimore. Vol. 1, p 288–310

Branham S E 1958 Reference strains for the serologic groups of meningococcus (*Neisseria meningitidis*). International Bulletin of Bacterial Nomenclature and Taxonomy 8: 1–15

Brodie E, Allan J L, Daly A K 1971 Bacterial endocarditis due to an unusual species of encapsulated *Neisseria*. American Journal of Diseases of Children 122: 433–437

Bygdeman S 1988 Polyclonal and monoclonal antibodies applied to the epidemiology of gonococcal infection. In:

Young H, McMillian A (eds) Immunological diagnosis of sexually transmitted diseases. Marcel Dekker, New York, p 117–165

Catlin B W 1970 Transfer of the organisms named *Neisseria catarrhalis* to *Branhamella* gen. nov. International Journal of Systematic Bacteriology 20: 155–159

Catlin B W 1973 Nutritional profiles of *Neisseria gonorrhoeae*, *Neisseria meningitidis* and *Neisseria lactamica* in chemically defined media and the use of growth requirements for gonococcal typing. Journal of Infectious Diseases 128: 178–194

Craven D E, Frasch C E 1979 Serogroup identification of meningococci by a modified antiserum agar method. Journal of Clinical Microbiology 9: 547–548

Doern G V, Morse S A 1980 *Branhamella* (*Neisseria*) *catarrhalis*: Criteria for laboratory identification. Journal of Clinical Microbiology 11: 193–195

Dossett J H, Appelbaum P C, Knapp J S, Totten P A 1985 Proctitis associated with *Neisseria cinerea* misidentified as *Neisseria gonorrhoeae* in a child. Journal of Clinical Microbiology 21: 575–577

Edwards E A, Driscoll W S 1967 Group specific haemagglutination test for *Neisseria meningitidis* antibodies. Proceedings of the Society for Experimental Biology and Medicine 126: 876–879

Exner A C, Skinner E N, Pace P J, Catlin B W 1982 Auxotypes and antibacterial resistance of gonococci with differing susceptibilities to vancomycin. British Journal of Venereal Diseases 58: 166–175

Fallon R J 1978. Meningococci. In: Reeves D A, Phillips I, Williams J D, Wise R (eds) Laboratory methods in antimicrobial chemotherapy. Churchill Livingstone, Edinburgh. p 99–102

Fallon R J 1983. Microbiological examination of cerebrospinal fluid. Association of Clinical Pathologists Broadsheet 108

Flynn J, Waitkins S A 1972 A serum-free medium for testing fermentation reactions in *Neisseria gonorrhoeae*. Journal of Clinical Pathology 25: 525–527

Frasch C E, Zollinger W D, Poolman J T 1985 Serotype antigens of *Neisseria meningitidis* and a proposed scheme for designation of serotypes. Reviews of Infectious Diseases 7: 504–510

Gini G A 1987 Ocular infection in a newborn caused by *Neisseria mucosa*. Journal of Clinical Microbiology 25: 1574–1575

Hodge D S, Ashton F E, Tesso R, Ali A S 1987 Organisms resembling *Neisseria gonorrhoeae* and *Neisseria meningitidis*. Journal of Clinical Microbiology 25: 1545–1547.

Jephcott A E 1981 Investigation of gonococcal infection. Association of Clinical Pathologists Broadsheet 100

Johnson A P 1983 The pathogenic potential of commensal species of *Neisseria*. Journal of Clinical Pathology 36: 213–223

Knapp J S, Totten P A, Mulks M H, Minshew B H 1984 Characterization of *Neisseria cinerea*, a nonpathogenic species isolated on Martin-Lewis medium selective for pathogenic *Neisseria* spp. Journal of Clinical Microbiology 19: 63–67

Maness M J, Sparling P F 1973 Multiple antibiotic resistance due to a simple mutation in *Neisseria gonorrhoeae*. Journal of Infectious Diseases 128: 321–330

Martin J E, Armstrong J H, Smith P B 1974 New system for cultivation of *Neisseria gonorrhoeae*. Applied Microbiology 27: 802–805

Martin J E, Jackson R L 1975 Biological environmental chamber for the culture of *Neisseria gonorrhoeae*. Journal of the American Venereal Disease Association 2: 28–30

Mazloum H et al 1986 An unusual *Neisseria* isolated from conjunctival cultures in rural Egypt. Journal of Infectious Diseases 154: 212–224

Mirret S, Reller L B, Knapp J S 1981 *Neisseria gonorrhoeae* strains inhibited by vancomycin in selective media and correlation with auxotype. Journal of Clinical Microbiology 14: 94–99

Odugbemi T O, McEntegart M G, Hafiz S 1978 A simple manganous chloride and Congo red disc method for differentiating *Neisseria gonorrhoeae* from *Neisseria meningitidis*. Journal of Clinical Pathology 31: 936–938

Riou J Y, Guibourdenche M, Popoff M Y 1983 A new taxon in the genus *Neisseria*. Annales de Microbiologie (Institut Pasteur) 134B: 257–267

Robertson D H H, McMillan A, Young H 1988 Gonorrhoea: diagnosis: laboratory and clinical procedures. Ch 15, in: Clinical practice in sexually transmissible diseases. Churchill Livingstone, Edinburgh

Ross C A C, Stevenson J 1962 Meningococcal 'aseptic' meningitis. Journal of Hygiene, Cambridge 60: 501–507

Sandström E, Danielsson D 1980 Serology of *Neisseria gonorrhoeae*. Classification with coagglutination. Acta Pathologica Microbiologica Scandinavica (B) 88: 27–38

Sng E H, Yeo K L, Rajan V S 1981 Simple method for detecting penicillinase-producing *Neisseria gonorrhoeae* and *Staphylococcus aureus*. British Journal of Venereal Diseases 57: 141–142

Stone J W, Das B C 1986 Investigation of an outbreak of infection with *Acinetobacter calcoaceticus* in a special care baby unit. Journal of Hospital Infection 7: 42–48

Tapsall J W, Cheng J K 1981 Rapid identification of pathogenic species of *Neisseria* by carbohydrate degradation tests: importance of glucose in media used for preparation of inocula. British Journal of Venereal Diseases 57: 249–252

Tronca E, Handsfield H H, Wiesner P J, Holmes K K 1974 Demonstration of *Neisseria gonorrhoeae* with fluorescent antibody in patients with disseminated gonococcal infection. Journal of Infectious Diseases 129: 583–586

Young H 1978a Identification and penicillinase testing of *Neisseria gonorrhoeae* from primary isolation cultures on modified New York City medium. Journal of Clinical Microbiology 7: 247–250

Young H 1978b Cultural diagnosis of gonorrhoea with modified New York City medium. British Journal of Venereal Diseases 54: 36–40

Young H, Reid K G 1988 Immunological diagnosis of gonococcal infection. In: Young H, McMillan A (eds) Immunological diagnosis of sexually transmissible diseases. Marcel Dekker, New York, p 77–116

Corynebacterium

The genus *Corynebacterium* comprises Gram-positive non-sporing rods, sometimes club-shaped and sometimes containing volutin granules, and growing in angular or palisade clusters; they are non-motile, non-capsulate and non-acid-fast, grow best aerobically though are facultatively anaerobic, are catalase positive and oxidase negative, and produce acid but not gas both fermentatively and oxidatively from carbohydrates. In the 8th edition of Bergey's Manual it has been included along with other genera with similar morphology in the 'Coryneform Group of Bacteria'. In clinical bacteriology it is convenient to apply the term 'diphtheroid' or 'coryneform' to any non-sporing Gram-positive rod thought to be a commensal not requiring definitive identification, but this practice has caused confusion in taxonomy. If difficulties in classification are to be overcome, consideration must be given to characters such as cell wall structure, antigenic composition, G+C ratio and the like.

The genus contains some species that are pathogenic to man and animals, and others, the 'diphtheroids', harmless commensals that include members of the normal flora of the human skin, throat and conjunctiva. Other species have their normal habitat in animals, plants or the soil.

Corynebacterium diphtheriae is the principal human pathogen and owes its pathogenicity to the production of a potent exotoxin active on a variety of tissues including heart muscle and peripheral nerves. Its infections typically cause an inflammatory lesion and membranous exudate on the mucosa of the upper respiratory tract. Occasionally it is implicated in wound and chronic skin infections.

Another pathogen is *C. ulcerans*, which generally causes localized ulceration of the throat, but occasionally a syndrome indistinguishable from diphtheria, and *C. haemolyticum* is thought to be a cause of severe sore throat and an itchy scarlatiniform rash in man. Other species such as *C. ovis* and *C. pyogenes* cause suppurative or granulomatous infections in animals.

Some diphtheroid bacilli, now termed the JK group of corynebacteria, have been implicated, like *Staphylococcus epidermidis*, in the causation of opportunistic infections in immuno-compromised patients and patients with malignant disease and in the colonization of Spitz-Holter valves.

CORYNEBACTERIUM DIPHTHERIAE

Morphology and staining

Gram-positive rods of varying length (average 3×0.3 μm) arranged in obtuse-angled pairs or parallel rows and often containing volutin (polyphosphate) granules. In older cultures they often show pleomorphism, with club-shaped, oval and globular forms, and stain only irregularly or weakly by Gram's method. With simple stains, e.g. methylene blue, the bacilli often have a beaded or barred appearance. With polychrome methylene blue or toluidine blue the volutin granules stain metachromatically a reddish purple. With special, double stains, e.g. Albert's (Ch. 3), the granules stand out purple-black against the lightly, e.g. green, counterstained cytoplasm. They are polar in short bacilli. Their observation helps to distinguish *C. diphtheriae* from most short non-pathogenic diphtheroids, which lack granules. However, some strains of *C. diphtheriae*, particularly those of the *intermedius* type, do not form granules and other strains may fail to form them on certain media. Thus, the same organism may show abundant volutin in films from a moist Loeffler serum slope, but none in films from a dry one. Morphology is atypical in films from cultures on tellurite-containing media. The organism is non-sporing, non-motile and non-capsulate.

Cultural characters

C. diphtheriae is an aerobe and facultative anaerobe, has an optimum temperature for growth of 37°C, but grows over the range 15–40°C, and grows best on media containing blood or serum, e.g. Loeffler's coagulated serum or blood agar containing fresh, lysed or heated blood. The addition of 0.03–0.04% potassium tellurite makes the medium selective for corynebacteria by inhibiting most other pathogenic and commensal bacteria, and imparts a black or grey colour to the colonies. It may retard the growth even of corynebacteria so that colonies may be very small after 24 h, and incubation should always be continued for 48 h. The size, shape and colour of the colonies on tellurite media such as McLeod's (Anderson et al 1931), Hoyle's (1941) or CTBA (cystine-tellurite-blood agar, Saragea et al 1979) differentiate *C. diphtheriae* into three biotypes termed *gravis, intermedius* and *mitis* on account of the differences originally observed in the severity of their infections. *Gravis* strains form relatively large, grey-black (slate-coloured), lustreless matt-surfaced colonies which in old cultures may have a radially striate, 'daisy head' appearance; they give a granular growth in broth. *Mitis* strains form convex, grey-black colonies with a matt but glistening surface, and give uniformly turbid growth in broth. *Intermedius* strains form small grey-black lustreless colonies with a 'poached egg' appearance and a remarkable uniformity in size.

Tinsdale's cystine-sodium thiosulphate-tellurite serum agar as modified by Billings (see Jellard 1971) or Meitert & Saragea (see Saragea et al 1979) has been found useful for the isolation and identification of *C. diphtheriae*, particularly in laboratories inexperienced in its recognition on earlier media such as Hoyle's. The colonies are grey-black and are surrounded by a dark brown halo. The halo is due to the formation of hydrogen sulphide from cystine (cystinase activity). It is formed only by *C. diphtheriae, C. ovis* and *C. ulcerans* among the corynebacteria.

On blood agar containing horse blood, but preferably rabbit blood, some *gravis* and all *mitis* strains form small zones of haemolysis under and around their colonies.

Biochemical reactions

C. diphtheriae produces acid from glucose and maltose, but not from lactose, mannitol, trehalose or, except for rare strains, sucrose. The fermentation of glucose but not sucrose distinguishes *C. diphtheriae* from the commonly met commensals, *C. hofmanni* which ferments neither sugar and *C. xerosis* which ferments both. *Gravis*, but not *intermedius* or *mitis* strains also ferment glycogen and starch. These and other reactions of corynebacteria are shown in Table 22.1 and details of methods are given at the end of the chapter.[*]

The fermentation tests are usually done by culture for 24 h at 37°C in Hiss's serum peptone water medium. Calf or rabbit serum should be used in the medium, for some batches of horse, ox and sheep serum contain a saccharolytic enzyme that gives rise to false-positive results. The serum in Hiss's medium is required to support growth of the bacillus, but its disadvantages can be avoided by use of a rapid, non-growth fermentation test in serum-free medium described by Rockhill et al (1981)[*].

Viability

The bacillus is readily killed by moist heat, e.g. in 10 min at 60°C, and the commonly used disinfectants. It dies rapidly in 0.85% NaCl solution, but remains alive for weeks in dust and on fomites when dry and protected from sunlight.

[*] Refer to *Methods* at end of this chapter.

Table 22.1 Biochemical reactions of some corynebacteria. Acid production from sugars in Hiss's medium is observed after 24 h at 37°C, except that by *C. ulcerans* from trehalose, which may take up to 14 days. Gelatin liquefaction at 22°C is similarly slow. *Key:* +/−, some strains positive, some negative.

Organism	Acid production from					Urease	Gelatin liquefied at 22°C	Cystinase[c]	Haemolysis on blood agar
	Glucose	Maltose	Sucrose	Trehalose	Starch				
C. diphtheriae									
gravis	+	+	−[a]	−	+	−	−	+	+/−
intermedius	+	+	−	−	−	−	−	+	−
mitis	+	+	−	−	−	−	−	+	+
C. ulcerans	+	+	−	+	+	+	+	+	+/−
C. haemolyticum[b]	+	+	+/−	+/−	+/−	−	+	−	+
C. pyogenes[b]	+	+	+/−	+/−	+/−	−	+	−	+
C. ovis	+	+	+/−	−	−	+	+/−	+	+
C. hofmanni	−	−	−	−	−	+	−	−	−
C. xerosis	+	+	+	−	−	−	−	−	−
JK group	+	+/−	−	+/−	−	−	−	−	−

[a] Rare strains of *C. diphtheriae* ferment sucrose.
[b] Only *C. haemolyticum* and *C. pyogenes* are catalase negative.
[c] H_2S production from cystine is observed in the formation of a brown halo around colonies on Tinsdale's medium or along a stab culture in Pisu's medium (Saragea et al 1979).

Antibiotic sensitivity

It is sensitive to many antibiotics, including penicillin, erythromycin and clindamycin, the latter two being used to treat patients allergic to penicillin. As well as having a role in the treatment of chronic carriers, the antibiotics are synergistic with antitoxin in the treatment of diphtheria, as they immediately stop the further production of toxin.

Toxigenicity

Strains of all three biotypes may produce the characteristic toxin and although the types were originally named according to the severity of the disease they then caused, these distinctions now have little clinical validity in Britain. Today, most strains isolated are of the *mitis* biotype and only about 10% are toxigenic. All toxigenic strains are lysogenic for a tox$^+$ phage, whose genome determines the ability of the bacillus to produce toxin under the appropriate growth conditions.

In view of the relative rarity of diphtheria in the immunized community and the clinical and epidemiological importance of quickly assessing the danger of any new isolate of *C. diphtheriae*, each such isolate should be tested for toxigenicity. Where animal facilities are not available the gel precipitation test of Elek (1949) as modified by Frobisher et al (1951) may be used.* However depending on the quality of the culture medium, antiserum and other factors, this and other in-vitro tests may be unreliable (Bickham & Jones 1972). Their use requires experience and careful control. For this reason, and particularly in laboratories rarely meeting with the infection, the isolates should be tested in vivo, if necessary by submission to a reference laboratory with animal facilities.

The guinea-pig is the preferred animal for toxigenicity tests. Where few isolates have to be tested, they should be subjected to the simple and reliable *subcutaneous toxigenicity test**, which requires the use of two animals, one protected with antitoxin as a control, for each culture. Where many isolates have to be tested, the experienced worker may economize in the use of animals by performing the *intradermal toxigenicity test**, in which up to 10 cultures may be tested on each pair of animals.

In the subcutaneous test, a toxigenic diphtheria culture causes death, usually in 1–2 days, in the unprotected animal but not in the animal protected with diphtheria antitoxin. In the intradermal test it causes an erythematous reaction within 48 h at the site of injection in the unprotected, but not the protected animal. *C. ulcerans*, which produces not only the diphtheria toxin but also another, antigenically distinct toxin, kills both animals in the subcutaneous test, though that protected by diphtheria antitoxin the more slowly, e.g. at 3–4 instead of 1–2 days. It causes intense inflammatory necrosis at the injection sites in both animals in the intradermal test.

Serotypes, phage types and bacteriocin types

For epidemiological studies, isolates of each of the three biotypes may be differentiated into a number of serotypes, phage types and bacteriocin types (Saragea et al 1979). Serotyping is done by agglutination tests, but there may be difficulty in obtaining stable bacterial suspensions, particularly of the non-toxigenic strains, and none of the various schemes proposed has been adopted internationally. Phage typing is the best developed method; the orginal scheme of Saragea & Maximescu (1969) was particularly successful in differentiating phage types among toxigenic *gravis* isolates in Rumania and the additional scheme of Maximescu et al (1972) has given good differentiation among *intermedius*, *mitis* and non-toxigenic *gravis* strains in many countries (for references, see Saragea et al 1979).

Laboratory diagnosis of diphtheria

The primary question of laboratory strategy to be settled is whether swabs from all patients with sore throats should be examined routinely for diphtheria bacilli as well as for *Streptococcus pyogenes* and other throat pathogens or whether examination for the bacilli should be selectively confined to cases in which there is a clinical or epidemiological indication of the likelihood of diphtheritic infection. Throat swabs will generally be cultured aerobically and anaerobically on blood agar for the common throat pathogens, and a thorough examination for diphtheria bacilli will incur the additional labour of preparing and reading cultures on at least two further media, e.g. Loeffler's serum and a tellurite blood agar

medium such as Hoyle's. If possible, these latter methods should always be applied in communities where diphtheria is prevalent, but in immunized communities, such as Britain today, where diphtheria is extremely rare, it is thought justifiable to confine examination for the bacilli to cases in which there is an indication of possible infection. The indicative criteria should be clearly determined, and then made known, e.g. in the bench manual, to all the laboratory staff concerned. They might specify (1) cases in which the clinician requests examination for diphtheria or mentions the possibility of the disease, (2) cases in which the clinical data on the Request form includes a mention of membrane in the throat, obstructed breathing, extreme toxicity, 'bull neck' or paralysis, e.g. difficulty in walking, talking or eating, and (3) cases in a family or community in which diphtheria has recently been diagnosed.

An intermediate laboratory policy for communities where diphtheria is infrequent but not very rare, would be to examine all throat swabs for the bacilli by the limited method of seeding them only on quarter of a plate of tellurite blood agar such as Tinsdale's, and perform the full examination only in indicated cases.

Specimens

In suspected cases, whether of faucial or nasal diphtheria, swabs should be taken both from the throat and from the nose, and preferably two swabs from the site most affected. Swabs should also be taken from skin lesions and wounds where diphtheritic infection is suspected, and both throat and nose swabs should be taken from suspected carriers.

Isolation and identification

It is best to proceed at once to culture from the swabs. Some workers attempt to get an earlier indication of the infection by microscopical examination of a smear made directly from the swab, but this procedure is rarely helpful, for *C. diphtheriae* does not form much volutin when growing in the throat and usually cannot be distinguished in the direct film from commensal diphtheroids, such as *C. xerosis*, which have a similar morphology and may produce a few volutin granules. Preliminary culture on Loeffler's serum or blood agar is required to induce the characteristic production of abundant granules in *C. diphtheriae*.

The swab should be rubbed over the surface of a wet slope of Loeffler's serum* and then be plated on blood agar and either Hoyle's or Tinsdale's tellurite blood agar*. Saragea et al (1979) recommend that if another swab is available it should be immersed and cultured in Calalb's egg-cystine-serum-tellurite liquid enrichment medium for plating next day on tellurite blood agar. The cultures should be incubated aerobically at 37°C.

1. *Loeffler culture*. After incubation for 6 h or overnight, make a smear of growth from all parts of the slope mixed in the condensation water, stain by the Albert-Laybourn method (Ch. 3) and look for the presence of slender green-stained bacilli containing the purple-black granules characteristic of *C. diphtheriae*. These bacilli will be mixed with various types of commensal bacteria from the throat or nose. If the finding is positive, at once warn the clinician of the possibility that the patient has diphtheria and tell him that confirmation by culture should be available in a day or two. Plate out the positive Loeffler culture on tellurite blood agar in case the primary culture on this medium fails to grow.

2. *Tellurite blood agar culture*. Inspect the plate after overnight incubation and then again after incubation for a further day. Growth is often poor at 24 h and the characteristic colonies are generally seen only after 48 h. On Hoyle's medium a dark, slate-grey colour and matt surface of the colonies is indicative of *C. diphtheriae*, and on Tinsdale's medium the presence of dark brown haloes around grey-black colonies is indicative of *C. diphtheriae* or *C. ulcerans*.

Prepare and examine a Gram film of a representative colony to confirm that it consists of corynebacteria. Then subculture three isolated characteristic colonies on to separate slopes of Loeffler's serum to provide inocula next day for identification tests. Also attempt earlier identification by inoculating a suspension of a well isolated colony into sugar fermentation media. It may be possible to determine the biotype of *C. diphtheriae* from the form of the colonies on the primary plate, but if that is in doubt, grow a culture for 48 h on a plate of CTBA* as described by Saragea et al (1979).

3. *Blood agar culture*. At 24 h look for pearly grey-white colonies with a slightly matt or granular surface and a form resembling that of one of the *C. diphtheriae* biotypes on tellurite blood agar. Look also for zones of haemolysis characteristic of *mitis* and some *gravis* strains. Keep the blood agar plate so that if diphtheria-like colonies are not seen on the tellurite blood agar at 48 h, colonies from the plain blood agar can be picked for identification. When diphtheria-like colonies are seen on the plain, but not the tellurite blood agar, the possibility that they are *C. haemolyticum* should be considered, for the growth of this organism is inhibited by 0.03% tellurite. *C. haemolyticum* may take 48 h to produce haemolysis on a blood agar plate made with human blood (Ryan 1972).

4. *Identification tests*. Film the Loeffler slope subcultures to check their coryneform morphology and plate them on blood agar to check their purity. Then inoculate from them into sugar fermentation media*, Elek plates* and guinea-pigs*. These identification tests must be adequately controlled. Thus, parallel fermentation tests should be made with known sucrose fermenting and non-fermenting and starch fermenting and non-fermenting strains of *C. diphtheriae* and a non-fermentative strain of *C. hofmanni*.

OTHER CORYNEBACTERIA

Other corynebacteria occasionally causing disease in man are *C. ulcerans*, *C. haemolyticum*, *C. ovis* (*C. pseudotuberculosis*) and the JK group of organisms (Lipsky et al 1982). *C. hofmanni* and *C. xerosis* are commonly present in man as commensals of the mouth, throat, nose, skin and conjunctiva, but there have been very few reports of cases, even in compromised hosts, in which they may have had a pathogenic role.

Corynebacterium ulcerans

This organism is primarily a parasite of animals but may occasionally infect man from an animal host. It can cause mastitis in cattle and has been found in milk responsible for sporadic cases or small outbreaks of ulcerative or exudative throat infection in man. Most of these human infections are mild, but in a few the patient suffers a serious illness resembling diphtheria with membrane formation and even cardiac and neurological complications. These toxic symptoms are due to a few strains producing diphtheria toxin in addition to the dermonecrotic toxin formed by most. The toxic illness should be treated with diphtheria antitoxin and erythromycin.

C. ulcerans grows well on Loeffler's serum, blood agar, on which large smooth opaque yellow-white colonies may be surrounded by small zones of haemolysis, and on Tinsdale's medium, on which large smooth black colonies are surrounded by wide brown haloes. In biochemical tests its ability to ferment trehalose, hydrolyse urea and liquefy gelatin distinguishes it from C. diphtheriae (see Table 22.1).

Corynebacterium haemolyticum

This organism, which is similar to the animal pathogen, C. pyogenes, is now accepted as an occasional human pathogen causing cases of pharyngitis, sometimes associated with cervical adenitis and often with a scarlatiniform rash. The condition may be mistaken for streptococcal or diphtheritic pharyngitis, but the disease is usually mild and resolves without treatment. Outbreaks have been reported in the USA, Europe and, more recently, Britain (Fell et al 1977). C. haemolyticum has also been isolated from chronic skin ulcers and occasionally from other lesions such as brain abscess and osteomyelitis (Coyle 1981).

Isolations of C. haemolyticum will be commoner when it is more widely appreciated that it will not grow on tellurite-containing media. On blood agar containing human blood it forms colonies like streptococci surrounded by wide zones of β-haemolysis, but on horse blood agar it shows no haemolysis at 24 h and only narrow zones at 48 h. It produces acid from glucose, maltose and, usually, lactose, sucrose and starch, and liquefies gelatin slowly. It is sensitive to penicillin and erythromycin. C. haemolyticum and C. pyogenes show important differences from other corynebacteria and it has been suggested they should be placed in a new genus, Arcanobacterium (Tompkins 1983).

Corynebacterium ovis

This organism, sometimes called C. pseudotuberculosis, causes a caseous lymphadenitis in animals, most commonly in sheep, in which it may also give rise to abscesses. A few human infections presenting as suppurative lymphadenitis have been reported in persons who have had contact with sheep.

C. ovis grows poorly on nutrient agar, but well on Loeffler's serum, forming opaque yellowish friable colonies within 24 h. On blood agar its colonies are surrounded by a zone of haemolysis. It ferments glucose, hydrolyses urea and may liquefy gelatin, but other biochemical activities are variable. It forms a dermonecrotic toxin that is antigenically distinct from diphtheria toxin.

JK group of corynebacteria

Within the last decade a group of corynebacteria with a special capacity for causing opportunistic infections in man has been recognized. Most of the infections are acquired in hospital and take place in immunocompromised patients with granulocytopenia associated with leukaemia or patients who have undergone cardiac surgery. About 10% of patients with bone marrow transplants suffer infections with these corynebacteria. The organisms are part of the normal commensal flora of the skin, particularly in the inguinal region, axilla and anus, and their carriage has been demonstrated in many hospital patients.

The JK corynebacteria grow on sheep blood agar to form very small, smooth white colonies of Gram-positive coccobacilli or longer bacilli.

They are relatively inert in biochemical reactions, but in serum media can ferment glucose and maltose slowly; they are catalase positive and urease negative. Vancomycin is the only antibiotic to which all strains are sensitive, but a few strains are also sensitive to erythromycin and tetracycline.

Laboratory diagnosis

The organisms may be isolated from a culture of the patient's blood or a swab from a septic lesion. They grow best on blood agar or other medium containing blood or serum. Incubation at 37°C may require to be continued for 48 h before adequate growth is present. Examination of a Gram smear will reveal the coryneform morphology, and biochemical tests the relative inertness. Sensitivity tests should be done for the commonly used antibiotics and vancomycin.

The problem confronting the microbiologist who isolates such a non-diphtheritic corynebacterium and the physician receiving the report is how to regard it. In the past these organisms would have been considered harmless contaminants from the skin, but as it is now accepted that they can cause opportunistic infections, their finding cannot be dismissed so easily. It is essential to determine the clinical history of the patient and factors affecting the state of his immune system. If it appears he may be immunodeficient or his resistance otherwise compromised, the organism's antibiotic sensitivities must be reported to the physician so that he may decide whether therapy should be given.

Corynebacterium hofmanni

This organism is a common commensal of the throat. It does not produce a toxin and hardly ever, if at all, acts as even an opportunistic pathogen. In films it appears as strongly Gram-positive short stout rods or coccobacilli arranged mainly in palisade formation. With methylene blue, an unstained middle area gives it the appearance of a diplococcus and with Albert's stain no volutin is seen. It grows aerobically on ordinary media without serum or blood, forming large smooth creamy white colonies, and on tellurite media forms smooth, greyish white opaque colonies. It is relatively inert biochemically, failing to ferment glucose and other carbohydrates, but it hydrolyses urea.

Corynebacterium xerosis

This organism is a commensal in the conjunctival sac and was originally wrongly thought to be the cause of xerosis conjunctivae. It is also found as a commensal in the ear, on the skin and occasionally in the throat, and probably is never pathogenic. Morphologically it resembles *C. diphtheriae*, though it is more strongly Gram-positive and shows fewer volutin granules. It grows to form small colonies on nutrient agar. On tellurite blood agar it forms small black colonies with a glossy surface which distinguishes them from the similarly sized colonies of the *intermedius* type of *C. diphtheriae*, which have a matt, granular surface. On Tinsdale's medium it forms dark colonies but without a brown halo. It is further distinguished from *C. diphtheriae* by its ability to ferment sucrose as well as glucose and maltose and by its lack of toxicity in laboratory animals.

Corynebacterium acnes

The organism formerly given this name is now placed in a separate genus as *Propionibacterium acnes*. It is part of the normal flora of the skin, where it breaks down sebum, and is found in acne pustules, but probably without any essential pathogenic role. Unlike corynebacteria, it is microaerophilic and forms propionic acid as a by-product of carbohydrate fermentation.

METHODS

Loeffler's serum slopes

Serum of ox, sheep or horse	300 ml
Nutrient broth, pH 7.6	100 ml
Glucose	1 g

1. Sterilize the serum by Seitz filtration.
2. Dissolve the glucose in the broth and sterilize by autoclaving at 115°C for 20 min.

3. Add the glucose broth to the serum with sterile precautions, mix thoroughly and distribute 2.5 ml amounts into sterile, screw-capped 6 ml bottles. Apply the caps tightly.

4. For inspissation, lay the bottles on their sides on a tray, sloped slightly to prevent the medium running up to the cap. Place the tray in a hot air oven. Raise the temperature slowly to 80°C and maintain it at 80°C for 2 h, when the serum will be coagulated to a yellow-white solid.

5. Allow the slopes to cool. They should have a moist surface and a small amount of condensation water at their foot. Properly capped against drying, they can be stored for long periods.

Hoyle's tellurite lysed-blood agar

Agar base

Meat extract (Oxoid Lab-Lemco)	10 g
Peptone (Difco proteose)	10 g
Sodium chloride, NaCl	5 g
Agar powder	15 g
Water	1 litre

Dissolve the ingredients, adjust to pH 7.8, distribute in 100 ml amounts in screw-capped bottles and autoclave at 121°C for 15 min.

Lysed horse blood. Obtain sterile horse blood. Lyse it by freezing and thawing four times and store in the cold, preferably frozen. Alternatively, lyse it with saponin (Young 1942) as follows:

1. Make a 10% solution of white saponin in water and sterilize it by autoclaving at 115°C for 15 min.

2. Incubate the blood at 37°C for 15 min. Then add 0.5 ml saponin solution to each 10 ml blood. Invert the bottle gently several times to mix without the formation of bubbles. Reincubate for a further 15 min. The lysed blood will have an 'inky' black appearance. It will keep for several months at 4°C.

Tellurite solution

Potassium tellurite, K_2TeO_3	0.7 g
Water	20 ml

Dissolve, autoclave at 115°C for 15 min and store in a tightly stoppered bottle in the dark.

Complete medium

Agar base	200 ml
Lysed blood	10 ml
Tellurite solution	2 ml

Melt the agar, cool it to 55°C, add the blood and tellurite, mix well without bubble formation and pour 15–20 ml amounts into sterile Petri dishes. After setting, dry off surface moisture.

Tinsdale's medium

Billings' modification of this cystine-thiosulphate-tellurite serum agar as described by Jellard (1971) is given. In the modification of Meitert & Saragea (1967, see Saragea et al 1979) LabLemco meat extract is substituted for half the peptone and a small amount of defibrinated sheep blood is added.

Agar base

Proteose peptone (Difco)	20 g
Sodium chloride, NaCl	5 g
Agar powder	19 g
Water	1 litre

Dissolve the ingredients, adjust to pH 7.4 and autoclave at 121°C for 15 min.

Enrichment. To 200 ml of melted agar base, cooled to 55°C, add aseptically, strictly in the following order, and mixing thoroughly after each ingredient:

1. Ox serum, Seitz filtered	20 ml
2. Sodium hydroxide, NaOH, 0.1 mol/litre	12 ml
3. L-Cystine, 0.4% in hydrochloric acid, HCl, 0.1 mol/l	12 ml
4. Potassium tellurite, K_2TeO_3, 1% in sterile water	6 ml
5. Sodium thiosulphate (anhydrous), $Na_2S_2O_3$, freshly made 2.5% solution in sterile water	3.4 ml

Preferably, solutions (2)–(5) should be first pasteurized at 60°C for 30 min. All should be stored at 4°C. As some batches of L-cystine are inhibitory to *C. diphtheriae*, each new batch should be tested before use.

Immediately after addition of the enrichments, 20 ml amounts of the melted medium should be poured into Petri dishes. The complete medium should be transparent and light yellow in colour. As it is not stable, the plates should be kept at 4°C and used within 4 days. Surface moisture should be dried off in the incubator, with their lids half open, for 10 min just before inoculation.

Commercial Tinsdale base and dried enrichment mixture are available (Difco).

CTBA medium

This cystine-tellurite-blood agar medium is recommended by Saragea et al (1979) for differentiation of the colonial biotypes of *C. diphtheriae*.

Cystine solution. Prepare a 1% solution of L-cystine by first dissolving 1 g anhydrous sodium carbonate (Na_2CO_3) in 10 ml distilled water, heating to 100°C and then adding 1 g L-cystine. Heat again and then add 90 ml distilled water while stirring well. Autoclave at 105°C for 20 min. Keep the solution in the dark at 4°C and use within 1 month. Discard it if its colour changes from light yellow.

Potassium tellurite solution. Dissolve 1 g K_2TeO_3 in 100 ml distilled water with heating. Autoclave at 105°C for 20 min.

Complete medium. To 100 ml melted nutrient agar, pH 7.4–7.6 at 45°C, add 10 ml sterile defibrinated sheep blood, 4 ml of the 1% potassium tellurite solution and 0.1 ml of the 1% L-cystine solution.

Hiss's serum sugar media

These media are used to test the fermentation reactions of nutritionally exacting bacteria such as diphtheria bacilli and streptococci. Hiss's serum water consists of 25% serum in distilled water adjusted to pH 7.5, and for the tests 1% of carbohydrate and an indicator dye are added.

Most workers, however, prefer to substitute dilute peptone water for the distilled water, as in the following formula.

Calf or rabbit (not horse) serum	200 ml
Peptone (0.5%) water, pH 7.6	800 ml
Test carbohydrate	10 g
Indicator solution, as below.	

Indicator. The indicator generally recommended is Andrade's 0.5% acid fuchsin neutralized to a yellow colour with just sufficient NaOH solution 1 mol/litre. 10 ml of this indicator is added to 1 litre of medium. It turns dark pink if acid is produced.

Alternatively, 50 ml of 0.2% phenol red solution (turns yellow at pH 6.8 and lower) or 12.5 ml of 0.2% bromothymol blue solution (yellow at pH 6.0 and lower) may be added per litre.

Sterilization. Preferably, sterilize the complete medium by filtration and distribute it aseptically in 2.5 ml amounts in sterile screw-capped 6 ml bottles.

Alternatively, if heat is used, care must be taken not to hydrolyse the test carbohydrate by overheating. Distribute the medium without carbohydrate in 2.5 ml amounts in screw-capped 6 ml bottles, apply the caps tightly and steam the batch at 100°C for 20 min on each of 3 successive days. Prepare 10% solutions of the test carbohydrates, sterilize them by filtration or steaming at 100°C for 60 min, and then with sterile precautions add them in 0.25 ml amounts to the bottles of 2.5 ml medium.

Starch medium. On standing in solution even in the cold, starch gradually becomes hydrolysed to glucose, which is fermented by all biotypes of *C. diphtheriae*. It is essential therefore to make up the starch solution only when required and add it to the serum water medium immediately before the test. To prepare 20–30 bottles of starch medium, proceed as follows. Weigh out 0.15 g of soluble starch and place it in a sterile Universal container. Add 5 ml of distilled water, screw on the cap and shake vigorously. Heat at 100°C for about 5 min, shaking at intervals to produce a homogeneous solution. Cool and then add 0.15 ml with a sterile pipette to each bottle of 2.5 ml serum medium. Use for tests within a few days.

Alternative serum sugar medium

Saragea et al (1979) recommend that the serum sugar media should be made up as follows.

Serum peptone water. Dissolve 7 g peptone and 1.4 g disodium hydrogen phosphate (Na_2HPO_4) in 1400 ml distilled water. Heat to 100 °C, filter through filter paper and autoclave at 121°C for 20 min. Cool and add 250 ml sterile ox serum. Steam at 100°C for 20 min. Add 11 ml of sterile Andrade's solution. Distribute aseptically in sterile bottles and store at 4°C.

Andrade's solution. To 100 ml distilled water add 0.5 g acid fuchsin and 10 ml of NaOH 1 mol/litre. Autoclave at 115°C for 30 min. Store at 4°C.

Carbohydrate solutions. Prepare 10% solutions of glucose, maltose, sucrose and glycogen and a 4% solution of starch. Sterilize by autoclaving at 105°C for 20 min. It is recommended that sucrose should instead be sterilized by filtration because it tends to hydrolyse on heating. It is also recommended that glycogen should be tested instead of starch, which gradually hydrolyses on standing.

Complete media. With sterile precautions, add 10 ml carbohydrate solution to 90 ml serum peptone water and distribute in 2.5 ml volumes. The final pH should be 8.1–8.2.

Rapid fermentation test

Rockhill et al (1981) have described a rapid, non-growth method of testing the fermentation reactions of *C. diphtheriae*, which avoids the need for serum in the medium and gives results within an hour. A dense suspension of the organism is incubated with a buffered solution of the test carbohydrate and phenol red as an indicator of acid production.

Buffer solution

Dipotassium hydrogen phosphate, K_2HPO_4 — 0.4 g

Potassium dihydrogen phosphate, KH_2PO_4 — 0.1 g
Potassium chloride, KCl — 8 g
Phenol red, 1% aqueous solution — 2 ml
Distilled water — 1 litre

Adjust pH to 7.2.

Carbohydrate media. Add glucose 2 g, maltose 2 g, sucrose 2 g and soluble potato starch 0.5 g to four separate 10 ml volumes of the buffer solution. Distribute 1 ml amounts in screw-capped tubes or bottles, store frozen at −20°C and hold at 5–8°C once thawed for use.

Method. 1. Grow a culture of the corynebacterium for 18–24 h on a plate of tryptic soy agar (Oxoid or Difco).

2. Make a dense suspension of the cultured bacteria in 1 ml of the buffer solution without carbohydrate.

3. Add one drop (0.05 ml) of each of the four carbohydrate media and one drop of buffer without carbohydrate (negative control) separately to five wells in a microtitre plate.

4. Then add one drop (0.05 ml) of the bacterial suspension to each well and incubate the plate at 37°C for 60 min.

A positive fermentation reaction is shown by the development of a distinct yellow colour, which should be absent from the well without carbohydrate.

Urease test

Inoculate solid culture material heavily on to a slope of Christensen's medium (Ch. 8), incubate for 24 h and look for the development of a purple-pink colour indicating urease activity.

Elek plate test for toxigenicity

This is a gel precipitation test done on a plate of a clear serum nutrient agar. Toxin diffusing from a streak culture of suspected *C. diphtheriae* is demonstrated by the formation of a white line of precipitate where it meets with diphtheria antitoxin diffusing from a strip of filter paper embedded in the agar (Fig. 22.1). That the

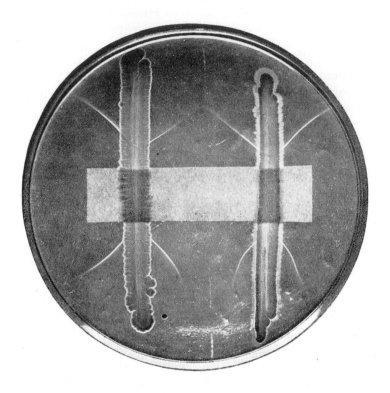

Fig. 22.1 Photograph showing the recognition of toxigenic strains of the diphtheria bacillus by the Elek method. In the centre is the horizontal strip of filter paper containing the antitoxin with the growths of the diphtheria bacillus at right angles to it. The fine white lines showing a positive reaction are well defined.

precipitation line consists of diphtheria toxin and antitoxin is shown by its fusing with a line formed by a parallel streak of a known toxigenic *C. diphtheriae* culture.

Success of the test is dependent on the quality of the medium and the antitoxin, which must be checked in preliminary tests. The strength of the antitoxin should be between 500 and 1000 units/ml.

Nutrient agar

Proteose peptone (Difco)	20 g
Meat extract (Difco)	5 g
Sodium chloride, NaCl	5 g
Agar powder (e.g. Bacto, Difco)	12 g

Dissolve at 100°C, adjust to pH 7.8, autoclave at 121°C for 15 min, remove any precipitate by filtering through paper or wadding, distribute in 12 ml volumes in 25 ml bottles and sterilize by autoclaving at 121°C for 10 min.

Normal serum. Use sterile horse or calf serum from a batch previously checked for suitability in the Elek test. Just before pouring the test plates, cool the melted nutrient agar to about 45°C, add 3 ml of the normal serum to 12 ml of the agar and mix gently to avoid the formation of bubbles.

Antitoxin strip. Prepare this in time to have it ready at the moment when the serum and agar are mixed. Soak a strip of sterile filter paper, 60 × 10 mm, in the diphtheria antitoxin 500–1000 units/ml, drain off excess antitoxin, lay the strip on the bottom of a sterile Petri dish and leave to dry at 37°C for 10 min.

Method. 1. Pour the melted serum nutrient agar into another sterile Petri dish and before it sets, lay the antitoxin-containing strip of paper across the middle of the plate on the surface of the agar. When the agar has set, dry off surface moisture by leaving the plate, with lid ajar, in the 37°C incubator for 30 min.

2. Streak a heavy inoculum of the culture to be tested across the plate in a narrow line at right angles to the paper strip. Parallel to this streak, at a distance of about 15 mm from it, streak a known toxigenic strain of *C. diphtheriae* on one side of the unknown strain and streak a non-toxigenic strain on the other side.

3. Incubate the plate aerobically at 37°C and examine after 24 h and 48 h with oblique lighting against a black background. A positive reaction is seen as a fine white line starting from the streak culture a few mm from the paper strip and passing obliquely away from it. At 24 h the line is best seen with the help of a hand lens; at 48 h it is more obvious. Look for continuity between the line from the unknown culture and that from the known toxigenic culture.

Modified method. For greater sensitivity, Saragea et al (1979) recommend applying the antitoxin in a 7 × 0.5 cm ditch cut in the agar in a 9 cm plate instead of in a paper strip. Antitoxin 0.5 ml is dropped in the ditch, the plate is left for 1–2 h at 37°C with the lid ajar and the ditch is then filled with more melted agar.

Subcutaneous toxigenicity test

Requisites. Two healthy guinea-pigs, e.g. 250 g body weight. Two sterile hypodermic syringes with needles. Diphtheria antitoxin of known potency, e.g. 1000 units/ml. Instruments for necropsy.

Method. 1. Grow a pure culture of the suspected diphtheria isolate on a slope of moist Loeffler's serum aerobically for 24 h at 37°C to be ready on the day of the test.

2. Mark the guinea-pigs to distinguish the one to be protected with antitoxin from the one to be left unprotected. Then inject 1000 units of diphtheria antitoxin intraperitoneally into the former animal.

3. After 2–3 h prepare a dense suspension of the Loeffler culture in 3 ml broth (not saline) and inject 1 ml of this suspension subcutaneously into the left thigh in each animal.

4. Observe the animals at intervals for up to 96 h.

5. Perform a necropsy on any animal dying within this period.

Results. If the culture is toxigenic *C. diphtheriae*, the animal unprotected by antitoxin will die, probably in 1–2 days, while the protected animal will survive. On necropsy of the former, gelatinous haemorrhagic oedema will be seen at the site of inoculation, blood-stained pleural and peritoneal exudates, and haemorrhagic inflammation of the adrenal glands, though the findings are not always wholly characteristic. If neither animal dies, the culture is non-toxigenic. If both animals die, the culture is virulent or toxigenic, but not *C. diphtheriae*.

A strain of *C. ulcerans* producing both diphtheria toxin and *C. ulcerans* dermonecrotic toxin will kill both animals, but the animal protected with diphtheria antitoxin will die later (e.g. at 3–4 days) than the unprotected animal (e.g. at 1–2 days), and although it will show local haemorrhagic oedema and haemorrhagic inflammation of the viscera, it will not show the characteristic haemorrhages in the adrenals. A strain of *C. ulcerans* not producing diphtheria toxin will kill both animals slowly, as if protected.

Intradermal toxigenicity test

Requisites. Two healthy, white guinea-pigs about 400 g body weight. Two sterile syringes and needles for intraperitoneal injections. A number of 1 ml sterile syringes and fine-bore needles (26 gauge, 2 cm long) to the number of cultures to be tested for the intradermal injections. A razor or depilating cream. A pencil with indelible dye to mark the depilated skin. Diphtheria antitoxin of known strength. A known toxigenic culture of *C. diphtheriae* as control.

Method. 1. Grow pure cultures of the unknown strains and control strain on moist slopes of Loeffler's serum for 24 h to be ready on the day of the test.

2. The day before the test, shave the skin of the abdomen and flanks of the two guinea-pigs. Alternatively, remove as much hair as possible with clippers, cover the area with depilating cream for a few minutes, then wash off with warm water and dry. Mark the animals to distinguish the one to be protected with antitoxin from the one to be left unprotected. Then inject 1000 units of antitoxin intraperitoneally into the former.

3. On the day of the test, first mark off the depilated area in each animal into a number of squares, up to 10, equal to the number of cultures to be tested. Make a plan of the squares showing the name or number of the culture to be injected into each.

4. From the Loeffler cultures, prepare suspensions in broth (not saline) to a density of about 10^9 bacilli/ml. Then inject 0.2 ml of each suspension intradermally into the centre of the appropriate square of skin in each animal. The inoculation must be intradermal, not subcutaneous; it should raise a small blister-like swelling. The injections should be made at least 2.5 cm apart from one another.

5. At about half an hour after the intradermal injections, inject 10 units of antitoxin (or 0.02 units/g body weight) intraperitoneally into the test animal previously unprotected with antitoxin. This small dose will prevent the animal dying without interfering with the skin reaction. Inspect the animals at 24, 48 and 72 h thereafter.

Results. Toxigenic *C. diphtheriae* produces at the site of injection in the test animal a well defined red area about 15 mm in diameter, which after the third or fourth day fades and leaves a necrotic patch with a scab surrounded by growing hair. In the control, protected animal, it produces no reaction beyond the small red puncture wound caused by the needle. Non-toxigenic *C. diphtheriae* causes no reaction in either animal. Any culture causing a reaction in both animals is toxigenic, but not *C. diphtheriae*; it may be *C. ulcerans*.

REFERENCES

Anderson J S, Happold F C, McLeod J W, Thomson J G 1931 On the existence of two forms of diphtheria bacillus – B. diphtheriae gravis and B. diphtheriae mitis – and a new medium for their differentiation and for the bacteriological diagnosis of diphtheria. Journal of Pathology and Bacteriology 34: 667–681

Bickham S, Jones W 1972 Problems in the use of the in-vitro toxigenicity test for C. diphtheriae. American Journal of Clinical Pathology 57: 244–246

Coyle M B 1981 Corynebacteria in Seattle. Clinical Microbiology Newsletter 3: 99–101

Elek S D 1949 The plate virulence test for diphtheria. Journal of Clinical Pathology 2: 250–258

Fell H W K, Nagington J, Naylor G R E, Olds R J 1977 Corynebacterium haemolyticum infections in Cambridgeshire. Journal of Hygiene, Cambridge 79: 269–274

Frobisher M Jr, King E O, Parsons E I A 1951 A test in vitro for virulence of Corynebacterium diphtheriae. American Journal of Clinical Pathology 21: 282–285

Hoyle L 1941 A tellurite blood-agar medium for the rapid diagnosis of diphtheria. Lancet 1: 175–176

Jellard C H 1971 Comparison of Hoyle's medium and Billings' modification of Tinsdale's medium for the bacteriological diagnosis of diphtheria. Journal of Medical Microbiology 4: 366–369

Lipsky B A, Goldberger A C, Tompkins L S, Plorde J J 1982 Infections caused by non-diphtheria corynebacteria. Reviews of Infectious Diseases 4: 1220–1235

Rockhill R C, Hadiputranto H, Sumarmo, Burhanudin Muslihun, Sjawitri P Siregar 1981 Rapid carbohydrate utilization test to identify Corynebacterium diphtheriae. South-East Asian Journal of Tropical Medicine and Public Health 12: 145–147

Ryan W J 1972 Throat infection and rash associated with an unusual corynebacterium. Lancet 2: 1345–1347

Saragea A, Maximescu P, Meitert E 1979 Corynebacterium diphtheriae: microbiological methods used in clinical and epidemiological investigations. In: Bergan T, Norris J R (eds) Methods in microbiology, vol 13. Academic Press, London. ch 4, p 61–176

Tompkins L S 1983 Corynebacterium haemolyticum (Editorial) Clinical Microbiology Newsletter 5: 29–30

Young M Y 1942 Diphtheria diagnosis with Hoyle's medium. Saponin and sodium-dioctyl-sulpho-succinate as haemolysing agents in the preparation of the medium. Journal of Pathology and Bacteriology 54: 253–256

Listeria: Erysipelothrix

The genera *Listeria* and *Erysipelothrix*, previously included in the family Corynebacteriaceae, have now been placed under the heading of Gram-positive Asporogenous Rod-shaped Bacteria as Genera of Uncertain Affiliation in the 8th Edition of Bergey's Manual of determinative bacteriology (Buchanan & Gibbons 1974). Although they share some biological features, these two genera are distinguished from one another by fundamental differences in their fatty acid composition, their cell wall contents and their lack of common antigens when tested by haemagglutination or immunodiffusion (Ewald 1981). They are common pathogens of animals and birds, both wild and domestic, and occasionally cause infections in man. Important characters of the two main species, *L. monocytogenes* and *E. rhusiopathiae* are shown in Table 23.1.

LISTERIA MONOCYTOGENES

Of the species in the genus *Listeria*, only *L. monocytogenes* is considered to be pathogenic, being consistently isolated from cases of the disease, listeriosis, which occurs worldwide in animals and man. The organism owes its name to the fact that its infection in rabbits causes a monocytosis (Murray et al 1926). Sporadic cases and epizootics occur in cattle, sheep, goats and swine, sometimes with a high mortality and usually manifest as a meningo-encephalitis. In cases of abortion in cattle and sheep, the listeria has been isolated from the fetus. It is also found in the blood, liver and myocardial abscesses in listeriosis in smaller animals such as rabbits and fowls.

Listeriosis in man

Twenty years ago listeriosis was considered to be an unusual cause of meningo-encephalitis in man and generalized infection in newborn babies. Since then an increasing number of sporadic cases and occasional small outbreaks, e.g. in hospitals, have been reported (Campbell et al 1981; Kachel & Lenard 1981; Isaacs & Liberman 1981). Human acquisition of listeriosis from animal sources has been shown to occur as an occupational hazard in farmers, butchers,

Table 23.1 Characters of *Listeria monocytogenes* and *Erysipelothrix rhusiopathiae.*

Character	L. monocytogenes	E. rhusiopathiae
Motility	+ 25°C	−
Growth at 4°C	+	−
Growth on MacConkey agar	+	−
Haemolysis on blood agar	+ β	− or weak α
Gas from glucose	−	−
Acid from:		
glucose	+	+
lactose	−[a]	+
trehalose	+	−
salicin	+	−
Catalase produced	+	−
Urease produced	−	−
Acetoin produced	+	−
Indole produced	−	−
Gelatin liquefied	−	−

[a] Lactose, sucrose, rhamnose and aesculin fermented only after 3–10 days or not at all; other biochemical results as at 24 h.

veterinary surgeons and others, but in most human cases an animal connection has not been demonstrated. An epidemic in Canada due to contaminated coleslaw has pointed to food as being a probable vehicle of transmission (Schlech et al 1983).

Three types of human disease have been described. (1) The commonest is a meningo-encephalitis, often with septicaemia, e.g. in an elderly adult compromised by a debilitating disease or treatment with immunosuppressive drugs. (2) In a mother with subclinical infection, intra-uterine infection may cause death of the fetus or the premature delivery of a neonate with pneumonic septicaemia and meningitis. (3) Adults may suffer an influenza-like illness accompanied by diarrhoea or, in females, with symptoms suggesting an infection of the genital tract.

Morphology and staining

Straight or slightly curved rods 2–3 × 0.5 μm, often in pairs lying at an acute angle end-to-end when taken from a smooth colony. When from a rough colony, especially from solid medium at room temperature, elongated filaments are present. Flagellate and actively motile in young broth cultures grown at 25°C, but poorly flagellate and very feebly motile in cultures grown at 37°C. Non-spore-forming. Gram-positive, but many Gram-negative bacilli are seen in older cultures. Non-acid-fast.

Cultural characters

Aerobe and facultative anaerobe. Optimum temperature for growth is 37°C, but the organism grows over a wide range of temperatures, with slow growth even at 4°C. Grows on ordinary media, e.g. nutrient agar, but growth is improved by the addition of blood, serum, liver extract or glucose.

After 24 h at 37°C colonies are small, 0.5–1.5 mm in diameter, smooth and translucent. By reflected light they have a blue-green colour. On horse blood agar they are surrounded by a narrow zone of β-haemolysis. There is growth but no liquefaction in a gelatin stab.

Biochemical reactions

Acid, but not gas, is produced from glucose and maltose in peptone water incubated for 24–48 h at 37°C. Lactose and sucrose are fermented after 3–10 days, if at all, whilst mannitol is not fermented. Catalase is produced.

Viability and antibiotic sensitivity

The organism can survive in tissues and other materials for several months at 4°C. It is sensitive in vitro to many antibiotics, including penicillin, ampicillin, erythromycin, cotrimoxazole, gentamicin and rifampicin. In clinical practice, listeriosis has been treated most successfully with ampicillin or ampicillin combined with gentamicin (Marklein & Häfelein 1981; Niels le Souëf & Walters 1981).

Antigens

A number of different O and H antigens have been recognized in different strains and some 12 serovars have been distinguished.

Animal pathogenicity

On experimental inoculation, the organism is pathogenic for mice, guinea-pigs and rabbits, but not for rats or pigeons. If one or two drops of an overnight broth culture are placed on the conjunctiva or rubbed over the eyelid of a guinea-pig or rabbit, a marked inflammatory reaction and purulent discharge are produced within 48 h. The intraperitoneal injection of bacilli from an overnight culture into a white mouse will cause death within 5 days and the organisms can be recovered from the blood, liver and spleen.

Laboratory diagnosis

Because listeriosis is relatively uncommon and positive findings are usually unexpected, the principal danger in diagnosis is that, when observed, the bacilli will be mistaken for contaminating commensal diphtheroids (corynebacteria) and disregarded. When, therefore, diphtheroid-like bacilli are seen in films of cerebrospinal fluid or a blood culture from a neonate, they should always be examined further to exclude the possibility that they are listeria. Blood cultures are quite often contaminated with skin corynebacteria and even when the cultures are from older children or adults, the colonies of any 'diphtheroids' grown in subculture on blood agar should be inspected carefully and, if resembling listeria colonies, be identified in further tests.

1. Examine cerebrospinal fluid, blood cultures and other materials from generalized lesions by Gram film, aerobic culture on a plate of horse blood agar at 37°C and other methods appropriate to the specimen. In meningitis, the cerebrospinal fluid may have a cell count of up to 2000 cells/mm^3 and show diphtheroid-like bacilli in a Gram film of its centrifuged deposit.

2. Look for small smooth transparent colonies with narrow zones of β-haemolysis on the horse blood agar plate and examine them in a Gram film to confirm their morphology and staining reactions.

3. Prepare a plate subculture on tryptone agar base plus 1% glucose and after 24 h at 37°C view the colonies by reflected light to detect the blue-green shining appearance characteristic of listeria.

4. Inoculate bacilli from the blood agar into a tube of peptone water, hold at room temperature or 20–25°C and after a few hours or overnight examine the culture microscopically in a wet film to detect the characteristic tumbling motility of *L. monocytogenes*.

Selective culture

The above methods are satisfactory for primary isolation from specimens such as cerebrospinal fluid or blood, in which the listeria is likely to be the only organism present, but selective methods of culture are generally required for specimens of faeces, tissues or exudates likely to contain a mixture of organisms. One such method is to inoculate the specimen into tryptose broth, incubate it at 4°C and subculture from it weekly over a period of several months. This 'cold storage' technique takes advantage of the exceptional ability of the listeria to multiply, though slowly, at a temperature so low as to be inhibitory to most other organisms that might be present.

Selective culture media have also been employed sucessfully. A medium containing thallous acetate and nalidixic acid in tryptose phosphate broth has an inhibitory effect on most Gram-positive and Gram-negative bacteria, but not listeria (Krammer & Jones 1969; Leighton 1979).

Typing

Isolates of *L. monocytogenes* can be typed by agglutination tests with type-specific sera. Serotypes 1 and 4b are the most commonly reported from human listeriosis. In Britain, strains for serotyping are commonly referred to the Central Public Health Laboratory, Colindale, London, NW9 5HT (Taylor 1980).

Isolates may also be differentiated by phage-typing. Though outbreaks of listeriosis due to case-to-case transmission are rare, some have been reported and phage-typing has been found a valuable tool in their investigation (Taylor et al 1981).

ERYSIPELOTHRIX RHUSIOPATHIAE

The only species in the genus *Erysipelothrix* is *E. rhusiopathiae*, the causative agent of swine erysipelas and of erysipeloid in man. Its distribution is worldwide and it causes disease in sheep, cattle, pigs, other domestic animals and birds. It has also been found in the slime on fish and in fish boxes.

Infection in man is mainly an occupational hazard of fish workers, butchers, poultry workers and others in contact with fish, shellfish, meat or poultry. It follows the introduction of the organism through the skin, e.g abraded skin, and causes the formation of a painful swollen purplish erythematous area which is slightly raised and extends peripherally. The fingers, hands or arms are the usual sites of infection.

Occasionally a septicaemia occurs and rare cases of endocarditis have been reported.

Morphology and staining

When examined from smooth colonies, the organisms are small, slightly curved slender rods, $1–2 \times 0.2–0.4$ μm, occurring either singly or in small groups. When taken from rough colonies, they present as filaments 50–60 μm long and occur in chains or tangled masses. They are non-motile, non-capsulate and non-sporeforming. They are Gram-positive in reaction, though easily decolourized, and non-acid-fast.

Cultural characters

The organism grows on ordinary media but growth is improved by the addition of serum or 0.5% glucose. It is non-haemolytic on blood agar. Though microaerophilic when first isolated, its later subcultures grow as well aerobically as anaerobically. The optimum temperature for growth is 37°C; it will grow slowly at room temperature, but not at all at 4°C.

Colonies on solid media are of two types: smooth colonies after 24 h at 37°C are very small, 0.5–1 mm in diameter, round, convex and smooth like drops of dew; rough colonies are larger, flatter, opaque and granular. In broth, two types of growth may be observed: a uniform turbidity associated with short rods and a floccular growth in which the organisms are filamentous.

Biochemical reactions

The organism ferments some carbohydrates, e.g. glucose, lactose and sucrose, with the formation of acid but not gas, whilst its reactions with others are variable (Sneath et al 1951). It does not produce catalase. In gelatin stabs it grows down the stab with lateral extensions ('pipe cleaner' effect), but does not cause liquefaction.

Viability and antibiotic sensitivity

Although non-sporing, *E. rhusiopathiae* can survive for long periods in a dried state and in the soil at low temperatures. Its viability is reduced by sunlight and high temperatures. It is resistant to sodium azide.

It is sensitive to penicillin and streptomycin, but resistant to sulphonamides. For treatment of erysipeloid, septicaemia or the rare cases of erysipelothrix endocarditis, penicillin is still the drug of choice (Muirhead & Reid 1980).

Animal pathogenicity

Mice are susceptible to intraperitoneal inoculation of a culture suspension and die from acute septicaemia in 4–5 days.

Laboratory diagnosis

1. Attempt to isolate the organism from the lesion. Take some tissue or tissue fluid from its edge and inoculate it into glucose broth as well as on to blood agar and other routine media. Swabbing a lesion is less likely to be successful.

2. Perform a blood culture when septicaemia is suspected.

3. Identify the organism by its morphology, absence of motility, colonial appearance, biochemical reactions, inability to grow at 4°C, ability to grow on Packer's (1943) sodium azide-crystal violet medium, and pathogenicity in a mouse.

4. When attempting isolation from specimens contaminated with other organisms, plate also on Packer's medium, which is selective for streptococci and erysipelothrix.

REFERENCES

Buchanan R E, Gibbons N E (1974) Bergey's manual of determinative bacteriology, 8th edn. Williams & Wilkins, Baltimore. p 593–597

Campbell A N, Sill P R, Wardle J K 1981 Listeria meningitis acquired by cross infection in a delivery suite. Lancet 2: 752–753

Ewald F W 1981 In: Starr M P, Stolp H, Trüper H P, Balows A, Schlegel H G (eds) The prokaryotes. Springer-Verlag, Berlin, ch 133, p 1695–1696

Isaacs D, Liberman M M 1981 Babies cross-infected with *Listeria monocytogenes*. Lancet 2: 940

Kachel W, Lenard H G 1981 Babies cross-infected with *Listeria monocytogenes*. Lancet 2: 939–940

Krammer P A, Jones D 1969 Media selective for *Listeria monocytogenes*. Journal of Applied Bacteriology 32: 381–394

Leighton I 1979 Use of selective agents for the isolation of *Listeria monocytogenes*. Medical Laboratory Sciences 36: 283–288

Marklein G, Häfelein J 1981 *In vitro* susceptibility of *Listeria monocytogenes* with special reference to newer Beta-lactam antibiotics. Zentralblatt für Bacteriologie I 25/A: 40–53. English summary

Muirhead N, Reid T M S 1980 *Erysipelothrix rhusiopathiae* endocarditis. Journal of Infection 2: 83–85

Murray E G D, Webb R A, Swann M B R 1926 A disease of rabbits characterized by a large mononuclear leucocytosis, caused by a hitherto undescribed bacillus, *Bacterium monocytogenes* (n.sp.). Journal of Pathology and Bacteriology 29: 407–439

Niels le Souëf P, Walters B N J 1981 Neonatal listeriosis: a summer outbreak. Medical Journal of Australia 2: 188–191

Packer R A 1943 The use of sodium azide (NaN$_3$) and crystal violet in a selective medium for streptococci and *Erysipelothrix rhusiopathiae*. Journal of Bacteriology 46: 343–349

Schlech W F et al 1983 Epidemic listeriosis – evidence for transmission by food. New England Journal of Medicine 308: 203–206

Sneath P H A, Abbott J D, Cunliffe A C 1951 The bacteriology of erysipeloid. British Medical Journal 2: 1063–1066

Taylor A G 1980 Listeriosis. Lancet 1:1136

Taylor A G, McLauchlin J, Green H T, Macaulay M B, Audurier A 1981 Hospital cross-infection with *Listeria monocytogenes* confirmed by phage-typing. Lancet 2:1106

Bacillus species: anthrax

The genus *Bacillus* comprises the Gram-positive rods that grow aerobically and form heat-resistant spores. The vegetative bacilli are large and straight, and often grow in filamentous chains. Most species are Gram-positive, but some are Gram-variable and some are Gram-positive only in the early stages of growth. Most are motile with lateral flagella. The spores in most species are oval in shape, centrally situated and do not distend the bacillus. Colonies are usually large, and irregular, rhizoid or spreading. Some species are facultative anaerobes and others strict aerobes. Most form catalase and most form acid but not gas from glucose.

Bacillus anthracis, the causative organism of anthrax, is the only true pathogen of higher animals. Anthrax is a zoonosis, primarily an infectious disease of wild and domestic herbivores, in which cutaneous, pulmonary or intestinal infection culminates in a fatal septicaemia. Man contracts the disease by coming into contact with infected animals or animal products. Anthrax is uncommon in Britain and North America, but relatively common in many other parts of the world.

Saprophytic species

The other species of *Bacillus*, e.g. *Bacillus cereus* and *Bacillus subtilis*, exist as saprophytes in soil, water, vegetation and foodstuffs. Their spores are ubiquitous, and commonly present in dust in hospitals, laboratories and other dwellings as well as out of doors. Small numbers of spores are often found contaminating clinical specimens and bacteriological cultures. The spores of some species, e.g. *B. subtilis*, are exceptionally resistant to heat, e.g. to boiling at 100°C for several hours, so that unless culture media are correctly autoclaved at 121°C for 15 min, they may become heavily contaminated due to the germination and growth of surviving spores.

Generally the presence of saprophytic species, or 'anthracoid bacilli', in cultures of clinical specimens is regarded as a contamination and of no clinical significance. Rarely, however, *B. cereus, B. subtilis* or some other species may act as an opportunistic pathogen in a debilitated or injured person, e.g. causing bacteriaemia, meningitis, endocarditis or pneumonia in cases of drug abuse, leukaemia, renal disease or immunosuppression; endophthalmitis after trauma or surgery of the eye; and meningitis after spinal anaesthesia. *B. cereus*, moreover, may cause food-poisoning after the consumption of cooked rice in which it has grown profusely and produced an enterotoxin.

BACILLUS ANTHRACIS

Morphology

Rods 4–8 × 1–1.5 μm and square-ended; arranged in chains in culture, but single or in pairs in animal's blood. Spores central, oval and non-bulging; not formed in animal tissues. Non-flagellate and non-motile. Capsule formed in the animal body, but in culture only on media with serum or bicarbonate in the presence of excess CO_2.

Staining reactions

Gram-positive, especially in tissues. Blue bacillus with irregular, purple granular surround when stained with polychrome methylene blue by McFadyean's method. Purple bacillus with red capsule when stained with Giemsa's stain. Non-acid-fast. Spores seen as unstained spaces in Gram-stained bacilli and, when free, faintly outlined with Gram counterstain.

Cultural characters

Aerobe and facultative anaerobe. Growth temperature range 12–45°C, optimum 37°C. Grows on all ordinary media. Sporulation requires aerobic conditions and is optimal at 25–30°C. Germination of spores requires fresh nutrients and aerobic conditions.

On nutrient agar, colonies are greyish, granular disks, 2–3 mm in diameter after 24 h at 37°C, with an uneven surface and wavy margin which gives them the 'medusa head' appearance. Each is a continuous, convoluted chain of bacilli and has a sticky, membranous consistency making it difficult to emulsify. Colonies of capsulate bacilli on bicarbonate media are smooth and mucoid. Colonies on blood agar produce very slight haemolysis.

In broth, growth develops as silky strands, a surface pellicle and a floccular deposit. In a gelatin stab, there is growth down the stab line with lateral spikes that are longest near the surface, giving the 'inverted fir tree' appearance; liquefaction is late and starts at the surface. Coagulated serum is partially liquefied.

Biochemical reactions

In glucose, maltose, sucrose, trehalose and dextrin, acid but not gas is formed. Nitrate is reduced to nitrite, catalase is formed and there is a weak lecithinase (egg-yolk) reaction.

Viability

In the dry state or in soil the spores may survive for many years. With moist heat, the vegetative bacilli are killed at 60°C in 30 min and the spores at 100°C in 10 min. With dry heat the spores are killed at 150°C in 60 min. The spores are also killed by 4% (w/v) formaldehyde or 4% (w/v) potassium permanganate in a few minutes.

Antibiotic sensitivity

The bacilli are sensitive to benzylpenicillin (0.02 mg/l), streptomycin (1 mg/l), tetracyclines (0.2 mg/l), chloramphenicol (5 mg/l) and sulphonamides.

Antigens

There are three main antigens observed in serological tests, the toxin complex (protein), the capsular polypeptide (of D-glutamic acid) and a somatic polysaccharide (N-acetylglucosamine and galactose).

Animal pathogenicity

Cattle, sheep, goats, pigs and other herbivores are naturally affected. Mice, guinea-pigs, rabbits, hamsters and monkeys are susceptible to experimental infection. There is usually septicaemia with marked splenic enlargement.

Other methods of identification

These include the bacteriophage susceptibility test of McCloy (1951a, 1951b) and the rapid immunofluorescence method of Cherry & Freeman (1959).

Laboratory diagnosis

In human anthrax, the bacillus is usually demonstrable in material from a malignant pustule, sometimes in sputum from pulmonary anthrax, and also in the blood in the septicaemic stage of all forms of the infection. Procedures should be carried out with the greatest care in an exhaust-ventilated safety cabinet.

Malignant pustule

The best specimen is fluid from an unbroken vesicle at the edge of the lesion. In early cases, fluid may be obtained by scraping the lesion with a needle. Take up the fluid on a swab.

1. Smear the material on two sterile slides and allow to dry. Stain one smear, unfixed, by Gram's method and the other, a thicker smear, imperfectly fixed by three rapid passes through a flame, by McFadyean's method* or with Giemsa's stain (Ch. 3). Provisionally identify as anthrax bacilli any large Gram-positive bacilli in the former smear and any blue-stained bacilli surrounded by irregular, red-purple capsular material in the latter. As spores may not be killed by the procedures of fixation and staining, stained smears must be autoclaved before being discarded.

2. Culture the exudate by plating on nutrient agar and blood agar, and also in broth. Incubate and store the cultures in a closed container, labelled 'anthrax', which can be autoclaved after use. After incubation for 18 h at 37°C, examine plates for the medusa-head colonies characteristic of *B. anthracis*. In broth, look for a pellicle and a deposit; the latter stirs up in a silky whirl when the tube is rotated.

Make films from the culture, stain by Gram's method and look for long, tangled chains of large Gram-positive bacilli, some of which have central, oval spores.

3. Confirm the identity of the culture by inoculating a small portion, e.g. 0.1 ml of 1 in 100 dilution of a broth culture, subcutaneously into a guinea-pig or mouse. Death of the animal in 24–72 h, the finding of many bacilli in the heart blood and spleen, and the post-mortem appearances are diagnostic of anthrax.

Perform the post-mortem examination with precautions to avoid contamination of the environment. Lay the animal on its back and peg it out on aluminium foil. Open the abdomen and chest and look for the characteristic appearances of anthrax: gelatinous, haemorrhagic oedema at the site of inoculation, petechial haemorrhages in the peritoneum, black blood slowly clotting when shed, and an enlarged, dark red spleen. Make smears from the heart blood and spleen, stain by Gram's and McFadyean's methods, and look for the large, typically stained bacilli, i.e.

blue bacilli surrounded by irregular, red-purple capsular material, some of which may be detached from the bacteria, in the McFadyean smear. Finally, wrap the foil round the animal, place the whole in an impervious pack and incinerate the pack.

Pulmonary anthrax

1. Collect sputum. Stain a film by Gram's method and examine for large Gram-positive bacilli. Culture the sputum on plates of nutrient agar, blood agar and Knisely's (1966)* selective medium and look for large, medusa-head colonies.

2. Make a blood culture by adding 5–8 ml of patient's blood to a broth medium for aerobic bacteria, incubate and then subculture on to a blood agar plate.

Diagnosis in domestic animals post mortem

Do not make the usual kind of post-mortem examination, for it is essential to avoid disseminating bacilli into the environment. Sporulation does not take place in the body, but the bacilli spore readily when exposed to air. (1) Prepare films of blood taken from a superficial vein in the ear, stain by Gram's and McFadyean's methods and look for the characteristic (non-sporing) bacilli. (2) Culture some of the blood on a nutrient agar plate and look for typical colonies.

Isolation of B. anthracis from contaminated materials

Special methods are required for the examination of materials, such as hide, hair, tissue and bone meal, that may be heavily contaminated with other kinds of bacteria. A 'wash' of the material is examined by culture and animal inoculation.

1. Prepare a 'wash' by shaking, e.g. 25 g of the material in 100 ml sterile water and allowing it to soak with occasional further shaking for 3 h. Allow the solid material to settle.

2. Collect the supernatant fluid and heat it for 10 min at 70°C to kill all non-spored organisms.

---

* Refer to *Methods* at end of this chapter.

3. Prepare several two- or four-fold dilutions of the heated fluid.

4. Culture each dilution by the pour-plate method in the unselective Yeastrel-peptone agar of Green & Jamieson (1958) or by spreading on a plate of selective medium, e.g. that of Pearce & Powell (1951), Morris (1955), Gillissen & Scholz (1961) or Knisely (1966)*. After 24 h at 37°C, look for characteristic colonies.

5. Provisionally identify suspect colonies by making a stab culture in the inner tube of a Craigie 'tube' (Ch. 29, *Methods*) containing semi-solid nutrient agar and incubating overnight at 37°C. *B. anthracis* appears as a fine, feathery growth down the length of the stab. Most other species of *Bacillus* are motile and therefore migrate through the agar and appear on the surface outside the inner tube. Confirm the identity of the culture by inoculating a small portion of it subcutaneously in a guinea-pig or mouse.

6. Also attempt to isolate *B. anthracis* by direct inoculation of the heat-treated 'wash' into an animal. Centrifuge the 'wash' for 15 min at about 1500 *g*, discard the supernate and inoculate the sediment intramuscularly into a guinea-pig that has been passively immunized 24 h previously with *Clostridium perfringens* antitoxin 1000 units, *C. septicum* antitoxin 500 units, *C. novyi* antitoxin 1000 units and tetanus antitoxin 1000 units, or into a mouse immunized with one-third these amounts of antitoxins. Death due to anthrax occurs in 2–3 days and a post-mortem examination will reveal the appearances described above for tests of cultures. Death may occur within 24 h from gas-gangrene caused by contaminating clostridial spores, but aerobic cultures made from the blood, spleen or injection site may still yield a few colonies of *B. anthracis*.

Isolation of B. anthracis from soil

The method of Manchee et al (1981) is recommended. Shake 10 g of soil in 10 ml of sterile water or 0.1 mol/litre phosphate buffer solution (pH 7.0) for 30 min, or on an orbital shaker at 300 r.p.m. for 3 min. Then heat for 60 min at 60°C to kill vegetative organisms. Allow the larger particles to settle, or remove them by filtration, and spread 0.2 ml volumes of the supernate or filtrate, and of several two-fold dilutions of it, on to each of five surface-dried plates of Knisely's selective medium* and incubate for 24 h at 37°C. Identify any colonies by film, stab subculture and either animal inoculation or the in-vitro McFadyean reaction*.

Serological diagnosis

It is not always possible to isolate *B. anthracis* from patients with cutaneous anthrax. The presence in patient's serum of antibodies to the anthrax toxin may be demonstrated by a gel diffusion test (Thorne & Belton 1957) or an in-vivo neutralization test in the rabbit (Darlow et al 1956). Antibodies are rarely found in uncomplicated cases of cutaneous anthrax, but these patients tend to develop antibodies after a single subsequent dose of anthrax vaccine instead of after three doses as in individuals with no history of anthrax (Darlow & Pride 1969).

OTHER SPECIES OF BACILLUS

For detailed differential features of the many saprophytic species of *Bacillus*, reference can be made to Bergey's Manual (Buchanan & Gibbons 1974). Some features of the commoner species, compared with those of *B. anthracis*, are shown in Table 24.1.

Morphology and staining

Large-celled species (width >0.9 μm), e.g. *B. cereus*, resemble *B. anthracis* except in that they are motile; they often contain unstained lipid granules. Other species, e.g. *B. subtilis*, are shorter and thinner (<0.9 μm) and have rounded ends. Most species are Gram-positive and form a single, centrally situated oval spore that does not bulge the containing bacillus. Some species, e.g. *B. polymyxa* and *B. stearothermophilus*, are Gram-variable and have bulging spores which may be situated centrally or terminally.

Table 24.1 Some differential features of species of *Bacillus*.
Key: Spore, C, central; T, terminal; ST, subterminal. Egg yolk reaction, +, wide zone of opacity around colony; ±, narrow zone of opacity just wider than colony; −, no zone of opacity.

Species classified by size of bacilli	Motility	Capsule	Spore	Pathogenicity for mouse	Optimum temp. for growth (°C)	Anaerobic growth	Egg yolk reaction
a. Large celled, 2–8 × 1–1.5 μm							
B. anthracis	−	+	C	High	35	+	±
B. cereus	+	−	C	Low	30	+	+
B. cereus var. *mycoides*	+	−	C	Low	30	+	+
B. megaterium	+	+/−	C	Low	35	−	−
b. Small celled, 1.5–5 × 0.5–0.8 μm							
B. subtilis	+	−	C	None	37	−	−
B. pumilis	+	−	C	None	37	−	−
B. licheniformis	+	−	C	None	37	+	−
B. polymyxa[a]	+	−	C/ST	None	35	+	−
B. stearothermophilus[a]	+	−	T	None	55	+/−	−

[a] Bacilli Gram-variable and distended by bulging, oval spores.

Cultural characters

Most species have an optimum temperature for growth between 30 and 37°C, but some are thermophilic, having an optimum temperature about 55°C and growing poorly, if at all, at 37°C, e.g. *B. stearothermophilus*. All species grow aerobically; some are facultative anaerobes, but others fail to grow anaerobically (Table 24.1). Most species grow profusely on all the ordinary culture media. Colonies are usually large, e.g. 2–5 mm in diameter, dull and greyish-white, and have an irregular edge and surface. Those of *B. cereus* usually resemble those of *B. anthracis*, though their edge is less wavy. Those of *B. cereus* var. *mycoides* are rhizoid and spreading. *B. subtilis* colonies may be irregular, spreading, or circular and smooth. Strains of *B. subtilis* and *B. licheniformis* that form a red pigment are sometimes called *B. globigi*. Colonies on MacConkey agar are pale, as most strains fail to ferment lactose. *B. cereus* colonies produce haemolysis on blood agar.

Egg yolk reaction

B. cereus and *B. anthracis* are distinguished from other species because they form a phospholipase that splits lecithin in egg yolk; their colonies on egg yolk agar* become surrounded by a circular zone of opacity in 1–5 days at 37°C (McGaughey & Chu 1948). The activity of *B. anthracis* is much weaker than that of *B. cereus*.

Animal pathogenicity

The saprophytic species are usually non-pathogenic on inoculation into laboratory animals, but *B. cereus* and *B. megaterium* may kill mice and guinea-pigs when injected intraperitoneally in large doses; in such cases, however, they do not give the appearances of anthrax infection or evidence of capsulated bacilli in the blood.

Laboratory diagnosis

The finding of a saprophytic species of *Bacillus* ('anthracoid bacilli') in a culture from a clinical specimen generally indicates that the culture or specimen has been contaminated from the environment, and it should not be reported, but in debilitated, traumatized or immunosuppressed patients, the possibility of an opportunistic infection should be considered. A pathogenic role would be suggested by the finding of bacilli in repeated blood cultures or in a fluid, e.g.

cerebrospinal fluid or aqueous humour, from a closed site not accessible to contamination from the environment. The finding of numerous bacilli in a film of sputum or wound exudate might also justify reporting the presence of the organism with its antibiotic sensitivities.

BACILLUS CEREUS FOOD-POISONING

This condition should be suspected in patients suffering from the onset of vomiting or diarrhoea within a few hours after eating cooked rice prepared in a commercial establishment. *B. cereus* may be cultured from the patient's faeces or vomit, or from an unconsumed portion of food. Large, irregular, pale colonies would be seen in a plating of faeces or vomit on MacConkey agar. *B. cereus* does not grow on deoxycholate citrate agar (DCA).

B. cereus in food

A quantitative method should be used in examining rice, milk or other food suspected of causing *B. cereus* food-poisoning. The causal role of the bacilli is indicated only if large numbers of them are found in the food, e.g. 10^8/g, for small numbers are commonly present as harmless contaminants.

1. Add 20 g rice to 180 ml quarter-strength Ringer's solution (Ch. 5) and mix in a 'Stomacher' (Seward) to obtain a 1 in 10 suspension.
2. Mix 10 ml of the suspension with 90 ml quarter-strength Ringer to obtain a 1 in 100 suspension, and repeat the dilution to obtain a 1 in 1000 suspension.
3. By the Miles and Misra technique (Ch. 12), inoculate three 0.02 ml drops of each dilution of the suspension on to plates of blood agar, milk agar (Ch. 16) and phenol-red egg-yolk poly-myxin agar.* Incubate for 48 h at 37°C.
4. Count the *B. cereus*-like colonies. On the phenol-red egg yolk polymyxin agar, *B. cereus* forms pink colonies surrounded by a large zone of pink opalescence in the medium. Identify pure subcultures and calculate the number of bacilli or spores per g of rice.

METHODS

McFadyean's stain

1. Make a fairly thick smear of blood, exudate or tissue fluid, dry in air and fix imperfectly by passing quickly three times through a flame. (The method is not applicable to cultures, except cultures in blood, see below.)
2. Stain with polychrome methylene blue (Ch. 3) for 30 s. Wash and dry.

Irregular pink-purple capsular material, both surrounding the blue-stained bacilli and some detached from them, is indicative of anthrax.

In-vitro McFadyean test

The McFadyean reaction is usually demonstrated in smears of blood or other material collected from a naturally or experimentally infected animal, but when large numbers of isolates have to be tested for identification as *B. anthracis*, the use of animals is inconvenient and expensive, and a simple, reliable in-vitro test should be used. Material from a colony of the isolate is inoculated into a tube containing a few millilitres of sterile heparinized horse blood and incubated for 6 h at 37°C. A smear of the blood culture material is then fixed by heat and stained with polychrome methylene blue as described above. The capsular material giving the characteristic reaction is formed and apparent in such blood cultures, though not in conventionally grown cultures.

Knisely's (1966) medium

This plating medium is selective for anthrax bacilli, inhibiting the growth of most strains of *B. cereus* and other *Bacillus* species, entero-bacteria and pseudomonads.

Heart infusion agar (Difco)	40 g
Thallous acetate	0.04 g
Disodium ethylenediamine-tetraacetate (EDTA)	0.3 g
Polymyxin	30 000 units
Lysozyme	0.04 g
Deionized water	1 litre

Dissolve the first three components in the

water with steaming, autoclave for 15 min at 121°C, cool to about 60°C and add the polymyxin and lysozyme in small volumes of solutions. Pour plates and dry their surfaces. The pH should be 7.35.

Phenol-red egg-yolk polymyxin agar

This medium (Baker et al 1980) is relatively selective for *B. cereus*. The colonies are recognized by their production of opacity in the egg yolk in the medium and their pink colouration with phenol red, showing their failure to ferment mannitol.

Peptone	10 g
Meat extract	1 g
Mannitol	10 g
Sodium chloride	10 g
Phenol red	0.025 g
Agar	15 g
Egg yolk emulsion	100 ml

Polymyxin B sulphate	0.01 g
Deionized water	1 litre

Dissolve the first six components in the water with mixing and steaming. Cool to about 60°C, dispense in 90 ml volumes into bottles and sterilize for 15 min at 121°C. The pH should be 7.2 exactly. When required for use, melt a 90 ml volume, cool to 50°C, add 10 ml of egg yolk emulsion and 1 ml of aqueous 1% (w/v) polymyxin B sulphate and pour plates.

Egg yolk agar

Prepare a 5% (w/v) suspension of egg yolk in nutrient broth, add 2 g kieselguhr per 100 ml, filter through paper pulp and sterilize by Seitz EK filtration. Add to an equal volume of nutrient agar containing a double-normal concentration of agar at 50°C and pour plates. Alternatively add 0.5 or 1 ml sterile commercial egg yolk emulsion to nutrient agar at 50°C, add 1% (w/v) NaCl and pour a plate.

REFERENCES

Baker F J, Breach M R, Leighton I, Taylor P 1980 Medical microbiological techniques. Butterworth, London. p 495

Buchanan R E, Gibbons N E 1974 Bergey's manual of determinative bacteriology 8th edn. Williams & Wilkins, Baltimore, p 529–550

Cherry W B, Freeman, E M 1959 Staining bacterial smears with fluorescent antibody. V The rapid identification of *Bacillus anthracis* in culture and in human and marine tissue. Zentralblatt für Bakteriologie (Orig A) 175: 582–604

Darlow H M, Belton F C, Henderson D W 1956 The use of anthrax antigen to immunize man and monkey. Lancet 2: 476–479

Darlow H M, Pride N B 1969 Serological diagnosis of anthrax. Lancet 2: 430

Gillissen G, Scholtz, H G 1961 Die Selektion von Milzbrandbazillen aus Flussigkerten mit Storker Verunreinigung durch *E. coli*. Zentralblatt für Bakteriologie (Orig A) 182: 232–236

Green D M, Jamieson W M 1958 Anthrax and bone meal fertilizer. Lancet 2: 153–154

Knisely R F 1966 Selective medium for *Bacillus anthracis*. Journal of Bacteriology 92: 784–786

McCloy E W 1951a Studies on a lysogenic bacillus strain. I A bacteriophage specific for *B. anthracis*. Journal of Hygiene, Cambridge 49: 114–125

McCloy E W 1951b Unusual behaviour of a lysogenic bacillus strain. Journal of General Microbiology 5:xiv (Proceedings, April 1951)

McGaughey C A, Chu H P 1948 The egg-yolk reactions of aerobic sporing bacilli. Journal of General Microbiology 2: 334–340

Manchee R J, Broster M G, Melling J, Henstridge R M, Stagg A J 1981 *Bacillus anthracis* on Gruinard Island Nature 294: 254–255

Morris E J 1955 A selective medium for *Bacillus anthracis*. Journal of General Microbiology 13: 456–460

Pearce T W, Powell E O 1951 A selective medium for *Bacillus anthracis*. Journal of General Microbiology 5: 387–390

Thorne C B, Belton F C 1957 An agar diffusion method for titrating *Bacillus anthracis* immunizing antigen and its application to a study of antigen production. Journal of General Microbiology 17: 505–516

Mycobacterium: tubercle bacilli

The genus *Mycobacterium* comprises the 'acid-fast bacilli', which are difficult to stain, but once stained resist decolourization with acid and alcohol. They are Gram positive, but some species are poorly coloured even after prolonged staining. They include the organisms of human tuberculosis, *Mycobacterium tuberculosis*, bovine tuberculosis, *M. bovis*, and avian tuberculosis, *M. avium*, and that of leprosy, *M. leprae*, which is not fully acid- and alcohol-fast.

The commoner species are classified in two groups: (1) the typical tubercle bacilli, *M. tuberculosis* and *M. bovis*, and (2) the atypical mycobacteria, including commensal, saprophytic and opportunistically pathogenic species. The term 'atypical' is not satisfactory, and other terms in use are anonymous, non-tuberculous or opportunist mycobacteria, and tuberculoid bacilli, of which the last seems the most appropriate. The typical, mammalian tubercle bacilli are described in this chapter, the tuberculoid and leprosy bacilli in Chapter 26.

M. TUBERCULOSIS AND M. BOVIS

Morphology and staining

Typically, the human tubercle bacilli are slender, straight or slightly curved rods which may show beading. Their size is generally about 3 × 0.3 μm, but varies with the cultural conditions. They are non-motile, non-sporing and non-capsulate. They remain uncoloured with simple stains, but show acid-fast staining with warm carbol fuchsin followed by 20% H_2SO_4 or by 3% HCl in 95% ethanol (Ziehl-Neelsen method,

Ch. 3). Bovine tubercle bacilli tend to be shorter and thicker than the human type.

Cultural characters

The tubercle bacillus is an obligate aerobe and grows at temperatures from 30–41°C, optimally at 35–37°C. Although primary isolation may be successful on a variety of media, only Löwenstein-Jensen with glycerol or sodium pyruvate* can be recommended. After several subcultures, the bacillus will grow in a simple salt solution with glycerol and asparagine.

Incubated at 37°C, growth on Löwenstein-Jensen medium is slow, so that colonies are not visible before 2–3 weeks. Incubation of negative slopes is continued for 6–8 weeks before discarding. *M. tuberculosis* colonies on LJ are rough, buff to yellowish in colour, and tough when picked off (eugonic growth). A bit of colony floated on to the surface of glycerol broth grows as a whitish wrinkled pellicle and granular deposit. Dispersed, uniform growth can be obtained by subculturing two or three times in Dubos and Davis liquid medium containing Tween 80 (polyoxyethylene sorbitan mono-oleate).* The addition of glycerol to Löwenstein-Jensen medium improves the growth of *M. tuberculosis*, but not that of *M. bovis*. Sodium pyruvate, on the other hand, increases the growth of *M. bovis* and some strains of drug-resistant *M. tuberculosis*.

M. bovis grows very slowly on Löwenstein-Jensen, taking 3 or more weeks to become

* Refer to *Methods* at end of this chapter.

visible as tiny transparent colonies which later become white. Growth is poor even when confluent (dysgonic growth). Pyruvate improves the growth of *M. bovis* over that on glycerol medium. Indeed, some strains will not grow in primary culture on Löwenstein-Jensen with glycerol.

Sensitivity to physical and chemical agents

Tubercle bacilli are killed by heat at 60°C in 15–20 min. They survive for many weeks in moist conditions in the dark and many days when dried in sputum smeared on clothing and in dust. They are killed fairly rapidly by sunlight and daylight, even through glass. They are relatively resistant to chemical disinfectants; e.g. sputum may require several hours' exposure to 5% phenol for disinfection. Specimens and cultures should be autoclaved before disposal. The organism is normally sensitive to a wide range of drugs, e.g. isoniazid, rifampicin and ethambutol.

Biochemical reactions

The tubercle bacilli are catalase positive. They do not produce acid in sugar-containing media. Biochemical tests are generally not used in their routine identification, but a variety of tests are employed for their definitive identification and that of the atypical mycobacteria, e.g. see Tables 25.1 and 26.1.

Antigenic characters

The human and bovine species cannot be distinguished antigenically, nor can the former be subdivided serologically. *M. avium* (Ch. 26) can be identified and divided into subtypes by serology (Birn et al 1967).

Phage-typing

In recent years the phage-typing of mycobacteria has progressed to the point where it is possible to identify several phage groups of *M. tuberculosis*, including types A, B and C (Redmond et al 1979). The method may make it possible to demonstrate the case-to-case spread of infection. It is also possible to identify certain mycobacteria by phage. For example, BCG may be identified by its resistance to phage 33D (Grange et al 1976; Grange & Redmond 1978).

Animal pathogenicity

The guinea-pig is highly susceptible to experimental infection with both *M. tuberculosis* and *M. bovis*, even in doses of as few as 10 bacilli. After subcutaneous injection of an infected specimen, a local swelling appears within a few days, which proceeds to caseate and finally ulcerate; neighbouring and, later, more distant lymph nodes become infected and swollen; the infection then spreads to produce yellowish tubercles, mostly 1–2 mm in diameter, in the spleen, liver and peritoneum, but few in the lungs and kidneys. The animal dies usually in 6–15 weeks. Mice are much less susceptible, but after intraperitoneal injection of a large dose of bacilli develop progressive generalized infection.

Rabbits are much less susceptible to *M. tuberculosis* than to *M. bovis*. After the intra-

Table 25.1 Distinguishing characters of tubercle bacilli.

Character	M. tuberculosis	M. bovis	M. africanum	BCG
Colonial growth on egg medium	Eugonic	Dysgonic	Dysgonic	Eugonic
Growth on PNB medium	−	−	−	−
Growth on TCH medium	+	−	−	−
Niacin production	+	−	+/−	−
Growth in semi-solid agar	Aerobic	Microaerophilic	Microaerophilic	Aerobic
Sensitivity to pyrazinamide	+	−	+	−
Nitrate reduction	+	−	±	−

Notes. (1) Refer to the *Methods* section of this chapter for the media and methods of the tests, except for those of the pyrazinamide test, which are given in the section on antibiotic sensitivities. (2) *M. africanum* gives a weak nitrate reduction reaction. Eugonic: abundant wrinkled growth. Dysgonic: poor flat growth.

venous injection of a suspension of 0.01–0.1 mg of surface growth from solid medium, *M. bovis* causes acute generalized tuberculosis, fatal usually in 3–6 weeks, whilst *M. tuberculosis* causes a chronic, often non-fatal infection with a few macroscopic lesions in the lungs and kidneys. But animal inoculation is rarely used nowadays for differentiation of the human from the bovine bacillus.

Monkeys, dogs and cats may be infected naturally with the human bacillus; cattle, monkeys, pigs, dogs, cats and badgers with the bovine bacillus; and cattle and pigs with the avian bacillus.

LABORATORY DIAGNOSIS

Diagnosis is generally done by demonstrating the presence of tubercle bacilli in a clinical specimen. The procedures for such demonstration will be described in detail. The value and limitations of serological diagnosis by the demonstration of antibodies to mycobacteria and those of demonstrating cell-mediated immunity by the tuberculin test will be described subsequently.

The specimen most commonly examined for the presence of tubercle bacilli is sputum, the processing of which will be described in detail. Other specimens are handled in the laboratory in broadly the same manner, so only the variations will be detailed.

The quality of the specimen is of particular importance in the examination for mycobacteria. When a patient is said to have purulent sputum and a specimen of saliva or mucoid material is received, another, better specimen should be requested. It is standard practice to examine several specimens of sputum or early morning urine taken from the patient on different days before accepting the result of the investigation as negative. Specimens of urine collected over 24 h are no longer considered necessary. Samples of pus are always preferable to swabs.

Methods for demonstration of tubercle bacilli

Three main methods are used to detect tubercle bacilli in sputum and other materials:

(1) microscopic examination for acid-fast bacilli in a Ziehl-Neelsen-stained or fluorochrome-stained film of unconcentrated or concentrated material; (2) culture on egg medium after decontamination and concentration; and (3) inoculation into a guinea-pig.

Microscopic examination has the advantage of giving a result at once, but is likely to be successful only if large numbers of bacilli are present, e.g. 10^5/ml or greater. The bacilli are more likely to be seen in smears of concentrated material than in direct smears of the original specimen. Culture and guinea-pig inoculation are much more sensitive methods and may detect as few as 10 bacilli/ml, but owing to the slow growth of the organism, give their results only after several weeks. Cultural isolation is necessary if species identification and drug-sensitivity tests are to be carried out.

Significance of findings

As tubercle bacilli are not found as commensals or in healthy carriers, their demonstration and identification in a specimen is diagnostic of tuberculosis. But the demonstration of acid- and alcohol-fast bacilli without species identification is not thus diagnostic, for other kinds of acid- and alcohol-fast bacilli are sometimes present. Urine specimens, in particular, may contain commensal *M. smegmatis* derived from the skin around the urethral orifice. Some strains of these smegma bacilli can be distinguished from tubercle bacilli because, though acid-fast, they are not also alcohol-fast. Other strains are both acid-fast and alcohol-fast and thus indistinguishable in morphology from tubercle bacilli. Fortunately, however, saprophytic or commensal mycobacteria are seldom found in sputum, so that the demonstration of acid-fast bacilli in sputum gives a fairly strong indication of the presence of pulmonary tuberculosis although in a few cases these bacilli may be tuberculoid, rather than tubercle bacilli.

Sputum

Sputum should be examined microscopically, firstly in a direct smear made from the untreated specimen and then again in a smear made from the centrifuged, concentrated deposit obtained after the specimen has been treated and homogenized by Petroff's* or other equivalent method. The smears should be stained by either the Ziehl-Neelsen or the fluorochrome method. The latter method facilitates the finding of scanty bacilli and saves time when numerous, mostly negative smears have to be examined, but until experience has been gained, any positive findings should be confirmed by Ziehl-Neelsen staining. The area of the smear showing the fluorescent bacilli can be marked and the smear then overstained by the Ziehl-Neelsen method.

Ziehl-Neelsen smear

1. Prepare a smear on a new slide from a purulent or mucopurulent portion of the sputum. A sterile swab may be used to make the smear if the sputum is thick and tenacious. Fix the smear by flaming.

2. Stain the fixed smear by the Ziehl-Neelsen method, using acid-alcohol as the decolourizer (Ch. 3). Dry with fresh blotting paper.

3. Examine the stained smear with the × 100 oil immersion lens for the presence of acid-fast (red-stained) bacilli on a background of non-acid-fast (blue-stained) material. If the background material is red-stained, the smear has not been properly decolourized and should be replaced by another. Continue the search for 10 min before accepting a smear as negative.

4. Make and stain a second smear from the deposit after concentration of the specimen by Petroff's method and repeat the examination.

Fluorochrome smear

1. Make and fix a smear of sputum as described for Ziehl-Neelsen staining. Stain it with auramine O and decolourize it with acid-alcohol (Ch. 3).

2. Using a microscope with an ultraviolet illuminant (e.g. a 200 W mercury vapour lamp or a quartz iodine lamp), scan the stained smear with a × 10 objective lens for the presence of bright yellow fluorescing bacilli. Confirm their presence with a × 40 objective.

3. Make and stain a second smear from the deposit after concentration of the specimen by Petroff's method and repeat the examination.

Avoidance of false findings

Care must be taken to avoid false-positive results from any of the following causes. (1) The transfer of stained bacilli to a negative smear by blotting paper used previously to dry a positive smear. Fresh blotting paper should be used for each smear. (2) The persistence of stained bacilli on a slide previously bearing a positive smear and reused after cleaning for a smear from a negative specimen. As it is scarcely possible to ensure that all bacilli are cleaned off a previously used slide, a *new* slide should be used for every specimen. (3) The spilling or spurting of material from a positive smear on to an adjacent area of the same slide used to make a negative smear. Smears of more than one specimen should not be made on the same slide. (4) The contamination of immersion oil on the microscope lens with stained bacilli detached from a previously examined smear. (5) Contamination with saprophytic acid-fast bacilli growing in a cold water tap when tap water is used to dilute material being smeared on a slide.

Report of microscopic findings

Because acid- and alcohol-fast bacilli in sputum occasionally are not tubercle bacilli, report positive findings on the following lines: 'Acid-fast bacilli morphologically resembling tubercle bacilli were seen in film. Cultures for tubercle bacilli have been set up and will be reported later.'

Culture on Löwenstein-Jensen medium

Specimens of sputum are always contaminated with numerous non-acid-fast commensal bacteria from the mouth and throat. These commensals grow much more quickly than tubercle bacilli so that if untreated sputum were inoculated on to a culture medium, their earlier growth would obscure or prevent the growth of tubercle bacilli. Before culture, therefore, sputa and other potentially contaminated specimens must be decontaminated by a procedure such as Petroff's, which kills non-acid-fast, but not acid-fast bacteria. The optimal medium for tubercle bacilli is Löwenstein-Jensen's solidified egg medium with glycerol (for *M. tuberculosis*) or pyruvate (for *M. bovis*). As tubercle bacilli are obligate aerobes, their cultures are grown on the surface of a slope of medium in a bottle also containing sufficient air to provide oxygen for their respiration. The bottle is kept sealed with a tightly applied screw cap to prevent the medium drying up during the long period of incubation.

1. Treat the specimen by Petroff's method* to decontaminate and homogenize it and concentrate the bacilli in a centrifuged deposit.

2. With a sterile swab, inoculate the deposit over the surface of a slope of Löwenstein-Jensen medium plus glycerol* and a second slope of Löwenstein-Jensen medium plus sodium pyruvate*. Cap the slopes tightly and incubate at 37°C.

3. Examine the slopes weekly for the appearance of growth. If abundant growth appears within the first week, or growth unlike that of tubercle bacilli, the culture is probably contaminated with a commensal mycobacterium, e.g. *M. smegmatis*, or a spore-forming bacillus that has survived the decontamination procedure. The morphology of the organism should be checked in a Ziehl-Neelsen smear, the contaminated culture discarded and culture for tubercle bacilli repeated on a fresh specimen. That contaminating mycobacteria are saprophytes may be confirmed by their rapid growth in subcultures, even on plain nutrient agar; and many are strongly pigmented.

4. Continue incubating negative cultures for 6–8 weeks before discarding.

5. Identify and report as 'a *Mycobacterium* species' any growth found in a Ziehl-Neelsen smear to consist of acid-fast bacilli. If the growth appears only after 2–3 weeks and resembles that of *M. tuberculosis* or *M. bovis*, report as 'Growth of a mycobacterium resembling the tubercle bacillus. Its identity and drug sensitivities will be reported later.'

6. Set up identification and sensitivity tests as described below or, preferably, send the culture

to a reference laboratory where these tests are done on a regular basis.

Inoculation into guinea-pig

Because modern methods of culture are so efficacious, inoculation of sputum into animals is now rarely indicated. When a first specimen gives negative results in culture, repeat specimens are readily obtained. If, however, inoculation of sputum or other specimen into animals is required, proceed as follows.

1. Decontaminate and concentrate the sputum by Petroff's method.* Draw up 0.5 ml of the neutralized, centrifuged deposit into a syringe. Discard the needle and fit a fresh one to minimize contamination of the animal's coat during injection and the probability of producing a discharging sore at the injection site.

2. Inject the material intraperitoneally into a guinea-pig. Alternatively, the injection may be made intramuscularly in the thigh, but this mode of inoculation may lead to the formation of a local abscess which later may ulcerate and discharge tubercle bacilli into the environment, with the risk of infecting attendants.

3. Examine the animal regularly, preferably every day but at least every few days. Wear protective clothing and gloves while doing so. As soon as signs of disease are present, e.g after 3–4 weeks, kill the animal. The earlier the animal is killed in the course of its infection the less likely it will be to disseminate tubercle bacilli into the environment, e.g. in its urine after involvement of the kidneys.

It is an advantage of intramuscular inoculation that the palpation of the local abscess or the swollen draining lymph node in the groin makes possible the earlier recognition of infection than after intraperitoneal inoculation.

4. If the guinea-pig remains apparently well, kill it at 6 weeks by exposure in a closed 'desiccator' jar on a wire mesh over a cotton-wool pad soaked in chloroform. Then perform a necropsy to detect any tuberculous lesions. Autoclave the vacated cage and bedding before cleaning and disposal.

5. *Necropsy.* The general methods are described in Chapter 14. For safety, wear a gown and

rubber gloves and perform the necropsy in a class 1 exhaust protective safety cabinet. Through its extended limbs, pin the animal on its back to a wooden board covered with a sheet of aluminium foil (for safe disposal) and then one of absorbent paper tissue (to soak up spilled blood). With scissors, cut the ventral skin from pubis to neck and with strong toothed forceps pull the skin edges apart to expose the abdominal and thoracic walls. With fresh sterile scissors, cut the muscular abdominal wall from pubis to sternum, then the thoracic cage up both sides of the sternum. Inspect the lungs, liver, spleen and kidneys for yellowish-white tubercles, 1–2 mm in diameter, and look for any enlarged abdominal lymph nodes. Tubercles are most likely to be seen in an enlarged spleen lying behind the stomach, and then in the liver. Cut out small portions of the tubercle-containing tissues and any enlarged lymph nodes and place these in separate sterile containers for transport to the laboratory.

Finally, look for a lesion, usually an abscess, at the site of inoculation. Dissect it out with care to avoid spilling pus and transfer it to a container for transport to the laboratory. Unpin the animal and wrap it in the paper tissue and aluminium foil, and place it in a plastic bag before taking it to the autoclave or incinerator for safe disposal. Sterilize instruments in a strong disinfectant, e.g. 20% lysol, or bag them for autoclaving.

If all the animal's tissues appear normal and tubercle-free to the naked eye, samples are not taken for filming and culturing. If, however, the animal has died spontaneously from a suspected intercurrent infection, identify the pathogen by culturing heart blood and portions of spleen and other tissues on blood agar and in cooked meat.

6. In the laboratory, make and examine Ziehl-Neelsen smears from the tissue samples to confirm the infection is with acid-fast bacilli and not *Pasteurella pseudotuberculosis*, salmonella, brucella or other pathogen causing a chronic, tuberculosis-like infection.

7. If direct culture from the sputum has failed, set up cultures from one of the samples of infected tissue. Store other samples from the same animal at −20°C in case culture from the chosen sample fails. Crush an infected lymph node or portion of tissue containing a tubercle against the wall of the container and, with a sterile swab, rub some of the crushed material over slopes of Löwenstein-Jensen medium. As the infected tissue is unlikely to be contaminated with commensal bacteria, decontamination by Petroff's method is unnecessary, but some of the material should be inoculated on aerobic and anaerobic blood agar plates to confirm the absence of contaminants.

Other specimens

Where sputum is absent or, if present, is being swallowed, material for culture may be obtained by a laryngeal swab, gastric lavage, bronchial lavage or bronchoscopy.

Laryngeal swab

The swab is borne on a wire about 20 cm long and 1.5 mm in diameter, bent at an angle of 120° about 3 cm from swab-bearing end. It is contained in a large, plugged tube and is sterilized by autoclaving.

1. Immediately before use, moisten the swab with sterile distilled water.

2. While the patient is seated and holding his tongue fully protruded with the help of a piece of gauze, pass the swab back through the mouth in the mid-line and downwards over the epiglottis into the larynx, where it should induce reflex coughing that will expel sputum on to the swab. The operator should take care not to be in the line of the cough spray.

3. Withdraw the swab and replace it in its tube for delivery to the laboratory.

4. In the laboratory, add enough 5% oxalic acid to the tube to cover the swab and leave it at room temperature for 30 min to kill non-acid-fast contaminants.

5. Squeeze the swab against the side of the tube to remove excess fluid. Then rub it over the surface of two slopes of Löwenstein-Jensen medium and incubate the slopes.

Gastric lavage

1. In the morning, before the patient has

eaten, but after a bout of coughing and swallowing, aspirate the fasting stomach contents with a Ryle tube.

2. At once neutralize the specimen by adding 4% sodium hydroxide until the colour of a little added indicator dye shows that the pH is about 7. If there is any delay in examining an unneutralized specimen, tubercle bacilli may be killed by the gastric acid.

Alternatively, place 15 ml gastric washings in a 25 ml bottle containing 5 ml of 15% trisodium phosphate, which will neutralize the acid; then cap and shake the bottle.

3. In the laboratory, homogenize and decontaminate the specimen by Petroff's method.* Centrifuge and examine the deposit in a Ziehl-Neelsen film and by culture on Löwenstein-Jensen medium.

Bronchoscopic specimens

When a bronchoscope, e.g. a flexible fibreoptic bronchoscope, is used for inspection of the bronchial tract and the collection of specimens, the instrument must be thoroughly disinfected between successive patients to prevent the transmission of mycobacteria. Vigorous mechanical cleaning followed by immersion for 30 min in 2% freshly activated alkaline glutaraldehyde (pH 8.0–8.5), e.g. Cidex (Surgikos), is recommended (Davis et al, 1984).

Urine

Special caution must be exercised in interpreting the finding of mycobacteria in urine, for samples may be contaminated with commensal *M. smegmatis* from the urethral orifice. The use of alcohol as well as acid for the decolourization of Ziehl-Neelsen films may be helpful in excluding the contaminants which, though acid-fast, are commonly decolourized by the alcohol. But in some specimens, the smegma bacilli resemble tubercle bacilli in being both acid- and alcohol-fast. The finding of such bacilli in a film of urine should therefore be reported in cautious terms, e.g. 'Film showed acid- and alcohol-fast bacilli which may be either tubercle bacilli or commensal mycobacteria. Cultures for tubercle

bacilli have been set up and will be reported later.'

In cultures on Löwenstein-Jensen medium, smegma bacilli are distinguished from tubercle bacilli by their faster growth. They usually give abundant wrinkled or smooth, creamy white or buff-coloured growth within 2–4 days, whilst a growth of tubercle bacilli is rarely visible before 10 days. Cultures should therefore be examined after 4–7 days to detect those contaminated with smegma bacilli.

If facilities for animal inoculation are available, it is helpful to inoculate the deposit from any urine showing acid- and alcohol-fast bacilli into a guinea-pig, so that the pathogenicity of the mycobacteria may be known as soon as possible.

Three or more early morning specimens of urine should be taken from the patient in preference to a 24 h collection. Each specimen should consist of about 40 ml distributed in two 25 ml Universal bottles.

1. Centrifuge the specimens as received in the Universal bottles at 1500 g for 30 min. Remove the supernatant liquid with a pipette and discard it gently into disinfectant. Pool the centrifuged deposits.

2. Treat the pooled deposit by Petroff's method.

3. Prepare and examine a Ziehl-Neelsen film of it.

4. Inoculate drops of deposit on to Löwenstein-Jensen slopes.

If the extra work can be done, it is preferable to culture each specimen separately, for if any one pooled specimen is contaminated the results for all will be lost.

Pleural and peritoneal fluids

As tubercle bacilli are usually scanty, a large specimen, e.g. 50–100 ml, should be obtained.

1. Centrifuge as large a volume as possible. Examine for contaminating bacteria or pathogens other than tubercle bacilli in a Gram film and blood agar culture from the deposit.

2. If the blood agar culture is sterile, inoculate drops of the deposit on to two Löwenstein-Jensen slopes, one with glycerol and the other with pyruvate.

3. If there is a growth of other organisms on blood agar, identify them. Then decontaminate the remainder of the deposit by Petroff's method and culture it on Löwenstein-Jensen slopes.

The method of Ives & McCormick (1956) may be used for fluids that are sterile on blood agar. Add 100 ml of the fluid to 100 ml of double-strength Sula's medium, incubate at 37°C and examine weekly for colonies in the clot that forms in the medium.

Cerebrospinal fluid

As large as possible a specimen should be collected, e.g. 3–4 ml, without causing the patient to suffer headache. In a typical case of tuberculous meningitis the count of leucocytes in the cerebrospinal fluid is moderately increased, e.g. 50–500/mm^3, and shows a preponderance of lymphocytes, but, particularly in the early stages of the disease, polymorphs may be in the majority. Glucose is moderately reduced and protein increased, but not as greatly as in pyogenic bacterial meningitis and findings may be atypical in some cases. The demonstration of acid-fast bacilli makes the diagnosis almost certain.

1. Make a count of leucocytes and, if any, erythrocytes in a film of the uncentrifuged fluid in a counting chamber (see Ch.39).

2. If a spider-web clot has formed in the fluid, transfer it carefully on to a slide, let it dry, fix by heat and stain by the Ziehl-Neelsen or fluorochrome method.

Alternatively, break up the clot by shaking with sterile glass beads before centrifuging the fluid.

3. Centrifuge the fluid and use the supernatant for glucose and protein estimations.

4. Make three films from the deposit. Stain one by Leishman's method to count the proportions of polymorphs and lymphocytes, a second by the Ziehl-Neelsen or fluorochrome method to detect acid-fast bacilli, and the third by Gram's method to detect any pyogenic bacteria.

5. Inoculate some deposit on to media, e.g. blood agar, for the detection of pyogenic or contaminating bacteria after overnight incubation.

6. If culture for tubercle bacilli is postponed until after the blood agar cultures are read next day, the deposit should meantime be stored in the refrigerator at 4°C to preserve the viability of the tubercle bacilli.

7. If pyogenic and contaminating bacteria are absent, inoculate the remainder of the deposit on to slopes of Löwenstein-Jensen media, one with glycerol, another with pyruvate.

8. If contaminating bacteria are present, treat the deposit by Petroff's method before culturing on Löwenstein-Jensen media.

9. If animal facilities are available, inoculate part of the uncentrifuged specimen into a guinea-pig.

In cases suspected of being tuberculous but in which acid-fast bacilli cannot be demonstrated, the bromide partition test of Naughton et al (1981) should be done; a ratio of serum bromide to cerebrospinal fluid bromide less than 1.6 to 1 supports the diagnosis of tuberculous meningitis.

ELISA test. Another test which may prove helpful when the diagnosis of tuberculous meningitis is in doubt is the detection of mycobacterial antigens in the cerebrospinal fluid by enzyme-linked immunosorbent assay (Sada et al 1983).

A latex particle agglutination test for mycobacterial antigens has also been developed for the diagnosis of tuberculous meningitis (Krambovitis et al 1984).

Pus

1. Examine in a Gram film and by culture on blood agar aerobically and anaerobically for bacteria other than tubercle bacilli.

2. Make a Ziehl-Neelsen smear and examine for acid-fast bacilli.

3. Refrigerate the remainder of the specimen overnight.

4. If the blood agar cultures are sterile, inoculate the pus on to Löwenstein-Jensen glycerol and pyruvate slopes.

5. If there is growth on the blood agar, decontaminate the pus by Petroff's method before inoculating on to Löwenstein-Jensen.

Tissue

Tissue taken from a patient at biopsy or

necropsy or from an experimental animal should be homogenized in half-strength Ringer's solution. A Colworth Stomacher (Seward) or a Griffith's tube may be used for this purpose and the procedure should be performed in a safety cabinet. The homogenized tissue is then examined by film and culture as described for pus.

Selective liquid medium

Specimens other than sputum may give improved cultural results if inoculated into selective liquid Kirchner medium* as well as on to Löwenstein-Jensen slopes (Mitchison et al 1983).

SENSITIVITY AND IDENTIFICATION TESTS

A laboratory isolating only a few dozen myco-bacterial cultures a year should send them to a reference laboratory where a complete range of identification and sensitivity tests is performed on a regular basis. A laboratory isolating several cultures a week should set up sensitivity tests for the drugs commonly used in its area, e.g. isoniazid, rifampicin and ethambutol, and send cultures to the reference laboratory for the other tests. The concentration of testing in a reference laboratory improves the reliability of results and reduces the danger of infection of staff in the local laboratories that isolate the cultures.

Sensitivity tests

Inoculum

1. Prepare the inoculum in a sterilized 6 ml screw-capped bottle containing 0.1 ml water and six 5 mm glass beads.
2. Take a large loopful of the culture and rub it on the inside of the bottle. Close the cap tightly and place the bottle in a mechanical shaker for 10 min. The shaker should be inside an exhaust protective safety cabinet and the bottle should not be opened for 10 min after the cessation of shaking.
3. Then add 0.4 ml sterile water to the suspension in the bottle and inoculate the test slopes with a loopful of suspension up the centre of each. A fresh disposable loop should be used for each antibiotic.

An alternative method of preparing the inoculum is first to inoculate heavily a bottle of Dubos and Davis liquid medium* and subculture the strain at 5 day intervals at 37°C in the same medium until a smoothly dispersed culture is obtained. A swab soaked in the smooth culture, or a disposable loop containing a loopful of it, may then be used to inoculate the sensitivity test slopes with a single stroke on each. It should be noted, however, that the manipulation of such dispersed liquid cultures creates a greater danger of infection of staff by aerosol formation.

Media

The tests are done on slopes of Löwenstein-Jensen glycerol medium each containing one of a series of different concentrations of the particular antibiotic. Slopes containing the antibiotics may be purchased commercially or may be made in the laboratory by adding the requisite amounts of antibiotic to bottles containing the liquid egg medium before it is sloped and solidified by heating at 75–80°C in the inspissator. Because the antibiotic potency of the slopes may be reduced by the heating, the results of tests are not expressed as absolute minimum inhibitory concentrations (MICs), but as *resistance ratios* comparing the MIC of the unknown culture to that of a standard sensitive control culture tested in parallel.

Löwenstein-Jensen pyruvate medium cannot be used in tests of *M. bovis*, for the pyruvate interferes with the effect of isoniazid. After subculture, however, the bovine bacilli usually grow well enough on the glycerol medium to make possible the reading of results.

Useful ranges of antibiotic concentrations are, e.g., for isoniazid, from 0.03–1 mg/litre, for ethambutol, from 1–6 mg/l, and for rifampicin, from 2–32 mg/l.

Controls

With each series of tests on unknown cultures, parallel sets of cultures should be inoculated with the H37Rv strain of *M. tuberculosis* and four to six recently isolated strains of *M. tuberculosis* of already tested and known sensitivity.

Reading results

After incubation for 3 weeks at 37°C, the slopes are examined for growth and the lowest concentration of antibiotic showing no more than 0–20 colonies is taken as the end-point, or nominal 'MIC'. The result is reported as the *resistance ratio*, i.e. the ratio of the 'MIC' of the test strain to the 'MIC' of the majority of the sensitive control strains. Thus, if the test strain is inhibited by 16 mg/l of rifampicin and the control strains by 4 mg/l, the resistance ratio of the test strain for rifampicin is 4. A resistance ratio of 8 is reported as unequivocally resistant. One of 4 is regarded as doubtfully resistant and the test should be repeated. A strain with a ratio of 2 or less is reported as sensitive.

Pyrazinamide sensitivity

M. tuberculosis and its variant *M. africanum* are the only mycobacteria sensitive to pyrazinamide, but they do not grow well at the pH of 5.5 or less at which the drug is active. Many methods to overcome this difficulty have been devised and that of Marks (1976) is recommended. The culture is inoculated on to three pairs of Löwenstein-Jensen slopes at pH values 5.4, 5.2 and 5.0, one slope of each pair containing pyrazinamide 40 μg/ml, the other drug-free. A sensitive strain will grow on the first two or all three of the drug-free slopes but not on the drug-containing slopes.

An alternative to the sensitivity test is a test for the presence of pyrazinamidase which produces ammonia from pyrazinamide (Bonicke 1962).

Rapid methods

The conventional methods of sensitivity testing involve a delay of three weeks before results are available. Rapid methods are being developed which measure the evolution of $^{14}CO_2$ from a radio-labelled substrate in the medium (Snider et al 1981); e.g. Bactec (Becton Dickinson).

Identification tests

When the sensitivity tests are being set up, inoculate the same bacterial suspension into the following identification test media, for preliminary differentiation of the mycobacterial species capable of growth at 37°C on Löwenstein-Jensen medium. Incubate at 37°C for at least 3 weeks.

1. Löwenstein-Jensen glycerol slope with para-nitrobenzoic acid (PNB) 500 mg/l.*
2. Löwenstein-Jensen glycerol slope with thiophen-2-carboxylic acid hydrazide (TCH) 10 mg/l.*
3. Löwenstein-Jensen glycerol slope for incubation in an incubator with a light for pigment production (Ch. 26).
4. Sauton agar with 0.2% picric acid (Ch. 26).
5. Dubos and Davis liquid medium* for the niacin test.*

All typical tubercle bacilli are sensitive to para-nitrobenzoic acid and fail to grow on the PNB medium. Among these, only strains of *M. tuberculosis* are resistant to thiophen-2-carboxylic acid hydrazide and can grow on the TCH medium. They may be identified on this basis without further tests. Any culture behaving differently should be tested further and identified by the reactions shown in Table 25.1. See also Tsukamura (1967).

Niacin test

M. tuberculosis produces niacin (nicotinic acid) in cultures and so differs from *M. bovis* and BCG, which are niacin negative. The niacin test* is therefore valuable in identifying the infrequent strains of *M. tuberculosis* that otherwise resemble *M. bovis* and BCG in being sensitive to TCH. As BCG gives a eugonic growth identical with that of *M. tuberculosis*, its distinction by the niacin test is critical.

There is a spectrum of variants between *M. tuberculosis* and *M. bovis*, which show atypical combinations of the usually distinctive characters. The name *M. africanum* is sometimes given to variants that resemble *M. tuberculosis* in their sensitivity to pyrazinamide, but resemble *M. bovis* in their dysgonic growth and sensitivity to TCH. These strains are variable in their niacin reactions.

Atmospheric requirements

These are tested by incubation at 37°C after dispersed inoculation of the culture into semi-solid medium.* The aerobic character of *M. tuberculosis* and BCG is shown by the confinement of their growth to the top 0.5–1 cm of the medium and the microaerophilic character of *M. bovis* and *M. africanum* by their growth extending well down into the medium, though with a band of maximum growth just below the surface.

Nitrate reduction

M. tuberculosis reduces nitrate, whilst *M. bovis* and BCG do not. *M. africanum* gives a weak reaction.

Tuberculoid bacilli

These 'atypical' mycobacteria are distinguished from tubercle bacilli by their resistance to both PNB and TCH, and thus by their ability to grow on media containing them. They are differentiated into species by their rate of growth on Löwenstein-Jensen glycerol medium, their ability to grow on Sauton's medium with 0.2% picric acid, the influence of light on the formation of pigment in their cultures, and other characters described in Chapter 26.

Mycobacteria not growing at 37°C

On primary isolation, *M. ulcerans* and *M. marinum* do not grow at 37°C on Löwenstein-Jensen media. If their presence is suspected, or if the material is from a skin lesion, cultures should be incubated at 30–33°C, as well as at 37°C. *M. leprae* does not grow on any inanimate medium at any temperature. These organisms are described further in Chapter 26.

IMMUNODIAGNOSIS

Serological tests

Antibodies to mycobacteria can be demonstrated in patient's serum by various techniques, e.g. the haemagglutination test of Middlebrook & Dubos (1948), but this test has not been found to be sufficiently specific or sensitive to be of clinical value (Hilson & Elek 1951). The presence or absence of the antibodies, or their titre when present, has shown little correlation with the clinical state of the patient, so that it is unlikely that tests of greater sensitivity, e.g. an enzyme-linked immunosorbent assay, will be any more valuable. Yet Daniel et al (1986) found that an ELISA test with antigen from a monoclonal immunoabsorbent had a sensitivity of 69% and a specificity of 88% in the diagnosis of tuberculosis in a population with a high prevalence of the disease.

Tuberculin test

The principal immunological response in tuberculosis is the development of cell-mediated immunity, which becomes detectable a few weeks after natural infection or BCG vaccination. It is demonstrated by the delayed hypersensitivity reaction which follows the intradermal inoculation of tuberculin, a preparation of protein antigens extracted from tubercle bacilli. A positive test in a person who has not been vaccinated with BCG indicates that tuberculous infection has taken place in the recent or distant past, but is not necessarily a sign of active disease. In the absence of BCG vaccination a positive reaction in children with symptoms suggestive of tuberculosis is valuable confirmatory evidence. The test is also useful in screening children who have been in contact with an open case of the disease. It should be borne in mind that the test may be negative in advanced or miliary infection. Two methods of testing are currently in use.

1. *Mantoux test*. This is the standard method with which all other methods are compared. A test dose of 0.1 ml of Purified Protein Derivative (PPD; e.g. from Evans) or Old Tuberculin (OT) containing 5 Tuberculin Units is injected intracutaneously into the skin of the volar aspect of the forearm. The site is examined and palpated 72 h later. The development of an area of palpable, firm induration greater than 10 mm in diameter is recorded as positive. The extent of

the accompanying erythema is irrelevant and should be ignored. If the reaction is completely negative, the test may be repeated by giving an injection of 100 Tuberculin Units.

2. *Heaf test*. This test is done with a multiple puncture apparatus with six needles that prick tuberculin 1–2 mm deep into the skin. A drop of undiluted PPD is spread on the area of skin selected for inoculation, the instrument is pressed against this area of skin and the needles are released. The site is inspected 72 h later, when a reaction comprising the presence of erythema and oedema or induration around at least four of the punctures is regarded as positive. Because of its ease of performance the Heaf test is principally used in epidemiological surveys and as a test for immunity before BCG vaccination. For diagnostic purposes the more accurate Mantoux test should be used. For further information, see Comstock et al (1971).

Because re-use of a multiple puncture apparatus on successive subjects might lead to the spread of hepatitis B or HIV infection, a fresh apparatus must be used for each person tested.

METHODS

Culture media

Detailed instructions for the preparation of media for optimal growth of clinically important mycobacteria are given by Stonebrink et al (1969).

Löwenstein-Jensen glycerol medium

This medium (Jensen 1954) has been modified from the original Löwenstein-Jensen medium by the omission of starch, which makes it more difficult to prepare and is unnecessary for the growth of tubercle bacilli. Malachite green has modest inhibitory effect on the growth of organisms other than mycobacteria and provides a colour contrast that facilitates the recognition of colonies which, especially when small, would be difficult to see on the medium without dye. The medium is recommended for the isolation of the human type of tubercle bacillus, whose growth is enhanced by glycerol, and for drug sensitivity tests. Colonial morphology allows the differentiation of the human and bovine types of bacillus, but the bovine bacilli may be inhibited by the glycerol and so may fail to grow on this medium.

Mineral salt solution

Potassium dihydrogen phosphate, KH_2PO_4 anhydrous	2.4 g
Magnesium sulphate, $MgSO_4$	0.24 g
Magnesium citrate, $Mg_3(C_6H_5O_7)_2.14H_2O$	0.6 g
Asparagine	3.6 g
Glycerol	12 ml
Water	600 ml

Dissolve the ingredients with heating. Autoclave at 121°C for 25 min to sterilize. The solution keeps indefinitely.

Malachite green solution. Prepare a 2% solution of malachite green in sterile water with sterile precautions. Allow the dye to dissolve by holding at 37°C in the incubator for 1–2 h. The solution keeps indefinitely but should be shaken before use.

Complete medium

Mineral salt solution	600 ml
Malachite green solution	20 ml
Egg fluid	1 litre

All utensils used to prepare the complete medium must be sterile. The eggs must be fresh, i.e. not more than 4 days old. About 20–22, depending on size, will be required to provide the litre of fluid. Wash them thoroughly in warm water with a brush and a plain alkaline soap, then rinse them in running water for 30 min. Drain off the water and allow the eggs to dry, covered with paper until the following day. Alternatively, dry them at once by sprinkling them with methylated spirit and burning it off. Crack the eggs with a sterile knife into a sterile beaker and beat them, whites and yolks together, with a sterile egg whisk until a uniform fluid mixture free from air bubbles is obtained. Add the mineral salt and malachite green solutions to the mixed egg fluid. Mix the complete medium thoroughly and distribute it in 5 ml amounts into 25 ml (McCartney) bottles and screw on the caps tightly. Lay the bottles horizontally in the inspissator and heat at 80°C for 1 h to coagulate and solidify the medium. As the medium has been prepared with sterile precautions, this final heating is to solidify, not to sterilize it.

A hot air oven fitted with a fan may be used for inspissation. Pre-heat the oven to 85°C. Then load it with shelves on which the bottles of medium have been laid horizontally. When the temperature reaches 80°C, adjust the thermostat to this level and continue heating for another 30 min.

The sloped medium will keep for some months in tightly closed, screw-capped bottles, but if slopes are made in test tubes they must be stored in the cold and used within a month.

Commercial medium. As preparation of the medium is complex, it is advantageous for laboratories with a small demand to obtain ready made slopes from a commercial supplier. Alternatively, a commercial basic mixture of mineral salts, asparagine and malachite green (e.g. Bacto-IUTM Base, Difco) may be used to make up a solution of 7.2 g base in 600 ml hot water containing 12 ml glycerol. Autoclave at 121°C for 15 min, cool to 50°C, then with aseptic precautions mix in 1000 ml sterile egg fluid without forming air bubbles and distribute into bottles for inspissation at 80°C in slopes.

Löwenstein-Jensen pyruvate medium

This medium is used for the primary isolation of *M. bovis*, to which the glycerol in the standard Löwenstein-Jensen medium is inhibitory. It is also preferable to the latter medium for the isolation of some drug-resistant strains of *M. tuberculosis*, but it should not be used for drug sensitivity tests, at least for those with isoniazid, for it interferes with the action of that drug.

The medium is made by substituting 7 g sodium pyruvate for the 12 ml glycerol in the 1600 ml of mineral salt and egg fluid mixture of the standard medium.

As an alternative, Stonebrink's (1957) medium containing 4.2 g/litre sodium pyruvate may be used.

Dorset's egg medium

This simple egg medium is suitable for the growth of laboratory strains of tubercle bacilli. In an emergency it may be used for isolations, when it would be advisable to add 1.25 ml of 2% malachite green per 100 ml, but the more enriched media give a greater number of positive cultures.

Mixed egg fluid (2 or 3 hen's eggs)	75 ml
Sterile nutrient broth	25 ml

Prepare the mixed white and yolk egg fluid free from bubbles, mix in the broth and dispense into bottles with sterile precautions for inspissation as for Löwenstein-Jensen medium.

Dubos and Davis medium

This liquid medium is used to give uniformly dispersed cultures to serve as inocula for drug-sensitivity and identification tests. The composition is as described by the Medical Research Council (1948). It should be noted that ordinary laboratory manipulations readily produce infective aerosols from dispersed liquid cultures, which should therefore be performed only in an exhaust ventilated safety cabinet.

Bovine albumin solution, 9%

Bovine albumin (fraction V, Armour)	4.5 ml
Water	45.5 ml

Mix and sterilize by filtration.

Complete medium

Potassium dihydrogen phosphate, KH_2PO_4	1 g
Disodium hydrogen phosphate, $Na_2HPO_4.12H_2O$	6.25 g
Sodium citrate, $C_6H_5Na_3O_7.2H_2O$	1.5 g

Magnesium sulphate,	
MgSO$_4$.7H$_2$O	0.6 g
Tween 80, 10% solution	5 ml
Casein hydrolysate, 20%	
solution	10 ml
Distilled water	1145 ml
Bovine albumin solution	40 ml

Dissolve each salt separately in portions of the water, then mix these solutions into the Tween and casein hydrolysate dissolved in the remaining water. The medium should be at pH 7.2. Distribute in culture containers, autoclave at 115°C for 10 min and add the bovine albumin with sterile precautions.

Commercial medium. A commercial medium is available from Difco, comprising Bacto Dubos broth base (0385–17–6) and Bacto Dubos medium albumin (0309–64–1).

Selective Kirchner medium

For improved cultural results with specimens other than sputum, use this selective liquid medium (Mitchison et al 1983) in addition to culture on Löwenstein-Jensen slopes.

Potassium dihydrogen phosphate,	
KH$_2$PO$_4$	2 g
Disodium hydrogen phosphate,	
Na$_2$HPO$_4$.12H$_2$O	19 g
Magnesium sulphate,	
MgSO$_4$.7H$_2$O	0.6 g
Sodium citrate, C$_6$H$_5$Na$_3$O$_7$.2H$_2$O	2.5 g
L-asparagine	5 g
Casein hydrolysate (Oxoid	
tryptone L42)	0.5 g
Glycerol	20 ml
Phenol red, 0.4% solution	3 ml
Distilled water	1 litre

Autoclave at 121°C for 15 min. The pH value should be between 6.9 and 7.2. Then add aseptically:

Polymyxin B	200 000 units
Carbenicillin	100 mg
Amphotericin	10 mg
Trimethoprim	10 mg
Sterile calf serum	100 ml

Distribute aseptically in 10 ml amounts into sterile 28 ml Universal containers.

Commercial medium. The complete medium with antibiotics is available from Difco (Code 9306–97).

Method. Only heavily contaminated specimens such as urine and faeces need to be decontaminated before inoculation. Centrifuge urine, treat the deposit with 1 ml of 5% (v/v) H$_2$SO$_4$ for 15 min, centrifuge again, resuspend the deposit in 15 ml sterile water, centrifuge yet again, resuspend the deposit in 1 ml sterile water and inoculate it into 10 ml medium. Extract faeces with ether and treat the interfacial material with 5% H$_2$SO$_4$ before inoculating it into the medium. Incubate the medium at 37°C and examine it weekly for microcolonies. If growth is detected, subculture it on to Löwenstein-Jensen slopes at once. If growth is not detected by 5 weeks, make subcultures then.

Decontamination of specimens

Before inoculation on to culture media, specimens such as sputum which are contaminated with bacteria other than mycobacteria must be treated by a method that kills the other bacteria but not the mycobacteria. Various methods of decontamination have been advocated, the most used of which have the additional advantages of homogenizing the specimen and concentrating the mycobacteria in a centrifuged deposit that serves as the inoculum for cultures. The concentrated deposit may also be examined microscopically in Ziehl-Neelsen stained film, wherein the probability of finding acid-fast bacilli is greater than in a 'direct' film of the unconcentrated specimen.

Petroff's method (modified)

1. Wearing rubber gloves and working in an exhaust ventilated safety cabinet, transfer up to 8–10 ml sputum into a 25 ml Universal container.
2. Add an equal volume of 4% sodium hydroxide, close the container tightly with a screw-cap fitted with an intact liner, and mix thoroughly by shaking.

Alternatively, where the sputum has been collected in a suitable wide-mouthed jar, the sodium hydroxide may be added directly to the jar and, after shaking and homogenization, the material transferred to a Universal container for centrifugation. The transfer of sputum is easier after it has been homogenized.

3. Place the container in an incubator at 37°C for 30 min, but remove briefly for further mixing by shaking at intervals.

4. In a sealed bucket, centrifuge the Universal container at about 1500 g for 30 min. Pipette off the supernatant fluid and discard it into strong disinfectant.

5. Add a drop of phenol red or Universal pH indicator to the deposit, then neutralize it to about pH 7 by adding 8% hydrochloric acid drop by drop. If too much acid is added, adjust the pH back to neutrality by adding 0.4% sodium hydroxide drop by drop.

6. With a hand operated pipette, transfer two or three drops of the deposit to each of two slopes of Löwenstein-Jensen medium, one with glycerol, the other with pyruvate, and another drop to a microscope slide for examination after Ziehl-Neelsen staining.

Use with acid media. Where an exhaust ventilated safety cabinet is unavailable, the danger to staff of infection by aerosol produced during the transfers made in the standard Petroff method may be reduced by use of modified methods employing acid media described by Zaher & Marks (1977). The specimen is treated with sodium hydroxide and incubated with shaking for 30 min as in the standard Petroff method, but the manipulations of neutralizing the alkaline mixture are avoided by the device of inoculating it on to an egg medium of an appropriate degree of acidity. Suitable acid egg media can be obtained from Oxoid.

If centrifugation of the treated specimen is to be avoided, 0.2 ml of it is inoculated on to a slope of Acid Egg Medium 1a (glycerol) and 0.2 ml on to a slope of Acid Egg Medium 1b (pyruvate). If the specimen can first be diluted 1 in 4 with distilled water and centrifuged, the deposit is inoculated on to slopes of the less acid Egg Media 2a and 2b.

Nassau's modification of Jungmann and Grushka's method

Solution A

| Ferrous sulphate, FeSO$_4$ | 20 g |
| Sulphuric acid, H$_2$SO$_4$ 20% (v/v) | 100 ml |

Solution B. Hydrogen peroxide, H$_2$O$_2$, 0.3% (1 volume).

Solution A can be made up in bulk and keeps indefinitely. Solution B must be made up freshly on each occasion from a standard 6% (w/v) solution kept in the dark.

1. Place 2 ml sputum in a Universal container. Add 1.2 ml solution A and 1.2 ml solution B. Close the container tightly.

2. Shake the container for 30 s and allow it to stand on the bench for 20 min, shaking at intervals.

3. Centrifuge the container in a sealed bucket at about 1500 g for 30 min and discard the supernate into strong disinfectant.

4. Fill the container to the shoulder with 5% sterile sodium citrate, shake vigorously and again centrifuge.

5. Remove and discard the supernate and inoculate the deposit on to slopes of Löwenstein-Jensen media.

Identification tests

These tests are conveniently set up at the same time, and seeded from the same culture suspension as the drug sensitivity tests (see above). Otherwise, inoculate a drop or large loopful of a freshly prepared suspension of a large loopful of culture from a Löwenstein-Jensen slope in 0.5 ml sterile water, homogenized by shaking with glass beads as described for drug sensitivity tests.

Sensitivity to para-nitrobenzoic acid (PNB)

Inoculate a large loopful of homogenized culture suspension on to a slope of medium containing PNB 500 mg/litre and observe for growth during incubation for 3 weeks at 37°C. *M. tuberculosis, M. bovis* and their variants are sensitive to PNB and fail to grow on the PNB medium. Tuberculoid bacilli are generally resistant and grow on the PNB medium.

Medium

Para-nitrobenzoic acid	0.2 g
Distilled water	15 ml
Sodium hydroxide, NaOH 1 mol/litre	2 ml

Shake to dissolve. Adjust the pH by adding about 0.8 ml hydrochloric acid, HCl 1 mol/litre until a precipitate just forms and then just redissolves. Make up the volume to 20 ml by adding water. Then add 5 ml of the mixture to 100 ml Löwenstein-Jensen glycerol medium, distribute in bottles, slope and inspissate.

Sensitivity to thiophen-2-carboxylic acid hydrazide (TCH)

Inoculate a large loopful of homogenized culture suspension on to a slope of medium containing TCH 10 mg/litre and observe for growth during incubation for 3 weeks at 37°C. Most strains of *M. tuberculosis* and tuberculoid bacilli are resistant to TCH and grow on the medium. *M. bovis*, *M. africanum* and BCG are sensitive and fail to grow.

Medium

Thiophen-2-carboxylic acid hydrazide	0.1 g
Distilled water	100 ml

Dissolve the TCH in the water and add 1 ml of the solution to 100 ml Löwenstein-Jensen glycerol medium. Distribute in bottles, slope and inspissate.

Niacin production

M. tuberculosis and some strains of *M. africanum* produce niacin (nicotinic acid) in their cultures. *M. bovis* and BCG are niacin negative.

1. Inoculate a large loopful of homogenized culture suspension into Dubos and Davis liquid medium (see above) and incubate for 3 weeks at 37°C.

2. Transfer 1 ml of the liquid culture to a tube or Universal container and insert a Bacto Niacin test strip (Difco).

3. Observe the fluid for the development of a yellow colour denoting that niacin has been produced.

Alternatively, the strip test may be performed on aqueous extract of a well grown culture on Löwenstein-Jensen medium. This method has the drawback of extracting a green colour from the medium which interferes with the detection of a weak reaction.

The strip methods of testing avoid the need to handle toxic chemicals as in the cyanogen bromide method (see 12th Edition of this book, Vol. 2, Ch. 7).

Atmospheric requirements

These are tested by dispersed culture in semi-solid medium.

Semi-solid medium

Disodium hydrogen phosphate, Na_2HPO_4	7.5 g
Potassium dihydrogen phosphate, KH_2PO_4	2 g
Magnesium sulphate, $MgSO_4.7H_2O$	0.6 g
Sodium citrate, $Na_3C_6H_5O_7.2H_2O$	2.5 g
Ferric ammonium citrate (green scales)	0.005 g
Tryptone (Oxoid)	5 g
Glycerol	20 ml
Distilled water to	1 litre
Ionagar (Oxoid, L28)	1 g

Dissolve the reagents except the agar in the water and adjust the pH to 7.3. Add the agar and dissolve it by steaming at 100°C. Sterilize the medium by autoclaving at 121°C for 5 min. Allow to cool to about 60°C, shake well and dispense 15 ml volumes into Universal containers. Autoclave at 121°C for 10 min. The medium has a shelf life of several months.

Method. 1. Heat at 100°C in a steamer to melt the agar and cool to about 55°C.

2. Add 0.5 ml sterile calf serum to the 15 ml medium in a Universal container.

3. Inoculate a drop of a suspension of the culture to be tested and mix it through the medium by repeated gentle inversion. Do not shake or cause the formation of bubbles.

4. Incubate for up to 3 weeks at 37°C.

Result. Aerobic requirement: growth almost confined to the top 0.5–1 cm of the medium.

Microaerophilic requirement: growth extends well down the medium, but there is a band of maximum growth just below the surface.

Nitrate reduction

M. tuberculosis reduces nitrate, whilst *M. bovis* and BCG do not. *M. africanum* reduces it weakly and different tuberculoid bacilli give different results (Ch. 26).

Medium

Sodium nitrate, NaNO₃, sterile
10% aqueous solution   10 ml
Dubos and Davis liquid
medium (see above), sterile   1 litre

Distribute aseptically in 7 ml volumes into Universal containers.

Method. 1. Inoculate the culture heavily into the test medium and incubate at 37°C for 14 days.

2. Add 1 ml of 0.8% sulphanilic acid in acetic acid 5 mol/litre.

3. Add 1 ml of 0.5% naphthylamine in acetic acid 5 mol/l.

4. Observe the mixture for the development of a red colour which denotes that nitrate has been reduced.

A parallel test should be done with *M. kansasi* as a positive control.

REFERENCES

Birn K J, Schaefer W B, Jenkins P A, Szulga T, Marks J 1967 Classification of *Myco. avium* and related opportunist mycobacteria met in England and Wales. Journal of Hygiene, Cambridge 65: 575–589

Bonicke R 1962 Identification of mycobacteria by biochemical methods. Bulletin of the International Union against Tuberculosis 32: 13–68

Comstock G W, Furcolow M L, Greenberg R A, Grzybowski S, Maclean R A, Baer H, Edwards P Q 1971 The tuberculin skin test. American Review of Respiratory Disease 104: 769–775

Daniel T M, de Murillo G L, Sawyer J A, Griffin A M, Pinto H, Debanne S M, Espinosa P, Cespedes E 1986 Field evaluation of enzyme-linked immunosorbent assay for the serodiagnosis of tuberculosis. American Review of Respiratory Disease 134: 662–665

Davis D, Bonekat H W, Andrews D, Shigeoka J W 1984 Disinfection of the flexible fibreoptic bronchoscope against *Mycobacterium tuberculosis* and *M. gordonae*. Thorax 39: 785–788

Grange J M, Collins C H, McSwiggan D 1976 Bacteriophage typing of *Mycobacterium tuberculosis* strains isolated in South East England. Tubercle 57: 59–66

Grange J M, Redmond W B 1978 Host phage relationships in the genus Mycobacterium and their clinical significance. Tubercle 59: 203–225

Hilson G R F, Elek S D 1951 The haemagglutination reaction in tuberculosis. Journal of Clinical Pathology 4: 158–172

Ives J C J, McCormick W 1956 A modification of Sula's method for the cultivation of tubercle bacilli from pleural fluid. Journal of Clinical Pathology 9: 177–178

Jensen K A 1954 Second Report of the Subcommittee on Laboratory Methods of the International Union against Tuberculosis. Bulletin of the International Union against Tuberculosis 24: 78–104. (See also vol. 25, p 89)

Krambovitis E, McIllmurray M B, Lock P E, Hendrickse W, Holzel H 1984 Rapid diagnosis of tuberculous meningitis by latex particle agglutination. Lancet 2: 1229–1231

Marks J 1976 A system for the examination of tubercle bacilli and other mycobacteria. Tubercle 57: 207–225

Medical Research Council 1948 Specific laboratory tests in streptomycin therapy. Lancet 2: 862–865

Middlebrook G, Dubos R J 1948 Specific serum agglutination of erythrocytes sensitized with extracts of tubercle bacilli. Journal of Experimental Medicine 88: 521–528

Mitchison D A, Allen B W, Devi Manickavasagar 1983 Selective Kirchner medium in the culture of specimens other than sputum for mycobacteria. Journal of Clinical Pathology 36: 1357–1361

Naughton E, Weindling A M, Newton R, Bower B D 1981 Tuberculous meningitis in children. Lancet 2: 973–975

Redmond W B, Bates J H, Engel H W B 1979 Methods for bacteriophage typing of mycobacteria. In: Bergan T & Norris J R (eds) Methods in microbiology, vol 13. Academic Press. London. ch VIII, p 345–376

Sada E, Ruiz-Palacios G M, López-Vidal Y, Ponce de León S 1983 Detection of mycobacterial antigens in cerebrospinal fluid of patients with tuberculous meningitis by enzyme-linked immunosorbent assay. Lancet 2: 651–652

Snider D E Jr et al 1981 Rapid drug-susceptibility testing

of *Myco. tuberculosis*. American Review of Respiratory Disease 123: 402–406

Stonebrink B 1957 Tubercle bacilli and pyruvic acid. Proceedings of the Tuberculosis Research Council 44: 67–74

Stonebrink B, Douma J, Manten A, Mulder R J 1969 A comparative investigation of the quality of various culture media used in the Netherlands for the isolation of Mycobacteria. Selected Papers. Royal Netherlands Tuberculosis Association 12:5

Tsukamura M 1967 Identification of mycobacteria. Tubercle 48: 311–338

Zaher F, Marks J 1977 Methods and media for the culture of tubercle bacilli. Tubercle 58: 143–145

Mycobacterium: tuberculoid and leprosy bacilli

The atypical mycobacteria, or tuberculoid bacilli, comprise most members of the genus *Mycobacterium* except the mammalian tubercle bacilli, *M. tuberculosis*, *M. bovis* and their variants. The term tuberculoid is not entirely satisfactory but has been preferred here because other terms, such as anonymous, atypical, and MOTT (mycobacteria other than tubercle) bacilli, are equally vulnerable to criticism.

These bacilli are acid- and alcohol-fast and may resemble or differ in morphology from the tubercle bacilli. They may be longer than the latter, or even filamentous, but a mycobacterium must not be identified as atypical solely on its appearance in a Ziehl-Neelsen film. They are distinguished from the tubercle bacilli by various cultural and biochemical characters, in particular by their ability to grow on media containing para-nitrobenzoic acid (PNB) and thiophen-2-carboxylic acid hydrazide (TCH), whereas none of the mammalian tubercle bacilli grows on PNB medium and only *M. tuberculosis* on TCH medium (Ch. 25 and Table 25.1). A mycobacterium that is sensitive to streptomycin, para-aminosalicylic acid and isoniazid cannot be a tuberculoid bacillus for such a bacillus is always resistant to at least one of these drugs.

Many tuberculoid bacilli are normally found in soil and water, but occasionally cause opportunistic infections in man indistinguishable clinically, radiologically and histologically from that caused by the human tubercle bacillus. Such infection is called mycobacteriosis and is not notifiable as tuberculosis. Generally there is no person-to-person transmission.

The isolation of a tuberculoid bacillus on a single occasion is not of itself sufficient evidence that it is the cause of the patient's illness; it may be a secondary invader or a contaminant. As soon as the presence of a tuberculoid bacillus is suspected, several further specimens from the patient should be requested for examination. In the case of sputum, three to six isolations of the organism are desirable before it is considered to be acting as a pathogen. Sometimes a tuberculoid bacillus colonizes a lung already damaged by the human tubercle bacillus and the possible additional presence of that more dangerous pathogen should not be overlooked.

When a tuberculoid bacillus, particularly *M. avium*, is the real pathogen, treatment is difficult and the disease may be fatal. Patients whose lungs are damaged by other conditions such as pneumoconiosis, or are immunodeficient, e.g. suffering from AIDS, or are being treated with immunosuppressive drugs are at risk from infection with tuberculoid bacilli. These infections have become much commoner in recent years (Woods & Washington, 1987).

Laboratory diagnosis

The microscopical and isolation procedures are as described for tubercle bacilli in Chapter 25. For skin lesions, however, two extra cultures should be set up on Lowenstein-Jensen slopes, one with glycerol, the other with pyruvate, and incubated at 30–33°C. If a laboratory encounters a cluster of atypical isolates from different patients, contamination should be suspected and the water supply and test reagents should be examined. To exclude the possibility that a human or bovine tubercle bacillus is also present in a culture of an atypical bacillus, the culture should be tested for niacin production and, if possible, be inoculated into a guinea-pig.

Identification tests

The initial, screening tests for the identification of a mycobacterium are as described in Chapter 25. They are for sensitivities to para-nitrobenzoic acid (PNB) and thiophen-2-carboxylic acid hydrazide (TCH), rate of growth on Lowenstein-Jensen medium, influence of light on the production of pigment (yellow or orange) in cultures, sensitivity to picric acid in Sauton's medium*, and the production of niacin.

They distinguish the tuberculoid bacilli, which grow in the presence of PNB, from the typical tubercle bacilli which do not. They also divide the tuberculoid bacilli into four groups: (1) photochromogens, (2) scotochromogens and (3) non-chromogens, all which groups are slow growing on egg media, taking 1–3 weeks for good growth, and (4) rapid growers, which grow well in 2–3 days. On nutrient agar the rapid growers grow freely, whilst the slow growers fail to grow or grow only very poorly. The rapid growers are also distinguished from the slow growers by their ability to grow on Sauton's agar with 0.2% picric acid.

Further tests, described in the *Methods* section below*, are required for identification of the species of the atypical bacilli. The distinguishing reactions of the commoner species are shown in Table 26.1. A smooth culture in Dubos and Davis liquid medium (Ch. 25) should be used to inoculate these additional tests as well as drug sensitivity tests. A laboratory isolating few atypical mycobacteria should send any isolate to a reference laboratory for both identification and sensitivity tests. For information on other species and additional tests, see Wayne (1985).

Photochromogens

This group of slowly growing tuberculoid bacilli form yellow or orange pigment when their cultures are grown with exposure to light, but not when they are kept in the dark. In the stan-

dard test for photochromogenesis two Lowenstein-Jensen slopes are seeded. One slope is wrapped in aluminium foil to exclude light from it and both are incubated for 14 days at 37°C in a lighted incubator.*

M. kansasi forms smooth, easily emulsified colonies that are yellow to orange when exposed to light. The bacilli may be long, e.g. 8–10 μm, or filamentous. Strains have been isolated from water. The organism may cause tuberculosis-like disease of the lungs, but strains that are catalase-weak are regarded as non-pathogenic. *M. kansasi* is resistant to isoniazid and para-aminosalicylic acid, and some strains are also resistant to streptomycin.

M. marinum (syn *M. balnei*, *M. platypoecilus*) forms rough colonies that are yellow when exposed to light. The bacilli may be long to filamentous. It is pathogenic for fish and has been isolated from swimming pool water and domestic fish tanks. In man it causes swimming pool granuloma. Isolation of a photochromogen from a skin ulcer in a culture incubated at 30°C but not in a culture at 37°C is almost diagnostic. *M. marinum* may also be distinguished from *M. kansasi* by its failure to reduce nitrate and failure to produce catalase, by thin layer chromatography (Szulga et al 1966) and by serological agglutination (Schaefer 1965). It is resistant to isoniazid and para-aminosalicylic acid, sometimes to streptomycin and rifampicin, and sensitive to ethambutol and ethionamide.

M. simiae, another photochromogen, was originally isolated from monkeys but has also been found in man. Conflicting accounts of its biochemical characters make its status doubtful (Buchanan & Gibbon 1974).

Scotochromogens

This second group of slowly growing tuberculoid bacilli form pigment in cultures incubated in the dark, though the intensity of the colour may increase on exposure to light.

M. scrofulaceum (syn. *M. marianum*, *M. paraffinicum*) forms smooth entire colonies that are yellow to orange in colour. The bacilli may be either short or long to filamentous. It is occasionally isolated from soil and is the

* Refer to *Methods* at end of this chapter.

Table 26.1 Distinguishing characters of tuberculoid bacilli.
Key: P, photochromogenic; S, scotochromogenic; N, non-chromogenic; a, growth only after adaptation to culture in laboratory; b, slight growth by some strains; $+^a$, also growth at 52°C; ±, weakly positive; +/−, some strains positive, some negative; . . ., no result given.

Species	Pigment formation	Growth at temperature (°C) 25	30	37	40	44	Nitrate reduction	Aryl sulphatase activity (3 days)	Tween hydrolysis (5 days)	Catalase production	Other reactions (see footnote)
Slow growers											
M. kansasi	P	+	+	+	+	−	+	−	+	+/±	1, 2
M. marinum	P	a	+	a	−	−	−	−	+	−	1, 2
M. gordonae	S	+	+	+	b	−	−	+	+	+	. . .
M. scrofulaceum	S	+	+	+	b	−	−	−	−	+	. . .
M. szulgai	S	+	+	+	b	−	+	+	+	+	. . .
M. ulcerans	S	a	+	a	−	−	+	−	. . .	±	2
M. xenopi	S	+	+	+	+	+	−	+	−	−	. . .
M. avium	N	b	+	+	+	b	−	−	−	−	3
M. intracellulare	N	b	+	+	+	b	−	−	−	±/−	3
M. gastri	N	+	+	+	+	−	−	+	+	−	3
M. malmoense	N	+	+	+	+	−	+/−	+	−	+	. . .
M. terrae	N	+	+	+	+	−	+	+	+	+	3
Rapid growers											
M. chelonae	N	+	+	+	+	−	−	+	−	. . .	2, 4
M. fortuitum	N	+	+	+	+	−	+	+	±	±	2, 4
M. phlei	S	+	+	+	+	$+^a$	+	−	+	+	4
M. smegmatis	N	+	+	+	+	+	+	−	+	±	2, 4

1, utilization of glucose – *M. kansasi* positive, *M. marinum* negative; 2, intraperitoneal inoculation in mouse – *M. kansasi* self-limiting lesions in liver and spleen, *M. marinum* ulceration of tail, paws and scrotum, *M. ulcerans* late ulceration of skin, *M. fortuitum* and some strains of *M. chelonae* and *M. smegmatis*, spinning disease; 3, reduction of tellurite – *M. avium* and *M. intracellulare* postitive, *M. gastri* and *M. terrae* negative; 4, degradation of salicylate – *M. chelonae* and *M. fortuitum* positive, *M. phlei* and *M. smegmatis* negative.

commonest cause of mycobacterial cervical lymphadenitis in children in Britain. When isolated from sputum or gastric lavage it is almost certainly a saprophytic contaminant, not the cause of lung infection. It is resistant to isoniazid and sensitive to cycloserine and ethionamide.

M. gordonae (syn. tap-water scotochromogen) forms smooth, yellow to orange colonies containing short bacilli. It has been isolated from soil and should be regarded as a saprophytic contaminant when isolated from sputum or gastric lavage.

M. szulgai is a scotochromogen in cultures grown at 37°C but a photochromogen in cultures grown at 25°C. Orange pigment formed at 37°C becomes more intense after exposure to light.

The bacilli are the same length as tubercle bacilli, but are stouter and may be banded. *M. szulgai* has been isolated from sputum, cervical adenitis and olecranon bursitis. A distinctive lipid can be demonstrated by chromatography (Marks 1976).

M. ulcerans (syn. *M. buruli*) grows slowly at 30–33°C, but not at all at 37°C in primary culture. It forms tiny transparent colonies which later become rough and yellow. The bacilli are fairly long. It was first reported in Australia as a cause of skin ulcers in man and later in other parts of the world, including Africa, where the disease is called Buruli ulcer. Isolation of a scotochromogenic mycobacterium in a culture grown at 30–33°C, but not in a culture at 37°C is practically diagnostic. *M. ulcerans* is sensitive to streptomycin, rifampicin and cycloserine, and variably sensitive to isoniazid and ethambutol.

M. xenopi (syn. *M. littorale*) grows at first as colourless smooth colonies that later become yellow. The bacilli are usually but not invariably long and filamentous. The organism is a saprophyte, but occasionally has been implicated as the cause of pulmonary or renal disease. It is sensitive to cycloserine, ethionamide and erythromycin, variably sensitive to streptomycin, and resistant to isoniazid and para-aminosalicylic acid.

Non-chromogens

M. avium is the important member of this group of slowly growing mycobacteria. It is similar in its reactions to *M. intracellulare*, which may be regarded as a variant of *M. avium* that is much less virulent in birds than typical strains of the latter. A mycobacterium is not *M. avium* if it does not grow on egg media at 42°C, is sensitive to thiacetazone or is resistant to cycloserine. Chromatographic analysis of the bacterial lipids and serotyping by agglutination (Birn et al 1967) are necessary for final identification.

M. avium and *M. intracellulare* are the commonest tuberculoid bacilli causing opportunistic infections in man. They frequently cause pulmonary, lymph node or disseminated infection and frequently infect patients with AIDS.

The colonies of both species, or variants, are smooth, white and easily emulsified. The bacilli are usually short, though under some conditions filamentous. *M. avium* and some strains of *M. intracellulare* are pathogenic in birds, cattle and pigs. They multiply in the rabbit and mouse without producing macroscopic lesions, that is, they produce Yersin type disease. Both organisms are resistant to isoniazid, para-aminosalicylic acid, streptomycin, rifampicin and ethambutol, and thus are difficult to treat.

M. gastri and *M. terrae* (syn. radish bacillus) grow as white, rough or smooth colonies. The bacilli are long or moderately so. Both species have been isolated from sputum, gastric lavage and soil, and are non-pathogenic.

M. malmoense. Recently, a mycobacterium that formerly would have been identified as *M. terrae* has been shown to be a cause of pulmonary disease and cervical adenitis (Jenkins & Tsukamura 1979). It has been named *M. malmoense.* It grows slowly as white rough colonies and is resistant to isoniazid and rifampicin, sometimes also to streptomycin and ethambutol. Lipid analysis distinguishes it from *M. terrae* and other non-chromogens.

Rapid growers

The rapidly growing mycobacteria are those species that from an inoculum giving well separated colonies show good growth within 5 days at 37°C, usually in 2–3 days. They are also distinguished from the slowly growing mycobacteria by their ability to grow on Sauton agar containing 0.2% picric acid.

M. chelonae (syn *M. abscessus. M. borstelense, M. runyoni*) forms white to cream-coloured colonies that are easily emulsified. The bacilli vary from coccoid to filamentous. It grows better at 25°C than at 37°C. Chromatography may be helpful in identification (Goodfellow & Minnikin 1981). Some strains are niacin positive and some are sensitive to picric acid. It has been isolated from abscesses at injection sites and occasionally from other lesions, but is found in the·soil and should not normally be regarded as a pathogen.

M. fortuitum (syn. *M. giae, M. minetti, M. ranae*) also grows as white to cream-coloured, easily emulsified colonies containing coccoid to filamentous bacteria. It is found in the soil and has been isolated from sputum and abscesses in man, but should not be regarded as a pathogen in such patients without further evidence. When inoculated intravenously in mice it causes 'spinning' ('rolling') disease and renal abscesses. It grows better at 37°C than at 25°C and grows to form red colonies on MacConkey agar.

M. phlei (syn. Timothy grass bacillus) grows as rough colonies that at first are buff coloured and later become yellow to orange. The bacilli are short rods. It differs from *M. smegmatis* and other rapidly growing mycobacteria by being capable of growth at 52°C. It is not pathogenic.

M. smegmatis (syn. smegma bacillus, *M. butyricum, M. stercoria*) forms rough colonies, white to buff in colour. The bacilli are slender rods, sometimes curved and beaded. It is not pathogenic. As it is present in smegma, a whitish secretion around the orifice of the urethra, it may be found in specimens of urine. Care must be taken not to mistake it for the tubercle bacillus. Some strains are less strongly acid-fast than the tubercle bacillus and are decolourized by alcohol, so that they are not seen in a Ziehl-Neelsen smear if acid-alcohol is used as decolourizer. Other strains are both acid- and alcohol-fast, and for this reason the appearance of acid- and alcohol-fast bacilli in a specimen of urine should not be reported as being *strongly* suggestive of tuberculous infection. The organism must be isolated and examined in culture, wherein its rapid growth distinguishes it from the tubercle bacillus. If possible, some centrifuged deposit of the urine, or some of the culture, should be inoculated into a guinea-pig, in which the smegma bacillus or other saprophytic acid-fast bacillus will be non-pathogenic.

Differential Mantoux tests

Tuberculin can be prepared from the different species of atypical mycobacteria and used in skin tests in the same way as tuberculin prepared from *M. tuberculosis*. If an atypical tuberculin produces a larger area of induration than the human-type tuberculin, support is given to the conclusion that the patient is suffering from an infection with the relevant atypical bacillus rather than from tuberculosis.

MYCOBACTERIUM LEPRAE

The leprosy bacillus was first observed microscopically in leprous tissue by Hansen in 1897, but has not yet been grown on inanimate culture media despite claims to the contrary. The bacillus is straight or slightly curved, about the same size as the tubercle bacillus, but not as strongly acid-fast. To demonstrate the organism, the Ziehl-Neelsen staining method should be modified by the use of a weaker decolourizer than used for tubercle bacilli; 5% H_2SO_4 should be used instead of 20% H_2SO_4, or 1% HCl in alcohol may be used.

Smears may be made from any ulcerated nodule on the skin. An unulcerated nodule may be slit with a scalpel and squeezed to exude fluid on to a slide. A smear made from a slit in the ear lobe may yield a positive result even when there is no obvious local lesion. Smears should always be made from scrapings or secretion from the nasal mucosa, for these may yield positive results when skin lesions are not apparent. The organism may also be present in sputum when the lungs are affected.

Two smears should be stained by the Ziehl-Neelsen method, the one with a strong acid decolourizer (e.g. 20% H_2SO_4), the other with a weak decolourizer (e.g. 5% H_2SO_4). The leprosy bacillus can thus be distinguished from tubercle bacilli and other mycobacteria because it may show acid-fast staining only in the latter smear.

The leprosy bacilli are typically found tightly packed within macrophages, but some extracellular bacilli can also be seen. In the examination of a smear from a patient under treatment, note should be taken of the relative numbers of well stained and poorly stained or fragmented bacilli. The morphological index (MI), i.e. the percentage of bacilli showing solid staining, can then be calculated. As poorly stained bacilli are probably dead, MI measurements may be used to monitor the effectiveness of treatment. A continuing fall in the MI is encouraging, but a fall succeeded by a rise indicates the onset of drug resistance in the bacteria or a failure by the patient to take the prescribed treatment.

Injection of material containing leprosy bacilli into the foot pads of mice induces a characteristic lesion. This animal model may be used for the testing of drug sensitivity in the bacillus and for assessing the value of new drugs. The armadillo has recently been found to be susceptible to widespread infection with *M. leprae* and can be used to produce large amounts of bacilli for research, the preparation of lepromin or the production of a vaccine.

Skin tests with lepromin prepared from infected human tissue and lepromin prepared from armadillo lesions produce similar reactions in man. A positive result does not aid diagnosis because many individuals not suffering from leprosy give positive reactions.

The intradermal inoculation of lepromin can elicit either of two types of reaction. The first is maximal at 48 h, is similar to a positive tuberculin reaction and is called the Fernandez reaction. The second, or Mitsuda reaction, appears 3–4 weeks after the injection in the form of a nodule that may proceed to ulcerate. The Fernandez reaction indicates that the patient has been infected at some time in the past, and can not be taken to indicate current disease activity. The Mitsuda reaction is associated with the tuberculoid type of leprosy and indicates some degree of immunity.

With the advent of the armadillo as an experimental animal there is hope that an effective vaccine may be produced from *M. leprae*. Meantime BCG has been tried as a vaccine against leprosy, but the results have been conflicting, good in Uganda but poor in Burma (Grange 1980).

METHODS

Sauton's medium

Asparagine	4 g
Citric acid	2 g
Glycerol	60 g
Dipotassium hydrogen phosphate, K_2HPO_4	0.5 g
Magnesium sulphate, $MgSO_4.7H_2O$	0.5 g
Ferric ammmonium citrate, green scales	0.05 g
Agar (Oxoid No. 3)	12 g
Distilled water	940 ml

Dissolve the reagents except the agar in the distilled water, add ammonium hydroxide, 20% NH_4OH solution, to adjust the pH to 7.2, add the agar and autoclave to dissolve and sterilize.

Picric acid medium

Picric acid is supplied as a suspension, 50% (w/w) in water. It should not be allowed to dry out as it then becomes explosive.

Picric acid suspension (50% in water)	4 g
Sauton's agar medium	1 litre

Autoclave to melt, mix and sterilize and distribute in 10 ml volumes as slopes in Universal containers. The complete medium contains 0.2% of picric acid. Inoculate moderately heavily and incubate at 37°C for up to 14 days before reading growth as negative.

Most of the rapidly growing tuberculoid bacilli, such as *M. chelonae*, *M. phlei* and *M. smegmatis*, give growth on this medium and are thereby distinguished from the slowly growing tuberculoid bacilli, which fail to grow in the presence of the picric acid.

Photochromogenesis test

Inoculate a suspension of the culture under test on to each of two Löwenstein-Jensen slopes. Wrap one slope in aluminium foil to exclude light from it and leave the other unwrapped. Incubate both slopes for 14 days at 37°C in an incubator containing a lighted 15 watt electric bulb shining on the slopes. If on removal from the incubator the unwrapped, but not the wrapped culture shows a yellow or orange pigment, the strain is a photochromogen. If both cultures are pigmented, it is a scotochromogen, and if neither is pigmented, it is a nonchromogen.

For laboratories that rarely isolate tuberculoid bacilli, a simpler but quite satisfactory method is to grow the culture fully in the dark in a conventional incubator, note the presence or absence of pigment immediately on removal from the incubator and note it again after the culture has been left for a day or two exposed to full daylight on a window sill.

Aryl sulphatase test

This test (Wayne 1961) identifies the presence of the enzyme aryl sulphatase in certain atypical mycobacteria by the ability of the organism to liberate phenolphthalein from potassium phenolphthalein disulphate.

Medium

Dubos oleic agar base (Difco) made according to manufacturer's instructions	100 ml
Glycerol	1 ml
Tripotassium phenolphthalein sulphate	65 mg

Mix and melt by autoclaving, distribute the melted medium in 3 ml amounts in small screw-capped bottles, autoclave at 121°C for 15 min, and allow the medium to cool and set in the sloped position.

Test. Inoculate 0.1 ml of liquid culture on to the slope and incubate for 3 days at 37°C. Then add 0.5 ml of 1 mol/litre sodium carbonate solution. The development of a pink or red colour denotes a positive aryl sulphatase reaction. A positive control culture of *M. fortuitum* should be set up in parallel with the test culture.

Alternative method

The method of Collins (1966) uses a simpler, liquid medium, but the test requires to be incubated for 14 days.

Medium

Potassium phenolphthalein disulphate	0.646 g
Distilled water	100 ml

Sterilize the solution by membrane filtration and add 10 ml of it to each 100 ml of Dubos and Davis liquid medium (Ch. 25). Distribute the medium aseptically in 3 ml volumes.

Test. Inoculate 0.1 ml of liquid test culture into 3 ml medium and incubate at 37°C for 14 days. Add 0.5 ml of 0.2 mol/litre sodium carbonate solution. The development of a red colour denotes a positive reaction. A positive control culture of *M. gordonae* should be set up in parallel with the test culture.

Tween hydrolysis test (Marks 1976)

Phosphate buffer, 0.067 mol/litre, pH 7.0

Disodium hydrogen phosphate, $Na_2HPO_4.12 H_2O$	5.75 g
Potassium dihydrogen phosphate, KH_2PO_4	3.5 g
Distilled water	1 litre

Medium

Tween 80, 10% solution	5 ml
Phosphate buffer solution, pH 7.0	100 ml

Check pH and adjust again to 7.0 if necessary. Then add 2 ml of fresh 0.1% neutral red solution. Dispense in 2 ml volumes. Autoclave at 121°C for 15 min. Cool and store in the refrigerator at about 4°C to keep for up to 4 weeks.

Test. Inoculate heavily, incubate at 37°C for 5 days, then read result. A red colour is a positive result. Put up a parallel test with a positive control culture of *M. kansasi.*

Catalase test

The reagent is a mixture of equal volumes of 1% Tween 80 and a 20 volume solution of hydrogen peroxide. Pour 5 ml of this reagent over the surface of a Löwenstein-Jensen slope culture of the strain to be tested and leave the slope in a horizontal position for 5 min. Then place upright and look for effervescence. A strongly positive control culture of *M. kansasi* should be set up in parallel.

Effervescence of more than 10 mm is strongly positive (+++); of 5–10 mm is moderately positive (++); of 1–5 mm is weakly positive (+); of under 1 mm is negative (−).

In Table 26.1, the +++ and ++ reactions are shown as + and the + reaction (weak) as ±.

Glucose utilization test (Tsukamura 1967)

Medium

Ammonium sulphate	2.64 g
Potassium dihydrogen phosphate, KH_2PO_4	0.5 g

Magnesium sulphate,
MgSO₄.7H₂O 0.5 g
Agar 20 g
Distilled water 990 ml

Mix, autoclave at 121°C for 15 min, cool and add 10 ml of 20% aqueous solution of glucose that has been sterilized by filtration. Dispense as slopes in Universal containers.

Test. Inoculate lightly and incubate at 37°C for 21 days. Put up a parallel positive control culture of *M. phlei*. Visible growth within 21 days denotes a positive result.

Salicylate degradation test (Tsukamura 1967)

Medium

Sodium salicylate 1 g
Sauton's agar medium 1 litre

Autoclave at 121°C for 15 min to melt, mix and sterilize. Distribute as slopes in Universal containers.

Test. Inoculate heavily and incubate at 37°C for 7 days. Growth with blackening of the medium is a positive result. Put up a parallel positive control culture of *M. fortuitum*.

Tellurite reduction test (Kilburn et al 1969)

The medium is Middlebrook 7H9 liquid medium (Difco) dispensed aseptically in 5 ml amounts. Inoculate the test culture heavily into the medium and incubate at 37°C for 7 days. Growth must be profuse if the result is to be valid. Then add two drops of 0.2% autoclaved aqueous solution of potassium tellurite and incubate at 37°C for another 3 days. Without shaking, examine the sediment. The presence of an intensely black precipitate denotes a positive result. A light grey or brown colouration is a negative result. Put up a parallel positive control culture of *M. fortuitum*.

REFERENCES

Birn K J, Schaefer W B, Jenkins P A, Szulga T, Marks J 1967 Classification of *Myco. avium* and related opportunist mycobacteria met in England and Wales. Journal of Hygiene, Cambridge 65: 575–589

Buchanan R E, Gibbon N E (eds) 1974 Bergey's Manual of determinative bacteriology, 8th edn. Williams & Wilkins, Baltimore. p 688

Collins C H 1966 Revised classification of anonymous mycobacteria. Journal of Clinical Pathology 19: 433–437

Goodfellow M, Minnikin D E 1981 Identification of *Myco. chelonei* by thin layer chromatographic analysis of whole organism methanolysates. Tubercle 62: 285–287

Grange J M 1980 Mycobacterial diseases. Arnold, London. Ch 6

Jenkins P A Tsukamura M 1979 Infections with *Mycobacterium malmoense* in England and Wales. Tubercle 60: 71–76

Kilburn J O, Silcox V A, Kubica G P 1969 Differential identification of mycobacteria. V. The tellurite reduction test. American Review of Respiratory Disease 99: 94–100

Marks J 1976 A system for the examination of tubercle and other mycobacteria. Tubercle 57: 207–225

Schaefer W B 1965 Serologic identification and classification of the atypical mycobacteria by their agglutination. American Review of Respiratory Disease 92: 85–93

Szulga T, Jenkins P A, Marks J 1966 Thin layer chromatography of mycobacterial lipids as an aid to classification; *Myco. kansasii* and *Myco. marinum* (balnei). Tubercle 47: 130–136

Tsukamura M 1967 Identification of mycobacteria. Tubercle 48: 311–338

Wayne L G 1961 Recognition of *Myco. fortuitum* by means of a three-day phenolphthalein sulphatase test. American Journal of Clinical Pathology 36: 185–187

Wayne L G 1985 The atypical mycobacteria: recognition and disease association. CRC Critical Reviews in Microbiology 12: 185–222

Woods G L, Washington J A 1987 Mycobacteria other than *Mycobacterium tuberculosis*: Review of microbiologic and clinical aspects. Reviews of Infectious Diseases 9: 275–294

W H O Report 1977 Fifth report of expert committee on leprosy. World Health Organization Technical Report Series No. 607

Actinomyces: Nocardia: Streptomyces

The actinomyces group of organisms are Gram-positive branching filamentous bacteria, mostly 0.6–1 μm in width, which may grow as a felted mass, or mycelium, or fragment into bacillary and coccoid forms. They are non-motile and slow growing. The genus *Actinomyces* comprises non-acid-fast, fragmenting species that are facultative, microaerophilic or obligatory anaerobes, live as commensal parasites in the mouth and intestine of man and animals, and occasionally cause actinomycosis, a chronic granulomatous disease. The genus *Nocardia* comprises strictly aerobic, fragmenting species, some of which are weakly acid-fast and some of which form fragmenting aerial hyphae; they are saprophytic inhabitants of the soil, but occasionally cause chronic infections such as mycetoma in man. The genus *Streptomyces* comprises aerobic species that form a non-fragmenting, non-acid-fast mycelium with aerial hyphae bearing chains of conidiospores; they are saprophytic inhabitants of the soil and rarely cause mycetoma in man. For a classification of the Actinomycetaceae, see Schofield & Schaal (1981).

ACTINOMYCES

In the infected body the actinomycetes grow as mycelia which appear in tissue and pus as granules. These granules are generally 0.3–1 mm in diameter and thus visible to the naked eye. They are white at first but become yellow later (sulphur granules) and in long-standing infections may eventually become dark brown. At their periphery the tips of the filaments may become expanded into Gram-negative, weakly acid-fast *clubs* which surround the granule like a ray of petals (ray fungus). The filaments have a marked tendency to fragment and many bacillary and coccoid forms are seen in films of crushed granules and cultures. Growth is improved by 5% CO_2.

Actinomyces israeli, a normal anaerobic inhabitant of the mouth and gut in man, occasionally acts as a pathogen and is the commonest cause of human actinomycosis. That disease is generally manifest as chronic suppurative lesions with discharging sinuses, though initially the lesions may appear as acute abscesses. The area most commonly affected is the face and neck, which become infected from the mouth. The lungs and abdomen are sometimes infected, and the uterus and cervix may be infected in women wearing an intrauterine contraceptive device (Traynor et al 1981). *A. bovis* is the cause of actinomycosis (lumpy jaw) in cattle but is not a pathogen in man.

A. naeslundi, *A. odontolyticus* and *A. viscosus* are common commensals in the mouth. They are found in saliva, but more particularly in dental plaque and the gingival crevice, and they may play a part in the causation of dental caries and gingivitis. *A. eriksoni* has been isolated from subcutaneous, pulmonary and abdominal actinomycotic abscesses, but is now considered to belong to the genus *Bifidobacterium*.

Laboratory diagnosis

Specimens

When pus is available it should be sent to the laboratory in preference to a swab. If discharge from a sinus is scanty, the gauze dressing should be obtained for examination. A tube or Universal container of pus should be rotated to allow the pus to flow over the inside of its walls, when any granules will be easily seen and can be picked off for examination. Otherwise, pus may be spread over the floor of a Petri dish to make the granules visible and accessible. If a soiled dressing is obtained it should be inspected for granules adhering to the fibres. When there is difficulty in collecting granules from pus, add the pus to sterile saline in a Universal container, cap tightly and shake. Then let the container stand until granules are seen to settle to the foot and collect them with a capillary pipette.

Microscopy

1. Place a granule in a drop of saline on a slide, press on a coverslip to flatten the granule and examine it with a × 40 dry objective. The centre of the granules will show interlacing, branching filaments and bacillary and coccoid forms, and the periphery may show radiating clubs.

2. Remove the coverslip, dry and heat-fix the smear on the slide and stain it by Gram's method. Alternatively, crush another granule between two slides, separate the slides, dry and heat-fix them, and stain one by Gram's method and the other by Ziehl-Neelsen. Examine with the × 100 oil-immersion objective. The presence of Gram-positive branching filaments, $0.6–1~\mu m$ in width, even if scantily present among a predominance of bacillary and coccoid forms, is strongly suggestive of the presence of an actinomycete.

3. Stain other crush preparations by the Ziehl-Neelsen and modified Ziehl-Neelsen methods with, respectively, 20% and 1% H_2SO_4 for 5 min as the decolourizer. Both preparations should show only non-acid-fast organisms if the infection is due to actinomyces. Organisms fast to 1% but not 20% H_2SO_4 are likely to be nocardias.

4. If there are no granules, make a Gram smear of the pus and look for Gram-positive branching filaments. Whilst most forms may be bacillary or coccoid, the presence of even short fragments of filaments showing true branching is suggestive of an actinomyces infection.

Culture

1. As actinomyces is slow growing and faster growing bacteria may be present as contaminants in the specimen, first wash the granules in saline to remove most of the contaminants. Mix some pus containing granules in 20 ml sterile saline in a Universal container, cap tightly and shake vigorously. Allow to stand until the granules settle, discard the supernate, replace with fresh saline and repeat this process about four times. Finally crush the granules in a small volume of saline with a sterile glass rod and inoculate the suspension into the culture media.

If granules are not available, make 10-fold dilutions of the pus from 1 in 10 to 1 in 100 000 and inoculate each dilution into culture media.

2. *Unselective media.* Inoculate a drop or loopful of the suspension on to each of the following unselective media. (a) A blood agar plate for incubation in air with 5% CO_2. (b) Two blood agar plates for anaerobic incubation, the one for examination after 48 h, the other for examination after 7 days. (c) A tube of thioglycollate broth. (d) A tube of cooked meat medium. (e) A tube of 1% glucose semi-solid agar which is rolled to give a uniform distribution of the inoculum (shake culture). Incubate all cultures at 37°C, (c)–(e) in air, and the fluid media for 2 weeks before discarding as negative.

3. *Selective media.* Blood agar containing a selectively inhibitory agent may be tried but may not always be successful. If selective media are used, unselective media should also be used in parallel (Willis 1977). The following agents have been recommended: colistin 10 mg/litre; kanamycin 7.5 mg/l (Ellner et al 1973); metronidazole 2.5 mg/l (Traynor et al 1981); nalidixic acid 15 mg/l (Ellner et al 1973); phenylethyl alcohol 25%; vancomycin 100 mg/l. An enriched gelatin agar containing metronidazole 10 mg/l and cadmium sulphate 20 mg/l has been described for the isolation of *A. naeslundi* and *A. viscosus* from dental plaque (Kornman & Loesche 1978).

Table 27.1 Distinguishing characters of *Actinomyces* species.
Key: ±, slight growth only; +/−, some strains positive, others negative

Character	A. israeli	A. bovis	A. naeslundi	A. viscosus	A. odontolyticus[a]	A. eriksoni
Growth						
in air	−	±	+	+	+	−
in air + CO_2	±	+	+	+	+	−
anaerobic + CO_2	+	+	+	+	+	+
Acid produced from						
glucose	+	+	+	+	+	+
mannitol	+/−	−	−	−	−	+
raffinose	+/−	−	+	+	+/−	+
starch	+/−	+	+/−	+/−	+	+
xylose	+	+/−	−	+/−	+/−	+
Catalase produced				+	−	−
Nitrate reduced	+/−	+/−	+	+	+	−

[a] Red colonies on blood agar.

4. *Results*. After 48 h examine the plates for small white colonies and, with a plate micro-scope, for microcolonies composed of branching filaments (spider colonies). Re-examine after 7 days, when colonies of *A. israeli* will be 0.5–3 mm in diameter, white, non-haemolytic, smooth and entire or lobulated (molar tooth form) or rough surfaced, and either hard or soft in texture.

At both examinations make Gram-stained smears of representative colonies. Subculture aerobically and anaerobically on blood agar any colony type seen to contain Gram-positive bacilli or filaments, even if without branching.

Observe the shake culture for maximal growth 10–20 mm below the surface, characteristic of microaerophilic *A. israeli*. Look for granules or turbidity in the liquid media. Examine in a Gram smear and subculture any growths of Gram-positive filaments or bacilli.

Identification

Prepare a homogenized suspension in saline from isolated colonies on the subculture plates and inoculate drops of it into the fermentation tests* and other tests listed in Table 27.1. For

* Refer to *Methods* at end of this chapter.

details of standardized procedures, see Slack (1968). The use of an API ZYM test kit may assist identification (Kilian 1978). Atmospheric requirements may be tested by shake culture in semi-solid agar as described under *Methods* in Chapter 25. Also send a subculture to a refer-ence laboratory. Meantime report as 'probably *Actinomyces israeli*' any isolate from a typical lesion consisting of slender branching Gram-positive filaments or bacilli that are anaerobic or microaerophilic, non-motile and catalase negative.

Fluorescent antibody techniques may be used to identify different species of *Actinomyces* and to separate *A. israeli* into two serotypes (Holm-berg & Forsum 1973). Other identification methods include thin-layer chromatography of the fatty acids produced in fermentation (Pala-suntheram et al 1977) and analysis of cell wall components (Boone & Pine 1968).

Antibiotic sensitivity

A. israeli is highly sensitive to a variety of drugs, including benzylpenicillin, cephaloridine, fusidic acid and lincomycin. Prolonged treatment may be required where penetration is poor. Because the actinomycetes are slow growing, sensitivities should be tested in a series of culture tubes containing different concentrations of the antibiotic, not by the disk diffusion method. The organism is resistant to metronidazole, which is incorporated in some selective media.

NOCARDIA

The nocardias are strictly aerobic and slow growing. A few days' incubation at 37°C is required before well sized colonies are formed. The Gram-positive branching filaments then tend to fragment into bacillary and coccoid forms. Though generally harmless saprophytes in the soil, some species occasionally cause opportunistic infections.

Nocardia asteroides, an acid-fast species, occasionally causes disease in previously healthy subjects, but the increasing use of steroids and cytotoxic drugs is predisposing to more frequent infections. As its normal habitat is the soil, inhalation of dust is the main mode of infection. It may cause severe pulmonary disease with cavitation and haematogenous dissemination, and it may also be found in cutaneous and subcutaneous abscesses, brain abscesses and renal lesions. Granules are not found in the pus or tissues. In culture, colonies usually appear in 2–3 days, but may take much longer to develop.

Actinomycotic mycetoma (Madura foot) is common in tropical and subtropical countries where people walk barefooted and commonly suffer the introduction of soil organisms through pricks and abrasions in the soles of their feet. It is a chronic suppurative disease of subcutaneous tissue and bone with multiple sinuses discharging pus containing pigmented granules. *N. madurae* (non-acid-fast), *N. brasiliensis* (acid-fast), other nocardias and various species of *Streptomyces*, e.g. *S. somaliensis* are found in this condition, either singly or in various combinations. Mycetoma is also caused by a variety of true fungi (Ch. 42).

Laboratory diagnosis

Specimens

Collect a sample of pus, sputum or other exudate. Swabs of exudate are unsuitable.

Microscopy

1. Make a Gram-stained smear of the specimen and look for slender Gram-positive branching filaments which may show beading. Their presence suggests actinomycosis or nocardiosis.

2. Make two further smears and stain them by the conventional and modified Ziehl-Neelsen methods, the one decolourized for 10 min with 20% H_2SO_4 (or 3% HCl in 95% ethanol) and the other for 5 min with 1% H_2SO_4 or 1% HCl. Some nocardias, e.g. *N. madurae* and *N. pelletieri*, are non-acid-fast with both the stronger and weaker decolourizers. Others, e.g. *N. asteroides* and *N. brasiliensis*, are acid-fast with the weaker but not the stronger one. Bacillary forms acid-fast with 20% H_2SO_4 are likely to be mycobacteria.

A provisional report of the presence of nocardia can be made if the smears show slender branching Gram-positive filaments that are non-sporing and weakly acid-fast.

Culture

1. Plate out the specimen on each of two plates of blood agar and two plates of Sabouraud agar (Ch. 42) not containing antibiotics or other selective agents. Incubate aerobically, one set at 37°C and the other at 40–42°C, for up to 14 days before discarding as negative. Contaminating bacteria are at a disadvantage at the higher temperature. Also inoculate into tubes of thioglycollate broth and cooked meat medium in case the organism is an actinomyces or other anaerobe.

Some acid-fast nocardias may survive treatment with NaOH by Petroff's method and grow on Löwenstein-Jensen medium. They may therefore be encountered on cultural examination for tubercle bacilli. Colonies of *N. asteroides* may closely resemble and be mistaken for those of *M. tuberculosis*.

2. Every day or so examine the plates for pigmented rough or smooth colonies with white aerial mycelium suggestive of a nocardia. Pigment, however, may be absent and aerial mycelium difficult to see. Colonies of *N.*

asteroides may be white or yellow or, on blood agar, orange with white aerial mycelium. Cultures of nocardias and streptomyces usually have an earthy odour.

3. Make a Gram film from each colony type and look for Gram-positive bacillary and coccoid forms as well as branching filaments, which may not be seen in older cultures. Also stain smears by the Ziehl-Neelsen and modified Ziehl-Neelsen methods to demonstrate the weakly acid-fast nocardias.

4. Set up slide cultures to demonstrate the branching of filaments. Look for aerial hyphae bearing long or short chains of conidiospores indicative of *Streptomyces*. The preparation may be set up as for the growth of dermatophytic fungi (Ch. 42). Various slide culture techniques are described by Williams & Cross (1971).

Identification

1. As the exact identification of a nocardial species is difficult, send a culture to a reference laboratory.

2. Set up and read the biochemical tests* shown in Table 27.2 for provisional identification of the more important species. The provisional identification of *N. asteroides* may be reported if the isolate is a Gram-positive branching filamentous or diphtheroid-like bacterium, not showing spores on slide culture, catalase-positive and not decomposing casein, tyrosine or xanthine.

Antibiotic sensitivity tests

The agar dilution method is more satisfactory

than the disk diffusion method (Wallace et al 1977). For further information, see Conant et al (1971) and Goodfellow (1971).

STREPTOMYCES

The streptomycetes are generally harmless saprophytes of the soil, though some species, e.g. *Streptomyces griseus* and *S. somaliensis*, have been found in cases of mycetoma. In the pus in such cases they form hard, smooth, yellowish red granules about 1 mm in diameter which are not dissociated by KOH. The increasing use of immunosuppressive drugs may lead to streptomycetes being isolated more frequently from the patients so compromised.

The streptomycetes are strictly aerobic actinomycetes which grow as non-fragmenting, branching Gram-positive filaments about 1 μm in width. Most species form aerial hyphae bearing long chains of, e.g. 10–50, conidiospores. Their morphology is best studied in slide cultures on yeast-malt or starch agar. They are distinguished from nocardias by their non-fragmenting mycelium, non-acid-fast character, and cell wall content of LL-, instead of meso-, diaminopimelic acid.

They grow slowly on blood agar, at first as small translucent colonies which later become opaque, rough and nodular and bear white or coloured aerial mycelium. The colonies are tough and adherent to the medium and cultures often have an earthy odour. Special media are needed to demonstrate the identifying characters of the different species, such as the colour of the colony and the morphology of the spore chain.

Table 27.2 Distinguishing characters of some nocardias.

| Species | Acid-fast with 1% H_2SO_4 | Catalase production | Decomposition of | | |
			Casein	Tyrosine	Xanthine
N. asteroides	+	+	−	−	−
N. brasiliensis	+	+	+	+	−
N. caviae	+	+	−	−	+
N. madurae	−	+	+	+/−	−
N. pelletieri	−	+	+	+	−

Speciation is a specialized procedure and an isolate thought to be a streptomycete should be referred to an expert. For an account of methods see Shirling & Gottlieb (1966) and, for a simple key, Küster (1972). For an identification matrix and details of methods, see Williams et al (1983).

METHODS

Optimal test methods for oxygen requirements and biochemical reactions of actinomycetes are described by Slack (1968).

Catalase test

Hold the culture for at least 30 min under aerobic conditions before testing. Pour a freshly prepared 3% solution of hydrogen peroxide in distilled water over a slant culture on brain heart infusion or similar agar medium. Look for the active production of bubbles.

Actinomyces fermentation tests

Media. The basal medium is thioglycollate broth (Ch. 6) without glucose or indicator. Yeast extract 0.2–0.5% may be added to enhance growth. Add filter-sterilized sugar solutions to a final concentration of 1% or, in the case of soluble starch, 0.4%. Distribute in tubes in 10 ml amounts.

Inoculum. Grow a culture of the actinomyces isolate for 3 or 4 days in thioglycollate broth. Mix the growth by drawing it in and out of a pipette.

Procedure. Add 0.1 ml of inoculum to each tube of carbohydrate medium. Incubate anaerobically, preferably in nitrogen with 5% (v/v) CO_2, for 48 h at 37°C. Add two drops of 0.4% bromothymol blue. The appearance of a yellow colour indicates acid production. Continue anaerobic incubation to 14 days. If the inoculum is heavy, the results may be readable at 48 h. If the colour of the indicator is equivocal, test with a pH meter and record a drop of one unit of pH as compared with uninoculated medium as indicative of acid production.

Decomposition of casein

Medium

Skim milk powder	75 g
Agar	20 g
Distilled water	1 litre

Add the milk powder a little at a time to a small volume of water to form a smooth paste, adding more water as required. Finally add water to 500 ml. Autoclave for 20 min at 115°C.

Dissolve the agar in another 500 ml water and autoclave. Cool both solutions to 60–65°C and pour the agar into the milk. Mix and pour 20 ml amounts into plates; allow to set and dry.

Method. Streak the test culture on a plate, incubate aerobically at 37°C for up to 14 days or until there is good growth. Examine for clearing around the streak, indicative of casein hydrolysis.

Decomposition of tyrosine and xanthine

Medium

Tyrosine	5 g
or xanthine	4 g
Nutrient agar, dehydrated	23 g
Distilled water	1 litre

Dissolve the nutrient agar powder in the water by autoclaving. Add the tyrosine or the xanthine and mix to distribute the crystals evenly. Adjust the pH to 7.0 and autoclave for 15 min at 121°C. Dispense 20 ml amounts in plates, keeping the bulk mixed to ensure even distribution of the crystals.

Method. Streak the test culture on the plate, incubate aerobically at 37°C for up to 14 days or until there is good growth. Examine for clearing around the streak, indicative of decomposition of the tyrosine or xanthine.

REFERENCES

Boone C J, Pine L 1968 Rapid method for the characterization of *Actinomyces israelii* by cell wall composition. Applied Microbiology 16: 279–284

Bowden G H, Hardie J M 1971 Anaerobic organisms from the human mouth. In: Shapton D A, Board R G (eds) Isolation of anaerobes. Society for Applied Bacteriology Technical Series No. 5. Academic Press, London. p 177–205

Conant N F, Smith D T, Baker R D, Callaway J L 1971 Manual of clinical mycology, 3rd edn. Saunders, London. ch 1, 2, 3

Ellner P D, Granato P A, May C B 1973 Recovery and identification of anaerobes. A system suitable for the routine laboratory. Applied Microbiology 26: 904–913

Goodfellow M 1971 Numerical taxonomy of some nocardioform bacteria. Journal of General Microbiology 69: 33–80

Holmberg K, Forsum U 1973 Identification of *Actinomyces, Arachnia, Bacterionema, Rothia* and *Propionibacterium* species by defined immunofluorescence. Applied Microbiology 25: 834–843

Kilian M 1978 Rapid identification of Actinomycetaceae and related bacteria. Journal of Clinical Microbiology 8: 127–133

Kornman K S, Loesche W J 1978 A new medium for isolation of *Actinomyces viscosus* and *Actinomyces naeslundii* from dental plaque. Journal of Clinical Microbiology 7: 514–518

Küster E 1972 Simple working key for the classification and identification of named taxa included in the international *Streptomyces* project. International Journal of Systematic Bacteriology 22: 139–148

Palasuntheram C, Drucker D B, Tuxford A F 1977 Feasibility of thin layer chromatography as an inexpensive alternative to gas liquid chromatography for the identification of some anaerobic Gram-positive nonsporing rods. Journal of Applied Bacteriology 42: 451–453

Schofield G M, Schaal K P 1981 A numerical study of members of the Actinomycetaceae and related taxa. Journal of General Microbiology 127: 237–259

Shirling E B, Gottlieb D 1966 Methods for the characterization of *Streptomyces* species. International Journal of Systematic Bacteriology 16: 313–340

Slack J M 1968 Subgroup on taxonomy of microaerophilic actinomycetes. Report on organization, aims and procedures. International Journal of Systematic Bacteriology 18: 253–262

Traynor R M, Parratt D, Duguid H L D, Duncan I D 1981 Isolation of *Actinomyces* from cervical specimens. Journal of Clinical Pathology 34: 914–916

Wallace R J Jr, Septimus E J, Musher D M, Martin R R 1977 Disc diffusion susceptibility testing of *Nocardia* species. Journal of Infectious Diseases 135: 568–576

Williams S T, Cross T 1971 Actinomycetes. In: Booth C (ed) Methods in microbiology, vol 4. Academic Press, London. ch 11

Williams S T, Goodfellow M, Wellington E M H, Vickers J C, Alderson G, Sneath P H A, Sackin M J, Mortimer A M 1983 A probability matrix for identification of some streptomycetes. Journal of General Microbiology 129: 1815–1830

Willis A T 1977 Anaerobic bacteriology: clinical and laboratory practice, 3rd edn. Butterworth, London

Enterobacteriaceae: Escherichia, Klebsiella, Proteus and other enterobacteria

ENTEROBACTERIACEAE

Definition of the family

The Enterobacteriaceae are Gram-negative bacilli that are either motile with peritrichous flagella or non-motile, grow both aerobically and anaerobically on simple laboratory media and on MacConkey bile-salt lactose agar (Ch. 6), are oxidase negative and, with few exceptions, catalase positive, and reduce nitrates to nitrites. They ferment glucose in peptone water with the production of either acid or acid and gas, and they break down glucose and other carbohydrates both fermentatively under anaerobic conditions and oxidatively under aerobic conditions, e.g. in the Hugh & Leifson test.

The above description defines the Enterobacteriaceae and separates the family from Gram-negative bacilli that might be confused with it. Of the many other genera of Gram-nega-tive bacilli some are easy to distinguish from the Enterobacteriaceae (e.g. *Brucella* and *Haemophilus* have exacting nutritional requirements; *Bacteroides* are strict anaerobes) but some which grow readily on simple laboratory media under aerobic conditions can give rise to problems in identification. Key differentiating characters of those most often encountered in medical microbiology are listed in Table 28.1. The taxonomy of the genera, and species within the genera, has been the subject of repeated changes partly because the organisms in this heterogeneous group are relatively inert in the common biochemical tests. For discussion see Cowan & Steel (1974) and Lennette et al (1980).

Genera of Enterobacteriaceae

Over the years there have been a number of confusing alterations in the nomenclature of the

Table 28.1 Differentiating characters of aerobic Gram-negative bacilli.
Key: pol, polar flagella; pt, peritrichous flagella; +, most or all members positive; −, most or all members negative; +/−, some members positive, some negative.

Genus	Motility	Flagella	Anaerobic growth	Catalase reaction	Oxidase reaction	Reaction with glucose[a]
Acinetobacter	−	...	−	+	−	O or −
Moraxella	−	...	−	+	+	−
Achromobacter	+	pt	−	+	+	O
Alkaligenes	+	pt	−	+	+	−
Pseudomonas	+	pol	−	+	+	O
Vibrio *Aeromonas* *Plesiomonas*	+	pol	+	+	+	F
Genera of Enterobacteriaceae	+/−	pt	+	+	−	F

[a] Reaction with glucose in the Hugh & Leifson test: F, acid produced under anaerobic conditions (fermentatively); O, acid produced only under aerobic conditions (oxidatively); −, acid not produced either fermentatively or oxidatively.

genera that constitute the family Entero-bacteriaceae. The genera recognized in this book are: *Citrobacter* (including the Ballerup-Bethesda group), *Edwardsiella, Enterobacter* (syn. *Cloaca*), *Erwinia, Escherichia* (including the Alkalescens-Dispar group), *Hafnia, Klebsiella, Proteus, Providencia, Salmonella* (including the Arizona group), *Serratia, Shigella* and *Yersinia*. These genera are differentiated by their biochemical characters (Table 28.2) and it is only within a genus that serological and other methods are employed for further subdivision.

Some members of the family of Entero-bacteriaceae, e.g. *Salmonella* spp. (Ch. 29), *Shigella* spp. (Ch. 30) and some strains of *Escherichia coli*, are primary pathogens for man and their precise identification is important both clinically and epidemiologically. The other entero-bacteria are essentially commensals or sapro-phytes, but some, e.g. *E. coli*, are also common pathogens in the urinary tract, in wounds and in organs associated with the gut, e.g. appendix and gall-bladder, and most enterobacteria occasionally act elsewhere as opportunistic pathogens in individuals with defective defences. Commensal and saprophytic enterobacteria may, therefore, be isolated from clinical specimens, but their precise identification, apart from the determi-nation of their antibiotic sensitivities, has little clinical significance, although it may sometimes assist in tracing the sources of outbreaks of infec-tion among patients in hospital.

The vernacular term 'coliform bacilli' is commonly used to refer to organisms resembling *E. coli*, but there is no general agreement on the definition and membership of the coliform group. Some authors use the term as being synonymous with the Enterobacteriaceae, others confine its use to the lactose-fermenting entero-bacteria (i.e. most species of *Escherichia, Kleb-siella, Citrobacter* and *Enterobacter*) and still others use it, as generally in this book, for the enterobacteria that are urinary-tract, wound and opportunistic pathogens (e.g. *Escherichia, Kleb-*

Table 28.2 Differentiating characters of the main genera of Enterobacteriaceae and some exceptional species. *Key*: +, most or all strains positive; −, most or all strains negative; +/−, some strains positive, some negative.

Genus	Acid from lactose	Gas from glucose	Motility	Urease	Citrate utilized[a]	Voges-Proskauer	Growth in KCN
Escherichia	+	+	+	−	−	−	−
Edwardsiella	−	+	+	−	−	−	−
Shigella	−	−	−	−	−	−	−
Citrobacter	+	+	+	+/−	+	−	+
Salmonella	−	+	+	−	+	−	−
Klebsiella	+	+	−	+	+	+	+
Enterobacter	+	+	+	+/−	+	+	+
Hafnia	−	+	+	−	+	+/−	+
Serratia	+/−	+/−	+	−	+	+	+
Proteus	−	+	+	+	+/−	−	+
Providencia	−	+	+	−	+	−	+
Erwinia	+/−	−	+	−	+	+/−	−
Yersinia	−	−	+/−	+/−	−	−	−

[a] Citrate utilization tested in Koser's or Simmons' medium (Ch. 8).
Notable exceptions: Alkalescens-Dispar organisms, like *Escherichia*, but non-lactose fermenting, non-gas producing and non-motile; Ballerup-Bethesda organisms, like *Citrobacter*, but non-lactose fermenting; *Salmonella arizonae*, most strains lactose-fermenting, some gelatin liquefying; *Salmonella typhi* is non-gas-producing and non-citrate utilizing; *Klebsiella rhinoscleromatis* is negative in all reactions tabled except that with KCN; *Klebsiella ozaenae* is late-lactose-fermenting and Voges-Proskauer negative; some strains of *K. ozaenae* are negative in the gas, citrate or urease tests.

siella and *Proteus*). *Pseudomonas aeruginosa*, which is not an enterobacterium, is sometimes regarded as a 'coliform bacillus' in this last sense.

Lactose fermentation

Reactions with lactose are of great practical importance for the primary isolation of enterobacteria from clinical specimens. The specimen, e.g. faeces, is usually plated on a lactose-containing medium, such as MacConkey's medium or deoxycholate citrate agar (DCA, Ch. 29), on which the colonies of lactose-fermenting bacteria are pink and those of non-lactose-fermenting bacteria are pale. This procedure makes possible an immediate presumptive distinction between colonies of the true intestinal pathogens, namely the salmonellae and shigellae, which do not ferment lactose, and colonies of the common intestinal commensals, *E. coli* and klebsiellae, which do ferment it. The identity of the pale colonies as salmonellae or shigellae must, however, be confirmed by further tests, because some commensal and saprophytic enterobacteria are non-lactose-fermenting, e.g. all *Proteus* and *Providencia* species and the Ballerup-Bethesda, Alkalescens-Dispar (A-D) and Hafnia groups of organisms (Tables 28.2, 28.3).

The term 'paracolon bacillus' was frequently used in the past to describe non-lactose-fermenting coliform bacilli that did not belong to the well defined, non-lactose-fermenting genera, *Salmonella, Shigella* and *Proteus*. These bacteria, however, are now regarded as being non-lactose-fermenting variants of organisms in genera that are characteristically lactose-fermenting, e.g. organisms of the Alkalescens-Dispar group as non-lactose-fermenting (and non-motile and anaerogenic) variants of *Escherichia*, organisms of the Ballerup-Bethesda group as non-lactose-fermenting variants of *Citrobacter* and organisms of the Hafnia group as non-lactose-fermenting variants of *Enterobacter*. Because their full identification is often difficult and because they are not important pathogens, many clinical bacteriologists do not identify paracolon bacilli further than to exclude

the possibility that they are salmonella, shigella, proteus or pseudomonas.

Other Gram-negative bacilli isolated from clinical material are morphologically, and sometimes culturally, similar to the enterobacteria although they do not belong to any genus in the family Enterobacteriaceae. They are distinguished by their non-conformation with the criteria defining the family and they include genera such as *Acinetobacter* (including 'Bacterium anitratum'), *Alkaligenes* and *Pseudomonas*. They may be observed initially as pale colonies growing on MacConkey medium.

Identification of genus and species

The effort necessary to identify a Gram-negative bacillus that grows readily on ordinary agar varies. Although some genera, e.g. *Proteus*, may be easy to recognize, others are particularly difficult. However, for the important intestinal pathogens, *Salmonella, Shigella* and the entero-pathogenic strains of *E. coli*, clear-cut methods are available and full identification is essential.

The genera of Enterobacteriaceae to be described in this chapter comprise *Escherichia, Edwardsiella, Klebsiella, Enterobacter, Hafnia, Serratia, Citrobacter, Proteus, Providencia* and *Erwinia*. Others, namely *Salmonella, Shigella* and *Yersinia*, are considered in Chapters 29, 30 and 34 respectively.

Morphology and staining

The bacteria of these 10 genera are alike in being Gram-negative bacilli, 2–4 × 0.6 μm, and non-sporing, but show differences in the presence or absence of motility (always due to peritrichous flagella), fimbriae and capsules.

Cultural characters

Members of most genera form 'coliform-type' colonies on simple solid media, i.e. circular, 1–3 mm in diameter, low convex, smooth surfaced, colourless to grey and translucent. On MacConkey agar the colonies may be *pink*, indicating that the organism ferments lactose

Table 28.3 Reactions of *Escherichia coli* and some other enterobacteria.

Key: +, result positive with at least 80% of strains; +/−, some strains positive, some negative; −, result negative with at least 80% of strains; (+), delayed positive result (e.g. 2–8 days); (+)/−, some strains delayed positive, some negative; ±, weak reaction; . . ., results not given.

Organism	Motility	Capsule	Glucose (gas)	Lactose (acid)	ONPG	Sucrose (acid)	Salicin (acid)	Adonitol (acid)	Dulcitol (acid)	Inositol (acid)	Mannitol (acid)	Indole	Methyl red	Voges-Proskauer	Citrate	Gelatin	Phenylalanine	Urease	Hydrogen sulphide	KCN[c]	Gluconate	Malonate	Lysine decarboxylase	Ornithine decarboxylase
Erwinia herbicola	+	−	−	−/+	+	+	+/−	−	−	−/+	+	−	−	−	+	+	+	−	−	−	−/+	+	−	−
Providencia stuarti	+	−	−	−	−	(+)	−	−	−	+	−	+	+	−	+	−	+	−	−	+	−	−	−	−
Providencia alcalifaciens	+	−	+	−	−	(+)/−	−	−	−	+	−	+	+	−	+	−	+	−	−	+	−	−	−	−
Proteus (Providencia) rettgeri	+	−	−	−	−	(+)	+/−	+	−	+	+	+	+	−	+	−	+	+	−	+	−	−	−	−
Proteus (Morganella) morgani	+	−	+	−	−	−	−	−	−	−	−	+	+	−	−	−	+	+	−	+	−	−	−	+
Proteus mirabilis	+	−	+	−	−	(+)	(+)/−	−	−	−	−	−	+	+/−	+/−	+	+	+	+	+	+/−	−	−	+
Proteus vulgaris	+	−	+	−	−	+	+	−	−	−	−	+	+	−	−/+	+	+	+	+	+	+	−	−	−
Citrobacter diversus	+	−	+	(+)/−	+	−/+	+	+	+	−/+	+	+	+	−	+	−	−	+/−	−	±	−	. . .	+	−
Citrobacter freundi	+	−	+	(+)/−	+	+/−	−	−	+/−	−	+	−	+	−	+	−	−	+	+	+	−	. . .	−	+/−
Serratia liquefaciens	+	−	+[a]	+/−	+	+	+	−	−	+	+	−	+	+/−	−[a]	+	−	+/−	−	+	+	−	+	+
Serratia marcescens	+	+/−	+/−	−	+	+	+	+/−	−	+/−	+	−	+	+	+	+	−	+/−	−	+	+	+/−	+	+
Hafnia alvei	+[a]	−	+[a]	−	+	+/−	+/−	−	−	−	+	−	−[a]	+[a]	+[a]	−	−	−	−	+	+	+/−	+	+
Enterobacter aerogenes	+	−	+	+	+	+	+	+/−	−	+	+	−	−	+	+	+/−	−	−	−	+	+	+	+	+
Enterobacter cloacae	+	−	+	+	+	+	+	−/+	+/−	+/−	+	−	−	+	+	(+)	−	+/−	−	+	+	+/−	−	+
Klebsiella species[b]	−	+	+/−	+/−	+/−	+	+	+/−	+/−	+	+	−	+/−	+/−	+/−	−	−	+/−	−	+/−	+/−	+	+/−	−
Edwardsiella tarda	+	−	+	−	−	−	−	−	−	−	+	+	+	−	−	−	−	−	+	−	−	−	+	+
A–D Group	−	−	−	+/−	+/−	+/−	+/−	−	+/−	−	+	+	+	−	−	−	−	−	−	−	−	+	+/−	+/−
Escherichia coli	+	−	+	+	+	+/−	+/−	−	+/−	−	+	+	+	−	−	−	−	−	−	−	−	−	+	+/−

Reaction

[a] Tests done at 25–30°C.
[b] See Table 28.5.
[c] Result for KCN: +, growth in KCN medium (Ch. 8); −, no growth.

rapidly, or *pale* (yellow-grey), indicating that it either does not ferment lactose or gives 'late' fermentation only after several days' incubation. Some genera, however, give characteristic appearances, e.g. the large mucoid colonies of klebsiella and the swarming colonies of proteus on non-inhibitory media.

Biochemical characters

Differences in biochemical activities provide the main means of differentiating the genera and species. Table 28.3 shows some of the most useful discriminating biochemical reactions along with the properties of motility and capsulation. In practice only a minority of laboratories are able to maintain stocks of all the media required to perform the full range of biochemical tests. Not only are some of the media difficult to prepare but the quality of each batch must be tested with organisms known to give both positive and negative results. The table should be considered in conjunction with the descriptions of the most constant differential features in the text below (see also Cowan & Steel 1974, p. 106–110). The results of the different tests are not given equal importance in the identification of a particular genus or species. Although equal weight is given to all characters in classification by the Adansonian principle, it is legitimate and, indeed, essential for diagnostic purposes to put different weightings on different characters (Cowan 1965). Thus, less weight should be given to a highly variable than to a more constant character. The representation of results by the notation '+', '−' and '+/−' in Table 28.3 is not sufficiently precise to indicate the amount of weighting to be given to a reaction, but the proper weighting can be assessed when the proportion of strains in the species that give a positive result is known. This information is available and enables identification to be done by the statistical expression of the results of a selected range of tests. Such an assessment may be done with the aid of a computer, as in certain reference laboratories (e.g. Computer Laboratory, Central Public Health Laboratory, Colindale Avenue, London). Commercially prepared 'kits' of tests embodying this principle can now be purchased and used in any laboratory; they enable a range of biochemical tests to be carried out simply and are issued with instructions on how the results should be interpreted (e.g. API 20E system, API, and Encise system, Roche).

Antigenic structure

Although much is known of the antigenic composition of the various genera (Kauffmann 1969; Edwards & Ewing 1972), this information is not generally used in ordinary diagnostic medical bacteriology. Where, however, it has a special value, e.g. in the identification of the enteropathogenic strains of *E. coli*, the necessary antisera are available from commercial sources.

ESCHERICHIA COLI

The genus *Escherichia* was formerly subdivided into a number of species by differences in sugar fermentation reactions, but nowadays only one species, *Escherichia coli*, is recognized and it is subdivided into serotypes and biotypes. The characters of *Escherichia* that distinguish it from other enterobacteria are that it is motile, forms gas from glucose, ferments lactose, produces indole, gives a positive methyl-red reaction and a negative Voges-Proskauer reaction, and does not utilize citrate, grow in KCN, decompose urea or liquefy gelatin (Table 28.3). Some strains differ from the typical in one or two of these characters, e.g. motility, gas formation, lactose fermentation or non-utilization of citrate, but are nevertheless accepted as *E. coli* (Sojka 1965).

Morphology

Gram-negative non-sporing bacilli. Most strains (about 80%) are motile, though motility is often feeble on primary isolation, and most strains (again about 80%) are fimbriate. The fimbriae in most of the fimbriate strains are type 1, i.e. haemagglutinating, adhesive for epithelial cells and mannose sensitive, but different kinds of fimbriae, type MRE, with mannose-resistant and eluting haemagglutinating and adhesive properties, are formed as well as type 1 fimbriae in some strains and in the absence of type 1 fimbriae in some others (Duguid et al 1955, 1979). (Chapter 8 gives methods for haemagglutination tests.) A few strains are capsulate and many others form abundant loose slime when grown on sugar-containing medium at 15–20°C (Duguid 1951).

Cultural characters

Since most strains ferment lactose rapidly, the colonies on MacConkey medium, which are smooth, glossy and translucent, are rose-pink in colour. On cystine-lactose-electrolyte deficient (CLED) medium with bromothymol blue,* much used for urinary bacteriology, colonies are smooth, circular, about 1–1.5 mm in diameter, and yellow opaque if lactose-fermenting, blue if non-lactose-fermenting. Growth is either impaired or totally inhibited on deoxycholate citrate agar (Ch. 29); any colonies that do grow are small, pink and opaque. On blood agar the colonies of some strains are surrounded by zones of haemo-lysis. Most strains are prototrophic and grow on simple synthetic media such as a glucose-ammonium-salts agar without supplementation with amino acids or vitamins, e.g. Davis & Mingioli medium (Ch. 6). *E. coli* is uninhibited by bile salt in MacConkey medium, but is inhi-bited by the citrate in Leifson's DCA medium and by sodium selenite, sodium tetrathionate, brilliant green and other substances used in media selective for salmonellae and shigellae (Ch. 29). It is also inhibited by 7% NaCl in salt media used for isolation of staphylococci.

Biochemical reactions

It is chiefly by the pattern of its biochemical reactions with certain substrates (Table 28.3) that *E. coli* is distinguished from other entero-bacteria and defined as a species. Carbohydrates are attacked fermentatively, with the production of acid and gas; a few strains are anaerogenic, producing acid but not gas. Traditionally, the prompt fermentation of lactose (within 24 h, and usually within 8 h) was a character essential for

* Refer to *Methods* at end of this chapter.

the identification of a strain as *E. coli*, but it is now accepted that the species includes some late-lactose-fermenting or lactose-negative strains.

For classifying enterobacteria isolated from drinking-water supplies, bacteriologists commonly use the so-called 'IMViC' reactions; thus the faecal coliform bacillus, *E. coli*, is distinguished from klebsiellae, enterobacters and other coli-forms derived from soil and vegetation by the pattern of reactions: indole positive, methyl-red positive, Voges-Proskauer negative and citrate-utilization negative. It is also distinguished from the other coliforms by its ability to form gas from lactose in Eijkman tests incubated at 44°C (see Report 1969).

For general purposes in clinical microbiology, the full range of tests (e.g. those in Table 28.3) necessary for the conclusive identification of an isolate's species as *E. coli* is rarely performed. A provisional identification based on the pattern of reactions in a restricted range of tests is usually considered sufficient: e.g. pink, non-mucoid colonies on MacConkey, fermentation of glucose and lactose, motility, indole production and non-utilization of citrate. If reliance is placed on still fewer tests, e.g. only on colony appearance and lactose fermentation, the isolate should be described as a 'coliform bacillus' rather than as *E. coli*.

Biotyping

Whilst the tests used to speciate an isolate are those in which most strains of the species give the same, characteristic pattern of reactions, tests in which different strains give different reactions may be used for the identification of individual strains. Such subspecies 'typing' may be required for the purpose of tracing the spread of a particular strain through the community or for distinguishing between its persistence and replacement in a chronically infected patient, e.g. one with recurrent urinary tract infection.

Substrates with which different strains of *E. coli* give different patterns of reactions include adonitol, aesculin, arginine, dulcitol, glutamic acid, glycerol, lactose, lysine, ornithine, raffinose, rhamnose, salicin, sorbose, sorbitol, sucrose and xylose (Sojka 1965; Crichton & Old

1979). Strains giving the same pattern of reactions with a selection of these substrates are said to belong to the same *biotype* and the determination of the biotype of a strain by such tests is called *biotyping*.

The tests to be selected for biotyping are those that are both reliable and discriminating. Reliability requires that the reactions are easy to read and that the tests give the same results on repeated testing of the same strain. Discriminativeness is the ability of the test to divide a large collection of strains into positively and negatively reacting groups both of which are numerous, and ideally about equal in number. Crichton & Old (1982) found that the most reliable and discriminating tests were those for reactions with raffinose, sorbose, ornithine and dulcitol, and distinguished the primary biotypes 1–16 by the 16 different combinations of positive and negative reactions in these four tests. Secondary tests, which distinguished subtypes a–z within the primary types, were for reactions with rhamnose, lysine and aesculin, motility, production of type-1 fimbriae, and requirements for growth factors.

For the finest possible discrimination of strains, *multiple typing* by a combination of different typing methods is required, e.g. biotyping plus serotyping (see below) or biotyping plus serogrouping, resistotyping, haemagglutinin typing and antibiotic sensitivity determination (Crichton & Old 1980). Strains that appear to be the same by one method of typing are commonly found to be different by another method.

The tests in the API 20E system have been selected primarily to identify the genus of an aerobic Gram-negative bacillus and not to differentiate types within a species. For that reason, the API profile of an *E. coli* strain should not be regarded as an adequately discriminative biotype, but since the API 20E system includes one highly (ornithine) and three less discriminative (lysine, rhamnose and sucrose) tests, its use supplemented by discriminative tests for fermentation of dulcitol, raffinose, sorbose and 5-ketogluconate, motility, and haemolysis on horse-blood agar has been recommended by Gargan et al (1982).

Antigenic structure

Three kinds of surface antigens demonstrable in agglutination tests are observed for the serotyping of *E. coli*: the O (somatic), K (capsular) and H (flagellar) antigens. Fimbrial antigens also take part in the agglutination reactions of bacilli that are phenotypically in the fimbriate phase; they are widely shared between strains of different serotypes, so that misleading cross-reactions may be obtained unless serotyping tests are done with bacilli from non-fimbriate-phase cultures (e.g. agar-grown cultures) or bacilli defimbriated by heating at 100°C for 1 h (Gillies & Duguid 1958; Duguid 1985).

Serotyping

In the Kauffmann–Knipschildt–Vahlne scheme for the serological classification of strains of *E. coli* the primary subdivision is made according to the specific character of the lipopolysaccharide O antigen of the cell wall. A different 'O group' of strains is defined by the presence of each different O antigen. The original scheme (Kauffmann 1947) included 25 O groups and O antigens, but over 160 such groups and antigens have now been described (Sojka 1965; Kauffmann 1969; Edwards & Ewing 1972). The O groups are subdivided into serotypes according to the K and H antigens present. At least 100 different K antigens and over 50 different H antigens are known. The serotype of a strain is defined by its full antigenic formula, i.e. its O, K and H antigens, e.g. *E. coli* O55:K59:H6.

The term K antigen is used to include three kinds of antigens that lie outside the cell wall and the O antigen; these are the L, A and B types of K antigen. The A type of K antigen is associated with the presence of a typical capsule visible in wet India ink films on bacteria from ordinary cultures; alternatively, the capsule may be seen by its 'swelling' with the homologous K antiserum in a wet film. Strains with L or B antigens generally show capsules only if grown on sugar-containing medium at 15–20°C. The properties of these three kinds of antigen differ also in the way they are affected by heat and treatment with chemicals. A knowledge of their differential susceptibilities is necessary for the preparation of pure antisera to the individual antigenic components and details are given by Sojka (1965), Kauffmann (1969) and Edwards & Ewing (1972). An important feature is that the ability of the L and B antigens to mask agglutination by the appropriate O antiserum is nullified by heating at 100°C for 1 h, whereas removal of the A antigen requires autoclaving at 121°C for 2.5 h.

Originally the K antigens of the L and A types wcrc numbered consecutively but the B antigens were numbered in a separate series. Subsequently the B antigens were renumbered so that they could be included in the same series as the other K antigens and both their old and new numbers are often shown in the designation of a strain's serotype, e.g. *E. coli* O55:K59(B5):H6. It should be noted that with few exceptions any one strain can possess only one of the three kinds of K antigen, i.e. L, A *or* B.

Studies of the immunoelectrophoretic patterns of water (60°C) extracts of the O and K antigens of *E. coli* strains in all known O groups suggest that only a minority of strains havc a polysaccharide K antigen separate from the O antigen, that most B antigen-containing strains lack such an independent K antigen and that some B antigens may represent labile material corresponding to part of the O antigen (Ørskov et al 1971; Ørskov & Ørskov 1972). These authors have proposed that the antigenic formula should ómit the K antigen designation in cases where an independent K antigen has not been demonstrated; e.g. serotypes O55:K59(B5):H6 and O111:K60(B4):H2 should instead be given as O55:H6 and O111:H2. They found that nearly all the strains possessing an independent K antigen were strains that possessed L type antigens and belonged to serotypes frequently found in the normal intestine and in extraintestinal disease such as septicaemia and urinary infections, e.g. O1:K51, O2:K56, O3:K2, O4:K3, O5:K4, O6:K2, O7:K7, O11:K10, O25:K19, O75:K?. These K antigens are acidic thermostable polysaccharides that appear to inhibit host

defence mechanisms such as phagocytosis and complement. Some thermolabile antigens outside, and tending to mask the O antigen are protein, e.g. the fimbrial and fimbria-like antigens, and their labile (L) and protein (P) characters may be indicated in their notation as, e.g. K88(L,P) and K99(L,P).

The O antigens of the commonly encountered O groups are predominantly cathodic (non-acid) in migration but those of some groups, including the groups associated with 'dysentery-like' disease, the enteroinvasive types of *E. coli* (O112ac, O124, O28 and O136) are wholly anodic (acidic). Most of the enteropathogenic serotypes associated with infantilc gastrocntcritis (e.g. O26, O55, O86, O111, O119, O127, O128 and O142) have wholly cathodic (non-acidic) O antigens and no independent K antigens.

For a recent review of methods of preparing diagnostic antisera and performing serological tests for the typing of *E. coli* and other enterobacteria, see Ørskov & Ørskov (1978).

Viability

E. coli is generally similar to other enterobactcria in its susccptibility to inimical agents and conditions, though it is slightly more resistant to heat, to some chemicals and to drying than are the salmonellae and shigellae. It is killed by moist heat at 60°C usually within 30 min, though occasionally some bacteria may survive pasteurization in milk at 62–63°C for 30 min. It can remain alive in water for several weeks or months, though it does not appear to grow in natural waters outside the body. It can survive for several days when dried on clothing or in dust, and pathogenic serotypes have been found to be viable and numerous in floor dust, in air and on clothing, napkins and ward equipment in hospitals containing infants with gastroenteritis (Rogers 1951; Hutchison 1957).

Antibiotic sensitivity

E. coli is similar to many other enterobacteria in its susceptibility to antibiotics and different strains differ markedly in the degree of their sensitivity to several of the drugs commonly used to treat coliform infections. Strains from the faeces of healthy persons or from infections, e.g. in the urinary tract, in patients outside hospitals are commonly sensitive to readily attainable concentrations of a variety of antimicrobial drugs, whilst strains causing infections in hospitals are often resistant to some of these drugs.

Penicillins. The earliest penicillin with clinically effective activity against *E. coli* was ampicillin (minimum inhibitory concentration 8 mg/litre) but soon after its introduction resistance due to drug hydrolysis by β-lactamases was recognized. This is now a major clinical problem and 30% or more of *E. coli* isolates are resistant. By far the most important enzymes are the TEM-type plasmid-mediated β-lactamases. Many *E. coli* strains are also sensitive to the extended spectrum penicillins, carbenicillin (4 mg/litre), ticarcillin (4 mg/l), mezlocillin (2 mg/l), piperacillin (2 mg/l) and azlocillin (8 mg/l) but all of these are unstable to several of the common clinically important β-lactamases. The addition of a β-lactamase inhibitor (e.g. clavulanic acid) to a penicillin theoretically confers β-lactamase stability on the previously susceptible drug and the first combination available for clinical use is Augmentin (amoxycillin and clavulanic acid).

Cephalosporins. Although *E. coli* was sensitive to the early cephalosporins (e.g. cephaloridine 4 mg/litre, cephalothin 8 mg/l) the newer agents in this group not only have much greater intrinsic activity but also are much more resistant to hydrolysis by β-lactamases. The minimum inhibitory concentration of the so-called second generation drugs (e.g. cefuroxime, cefamandole, cefoxitin) is of the order of 0.5–2 mg/litre and of the third generation drugs (e.g. cefotaxime, latamoxef, ceftriaxone, ceftazidime) 0.05–1 mg/l.

Aminoglycosides. These antibiotics are the drugs of choice for serious infections due to *E. coli* and resistance to them is uncommon in Britain. The minimum inhibitory concentration of gentamicin, tobramycin and netilmicin is 0.1–1 mg/litre and of amikacin 1–4 mg/l.

Other antimicrobial agents. In clinical practice these are used mainly, in fact almost exclusively, to treat urinary tract infections. Orally adminstered drugs active against *E. coli* include sulphonamides (although resistance is common), trimethoprim, cotrimoxazole (the combination of a sulphonamide with trimethoprim), tetracyclines, ciprofloxacin, nitrofurantoin and nalidixic acid.

Occurrence of E. coli serotypes

Strains of *E. coli* differ in their pathogenic potential and those of certain serotypes have a special potential for causing particular types of infection, e.g. in the intestine, where most serotypes are merely commensal. The identification of the serotype of an isolate may therefore help to determine its probable pathogenic significance in the patient.

E. coli in the healthy intestine

E. coli strains predominate among the aerobic commensal bacteria present in the healthy gut. Strains of any O group may be present as commensals, though some groups, e.g. O1, O2, O4, O6, O7, O18 and O75, appear to occur more commonly than others. Many serotypes may be present in an individual's intestine at any one time, but over a period the types change. Some types ('residents') persist for relatively long periods, e.g. many months, whereas others ('transients') persist for only a few days or weeks (Sears et al 1950). Most workers have found that a strain of a new serotype deliberately swallowed in large numbers rarely becomes established as a resident (for discussion, see Cooke 1974).

E. coli in infections

The intestinal commensal strains of *E. coli* commonly cause opportunistic infections in other parts of the body where there is some abnormality or impairment of defences. They are the commonest cause of urinary tract infections (cystitis, pyelitis and pyelonephritis) and are commonly present in appendix abscess, peritonitis, cholecystitis, septic wounds and bedsores. They may infect the lower respiratory passages or cause bacteraemia and endotoxic shock, particularly in surgical or otherwise debilitated patients being treated with antibiotics to which they are resistant, and they occasionally cause meningitis in neonates. The commensal strains, however, do not act as primary pathogens in the intestine and are not known to cause gastroenteritis.

Due to contamination with traces of faeces, *E. coli* bacilli are commonly present on the skin and so come to contaminate many diagnostic specimens, such as midstream urines and wound exudates, in cases in which they have no pathogenic role. When attempting to decide the significance of their finding, the microbiologist may be guided by the probability that they have a pathogenic role if they are numerous but that they are insignificant contaminants if scanty.

E. coli diarrhoea

Strains of certain serotypes of *E. coli* have a primary pathogenicity in the intestine and cause gastroenteritis. They fall into three distinct groups associated with different disease syndromes (Table 28.4): the enteropathogenic strains (EPEC), the enterotoxigenic strains (ETEC) and the enteroinvasive strains (EIEC).

Enteropathogenic E. coli (EPEC). Formerly in Britain and other countries EPEC strains caused epidemics of diarrhoea in infants under 2 or 3 years of age. Outbreaks in the community mainly affected bottle-fed babies in the lower socio-economic groups and outbreaks in hospital were due to cross-infection through contaminated feeding bottles, bathing equipment and other vehicles. The mortality rate was high. But since 1960 there has been a marked decrease in the incidence and mortality of these infections in developed countries, probably due to improvements in hygiene and clinical management. The disease is still common in developing countries among babies in the second 6 months of life when they are being weaned from breast feeding, which is highly protective. Strains of serotypes O111:K58(B4) and O55:K59(B5) were the first to be incriminated and these were followed by strains of the other EPEC serotypes listed in Table 28.4.

Not all strains in the EPEC serotypes are able to cause gastroenteritis. Thus, in a nursery studied by McDonald & Charter (1956), no illness was caused during waves of colonization of the infants with strains of O groups 26, 111, 125 and 126. Such strains presumably lack a pathogenic factor possessed by the diarrhoeal strains of the same serotypes, but what this factor may be is unknown. Most of the classical EPEC strains lack the enterotoxins and mannose-

Table 28.4 Association of *Escherichia coli* with diarrhoeal disease.

E. coli strains	O serogroup	Age affected	Associated disease	Pathogenesis	Strain identification
Enteropathogenic strains (EPEC)	26, 55, 86, 111, 114, 119, 125, 126, 127, 128, 142	Infants, rarely adults	Infantile diarrhoea	Unknown	Typing with specific antisera
Enterotoxigenic strains (ETEC)	6, 8, 15, 25, 27, 63, 78, 115, 148, 153, 159	All ages	Infantile and adult diarrhoea in the third world. Traveller's diarrhoea	Production of enterotoxin (LT, ST or LT/ST). Colonization factor antigen (mannose-resistant adhesin)	*Provisional*: typing with specific antisera *Definitive*: demonstration of toxin LT: Y_1 mouse adrenal assay, CHO assay, Biken test, ELISA ST: Infant mouse assay, ELISA
Enteroinvasive strains (EIEC)	28ac, 112ac, 124, 136, 143, 144, 152, 164	All ages	Dysentery-like diarrhoea	Epithelial cell invasion	*Provisional*: typing with specific antisera. Recognition of atypical biochemical reactions *Definitive*: Serény test, HeLa or HEp-2 cell assay

resistant adhesins of ETEC strains and the epithelial invasiveness of EIEC strains. Most do form type 1 fimbriae bearing a mannose-sensitive adhesin for epithelium, which might promote the characteristic profuse proliferation of EPEC bacilli in the upper small intestine, from which they would otherwise be flushed. But as this adhesin is also present in most non-enteropathogenic strains of *E. coli*, it cannot be the specific pathogenic factor.

The demonstration that a strain of *E. coli* isolated from diarrhoeal faeces belongs to an EPEC serotype suggests that it may be the cause of the diarrhoea, but since some strains in EPEC serotypes are non-enteropathogenic, this does not prove either its enteropathogenicity or its causative role. If, however, the same strain is isolated from many cases in an outbreak of diarrhoea, a causative role is strongly indicated. At present there is no established laboratory test for the pathogenicity of strains of EPEC serotypes.

Because EPEC diarrhoea has become less common and because serotyping does not prove enteropathogenicity, many laboratories no longer undertake the laborious work of attempting to isolate EPEC strains from sporadic cases of infantile diarrhoea, though they do so from cases in outbreaks. EPEC strains rarely cause diarrhoea in adults, though a few food-poisoning outbreaks have been recorded and diarrhoea may be produced by oral feeding of large doses to volunteers. A search should therefore be made for EPEC in food-poisoning outbreaks from which no other pathogen has been isolated.

The antibody response to clinical or subclinical EPEC infection can be detected by an indirect haemagglutination test in which the patient's serum is reacted with red blood cells coated with the specific O antigen (Neter et al 1952), but the significance of a positive result is likely to be uncertain and the test is not generally used for diagnostic purposes.

Enterotoxigenic E. coli (ETEC). Enterotoxin producing strains of *E. coli*, first recognized about 15 years ago, are a common cause of acute watery diarrhoea in the tropics, particularly in infants under 2 years old, but also not infrequently in adults. They are rarely respon-sible for diarrhoea in temperate countries with good hygiene, but cause perhaps about half of the episodes of diarrhoea in travellers from these countries to the third world (Gross et al 1979). The illness may be mild or so severe it resembles cholera. Because ETEC strains are unlikely to be the cause of outbreaks of infantile diarrhoea in Britain, they are generally not sought in specimens submitted to diagnostic laboratories. If, however, no EPEC or other enteric pathogen can be demonstrated in an outbreak, the predominant *E. coli* strain isolated from cases should be sent to a reference laboratory to be examined for enterotoxin production (Rowe et al 1978).

Two distinct enterotoxins are recognized, a heat-labile toxin (LT) and a heat-stable toxin (ST), of which an ETEC strain may produce one, other or both. A general but laborious way of demonstrating either toxin is by the induction of fluid accumulation in ligated ileal loops in rabbits injected with the culture (Smith & Halls 1967). LT may be identified in tests with specific anti-LT serum, including the Biken agar gel diffusion test (Honda et al 1981) and an ELISA test (De Mol et al 1982) and recently an ELISA test has also been described for ST (De Mol et al 1983). A kit to detect LT by reversed passive latex agglutination is available from Oxoid. Gene probes may be used to detect the genes for toxin production (Ch. 48).

Enterotoxin production is plasmid mediated and transferable in vitro to recipient strains. Although strains of any serotype might thus become toxigenic, the distribution of ETEC among the various O serogroups is not random; a restricted range of groups, notably O6, O8, O25, O78, O148 and O159, appear to be specially adapted as carriers of the enterotoxin plasmids (Table 28.4). Thus, a polyvalent O antiserum could be used for provisional identi-fication of ETEC (Merson et al 1980).

Infection with an ETEC strain causes only mild symptoms unless, as well as enterotoxin, the strain forms a *colonization factor antigen* (CFA), which is a fimbrial mannose-resistant adhesin that promotes attachment of the bacteria to the intestinal epithelium and thus a profuse colonization of the small intestine. Two such antigens involved in human infections, CFA/I and CFA/II, have been identified by their serological and haemagglutination reactions (Satterwhite et al 1978; Evans et al 1980), but tests for them have not yet come into general diagnostic use.

Enteroinvasive E. coli (EIEC). Certain serogroups of *E. coli*, especially O124, O136, O144 and O164, have been implicated as a cause of dysentery-like diarrhoea with blood and mucus in the stools. The strains causing this syndrome are called enteroinvasive (EIEC) and, like the shigellae, they penetrate into and multiply within the cells of the intestinal epithelium, kill them and so cause ulceration. They do not form enterotoxins like the ETEC.

Since the EIEC belong to a limited number of O serogroups (Table 28.4), it has been suggested that pooled and monovalent typing antisera might be used for their provisional identification. Strains are often non-motile and atypical in their biochemical reactions. Many are late- or non-fermenters of lactose, fail to produce gas in carbohydrate fermentation tests and fail to decarboxylate lysine. In these reactions they resemble shigellae. Moreover, EIEC commonly share antigens with shigellae; for example, the somatic antigen of *E. coli* O124 is identical with that of *Shigella dysenteriae* serotype 3.

The recognized test for epithelial invasiveness is the Serény test for the production of keratoconjunctivitis in the guinea-pig eye (Day et al 1981), but simpler tests have also been described using HeLa cells (Du Pont et al 1971) or HEp2 cells (Day et al 1981).

E. coli urinary tract infection

E. coli is by far the commonest cause of urinary tract infection and the serogroups most often responsible are O1, O2, O4, O6, O7, O9, O11, O18, O39 and O75 (Grüneberg & Bettelheim 1969). The serogroups associated with urinary tract infection correspond to those that predominate in the faeces and this correlation led to the 'prevalence theory' that a limited number of O groups were involved simply because they were dominant in the colon which is the reservoir of the infecting organisms. The alternative, 'special pathogenicity theory' postulates that the *E. coli* strains which cause infection, in addition to being prevalent, are specially equipped to colonize the periurethral area and subsequently invade the urinary tract. The possession of one or both of two different structures (K antigens; fimbriae) has been demonstrated with increasing frequency in strains that cause asymptomatic bacteriuria, cystitis and pyelonephritis (70–90% of strains), in that order, and least often in faecal strains. This correlation has been best documented in childhood disease.

K antigens are thought to increase virulence because they inhibit phagocytosis and the bactericidal effect of complement. K-rich strains are more pathogenic (Glynn et al 1971) but the type as well as the amount of K antigen is important. *E. coli* strains containing antigens K1 and K12 are said to be most invasive (Kaijser et al 1977). Fimbriae that produce mannose-resistant haemagglutination of erythrocytes cause *E. coli* to adhere to urinary tract epithelium. This adhesion is not mediated by mannose-sensitive (type 1) fimbriae which the bacteria may also possess. The binding site of most (the P-fimbriae) but not all of these mannose-resistant fimbriae is a carbohydrate moiety that forms part of the structure of the glycosphingolipids of the P blood group antigens carried on many human cells including uroepithelium (Väisänen et al 1981; Kallenius et al 1981). However, Harber et al (1982) do not believe that adhesion is a virulence factor for bacteria within the urinary tract.

Serotyping of *E. coli* from the urinary tract is done only in special circumstances, e.g. in epidemiological studies of cross-infection in urological or gynaecological wards or in the prospective investigation of patients with chronic infection in whom it is wished to distinguish reinfection with a new strain from relapsing infection with the strain formerly present. Although commercially prepared antisera are available, the range that a laboratory can be expected to stock is restricted by cost. In addition a proportion of strains are autoagglutinable and, therefore, untypable. With antisera to eight of the commonest urinary O serotypes only about half of the *E. coli* isolates can be identified. The limited discrimination provided by a partial O serotyping scheme can be extended if biotyping is also carried out. Strains of the same O serotype may belong to different biotypes (Crichton & Old 1982).

The determination of the site of infection within the urinary tract is often difficult to make and the value of laboratory tests is disputed (for discussion see Maskell 1982). The demonstration in a bacterial (Widal-type) agglutination test that the serum of a patient contains a significant (e.g. > 64) or rising titre of O antibodies to the strain of *E. coli* isolated from the urine is considered to be evidence of involvement of the kidney in a urinary tract infection (Brumfitt & Percival 1964). The other test that has been most widely assessed visualizes by direct immunofluorescence antibody-coated bacteria in urine. The presence of these antibody-coated bacteria is said to indicate upper urinary tract infection (Thomas et al 1974).

ALKALESCENS-DISPAR (A–D) ORGANISMS

The A–D group of organisms includes non-motile anaerogenic enterobacteria that ferment lactose late (Bacillus dispar) or not at all (Bacillus alkalescens), but otherwise resemble *E. coli* in their biochemical reactions. Many members of the group have the same O and K antigens as typical strains of *E. coli* and they are now classified in this species. In their biochemical reactions they are easy to confuse with *Shigella* (see Ch. 30). They resemble *E. coli* in occurring in the intestine in healthy persons and in some cases of urinary tract infection.

EDWARDSIELLA

Although recognized, with reluctance, as a separate genus by Cowan & Steel (1974) this genus is separated from *Escherichia* by its ability to produce hydrogen sulphide in triple sugar iron agar. *Edwardsiella tarda* as the name suggests is

much less active in fermenting carbohydrates than *Escherichia coli* (Table 28.3).

KLEBSIELLA

The genus *Klebsiella* is a group of coliform bacteria which has given rise to many problems in classification. The scheme adopted in this book is that proposed by Cowan et al (1960) which excludes motile and gelatin-liquefying forms. The characters that distinguish *Klebsiella* from other enterobacteria are that all klebsiella strains are non-motile, do not liquefy gelatin and do not produce ornithine decarboxylase or phenylalanine deaminase and that most strains are capsulate, produce gas from glucose, ferment lactose, adonitol and inositol, do not produce indole but give positive reactions in the Voges-Proskauer, citrate, urease and KCN tests (see Table 28.3).

The majority of strains isolated from vegetation, soil, water and faeces form a biochemically homogeneous group, *Klebsiella aerogenes*, which traditionally has been recognized as being lactose-fermenting and having the IMViC reactions: indole negative, methyl-red negative, Voges-Proskauer positive and citrate positive. Indole-producing strains that are like *K. aerogenes* in other respects are sometimes classified in a separate species as *K. oxytoca*. Motile enterobacteria with similar reactions, many of which liquefy gelatin, are now placed in the genus *Enterobacter*, but one motile species, *Enterobacter aerogenes*, so closely resembles *K. aerogenes* in most of its characters that it has been classified as a species of *Klebsiella, K. mobilis*. Klebsiellae isolated from the healthy or diseased respiratory tract are more heterogeneous in their reactions. Some give reactions identical with those of *K. aerogenes* and others show several differences. The species other than *K. aerogenes* recognized by Cowan et al are *K. pneumoniae, K. ozaenae, K. rhinoscleromatis, K. edwardsi* var. *edwardsi* and *K. edwardsi* var. *atlantae*; for convenience, the last two of these species are named in this book *K. edwardsi* and *K. atlantae* respectively. The distinguishing reactions of these species are shown in Table 28.5.

Table 28.5 Distinguishing reactions of *Klebsiella* species.
Key: +, result positive with at least 80% of strains; −, result negative with at least 80% of strains; +/−, some strains positive, some negative; −‡, negative at 24 h, delayed positive at 2–8 days.

Reaction	K. aerogenes	K. pneumoniae	K. edwardsi	K. atlantae	K. ozaenae	K. rhinoscleromatis
Fimbriae (type)	+ (1,3)	+(1)	−	−	− or +(6)	−
Glucose (gas)	+	+	−	+	+/−	−
Lactose (acid)	+	+	−‡	−‡	−‡	−
ONPG	+	+	+	+	+	−
Sucrose (acid)	+	+	+	+	+/−	+
Dulcitol (acid)	+/−	+	−	−	−	−
Methyl red	−	+	+/−	+	+	+
Voges-Proskauer	+	−	+	+/−	−	−
Citrate	+	+	+/−	+	+/−	−
Urease	+	+	+	+	+/−	−
KCN[a]	+	−	+	+	+	+
Gluconate	+	+/−	+	+/−	−	−
Malonate	+	+	+/−	−	−	+
Lysine decarboxylase	+	+	+	+	+/−	−
Capsule serotypes	1–72	3	1, 2	1	3–6	3

[a] Result for KCN: +, growth in KCN medium (Ch. 8); −, no growth.

This classification of klebsiellae, which is used for its clinical convenience, is no longer accepted as taxonomically valid. Correctly, but confusingly, the name *K. pneumoniae* is now used in a broad sense for the saprophytic klebsiellae formerly called *K. aerogenes*, as well as for varieties more commonly associated with infections of the respiratory tract, namely *K. pneumoniae senso strictu*, *K. atlantae* and *K. edwardsi*. The varieties must therefore be distinguished by naming them as subspecies or biovars: *K. pneumoniae* subspecies *aerogenes*, *K. pneumoniae* subspecies *pneumoniae*, *K. pneumoniae* biovar *atlantae*, and *K. pneumoniae* biovar *edwardsi*.

K. ozaenae and *K. rhinoscleromatis* remain recognized as distinct species. Some recently identified saprophytic species, including *K. planticola*, *K. terrigena* and *K. trevisani*, are so seldom isolated from clinical specimens that they are not dealt with in this book.

Morphology

Gram-negative non-sporing non-motile bacilli which tend to be short and thick, e.g. 1–2 × 0.8 μm. Virtually all freshly isolated strains form a well defined polysaccharide capsule which is readily visible in wet India ink films or by its 'swelling' reaction in films with homologous antiserum; the capsule is largest in cultures on sugar-containing media, especially those with a high ratio of sugar to other nutrients. Some of what appears to be the same extracellular polysaccharide is secreted from the bacteria as a loose, soluble slime, and it is the accumulation of the loose slime that gives colonies their large 'mucoid' form (Duguid 1951; Wilkinson et al 1954). The power to form capsules and slime is generally well preserved in laboratory cultures, but non-capsulate non-slime-forming mutants appear from time to time and can be recognized by the smaller, non-mucoid appearance of their colonies. Rarely, a non-capsulate but still slime-forming mutant is produced and such a mutant forms mucoid colonies.

Fimbriae of one or more of three types, 1, 3 and 6, are present in a majority of strains (Duguid 1959; Thornley & Horne 1962; Duguid 1968, Table 1). Most strains of *K. aerogenes* produce both type 1 fimbriae (mannose-sensitive, haemagglutinating, about 7 nm in width) and type 3 fimbriae (mannose-resistant, haemagglutinating only with tannic-acid-treated erythrocytes, about 5 nm in width), though in different phases of their growth they may form only the one type or the other or neither. A few strains of *K. aerogenes* form only type 1 fimbriae and a few form only type 3. *K. pneumoniae* forms only type 1 fimbriae, whereas *K. edwardsi*, *K. atlantae*, *K. rhinoscleromatis* and *K. ozaenae* are non-fimbriate with the exception of a few *K. ozaenae* strains which form the non-haemagglutinating type 6 fimbriae (Duguid 1968). Chapter 8 gives methods for haemagglutination tests.

Cultural characters

Grow well on ordinary nutrient media and on glucose-ammonium-salts agar unsupplemented with growth factors. Temperature range for growth is 12–43°C, optimum 37°C. Colonies are large, raised, moist and viscid, i.e. 'mucoid'; the degree of mucoidness depends on the amount of loose slime produced and this depends on the amount of carbohydrate in the culture medium as well as varying from strain to strain. The colonies of non-capsulate non-slime-forming mutants resemble those of other non-capsulate coliform bacteria. Most strains ferment lactose and their colonies on MacConkey medium are pink, though this colour may not be clearly apparent in very mucoid colonies.

Biochemical reactions

The reactions of the different species of *Klebsiella* are shown in Table 28.5. All species fail to liquefy gelatin and none produces ornithine decarboxylase or phenylalanine deaminase. Most species hydrolyse urea but do so much more slowly than *Proteus* species. *K. aerogenes* is the most active fermenter among the klebsiellae and it produces acid and gas from the widest range of carbohydrates; its IMViC reactions are indole negative, methyl-red negative, Voges-Proskauer positive and citrate positive. *K. pneumoniae*, all strains of which appear to ferment dulcitol and belong to capsule serotype 3, differs from *K. aerogenes* in being methyl-red positive, Voges-Proskauer negative and KCN negative. *K. edwardsi* and *K. atlantae*, which form large capsules and very mucoid colonies even on media not containing added sugar, differ from *K. aerogenes* in usually giving only delayed fermentation of lactose, a positive methyl-red reaction and a negative malonate reaction; *K. edwardsi* is anaerogenic. *K. ozaenae* is also a late fermenter of lactose; it is methyl-red positive, Voges-Proskauer negative, gluconate negative and malonate negative. *K. rhinoscleromatis* is the least active biochemically; it is anaerogenic, fails to ferment lactose, is methyl-red positive, Voges-Proskauer negative, citrate negative but malonate positive.

Antigenic structure

O and R somatic (cell wall) antigens have been recognized in smooth and rough variant strains of klebsiellae. Five different O antigens have been distinguished, four of which, O1, O3, O4 and O5, are related to *Escherichia coli* O antigens 19b, 9, 20 and 8 respectively. These O antigens occur in different combinations with K antigens in different strains (see Table 37, Kauffmann 1969). The O antigens are masked by the K antigens in capsulate strains and because the K antigens are heat-stable at 100°C for 2.5 h, the O antigens are identifiable only in non-capsulate mutants. Because of this difficulty in demonstrating them, they are not observed in ordinary typing studies.

K antigens. The klebsiellae are differentiated into 72 capsule serotypes by the identification of their K antigens (no. 1–72), which is usually done by the microscopical demonstration of capsule 'swelling' in wet films with capsular antiserum (Edwards & Ewing 1972). Slide and tube agglutination tests and precipitation tests may also be used to determine the K antigen of a strain, but the O antigens may participate in these reactions and K antisera absorbed free from O antibodies are required for such tests.

The six species of *Klebsiella* determined by biochemical reactions were found by Cowan et al (1960) to contain strains of different capsular serotypes as follows: *K. aerogenes*, all 72 serotypes; *K. pneumoniae*, type 3; *K. edwardsi*, types 1 and 2; *K. atlantae*, type 1; *K. rhinoscleromatis*, type 3; *K. ozaenae*, types 3, 4, 5 and 6.

M antigen. This term has sometimes been used

for the loose-slime polysaccharide antigen that can be demonstrated in bacteria-free culture supernates by precipitation with capsular antiserum. It appears to have the same chemical composition and antigenic specificity as the K antigen of the same strain (Edwards & Fife 1952; Wilkinson et al 1954).

ENTEROBACTER (CLOACA) AND HAFNIA

These are motile organisms that otherwise resemble *K. aerogenes* in many of their biochemical characters. Enterobacter strains are mostly fimbriate (type 1 fimbriae) and slime-forming; they generally do not show defined capsules in wet India ink films, but K antigens often render them O-inagglutinable. They have the same IMViC reactions as *K. aerogenes*, but differ from that species in producing ornithine decarboxylase, in generally failing to form urease and in commonly liquefying gelatin (Table 28.3).

Two species of *Enterobacter* are recognized: *E. cloacae* (Cloaca A), which always liquefies gelatin, but only slowly (after 7 days at 22°C), and fails to produce gas in glycerol and inositol, and *E. aerogenes* (Cloaca B); which commonly fails to liquefy gelatin even slowly.

The independent status of the genus *Hafnia*, with its type species *Hafnia alvei*, is in doubt. These organisms are probably best regarded as being non-lactose-fermenting members of the genus *Enterobacter*, i.e. as *E. hafnia*. They resemble *Serratia liquefaciens* in having a low optimum temperature for growth and they give regular, characteristic results in motility and biochemical tests only when incubated at 25–30°C. They do not liquefy gelatin. Some strains of hafnia form type 1 fimbriae and many strains have an O antigen related to those of *Salmonella basel* ($58:1,z_{13},z_{28}:1,5$) and *Shigella flexneri* serotype 4a (Sedlák & Kertészová 1968). Many strains possess the thermolabile surface alpha-antigen of Stamp and Stone (Emslie-Smith 1961) and since many rabbit sera have a high natural titre of alpha-agglutinins, agglutination tests with live hafnia bacteria commonly give false-positive reactions.

Enterobacter and hafnia organisms are sapro-

phytes found in water, soil and vegetation, but sometimes also in human faeces and infections.

SERRATIA

Members of the genus *Serratia* are motile enterobacteria which resemble *Enterobacter* organisms in many of their biochemical reactions. For example members of both genera produce ornithine decarboxylase and are gluconate positive, indole negative and citrate positive but *Serratia* species differ from *Enterobacter* species in liquefying gelatin *rapidly*, in failing to ferment rhamnose and in producing deoxyribonuclease. Like *Hafnia* the most reliable biochemical test results are obtained at 25–30°C (Table 28.3).

The best characterized species is *Serratia marcescens* which when isolated as a saprophyte from soil and water classically forms a non-diffusible red pigment. However, almost all strains associated with human infections are non-pigmented and the importance of *S. marcescens* as a pathogen, which may have been underestimated in the past, is increasing (Platt & Sommerville 1981).

S. marcescens is a small Gram-negative coccobacillus $0.7–1.5 \times 0.7$ μm with peritrichous flagella and fimbriae (types 1 and 3); it may form a capsule on sugar-containing medium.

Most saprophytic strains form a red pigment, prodigiosin, which is insoluble in water and does not diffuse away from the colonies on agar medium; these, therefore, are pink or red. The optimum temperature for growth is 30–37°C, but pigmentation may be poor at such temperatures and may be strong only in cultures grown at lower temperatures, e.g. 15–20°C. The pigment is formed only in cultures grown aerobically and in some strains it may be inapparent in cultures grown on ordinary media. Non-pigmented variant strains may originate by mutation in laboratory cultures but non-pigmented clinical isolates do not produce pigmented variants.

S. liquefaciens, a less common species, was previously classified as *Enterobacter liquefaciens*. It never forms pigmented colonies and also differs from *S. marcescens* in fermenting arabinose and raffinose.

Although *Serratia* species are ONPG positive many strains fail to ferment lactose and, unless pigment is produced, form pale colonies on MacConkey agar.

CITROBACTER

Members of the genus *Citrobacter* are motile enterobacteria that have been confused with both *Escherichia* and *Salmonella*. The type species, *Citrobacter freundi*, is a rapid fermenter of lactose and it corresponds to the organisms known to water bacteriologists as 'intermediate coliform bacilli'; formerly it was called *Escherichia freundi*. It is distinguished from *E. coli* by being citrate positive, KCN positive, hydrogen sulphide positive, lysine decarboxylase negative and usually indole negative (Table 28.3).

Late-lactose-fermenting and non-lactose-fermenting strains of *C. freundi* constitute the Bethesda-Ballerup group. Because they form pale colonies on MacConkey and DCA media and share somatic antigens with salmonellae, they may be mistaken for salmonellae when they are encountered in cultures of faeces. They are distinguished, however, by their negative lysine decarboxylase and positive KCN reactions. Certain strains possess a K antigen closely related to the Vi antigen of *Salmonella typhi* and *S. paratyphi C* (see Ch. 29), but they are saprophytes and lack the pathogenicity of salmonellae.

Of the other species that have been recognized within the genus the best characterized is *C. diversus*. It differs from *C. freundi* by being hydrogen sulphide negative, indole positive, KCN negative and producing acid in adonitol (Table 28.3).

PROTEUS

The genus *Proteus* consists of highly motile ('swarming') enterobacteria that are urease positive, phenylalanine deaminase positive and KCN positive. Four species are recognized, *Proteus vulgaris*, *P. mirabilis*, *P. morgani* and *P. rettgeri*. However, there is controversy over classification. It has been proposed that *P. morgani* should be placed in a separate genus *Morganella* as *Morganella morgani* and that *P. rettgeri* should be assigned to the genus *Providencia* as *Providencia rettgeri* (Table 28.3). By far the commonest species encountered in clinical bacteriology is *P. mirabilis*. This and the other species of *Proteus* are free-living saprophytes in soil, vegetation, water and sewage, and are found in the intestine in many healthy persons. They occur also in infections of the urinary tract, wounds and other sites.

Morphology

Non-capsulate Gram-negative rods varying in length from short coccobacilli to long filaments; filamentous cells are common in young swarming cultures on agar media. Most strains are highly motile and richly flagellated, but non-flagellate non-motile variant strains are encountered. All four species are fimbriate (types 1, 3 and/or 4 fimbriae; Duguid & Old 1980).

Cultural characters

Proteus organisms are usually first recognized by their fishy smell and their swarming appearance when grown on non-inhibitory solid media such as nutrient agar and blood agar. *P. morgani* differs from the other species of *Proteus* by failing to swarm on the conventional agar media, though it does swarm on 'soft' agar media with a reduced content of agar. Swarming appears as a thin, colourless, transparent film extending from the margins of a young colony and spreading in several waves demarcated by a raised margin until most or all of the surface of the culture plate is covered. Colonies of other organisms on the plate are covered and contaminated by the film of proteus growth, which sometimes is so thin that its presence may at first be overlooked. The fishy smell draws attention to the likelihood that proteus is present and if the apparently clean surface of the medium is stroked lightly with an inoculating loop, material from the inapparent film of growth will be seen to accumulate on it.

When the presence of proteus in a clinical specimen makes it difficult to isolate in pure culture another organism such as *Streptococcus pyogenes* or *Staphylococcus aureus*, the specimen should be plated on a medium that inhibits swarming, e.g. PNPG medium (Kopp et al 1966; Senior 1978), which is blood agar containing 0.215 g *p*-nitrophenylglycerol added to each 500 ml of the nutrient agar base before autoclaving. Alternatively, blood agar containing two to three times the usual concentration of agar may be used, but on such concentrated medium colonies of different bacteria are smaller than usual and often atypical in appearance. Swarming is inhibited and compact 'pale' (non-lactose-fermenting) colonies are formed on MacConkey medium and deoxycholate citrate agar. It is simple, therefore, to separate from proteus the other enterobacteria that grow on these bile-salt media.

Dienes phenomenon. When two identical proteus cultures are inoculated at different points on the same plate of non-inhibitory medium the resulting swarms of growth coalesce without signs of demarcation. When, however, two different strains of a *Proteus* species are inoculated, the spreading films of growth fail to coalesce and remain separated by a narrow, easily visible furrow. The observation of this appearance, the 'Dienes phenomenon', has been used to determine the identity or non-identity of strains in epidemiological studies (Skirrow 1969).

Biochemical reactions

Two tests serve to distinguish a culture of a *Proteus* species from other enterobacteria: (1) the demonstration of its ability to hydrolyse urea rapidly (within a few, e.g. 2–4 hours) and (2) the demonstration of its ability oxidatively to deaminate phenylalanine to phenylpyruvic acid. Proteus shares the latter property with species of *Providencia*. Reactions differentiating the four species of *Proteus* are shown in Table 28.3. In fermenting glucose and other carbohydrates all species except *P. rettgeri* usually produce gas. *P. vulgaris* is alone in fermenting maltose, only *P. mirabilis* fails to form indole and only *P. rettgeri* ferments mannitol.

Antigenic structure

Strains of *P. vulgaris* and *P. mirabilis* have been classified by their O antigens into 49 O groups and the groups subdivided according to different H antigens into a large number of serotypes (see Kauffmann 1969, Table 40). Similarly, 57 serotypes of *P. morgani* and 45 serotypes of *P. rettgeri* have been described.

Determination of the O serotype of isolates provides a useful means of recognizing whether they belong to the same or different strains. A method of O serotyping isolates in epidemiological studies has been described by Larsson & Olling (1977) and Senior & Larsson (1983).

Certain types of proteus are agglutinated by the serum of patients with typhus fever. This reaction, the Weil-Felix reaction, is used as a diagnostic test (Ch. 44). The strain employed, *Proteus* X19 has the biochemical reactions of *P. vulgaris*. The Weil-Felix reaction is dependent on a close relationship between the specific O antigen of *Proteus* X19 and a somatic antigen in *Rickettsia prowazeki*, the causative organism of typhus fever.

Another proteus type designated XK (biochemically *P. mirabilis*) is agglutinated by the serum of patients with 'scrub typhus', an infection due to *Rickettsia tsutsugamushi*. A diagnostic agglutination test similar to the Weil-Felix test is based on this antigenic relationship.

Proticin production and sensitivity

Many strains of *P. mirabilis* and *P. vulgaris* produce bacteriocins (proticins), to the lethal action of which other strains are sensitive. Senior (1977) has described a highly discriminating method of typing strains by determination of their proticin production and sensitivity (P–S typing) and the method is made even more discriminating when used in combination with O serotyping (Senior & Larsson 1983).

PROVIDENCIA

Members of the genus *Providencia* are motile, non-lactose-fermenting Gram-negative bacilli which resemble *Proteus* in their ability to deaminate phenylalanine but differ from *Proteus* by failing to hydrolyse urea. They do not swarm on ordinary agar media but can swarm on soft agar media containing half the usual concentration of agar. They occur in some infections of the urinary tract.

Two biotypes and many serotypes are recognized. The biotypes are regarded by some authors as distinct species. *Providencia alcalifaciens* (Providence I, Providence A) produces gas from glucose and acidifies adonitol but not inositol; *Providencia stuarti* (Providence II, Providence B) is anaerogenic and acidifies inositol but not adonitol.

ERWINIA

A genus with characters that relate it to both *Citrobacter* and *Enterobacter*. Members are classically associated with plant disease but it is now recognized that there are human and animal strains in the genus. The type species is *Erwinia herbicola* (Table 28.3).

LABORATORY DIAGNOSIS OF COLIFORM INFECTIONS

Miscellaneous coliform infections

Escherichia coli, klebsiella, proteus, pseudomonas or other coliform bacillus may be found as the only organism present in a blood culture, cerebrospinal fluid or exudate from a closed site, in which case its pathogenic role and clinical significance is obvious and its elimination by appropriate antibiotic therapy should be recommended. Often, however, a coliform bacillus is found in a specimen of sputum or urine, or a swab from an open site such as the throat, ear, vagina, a wound or a skin lesion, in which it is accompanied by other commensal or potentially pathogenic bacteria such as staphylococci, streptococci, pneumococci, haemophili, neisseriae and diphtheroid bacilli. In these cases its clinical significance and the need for its elimination by antibiotic therapy are difficult to determine.

Although in some cases the coliform bacilli found in a specimen from an open site with a mixed flora may have an important pathogenic role, in other cases they may be present only as harmless contaminants. Thus, they may be found

in mid-stream urine as a result of having contaminated the passing urine from a site of commensal growth in the intestine, perineum or urethral meatus. They may be present in sputum as a result of contamination with throat secretion, particularly when they have been growing profusely in the throat in a patient whose normal throat flora has been eliminated by antibiotic therapy, and they may be present as harmless superficial contaminants in wounds subject to serious deep infection with some other organism. In such cases their elimination with antibiotics is unnecessary.

The bacteriologist should attempt to assess the likely clinical significance of coliform bacilli found in a specimen with a mixed flora so that he may be in a position to advise the physician on the need for anti-coliform chemotherapy. Among the factors to be considered are the absolute and relative numbers of coliform bacilli in the specimen and the presence or absence of more virulent potential pathogens. The likelihood that the coliform bacilli are exerting a pathogenic effect will be greatest if they are present in large numbers, if they outnumber the other organisms present and if no other, more virulent organism is present. If there are only a few coliform bacilli in the specimen and the circumstances suggest they are merely harmless contaminants, it will probably be best for the bacteriologist to omit testing their antibiotic sensitivities and omit reporting their presence.

Isolation and identification

Specimens from closed sites, e.g. cerebrospinal fluid, should be examined microscopically, as the presence of Gram-negative bacilli may be demonstrated and the possibility suggested that they may be coliform bacilli. A Gram film is less helpful when the specimen is from a site with a mixed commensal flora, though the finding that Gram-negative bacilli are predominant in the flora may help to indicate that their presence is clinically significant.

Coliform bacilli usually grow well and form large colonies on most kinds of culture media. Their colonies are easily seen and recognized even on unselective media, such as blood agar, and even in the presence of much larger numbers of other bacteria which form smaller colonies. Indeed, care must be taken not to allow the impression of their large size to lead to an over-estimate of their relative numbers on a culture plate. When unusually small, as from crowding, the colonies of *E. coli* and similar coliforms can still be distinguished from similarly sized colonies of staphylococci by their lesser opacity.

When a coliform infection is suspected, a specimen likely to contain a mixed flora should be cultured on MacConkey agar as well as blood agar. In the MacConkey culture the lactose-fermenting and non-lactose-fermenting coliforms are distinguished by their colony colour, the mucoid character of klebsiella is enhanced, the troublesome spreading of proteus prevented and the growth of many non-coliform bacteria inhibited.

Most clinical purposes will be served by the provisional identification of *E. coli*, klebsiella, proteus and pseudomonas, and their separation from other coliforms, for which only a limited number of tests need be done. Thus it might suffice to inoculate the coliform isolate into a soft tryptone agar stab to test it for motility and indole production, into glucose peptone water to test for the production of acid and gas, on to a Simmons slope to test for citrate utilization, into urea broth to test for urease production and on to a MacConkey plate to confirm the purity of the inoculated culture. Performance of the oxidase test by the filter paper method conveniently facilitates the recognition of colonies of pseudomonas.

Only in exceptional circumstances is a full species identification likely to have real clinical value. If such identification is required, it will be necessary to expose the isolate to an extended range of biochemical tests, as shown in Table 28.3. For convenience, these may be done in a commercial, multi-test kit, e.g. API 20E.

Antibiotic sensitivity tests

The suspension of the coliform isolate used as inocula for the identification tests may also be used to seed plates for antibiotic sensitivity tests by a method ensuring that this inoculum is not too heavy. It is advisable thus to set up the sensitivity tests at the same time as the identification tests, rather than only after the results of the latter have become known, for the sensitivities as well as the identity of the organism may then be reported to the physician a day earlier.

When for this reason the sensitivity tests are set up before the identity of the coliform isolate has been determined, it is necessary to test a range of antibiotics that includes some likely to be effective against each of the common coliform genera. Six antibiotics that might be tested routinely are sulphonamide; trimethoprim; cephalexin or cephradine; amoxycillin or ampicillin; gentamicin or netilmicin; and cefuroxime or cefotaxime. The first four, and less expensive of these drugs would be suitable for the oral treatment of the less serious, sensitive infection, and the last two for parenteral treatment of the more serious infections.

If the specimen is from a site, e.g. ear or eye, where topical treatment is applicable, chloramphenicol, colistin, neomycin and sulphonamide might be tested. If the specimen is a blood culture and the possibility that the isolate is a salmonella has not yet been excluded, chloramphenicol should be tested in addition to the routine set, and if in a serious infection the possibility that the isolate is a pseudomonas has not yet been excluded, tobramycin, amikacin, azlocillin and piperacillin, or equivalent anti-pseudomonas drugs should also be tested.

Urinary tract infections

Laboratory methods for the diagnosis of urinary tract infections are discussed in Chapter 39. 'Clean-catch' specimens of mid-stream urine, fresh or refrigerated, are examined by semi-quantitative culture on MacConkey or CLED* agar. As *E. coli* is commonly present as a harmless colonist of the perineum and urethral meatus, it often contaminates mid-stream urine in numbers up to 10 000 /ml, when its presence is not regarded as signifying infection within the urinary tract. In infections of the bladder or kidney, the urine usually contains about or more than 100 000 bacilli/ml and only counts of that order are taken to indicate clinically significant bacteriuria. If the specimen of urine has been obtained by supra-pubic stab or aseptic catheterization, lower counts may be regarded as clinically significant.

The predominant colony type in cultures with significant count should be picked for provisional identification, as described above for miscellaneous infections, and sensitivity tests against appropriate antibiotics, e.g. amoxycillin or ampicillin, cephalexin or cephradine, cotrimoxazole or trimethoprim, sulphonamide, nalidixic acid, and nitrofurantoin.

Infantile gastroenteritis

Faeces from patients under 5 years old involved in institutional outbreaks of diarrhoea should be examined for enteropathogenic serotypes of E. coli as well as for other enteric pathogens. Unfortunately there is no selective medium that will grow only the enteropathogenic strains of E. coli, so that unselective culture media have to be used, but isolation is commonly successful because during acute infections the enteropathogenic strain is very numerous in the faeces.

1. *On the first day* plate out the specimen thinly on a whole MacConkey plate as well as on the other media used for the isolation of salmonella (Ch. 29), shigella (Ch. 30) and campylobacter (Ch. 32).

2. *On the second day* test separately by slide agglutination a minimum of five pink (lactose-fermenting) colonies from the MacConkey plate. Ensure that all morphologically different colonial types are examined. For each colony prepare a slide with three drops of saline on different areas. Take up about *half* of the colony on a wire loop and touch portions of it on to the glass close to each of the three drops. Rub the third portion into its drop to form a uniform milky suspension, then the second portion into its drop and then the first into its drop. With a small (2 mm) loop, flamed and cooled between each transfer, add in turn a loopful of one of the three different polyvalent E. coli typing antisera (see below) to each of the three bacterial suspensions. Tilt the slide to and fro while viewing under a good light against a dark background. Read as positive only if distinct agglutination takes place with one serum pool within 30 s and there is no agglutination with the other two pools.

Subculture the remaining half of any colony giving a positive reaction with a serum pool on to a nutrient agar plate.

3. *On the third day* inspect well separated colonies on the nutrient agar plate for purity of the culture as shown by uniformity of colonial appearance. Now suspend several colonies from the plate in a tube of 2 ml sterile (0.85%) saline until distinctly milky. Carry out slide agglutination tests on this suspension first with the polyvalent antiserum that gave a positive result on the previous day and then, if this test is positive, with each of the monovalent (single factor) antisera contained in that pool.

Any positive slide reaction *must* be confirmed by slide and tube agglutination tests on a heated suspension, because antisera contain agglutinins to both O and K antigens and a positive slide reaction with a living culture is generally due to reaction with the surface K antigen. Biochemical tests should also be set up to establish that the lactose-fermenting coliform is E. coli; confusing positive agglutination tests may be observed with other genera because of the wide sharing of antigenic components within the Enterobacteriaceae.

Tests with a heated suspension. Steam at 100°C for 1 h the suspension of living organisms to destroy the K antigen. Repeat the slide agglutination test with the monovalent antiserum that previously gave a positive result with the unheated suspension. If the test is still positive, issue provisional report of the isolation of an enteropathogenic E. coli.

Dilute the remainder of the steamed suspension with sterile saline until it is only slightly turbid (a density of about 10^8 bacteria /ml as judged by comparison with an opacity standard). Prepare dilutions of the antiserum that reacted in the slide test from 1 in 10 to 1 in 640 in 0.5 ml volumes. Add 0.5 ml of the bacterial suspension to each tube and to a control tube containing 0.5 ml saline. Incubate the tubes overnight in a waterbath at 50°C. Read the test as positive if agglutination has taken place to the correct titre for the antiserum as stated on the bottle. This test set up on the third day is *read on the fourth day*. (The tube agglutination method is described in greater detail in Ch. 29.)

Antisera. Sera for the identification of enteropathogenic *E. coli* are laborious to prepare and so are usually purchased from commercial sources (e.g. Wellcome). Pools of polyvalent sera should be stocked in the diagnostic laboratory and if large numbers of specimens are to be examined, monovalent sera should also be kept. Wellcome provide the following sera:

Escherichia coli Polyvalent 2 (Types O26:K60, O55:K59, O111:K58, O119:K69, O126:K71).

Escherichia coli Polyvalent 3 (O86:K61, O114:K90, O125:K70, O127:K63, O128:K67).

Escherichia coli Polyvalent 4 (O18:K77, O44:K74, O112:K66, O124:K72, O142:K86). Some of the serotypes in this pool are associated with enteroinvasive disease (Table 28.4).

Monovalent sera to types O18:K77, O26:K60, O44:K74, O55:K59, O86:K61, O111:K58, O112:K66, O114:K90, O119:K69, O124:K72, O125:K70, O126:K71, O127:K63, O128:K67, O142:K86.

Confirmatory biochemical tests. Pick an isolated colony from the nutrient agar plate into a tube containing 0.5 ml sterile saline and another containing 3 ml of peptone water. Inoculate a drop of the saline suspension on to a slope of Simmons citrate agar. Incubate the peptone water culture for 4 h at 37°C and with a sterile Pasteur pipette then inoculate single drops of it into each of the following media: inositol and gluconate peptone waters, Christensen's urea medium, peptone water (for indole test) and glucose phosphate peptone water (for methyl red and Voges-Proskauer tests) (Ch. 8). Incubate the tests for 48 h at 37°C. Read the

Table 28.6 Reactions of *Escherichia coli*.

Test	Typical reactions of *E. coli*
Inositol to acid	−
Oxidation of gluconate	−
Urease	−
Indole	+
Methyl red	+
Voges-Proskauer	−
Growth on citrate	−

results and identify the organism by the reactions in Table 28.6.

These biochemical tests set up on the third day are *read on the fifth day*, when a final report may be issued.

METHODS

Most of the media and methods referred to in this chapter are given in chapters 6, 8 and 29.

Cystine lactose electrolyte deficient (CLED) medium

This medium (Mackey & Sandys 1966) is considered preferable to MacConkey's bile salt-lactose medium for the culture of coliform and other bacteria from infected urine. Like MacConkey medium, it distinguishes between lactose-fermenting (yellow) and non-lactose-fermenting (blue, grey or green) colonies, inhibits swarming of proteus and shows the greenish colour, matt surface and rough periphery of pseudomonas colonies. It has the advantage in supporting the growth of certain staphylococci, streptococci and candida strains that fail to grow on MacConkey. *E. coli* forms yellow opaque colonies usually 1–1.5 mm in diameter, klebsiella mucoid yellow to whitish blue colonies, *Staphylococcus aureus* deep yellow opaque colonies, other staphylococci yellow to white opaque colonies, and *Streptococcus faecalis* yellow to white translucent colonies about 0.5 mm in diameter.

Ingredients

Peptone	4 g
Tryptone	4 g
Lab-Lemco meat extract powder	3 g
Lactose	10 g
L-cystine	0.128 g
Bromothymol blue	0.02 g
Agar	15 g
Water	1 litre

Preparation. Suspend the ingredients in the water, bring to the boil to dissolve, sterilize for 15 min at 121°C and mix well before pouring.

REFERENCES

Brumfitt W, Percival A 1964 Pathogenesis and laboratory diagnosis of non-tuberculous urinary tract infection: a review. Journal of Clinical Pathology 17: 482–491

Cooke E M 1974 *Escherichia coli* and man. Churchill Livingstone , Edinburgh. p 20–24

Cowan S T 1965 Principles and practice of bacterial taxonomy – a forward look. Journal of General Microbiology 39: 143–153

Cowan S T, Steel K J 1974 Manual for the identification of medical bacteria, 2nd edn. University Press, Cambridge

Cowan S T, Steel K J, Shaw C, Duguid J P 1960 A classification of the klebsiella group. Journal of General Microbiology 23: 601–612

Crichton P B, Old D C 1979 Biotyping of *Escherichia coli*. Journal of Medical Microbiology 12: 473–485

Crichton P B, Old D C 1980 Differentiation of strains of *Escherichia coli*: multiple typing approach. Journal of Clinical Microbiology 11: 635–640

Crichton P B, Old D C 1982 A biotyping scheme for the subspecific discrimination of *Escherichia coli*. Journal of Medical Microbiology 15: 233–242

Day N P, Scotland S M, Rowe B 1981 Comparison of an HEp-2 tissue culture test with the Serény test for detection of entero-invasiveness in *Shigella* spp. and *Escherichia coli*. Journal of Clinical Microbiology 13: 596–597

De Mol P, Hemelhof W, Papa-Kango E, Butzler J P, Bravo N, Honda T 1982 Detection of *Escherichia coli* producing heat-labile toxin: comparison between Y_1 adrenal cell assay, ganglioside-ELISA, and Biken tests. Lancet 1: 739–740

De Mol P, Van Wijnendaele F, Hemelhof W, Corrazza Y 1983 Possible field test for ST-producing *Escherichia coli*. Lancet 1: 524–525

Duguid J P 1951 The demonstration of bacterial capsules and slime. Journal of Pathology and Bacteriology 63: 673–685

Duguid J P 1959 Fimbriae and adhesive properties in klebsiella strains. Journal of General Microbiology 21: 271–286

Duguid J P 1968 The function of bacterial fimbriae. Archivum Immunologiae et Therapiae Experimentalis 16: 173–188

Duguid J P 1985 Antigens of type-1 fimbriae. In: Stewart-Tull D E S & Davies M (eds) Immunology of the bacterial cell envelope. John Wiley & Sons, Chichester. Ch. 11, p 301–318

Duguid J P, Clegg S, Wilson M I 1979 The fimbrial and non-fimbrial haemagglutinins of *Escherichia coli*. Journal of Medical Microbiology 12: 213–227

Duguid J P, Old D C 1980 Adhesive properties of Enterobacteriaceae. In: Beachey E H (ed) Bacterial adherence, Receptors and Recognition series B, Vol 6, Chapman and Hall, London. Ch 7, p 187–217

Duguid J P, Smith I W, Dempster G, Edmunds P N 1955 Non-flagellar filamentous appendages ('fimbriae') and haemagglutinating activity in *Bacterium coli*. Journal of Pathology and Bacteriology 70: 335–348

Du Pont H L, Formal S B, Hornick R B, Snyder M J, Libonati J P, Sheahan D G, La Brec E H, Kalas J P 1971 Pathogenesis of *Escherichia coli* diarrhoea. New England Journal of Medicine 285: 1–9

Edwards P R, Ewing W H 1972 Identification of Enterobacteriaceae, 3rd edn. Burgess, Minneapolis

Edwards P R, Fife M A 1952 Capsule types of klebsiella. Journal of Infectious Diseases 91: 92–104

Emslie-Smith A H 1961 *Hafnia alvei* strains possessing the alpha antigen of Stamp and Stone. Journal of Pathology and Bacteriology 81: 534–536

Evans D J Jr, Clegg S, Evans D G 1980 Fimbrial antigens and pathogenic *Escherichia coli*. Lancet 1:201

Gargan R, Brumfitt W, Hamilton-Miller J M T 1982 A concise biotyping system for differentiating strains of *Escherichia coli*. Journal of Clinical Pathology 35: 1366–1369

Gillies R R, Duguid J P 1958 The fimbrial antigens of *Shigella flexneri*. Journal of Hygiene, Cambridge 56: 303–318

Glynn A A, Brumfitt W, Howard C J 1971 K antigens of *Escherichia coli* and renal involvement in urinary-tract infections. Lancet 1: 514–516

Gross R J, Scotland S M, Rowe B 1979 Enterotoxigenic *Escherichia coli* causing diarrhoea in travellers returning to the United Kingdom. British Medical Journal 1:1463

Grüneberg R N, Bettelheim K A 1969 Geographical variation in serological types of urinary *Escherichia coli*. Journal of Medical Microbiology 2: 219–224

Harber M J, Chick S, MacKenzie R, Asscher A W 1982 Lack of adherence to epithelial cells by freshly isolated urinary pathogens. Lancet 1: 586–588

Honda T, Akhtar Q, Glass R I, Golam Kibriya 1981 Simple assay to detect *Escherichia coli* producing heat labile enterotoxin: Results of a field study of the Biken test in Bangladesh. Lancet 2: 609–610

Hutchison R I 1957 *Escherichia coli* (O-types 111, 55 and 26) and their association with infantile diarrhoea: a five year study. Journal of Hygiene, Cambridge 55: 27–44

Kaijser B, Hanson L A, Jodal U, Lindin-Janson G, Robbins J B 1977 Frequency of *E. coli* K antigens in urinary-tract infections in children. Lancet 1: 663–664

Källenius G, Möllby R, Svenson S B, Helin I, Hultberg H, Cedergren B, Winberg J 1981 Occurrence of P-fimbriated *Escherichia coli* in urinary tract infections. Lancet 2: 1369–1372

Kauffmann F 1947 The serology of the Coli-group. Journal of Immunology 57: 71–100

Kauffmann F 1969 The bacteriology of enterobacteriaceae, 2nd edn. Munksgaard, Copenhagen

Kopp R, Müller J, Lemme R 1966 Inhibition of swarming *Proteus* by sodium tetradecyl sulfate, β-phenylethyl alcohol, and *p*-nitrophenylglycerol. Applied Microbiology 14: 873–878

Larsson P, Olling S 1977 O antigen distribution and sensitivity to the bactericidal effect of normal human serum of *Proteus* strains from clinical specimens. Medical Microbiology and Immunology 163: 77–82

Lennette E H, Balows A, Hausler W J, Truant J P 1980 Manual of clinical microbiology, 3rd edn. American Society for Microbiology, Washington DC

McDonald J C, Charter R E 1956 *Escherichia coli* serotypes in a nursery. Proceedings of the Royal Society of Medicine 49: 85–88

Mackey J P, Sandys G H 1966 Diagnosis of urinary infections. British Medical Journal 1:1173

Maskell R 1982 Urinary tract infection. Edward Arnold, London. p 42–46

Merson M H, Rowe B, Black R E, Huq I, Gross R J, Eusof A 1980 Use of antisera for identification of enterotoxigenic Escherichia coli. Lancet 2: 222–224

Neter E, Bertram L F, Arbesman C E 1952 Demonstration of Escherichia coli O55 and O111 antigens by means of a haemagglutination test. Proceedings of the Society for Experimental Biology and Medicine, New York 79: 255–257

Ørskov F, Ørskov I 1972 Immunoelectrophoretic patterns of extracts from Escherichia coli O antigen test strains O1 to O157, examinations in homologous OK sera. Acta pathologica microbiologica scandinavica, Section B 80: 905–910

Ørskov F, Ørskov I 1978 Serotyping of Enterobacteriaceae, with special emphasis on K antigen determination. In: Bergan T, Norris J R Methods in microbiology, vol 11. Academic Press, London. Ch 1, p 1–77

Ørskov F, Ørskov I, Jann B, Jann K 1971 Immunoelectrophoretic patterns of extracts from all Escherichia coli O and K antigen test strains, correlation with pathogenicity. Acta pathologica microbiologica scandinavica, Section B 79: 142–152

Platt D J, Sommerville J S 1981 Serratia species isolated from patients in a general hospital. Journal of Hospital Infection 2: 341–348

Reports on Public Health and Medical Subjects No. 71 1969 The bacteriological examination of water supplies. Her Majesty's Stationery Office, London

Rogers K B 1951 The spread of infantile gastro-enteritis in a cubicled ward. Journal of Hygiene, Cambridge 49: 140–151

Rowe B, Gross R J, Scotland S M, Wright A E, Shillom G N, Hunter N J 1978 Outbreak of infantile enteritis caused by enterotoxigenic Escherichia coli O6:H16. Journal of Clinical Pathology 31: 217–219

Satterwhite T K, Evans D G, DuPont H L, Evans D J Jr 1978 Role of Escherichia coli colonisation factor antigen in acute diarrhoea. Lancet 2: 181–184

Sears H J, Brownlee I, Uchiyama J K 1950 Persistence of individual strains of Escherichia coli in the intestinal tract of man. Journal of Bacteriology 59: 293–301

Sedlák J, Kertészová V 1968 On the taxonomy of the genus Hafnia. Archivum Immunologie et Therapiae Experimentalis 16: 243–251

Senior B W 1977 Typing of Proteus strains by proticine production and sensitivity. Journal of Medical Microbiology 10: 7–17

Senior B W 1978 P-Nitrophenylglycerol–a superior antiswarming agent for isolating and identifying pathogens from clinical material. Journal of Medical Microbiology 11: 59–61

Senior B W, Larsson P 1983 A highly discriminatory multi-typing scheme for Proteus mirabilis and Proteus vulgaris. Journal of Medical Microbiology 16: 193–202

Skirrow M B 1969 The Dienes (mutual inhibition) test in the investigation of proteus infections. Journal of Medical Microbiology 2: 471–477

Smith H W, Halls S 1967 Observations by the ligated intestinal segment and oral inoculation methods on Escherichia coli infections in pigs, calves, lambs and rabbits. Journal of Pathology and Bacteriology, 93: 449–529

Sojka W J 1965 Escherichia coli in domestic animals and poultry. Commonwealth Agricultural Bureaux, Farnham Royal, Bucks, England

Thomas V, Shelokov A, Forland M 1974 Antibody-coated bacteria in the urine and the site of urinary tract infection. New England Journal of Medicine 290: 588–590

Thornley M J, Horne R W 1962 Electron microscope observations on the structure of fimbriae, with particular reference to klebsiella strains, by the use of the negative staining technique. Journal of General Microbiology 28: 51–56

Väisänen V, Elo J, Tallgren L G, Siitonen A, Mäkelä P H, Svanborg-Edén C, Källenius G, Svenson S B, Hultberg H, Korhonen T 1981 Mannose-resistant haemagglutination and P antigen recognition are characteristic of Escherichia coli causing primary pyelonephritis. Lancet 2: 1366–1369

Wilkinson J F, Duguid J P, Edmunds P N 1954 The distribution of polysaccharide production in aerobacter and escherichia strains and its relation to antigenic character. Journal of General Microbiology 11: 59–72

Salmonella

Definition of genus Salmonella

Enterobacteria (i.e. fermentative, facultatively anaerobic, oxidase-negative Gram-negative rods) that generally are motile, aerogenic, non-lactose-fermenting, urease-negative, citrate-utilizing, acetylmethylcarbinol-negative and KCN-negative (i.e. KCN-sensitive).

Morphology

Gram-negative bacilli, 2–4 × 0.6 μm, non-acid-fast, non-capsulate and non-sporing. Most serotypes (or 'species') are motile with peritrichous flagella, but *S. gallinarum* and *S. pullorum* are non-motile and non-motile variants (OH → O variation) are occasionally found in other serotypes. Most strains of most serotypes form type 1 (mannose-sensitive, haemagglutinating) fimbriae; *S. gallinarum*, *S. pullorum* and a few strains in other serotypes either form type 2 (non-haemagglutinating) fimbriae or are non-fimbriate; most strains of *S. paratyphi A* are non-fimbriate (Duguid et al 1966).

Culture

Aerobic and facultatively anaerobic. Grow on simple laboratory media in the temperature range 15–45°C, optimally at 37°C. Many strains are prototrophic, i.e. capable of growing on a glucose-ammonium minimal medium such as that of Davis & Mingioli, but some strains are auxotrophic and require enrichment of the minimal medium with one or more amino acids or vitamins, e.g. cysteine or nicotinamide; most *S. typhi* strains require tryptophan.

Nutrient agar and blood agar. After 24 h at 37°C, colonies of most strains are moderately large (e.g. 2–3 mm in diameter), grey-white, moist, circular disks with a smooth convex surface and entire edge, thus resembling the colonies of many other enterobacteria. Their size and degree of opacity varies with the serotype, e.g. those of *S. paratyphi A, S. abortus-ovis, S. pullorum, S. sendai* and *S. typhi-suis* are relatively small. 'Rough', non-virulent variant strains (S → R variation) form opaque granular colonies with an irregular surface and indented edge. Many strains of *S. paratyphi B* and a few of other serotypes form large mucoid colonies, or colonies surrounded by a thick mucoid 'slime wall', when plates are left at room temperature for a few days after incubation for 24 h at 37°C; the mucoid character is due to the formation of loose polysaccharide slime.

Peptone water and nutrient broth. In liquid media most strains give abundant growth with uniform turbidity. A thin surface pellicle usually forms on prolonged incubation. 'Rough' (R) variants, which have a hydrophobic surface and tend to autoagglutinate, produce a granular deposit and sometimes a thick pellicle.

Differential and selective solid media.

These media are valuable for the isolation of salmonellae from faeces and other materials contaminated with many bacteria of other kinds. They include:

1. *MacConkey bile-salt lactose agar* (Ch. 6). After 18–24 h at 37°C the colonies are pale yellow or nearly colourless, 1–3 mm in diameter,

and easily distinguished from the pink-red colonies of lactose-fermenting commensal coliform bacilli, e.g. *Escherichia coli*, which also grow well on this *unselective* differential (indicator) medium.

2. *Brilliant green MacConkey agar.* The addition to MacConkey agar of brilliant green 0.004 g/litre, which is inhibitory to *E. coli*, *Proteus* species and other commensal enterobacteria likely to outnumber the salmonellae in faeces, makes this an excellent selective as well as differential medium for salmonellae except *S. typhi*, which does not grow well on it. Salmonellae appear as low convex, pale-green translucent colonies 1–3 mm in diameter. Lactose-fermenting bacteria, including those of *Salmonella* subgenus III (see Table 29.1), produce blue-purple colonies.

3. *Leifson's deoxycholate-citrate agar (DCA).* The colonies of salmonellae on DCA are similar to or slightly smaller in size than those on MacConkey agar. They are pale, nearly colourless, smooth, shiny and translucent. Sometimes they have a black centre and sometimes they are surrounded by a zone of cleared medium, but these characters may require 48 h of incubation for their development. Salmonellae are easily distinguished from the opaque pink colonies of lactose-fermenting coliform bacilli, which are largely inhibited on this *selective* differential medium. DCA is also selective for shigellae, which give colonies similar to those of salmonellae, and for this reason is probably the most widely used plating medium for the isolation of intestinal pathogens from faeces. Unfortunately, *Proteus* species grow well on DCA and produce colonies that may be mistaken for salmonellae or shigellae.

4. *Wilson & Blair's brilliant-green bismuth sulphite agar (BBSA).* This medium is particularly valuable for the isolation of *S. typhi*. Cultures should be examined after 24 h, then again after 48 h. Crowded colonies about 1 mm in diameter may take up the dye from the medium and appear

* Refer to *Methods* at end of this chapter.

green or pale brown. Larger, discrete colonies have a black centre and a clear edge. All salmonellae may produce hydrogen sulphide which causes the colony to be surrounded by a metallic sheen. The medium is highly selective for salmonellae, being inhibitory to coliforms, proteus and shigellae; occasional strains of coliforms grow to form dull green or brown colonies, but without a surrounding metallic sheen.

5. *Taylor's xylose lysine deoxycholate (XLD) agar.* XLD was developed by Taylor (1965) as a selective medium for shigellae because he found that *Shigella dysenteriae* and *Shigella flexneri* were liable to be inhibited by the concentrations of deoxycholate, brilliant green, selenite and tetrathionate in the selective media most used for salmonellae. Sodium deoxycholate is incorporated in XLD to restrain the growth of *E. coli* and prevent spreading by proteus, but at a concentration of only 0.1 or 0.25%, instead of at 0.5% as in DCA.

XLD has other advantages to make it the preferred medium for the primary plating of faeces from suspected salmonella and shigella infections. It gives colony appearances that distinguish salmonellae from shigellae, and these pathogens from the many non-lactose-fermenting strains of non-pathogenic enterobacteria which form pale colonies similar to theirs on MacConkey and DCA.

Colonies of salmonellae and shigellae are red (alkaline to phenol red) because shigellae do not form acid from the xylose, lactose and sucrose in the medium within 24 h and because salmonellae neutralize the acid they form from the limited amount of xylose by decarboxylating the lysine.

Most salmonellae (and edwardsiellae) are distinguished from the shigellae because they produce hydrogen sulphide which reacts with ferric ammonium citrate in the medium to produce black centres in their red colonies. The shigellae, H_2S-negative salmonellae, e.g. *S. paratyphi A*, and providenciae form red colonies without black centres.

Yellow (acid) colonies are formed by most other enterobacteria, namely (1) those, e.g. *E. coli*, that form so much acid from the lactose and sucrose as not to be neutralizable by the decarboxylation of lysine, and (2) those, e.g. *Citrobacter* and *Proteus*, that do not ferment lactose or sucrose, but from failing to decarboxylate lysine do not neutralize the acid they form from the xylose. The acid reaction delays blackening of the colonies of H$_2$S-producing strains of *Citrobacter* and *Proteus* until after the time for reading at 18–24 h.

Enrichment media

These are liquid media used to assist the isolation of salmonellae from faeces, sewage, foodstuffs and other materials containing a mixed bacterial flora. A larger amount of the material can be inoculated into an enrichment medium than on to an agar plate, so facilitating the isolation of salmonellae when these are present only in small numbers. During incubation, any salmonellae multiply rapidly, while *E. coli* and most other bacteria are inhibited. After 18–24 h the enriched culture is plated on to a differential agar medium, e.g. MacConkey or DCA, on which the production of salmonella-like colonies may be observed. Proteus, which is commonly present in faeces and sewage, is often able to grow in the salmonella-enrichment media and, when it does so, will produce salmonella-like colonies in the platings on MacConkey or DCA. Such colonies, therefore, must be subjected to tests for their identification. Good enrichment media include:

1. *Tetrathionate broth** enriches salmonellae, including *S. typhi*, and sometimes shigellae, but permits the growth of *Proteus* species, which may reduce the tetrathionate and thus impair the selectivity for salmonellae.

2. *Kauffmann-Müller tetrathionate broth with brilliant green**. The addition of brilliant green inhibits the growth of proteus and so improves the selectivity of the tetrathionate broth, but also makes it rather too inhibitory to *S. typhi* and shigellae. As an alternative to brilliant green, the addition of 40 mg novobiocin /litre of medium before the addition of iodine serves to overcome interference by proteus (Jeffries 1959).

3. *Selenite F broth** is probably the most used enrichment medium for specimens that may contain either salmonellae or shigellae. It is excellent for *S. typhi* and *S. dublin*, but some salmonellae, e.g. *S. paratyphi A* and *S. choleraesuis*, and some shigellae may fail to multiply.

4. *Rappaport's malachite green magnesium chloride broth** has been reported to be more efficient than other enrichment media for the isolation of salmonellae from faeces, water and foodstuffs (Iveson et al 1964).

5. *Strontium chloride broth* was found by Iveson & Mackay-Scollay (1969) to be superior to selenite F broth for the isolation of a wide range of salmonellae from faeces and sewage.

Although enriched cultures are generally subcultured on to plates after incubation for 18–24 h, more positive results can be obtained if they are also plated after 6 h and 48 h. Many salmonellae can multiply at higher temperatures than common contaminants and for this reason the selectivity of brilliant-green tetrathionate broth and selenite F broth, except for *S. typhi*, may be improved by incubation at 42–43°C instead of 37°C (Public Health Laboratory Service 1974).

Biochemical reactions

Although most species and strains conform with the pattern of reactions shown for *Salmonella* in Table 28.2, the decision that a bacterium is not a salmonella should not be based on the result of only a single test. Some strains show exceptional reactions in particular tests and it is necessary to consider the general pattern of the reactions in a group of tests. For biochemical test methods, see Chapter 8.

1. *Fermentation tests*. Carbohydrates are generally fermented with the production of acid and gas. *S. typhi*, *S. gallinarum* and rare anaerogenic variants in other serotypes, e.g. *S. typhimurium*, form only acid. Typically, glucose, mannitol, arabinose, maltose, dulcitol and sorbitol are fermented, but not lactose, sucrose, salicin or adonitol; the ONPG test for β-galactosidase is negative. Among exceptional strains, *S. cholerae-suis* and some strains of *S. typhi* do not ferment arabinose, whereas *S. cholerae-suis*, *S. pullorum*, most strains of *S. typhi*

and some strains of *S. paratyphi A* and *S. paratyphi B* do not ferment dulcitol.

When reading the results of fermentation tests, the different types of reaction should be borne in mind. Most strains fermenting a particular sugar give 'strong' fermentation; they show acid production in sugar peptone water within 6–10 h at 37°C and can grow on a defined medium with the sugar as sole source of carbon and energy. Some strains, deficient in the uptake mechanism, give 'weak' fermentation, showing acid production in sugar peptone water only after 10–20 h and fail to grow on a defined medium with the sugar as sole carbon and energy source. Thus, biotypes 1–16 of *S. typhimurium* give strong fermentation of D-xylose and biotypes 17–32 weak fermentation (Duguid et al 1975). Non-fermenting strains may give rise to fermenting mutants and show acid production in a proportion of sugar peptone water cultures after incubation for two or more days; they might be misread as fermenters unless the definitive reading time of 24 h is adhered to.

The fermentation of *d*-tartrate is observed to distinguish *S. java* (positive) from *S. paratyphi B* (negative) and between biotypes of *S. typhimurium*. The reaction is not demonstrable by acid production, but by the promotion of growth due to utilization of the tartrate. The *d*-tartrate dehydrase of positive strains is oxygen sensitive and the test should be done under the poorly aerobic conditions of static culture in a deep tube of *d*-tartrate peptone water, in which positive strains give several times as much growth and turbidity as negative ones (Duguid et al 1975; Barker 1985)*. Alternatively, positive reactions may be demonstrated by the appearance of growth on a defined *d*-tartrate medium in plates incubated anaerobically for 2 days (Barker 1985).

2. *Decarboxylase tests.* Salmonellae decarboxylate the amino acids, lysine, ornithine and arginine, but not glutamic acid. *S. typhi* is exceptional in lacking ornithine decarboxylase and *S. paratyphi A* in lacking lysine decarboxylase.

3. *Other biochemical tests.* Most salmonellae have the following reactions. Indole not produced. Methyl-red positive. Acetyl methyl carbinol not produced (i.e. Voges-Proskauer negative). Citrate utilized, except by *S. typhi* and *S. paratyphi A*. Malonate not utilized. Gluconate not utilized. Urease not produced. Phenylalanine deaminase not produced. Hydrogen sulphide produced in ferrous chloride-gelatin medium, except by *S. paratyphi A*, *S. cholerae-suis*, *S. typhi-suis* and *S. sendai*. No growth in KCN medium. Gelatin not liquefied.

Subgenera of Salmonella. A minority of serotypes give atypical biochemical reactions. Kauffmann (1969) has divided the genus *Salmonella* into four subgenera (Table 29.1); subgenus I, which contains all the serotypes commonly infecting man and mammals, gives the typical reactions in the six definitive tests, and the other subgenera give atypical reactions. Within each subgenus a few strains give exceptional reactions, e.g. gelatin is liquefied by *S. abortus-bovis*, *S. azteca*, *S. schleissheim* and *S. texas* in subgenus I, and dulcitol is not fermented by most strains of *S. typhi* and some of *S. paratyphi A* and *S. paratyphi B*.

Table 29.1 Biochemical reactions of subgenera of *Salmonella*.

Test	Subgenus			
	I	II	III	IV
Dulcitol fermentation	+	+	−	−
Lactose fermentation	−	−	+	−
Salicin fermentation	−	−	−	+
Malonate utilization	−	+	+	−
KCN, growth in	−	−	−	+
Gelatin liquefaction	−	+	+	+

Arizona group. This group was originally named *Salmonella arizonae*. It is classified as subgenus III of *Salmonella* by Kauffmann (1969), though some authors give it the status of a separate genus, *Arizona*. The arizonae have been found mainly in reptiles and birds, being responsible for heavy losses in turkey flocks in the USA, but also occasionally in human patients with diarrhoea or septicaemia.

Arizonae exhibit important biochemical differences from typical salmonellae. Most strains ferment lactose promptly and others ferment it after several days' incubation of the test. The ONPG test is positive, dulcitol is not fermented, malonate is usually utilized and gelatin is commonly liquefied after 7–10 days at 22°C.

Like the salmonellae, the arizonae are divided into numerous serotypes by differences in their O and H antigens, many of which resemble particular salmonella antigens though designated with different numbers (Edwards & Ewing 1972).

Antigenic structure

In the Kauffmann-White classification the genus *Salmonella* is subdivided into more than a thousand serotypes containing different combinations of antigens. The identification of these serotypes depends on detection of the O (somatic) and H (flagellar) antigens by means of agglutination tests with specific antisera. Many different serotypes have one or more of their O or H antigens in common and their distinctive antigens have to be demonstrated in tests with 'single-factor' antisera which have been absorbed with heterologous bacteria to free them from antibodies to the shared antigens (Edwards & Ewing 1972; Ørskov & Ørskov 1978).

Salmonella antigens are also found in some members of other genera. The frequent sharing of O and H antigens with arizonae has already been mentioned and salmonella O antigens are also found in some strains of *Escherichia, Shigella, Citrobacter* and *Proteus*.

O antigens. These somatic antigens represent the side-chains of repeating sugar units projecting outwards from the lipopolysaccharide layer on the surface of the bacterial cell wall. They are hydrophilic and enable the bacteria to form stable, homogeneous suspensions in saline (0.85% NaCl) solution. Over 60 different O antigens have been recognized and they are designated by arabic numerals. The O antigens are heat-stable, being unaffected by heating for 2.5 h at 100°C, and alcohol-stable, withstanding treatment with 96% ethanol at 37°C for 4 h. The former procedure destroys flagellar and fimbrial antigens, whilst the latter detaches the flagella from the bacteria. Either method can be used to

prepare bacterial suspensions susceptible to agglutination by O antibodies but insusceptible to agglutination by H antibodies. The O antigens are unaffected by suspension of the bacteria in 0.2% formaldehyde, but if flagella are present, their fixation by the formaldehyde renders the bacteria inagglutinable by O antibodies. As will be discussed later, the O antigens are liable to be changed in character by *form variation* and *lysogenic conversion*, and to be lost from the bacteria in $S \rightarrow R$ *mutation*.

H antigens. These antigens represent determinant groups on the flagellar protein. They are heat-labile and alcohol-labile, but are well preserved in 0.04–0.2% formaldehyde. Heating at temperatures above 60°C detaches the flagella from the bacteria and detachment of all flagella is achieved by heating for 30 min at 100°C. The deflagellated bacteria are inagglutinable by H antibodies but the detached flagella remain immunogenic, and suspensions of bacteria to be used for the production of O antisera should be freed from detached flagella by centrifugation and washing or by inactivation by heating for 2.5 h at 100°C.

In many but not all salmonellae the production of flagellar antigens is diphasic, each strain varying spontaneously and reversibly between two phases with different sets of H antigens. In *phase 1*, the 'specific phase', the bacteria form flagella with one or more antigens from a set of over 70 H antigens designated by the small letters of the alphabet, a to z, then as z_1, z_2, z_3, etc. In *phase 2*, the 'group phase', the bacteria form flagella with one or more antigens from a mainly different set of H antigens. The first discovered of these were designated by arabic numerals (not implying any relationship with the similarly numbered O antigens), but later, certain phase-1 antigens, especially e, n, x, z, 1, and w, were found in the phase 2 of some serotypes. Phase 2 is termed the 'group' or 'nonspecific' phase because numerous serotypes of salmonellae share the same antigens when in this phase. The presumptive identification of serotypes therefore mainly depends on the identification of the H antigens in phase 1, which are relatively 'specific'.

A given culture of diphasic salmonella may consist almost entirely of bacteria in the one or other phase. A colony or a first subculture of a colony is likely to be mainly in one phase because it consists only of the recent progeny of a single bacterial cell. Other cultures may contain numerous bacteria of each phase. Thus, when a culture in one phase is subcultured serially by mass inoculation, variants into the other phase multiply until they comprise a substantial equilibrating proportion of the population (Stocker 1949).

The definitive identification of a diphasic salmonella always requires the identification of the H antigens of both phases. It is therefore necessary to obtain a culture in the different phase from that first isolated from the patient. The alternative phase may be obtained by selective cultivation of the isolate in semi-solid agar containing monophasic antiserum to the original phase antigens, e.g. by the modified Craigie tube method* or Jameson strip methods.*

A few serotypes of salmonella are monophasic, forming flagella with antigens only of the phase-1 or, rarely, phase-2 series, and a few serotypes are triphasic, especially those that express a higher numbered z antigen in one of their phases.

Flagella and their antigens may be lost from a strain of salmonella by a rare spontaneous mutation, termed $OH \rightarrow O$ variation. This variation is usually irreversible, but it is sometimes possible to select motile and flagellated back-mutants by stab culture in semi-solid agar in a Craigie (1931) tube; the non-motile bacteria remain at the site of inoculation while the motile mutants swarm away through the agar and may be picked up at a distance for subculture. One or two subcultures by this method can also yield richly flagellated variant cultures from strains that are poorly flagellated by their genotype when first isolated. The abundance of flagella varies with the conditions of culture as well as with the genotype; it is maximal in young (6 h) broth cultures and minimal in older (24 h) cultures on thin, firm agar plates.

Kauffmann-White classification. This scheme, first developed in 1934, classifies the salmonellae

into different *O groups*, or *O serogroups*, each of which contains a number of serotypes possessing a common O antigen not found in other O groups. The O groups first defined were designated by capital letters A to Z and those discovered later by the number (51–67) of the characteristic O antigen. Group A, for example, is characterized by O antigen 2, group B by O antigen 4, and group D by O antigen 9. Some groups are divided into subgroups whose members are distinguished by a second O antigen, e.g. group C_1 is characterized by O antigens 6 and 7, and group C_2 by O antigens 6 and 8. O antigen 29 is characteristic of the genus *Citrobacter* and O antigens 61–64 of *Arizona* (*Salmonella* subgenus III). Groups A–E contain nearly all the salmonellae that are important pathogens in man and animals.

Within each O group the different serotypes are distinguished by their particular H antigen or combination of H antigens. The antigenic formulae of some representative salmonellae are shown in Table 29.2, which includes the serotypes most virulent in man, those commonest in Britain and those most likely to be confused with the virulent and common serotypes. Fuller tables of serotypes are given by Kauffmann (1969) and Edwards & Ewing (1972). It should be noted that although O antigens 6 and 12 are shown in the table as single entities, antigen 6 is a complex of two factors, 6_1 and 6_2, and antigen 12 is a complex of three factors, 12_1, 12_2, and 12_3.

Differentiation of antigenically similar strains. As may be seen from examples in Table 29.2, not all named serotypes have a unique antigenic structure. Thus, *S. paratyphi B*, a cause of enteric fever in man, has the same antigens as *S. java*, an animal parasite of lesser virulence for man, in whom it causes gastroenteritis but not enteric fever. *S. paratyphi C* has the same O and H antigens as *S. cholerae-suis*, *S. decatur* and *S. typhi-suis*. *S. sendai*, a rare cause of enteric fever, has the same antigens as the less virulent *S. miami*, and *S. gallinarum* has the same antigens as *S. pullorum*.

The serotypes that share the same antigenic formula are distinguished from one another by biochemical tests. *S. paratyphi B* forms mucoid

Table 29.2 Antigens of some representatives of the genus *Salmonella* (Kauffmann-White classification).

O group	Serotype ('species')	O antigens[a] (and Vi)[a]	H antigens Phase 1	H antigens Phase 2
A	*S. paratyphi A*	1, **2**, 12	a	—
	S. paratyphi A var. *durazzo*	**2**, 12	a	—
B	*S. paratyphi B*	1, **4**, 5, 12	b	1, 2
	S. paratyphi B var. *odense*	1, **4**, 12	b	1, 2
	S. java	1, **4**, 5, 12	b	(1, 2)
	S. limete	1, **4**, 12, 27	b	1, 5
	S. typhimurium	1, **4**, 5, 12	i	1, 2
	S. typhimurium var. *copenhagen*	1, **4**, 12	i	1, 2
	S. agama	**4**, 12	i	1, 6
	S. abortus-equi	**4**, 12	—	e, n, x
	S. abortus-ovis	**4**, 12	c	1, 6
	S. agona	**4**, 12	f, g, s	—
	S. brandenburg	**4**, 12	*l*, v	e, n, z_{15}
	S. bredeney	1, **4**, 12, 27	*l*, v	1, 7
	S. derby	1, **4**, 5, 12	f, g	—
	S. heidelberg	1, **4**, 5, 12	r	1, 2
	S. saint-paul	1, **4**, 5, 12	e, h	1, 2
	S. salinatis	**4**, 12	d, e, h	d, e, n, z_{15}
	S. stanley	**4**, 5, 12	d	1, 2
C_1	*S. paratyphi C*	**6, 7** (Vi)	c	1, 5
	S. cholerae-suis	**6, 7**	c	1, 5
	S. cholerae-suis var. *kunzendorf*	**6, 7**	(c)	1, 5
	S. decatur	**6, 7**	c	1, 5
	S. typhi-suis	**6, 7**	c	1, 5
	S. bareilly	**6, 7**	y	1, 5
	S. infantis	**6, 7**	r	1, 5
	S. menston	**6, 7**	g, s, t	—
	S. montevideo	**6, 7**	g, m, s	—
	S. oranienburg	**6, 7**	m, t	—
	S. thompson	**6, 7**	k	1, 5
C_2	*S. bovis-morbificans*	**6, 8**	r	1, 5
	S. newport	**6, 8**	e, h	1, 2
D	*S. typhi*	**9**, 12, (Vi)	d	—
	S. ndolo	**9**, 12	d	1, 5
	S. dublin	1, **9**, 12, (Vi)	g, p	—
	S. enteritidis	1, **9**, 12	g, m	—
	S. gallinarum	1, **9**, 12	—	—
	S. pullorum	(1),**9**, 12	—	—
	S. panama	1, **9**, 12	*l*, v	1, 5
	S. miami	1, **9**, 12	a	1, 5
	S. sendai	1, **9**, 12	a	1, 5

Table 29.2 (cont'd).

O group	Serotype ('species')	O antigens[a] (and Vi)[a]	H antigens Phase 1	Phase 2
E_1	S. anatum	**3, 10**	e, h	1, 6
	S. give	**3, 10**	l, v	1, 7
	S. london	**3, 10**	l, v	1, 6
	S. meleagridis	**3, 10**	e, h	l, w
E_2	S. cambridge	**3, 15**	e, h	l, w
	S. newington	**3, 15**	e, h	1, 6
E_3	S. minneapolis	(3), (15), **34**	e, h	1, 6
E_4	S. senftenberg	1, **3, 19**	g, s, t	—
	S. simsbury	1, **3, 19**	—	z_{27}
F	S. aberdeen	**11**	i	1, 2
G	S. cubana	1, **13**, 23	z_{29}	—
	S. poona	**13**, 22	z	1, 6
H	S. heves	**6, 14**, 24	d	1, 5
	S. onderstepoort	1, **6, 14**, 25	e, h	1,5
I	S. brazil	**16**	a	1, 5
	S. hvittingfoss	**16**	b	e, n, x
Others	S. kirkee	**17**	b	1, 2
	S. adelaide	**35**	f, g	—
	S. locarno	**57**	z_{29}	z_{42}

[a] Numbers in bold type indicate the antigens characterizing the O group.
Numbers in brackets are antigens that are not always present.

colonies on prolonged incubation and usually does not ferment d-tartrate, whereas S. java is non-mucoid and usually ferments d-tartrate. S. paratyphi C ferments d-tartrate and trehalose within 2 days, but not Stern's glycerol*; S. cholerae-suis ferments d-tartrate, but not trehalose or Stern's glycerol; S. decatur ferments all three substrates and S. typhi-suis only trehalose. S. sendai ferments arabinose but not Stern's glycerol, whereas S. miami ferments Stern's glycerol but not arabinose. S. gallinarum is anaerogenic and ferments d-tartrate and dulcitol, whilst S. pullorum forms gas from glucose but fails to ferment d-tartrate or dulcitol.

Other surface antigens. Although the serotype of an enterobacterium is defined mainly by its O and H antigens, there may be other antigens at the bacterial surface that determine agglutination with homologous antibodies. These include the capsular, or K antigens (Kauffmann 1969;

Ørskov et al 1977), including the Vi antigen; the slime (mucus), or M antigen; and the fimbrial, or F antigens (Duguid & Campbell 1969; Ørskov et al 1977). Such antigens may cause difficulty in the serological identification of bacteria either by masking the O antigens so that the bacteria are inagglutinable by O antibodies or by causing non-specific cross-reactions due to their presence in unrelated bacteria.

Vi antigen. Almost all recently isolated strains of S. typhi form Vi antigen as a covering layer outside their cell wall. This antigen is an acidic polysaccharide. When fully developed it renders the bacteria agglutinable by Vi antibody and inagglutinable by O antibody. Antigens identical with or closely related to the Vi antigen of S. typhi have been found in S. paratyphi C, S. dublin and some strains of Escherichia and Citrobacter (Ballerup-Bethesda group). Freshly isolated strains of S. typhi rich in Vi antigen (V forms) produce more opaque colonies than strains lacking Vi antigen (W forms). Vi rich strains maintained by subculture on conventional media are rapidly replaced by spontaneously originating Vi deficient mutants (V → W variation).

The Vi antigen is heat-labile. It can be removed from the bacteria by heating a suspension for 1 h at 100°C and centrifuging the bacteria from the Vi-containing fluid. Even without heating, Vi antigen gradually separates from the bacteria in a saline suspension. Tests for Vi antigen are therefore best done with a bacterial suspension freshly made from an agar culture grown from a V form colony.

M antigen. This antigen is a loose extracellular polysaccharide slime consisting of colanic acid. It occurs in a serologically similar form in various unrelated enterobacteria, including *S. paratyphi B* and other serotypes of salmonella and many strains of *E. coli.* Salmonellae form it most abundantly when, after incubation for 1 day at 37°C, plate cultures are held for several days at ambient temperature; on such plates it causes the colonies to become mucoid, particularly at their margins, which then appear as a 'slime wall'. Although of different antigenic specificity from the Vi antigen, it resembles the Vi antigen in preventing agglutination by O antibodies. Heating for 2.5 h at 100°C removes the M antigen and renders the bacteria agglutinable by O antiserum. A motile, non-mucoid mutant can sometimes be selected by serial passage through semi-solid agar (M → N variation). The M antigen cross-reacts serologically with some type-specific K antigens, such as the K 30 and K 39 antigens of *E. coli* and the K 8 and K 13 antigens of *Klebsiella aerogenes.*

Fimbrial antigens. Type 1 fimbriae, which are formed by most strains of salmonellae, bear antigens that determine agglutination by sera containing anti-fimbrial antibodies (Duguid & Campbell 1969; Duguid 1985). The bacteria vary reversibly between a fimbriate phase, which predominates in 24–48 h broth cultures, and a non-fimbriate phase which predominates in young (6 h) broth cultures and 24 h agar plate cultures (fimbrial phase variation, F ⇌ N). A common antigen is present in the fimbriae of different salmonella serotypes and strains of arizona and citrobacter, but there is no sharing of fimbrial antigens with *Escherichia, Shigella, Klebsiella* and *Enterobacter.*

The sharing of fimbrial antigens among different serotypes of salmonella gives rise to confusing cross-reactions if agglutination tests are done with bacteria from fimbriate-phase cultures and sera containing fimbrial antibodies. Such cross-reactions are best avoided by the use of non-fimbriate-phase cultures for the preparation of agglutinable bacterial suspensions, e.g. broth cultures grown for only 6 h, glucose broth cultures grown for 12 h or thin agar plate cultures grown for 24 h.

Like the flagellar antigens, the fimbrial antigens are preserved in bacteria held in 0.1 or 0.2% formaldehyde. They are detached from the bacteria by heating for 30 min at 100°C and are inactivated by heating for 15 min at 121°C. Agglutination by fimbrial antibodies is best tested with formaldehyde-killed bacteria from a 48 h broth culture. Fimbrial antiserum is prepared by injecting such fimbriate bacteria into rabbits and may be absorbed free from O and H antibodies with non-fimbriate bacteria grown in glucose broth or on agar plates.

R antigens. In S → R mutation the O antigens are lost and new 'R' antigens are revealed at the bacterial surface. Mutational loss of an enzyme required for the formation of one of the links in the polysaccharide core or side chains of the cell-wall lipopolysaccharide leads to an absence of the hydrophilic side chains that determine O antigen specificity. The exposed incomplete (R_I) or complete (R_{II}) core polysaccharide constitutes the R antigen. The R antigens are the same in the R variants from different salmonella serotypes, though different from the R antigens of other enterobacteria.

The R variant bacteria tend to outgrow the parental S bacteria during serial culture in the laboratory. They form rough colonies, and are autoagglutinable in saline and sensitive to killing by complement. Because they are autoagglutinable and lack serotype specificity, they are unsuitable for serological tests. R cultures can be recognized by the rapid agglutination caused when a dense suspension of the bacteria is mixed with a drop of 0.2% acriflavine in 0.85% NaCl solution. This test will detect minor degrees of 'roughness' not revealed either by colonial morphology or by inability to form a uniform suspension in saline.

Antigenic variations. The mutations V → W, M → N, S → R and OH → O, and the phase variations of flagellar (phase 1 ⇌ phase 2) and fimbrial (F ⇌ N) antigens have been described above.

Form variation is a spontaneous reversible variation in the amount of one of the O antigens, e.g. factor 1, 6_1, 12_2, 22, 23, 24 or 25. Different amounts of the antigen are found in different colonies in a plating from the culture.

Lysogenic conversion may cause gain, loss or change of an O antigen. Thus, in *S. typhimurium* and other members of O groups A, B, D, G, R and T, the formation of O antigen 1 is dependent on the presence in the bacterium of the genome of a temperate A-type phage, such as P22. Strains gain or lose O antigen 1 when they are lysogenized or delysogenized with the phage. By a similar process, *S. anatum* (O-3,10; H-e,h:1,6) forms O antigens 3 and 15 and so comes to resemble *S. newington* (O-3,15; H-e,h:1,6) when it is lysogenized with phage epsilon[15] derived from *S. newington*. It forms O antigens 3, 15 and 34 when it is further lysogenized with phage epsilon[34] derived from a group-E_3 serotype such as *S. minneapolis*.

Bacteriophage typing

Strains within a particular serotype may be differentiated into a number of *phage types* by their patterns of susceptibility to lysis by members of a series of phages with different specificities. The determination of the phage type of strains isolated from different patients, carriers, other sources or vehicles is valuable in the epidemiological study of infections because it helps to define groups of persons who have been infected with the same strain from the same source. Serotypes that are subdivided in existing systems of phage typing include *S. typhi*, *S. paratyphi A*, *S. paratyphi B*, *S. typhimurium* and *S. enteritidis*. Thus, over 80 different phage types of *S. typhi* and over 200 phage types of *S. typhimurium* are distinguished.

The phage typing of *S. typhi* is done by determining the sensitivity of the culture to a series of variants of a single phage, Vi-phage II, which have been adapted to the different types of typhoid bacillus. The specific phage-sensitivity, and thus the phage type of the bacterium is determined partly by its content of particular 'type-determining' symbiotic phages and partly by other heritable traits. In other serotypes the phage typing is done with sets of unrelated O-phages collected from a variety of sources. The techniques of phage typing are complicated and it is usual for cultures to be sent for typing at a reference laboratory (Guinée & van Leeuwen 1978).

Biotyping

Strains in a particular serotype may be differentiated into a number of biotypes by the pattern of their fermentative and biosynthetic reactions with a series of substrates. In *S. typhimurium*, for example, a typing system with 15 tests differentiated over 144 different biotypes (Duguid et al 1975). Strains of the same phage type may be subdivided into different biotypes and strains of the same biotype into different phage types, so that a combination of the two methods gives a finer discrimination of strains than either method alone (Anderson et al 1978). The tests and substrates used to biotype *S. typhimurium* are also useful in biotyping *S. paratyphi B* and some other serotypes. In *S. typhi*, different biotypes may be distinguished by reactions with arabinose, dulcitol and xylose. For reliability in biotyping it is essential to use standardized methods, media and inocula. It is also necessary to read the results of tests only after a 'definitive' time of incubation which is chosen to distinguish between strains that are genotypically capable of giving the reaction in question and strains that are genotypically 'negative' but able on prolonged incubation to give rise to 'positive' mutants.

Viability

Salmonellae are readily killed by moist heat, e.g. in 1 h at 55°C or 15 min at 60°C, and most strong disinfectants. Cultures on slopes of Dorset's egg kept tightly capped to prevent drying and stored in the dark at room temperature usually remain viable for at least 10–20 years. *S. typhi* and other salmonellae gradually die in contaminated moist natural environments outside the body, but some bacilli may survive for over 4 weeks in, for example, sewage-polluted water or moist soil. They die more quickly when dried, *S. typhi* often within a few hours, so that spread is less likely to take place by dust or dry fomites than by water or moist foodstuffs. Many salmonellae, however, survive for fairly long periods when dried in foodstuffs, e.g. in dried egg, milk or coconut, and infections have been carried in such products from one country to another.

Antibiotic sensitivity

Most strains are sensitive to chloramphenicol (MIC 2 mg/litre), ampicillin (MIC 1–8 mg/l), gentamicin (MIC 0.25 mg/l), tetracycline (MIC 1 mg/l), cotrimoxazole and some other antibiotics. Chloramphenicol is considered to be the most effective agent for the treatment of typhoid fever; the alternative drug is cotrimoxazole. Ampicillin has been disappointing in treatment of the fever, but has shown some success in elimination of the carrier state. Some strains of salmonella are highly resistant to certain of these drugs and it is necessary to test the antibiotic sensitivities of any strain isolated from a septicaemic illness.

Salmonella food-poisoning uncomplicated by septicaemia should not be treated with antibiotics, for there is evidence that such treatment by its effect on the normal intestinal flora may paradoxically prolong the excretion of salmonellae and fail to give any clinical benefit. It is, however, useful to determine the sensitivities of food-poisoning strains so that prompt treatment may be given in the rare cases that become septicaemic.

LABORATORY DIAGNOSIS OF INFECTIONS

Laboratory diagnosis of salmonella infections depends mainly on the isolation and identification of the causal salmonella from a specimen of the patient's blood, faeces, urine or vomit.

Testing the patient's serum for salmonella antibodies is useful only in the diagnosis of enteric fever (Widal reaction) and even for this condition the significance of the results of the test is often doubtful. For the diagnosis of pyrexial illnesses, physicians should be advised to submit blood cultures and faeces to the laboratory and not to rely on the fallible serological tests. If a blood culture cannot be obtained, the bacteriologist may culture the clot taken from a blood specimen submitted for serology.

Isolation of a salmonella by blood culture is proof that the patient has a salmonella septicaemia. Isolation from the faeces is of less certain significance; in illnesses resembling enteric fever or gastroenteritis such an isolation strongly suggests that salmonella infection is the cause, but since salmonellae may be present in the faeces of carriers it does not amount to proof of a causal role.

The clinical value of identifying the serotype of a salmonella isolate lies in distinguishing the serotypes that cause enteric fever in man, namely *S. typhi, S. paratyphi A, S. paratyphi B* and *S. sendai*, from the other serotypes, which in man commonly cause gastroenteritis (food-poisoning) but rarely septicaemic infections. The value of identifying the serotype of a 'non-enteric-fever' salmonella is mainly epidemiological; knowledge of the serotype helps to define the sources and vehicles of infection in outbreaks of food-poisoning. Phage typing and biotyping may be used to obtain more precise information for this purpose.

Specimens for isolation of salmonellae

Faeces is the specimen most commonly submitted. It should be collected in a faeces container, or 'outfit', a 25 ml cylindrical glass or plastic jar with a screw cap bearing on its under side a small 'spoon'. A 'spoonful' of faeces should be taken from stool that has been passed into a clean bedpan or collected on toilet paper. The 'spoon' should then be replaced in the container, taking care not to soil the rim or outside of the container, and the screw cap should be firmly applied. No attempt should be made to collect several spoonfuls of faeces or to fill the container. If delay in transport of the specimen to the laboratory is inevitable, and especially if the weather is warm, the faeces should be placed in a container with about 6 ml of buffered glycerol saline transport medium (Ch. 6).

Rectal swabs are convenient to collect, but compare unfavourably with faeces in their yield of isolations. *Faecal swabs*, which are swabs dipped into and heavily charged with faeces after it has been passed, are good specimens. If delay in transit of swabs to the laboratory is inevitable, they should be placed and submitted in Stuart's transport medium (Ch. 6). Pus swabs should be treated as rectal or faecal swabs. Specimens of urine, vomit or bile should be centrifuged and the deposit cultured.

Blood culture. The isolation of salmonella from the blood by blood culture follows the methods described in Chapters 7 and 39. Usually blood cultures are subcultured only on to a non-selective medium such as blood agar on which salmonella colonies look like coliforms and lack distinctive features. It is imperative, therefore, that all Gram-negative bacilli isolated from blood are fully identified. When in the absence of blood cultures, clotted blood is submitted for serological examination (Widal test), it is useful to culture the clot by transferring it into 15 ml bile salt streptokinase broth* and subculturing after incubation for one or more days. *Clot culture* is carried out in many laboratories serving populations with a high incidence of enteric fever, but is not used routinely in Britain.

Isolation and identification of salmonella from faeces

The faeces is cultured on plates of one or more kinds of selective media, both directly and after preliminary culture in a liquid enrichment medium, and the plates are observed for the presence of salmonella-like colonies. A well separated colony is picked to obtain a pure culture and the pure culture is identified first by a selection of biochemical tests and finally by agglutination tests with specific antisera. The choice of culture media and biochemical tests

differs in different laboratories, but the following scheme of procedures for isolation and identification can be recommended as being both effective and relatively economical in labour. If as is often the case, the presence of enteropathogenic bacteria other than salmonellae is possible, e.g. *Staphylococcus aureus, Bacillus cereus*, entero-pathogenic *Escherichia coli*, shigellae, campylo-bacters, vibrios and clostridia, additional media and tests may have to be included (Chs 16, 24, 28, 30, 32 and 38).

1. *On the first day*, inoculate a large loopful of faeces on to a DCA or XLD plate and several loopfuls into selenite F broth or, if *S. typhi* need not be expected, tetrathionate broth. If the faeces is solid, emulsify it to form a dense suspension in peptone water and use this suspension for the inoculations. When plating on DCA or XLD, spread the loopful of faeces uniformly over an area at one side of the plate amounting to about one-fifth of the whole. Flame the loop, cool it in the edge of the agar and recharge it by rubbing it over the seeded area. Then, without further flaming or recharging, plate out the inoculum on the remainder of the plate by making about eight strokes across it in each of three directions. Because DCA and XLD are selective, they can be thus heavily inoculated and yet yield separate colonies.

DCA, XLD and other plating media are not absolutely selective for salmonellae and shigellae, but generally permit the growth of many commensal bacteria. Good plating technique, yielding many (e.g. 100–200) separate colonies, is therefore needed to maximize the chances of isolating a pathogen present in the faeces in only small or moderate numbers. If, for instance, a pathogen constitutes only 1 or 2% of the faecal bacteria able to grow on the medium, it is likely to be missed in a plating that yields only 20 or 30 separate colonies.

If the specimen is a swab, rub it heavily over half of the DCA or XLD plate and stroke out with the loop over the other half. Then inoculate the swab into the liquid enrichment medium, rotating it to disperse the faecal material.

Incubate the plate and the enrichment broth overnight at 37°C. The chance of isolating a salmonella may be slightly increased if other plates, e.g. MacConkey or Wilson & Blair's BBSA,* and enrichment media, are used as well as DCA, XLD and selenite broth. It is also increased (a) if the selenite broth is incubated at 43°C instead of 37°C (except for *S. typhi*) and (b) if the broth is examined by plate subculture after 6, 48 and 72 h as well as after 18–24 h (Chattopadhyay & Pilfold 1976).

2. *On the second day*, proceed as follows: (a) Subculture the enrichment, e.g. selenite, culture by plating thinly, for separate colonies, on to DCA or XLD. Do not first shake the broth, because the greater motility of salmonellae as compared with *E. coli* results in there being a greater concentration of salmonellae at its undisturbed surface. If it is considered important to detect rare, lactose-fermenting variants of salmonellae, also subculture the enrichment broth on to a plate of BBSA; these variants give pink colonies indistinguishable from *E. coli* on DCA, but can be recognized by their black colonies on BBSA. Incubate the plates overnight at 37°C.

(b) Examine the primary DCA plate and any other primary plate for salmonella-like colonies, i.e. 'pale', non-lactose-fermenting colonies on DCA and red, black-centred colonies on XLD. If there are no salmonella-like colonies on the primary plate, discard this plate and next day (*third day*) examine the plate subculture(s) from the enrichment broth for salmonella-like colonies. If there are salmonella-like colonies on any of the plates, examine and identify one of them as from (3) below.

3. Select for pure subculture and biochemical tests a salmonella-like colony that is well separated from other colonies. With a straight inoculating wire, pick material from it, inoculate it into 2 ml urea broth (Christensen's medium without agar, Ch. 8) and incubate for 5–6 h in a waterbath. If there are different types of salmonella-like colonies, pick one of each type into separate urea broths.

If all the salmonella-like colonies on the plates are crowded and touching other colonies, do not subculture any of them into urea broth. Instead,

pick one as cleanly as possible and streak it out thinly on a MacConkey plate with the aim of getting well separated colonies. Incubate this plate overnight at 37°C and then select a well separated colony for subculture into urea broth. When this procedure is necessary, it delays the examination of the specimen by a day.

It is unwise to make serological agglutination tests on bacteria from a colony, even a well separated one, on a selective medium, for such bacteria often give unstable or mixed suspensions. If there is great urgency in obtaining a serological identification, subculture a well separated colony on to a moist agar slope and attempt slide agglutination tests after incubation for 4 h.

4. Examine each *urea broth* after 5–6 h. If it is pink, it is strongly urease positive and probably proteus; discard it and regard the culture as negative for salmonella and shigella. If it is still colourless, i.e. probably urease negative, use it to inoculate the primary identifying tests described in (5) below and further incubate its residue along with these tests.

5. *Set up primary identifying tests* from the 5–6 h urea broth culture (late on the same day as that on which the culture was grown). With a sterile Pasteur pipette, inoculate single drops of the urea broth culture into each of the following test media and incubate overnight at 37°C: glucose, lactose, sucrose and mannitol peptone waters (Ch. 8), semi-solid tryptone agar (Ch. 6; stab down 2 cm), a nutrient agar slope (run 3–4 drops over it) and a MacConkey plate (stroke out thinly for separate colonies). Before inoculating, check that the sugar media are not turbid (i.e. contaminated) and that the Durham tube in the glucose medium does not contain a bubble of air. The MacConkey plate ('primary purity plate') serves to check whether the urea broth used to inoculate the tests was a pure culture.

6. *Read the primary identifying tests* the next day, i.e. on the third or fourth day of the examination.

(a) Confirm that the reincubated urea broth

shows both *bacterial growth* (turbidity) and a *negative reaction* (colourless). If the urease reaction has become positive, discard the other tests, seed another urea broth from a pale colony on the purity plate and repeat the examinations from (3) above. Otherwise proceed as follows.

(b) Inspect the primary purity plate to confirm that only a *single type* of colony is present on it and that this is *pale*, i.e. non-lactose-fermenting. If so, retain the plate for later inoculation of the secondary identifying tests (see 9 below). If not, discard the primary tests, seed another urea broth from a pale colony on the purity plate and repeat the examinations from (3) above.

(c) Read the semi-solid tryptone agar for *motility* (haze spreading from stab line) or *non-motility* (growth confined to stab). Then add 2–3 drops of Kovac's rosindole reagent (Ch. 8) and watch a few minutes for the development of a pink colour denoting a positive *indole reaction*.

(d) Read the sugar media for the production of *acid* (colour change) and the glucose medium also for the production of *gas* (bubble in Durham tube).

(e) Provisionally identify the organism by the reactions in the primary tests as shown in Table 29.3. Discard if neither salmonella nor shigella.

7. *Slide agglutination tests*. If the primary biochemical tests have identified the organism as a possible salmonella, attempt to identify the serotype by slide agglutination tests with salmonella antisera.

(a) Prepare a milky bacterial suspension from the overnight slope culture by placing 0.5 ml sterile (0.85%) saline in a test-tube and, with the same pipette, adding several drops of the bacteria-containing fluid from the foot of the slope. Retain the pipette in the tube of suspension for transferring drops on to slides.

(b) Place a drop of the bacterial suspension on a clean slide. Do no more than two tests on the same slide. With a 2 mm *platinum* wire loop that has been flamed and cooled in air for at least 20 s, take a small, bulging loopful of the diagnostic serum and rub it into the bacterial suspension. Mix by tilting to and fro for 30–60 s while viewing under a good light against a dark background with the naked eye. Distinct clumping within 60 s is a positive result. At once discard the used slide into disinfectant. Take care not to contaminate the fingers or bench with the live bacterial suspension.

For salmonella isolated for the first time, test the following sera* in the order (i) to (vi):

(i) Salmonella polyvalent O (groups A–G) serum on one half of the slide. Test the suspension alone on the other half as a control to exclude saline autoagglutinability.

(ii) Salmonella mixed specific and non-specific H (i.e. polyvalent phases 1 and 2) serum and salmonella mixed non-specific H (i.e. polyvalent phase 2) serum on separate halves of a slide. If the polyvalent O and polyvalent H reactions are negative, do no further slide tests for salmonella except, if the isolate is anaerogenic, to exclude *S. typhi* (see vi), but proceed to the secondary identifying biochemical tests (see 9 below). If the polyvalent O or polyvalent H reactions are

Table 29.3 Reactions of salmonellae and shigellae in primary tests.
Key: +, positive; −, negative; . . ., result not given

Test	Typical reactions of salmonellae	% salmonellae giving atypical reaction	Typical reactions of shigellae
Urease	−	0	−
Motility	+ (rarely −)	. . .	−
Indole	−	3	− or +
Gas from glucose	+ (*S. typhi* −)	. . .	− (rarely +)
Glucose to acid	+	0	+
Lactose to acid	−	1	−
Sucrose to acid	−	1	−
Mannitol to acid	+	1	+ (*S. dysenteriae* −)

positive for salmonella, proceed to the slide tests (iii)–(v).

(iii) Individual Salmonella O-group sera A–G in separate tests. Test each of these group-specific sera and do *not* stop the examination when a positive result is obtained with one of them.

(iv) If the culture is in the specific phase, i.e. reacts positively with mixed phase 1 and 2 H-serum and negatively with mixed phase 2 H-serum (see ii above), and if it reacts positively with any single O-group serum, test it with the single factor H sera (a, b, d, i, etc), beginning with the 'i' serum if the culture is in O-group B (O antigen 4).

(v) If the culture is in the non-specific phase, i.e. reacts positively with the mixed phase 2 serum, pass it overnight through a Craigie tube* or Jameson strip* containing phase 2 (non-specific) H serum to change its phase. Then re-examine with phase-1 H sera as in (iv) above.

(vi) *S. typhi* may fail to agglutinate with group D (O9) serum because the bacilli are coated with Vi antigen. If an anaerogenic culture is found negative with the O-group sera, test it with Vi serum. If Vi positive, make a suspension of the bacteria in 0.5 ml saline, heat for 30 min at 100°C, cool and re-test with O9 serum.

8. *Provisional report*. If clear-cut positive results have been obtained at this stage, i.e. on the third or fourth day (48–72 h after receipt of specimen), inform the clinician or health officer without delay.

9. *Secondary identifying tests and sensitivity tests*. Do these tests on all first isolates from a patient of a bacterium provisionally identified by the primary biochemical tests as a possible salmonella. The secondary identifying tests should be done regardless of whether positive or negative results are obtained in the slide agglutination tests, for these slide tests are not fully reliable.

Prepare an inoculum by picking *one* well separated pale colony from the primary MacConkey purity plate and suspending it in 2 ml sterile saline. With a sterile pipette,

inoculate single drops of this suspension into the following test media (Ch. 8) and incubate overnight: citrate agar slope, lysine decarboxylase medium, decarboxylase medium without lysine as a control, salicin peptone water, ONPG medium, MacConkey secondary purity plate (streak out thinly for separate colonies), nutrient agar slope (several drops), and a sensitivity agar plate. Spread the inoculum uniformly over the sensitivity plate and apply an appropriate range of antibiotic disks, e.g. chloramphenicol, ampicillin, sulphonamide, trimethoprim, mecillinam and cefotaxime. Alternatively, for identification, use a multi-test system such as API 20E.

10. Next day, read the secondary identifying and sensitivity tests. First inspect the MacConkey plate to confirm that only one type of colony is present and thus that the inoculum was pure. Then read the antibiotic sensitivities and the other tests. Re-incubate the lysine decarboxylase test and read again after another day. Identify a salmonella by the reactions as shown in Table 29.4.

11. *Confirmatory agglutination tests*. Do slide agglutination tests on bacteria from the secondary agar slope culture to confirm the results obtained for the primary slope culture or to identify the serotype if the previous slide tests were inconclusive (see 7 above).

If the secondary tests confirm that the isolate is a pure culture of a salmonella, seed it on to two Dorset egg slopes and send one to a Salmonella Reference Laboratory for final serotyping.

Table 29.4 Reactions of salmonellae and shigellae in secondary tests.
Key: +, positive; −, negative; . . ., result not given.

Test	Typical reactions of salmonellae	% salmonellae giving atypical reaction	Typical reactions of shigellae
Growth on citrate	+	25	−
Lysine decarboxylase	+	4	−
Salicin to acid	−	0	−
ONPG reaction	−	2	. . .

Send the clinician or health officer a confirmatory report, which should include the results of the antibiotic sensitivity tests if the illness is enteric fever or septicaemic. If the illness is simple gastroenteritis, the sensitivity results may be withheld, unless specially requested, so as not to encourage unnecessary therapy which may be disadvantageous to the patient.

The identification scheme just described is adequate for use in laboratories that send cultures of presumptive or partially identified salmonellae to a reference laboratory. It is wasteful of reagents for a general hospital laboratory to hold stocks of a wide range of single-factor typing sera. For the full and certain identification of a salmonella serotype it is necessary (a) to identify *both* phases of the H antigen, i.e. conversion to the alternate phase is always necessary, and (b) to confirm the results of H antigen identification with a tube agglutination test. Confirmation by tube tests is not normally required for recognition of the O and Vi antigens.

Tube agglutination tests

Bacterial suspensions for testing for O, H and Vi antigens are prepared as follows.

H antigens. Inoculate bacteria from a single colony in the required H phase into broth and incubate for 6 h. View a drop of the culture in a wet film to confirm that most of the bacteria are motile and therefore sufficiently flagellated for the tests. Kill the culture by adding formaldehyde to a concentration of 0.2% and incubating for several hours at 37°C. If the broth culture is found to be poorly motile, select a highly motile variant by passing subcultures once or twice through semi-solid agar in a Craigie tube (without antiserum) or by stab-culturing in a plate of semi-solid agar and subculturing from the periphery of the swarm.

O antigens. Suspend the bacteria from an agar culture in saline and heat for 30 min at 100°C to remove flagella and fimbriae. Centrifuge to separate the bacteria from the detached flagella and fimbriae and resuspend the bacteria in saline. Alternatively, remove the flagella by

mixing a dense saline suspension of the bacteria with an equal volume of 96% ethanol and incubating for 20 h at 37°C; before use, dilute in saline to a suitable density.

Vi antigen. Prepare a fresh suspension of live bacteria from an opaque (Vi-rich) colony just before testing. Take care in handling and testing this suspension to avoid spreading infection.

Method. 1. Dilute the antigens with saline to a density of about 2×10^8 bacteria/ml, as judged by comparison with an opacity standard.

2. Perform the tests in small tubes containing 0.4 ml of mixtures of the bacterial suspension with different dilutions of the diagnostic antiserum. Prepare six or so doubling dilutions of the serum in saline, starting at a 1 in 10 dilution for O and Vi agglutinations and at a 1 in 50 dilution for H agglutination. Add equal volumes of the bacterial suspension (0.2 ml) to the diluted serum (0.2 ml) in each tube and to a control tube containing only saline (0.2 ml).

3. Incubate the tubes in a waterbath, immersed so that the surface of the water in the bath is level with the mid-point of the columns of fluid within them. This arrangement ensures convectional mixing of the contents. Incubate H agglutinations for 2 h at 50°C or 4 h at 37°C, O agglutinations for 20 h at 50°C or for 6 h at 37°C followed by refrigeration overnight, and Vi agglutinations for 2 h at 37°C followed by refrigeration overnight.

4. Read the results by viewing the tubes under good light against a dark background with the aid of a × 2 magnifying lens. If necessary, rotate the tubes to swirl up granules from the deposit, but do not shake them. Take the titre of the serum as the greatest dilution giving visible agglutination. Thus, if the limiting dilution is 1 in 200 (i.e. 200-fold), the titre is 200 (not 1/200). The tube test is positive only if the titre is equal to or greater than the titre stated on the bottle of the typing serum.

Isolation and identification from other sources

Vomit, urine, pus and blood. The methods of isolation and identification of salmonellae from these specimens from patients mainly follow the methods just outlined for the examination of faeces. But for those specimens, e.g. pus and blood, unlikely to be contaminated with other organisms, unselective plating media such as blood agar and MacConkey agar are used instead of the selective DCA and BBSA media.

Faeces of healthy carriers. The number of salmonellae in the faeces of an asymptomatic carrier may be far fewer than that in the faeces of a patient. When, therefore, a search is being made among healthy persons for an unknown carrier who has been a source of infection in others, it may be necessary to examine repeated specimens of faeces from the suspected individuals, to use more than one plating medium and one enrichment medium, and to increase the efficiency of enrichment by incubating the enrichment media at 43°C and subculturing from them after 72 h as well as after 24 h.

When the faeces of known convalescent carriers are being examined as a test of cure before return to normal employment, it is generally unnecessary to use the more exacting methods for isolation, for there is little risk of an individual disseminating infection when only a small number of salmonellae is present in a formed, solid stool. It is a matter of judgement when a food-handler should be allowed to return to work (Pether & Scott 1982).

Isolation from foodstuffs. The following points are important in the isolation of salmonellae from food (Public Health Laboratory Service 1974). For alternative methods, see van Leusden et al (1982) and Harvey & Price (1982); see also Chapter 11.

1. Relatively small numbers of several different salmonella serotypes may be present in the same foodstuff and the sample should be partitioned to increase the chance of isolation of each of them. Examine at least two, preferably four, 25 g amounts.

2. Do not attempt direct plating of the foodstuff, but add each 25 g sample to 100 ml nutrient broth and incubate overnight at 37°C. Because the salmonellae are often of diminished viability, they may fail to grow if the sample is placed directly into an enrichment medium containing selectively toxic chemicals.

3. After the pre-enrichment culture in nutrient broth, add aliquots of that culture to an equal volume of each of two double-strength enrichment media. The use of only one enrichment medium may selectively promote the growth of only one of the serotypes present. Choose two of the following media: selenite F broth*, tetrathionate broth* and Rappaport broth.* Incubate at 43°C.

4. Subculture the enrichment cultures after incubation for 24 h, and again after 48 h, by plating on to DCA and brilliant green MacConkey agar* and incubating overnight at 37°C. Examine the plates for salmonella-like colonies.

Serological diagnosis by the Widal test

Tests for the presence of salmonella antibodies in the patient's serum may be of value in the diagnosis of enteric fever, but are of little help in that of salmonella food-poisoning. The patient's serum is tested by tube agglutination for its titres of antibodies against H, O and Vi suspensions of the enteric fever bacteria likely to be encountered, e.g. *S. typhi* and *S. paratyphi B* in Britain. These suspensions may be prepared from suitable stock laboratory cultures by the methods described above for suspensions for tube agglutination tests, but commercially prepared suspensions are generally used.

Method. 1. Test the patient's serum in a series of dilutions against each of the different salmonella suspensions. For each series use seven small (7 × 1 cm) test tubes, six for six serum dilutions and the seventh for a saline, non-serum control.

2. Place 0.4 ml saline (0.85% NaCl) in each of tubes 2–7. Make up a 1 in 15 dilution of the patient's serum in saline and with a fresh graduated pipette add 0.4 ml of the diluted serum to each of tubes 1 and 2. Tube 2 will then contain 0.8 ml of serum diluted 1 in 30.

3. Mix the fluid in tube 2 by pipetting up and down several times, then transfer 0.4 ml into tube 3. With the same pipette similarly mix the 0.8 ml contents of tube 3 and then transfer 0.4 ml to tube 4. Repeat the process to tube 6, from which, after mixing, discard 0.4 ml. Each

tube then contains 0.4 ml fluid, tubes 1–6 containing serum dilutions of 15, 30, 60, 120, 240 and 480, and tube 7 only saline.

4. With a fresh pipette, then add 0.4 ml bacterial suspension to each tube, starting at tube 7 and working backwards to tube 1. The serum dilutions in tubes 1–6 are now 30–960.

5. With a capillary pipette, transfer the mixtures to narrow agglutination tubes, starting at tube 7 and working backwards to tube 1.

6. Incubate H agglutinations for 2 h at 37°C and read after standing on the bench for half an hour. Incubate O agglutinations for 4 h at 37°C and read after refrigeration overnight at 4°C. Use a waterbath for incubation. Read the tests by viewing them under a good light against a dark background. The large flakes of H agglutination are easily visible with the naked eye, but a × 2 magnifying lens should be used to detect the small granules of O agglutination after raising these by rotating the tube.

Vi agglutinations. Test these in doubling serum dilutions from 1 in 10 to 1 in 640 in 7 × 1 cm test tubes. Incubate these tubes for 2 h at 37°C, stand at room temperature overnight and then read with a lens. In the control, the bacteria will be sedimented to a small compact deposit. If agglutination has occurred a granular deposit is scattered over the foot of the tube.

Interpretation. The titre of the patient's serum for each salmonella suspension is read as the highest dilution of serum giving visible agglutination, e.g. if this dilution is 1 in 240, the titre is 240. A positive reaction is first detected about the seventh to tenth day of the illness in enteric fever, so that a negative result at an early stage is inconclusive. The strength of the reaction for the infecting serotype increases progressively to a maximum about the end of the third week and the demonstration of such a *rising titre*, e.g. four-fold or greater rise, between tests made in the first and third weeks is highly significant.

Positive results in a single test by no means prove the presence of enteric fever nor negative results its absence. From an extensive study of sera collected from patients during and after the outbreak of typhoid fever in Aberdeen in 1964, Brodie (1977) concluded that the value of the Widal reaction as an aid to diagnosis was very limited. In contradiction of generally held opinion, he found that the H antibody titre was a more reliable indicator of infection than the O antibody titre. However, Pang & Puthucheary (1983) in a detailed study in Malaysia demonstrated the diagnostic value of the Widal test in an area where typhoid is endemic.

In interpreting results the following points should be borne in mind:

1. The serum of some 'normal' (uninfected) persons agglutinates salmonella suspensions at dilutions of up to about 1 in 50, so that titres cannot be taken as significant unless they are greater than about 100.

2. Persons who have received TAB vaccine may show high titres to each of the salmonellae in the vaccine and only if a marked rise of titre to one serotype is observed can the result be regarded as diagnostically significant. H agglutinins tend to persist for many months after vaccination but O agglutinins tend to disappear sooner, e.g. within 6 months.

3. For determining the serotype of the infecting organism, the H reaction is more reliable than the O reaction because the different serotypes have some O antigens in common.

4. Non-specific antigens, such as fimbrial antigens, may be present in the test suspensions and then give false-positive results by reacting with a homologous agglutinin present in the serum of some uninfected individuals.

5. The Widal reaction is positive in many healthy carriers, and such a carrier may suffer a pyrexial illness due to a different, non-salmonella infection. Although a negative reaction does not exclude the carrier state, a positive reaction, particularly a Vi titre of 10 or greater, is said to be helpful for its recognition. Brodie (1977), however, found such Vi titres in patients who were not *S. typhi* excretors a year or more after recovery and in healthy persons some but not all of whom had received TAB vaccine.

Serological diagnosis by counterimmunoelectrophoresis

Counterimmunoelectrophoresis of patient's serum with a Veronal buffer extract of *S. typhi* was found by Tsang & Chau (1982) to give a higher proportion of positive reactions (96%) in typhoid patients and a lower proportion of 'false-positive' reactions (0%) in uninfected subjects than the Widal test (73 and 16%, respectively).

METHODS

Deoxycholate citrate agar (DCA)

Hynes' (1942) modification of Leifson's (1935) medium is particularly suitable for the isolation of dysentery bacilli, food-poisoning salmonellae and *S. paratyphi B*, and less so, but superior to MacConkey agar, for *S. typhi*. In the medium described here, Hynes' change to ferric citrate from the ferric ammonium citrate of Leifson's medium is not adopted because there is less precipitation of solution A and the medium is slightly less inhibitory, providing a better chance of recovering scanty pathogens at the expense of some growth of *Escherichia coli*. Various modifications of DCA medium are commercially available.

Neutral red lactose agar

Meat extract (Lab-Lemco, Oxoid)	20 g
Peptone (Difco proteose)	20 g
Agar	90 g
Neutral red 2% in 50% ethanol	5 ml
Lactose	40 g
Water	4 litre

Dissolve the meat extract in 200 ml water over a flame. Make just alkaline to phenolphthalein by addition of sodium hydroxide, boil at 100°C and filter through filter paper. Adjust the pH to 7.4, make up the volume to 200 ml and add the peptone. Dissolve the agar in 3800 ml water by steaming for 1 h at 100°C. Filter if necessary to clarify. Add the meat extract and peptone solution to the agar solution and mix well. Add the neutral red and lactose, mixing again. Bottle in accurate 100 ml lots and heat for 1 h in free steam at 100°C, then without intermediate cooling, autoclave for 15 min at 115°C.

Solution A

Sodium citrate ($Na_3C_6H_5O_7.2H_2O$)	17 g
Sodium thiosulphate ($Na_2S_2O_3.5H_2O$)	17 g
Ferric ammonium citrate	4 g
Sterile water	100 ml

Solution B

Sodium deoxycholate	10 g
Sterile water	100 ml

Prepare solutions A and B with sterile precautions, heating for 1 h at 60°C to facilitate solution.

Complete medium

Neutral red lactose agar	100 ml
Solution A	5 ml
Solution B	5 ml

Melt the agar and add solutions A and B with separate pipettes, in that order and mixing well between additions. Pour plates *immediately*, allow to cool and dry their surfaces. Any delay in pouring and cooling after addition of the deoxycholate makes the medium very soft. The deoxycholate must be pure and should be tested with known positive specimens before purchase because batches vary in their inhibitory capacity. The finished medium is pale pink in colour and should be quite clear.

DCA is a *heat-sensitive* medium. It must not be autoclaved or remelted. When prepared from a commercial powder containing the deoxycholate, the powder must be dissolved and 'sterilized' with only the shortest period of heating at 100°C, with stirring, necessary for complete solution.

Addition of *sucrose* (1%) as well as lactose to the medium is advantageous in causing non-pathogenic coliform bacteria that ferment sucrose but not lactose, e.g. *Proteus vulgaris* and some strains of *E. coli*, to form pink colonies distinguishable from the pale colonies of salmonellae and shigellae, which do not ferment sucrose.

Wilson & Blair's BBSA

The use of this brilliant green bismuth sulphite agar (Wilson 1938) depends on the reduction of sulphite to sulphide by *S. typhi* and *S. paratyphi B*, which thereby form black colonies, and the inhibition of *E. coli* by brilliant green and by bismuth sulphite in the presence of excess sulphite.

Bismuth sulphite glucose phosphate mixture

Bismuth ammonio-citrate scales	30 g
Sodium sulphite (Na_2SO_3)	100 g
Disodium hydrogen phosphate ($Na_2HPO_4.12H_2O$)	100 g
Glucose	50 g
Sterile water	1 litre

With sterile precautions dissolve the bismuth ammonio-citrate in 250 ml boiling water, and the sodium sulphite in 500 ml boiling water. Mix the solutions and while the mixture is boiling add the disodium hydrogen phosphate. When the mixture is cool, add the glucose previously dissolved in 250 ml boiling water and cooled. This mixture will then keep for months.

Iron citrate brilliant green mixture

Ferric citrate, brown scales	2 g
Brilliant green	0.25 g
Sterile water	225 ml

With sterile precautions mix (a) a solution of the ferric citrate in 200 ml water with (b) a solution of the brilliant green in 25 ml water. This mixture will keep for months.

Complete medium

Sterile nutrient agar	100 ml
Bismuth sulphite glucose phosphate mixture	20 ml
Iron citrate brilliant green mixture	4.5 ml

Melt the agar and cool to 60°C. Add the other ingredients with sterile precautions and pour plates.

When preparing the medium from a commercial powder, follow the manufacturer's instructions for dissolving and 'sterilizing' it with a minimal period of heating at 100°C.

After 18 h salmonella colonies may be clear, green, black-centred or black, but after 48 h are uniformly black and surrounded by a dark zone and metallic sheen. Other organisms are usually inhibited, but may form green or brown colonies without a dark halo or metallic sheen.

Brilliant green MacConkey agar

The medium is prepared as MacConkey agar (Ch. 6), but with the addition of 0.004 g brilliant green/litre. The brilliant green is inhibitory to *E. coli* and renders the medium selective for salmonellae, which form pale colonies.

More complex brilliant green plating media, containing both lactose and sucrose, and phosphate buffer, are available commercially in powdered form and can be recommended. Where phenol red is used as the indicator of acid production, salmonella colonies are red and the colonies of lactose- or sucrose-fermenting organisms are yellow.

Xylose lysine deoxycholate (XLD) agar

Taylor's (1965) formula is as follows:-

Yeast extract	3.0 g
Xylose	3.75 g
Lactose	7.5 g
Sucrose	7.5 g
L-Lysine HCl	5.0 g
Sodium chloride	5.0 g
Sodium deoxycholate	2.5 g
Sodium thiosulphate	6.8 g
Ferric ammonium citrate	0.8 g
Phenol red	0.08 g
Agar	15 g
Water	1 litre

Except for the deoxycholate, thiosulphate and ferric ammonium citrate, dissolve the ingredients in the water by autoclaving. Cool to 50°C and add, per litre, 20 ml of a solution of sodium thiosulphate 34% and ferric ammonium citrate 4%, and 25 ml of a solution of sodium deoxycholate 10%. Mix, adjust the pH to 6.9 and at once pour in plates. Read after the seeded plates have been incubated at 37°C for only 18–24 h.

Complete medium in powdered form is available commercially, e.g. Oxoid CM469, which contains only 0.1% of the deoxycholate and 1.25% of agar. Suspend 53 g of CM469 in 1 litre distilled water. Heat with agitation to boiling point to dissolve. Avoid prolonged heating. Cool to 50°C in a waterbath, adjust the pH to 7.4 and at once pour in plates.

Red colonies with black centres: most strains of *Salmonella*, the Arizona group and *Edwardsiella*.

Red colonies without black centres: *Shigella*, *Providencia*, H$_2$S-negative serovars of *Salmonella*, and some strains of *Proteus morgani*, *Proteus rettgeri* and *Pseudomonas*.

Yellow colonies: most strains of *E. coli*, *Klebsiella*, *Enterobacter*, *Citrobacter*, *Proteus* and *Serratia*.

Selenite F broth

The selenite in this enrichment medium (Leifson 1936) inhibits coliform bacilli while permitting salmonellae and many shigellae to grow.

Sodium hydrogen selenite (NaHSeO$_3$)	4 g
Peptone	5 g
Lactose	4 g
Disodium hydrogen phosphate (Na$_2$HPO$_4$.12H$_2$O)	9.5 g
Sodium dihydrogen phosphate (NaH$_2$PO$_4$.2H$_2$O)	0.5 g
Sterile water	1 litre

Dissolve the ingredients with sterile precautions and distribute the yellowish solution in about 10 ml amounts into screw-capped Universal bottles or to a depth of 5 cm in test tubes. Steam for 20 min at 100°C. Do not autoclave, for excessive heating spoils the medium. The amount of red precipitate should be very slight. The pH of the completed medium should be 7.1 and, if necessary, the proportions of the two phosphate salts should be slightly adjusted to attain this value.

Care must be taken in the preparation and use of the medium, for selenium salts are toxic and teratogenic, and volatile derivatives, including hydrogen selenide, are toxic when inhaled.

The selectivity of the medium is diminished if an excessive amount of organic material is inoculated into it. When attempting to isolate salmonella from foodstuffs, either inoculate from a pre-enrichment broth culture as described above in this chapter or inoculate about 1 ml of the supernate of a suspension of about 3 g specimen in 15 ml saline after the debris has settled on standing.

Tetrathionate broth

Thiosulphate solution

Sodium thiosulphate (Na$_2$S$_2$O$_3$.5H$_2$O)	24.8 g
Sterile water to	100 ml

Mix the salt and the water with sterile precautions and steam for 30 min at 100°C. This gives a 1 mol/litre solution.

Iodine solution

Potassium iodide (KI)	20 g
Iodine (I)	12.7 g
Sterile water to	100 ml

With sterile precautions dissolve the potassium iodide in about 50 ml warm water, add the iodine and make up the volume to 100 ml. This gives a 0.5 mol/litre solution.

Complete medium

Calcium carbonate (CaCO$_3$)	2.5 g
Nutrient broth	78 ml
Thiosulphate solution	15 ml
Iodine solution	4 ml
Phenol red, 0.02% in 20% ethanol	3 ml

Add the calcium carbonate to the broth and sterilize it by autoclaving for 20 min at 121°C. When cool, add the thiosulphate, iodine and phenol red solutions with sterile precautions. Distribute 10 ml amounts in sterile screw-capped bottles or test tubes. Even in the refrigerator the completed medium does not keep for more than about 1 week. It is convenient to keep the stock solutions and prepare the complete medium as required (Knox et al 1942). Ideally the medium should be used within a few hours of adding the iodine solution to the other reagents.

Brilliant green tetrathionate broth

This medium is more selective for most salmonellae than the original tetrathionate broth because the brilliant green in it checks the growth of proteus, but it is too inhibitory to *S. typhi* and shigellae.

Thiosulphate solution

Sodium thiosulphate ($Na_2S_2O_3.5H_2O$)	50 g
Sterile water	100 ml

Mix the salt and water with sterile precautions and steam for 30 min at 100°C.

Iodine solution

Potassium iodide (KI)	25 g
Iodine (I)	20 g
Sterile water	100 ml

With sterile precautions dissolve the potassium iodide and add the iodine.

Ox bile solution

Desiccated ox bile	0.5 g
Sterile water	5 ml

Dissolve with sterile precautions.

Complete medium

Nutrient broth, pH 7.4	90 ml
Calcium carbonate ($CaCO_3$)	5 g
Brilliant green, 1 in 1000 aqueous	1 ml
Thiosulphate solution	10 ml
Iodine solution	2 ml
Ox bile solution	5 ml

Add the calcium carbonate to the broth and sterilize it by autoclaving for 20 min at 121°C. When cool, add the other solutions and distribute with sterile precautions in about 10 ml amounts. Heat these once for 10 min at 100°C in the steamer.

Rappaport's malachite green magnesium chloride broth

This efficient enrichment medium for salmonellae is recommended by Iveson et al (1964).

Solution A

Tryptone	5 g
Sodium chloride (NaCl)	8 g
Potassium dihydrogen phosphate (KH_2PO_4)	1.6 g
Distilled water to	1 litre

Prepare the solution on the day of use by boiling the ingredients in the distilled water to dissolve them. No further sterilization is necessary.

Solution B

Magnesium chloride ($MgCl_2.6H_2O$)	40 g
Distilled water	100 ml

Solution C

Malachite green	0.4 g
Distilled water	100 ml

Complete medium

Solution A	1 litre
Solution B	100 ml
Solution C	30 ml

Mix the three solutions, distribute 10 ml amounts in screw-capped containers and sterilize by steaming for 30 min at 100°C. The complete medium may be held without deterioration for a month at room temperature, but preferably should be stored at 4°C.

Bile salt streptokinase broth

This medium is used to culture blood clots from patients with suspected enteric fever.

Nutrient broth, sterile	1 litre
Sodium taurocholate	5 g
Streptokinase solution (Calbiochem), 100 000 units/ml, sterile	1 ml

Adjust the pH of the broth to 7.6 and dissolve the bile salt in it. Autoclave for 15 min at 108°C. Cool and add the streptokinase with sterile precautions. Distribute in 15 ml amounts with sterile precautions.

d-Tartrate fermentation test

This test distinguishes *S. java* (positive) from *S. paratyphi B* (negative) and between certain other salmonella biotypes. It is best done by the turbidity method of Alfredsson et al (see Barker 1985).

Medium

Peptone, e.g. Oxoid L37	10 g
Potassium *d*-tartrate	10 g
Sodium chloride	3.3 g
Water, deionized	1 litre

Make 2 litres of peptone water from the peptone and sodium chloride, adjust the pH to 7.0 and autoclave at 121°C for 15 min. Keep 1 litre for control cultures without *d*-tartrate. To the other litre, add 110 ml of sterile (autoclaved) 10% solution of potassium *d*-tartrate to give a final tartrate concentration of 10 g/litre. Check and if necessary adjust the pH to 7.0. Dispense the two media in 8 ml amounts in cotton-wool stoppered test tubes (12 × 1 cm)

The test is unreliable if the tartrate medium is more alkaline than pH 7.2 and as autoclaving tends to raise the pH, the reaction should be checked just before use.

Method

From a slope culture of the strain to be tested, prepare a suspension of about 10^9 bacteria/ml in saline. Inoculate 0.05 ml amounts of the suspension into a tube of the peptone water with *d*-tartrate and a tube of the peptone water without *d*-tartrate. Incubate the tubes for 24 h at 37°C under aerobic static conditions, i.e. in air, but without movement or artificial aeration.

To read, mix the contents in each tube and compare their turbidities. Fermenting strains give at least twice, and usually three to five times as much growth in the medium with *d*-tartrate as in that without. Non-fermenting strains give about the same amount of growth in the two media (difference usually under 30%).

Stern's glycerol reaction

This reaction is used in the biotyping of salmo-nellae. It shows the ability of the organism to convert glycerol into an aldehyde that recolourizes fuchsin-sulphite.

Medium. To 1 litre of broth (1% meat extract, 2% peptone, pH 8.0) add 2 ml of a saturated (10%) alcoholic solution of basic fuchsin, 16.6 ml of a fresh 10% aqueous solution of sodium sulphite and 10 ml glycerol. Tube to a depth of about 5 cm and sterilize at 121°C for 15 min.

Method. Inoculate bacteria from a culture on agar and incubate at 37°C. The development of a deep red colour within 2 days indicates a positive reaction. An unseeded tube incubated in parallel should remain uncoloured or become only faintly pink.

Sera for the identification of salmonellae

Diagnostic antisera can be prepared in the laboratory by immunizing rabbits with the appropriate antigens, but agglutinating antibodies to cross-reacting antigens must be removed by absorption and the method (see Edwards & Ewing 1972) is not only tedious but also requires considerable expertise. It is usual, therefore, to employ commercially prepared antisera (e.g. from Wellcome). The choice of sera to be held in the laboratory will vary with the type of specimens received, but the following sera would be suitable for a large hospital or public health laboratory.

O antisera

Polyvalent-O, groups A–G
2-O, group A
4-O, group B
6,7-O, group C_1
8-O, group C_2
9-O, group D
3,10,15,19-O, group E
11-O, group F
13,22-O, group G

Vi antiserum

H antisera

Polyvalent-H, specific and non-specific

Polyvalent-H, non-specific, factors 1,2,5,6,7
a-H (*S. paratyphi A*-H)
b-H (*S. paratyphi B*-H specific)
c-H (*S. paratyphi C*-H specific)
d-H (*S. typhi*-H)
e,h-H (*S. newport*-H specific)
f,g-H (*S. derby*-H)
g,m-H (*S. enteritidis*-H)
i-H (*S. typhimurium*-H specific)
k-H (*S. thompson*-H specific)
l,v-H (*S. london*-H specific)
m,t-H (*S. oranienberg*-H)
r-H (*S. bovis-morbificans*-H specific)

As an alternative to holding a range of H antisera, a laboratory that isolates salmonellae infrequently may choose to use the three so-called *rapid diagnostic sera*, with the addition of i-H serum.

Rapid diagnostic 1-H (factors b,d,E,r)
Rapid diagnostic 2-H (factors b,E,k,L)
Rapid diagnostic 3-H (factors d,E,G,k)
    E = polyvalent for e,h and e,n,x, etc.
    G = polyvalent for g,m and g,p, etc.
    L = polyvalent for l,v and l,w, etc.

Antigens for production of antisera. O antigens should consist of agar-grown bacteria heated for 2.5 h at 100°C, separated by centrifugation, treated with 96% ethanol for 4 h at 37°C, centrifuged and resuspended in saline. H antigens should consist of bacteria from a young (6 h) broth culture grown from a colony of the required phase and killed by the addition of formaldehyde to a concentration of 0.2%.

Craigie tube method for changing H phase

1. Prepare tubes or bottles containing 5–10 ml semi-solid nutrient agar (e.g. 0.2–0.3% agar, according to quality) and a small inner tube open at both ends with the upper end projecting well above the agar.

2. Melt the medium, cool to 50°C and add 0.5 ml of a 1 in 5 dilution of non-specific-phase H serum to one tube and 1 ml of the same dilution to another tube. (The serum is previously sterilized by filtration.) Allow to cool and solidify.

3. When the medium has solidified, inoculate the non-specific-phase culture with a straight wire into the agar *inside* the inner tube. Take care not to spill any inoculum outside this tube. Incubate at 37°C.

4. After the shortest period, e.g. 8–16 h, required for swarming, take material for subculture from the agar *outside* the inner tube. Specific-phase variant bacteria can swarm freely from the inner tube, but the parental, non-specific-phase bacteria are immobilized at the site of inoculation by the non-specific-phase antibodies.

5. Prepare subcultures on agar slopes and in nutrient broth, and confirm the change of phase by demonstrating the absence of agglutination with polyvalent-H non-specific serum. Then use the subculture for identification of the specific-phase H antigens.

Jameson strip method for changing H phase

1. Cut and remove a ditch 1 cm wide from a nutrient agar or blood agar plate. The concentration of agar should be just enough to allow removal of the block of agar without collapse of the rest of the medium.

2. Place across the ditch a strip of Whatman No 1 filter paper (4 × 0.5 cm) previously sterilized by dry heat. Without delay, add one drop of undiluted non-specific-phase H serum from a fine pipette to the centre of the strip before it has become moist by absorption of fluid from the agar.

3. Inoculate the non-specific-phase culture on one end of the paper strip and the adjacent medium. Incubate the plate in the uninverted position until bacterial growth is visible at the other end of the strip (usually 6–8 h).

4. Scrape off some growth from the newly colonized end of the strip and prepare subcultures on agar slopes and in nutrient broth.

5. Confirm the change of phase by demonstrating the absence of agglutination of bacteria from a subculture in a test with polyvalent-H non-specific serum. Then use the subculture for identification of the specific-phase H antigens.

Note. Either the Craigie tube or Jameson strip method may be used to change the specific to the non-specific phase. For this purpose, add homologous specific-phase H serum to the semi-solid agar or filter paper strip.

Phase change is not always achieved at the first attempt. When necessary, repeat the procedure at least three times before concluding that the salmonella has no alternate phase.

REFERENCES

Anderson E S, Ward L R, De Saxe M J, Old D C, Barker R, Duguid J P 1978 Correlation of phage-type, biotype and source in strains of *Salmonella typhimurium*. Journal of Hygiene, Cambridge 81: 203–217

Association of Clinical Pathologists 1967 Broadsheet 58, October 1967. The isolation and identification of salmonellae. From Publishing Manager, Journal of Clinical Pathology, BMA House, Tavistock Square, London WC1H 9JR

Barker R M 1985 Utilization of *d*-tartaric acid by *Salmonella paratyphi B* and *Salmonella java*: comparison of anaerobic plate test, lead acetate test and turbidity test. Journal of Hygiene, Cambridge 95: 107–114

Brodie J 1977 Antibodies and the Aberdeen typhoid outbreak of 1964. Journal of Hygiene, Cambridge 79: 161–192

Chattopadhyay B, Pilfold J N 1976 The effect of prolonged incubation of selenite F broth on the rate of isolation of Salmonella from faeces. Medical Laboratory Sciences 33: 191–194

Cowan S T, Steel K J 1974 Manual for the identification of medical bacteria, 2nd edn. Cambridge University Press

Craigie J 1931 Studies on the serological reactions of the flagella of *B. typhosus*. Journal of Immunology 21: 417–511

Duguid J P 1985 Antigens of type-1 fimbriae. In: Stewart-Tull D E S & Davies M (eds) Immunology of the bacterial cell envelope. John Wiley & Sons, Chichester. Ch 11, p 301–318

Duguid J P, Anderson E S, Alfredsson G A, Barker R, Old D C 1975 A new biotyping scheme for *Salmonella typhimurium* and its phylogenetic significance. Journal of Medical Microbiology 8: 149–166

Duguid J P, Anderson E S, Campbell I 1966 Fimbriae and adhesive properties in salmonellae. Journal of Pathology and Bacteriology 92: 107–138

Duguid J P, Campbell I 1969 Antigens of type-1 fimbriae of salmonellae and other enterobacteria. Journal of Medical Microbiology 2: 535–553

Edwards P R, Ewing W H 1972 Identification of Enterobacteriaceae, 3rd edn. Burgess, Minneapolis

Gillies R R, Duguid J P 1958 The fimbrial antigens of *Shigella flexneri*. Journal of Hygiene, Cambridge 56: 303–318

Guinée P A M, van Leeuwen W J 1978 Phage typing of *Salmonella*. In: Bergan T, Norris J R (eds) Methods in microbiology, vol 11. Academic Press, London. ch IV, p 157–191

Harvey R W S, Price T H 1982 Salmonella isolation and identification techniques alternative to the standard method. In: Corry J E L, Roberts D, Skinner F A (ed) Isolation and identification methods for food poisoning organisms. Academic Press, London. p 51–72

Hynes M 1942 The isolation of intestinal pathogens by selective media. Journal of Pathology and Bacteriology 54: 193–207

Iveson J B, Kovacs N, Laurie W 1964 An improved method of isolating salmonellae from contaminated desiccated coconut. Journal of Clinical Pathology 17: 75–78

Iveson J B, Mackay-Scollay E M 1969 Strontium chloride and strontium selenite enrichment broth media in the isolation of salmonella. Journal of Hygiene, Cambridge 67: 457–464

Jameson J E 1961 A simple method for inducing motility and phase change in salmonella. Monthly Bulletin of the Ministry of Health and the Public Health Laboratory Service 20: 14–16

Jeffries L 1959 Novobiocin-tetrathionate broth: a medium of improved selectivity for the isolation of salmonellae from faeces. Journal of Clinical Pathology 12: 568–571

Kauffmann F 1969 The bacteriology of Enterobacteriaceae, 2nd edn. Munksgaard, Copenhagen

Knox R, Gell P G H, Pollock M R 1942 Selective media for organisms of the salmonella group. Journal of Pathology and Bacteriology 54: 469–483

Leifson E 1935 New culture media based on sodium desoxycholate for the isolation of intestinal pathogens and for the enumeration of colon bacilli in milk and water. Journal of Pathology and Bacteriology 40: 581–599

Leifson E 1936 New selenite enrichment media for the isolation of typhoid and paratyphoid (*Salmonella*) bacilli. American Journal of Hygiene 24: 423–432

Mushin R 1949 A new antigenic relationship among faecal bacilli due to a common β antigen. Journal of Hygiene, Cambridge 47: 227–235

Ørskov F, Ørskov I 1978 Serotyping of Enterobacteriaceae, with special emphasis on K antigen determination. In: Bergan T, Norris J R (ed) Methods in microbiology vol 11. Academic Press, London. ch I, p 1–77

Ørskov I, Ørskov F, Jann B, Jann K 1977 Serology, chemistry and genetics of O and K antigens of *Escherichia coli*. Bacteriological Reviews 41: 667–710

Pang T, Puthucheary S D 1983 Significance and value of the Widal test in the diagnosis of typhoid fever in an endemic area. Journal of Clinical Pathology 36: 471–475

Pether J V S, Scott R J D 1982 Salmonella carriers: are they dangerous? A study to identify finger contamination with salmonellae by convalescent carriers. Journal of Infection 5: 81–88

Public Health Laboratory Service 1974 Isolation of salmonellas. Monograph Series No 8. Her Majesty's Stationery Office, London

Stamp Lord, Stone D M 1944 An agglutinogen common to certain strains of lactose and non-lactose fermenting coliform bacilli. Journal of Hygiene, Cambridge 43: 266–272

Stocker B A D 1949 Measurements of rate of mutation of flagellar antigenic phase in *Salmonella typhimurium*. Journal of Hygiene, Cambridge 47: 398–413

Taylor W I 1965 Isolation of shigellae 1. Xylose lysine agars; New media for isolation of enteric pathogens. American Journal of Clinical Pathology 44: 471–475

Tsang R S W, Chau P Y 1982 Serological diagnosis of typhoid fever by counterimmunoelectrophoresis. British Medical Journal 282: 1505–1507

van Leusden F M, van Schothorst M, Beckers H J 1982 The standard salmonella isolation method. In: Corry J E L, Roberts D, Skinner F A (ed) Isolation and identification methods for food poisoning organisms. Academic Press, London. p 35–49

Wilson W J 1938 Isolation of *Bact. typhosum* by means of bismuth sulphite medium in water- and milk-borne epidemics. Journal of Hygiene, Cambridge 38: 507–519

Shigella

Biological characters

Definition of genus Shigella

Enterobacteria (fermentative, facultatively anaerobic, oxidase-negative Gram-negative rods) that are non-lactose-fermenting, non-motile, mostly anaerogenic, urease negative, non-citrate-utilizing and KCN sensitive.

Morphology

Like salmonellae, they are non-sporing non-capsulate Gram-negative rods, 2–4 × 0.6 μm, but unlike most salmonellae, they are non-motile and non-flagellate. Fimbriae (type 1) are found only in *Shigella flexneri*, though not in serotype 6 and some strains in other serotypes (Duguid & Gillies 1957).

Culture

Aerobic and facultatively anaerobic. Optimal growth temperature is 37°C; *Shigella sonnei* grows well even at 10°C and 45°C. Grow well on conventional media, but none can grow on a simple glucose-ammonium salts medium without supplementation with nicotinic acid; some strains also require other growth factors.

1. *Nutrient agar and blood agar.* Smooth, greyish or colourless, translucent colonies, often 2–3 mm in diameter, resembling those of salmonellae. Those of *S. sonnei* are slightly larger and more opaque than those of other shigellae. *S. sonnei* has two antigenic forms, sometimes incorrectly called 'phases', a term that should be reserved for reversible (e.g. H antigen) variation, as in salmonellae. Form 1 colonies, which predominate in primary platings, are like the colonies of other shigellae. Form 2 colonies, which arise by irreversible variation from form 1 and are seen in early subcultures from primary isolates, are larger and less opaque and have an irregular, matt surface and a crenated edge. This variation probably corresponds to S → R variation in salmonellae.

2. *MacConkey agar.* Colonies are pale and yellowish (non-lactose-fermenting) and resemble those of salmonellae. Colonies of *S. sonnei*, a late fermenter of lactose, become pink when incubation is prolonged beyond 24 h.

3. *Deoxycholate citrate agar.* DCA (Ch. 29) is an excellent selective plating medium for the isolation of shigellae from faeces. Colonies are pale and similar to, though usually slightly smaller, e.g. 1–1.5 mm in diameter, and more translucent than those of salmonellae. They do not form a black centre. On prolonged incubation, those of *S. sonnei* form pink papillae.

4. *Wilson and Blair's brilliant green bismuth sulphite medium.* Shigellae do not grow on this medium (Ch. 29).

5. *Xylose lysine deoxycholate* XLD (Ch. 29) is probably the best selective medium for shigellae, being less inhibitory to *S. dysenteriae* and *S. flexneri* than DCA. Colonies are red and, unlike those of most salmonellae, without black centres.

6. *Peptone water and nutrient broth.* Good growth with uniform turbidity on incubation overnight at 37°C. Some strains, especially fimbriate ones, form a surface pellicle on longer incubation.

7. *Selenite F broth.* This medium (Ch. 29) will grow and enrich *S. sonnei* and *S. flexneri*

serotype 6, but is inhibitory to other shigellae. Tetrathionate broth and brilliant green media (Ch. 29) are inhibitory and unsuitable for enrichment cultures.

Biochemical reactions

The shigellae are divided into four groups, or species, by their biochemical reactions (in tests described in Ch. 8) and antigenic structure (Table 30.1). The groups A, B, C and D correspond to the species *S. dysenteriae, S. flexneri. S. boydi* and *S. sonnei.*

1. *Fermentation of carbohydrates.* Most strains attack sugars with the production of acid but not gas, though some strains in two serotypes, *S. flexneri* serotype 6 (Newcastle and Manchester varieties) and *S. boydi* serotype 14, form gas. Glucose is fermented by all strains.

Lactose is not fermented within 24 h by any strain nor on longer incubation by the majority. Most strains of *S. sonnei*, however, ferment lactose after several days and some strains of *S. dysenteriae* type 1 also produce acid on prolonged incubation.

The ONPG test for β-galactosidase is usually negative in groups A, B and C, but positive reactions are given by 15% of strains of *S. dysenteriae* (especially type 1), 8% of strains of *S. boydi* (regularly by type 5 strains) and all strains of *S. sonnei.*

Mannitol reactions are important because they distinguish group A strains, which do not ferment mannitol, from groups B, C and D, most strains of which do ferment it. There are, however, some mannitol-negative strains in nearly all serotypes, e.g. the Newcastle variety of *S. flexneri* serotype 6 and the biotype 'S. rabaulensis' of *S. flexneri* serotype 4a.

Dulcitol is not fermented by the majority of shigellae, but the Newcastle and Manchester varieties of *S. flexneri* serotype 6 and strains of *S. dysenteriae* serotype 5 and *S. boydi* serotypes 2, 3, 4, 6 and 10 are dulcitol fermenters.

Sucrose is not fermented except by *S. sonnei* and some strains of *S. flexneri* when incubation is prolonged for several days. Xylose is not fermented except by the mannitol-negative biotype of *S. flexneri* type 4a and some strains

of *S. boydi* and *S. sonnei.* Salicin is not fermented except by rare strains of *S. sonnei.* Adonitol and inositol are not fermented.

2. *Indole production. S. dysenteriae* serotype 1. *S. flexneri* serotype 6 and *S. sonnei* are always indole negative. Strains of other serotypes differ in their reactions.

3. *Catalase test.* The general finding that enterobacteria produce catalase has important exceptions in *S. dysenteriae* serotype 1 and a few strains of *S. flexneri* (mostly in serotype 4a) which are catalase negative.

4. *Decarboxylase tests.* Members of groups A, B and C fail to decarboxylate lysine and ornithine. *S. sonnei* decarboxylates ornithine but not lysine.

5. *Other biochemical tests.* Urease negative. Methyl red positive. Voges-Proskauer negative. Citrate not utilized. KCN broth negative. Gluconate not utilized. Malonate not utilized. Phenylalanine deaminase negative. Gelatin not liquefied. H_2S not produced. See Table 28.2.

Antigenic structure

Shigellae are differentiated by their somatic (O) antigens into serotypes identified by agglutination tests with absorbed specific antisera (Kauffmann 1969; Edwards & Ewing 1972). Some serotypes may be identified by agglutination with unabsorbed sera, but absorbed sera must be used for other serotypes between which minor antigens are shared.

Group A. S. dysenteriae contains 10 serotypes, each characterized by a different type antigen. Serotypes 1 and 2 are the organisms formerly called *S. shiga* and *S. schmitzi.* Serotype 2 shares a minor antigen with serotype 10.

Group B. For more than 50 years *S. flexneri* was known to have a complex antigenic structure. This structure was elucidated by Boyd in the decade 1930–40 (see Wilson & Miles 1975). A simplified antigenic scheme for the six serotypes and two variants is set out in Table 30.2. Serotypes 1–6 are characterized by their possession of different specific *type antigens*, designated I–VI. They share other, *group antigens* from a series designated 1–8. The serotypes 1–4 are each divided into subserotypes by the

Table 30.1 Biochemical reactions of *Shigella* species and serotypes.
Key: +, positive reaction (sugars fermented in 24 h); late positive at 2–8 days; +/–, some strains positive, others negative; (e), see text for exceptions.

Group	Species, serotype and variety	Gas from glucose	Acid produced in fermentation of					Indole production	Catalase reaction	Lysine decarboxylase	Ornithine decarboxylase
			lactose	mannitol	dulcitol	xylose	sucrose				
A	*S. dysenteriae*										
	1 (S. shiga)	–	–(e)	–	–	–	–	–	–	–	–
	2 (S. schmitzi)	–	–	–	–	–	–	+	+	–	–
	3–10	–	–	–	–(e)	–	–	+/–	+	–	–
B	*S. flexneri*										
	1–5, X and Y	–	–	+(e)	–	–(e)	–(e)	+/–	+(e)	–	–
	6, variety 88	–	–	+	+/–	–	–(e)	–	+	–	–
	6, variety Newcastle	+	–	–	–^{a}	–	–(e)	–	+	–	–
	6, variety Manchester	+	–	+	–^{a}	–	–(e)	–	+	–	–
C	*S. boydii*										
	1–15	–(e)	–	+	+/–	+/–	–	+/–	+	–	–
D	*S. sonnei*	–	–^{a}	+	–	+/–	–^{a}	–	+	–	+

Table 30.2 Antigens of *Shigella flexneri* serotypes.

Serotype	Subserotype	Type antigen	Group antigens[a]
1	1a	I	1, 2, 4
	1b	I	1, 2, 4, 6
2	2a	II	1, 3, 4
	2b	II	1, 7, 8
3	3a	III	1, 6, 7, 8
	3b	III	1, 3, 4, 6, 7, 8
	3c	III	1, 6
4	4a	IV	1, 3, 4
	4b	IV	1, 3, 4, 6
5	. . .	V	1, 7, 8
6	. . .	VI	1, 2, 4
X variant	. . .	—	1, 7, 8
Y variant	. . .	—	1, 3, 4

[a] Not all group antigens are listed.

nature of their group antigens. Variants X and Y have lost their type antigens and are distinguished by their different group antigens.

The O antigens of *S. flexneri* represent the structure of the O-specific side chains of repeating sugar units of the cell-wall lipopolysaccharide. The type antigens reflect the nature of the linkages of secondary α-glucosyl side-chains, which differ among the serotypes, and the group antigens reflect common sequences in the primary side-chains (Simmons 1971). The type antigens are determined by specific prophages and the serotype of a strain may be changed by lysogenization. The group antigens appear to be determined by genes on the bacterial chromosome.

Although serotype 6 strains are classified as *S. flexneri* because they share group antigens with other *S. flexneri* serotypes, they show differences that would justify their classification in a separate genus; their cell-wall lipopolysaccharide has a very different basal (core) structure from that common to the other serotypes of *S. flexneri* (Simmons 1971) and their gas-producing property and lack of fimbriae are also distinctive.

Group C. Fifteen different serotypes of *S. boydi* are recognized. Sharing of antigenic components among serotypes 1, 4 and 11, between serotypes 10 and 11 and between serotypes 9 and 13 makes the use of absorbed sera necessary for their identification.

Group D. S. sonnei is antigenically homo-

geneous, but the form-2 (R) variant is antigenically different from the form-1 (S) variant.

Cross-reactions between groups. There are close relationships between the O antigens of many shigella serotypes and those of serotypes in other *Shigella* species and certain serotypes of *Escherichia coli* and the Alkalescens-Dispar group of organisms. For example, the O antigen of *S. dysenteriae* serotype 1 is related to the O antigens of *E. coli* O-group 1 and A–D group 1; that of *S. dysenteriae* serotype 2 to those of *S. boydi* serotype 15 and *E. coli* O112a, O112c; that of *S. dysenteriae* serotype 3 to that of *E. coli* O124; those of *S. flexneri* serotypes 2, 3 and 4 to that of *E. coli* O13; that of *S. flexneri* serotype 6 to those of *S. boydi* serotype 5, *E. coli* O19a and A–D group 2; those of *S. boydi* serotypes 1 and 4 to that of A–D group 1 (also Boyd 1 to *E. coli* O2 and Boyd 4 to *E. coli* O53); and that of *S. boydi* serotype 6 to that of *S. sonnei* form-2 (R). The O antigen of *S. sonnei* form-1 (S) is unrelated to the O antigens of other enterobacteria, including *E. coli* O-groups 1–145, but is identical with that of a polar-flagellated oxidase-positive Gram-negative rod previously designated 'paracolon C27' and now classified as *Plesiomonas shigelloides* (Ch. 32). The relationships of some shigellae, particularly of *S. boydi* serotypes, with Alkalescens-Dispar organisms are of particular importance because the latter organisms resemble shigellae in being nonmotile, anaerogenic and, in many strains, nonlactose-fermenting. More recently the enteroinvasive *E. coli* (e.g. *E. coli* serotype O124 and others) have been noted to exhibit antigen sharing with, and biochemical similarity to, shigellae. A full range of biochemical tests and tests with carefully absorbed sera are necessary to differentiate these organisms from shigellae.

K antigens. Some strains in many shigella serotypes are inagglutinable by homologous O antisera because they possess a K antigen, which may or may not be visible as a capsule and which covers their O antigen. The K antigen in each O serotype appears to be specific for that serotype and different from those in other serotypes; exceptions are the related K antigens of *S. boydi* serotypes 10 and 11. In cases where the same O antigen is present in a shigella serotype and an

E. coli O-group, the K antigens of the organisms are also similar. Like the B variety of K antigen in *E. coli*, the K antigens of shigellae are heat-labile and the cultures possessing them can be rendered agglutinable by O antisera by heating at 100°C for 1 h.

Fimbrial antigens. Fimbriate strains in the different serotypes of *S. flexneri* form identical fimbrial antigens (Gillies & Duguid 1958). Richly fimbriated cultures obtained by prolonged or serial culture in broth, e.g. 3 passages at 37°C for 48 h periods, are agglutinable by antisera raised to fimbriate cultures of any serotype. Minor antigens are shared between the fimbriae of *S. flexneri* and those of *E. coli* and *Klebsiella aerogenes*, but there is no sharing with salmonella fimbriae. Antibodies to the shared coliflexneri fimbrial antigens are present in the sera of many persons and some unimmunized rabbits. Fimbriae may be removed from the bacteria by heating at 100°C for 30 min and washing by centrifugation, but misleading cross-agglutination reactions are best avoided by using only agar-grown non-fimbriate-phase cultures for the preparation of agglutinable bacterial suspensions and immunizing antigens.

Typing of strains for epidemiological purposes

Within groups A, B and C the determination of serotype has an epidemiological value and subdivision of the serotype is rarely attempted. The subdivision of *S. flexneri* by the method of phage typing distinguishes a number of different phage types within each serotype and a total of 123 phage types have been identified by Milch et al (1968). *S. sonnei* consists of only a single serotype and it is in this species that there is the greatest requirement for subdivision by some other typing method. Phage typing has been attempted in *S. sonnei*, but instability of type and the predominance of strains of one phage type did not encourage its use (Tee 1955); the method has, however, been found useful and reliable over a long period in Sweden where up to 21 out of about 100 recognized phage types were distinguished in a single year (Kallings et al 1968). In most centres, however, the method of colicin typing* is used for the subdivision of *S.*

sonnei strains because the method is simpler than that of phage typing and the typing characters are more stable.

Viability

Cultures retain their viability well, e.g. for many years on Dorset's egg. All types are killed by moist heat at 55°C in 1 h and fairly readily by strong disinfectants, e.g. by 1% phenol in 15 min. The bacilli tend to die within a few hours in faeces allowed to become acid due to the growth of commensal bacteria, but can survive for some days in faeces kept non-acid in buffered glycerol solution or preserved at 4°C. They mostly die within a few hours if dried, but under some circumstances survive for several (e.g. 5–20) days, for example in faeces dried on cloth, or on soiled lavatory seats and other fomites, in cool, damp, dark conditions. *S. sonnei* is more resistant and survives better in the environment than the other species of *Shigella*, a difference that may explain why Sonne dysentery has not been as readily controlled by improvements in community hygiene as the other types of bacillary dysentery.

Antibiotic sensitivity. Different strains of a serotype differ in their sensitivity to sulphonamide, chloramphenicol, tetracycline, streptomycin, neomycin and other antibiotics, and some show multiple resistance due to the acquisition of a transmissible resistance plasmid. Therapy with antibiotics tends to prolong the excretion of shigellae and is best avoided except in severe illnesses, when it should be based on the results of an antibiotic sensitivity test made on a culture isolated from the patient.

Laboratory diagnosis of shigella dysentery

Shigellae are rarely present in the body other than in the intestine and the laboratory diagnosis of bacillary dysentery can be made only by the isolation of a shigella from the faeces. A positive finding in a case of diarrhoeal illness is practically diagnostic of shigella dysentery. Shigellae may, however, be present in the faeces of

---

* Refer to *Methods* at end of this chapter.

chronic carriers and so may occasionally be found in the faeces of a patient with diarrhoea due to a cause other than shigellosis, but mistakes due to such a coincidence are likely to be rare.

Shigellosis is very infectious and in a study of Sonne dysentery in general practice, Thomas & Tillett (1973) reported that 30% of all contacts were infected.

Determination of the serotype of an isolate is necessary to confirm its identity as a shigella and has a further, epidemiological value in defining groups of patients infected with the same serotype from a common source. Phage typing or colicin typing of strains within a scrotype defines even more precisely the similarities and differences between strains from different sources.

Isolation of shigellae from faeces

Specimen collection and method of examination are identical to those described in Chapter 29 for the isolation of salmonellae. The scheme of investigation follows that set out in Chapter 29 for salmonellae, but there are some important points that apply specifically to thc diagnosis of shigella infections.

1. *Microscopy.* In severe shigellosis the diarrhoeal faeces may be blood stained and it is necessary to exclude amoebic dysentery. Makc a wet film of a suspension of the faeces in saline. This will show numerous erythrocytes and polymorphs and some macrophages. Care must be taken not to mistake the macrophages for the vegetative forms of *Entamoeba histolytica*, which have relatively smaller nuclei and are usually motile in warm fresh specimens (see Ch. 43).

2. *Plate cultures.* Recognition and further examination of pale (i.e. non-lactose fermenting) colonies on the primary DCA and MacConkey plates, or red colonies on XLD, is the most reliable method for isolating shigellae.

3. *Enrichment media.* Preliminary culture in liquid enrichment media, which greatly increases the isolation of salmonellac, is much less helpful in the diagnosis of shigellosis. Iveson (1973) reported that direct plating on DCA was superior to a variety of enrichment methods for

the isolation of shigellae. Price (1976) found that Selenite F broth, the only enrichment medium that may be of value, significantly increased the recovery of *S. sonnei* from fresh specimens, but not from faeces sent to the laboratory by post.

4. *Primary identifying biochemical tests.* These are the same as those for a suspect salmonella (see Table 29.3). The typical biochemical reactions of *Shigella* species are:

Urease   —
Motility   —
Indole   — or +
Gas from glucose   — (rarely +)
Glucose to acid   +
Lactose to acid   — (S. sonnei + on extended incubation for 2–8 days)
Sucrose to acid   —
Mannitol to acid   + (S. dysenteriae —)

5. *Slide agglutination.* If the organism is a possible shigella, carry out serological slide agglutination tests (with sera specified below*) on a suspension of about 10^{10} bacteria/ml saline in the following order:

a. *S. sonnei* (form 1 and 2) serum on one half of a slide; test the suspension without serum on the other half to exclude autoagglutinability in saline. If positive, test no further sera. If negative, test:

b. *S. flexneri* polyvalent. If positive, test in turn *S. flexneri* types 1–6, X, Y. If negative, test:

c. *S. boydi* polyvalent.

d. *S. dysenteriae* polyvalent.

e. If a shigella-like organism is not agglutinated by O antisera in the tests above suspect the presence of a masking K antigen. Make a suspension of the culture in 0.5 ml saline (about 10^9 bacteria/ml), heat at 100°C for 1 h, cool and re-test with the range of O antisera.

6. *Secondary identifying biochemical tests.* These differ from those for a suspect salmonella (see Table 29.4) in that melibiose peptone water is inoculated instead of ONPG medium. The typical reactions of shigellae are:

Growth on citrate   —
Lysine decarboxylase —
Salicin to acid   —
Melibiose to acid   — (S. flexneri and S. boydi may be +)

7. *Tube agglutination*. Tube tests should be done if there is any doubt about the results of the slide agglutination tests or if the biochemical reactions of the isolate are atypical. Reference laboratories that stock the full range of single factor sera use these to extend the presumptive identification made with polyvalent (composite) sera: positive slide agglutination results are confirmed by tube agglutination.

Prepare the antigen for tube agglutination tests by suspending the growth from a nutrient agar slope or plate either in saline containing 0.2% formaldehyde or in mercuric iodide solution* to a density of approximately 4×10^8 bacteria/ml. If the strain is thought to contain a masking K antigen suspend the growth in saline, heat at 100°C for 1 h, centrifuge and resuspend the deposit in formaldehyde-saline. Do not use broth cultures because *S. flexneri* when grown in broth may form fimbrial antigens which interfere with the test. Set up the test as for salmonella tube agglutinations (Ch. 29) with the dilution of antiserum in the first tube 1 in 10, i.e. a final serum dilution of 1 in 20 when an equal volume of antigen suspension has been added to it. Incubate the tubes at 50°C for 4 h and read the results. Identification depends on agglutination occurring at the stated titre of the serum.

Bacteria that may be confused with shigellae

Gram-negative bacilli of several other genera share many biochemical reactions with the shigellae and some share antigens with particular shigella serotypes. These bacteria may be mistaken for shigellae, particularly because some strains of shigella differ in one or more of their biochemical reactions from the pattern typical of their serotype.

(i) *Salmonella*. Anaerogenic and non-motile strains of salmonellae may be mistaken for shigellae if only a limited range of biochemical tests is carried out. The tests of most value for the differentiation of such salmonellae from shigellae are those for citrate utilization, H_2S production, decarboxylation of lysine and ornithine, and agglutination with polyvalent salmonella O and H sera (see Ch. 29).

(ii) *Alkalescens-Dispar group*. These non-motile

anaerogenic non-lactose-fermenting members of the genus *Escherichia* may mimic shigellae in the initial biochemical tests and some strains share antigens with particular shigella serotypes. They can be differentiated in tests of bacteria heated at 100°C for 0.5 to 1 h with absorbed type-specific sera for the different shigella and Alkalescens-Dispar serotypes (see Ch. 28). Some A–D strains are distinguished by their decarboxylation of lysine.

(iii) *Hafnia*. Hafnia organisms are non-lactose-fermenting bacilli that otherwise resemble organisms in the genus *Enterobacter*. They are distinguished from shigellae by their motility and their positive gluconate, malonate, ornithine-decarboxylase and citrate-utilization reactions (see Ch. 28). Some hafnia strains share O antigens with certain shigella serotypes, e.g. *S. flexneri* type 4a, and *S. boydi* type 11.

(iv) *Providencia*. These non-lactose-fermenting organisms are distinguished from shigellae by their motility and their ability to deaminate phenylalanine (see Ch. 28).

(v) *Plesiomonas shigelloides*. This Gram-negative bacillus, which shares antigens with *S. sonnei* form 1 and resembles it in being anaerogenic and non-lactose-fermenting, is distinguished by its motility, positive oxidase reaction, positive indole reaction and failure to ferment mannitol (see Ch. 32).

Tests for shigella antibody in patient's serum

Antibody production is irregular in bacillary dysentery and tests for it have no part to play in the diagnosis of the disease.

METHODS

Sera for the identification of shigellae

Typing sera should be purchased from commercial sources (e.g. Wellcome) because laborious absorptions are required to make sera sufficiently specific (Edwards & Ewing 1972). The set of antisera held should comprise at least those for *S. dysenteriae* (polyvalent for serotypes 1–10), *S. flexneri* (polyvalent for serotypes 1–6 and variants X and Y), *S. boydi* (polyvalent for serotypes 1–15) and *S. sonnei* (forms 1 and 2). Additional monovalent sera for the different *S. dysenteriae*, *S. flexneri* and *S. boydi* types should be kept if the laboratory examines many faecal specimens and is situated in an area where bacillary dysentery due to these serotypes is prevalent.

Mercuric iodide solution for use in tube agglutination tests

Mercuric iodide	0.1 g
Sodium chloride	0.45 g
Formalin (40% HCHO)	0.2 ml
Potassium iodide	0.4 g
Distilled water to	100 ml

Store at room temperature.

Colicin typing of S. sonnei

The majority of strains of *S. sonnei* are colicinogenic and different strains produce colicins active against different susceptible 'indicator' strains of *S. sonnei* and other enterobacteria. The ability of a strain to produce a particular colicin is a fairly stable character and strains are therefore typed by identifying the colicins they produce by a test of their ability to inhibit the growth of a set of selected indicator strains. The sensitivity of *S. sonnei* strains to colicins is a less stable character, so that a system of typing based on observations of the sensitivity of the strains to standard colicins is unsatisfactory.

The method of typing *S. sonnei* by observation of colicin production recommended by Gillies (1964) is based on that of Abbot & Shannon (1958).

Indicator strains. 15 strains are usually used, e.g. *S. sonnei* strains 2, 56, 17, 2M, 38, 56/56, 56/98, R1, R6; *S. schmitzi* M19; *S. sonnei* 2/7, 2/64, 2/15, R5; *E. coli* strain Row. These are the indicator strains no. 1–15, respectively, as used by Gillies & Brown (1966) and in the scheme shown in Table 30.3.

Medium. Tryptone soya (TS) agar (Oxoid) is reconstituted according to the manufacturer's instructions and horse blood is added to give a final concentration of 2.5% (v/v). It is poured in Petri dishes in a layer about 3–4 mm thick.

Method. The strain to be typed is inoculated as a single streak across the diameter of a TS agar plate and the plate is incubated at 35°C (*not* 37°C) for 24 h. The growth is removed with the edge of a glass slide and 2–3 ml CHCl₃ is put into the lid of the plate and the medium-containing dish, medium side downwards, is placed on top of it. After exposure to the chloroform vapour for a period of 10–15 min, sufficient for the killing of all bacteria, the chloroform is decanted and the plate exposed to air for a further 10–15 min. The indicator strains, which have been grown overnight in nutrient broth, are inoculated on to the plate in parallel

Table 30.3 Inhibition patterns given by 17 colicin-type strains of *S. sonnei* against 15 indicator strains.
Key: +, indicator strain inhibited by colicin-type strain; −, indicator strain not inhibited; v, variable reaction.

Indicator strain	Inhibition caused by producer strain colicin type																
	1a	1b	2	3	3a	4	5	6	7	8	9	10	11	12	13	14	15
1	+	+	−	+	+	+	+	−	−	+	+	+	−	+	−	+	+
2	+	+	+	+	+	+	+	+	−	−	+	+	−	+	+	+	−
3	+	+	+	+	+	+	+	−	+	+	+	+	−	−	+	+	+
4	−	−	−	−	−	v	v	−	−	−	−	−	−	−	−	v	+
5	−	−	−	+	+	+	+	−	−	+	v	+	−	+	−	+	+
6	+	+	−	+	+	−	+	+	−	−	+	+	−	+	+	+	−
7	+	+	−	+	+	−	+	+	−	−	+	+	−	+	+	+	−
8	−	−	−	+	+	+	+	−	−	+	+	+	−	+	−	+	+
9	−	+	+	+	+	+	+	+	−	−	+	+	−	+	+	+	−
10	+	+	−	+	−	+	−	−	−	−	+	−	−	−	−	−	−
11	−	−	−	+	+	+	+	−	−	−	−	−	−	−	−	+	+
12	−	−	−	+	+	+	+	−	−	−	−	−	−	−	−	−	−
13	−	−	−	+	+	+	+	−	−	+	+	+	−	+	−	+	+
14	−	−	−	+	+	−	−	−	−	−	−	−	−	−	−	−	+
15	+	+	+	+	+	+	+	+	−	+	+	+	+	+	+	+	+

streaks at right angles to the line of the original growth. The plate is then incubated at 37°C for 8–12 h and observed for any inhibition of the streak-growths of the indicator strains.

Interpretation of results. More than 17

colicin-types of *S. sonnei* are distinguished according to the different combinations of the indicator strains inhibited by their colicins (Table 30.3).

REFERENCES

Abbott J D, Shannon R 1958 A method of typing *Shigella sonnei* using colicine production as a marker. Journal of Clinical Pathology 11: 71–77

Association of Clinical Pathologists Broadsheet 60: January 1968 Identification of shigella. From Publishing Manager Journal of Clinical Pathology, BMA House, Tavistock Square, London WC1H 9JR

Duguid J P, Gillies R R 1957 Fimbriae and adhesive properties in dysentery bacilli. Journal of Pathology and Bacteriology 74: 397–411

Edwards P R, Ewing W H 1972 Identification of Enterobacteriaceae, 3rd edn. Burgess, Minneapolis

Gillies R R 1964 Colicine production as an epidemiological marker of *Shigella sonnei*. Journal of Hygiene, Cambridge 62: 1–9

Gillies R R, Brown D O 1966 A new colicine type (type 15) of *Shigella sonnei*. Journal of Hygiene, Cambridge 64: 305–308

Gillies R R, Duguid J P 1958 The fimbrial antigens of *Shigella flexneri*. Journal of Hygiene, Cambridge 56: 303–318

Iveson J B 1973 Enrichment procedures for the isolation of salmonella, arizona, edwardsiella and shigella from faeces. Journal of Hygiene, Cambridge 71: 349–361

Kallings L O, Lindberg A A, Sjoberg L 1968 Phage typing of *Shigella sonnei*. Archivum Immunologiae et Therapiae Experimentalis 16: 280–287

Kauffmann F 1969 The bacteriology of the Enterobacteriaceae, 2nd edn. Munksgaard, Copenhagen

Milch H, Laszlo G, Slopek S, Mulczyk M 1968 Lysotypes of *Shigella flexneri*. Archivum Immunologiae et Therapiae Experimentalis 16: 265–279

Price T H 1976 Isolation of *Shigella sonnei* by fluid media. Journal of Hygiene, Cambridge 77: 341–348

Simmons D A R 1971 Immunochemistry of *Shigella flexneri* O-antigens: a study of structural and genetic aspects of the biosynthesis of cell-surface antigens. Bacteriological Reviews 35: 117–148

Tee G H 1955 Bacteriophage typing of *Shigella sonnei* and its limitations in epidemiological investigations. Journal of Hygiene, Cambridge 53: 54–62

Thomas M E M, Tillett H E 1973 Dysentery in general practice: a study of cases and their contacts in Enfield and an epidemiological comparison with salmonellosis. Journal of Hygiene, Cambridge 71: 373–389

Wilson G S, Miles A A 1975 Principles of bacteriology, virology and immunity, 6th edn. Arnold, London. ch 28, p 908

Pseudomonas

Members of this large diffuse genus of aerobic, Gram-negative, non-fermentative bacilli are widely distributed in nature as saprophytes or as commensals and pathogens for man, plants, animals and insects. In medical microbiology, the genus can be divided into three groups. (i) Species which are opportunist pathogens in patients immunologically compromised by disease or treatment; in this group *P. aeruginosa* (*P. pyocyanea*) is pre-eminent, followed by *P. maltophilia, P. fluorescens, P. putida, P. cepacia* and *P. stutzeri*. (ii) Two species, *P. pseudomallei* and *P. mallei* (both previously known under the generic title *Loefflerella*) cause severe and often fatal infections in healthy persons or animals and must be processed with extreme caution in the laboratory. (iii) The remaining members of the genus, over 100 species, have little or no role as commensals or pathogens for man or animals. Some are plant pathogens or are associated with particular plant hosts, e.g. *P. tomato*; others are of interest because of particular physiological properties. Some species are of doubtful taxonomic status since the genus, in the past, has often served as a convenient dumping ground for taxonomically difficult organisms.

All pseudomonads are aerobic Gram-negative bacilli; motile (except *P. mallei*), with polar flagella, mono- or multi-trichous; oxidase positive (except *P. maltophilia*) and catalase positive. Typically the breakdown of carbohydrates is oxidative. Many species produce characteristic water-soluble pigments. The fluorescent pseudomonads produce fluorescein, a yellow fluorescent pigment, whilst *P. aeruginosa* strains, in addition to fluorescein, can also produce pyocyanin (blue), pyorubrin (red) and pyo-melanin (brown). Characteristics that distinguish the species of greatest importance in medicine are listed in Table 31.1.

PSEUDOMONAS AERUGINOSA

P. aeruginosa is a classic opportunist pathogen with innate resistance to many antibiotics and disinfectants. It flourishes as a saprophyte in warm moist situations in the human environment, including sinks, drains, respirators, humidifiers and disinfectant solutions. Isolation of *P. aeruginosa* from healthy carriers or environmental sites is significant only when there is a risk of transfer to compromised patients, e.g. by nurses' hands or respirators. Normally, human faecal carriage of *P. aeruginosa* is low, around 3%; however, carriage increases with the length of stay in hospital, reaching 30% after 3 weeks, and thus can present a distinct risk of endogenous infection.

In patients with no clinical evidence of infection isolation of *P. aeruginosa*, particularly in association with other resistant organisms such as *Candida*, can be a consequence of selection by antibiotic therapy and of little clinical relevance. Infections due to *P. aeruginosa* are seldom encountered in healthy adults but in the last two decades the organism has become increasingly recognized as the aetiological agent in a variety of serious infections in hospitalized patients with impaired immune defences (Neu 1983). Susceptibility to infection with *P. aeruginosa* may also be occupational, e.g. ear infections in divers, or recreational, e.g. whirlpool-associated (jacuzzi) rash (Vogt et al 1982).

Table 31.1 Distinguishing characters of clinically relevant *Pseudomonas* species.

Methods. Arginine dihydrolase after Thornley (1960) or in Stewart's AG medium (1972); maltose and lactose utilization in ammonium salt medium (Cowan 1974, p 109); accumulation of poly β-hydroxybutyrate after Stanier et al (1966); other tests included in API strips or Flow N/F system.

Note. All species motile except *P. mallei*; all species oxidase positive except most strains of *P. maltophilia* and *P. mallei*.

Key: . . ., no result given

	Pyocyanin	Fluorescein	Growth at 42°C	Arginine dihydrolase	Lysine decarboxylase	Gelatinase	Aesculin hydrolysis	Lactose (oxidative)	Maltose (oxidative)	Poly-β- hydroxybutyrate	NO$_3$ reduction to N$_2$
P. aeruginosa	+	+	+	+	–	+	–	–	–	–	+
P. fluorescens	–	+	–	+	–	+	–	–	–	–	–
P. putida	–	+	–	+	–	–	–	–	–	–	–
P. maltophilia	–	–	+	–	+	+	+	–	+	–	–
P. stutzeri	–	–	+	–	–	–	–	–	+	–	+
P. cepacia	–	–	+	–	+	+	+	+	+	+	–
P. pseudomallei	–	–	+	+	–	+	+	+	+	+	+
P. mallei	–	–	+	+	–	+	. . .	. . .	+/–	+	+

Despite the emphasis on caution in assessing the clinical significance of *P. aeruginosa*, there are undoubtedly occasions when *P. aeruginosa* causes serious infection. Panophthalmitis can result in partial blindness or loss of an eye. Acute otitis media in the saturation conditions necessary for deep water diving is painful and socially debilitating. Endocarditis and septicaemia are relatively rare but carry a high mortality rate, exceeding 70% in patients compromised by severe burns, cancer or drug addiction. Perhaps the most significant and troublesome pathogenic role for *P. aeruginosa* at the present time is in the chronic debilitating respiratory infections due to mucoid strains that are now a major cause of death in patients with cystic fibrosis. Quantitative estimates of the number of *P. aeruginosa* present in these respiratory infections can be used to indicate the progression from early colonization to infection (10^7 orgs/ml), and to follow the results of antibiotic treatment.

Assessment of the significance of a particular episode or outbreak of infection and the most appropriate management procedures require knowledge and appreciation of both the organism and the host. This can best be achieved by consultations between microbiologist and clinician which take account of the patient's clinical status, the factors responsible for susceptibility to the infection and any virulence factor exhibited by the particular strain of *P. aeruginosa*. Putative virulence factors, known to be produced in vitro and in vivo, include the most active factor, toxin A, but also elastase and other proteases that are of importance in corneal infection and the alginate-like polysaccharide produced by mucoid strains from patients with cystic fibrosis. Typing methods are important in epidemiological studies to determine sources of infection and methods of spread.

Morphology and staining

Gram-negative, non-sporing rods; motile, usually with a single polar flagellum. Fimbriae may be present and are usually polar and non-haemagglutinating. Some *P. aeruginosa*, notably from respiratory tract infections in patients with cystic fibrosis, produce large amounts of alginate, an exopolysaccharide consisting of mannuronic and guluronic acids which gives rise to strikingly mucoid colonies. When such strains are examined in vitro with the India ink technique the exopolysaccharide may appear as a discrete capsule but usually as a loosely bound extracellular matrix. It should be emphasized that the alginate produced by these mucoid colonial forms of *P. aeruginosa* is distinct from pseudomonas slime, a heterogeneous mixture of hexoses which is produced by all strains of the species on prolonged incubation in media with high carbon, low nitrogen content.

Cultural characters

Grows readily on simple media. *P. aeruginosa*, like other members of the genus, is extremely adaptable in nutritional terms and can utilize a very wide range of organic substrates as sources of C and N. Cultures produce a characteristic sweet, musty smell of aminoacetophenone. Strict aerobe, although NO_3 can be used as an electron acceptor to permit anaerobic growth. Colonies are usually very small or extremely flat if growth occurs at all on anaerobic plates. Temperature range 5–42°C, optimum 37°C; *P. aeruginosa*, unlike most other *Pseudomonas* species, will grow in serial subculture at 42°C. Optimum pH 7.4–7.6.

After aerobic incubation on nutrient agar for 24 h at 37°C six distinct colonial types of *P. aeruginosa* are encountered (Phillips 1969). Type 1 is the most common and easily recognized; the colonies are large, low convex, rough in appearance and often oval with the long axis in the line of the inoculum streak; sometimes they are surrounded by a thin serrated 'skirt' of growth. Type 2 colonies are small, domed and smooth in appearance and described as coliform-like. Colony types 3 and 4 are also small and appear rough and rugose respectively. The mucoid alginate-producing type 5 colony is very striking; the large amounts of exopolysaccharide produced during overnight incubation often result in merging colonial growth, and on further incubation the copious exopolysaccharide may drip on to the lid of the inverted Petri dish. The dwarf colony type 6 is the smallest colony form of *P. aeruginosa*; dwarfs are usually variants of the mucoid colonial form and may appear slightly mucoid.

Colonial dissociation from one colony type to another is frequently observed both on subculture and in primary diagnostic plates and does not necessarily indicate the presence of more than one strain of the species. Dissociation is most frequently observed between colony types 1 and 2 and these forms, together with the dwarf type 6, are often seen as non-mucoid revertants of the mucoid type 5 form. Attempts have been made to associate particular colonial types with environmental or infectious loci. The only generally accepted associations, however, are the frequent isolation of coliform type 2 forms from environmental sources and the very characteristic isolation of mucoid type 5 strains in the course of chronic respiratory infections in patients with cystic fibrosis.

Many strains exhibit the phenomenon known as iridescence, which is observed as a moth-eaten type of colonial lysis with a metallic sheen. Although the phenomenon resembles lysis due to bacteriophage it actually has no association with phage activity. Colonies on blood agar may be surrounded by a zone of haemolysis. On MacConkey agar, *P. aeruginosa* colonies are pale, i.e. non-lactose-fermenters, and, as on blood agar, the characteristic pigments are often poorly observed.

Production of pigments

Demonstration of the presence of the blue pigment pyocyanin is absolute confirmation of a strain as *P. aeruginosa* and thus the major diagnostic test. Pigment-enhancing media should be used (see below). The yellow pigment fluorescein is also produced by many strains, giving the characteristic blue-green appearance of infected pus or cultures. Pyocyanin, fluorescein and the more rarely observed pyomelanin and pyorubrin are easily identified on nutrient or sensitivity test agars, particularly after prolonged incubation.

Biochemical reactions

In general, *P. aeruginosa* appears inert in the usual tests (including API 20E reactions) used for the fermentative Gram-negative bacilli, e.g. indole and H_2S are not produced, Voges-Proskauer and methyl red reactions are negative. Tests that may be used to characterize *P. aeruginosa*, particularly when pyocyanin production is absent or doubtful, are shown in Table 31.1.

Sensitivity to chemical and physical agents

P. aeruginosa survives well in wet environments but is not very resistant to drying and is easily killed by heat. *P. aeruginosa* has exceptional resistance to chemical antibacterials. Consequently the species is a very significant contaminant of pharmaceuticals and cosmetics and its presence in such products must be avoided to prevent inactivation of the medicaments as well as direct damage to the user. In the preservation of ophthalmic solutions, phenylethanol is recommended for use in combination with a suitable broad spectrum antibacterial such as benzalkonium chloride, or chlorocresol, or to a lesser extent chlorhexidine. Other effective combinations include EDTA-benzalkonium and EDTA-chlorocresol.

To reduce surface contamination due to *P. aeruginosa* on instruments and in hospital sinks and drains, care is required in the choice and use of disinfectants. *P. aeruginosa* is resistant to many disinfectants including quaternary ammonium compounds; indeed Dettol and cetrimide can be incorporated in selective media for isolation of pseudomonads. Cidex (a 2% aqueous alkaline solution of glutaraldehyde) is suitably active against *P. aeruginosa* but great care must be taken to avoid accidental over-dilution and to follow the manufacturer's instructions for the preparation and replacement of in-use dilutions.

Antibiotic sensitivity and resistance

P. aeruginosa has high intrinsic resistance to many antibiotics at levels attainable in body tissues. Those antibiotics likely to be most effective are gentamicin, tobramycin and amikacin, carbenicillin and ticarcillin, and the newer ureido-penicillins, azlocillin and piperacillin. Most first and second generation cephalosporins are poorly active against *P. aeruginosa* but some of the more recent derivatives, e.g. cefsulodin and ceftazidime, may prove useful non-toxic alternatives to the aminoglycosides. Current clinical trials with ciprofloxacin, a new 4-quinolone derivative, suggest that it may provide a major advance as the first highly active anti-pseudomonal effective by oral administration.

Despite the significant improvements in the anti-pseudomonal activity of these antibiotics, larger than normal doses are necessary in severe infections. A further problem with *P. aeruginosa* is that many strains do not respond clinically although apparently sensitive to the antibiotic in vitro. With aminoglycosides this is partly explained by tissue antagonism, the effect of ionized divalent cations and poor entry into tissues. The exopolysaccharide produced by mucoid *P. aeruginosa* gels rapidly in the presence of physiological levels of divalent cations; thus with mucoid *P. aeruginosa* the phenomenon may be partly explained by aggregation of bacteria in vivo as microcolonies embedded within a gelled ionized matrix.

Acquired additional resistance superimposed on natural resistance is also a problem. Plasmid mediated resistance involving modifying enzymes is particularly associated with topical antibiotic use and with sites, e.g. bladder, where high levels of antibiotic are achieved. An additional form of acquired resistance does not involve modifying enzymes but is apparently the result of reduced permeability associated with a change in outer membrane proteins.

Although *P. aeruginosa* is often initially recognized as an organism that appears resistant to commonly used antibiotic disks on primary culture plates, it should be appreciated that this is not always a reliable screening test. A considerable percentage of respiratory tract isolates express a 'hypersensitive' mutation which results in a zone of inhibition with such unlikely anti-pseudomonal antibiotics as ampicillin, trimethoprim, nalidixic acid and cefuroxime, and a larger than normal zone of inhibition with carbenicillin. The MIC values of carbenicillin for hypersensitive *P. aeruginosa* are less than 1 μg/ml, compared with a normal range of 20–60 μg/ml. Hypersensitivity does not include the aminoglycosides and the phenomenon is almost exclusively observed in *P. aeruginosa* strains isolated from chronic respiratory infections (Irvin et al 1981; Fyfe & Govan 1984).

Antigenic characters

17 distinct group-specific heat-stable O antigens and at least 2 heat-labile H antigens are recognized on the basis of standard slide agglutination procedures (Liu et al 1983). Serological characterization is primarily used as an epidemiological typing technique rather than for diagnostic confirmation of species identity.

Bacteriocin production

The bacteriocins of *P. aeruginosa* are called aeruginocins, or more usually *pyocins* after the former species nomenclature, *P. pyocyanea*. Pyocinogeny, the ability to produce pyocins, is found in over 90% of *P. aeruginosa* strains. Four distinct types of pyocin are recognized. R pyocins resemble the tails of contractile phages (Ishii et al 1965; Govan 1974a,b), whilst morphologically distinct rod-shaped, flexuous F pyocins resemble the tails of non-contractile phages (Takeya et al 1969; Govan 1974b). Low molecular weight S pyocins (*c.* 10^5 daltons) also occur; two categories have been described, trypsin-sensitive (Ito et al 1970) and trypsin-resistant (Govan 1978). Within each category of pyocin a variety of individual pyocins can be recognized on the basis of their spectrum of activity against different strains of *P. aeruginosa*. Strains are immune to their own pyocin, but sensitive cells are killed following attachment of pyocin to specific receptors on the cell surface. Individual strains of *P. aeruginosa* may produce more than one category of pyocin and also possess receptors for several different pyocins (Govan 1974b, 1978). Characterization of bacteriocin production is used in epidemiological typing of *P. aeruginosa* strains.

Laboratory diagnosis of P. aeruginosa infection

P. aeruginosa grows well on all normal laboratory media but specific isolation of the organism from environmental sites or from human, animal or plant sources is best carried out on a medium which contains a selective agent and also constituents to enhance pigment production. Most selective media depend upon the intrinsic resistance of the species to various antibacterial agents, e.g. nalidixic acid, and the organism's ability to withstand and even flourish in the use-dilution of common hospital disinfectants, e.g. Dettol, cetrimide. In our experience one of the most satisfactory media is Pseudomonas Isolation Agar (PIA; Difco) which contains pigment-enhancing components and the selective agent irgasan. An alternative commercially produced selective medium is the cetrimide-containing Pseudosel Agar (BBL); in our experience this has proved too inhibitory and gives a significantly lower yield than PIA. For isolation of *P. aeruginosa* from clinical sources a selective medium, e.g. PIA, can be used alone as the primary medium but superior isolation rates, particularly from nose, throat and faeces, have been reported with the use of an acetamide enrichment broth (Kelly et al 1983).*

Most strains of *P. aeruginosa* are easily recognized on conventional laboratory media by their typical colonial appearance, the characteristic sweet musty odour and the distinctive blue-green appearance produced in the medium by the pigments fluorescein and pyocyanin. In cases when colonies that might be pseudomonas are seen in primary culture, an oxidase test should be done; a positive result is then suggestive of their identity.

When primary culture has been on diagnostic media not conducive to pigment production, e.g. MacConkey medium, colonies may subsequently be recognized as *P. aeruginosa* when antibiotic sensitivity testing is carried out; pigment production is enhanced on sensitivity test agars. The possible presence of *P. aeruginosa* may also be indicated by characteristic resistance to most of the commonly used antibiotics. However, caution should be exercised to recognize hypersensitive variants of *P. aeruginosa* that may be encountered in the respiratory tract (see above).

Demonstration that the organism produces the pigment pyocyanin confirms the identity of a pseudomonad as *P. aeruginosa**. However, a small proportion of strains, usually less than 10%, do not produce any pigment on first isolation, or lose the property on repeated subculture, and thus require further confirmation of identity, e.g. by the tests shown in Table 31.1. The oxidase test (Kovacs 1956), the oxidation-fermentation test (Hugh & Leifson 1953) and the arginine dihydrolase test are of great value in distinguishing non-pigment-producing *P. aeruginosa* and other pseudomonads from *Aeromonas*, *Achromobacter* and Enterobacteriaceae. In such cases a positive diagnosis is aided by noting such reactions as motility, growth in serial subculture at 42°C but not 4°C and ability to reduce nitrate to nitrogen gas. Failure to exhibit any one of these characteristics should cast doubt that the strain is *P. aeruginosa*.

In addition, because of the high percentage of strains that are typable with the serotyping and pyocin typing systems (see below), organisms that do not produce pyocyanin and that neither agglutinate with any of the 17 somatic sera nor produce detectable pyocin activity should be examined carefully and identified as *P. aeruginosa* only if the species characteristics outlined in Table 31.1 are satisfied.

Discriminatory tests have been incorporated in several schemes for the identification of *P. aeruginosa*. A useful single tube composite medium for the characterization of *P. aeruginosa* and other clinically relevant pseudomonads was described by Stewart (1972)*; another suitable scheme is that described by King & Phillips (1978). The rapid (4 h) identification test specific for *P. aeruginosa* described by Davis et al (1983) is based on ability to produce turbid growth in the presence of 50 μg/ml 9-chloro-9-(4-diethylaminophenyl)-10-phenylacridan (C-390; Norwich-Eaton). Alternatively, commercially produced multisystems are now available for the accurate identification of pseudomonads, e.g. the N/F two tube screen (Flow) or the more multipurpose API 20E test strip; recommendations regarding the use of multisystems are given below in the section dealing with the identification of pseudomonads other than *P. aeruginosa*.

* Refer to *Methods* at end of this chapter.

Epidemiological typing methods for Pseudomonas aeruginosa

Several biological characters have been assessed for typing purposes, including colonial morphology, pigment production, antibiograms and phage sensitivity; the two most reliable and generally accepted methods are serotyping and bacteriocin typing.

Serotyping. Identification of group-specific heat-stable lipopolysaccharide antigens by agglutination forms the basis of O serotyping procedures. Several systems have been described and their use has been reviewed (Lanyi & Bergan 1978; Brokopp & Farmer 1979; Pitt 1980; Pitt 1988). The major disadvantage of serotyping is its limited discriminating power; only nine serotypes account for over 90% of isolates (Brokopp et al 1977).

Serotyping based on H antigens is also possible. Used alone, H typing is not satisfactory for routine use as nearly 50% of strains share the same H antigen; however, in combination with O grouping it has proved useful for subdividing common O groups (Pitt 1981). Unfortunately the procedures for H antigen typing, namely immunofluorescence, immobilization or agglutination with sera prepared against purified flagella, are outwith the scope of many laboratories.

Although more than 90% of clinical strains can be typed by O serotyping, this technique is unsatisfactory for typing mucoid strains of *P. aeruginosa* since O antigens are masked. It is also unsuitable for comparisons of colonial dissociants, because antigenic changes are observed within a single culture, and for typing polyagglutinable *P. aeruginosa*, i.e. strains that are agglutinated by more than one serum in patterns that are outside the established cross-reactions of the serotype strains. Polyagglutinable and mucoid strains of *P. aeruginosa* form less than 5% of general isolates but are frequently observed in patients with cystic fibrosis.

Bacteriocin typing. Typing of *P. aeruginosa* based on pyocin production is the most popular method for typing *P. aeruginosa* in the hospital laboratory (Pitt 1980). Pyocin typing offers greater discriminating power than serotyping whilst retaining simplicity and reliability. A number of methods have been described but comparative experience (Lanyi & Bergan 1978; Brokopp & Farmer 1979) has indicated that the best method is the standard technique described by Govan & Gillies (1969) as amended by Govan (1978). Subsequently, Govan and colleagues have made further improvements to this method and the revised technique* (Fyfe et al 1984) is now recommended; it is less time-consuming and offers other advantages, particularly in strain discrimination and in typing mucoid strains.

Both serotyping and pyocin typing can contribute significantly to epidemiological studies and in the author's laboratory each system is used when appropriate. Serotyping provides a rapid screening procedure to detect whether antigenic differences are present in strains from an epidemic situation, whilst within 24 h the greater discriminating power of pyocin typing provides a more confident basis for epidemiological interpretations. Pyocin typing is the more suitable method for typing mucoid *P. aeruginosa* or polyagglutinable strains, and for comparisons of colonial disssociants.

In the UK the reference centre for serotyping and phage typing is maintained by Dr T. L. Pitt, at the Central Public Health Laboratory, Colindale, London NW9 5HT; for pyocin typing, indicator strains and information can be obtained from Dr J. R. W. Govan, Department of Bacteriology, University of Edinburgh Medical School, Teviot Place, Edinburgh EH8 9AG.

PSEUDOMONAS MALLEI AND P. PSEUDOMALLEI

Human laboratory-acquired infection with *P. mallei* and *P. pseudomallei* is a hazard and few other organisms are so dangerous to work with (Schlech et al 1981). Both species were categorized by the Howie Report of 1978 as category A pathogens; they are now categorized in containment category 3 and require to be handled with the greatest care and under strict and designated isolation conditions (see Ch. 15).

Pseudomonas mallei

This organism, which has also been known as *Malleomyces mallei* and *Loefflerella mallei*, causes equine glanders, a disease characterized by the formation of nasal abscesses and cutaneous and lymphatic nodules ('farcy buds') and abscesses. Human disease may take the form of an acute fulminant febrile illness or a chronic indolent infection producing abscesses in the respiratory tract or skin. It is not common and almost totally restricted to persons handling horses in those countries from which the disease has not been eradicated, principally in Asia and South America. In its morphology and biochemical reactions *P. mallei* closely resembles *P. pseudomallei* (see Table 31.1) but shows a number of negative differences; it is non-motile, has a narrower range of carbon and energy sources, does not grow on MacConkey medium and is usually oxidase negative. It has been suggested by Redfearn et al (1966) that the two species share a common ancestor, and that the negative differences of *P. mallei* are the result of functional and structural loss-adaptation to a strictly parasitic mode of existence.

Guinea-pigs are susceptible. Intraperitoneal injection of small amounts of a pure culture causes testicular swelling in 2–3 days due to bacillary invasion of the tunica vaginalis, which increases up to the tenth day. The 'Strauss reaction' may be followed by death of the animal.

Pseudomonas pseudomallei

P. pseudomallei (*Malleomyces pseudomallei*, *Loefflerella pseudomallei*) is the causal agent of melioidosis, a disease of rodents. Man is seldom infected and then usually by eating food contaminated with infected rodent excreta or by direct contact with infected animals. Originally the disease was restricted to SE Asia, but it became of increased importance in the USA as a result of military personnel returning from the Vietnam war. Exacerbations of melioidosis can occur a considerable time after exposure (the disease has been referred to as the Vietnam time bomb) and thus laboratory differentiation from other pseudomonads is important in patients returning from endemic areas. Clinically, the human disease, which is difficult to treat and often fatal, may be a chronic indolent infection resembling glanders (see *P. mallei*) with the formation of caseous nodules, round embolic foci and multiple abscesses in the skin, bone and internal organs, or it may present as a fulminating septicaemia.

On nutrient agar *P. pseudomallei* produces unusual and distinctive rough 'corrugated' colonies (Lapage et al 1968). Biochemically *P. pseudomallei* broadly resembles other pseudomonads but does not produce a definite pigment on nutrient agar and cultures do not fluoresce on media designed to enhance fluorescein production. Like *P. aeruginosa* it grows well at 42°C. Tests for differentiation are shown in Table 31.1.

It should be noted that *P. stutzeri* has a colonial appearance similar to that of *P. pseudomallei* and the two species can be confused as they give similar results in biochemical tests. Both species are motile but *P. stutzeri* has a single polar flagellum whilst *P. pseudomallei* has several polar flagella. Useful differential tests, positive for *P. pseudomallei* but negative for *P. stutzeri*, include gelatin liquefaction, arginine dihydrolase and intracellular accumulation of poly-β-hydroxybutyrate.

Strains of *P. pseudomallei* contain common agglutinating components that are also present in strains of *P. mallei*. Suspect cultures can be identified serologically by agglutination tests, employing rapid slide or tube agglutination techniques. Antisera for these tests and for fluorescent antibody studies, which should be used to confirm the identification of all *P. pseudomallei* isolates, are available from Difco. Recently, Ismail et al (1987) have described a very sensitive method for detecting *P. pseudomallei* exotoxin by an ELISA test based on a monoclonal antitoxin; this test is potentially useful in research and diagnosis of melioidosis.

OTHER PSEUDOMONAS SPECIES

A number of other species, principally *P. maltophilia (Xanthomonas maltophilia), P. putida, P. stutzeri, P. fluorescens* and *P. cepacia*, are capable of causing opportunist infection in immunologically compromised patients (Gilardi 1972). It should be appreciated that the genus *Pseudomonas* contains an uncomfortably large and heterogeneous group of bacteria. The taxonomic status of many of the 171 species named in Bergey's Manual (1984) is debatable. A dogmatic approach to species identification is usually unnecessary in clinical microbiology but there are circumstances when accurate species identification within the pseudomonads is desirable. Thus *P. cepacia* was originally found as a plant pathogen causing soft rot in onions but is now isolated with increasing frequency from human infections. It causes a distinctive form of trench foot in troops training in swamps (Taplin et al 1971), and in the last 10 years has been implicated in acute and fatal exacerbations of respiratory infection in patients with cystic fibrosis. At present, the problem seems restricted to a few North American clinics treating such patients and it remains to be determined whether *P. cepacia* will emerge as a major pathogen in cystic fibrosis generally or whether the present situation is the result of cross-infection within particular clinics. Previously, epidemiological investigations and judgments have been hampered by a lack of suitable typing methods for *P. cepacia*. The recent development and validation of a bacteriocin typing system for *P. cepacia* (Govan & Harris 1985), based on the technique used successfully for pyocin typing of *P. aeruginosa*, provides a useful aid for future epidemiological studies.

A further reason for careful identification of a pseudomonad arises because of the risk of laboratory-acquired melioidosis. A particularly instructive episode was described by Schlech et al (1981). In this case a technician acquired melioidosis while involved in the isolation of aminoglycoside-degrading enzymes from an organism identified as *P. cepacia* in a local hospital. Further enquiries revealed that the patient from whom the organism had been isolated had been treated for a febrile illness in Vietnam 10 years previously. The patient had died from his undiagnosed illness, and the organism was subsequently identified as *P. pseudomallei*.

Laboratory identification of other Pseudomonas species

Gram-negative non-glucose-fermenting bacilli often grow slowly with optimum growth temperatures less than 37°C and are relatively inert biochemically. Thus, traditional identification schemes are time consuming, requiring prolonged incubation with special media in order to perform the tests listed in Table 31.1.

Within the last decade, however, several commercial manual and automated microsystems have become available, including the API 20E and 20NE test strips, the N/F system (Flow), and the Oxi/Ferm Tube (Roche). No two systems use the same range of tests and none offers ideal identification of all clinically relevant pseudomonads.

All four systems provide excellent identification of *P. aeruginosa*, including non-pigment-producing strains, but accuracy is reduced to 70–95% with other pseudomonads. Comparison of reports in the literature is made difficult by the different collections of strains tested, with occasional reliance on a single species representative. In general, the widely used API 20E system, designed predominantly for the Enterobacteriaceae offers good identification of *P. aeruginosa* and *P. maltophilia* but is less accurate for the other species included in the manufacturer's index, *P. fluorescens*, *P. putida*, *P. cepacia* and *P. putrefaciens*. Koestenblatt et al (1982) found the N/F system, developed specifically for non-fermenters, to be more accurate than the Oxi/Ferm system.

It is the author's experience that the N/F system and the more recently introduced API 20NE are the most appropriate systems presently available for identification of the pseudomonads. The N/F system consists of a two tube N/F screen and a plate (Uni-N/F-Tek) containing a number of sealed wells. The two tube screen allows determination of five reactions; 42°C growth tolerance, pyocyanin production, fluorescent pigments, glucose oxidation and N_2 production. The plate, constructed in the shape of a wheel containing independently sealed wells, allows determination of 13 different biochemical parameters. The N/F system shows good ability to identify individual species, including *P. aeruginosa*, *P. pseudomallei*, *P. fluorescens* (grouped with *P. putida*), *P. maltophilia*, *P. cepacia* and 12 other less common species. The API 20NE system is similar in format to the well known API 20E strips but with tests designed for identification of non-fermenting Gram-negative bacilli; these are not identical to those in the N/F system. In the author's laboratory a comparative investigation of both systems for identification of over 200 pseudomonads suggested that neither system has a clear advantage, although in practice the N/F system was found to be easier to set up and interpret.

Ultimately, the choice of approach, be it manual or automatic, composite multitest system or conventional individual tests, depends upon the facilities and finances available and the degree of accuracy required by clinical circumstances. A compromise, but realistic, approach suitable for the average diagnostic laboratory would be to identify *P. aeruginosa* conventionally by production of pyocyanin and to use the multipurpose API 20E system for confident identification of *P. maltophilia* and non-pigment-producing *P. aeruginosa*. Strains presumptively identified as belonging to other pseudomonas species are then best examined by a system specifically designed for non-fermenters, e.g. the N/F wheel or the API 20NE system, or alternatively sent to a reference laboratory. These commercial systems are relatively expensive. If large collections of strains are to be screened we have found that the single tube composite arginine glucose (AG) medium* (Stewart 1972) gives excellent discrimination between the *P. aeruginosa/P. fluorescens/P. putida* group, *P. maltophilia*, *P. stutzeri* and *P. cepacia*.

METHODS

Pseudomonas enrichment broth (Kelly et al 1983)

NaCl	5 g
MgSO$_4$	0.2 g
NH$_4$H$_2$PO$_4$	1 g
K$_2$HPO$_4$	1 g
Acetamide, CH$_3$CONH$_2$	20 g
Distilled water	1 litre

Dissolve the acetamide and other ingredients in the distilled water and autoclave at 121°C for 10 min. Incubate swabs or specimens in this medium for 18 h at 37°C and then subculture to Pseudomonas Isolation Agar (PIA; Difco).

Stewart's arginine glucose (AG) medium (Stewart 1972)

Indicator mixture. This contains 0.03 g cresol red (BDH) and 0.02 g bromothymol blue (BDH), dissolved together with heating in 100 ml of 0.01 mol/litre NaOH. Filter the solution after cooling.

Medium

Nutrient broth granules, (Oxoid No. 2)	2 g
L-arginine HCl	1 g
Glucose	10 g
Indicator mixture	60 ml
Agar No. 3 (Oxoid)	8 g
Distilled water	1 litre

Dissolve the ingredients in the water; the pH should be 7.4 before autoclaving. Distribute the melted medium in 9 ml amounts in test tubes (152 × 16 mm) closed with loose metal or plastic caps. After autoclaving at 121°C for 10 min allow the medium to gel with a slope 4 cm long and a butt *c.* 4 cm deep.

Inoculation of AG medium. With a straight wire remove a fleck of culture from nutrient agar

Table 31.2 Reactions produced by *Pseudomonas* species and Enterobacteria in Stewart's Arginine Glucose medium after 24–72 h at 30°C.
Key: Y, yellow (acid production); G, green (pH unaltered); B, blue (slight alkali production); V, violet (strong alkali production).

Organism	Colour of	
	Slope	Butt
P. aeruginosa *P. putida* *P. fluorescens*	Y	V
P. maltophilia *P. stutzeri*	B	G
P. cepacia	Y	G
Enterobacteria[a]	Y	Y + gas

[a] *Escherichia coli*, *Klebsiella aerogenes*, *Salmonella* spp., *Proteus vulgaris*, *Serratia marcescens*.

plates incubated for 24–48 h at 30°C. Stab this inoculum 4 or 5 times to the foot of the tube of AG medium and then streak the slope well with the tip of the wire. Incubate the cultures at 30°C for 24–72 h. Use the reaction patterns shown in Table 31.2 to identify the organisms.

Production and identification of pseudomonas pigments

Pyocyanin and fluorescein

Most pigment-enhancing media are based on Media A and B described by King et al (1954), for production of the major pigments pyocyanin and fluorescein respectively. Most strains of *P. aeruginosa* produce both pigments and the media were developed to enhance production of one pigment whilst suppressing the other.

Various commercial forms of these media are available, e.g. Medium P (Difco) which enhances production of pyocyanin. Pseudomonas Isolation Agar (PIA; Difco) combines the pyocyanin-enhancing properties of Medium P with the selective agent irgasan (2,4,4 trichloro-2-hydroxyphenylether) and is recommended for demonstration of pyocyanin production in normal practice. Production of fluorescein is best achieved by the use of Medium F (Difco) or of the original King's Medium B. The recipes for the Difco media P, F and PIA, are given below.

Pyocyanin is blue in colour and non-fluorescent; it is formed best in peptone media and is soluble in both chloroform and water. In liquid cultures of *P. aeruginosa* grown without agitation a pyocyanin-containing layer can often be observed in the upper part of the broth at the air/liquid interface. Fluorescein is yellow and fluorescent; it is formed only in the presence of phosphate and is soluble in water but not in chloroform. When pyocyanin is produced in small amounts, or its presence is obscured by other pigments, it can be more readily observed by shaking a few millilitres of chloroform in a broth culture or on an agar slope culture; on standing, pyocyanin (but not fluorescein) will appear in the $CHCl_3$ once the phases have separated out. Fluorescein is best observed by use of a suitable dark chamber, with the cultures illuminated with UV light.

Pyorubrin and pyomelanin

A small percentage of strains of *P. aeruginosa* also produce the red pigment pyorubrin or the brown pyomelanin. Caution should be exercised in the identification of these pigments since acidification of pyocyanin produces a red colour and prolonged exposure of pyocyanin to air produces a brownish oxidation product. Identification of pyorubrin and pyomelanin is aided by the use of specific culture media. Growth in 1% DL-glutamate allows pyorubrin but not pyomelanin production. Davis & Mingioli's minimal salts medium supplemented with 1% tyrosine enhances pyomelanin production but not pyorubrin. Alternatively, Furunculosis Agar (tryptone, 10 g; yeast extract, 5 g; L-tyrosine, 1 g; NaCl, 2.5 g; agar, 15 g/ litre) can also be used to detect pyomelanin production (Ogunnariwo & Hamilton-Miller 1975).

Difco P and F media

Difco medium P

Bacto peptone	20 g
Magnesium chloride	1.4 g
Potassium sulphate	10 g
Bacto agar	15 g
Distilled water	980 ml

Difco medium F

Bacto tryptone	10 g
Bacto proteose peptone No. 3	10 g
Dipotassium phosphate	1.5 g
Magnesium sulphate	1.5 g
Bacto agar	15 g
Distilled water	980 ml

Preparation of media

Dissolve either medium (46.4 g Medium P or 38 g Medium F) in the water and add 20 ml Bacto glycerol. Heat to boiling to dissolve the medium completely. Autoclave for 15 min at 121°C.

Pseudomonas isolation agar (PIA)

Bacto peptone	20 g
Magnesium chloride	1.4 g

Potassium sulphate	10 g
Irgasan, 2,4,4 trichloro-2-hydroxy phenylether	0.025 g
Bacto agar	13.6 g
Distilled water	980 ml

Method. Dissolve 45 g medium in the water and add 20 ml Bacto glycerol. Heat to boiling to dissolve the medium completely. Autoclave for 15 min at 121°C. Final pH 7.0 ± 0.2 at 25°C.

Pyocin typing

The standard procedure (Govan 1978) used a cross-streaking technique in which pyocin production by the test strain was detected by inhibitory activity against a standard set of 13 indicator strains of *P. aeruginosa*. The main disadvantages of the technique are the 72 h period required for a result, the need to remove producer strain growth, the poor recognition of S pyocin activity and the difficulty of typing mucoid strains of *P. aeruginosa*. These problems have been overcome by the development of a revised spotting procedure (Fyfe et al 1984) which retains the use of the same 13 indicator strains and the same typing pattern list as previously. The revised procedure is described below.

1. Grow the strains of *P. aeruginosa* to be typed on nutrient agar (Columbia Agar Base, Oxoid) at 37°C overnight. Use individual colonies of each test strain to prepare bacterial suspensions of 10^8–10^9 organisms in 1 ml of sterile physiological saline (absorbance at 550 nm = 0.5).

2. Use a multipoint inoculator (e.g. Model A400, Denley; this incorporates 21 stainless steel pins of 2 mm diameter set 16 mm apart) to dispense 1 μl volumes of the bacterial suspensions on to a set of 13 plates (diameter 90 mm) each containing 10 ml Tryptone Soya Agar (Oxoid). In this way 20 test strains (1 pin being a marker) can be typed simultaneously against each indicator strain. After the spots have dried, usually within a few minutes, incubate the plates at 30°C for 6 h.

3. Impregnate filter-paper disks (5 cm; Whatman) with chloroform and place the plates over the disks for 15 min to allow chloroform vapour to kill the bacteria. Expose the plates to air for an additional 15 min to eliminate residual chloroform vapour.

4. Prepare cultures of the indicator strains in Nutrient Broth (Oxoid, No. 2) without agitation for 4 h at 37°C to a population size of *c*. 10^7 orgs/ml.

5. Apply a separate indicator strain to each plate by adding 0.1 ml of each bacterial indicator culture to 2.5 ml of molten semi-solid agar (1% Peptone, Difco, in 0.5% agar, Oxoid Lll, held at 45°C); then pour it as an overlay. When the overlays have set, incubate the plates for 18 h at 37°C.

6. Determine the pyocin types of the test strains, as with the cross-streaking method, on the basis of the patterns of inhibition observed against the 13 indicator strains (Govan 1978). Note that with the revised technique the sizes of

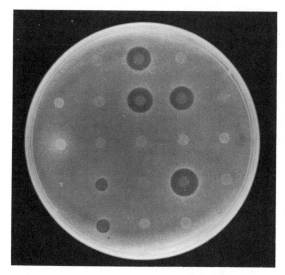

Fig. 31.1 Typical routine typing plate obtained by the revised spotting method for pyocin typing (Fyfe et al 1984). The agar overlay incorporates indicator strain 5. The plate shows the reactions produced by 20 test strains of *P. aeruginosa*. Four strains are surrounded by extensive S pyocin activity; 2 strains show restricted zones of inhibition characteristic of R and F pyocins; the remaining strains have produced no activity against this particular indicator strain.

the inhibition zones are also taken into account for the purpose of more detailed strain comparison, and determination of S pyocin activity is incorporated into the typing results as in the original cross-streaking method (see Fig. 31.1).

REFERENCES

Bergey 1984 In: Holt J G, Krieg N R (eds) Bergey's Manual of systematic bacteriology. vol 1. Williams & Wilkins Company, Baltimore. section 4, p 141–198

Brokopp C D, Farmer J J 1979 Typing methods for *Pseudomonas aeruginosa*. In: Doggett R (ed) *Pseudomonas aeruginosa*, clinical manifestations of infection and current therapy. Academic Press, New York. p 90–131

Brokopp C D, Gomez-Lus R, Farmer J J 1977 Serological typing of *Pseudomonas aeruginosa*: use of commercial antisera and live antigens. Journal of Clinical Microbiology 5: 640–649

Cowan S T 1974 Cowan and Steel's Manual for identification of medical bacteria, 2nd edn. University Press, Cambridge.

Davis J R, Stager C E, Araj G F 1983 4-h identification of *Pseudomonas aeruginosa* with 9-chloro-9-(4-demethylaminophenyl)-10-phenylacridan. Journal of Clinical Microbiology 17: 1054–1056

Fyfe J A M, Govan J R W 1984 Chromosomal loci associated with antibiotic hypersensitivity in pulmonary isolates of *Pseudomonas aeruginosa*. Journal of General Microbiology 130: 825–834

Fyfe J A M, Harris G, Govan J R W 1984 Revised pyocin typing method for *Pseudomonas aeruginosa*. Journal of Clinical Microbiology 20: 47–50

Gilardi G L 1972 Infrequently encountered *Pseudomonas* species causing infection in humans. Annals of Internal Medicine 77: 211–215

Govan J R W 1974a Studies on the pyocins of *Pseudomonas aeruginosa*: Morphology and mode of action of contractile pyocins. Journal of General Microbiology 80: 1–15

Govan J R W 1974b Studies on the pyocins of *Pseudomonas aeruginosa*: production of contractile and flexuous pyocins in *Pseudomonas aeruginosa*. Journal of General Microbiology 80: 17–30

Govan J R W 1978 Pyocin typing of *Pseudomonas aeruginosa*. In: Bergan T, Norris J R (eds) Methods in microbiology, vol 10. Academic Press, London. p 61–91

Govan J R W, Gillies R R 1969 Further studies in the pyocin typing of *Pseudomonas pyocyanea*. Journal of Medical Microbiology 2: 17–25

Govan J R W, Harris G 1985 Typing of *Pseudomonas cepacia* by bacteriocin susceptibility and production. Journal of Clinical Microbiology 22: 490–494

Hugh R, Leifson E 1953 The taxonomic significance of fermentative versus oxidative metabolism of carbohydrates by various Gram negative bacteria. Journal of Bacteriology 66: 24–26

Irvin R T, Govan J R W, Fyfe J A M, Costerton J W 1981 Heterogeneity of antibiotic resistance in mucoid isolates of *Pseudomonas aeruginosa* obtained from cystic fibrosis patients: role of outer membrane proteins. Antimicrobial Agents and Chemotherapy 19: 1056–1063

Ishii S, Nishi Y, Egami F 1965 The fine structure of a pyocin. Journal of Molecular Biology 13: 428–431

Ismail G, Noor Embi M, Omar O, Allen J C, Smith C J 1987 A competitive immunosorbent assay for detection of *Pseudomonas pseudomallei* exotoxin. Journal of Medical Microbiology 23: 353–357

Ito S, Kageyama M, Egami F 1970 Isolation and characterisation of pyocins from several strains of *Pseudomonas aeruginosa*. Journal of General Applied Microbiology 16: 205–214

Kelly N M, Falkiner F R, Keane C T 1983 Acetamide broth for isolation of *Pseudomonas aeruginosa* from patients with cystic fibrosis. Journal of Clinical Microbiology 17: 159

King A, Phillips I 1978 The identification of pseudomonads and related bacteria in a clinical laboratory. Journal of Medical Microbiology 11: 165–176

King E O, Ward M I C, Raney D E 1954 Two simple media for the demonstration of pyocyanin and fluorescein. Journal of Laboratory and Clinical Medicine 44: 301–307

Koestenblatt E K, Larone D H, Pavletich K J 1982 Comparison of the Oxi/Ferm and N/F systems for identification of infrequently encountered nonfermentative and oxidase-positive fermentative bacilli. Journal of Clinical Microbiology 15: 384–390

Kovacs N 1956 Identification of *Pseudomonas pyocyanea* by the oxidase reaction. Nature, London 178:703

Lanyi B, Bergan T 1978 Serological characterisation of *Pseudomonas aeruginosa*. In: Bergan T, Norris J R (eds) Methods in microbiology, vol 10. Academic Press, London. p 93–168

Lapage S P, Hill L R, Reeve J R 1968 *Pseudomonas stutzeri* in pathological material. Journal of Medical Microbiology 1: 195–202

Liu P V, Matsumoto H, Kusama H, Bergan T 1983 Survey of heat-stable, major antigens of *Pseudomonas aeruginosa*. International Journal of Systematic Bacteriology 33: 256–264

Neu H C 1983 The role of *Pseudomonas aeruginosa* in infections. Journal of Antimicrobial Chemotherapy 11: Suppl B, 1–13

Ogunnariwo J, Hamilton-Miller J M T 1975 Brown- and red-pigmented *Pseudomonas aeruginosa*: differentiation between melanin and pyorubrin. Journal of Medical Microbiology 8: 199–203

Phillips I 1969 Identification of *Pseudomonas aeruginosa* in the clinical laboratory. Journal of Medical Microbiology 2: 9–16

Pitt T L 1980 State of the art: typing of *Pseudomonas aeruginosa*. Journal of Hospital Infection 1: 193–199

Pitt T L 1981 A comparison of flagellar typing and phage typing as means of subdividing the O groups of *Pseudomonas aeruginosa*. Journal of Medical Microbiology 14: 261–270

Pitt T L 1988 Epidemiological typing of *Pseudomonas aeruginosa*. European Journal of Clinical Microbiology *in press*

Redfearn M S, Palleroni N J, Stanier R Y 1966 A comparative study of *Pseudomonas pseudomallei* and *Bacillus mallei*. Journal of General Microbiology 43: 293–313

Schlech W F, Turchik J B, Westlake R E, Klein G C, Band J D, Weaver R E 1981 Laboratory-acquired infection with *Pseudomonas pseudomallei* (melioidosis). New England Journal of Medicine 305: 1133–1135

Stanier R Y, Palleroni N J, Doudoroff M 1966 The aerobic pseudomonads: a taxonomic study. Journal of General Microbiology 43: 159–271

Stewart D J 1972 A composite arginine glucose medium for the characterisation of *Pseudomonas aeruginosa* and other Gram-negative bacilli. Journal of Applied Bacteriology 34: 779–785

Takeya K, Minamishima Y, Ohnishi Y, Amako K 1969 Rod-shaped pyocin 28. Journal of General Virology 4: 145–149

Taplin D, Bassett D C, Mertz P 1971 Foot lesions associated with *Pseudomonas cepacia*. Lancet 2: 568–571

Thornley M J 1960 The differentiation of *Pseudomonas* from other Gram-negative bacteria on the basis of arginine metabolism. Journal of Applied Bacteriology 23: 37–52

Vogt R, LaRue D, Parry M F, Brokopp C D, Klaucke D, Allen J 1982 *Pseudomonas aeruginosa* skin infections in persons using a whirlpool in Vermont. Journal of Clinical Microbiology 15: 571–574

Vibrio: Aeromonas: Plesiomonas: Spirillum: Campylobacter

The genus *Vibrio*, previously defined as the curved Gram-negative rods with polar flagella, was included in the family Spirillaceae, but after a change in its definition, only a few species were found to conform to the required criteria and retained within it. It has been removed from the Spirillaceae and placed in a family, Vibrionaceae, along with the genera *Aeromonas*, *Plesiomonas* and *Photobacterium* (Sakazaki & Balows 1981). Certain marine vibrios for which the genera *Beneckea* and *Lucibacterium* had been proposed, are now also included in the genus *Vibrio*. On the other hand, the microaerophilic bacteria formerly included in the genus, namely *Vibrio foetus*, *V. sputorum* and *V. faecalis*, are now grouped in the genus *Campylobacter* in the family Spirillaceae.

The Vibrionaceae are rigid Gram-negative rods, motile by a single polar flagellum, though some species develop peritrichous flagella on certain media; they are non-sporing, aerobic and facultatively anaerobic, non-exacting in nutritional requirements, catalase positive, oxidase positive in most species, and able to reduce nitrate to nitrite.

VIBRIO

The genus *Vibrio* consists of curved Gram-negative rods, motile by a single polar flagellum, which ferment carbohydrates with the production of acid but not gas; some species are halophilic, requiring sodium chloride for growth, and most produce a variety of extracellular enzymes, including amylase, chitinase, gelatinase, lecithinase and lipase. Some species are pathogenic to man, some are potential pathogens and others non-pathogens. Of prime importance is the causative agent of classical cholera, *V. cholerae*, and its biovar El Tor, both of which are non-halophilic. The El Tor vibrio was responsible for the last pandemic of cholera and is now a commoner cause of outbreaks than the classical *V. cholerae* biovar.

Other non-halophilic vibrios which share the H antigen but not the O antigen with *V. cholerae* are called 'non-cholera vibrios'; they are associated with diarrhoeal illnesses, though usually much less severe than classical cholera. Confusingly, these non-cholera vibrios are classified as *V. cholerae* serovars O2–O84, whilst the classical cholera vibrio is classified as *V. cholerae* serovar O1.

Among halophilic species, *V. parahaemolyticus* causes a type of food-poisoning, and *V. fluvialis*, a recently described species, may cause enteritis. Other vibrio species appear to be non-pathogenic in man, though *V. vulnius* may rarely cause a septicaemia. The habitats of these vibrios are river, surface and sea waters and sediments, sewage, prawns and other sea foods, and human and animal intestines.

Vibrio cholerae

Morphology and staining

Short Gram-negative rods which in young cultures are curved like a comma with rounded or pointed ends, and about 2×0.5 μm. In liquid media they are often seen in pairs or short chains, giving an S-shaped or spiral appearance. In older cultures pleomorphic involution forms are present. They have a very rapid, darting motility, are non-sporing and non-capsulate.

Cultural characters

Aerobic and only very slight growth under anaerobic conditions. Optimum temperature for growth 37°C, range 16–40°C. Grows well on ordinary culture media, e.g. rapidly as a surface pellicle on peptone water, visible in 6–9 h. Optimum pH for growth is 8.2 and growth occurs freely between pH 7.4 and pH 9.6, but is inhibited by acid reactions at pH values below 6.8.

After 12–18 h at 37°C on nutrient agar, colonies are glistening translucent disks 1–2 mm in diameter with a bluish or greenish appearance in obliquely transmitted light. Colonial variants are opaque, mucoid or rugose. *V. cholerae* grows well on MacConkey's lactose bile-salt medium; after 24 h the colonies are colourless and rather smaller than on nutrient agar, but when incubation is continued for a few days they become pink and finally dark red. Non-pathogenic vibrios grow poorly on MacConkey medium. Deoxycholate citrate agar (Ch. 29) is more inhibitory and not all strains of *V. cholerae* grow on it. On horse blood agar, zones of haemolysis are produced around the colonies by the El Tor biovar and other haemolysin-producing vibrios, but zones of clearing (pseudo-haemolysis) may also be formed by classical *V. cholerae* and other vibrios that do not form a haemolysin. In a gelatin stab, there is a white line of growth along the track of the wire; liquefaction begins at the top and spreads downwards in funnel-shaped form.

Selective media. The tolerance of vibrios for alkaline conditions is exploited in the formulation of selective media. Alkaline peptone water pH 8.6* is useful for preliminary enrichment of vibrios from faeces or other contaminated material. Dieudonné's (1909) blood alkali agar* was a selective plating medium much used in the past. Nowadays probably the most used selective plating medium is thiosulphate citrate bile

* Refer to *Methods* at end of this chapter.

sucrose (TCBS) agar* (Kobayashi et al 1963); it has some of the inhibitory properties of deoxycholate citrate agar, but its pH is 8.6 and it is much more favourable to the growth of vibrios. *V. cholerae*, its El Tor biovar and other sucrose-fermenting vibrios form yellow colonies, whilst *V. parahaemolyticus* and non-sucrose-fermenting vibrios form blue or green colonies. Another useful alkaline plating medium is Monsur's (1963) tellurite taurocholate gelatin agar.* These media are used routinely for the isolation of *V. cholerae* from the faeces of cholera patients, but they are also very useful for the isolation of vibrios from the faeces of carriers and the isolation of *V. parahaemolyticus* from foodstuffs.

Salt requirements. V. cholerae is a non-halophilic vibrio; it cannot grow in media with a concentration of sodium chloride greater than 5 or 6% and it is able to grow in media lacking any NaCl. Vibrios designated halophilic can grow in media containing up to 7–10% NaCl, grow best in media with about 3% NaCl and cannot grow in media, e.g. peptone water, lacking NaCl. A convenient way of determining whether a vibrio is halophilic or non-halophilic is to inoculate it on cystine lactose electrolyte-deficient (CLED) medium, pH 7.5, with Andrade's indicator (Ch. 28, *Methods*), on which non-halophilic organisms will grow, but not halophilic ones (Furniss et al 1978). Otherwise, tests should be made in peptone waters with different concentrations of sodium chloride*.

Sensitivity to physical and chemical agents

Killed by moist heat at 56°C in 30 min. Dies quickly on dry fomites and in sewage-polluted water, but survives for 1–2 weeks in clean, non-acid fresh or sea water. In faeces, dies within 24 h at high atmospheric temperatures, but survives several weeks at temperatures near freezing. May survive up to a few days on moist fruit, vegetables, fish and cooked foods.

Both the classical and El Tor biovars are sensitive to a wide range of antimicrobial drugs, including the sulphonamides, chloramphenicol, tetracyclines, ampicillin, kanamycin and trimethoprim, though in recent years strains resistant to one or more of these drugs have appeared. The El Tor biovar is resistant to polymyxin and this property is a useful taxonomic marker. Most vibrios are sensitive to compound 0/129 (2:4 diamino 6,7 diisopropyl pteridine), though some halophilic vibrios are less so; *Aeromonas* strains, with which vibrios may be confused, are resistant to this drug. Tests for sensitivity to polymyxin and compound 0/129 are described below*.

Biochemical reactions

The cholera vibrios ferment glucose, maltose, mannose, sucrose and mannitol within 24–48 h, producing acid but not gas, and ferment lactose only after several days; they do not ferment arabinose and dulcitol. They produce indole, reduce nitrate to nitrite, and give the cholera-red reaction,* i.e. the development of a red colour when sulphuric acid is added to a culture that has formed indole and nitrite. They are catalase positive, oxidase positive, urease negative and gelatin liquefying, and form decarboxylases for lysine and ornithine but not arginine. Many non-cholera vibrios differ from *V. cholerae* in some of these reactions, e.g. in fermenting arabinose, not fermenting mannose, not forming indole, or forming arginine decarboxylase.

Properties of biovars

Both the classical and El Tor biovars produce the diffusible enterotoxin that induces the excessive outpouring of isotonic fluid by the intestinal mucosal cells causing the profuse watery diarrhoea characteristic of cholera (Field 1971). They also produce in peptone water cultures an apparently identical exotoxin which causes increased tissue permeability when injected intradermally in rabbits. This test, however, is not used for diagnostic purposes.

The biovars can be distinguished from each other by a number of properties. The El Tor biovar produces acetoin in the Voges-Proskauer test (Barritt method, Ch. 8), agglutinates fowl erythrocytes (Finkelstein & Mukerjee 1963),* lyses sheep erythrocytes in a heart infusion broth with glycerol (Sakazaki et al 1971) and grows in

the presence of polymyxin B (50 unit disk, Han & Khie 1963),* whilst the classical biovar does not produce acetoin, agglutinate fowl erythrocytes, lyse sheep erythrocytes or grow in the presence of polymyxin. The classical, but not the El Tor biovar is sensitive to Mukerjee's (1961) group IV phage, and the El Tor but not the classical biovar is sensitive to the group V phage of Basu & Mukerjee (1970).

Antigenic characters

The species *V. cholerae* is now divided into 84 serovars by differences in their O antigens. The two biovars, classical and El Tor, causative of cholera, share the same O antigen, O1, which is limited to them alone and is thus their cardinal identifying character. They are agglutinated by *V. cholerae* O1 antiserum and termed *V. cholerae* O1. The serovars O2–O84 are found among the non-cholera vibrios and termed non-O1 *V. cholerae*, meaning not agglutinated by O1 antiserum. To physicians, however, they are better referred to as 'non-cholera vibrios', for the term 'non-O1 *V. cholerae*' may mislead them into thinking that an isolate so reported is a cholera organism.

The non-cholera vibrios are biochemically similar or identical to the classical and El Tor biovars and the close relationship is confirmed by DNA homology studies. They can cause symptoms similar to those of cholera and are believed to have been responsible for epidemics of enteritis, but they are generally much less pathogenic than the O1 strains. They are more often found in Britain than the latter and are now recognized as being indigenous in Northern Europe.

The classical and El Tor vibrios agglutinated by O1 antiserum can be divided by tests with absorbed sera into two subtypes, Inaba and Ogawa. Rare strains agglutinated by both the Inaba and Ogawa sera are known as Hikojima strains. Variation from the Ogawa to the Inaba serotype occasionally takes place during excretion by an individual or in the course of a localized outbreak (Sakazaki & Tamura 1971).

A heat-labile flagellar H antigen is common to all O-serovars of *V. cholerae*, identical in the cholera (O1) and non-cholera (O2–O84) vibrios. Its observation thus plays no part in distinguishing the former from the latter organisms, but it may be useful in the routine laboratory for the recognition of non-cholera vibrios by distinguishing these, with *V. cholerae*, from all other vibrios. The isolate so recognized by the H-antigen test* may then be sent to a reference laboratory for identification of its O-serovar.

Phage typing

Strains of the classical biovar of *V. cholerae* O1 can be divided into five phage types by tests with phages of the four groups, l–IV, of Mukerjee (1961), but now that classical strains are uncommon the method is little used. A scheme for phage typing El Tor strains (Basu & Mukerjee 1968) has been extended at the PHLS laboratory at Maidstone, UK, to distinguish strains with 25 different sensitivity patterns. It may prove possible eventually to have one scheme that embraces the non-cholera vibrios as well as the classical and El Tor biovars (Furniss et al 1978).

Laboratory diagnosis of cholera

Cholera has not been endemic in Britain and other developed countries for over a century, but the possibility of its occurring in a patient returning with diarrhoea from a visit to a country with endemic or epidemic infection should be borne in mind. When a faecal specimen is received from such a patient, it should be inoculated on to selective media for vibrios as well as on to those for the common enteropathogens.

Specimens

Faecal specimens from early acute cases should be collected into a sterile container, e.g. Universal container, preferably through a rubber catheter (No. 24–26) or, if they can be plated without delay, on to a rectal swab. Collection from a bedpan should be avoided because of the risk of contamination or the presence of disinfectant. Moistened rectal swabs may be taken conveniently from convalescent cases and suspected carriers. If there is likely to be a delay of more than 6 h in specimens reaching the laboratory, faeces or rectal swabs should be placed in a liquid alkaline *V. cholerae* transport medium to prevent overgrowth of the vibrios by other organisms; 1–3 ml faeces may be added to 10 or 20 ml transport medium, e.g. alkaline salt medium with boric acid* or taurocholate peptone medium with tellurite.*

Microscopy

If a specimen is obtained on the first day of the illness the vibrios are likely to be present in enormous numbers, e.g. $10^7–10^9$/ml, and it is then possible, in urgent cases, to make a provisional diagnosis by direct microscopical examination of a film of the faeces, preferably by dark-ground illumination. The vibrios should be seen darting about and to be immobilized when specific antiserum is added to the film.

Culture

1. Inoculate about 2 ml of faeces into 20 ml of alkaline peptone water and spread a large loopful of faeces over a plate of TCBS medium.* The classical biovar does not grow as freely on TCBS as the El Tor and other vibrios, so if its presence is possible, also seed a plate of non-selective nutrient agar or Monsur's selective tellurite taurocholate gelatin agar.* Incubate aerobically at 37°C.

2. After incubation for about 5 h, subculture a loopful from the surface of the alkaline peptone water on to a second plate of TCBS medium and a 1 ml volume into a second bottle of 20 ml alkaline peptone water. Also make a wet film from the alkaline peptone water and examine it microscopically for motile vibrios. Reincubate the original cultures along with the subcultures overnight.

3. Next day, first subculture a loopful from the surface of the second alkaline peptone water on to a third plate of TCBS medium. Then examine the first and second TCBS plates and

any other plate cultures for the presence of vibrio colonies. *V. cholerae* O1 and and other sucrose-fermenting vibrios, including non-O1 *V. cholerae*, form yellow colonies 2–3 mm in diameter, whilst *V. parahaemolyticus*, *V. vulnificus* and other non-sucrose-fermenters form blue-green colonies 2–5 mm in diameter.

4. Test bacteria from yellow colonies on TCBS or suspect colonies on other media for slide agglutination with *V. cholerae* O1 antiserum (Inaba-Ogawa bivalent). If the test is negative or if the bacteria are autoagglutinable, subculture the organism on salt-free nutrient agar and repeat the slide agglutination test. Confirm the identity of O1-agglutinating organisms as *V. cholerae* O1 by demonstrating they are Gram negative, motile, sucrose fermenting and oxidase positive; then report the presence of 'cholera vibrio' to the physician. The biovar may be determined by the Voges-Proskauer, haemagglutination, haemolysin, polymyxin and phage sensitivity tests as described above.

5. If vibrio colonies are found not to be *V. cholerae* O1, test bacteria from them in a slide agglutination test with *V. cholerae* H-antiserum so that non-cholera vibrios (*V. cholerae* O2–O84) may be recognized by their positive reaction. Finally attempt culture on CLED medium, so that halophilic vibrios, such as *V. parahaemolyticus*, may be recognized by their failure to grow.

6. *Serological diagnosis*. This can be done by the demonstration of a rising titre of agglutinins or vibriocidal antibodies in paired sera, one taken in the first 3 days of illness and the other after 7–10 days (Holmgren et al 1971).

For fuller details of diagnostic procedures see WHO Bacterial Diseases Unit (1974) and Furniss et al (1978). Characters distinguishing cholera vibrios from related organisms are shown in Table 32.1. Isolates should be sent to a reference laboratory for confirmation of identity and O-serotyping.

Vibrio parahaemolyticus

This halophilic vibrio was first identified in Japan as a cause of food-poisoning and is now recognized as being responsible world-wide for outbreaks of gastroenteritis associated with the eating of crabs, prawns, shrimps and other seafoods. It has been isolated from shell-fish and other fish in the warm coastal and estuarine waters of many countries and is quite common in waters around Britain, particularly in the summer (Ayres & Barrow 1978). The clinical infection is characterized by a sudden onset of acute gastroenteritis after an incubation period of 10–20 h (range 2–40 h) and lasts only a few days. The vibrios are very numerous in the faeces during the illness, but rapidly disappear on recovery (Peffers et al 1973).

Table 32.1 Distinguishing characters of species of *Vibrio*, *Aeromonas* and *Plesiomonas*.
Key:+/−, some strains positive, some negative; ±, weakly positive.
Note. All shown species are oxidase positive. Only *V. cholerae* O1 is agglutinatined by a *V. cholerae* O1 antiserum.

Species	Growth on TCBS agar[a]	Growth in peptone water with added NaCl					Acetoin formed in VP test	Acid formed from		Sensitivity to 0/129	
		0%	3%	6%	8%	10%		Arabinose	Sucrose	10 μg	150 μg
V. cholerae O1	Y	+	+	±	−	−	+/−	−	+	+	+
V. cholerae non-O1	Y	+	+	±	−	−	+/−	−	+	+	+
V. parahaemolyticus	G	−	+	+	+	−	−	+/−	−	−	+
V. fluvialis	Y	+/−	+	+	±	−	−	+	+	−	+
V. vulnificus	G	−	+	+	−	−	−	−	−	+	+
V. alginolyticus	Y	−	+	+	+	+	+	−	+	−	+
Aeromonas species	Y/−	+	+	−	−	−	+/−	+/−	+	−	−
P. shigelloides	−	+	+	−	−	−	−	−	−	+	+

[a] On TCBS: Y, growth of yellow colonies; G, growth of green colonies; −, no growth.

Biological characters

In morphology and staining it resembles *V. cholerae* and is actively motile in fluid cultures. It grows overnight at 37°C on selective TCBS agar to form large, smooth dome-shaped colonies with an opaque centre and a greenish-blue colour, the films from which show pleomorphic Gram-negative bacilli. It is halophilic and fails to grow in peptone water without NaCl or on electrolyte-deficient CLED medium, but grows well in peptone water with 8% NaCl, though not in similar medium with 10% NaCl. It is β-haemolytic on sheep blood agar and grows on MacConkey agar as pale, non-lactose-fermenting colonies. It is sensitive to the same vibriocidal drugs as *V. cholerae*, though less so to compound 0/129. See Table 32.1.

It ferments glucose with the production of acid but not gas, and usually also arabinose and mannose, but neither lactose nor sucrose. It does not produce acetoin in the Voges-Proskauer test, is catalase positive and oxidase positive, and decarboxylates lysine and ornithine but not arginine. Strains isolated from gastroenteritis lyse human erythrocytes in the Kanagawa test (Miyamoto et al 1969). Numerous serovars are distinguished by the possession of different O and K antigens.

Laboratory diagnosis of Vibrio parahaemolyticus

The procedures for isolation and identification are similar to those already described for the cholera vibrio. *V. parahaemolyticus* is identified by the finding of a Gram-negative vibrio from green-blue colonies on TCBS medium that grows in alkaline peptone water with 8% NaCl but not in peptone water without NaCl or on CLED medium, and is not agglutinated by *V. cholerae* O1 antiserum. Isolates may be serotyped at a reference laboratory.

Vibrio fluvialis

These halophilic vibrios, previously called group F vibrios, are widely distributed in the sea and estuaries around Britain. They have been isolated from the faeces of patients with diarrhoea and were associated with an outbreak of enteritis in Bangladesh. So far they have not been found in the faeces of healthy individuals.

The organism grows well and forms yellow colonies on TCBS medium. It ferments glucose, sucrose, lactose and arabinose with the production of acid but not gas, though some non-human isolates may form gas from arabinose (Von Graevenitz 1983). It is oxidase positive, indole negative, acetoin negative and arginine decarboxylase positive, and it is not agglutinated by *V. cholerae* O1 antiserum.

Vibrio vulnificus

This halophilic vibrio is phenotypically similar to *V. parahaemolyticus*, forming green, non-sucrose-fermenting colonies on TCBS medium, but differs in fermenting lactose and growing in the presence of a 300 unit disk of polymyxin. It has been found in septicaemias in the USA following the eating of raw oysters (Ellington et al 1982). Septicaemias have also followed wound infection after exposure to sea water or injury in handling crabs.

Vibrio alginolyticus

This sucrose-fermenting halophilic vibrio is the commonest vibrio found in the sea around Britain. It is similar biochemically to *V. parahaemolyticus*, but differs in fermenting sucrose and producing acetoin. It may act as an opportunist pathogen by infecting the ear or a wound after sea-bathing.

AEROMONAS

The taxonomy of this genus is still uncertain. Most strains are grouped in a single species, *A. hydrophila*, probably composed of several biovars. Strains of the fish pathogen, *A. salmonicida*, differ from *A. hydrophila* in being non-motile and unable to grow at 37°C (Gilardi 1983).

Aeromonas hydrophila

The organisms are straight Gram-negative rods with rounded ends, about 4.5 × 1 μm, with some filaments. The bacilli may be single, in pairs or in chains. They are motile with a single polar flagellum, though some strains are non-motile.

The temperature range for growth is 20–37°C, with the optimum about 30°C (*A. salmonicida* range 5–32°C, optimum 20°C), and the pH range 5.5–9. They grow well on nutrient agar, blood agar (giving wide β-haemolysis), MacConkey agar (colonies pale at 24 h, pink later), deoxycholate citrate agar and CLED agar, but growth is variable on TCBS medium, on which colonies are usually yellow. They are not halophilic. They produce acid and usually gas from glucose, maltose, starch and, usually, arabinose and sucrose, and form a variety of enzymes, e.g. amylase, arginine hydrolase, chitinase, deoxyribonuclease, gelatinase, lecithinase and lipase. They are resistant to agent 0/129. See Table 32.1.

Strains are found in fresh and sea water and in the soil. They are opportunistic pathogens and may cause septicaemia in immunodeficient subjects and patients with chronic disease. They are found in ears and wounds infected perhaps from water or soil and have been isolated from faeces from patients with enteritis in which they may act as primary pathogens (Gracey et al 1982). They are not part of the normal flora of the human intestine.

Laboratory diagnosis of Aeromonas hydrophila

The organism is readily isolated on ordinary media from blood cultures and infected wounds. In the past its isolation from faeces has been hindered by the absence of a good selective medium. But evaluations of different selective media have recently been reported (Moulsdale 1983; Von Graevenitz & Bucher 1983). Agger et al (1985) recommend the use of sheep blood agar with ampicillin 15 mg/litre which grows aeromonas colonies identifiable by narrow zones of haemolysis and, after flooding with oxidase reagent, by a purple-black reaction.

PLESIOMONAS

Plesiomonas shigelloides is the only species in this genus and gained its name *shigelloides* because strains originally isolated from faeces

formed pale colonies on MacConkey and DCA media and some were agglutinated by antiserum to *Shigella sonnei* form 1, with which they shared the O antigen. They differ from shigellae in being oxidase positive and motile with polar flagella, which, with other characters, relate them to *Vibrio* and *Aeromonas*.

The organisms are straight Gram-negative bacilli, about 0.8×3 μm, which grow singly, in pairs and in short chains and bear polar flagella. Growth is good at 37°C, though better at 30°C. They are facultative anaerobes and grow well on ordinary media, MacConkey, DCA and CLED, but usually not on TCBS. They are non-haemolytic on blood agar and non-halophilic, failing to grow in media with more than 6 or 7% NaCl.

They ferment glucose, maltose, trehalose, glycerol and inositol with the production of acid but not gas, but do not ferment sucrose or starch. Some strains ferment lactose in 24 h, but most do so only after a few days. Like aeromonads they are catalase and oxidase positive, but differ from them not only in failing to ferment sucrose and starch, but also in not liquefying gelatin, being non-haemolytic on blood agar and being sensitive to compound 0/129 (Table 32.1). They decarboxylate lysine, ornithine and arginine, are urease negative, indole positive and fail to grow in KCN medium (Ch. 8).

Strains have been isolated from fresh and river water, ponds and mud, freshwater fish, newts, dogs, cats and the faeces of patients with diarrhoea. Their finding in sporadic cases and outbreaks of diarrhoea in many countries (Tsukamoto et al 1978; Mandal et al 1982) has led to the recent recognition of their enteropathogenicity. They usually form pale colonies on MacConkey and DCA medium, like those of *S. sonnei*, but a few strains form pink colonies like those of *Escherichia coli*. In either case the demonstration that they are oxidase positive will prevent their misidentification.

SPIRILLUM

Members of this genus are rigid spiral Gram-negative filamentous cells that are motile with bipolar flagella, oxidase positive and able to grow on ordinary bacteriological media. They are found mainly in fresh or sea water and with one exception are non-pathogenic to man and animals. The exception is *Spirillum minus*, a natural parasite of rats which cannot be grown on artificial culture media and which may be more closely related to *Campylobacter* than to other members of the genus *Spirillum* (Krieg 1981).

Spirillum minus

S. minus is the cause of one type of rat bite fever in man (Sodoku). It is a spiral Gram-negative organism, generally short, e.g. 2–5 μm in length, but sometimes up to 10 μm, with regular tight coils about 1 μm across. It has bipolar tufts of 1–7 flagella at each end and has a very active, darting motility unlike the undulatory movement of spirochaetes. The motility and flagella are best seen with the darkground microscope. It stains well with Romanowsky dyes such as Leishman's. Rats act as healthy carriers, whilst guinea-pigs, white rats and mice can be infected experimentally; guinea-pigs develop a slowly progressive septicaemic disease and die after several weeks. In man there is local inflammation at the site of the rat bite, swelling of the regional lymph nodes, a macular skin eruption and fever, these symptoms fluctuating in parallel. The infection responds to penicillin and the tetracyclines.

Laboratory diagnosis. Attempt to demonstrate the spirilla in exudate from the local lesion, in aspirate from the swollen lymph nodes and in a sample of venous blood. Examine films of the specimens by darkground microscopy. Also inoculate portions of the specimens, e.g. 1 ml of venous blood, intraperitoneally in a mouse. The mouse will show no signs of illness, but after 5–14 days small numbers of spirilla may be demonstrated microscopically in its blood and peritoneal fluid. A further inoculation may be made into a guinea-pig.

CAMPYLOBACTER

The campylobacters are small curved Gram-negative rods with polar flagella, generally single, and were formerly classified in the genus

Vibrio. They have long been known as pathogens of animals, e.g. '*Vibrio fetus*' as a cause of abortion in cattle and sheep and '*V. jejuni*' as a cause of diarrhoea in cattle and pigs. But two species, *Campylobacter jejuni* and *C. coli*, are now among the commonest identified causes of enteritis in man, responsible for about 7% of all cases in Britain. It was due to the former lack of a selective culture medium for their isolation from faeces that their role as human pathogens was not recognized before the last decade. They are found in the intestine in only very few (under 0.5%) persons without diarrhoea.

Recently, a campylobacter-like organism, *C. pylori*, formerly named *C. pyloridis*, has been found on the mucosa of the gastric antrum in a large proportion of patients with gastritis, duodenitis and peptic ulcers, and is thought to have a role in the causation of these conditions. The symptoms and histological signs of the inflammation disappear when the organism is eliminated by treatment with a locally active antibacterial drug such as amoxycillin or bismuth salicylate (McNulty et al 1986).

The campylobacters resemble vibrios in their morphology, polar flagellation and oxidase-positive character, but differ in being micro-aerophilic, not fermenting sugars and having a lower DNA guanidine-cytosine content (30–35 moles % as against 40–50 moles % in vibrios), characters that determine their classification in the separate genus, *Campylobacter*. Their exceptionally small size enables them to pass through filters fine enough to retain most other kinds of bacteria, e.g. a Millipore filter with a mean pore diameter of 0.65 μm, a property exploited in early methods for their isolation from contaminated materials.

The genus is divided into two groups of species, the one producing catalase, the other not. The catalase-negative group includes *C. sputorum* subspp. *sputorum, bubulus* and *mucosalis*, none of which is pathogenic to man, though they are occasionally found in human faeces unassociated with diarrhoea. The catalase-positive group includes the animal and human pathogens, *C. fetus, C. coli, C. jejuni* and *C. laridis. C. fetus* has two subspecies that cause abortion in cattle and sheep, *C. fetus* subsp. *venerealis*, which is not found in human disease, and *C. fetus* subsp. *fetus*, which can act as an opportunistic pathogen in patients with chronic or debilitating disease and may be isolated from their blood and body fluids. Of more importance in human medicine are *C. jejuni* and *C. coli*, which cause diarrhoea in cattle and pigs respectively, but also often cause diarrhoea, sometimes with septicaemia, in man. These two species, which have sometimes been named together as *C. jejuni*, correspond to the 'related campylobacters' found by King (1957, 1962) to be associated with enteritis in man, but isolated by her only from blood cultures for want of a selective method for isolation from faeces (Skirrow 1977; Butzler & Skirrow 1979). Another species closely related to them is *C. laridis*, which has been isolated from the intestinal tract of seagulls as well as from man and animals. The taxonomy of *Campylobacter* has undergone a number of changes in recent years as a result of investigations that have confirmed the identity of putative species and established new ones (Buck 1984).

Campylobacter jejuni

Morphology and staining

Gram-negative slender, curved or spiral rods, $0.2–0.5 \times 1.5–5\ \mu m$, appearing in comma, S-shaped or 'gull-wings' forms. Old cultures show long spiral filaments with some coccoid and spherical forms. Motility is of the darting type, with a corkscrew-like movement, and when recently passed stools are examined by dark-ground microscopy, campylobacters can be recognized by their peculiar motility.

Cultural characters

C. jejuni is microaerophilic, requiring a reduced concentration of oxygen, about 6%, in the atmosphere and, preferably, about 10% of added carbon dioxide. It is also thermophilic, growing at 37°C, but better at 42–43°C and not at all at 25°C. *C. coli* and *C. laridis* resemble it in these respects, but *C. fetus* subspecies differ in growing at 25°C and 37°C but not at 42°C (Table 32.2). Campylobacters grow well on a good quality nutrient agar, e.g. Oxoid Blood Agar Base No 2, but growth is slow and may take 2–5 days to develop fully. On solid medium the colonies are flat, moist and translucent, like droplets of water when young. They commonly range from 0.5–2 mm in diameter and tend to become confluent along the streaks made by the inoculating wire. Colonies of *C. coli* spread out less than those of *C. jejuni*. On blood agar they are non-haemolytic. Various selective plating media have been used for the isolation of *C. jejuni* from faeces, that of Skirrow (1977) containing vancomycin, polymyxin and trimethoprim in lysed-blood agar, that of Butzler & Skirrow (1979) bacitracin, cephazolin, colistin, cycloheximide and novobiocin, and that of Bolton & Robertson (1982) cycloheximide, polymyxin, rifampicin and trimethoprim.

Biochemical reactions

C. jejuni, *C. coli* and *C. laridis* are catalase positive, oxidase positive, non-proteolytic and unable to attack carbohydrates. They can be differentiated from one another and from other *Campylobacter* species by tests of further

Table 32.2 Distinguishing characters of some *Campylobacter* species and subspecies. Key: . . ., result not given.

Species or subspecies	Growth at			Sensitivity to nalidixic acid, 30 μg disk	Hippurate hydrolysis	Growth on medium containing		
	25°C	37°C	42°C			0.4 g/l TTC[a]	1.5% NaCl	1% glycine
C. fetus ssp. *fetus*	+	+	−	−	−	−	−	+
C. fetus ssp. *venerealis*	+	+	−	−	−	−	−	−
C. jejuni	−	+	+	+	+	−	−	+
C. coli	−	+	+	+	−	+	−	+
C. laridis	−	+	+	−	−	−	+	. . .

[a] 2,3,5-triphenyltetrazolium chloride.

reactions and their ability to grow at different temperatures (Skirrow & Benjamin 1980a; Table 32.2). Thus, *C. jejuni* and *C. coli* are sensitive to nalidixic acid in a plate test with a 30 μg disk, whereas *C. fetus* subspecies and *C. laridis* are resistant to it. *C. laridis*, which was originally designated NARTC (nalidixic acid resistant thermophilic campylobacter), resembles *C. jejuni* in its failure to grow at 25°C but differs from it both in being resistant to nalidixic acid and in growing on a basal medium containing 1.5% sodium chloride. *C. coli* differs from *C. jejuni* in giving growth on a medium with 0.4 g/litre 2,3,5-triphenyltetrazolium chloride (TTC) and in failing to lyse sodium hippurate (Skirrow & Benjamin 1980b). *C. fetus* differs in the guanidine-cytosine content of its DNA from the thermophilic campylobacters, while tests of DNA sequence relatedness among the latter have confirmed the differentiation of *C. jejuni*, *C. coli* and *C. laridis* as separate species (Owen 1983).

Viability

C. jejuni can multiply in human bile at 37°C and survive in it for up to 2 months. Campylobacters survive better at 4°C than at 25°C and higher temperatures. They may survive for 3 weeks in milk or faeces at 4°C and for 4–5 weeks in water or urine, so that when these materials are contaminated they may act as reservoirs of infection (Blaser et al 1980). Outbreaks of infection have followed the drinking of untreated water from rivers, streams and lakes, and raw or improperly pasteurized milk from cows that have contaminated it from their faeces or infected udders (Robinson & Jones 1981). Campylobacters also survive well on raw meat, pork or poultry derived from infected animals, which may cause infection when eaten only lightly cooked, salted or smoked. Persons handling or preparing the raw flesh may infect themselves (Skirrow 1982).

Antibiotic sensitivity

C. jejuni strains are sensitive in vitro to aminoglycosides, chloramphenicol, clindamycin, erythromycin and tetracyclines, but resistant to penicillin, cephalosporins, polymyxin, trimethoprim and vancomycin. Erythromycin is the drug of choice for treatment of the few cases that require antibacterial therapy, namely those with long persistence of symptoms, frequent bloody diarrhoea or high fever. An in-vitro test for sensitivity to erythromycin should be done on all isolates because a small minority of strains are resistant to this drug; in such cases clindamycin or tetracycline may be used.

Antigenic characters

The availability of a simple, reliable serotyping method for the differentiation of strains would greatly facilitate studies of the epidemiology of campylobacter infections, but though many serological methods have been tested, none is yet accepted for general application; some are of limited value and others are laborious and costly.

A slide agglutination method distinguishing thermolabile antigens has been developed by Lior et al (1982). The antisera to reference strains are absorbed with a heated suspension of the homologous strain and, in some cases, also with a heterologous strain. The method has been extended to identify over 53 serogroups, some of which contain strains of both *C. jejuni* and *C. coli*, and some also strains of *C. laridis*. Its application has enabled most human isolates to be typed.

Another method employs the passive haemagglutination technique to identify thermostable lipopolysaccharide antigens (Penner & Hennessy 1980) and has demonstrated 41 serotypes of *C. jejuni* and 18 of *C. coli*. A further 10 and 8 serotypes, respectively, of these two species may be identified in a supplementary scheme.

If either the Lior or the Penner scheme is used to type a batch of strains, it is found that use of the other scheme supplements that primarily employed and increases the total number of strains that can be typed. Moreover, a biotyping study of temperature, biochemical and resistance characters may make possible a further differentiation of strains within a single serotype (Jones et al 1984). A phage-typing scheme is under investigation but is not yet a practical proposition.

Patients infected with *C. jejuni* acquire serum antibodies which are demonstrable by agglutination and complement-fixation tests. Bactericidal antibodies may also be shown in convalescent serum.

Pathogenesis

The infecting dose of *C. jejuni* is not known, but one volunteer developed campylobacter enteritis after ingesting 500 bacteria (Robinson 1981). The bacteria that escape killing by the gastric acid multiply rapidly in the near neutral, microaerophilic environment of the small intestine, so that the stools of patients may contain $10^6–10^9$ campylobacters/g. They produce an oedematous exudative enteritis of the jejunum, ileum and colon, with cellular infiltration and ulceration of the mucosa. How they produce the damage is unclear (Butzler & Skirrow 1979; Blaser & Reller 1981). They appear to enter, multiply in and damage the mucosal cells and thence gain access to the blood stream. *C. jejuni* produces two exotoxins: a heat-labile cytotonic or enterotoxin (CJT) and a cytotoxin. The CJT induces secretory diarrhoea by stimulating adenylate cyclase activity in the intestinal mucosa.

Laboratory diagnosis of campylobacter enteritis

The isolation of campylobacters from faeces requires the use of selective media and the correct atmospheric conditions. The original method of isolation on non-selective blood agar involved a preliminary filtration of the specimen through a membrane that allowed the small campylobacters to pass but retained most other faecal bacteria. This method, however, was costly and time-consuming, and it was the introduction of selective media that made possible the routine examination of faeces for campylobacters.

The selective medium of Skirrow (1977)* has been much used and found very successful, though advantages have been claimed for other media, e.g. that of Lauwers et al (1978). The Preston medium of Bolton & Robertson (1982)* has been found to give the maximum rate of isolation of campylobacters from all types of specimens and to be more selective than the

other media tested (Bolton et al 1983). These media are commercially available in the form of supplements to be added to lysed blood agar (e.g. from Oxoid). Fresh specimens of faeces, within 24 h of collection and likely to contain numerous campylobacters should be plated directly on the selective plating medium, but older specimens and those likely to contain few campylobacters should first be enriched by culture for 24 h in a liquid medium such as the Preston campylobacter enrichment broth* before plating out on the selective agar medium.

The temperature of incubation should be 42°C to favour growth of the thermophilic campylobacters over that of other faecal bacteria. If, however, the presence of *C. fetus* is suspected, additional plates should be incubated at 37°C to allow growth of this non-thermophile.

Incubation must be under microaerophilic conditions, preferably in an atmosphere containing 5–6% (v/v) oxygen, 7–10% carbon dioxide and the rest nitrogen or hydrogen. Place the plates in an anaerobic-type jar without a catalyst, seal tightly, extract 65–70% of the air by drawing a vacuum of 500–550 mm Hg (i.e. to a residual pressure of about 250 mm Hg) and let the jar refill to atmospheric pressure (760 mm Hg) with a mixture of 10% carbon dioxide and 90% nitrogen or hydrogen. Alternatively, use a commercial gas-generating kit (see Ch. 7).

If such precise means for obtaining microaerophilic conditions are not available, plates may be incubated in a candle jar or sealed over a second plate seeded with an oxygen-utilizing and carbon dioxide-producing organism like *Serratia marcescens*. In that case the campylobacter plating medium should be supplemented with a mixture of ferrous sulphate, sodium metabisulphite and sodium pyruvate* to increase the aerotolerance of the bacteria.

Procedure

1. For fresh (<24 h old) diarrhoeal faeces, plate out a loopful thinly on a plate of Skirrow's medium* or the Preston medium of Bolton & Robertson*. For older (>24 h) specimens or formed stools, inoculate a loopful of the specimen in a tube of 10 ml selective enrichment

broth* and incubate aerobically for 24 h at 42–43°C; then plate out a loopful from this culture on Skirrow or Preston medium.

2. Incubate the plate for 48 h at 42–43°C in a microaerophilic atmosphere obtained as described above.

3. Examine the plates for the characteristic effuse droplet-like colonies.

4. Confirm the colonies are campylobacters as follows. (a) In a Gram smear counterstained with dilute carbol fuchsin for 5 min, demonstrate small curved or spiral Gram-negative bacteria. (b) Demonstrate darting motility in a wet film or hanging drop of a suspension or subculture in liquid medium. (c) Perform an oxidase test on the colonies by the filter paper method (Ch. 8) to demonstrate the positive reaction of campylobacters.

5. Test the isolate for sensitivity to erythromycin. Plate out material from one or two characteristic colonies on a suitable nutrient agar, e.g. Oxoid Blood Agar Base No. 2, or blood agar, and place a disk with 15 μg erythromycin on the confluently inoculated 'well' area. Incubate under microaerophilic conditions for 18–24 h at 37°C. Read a clear zone of inhibition as denoting sensitivity. Check by inspection of the area with separate colonies that the inoculum was pure.

6. The organism isolated and identified by the above procedures will almost certainly be *C. jejuni* or *C. coli*, and that information should suffice for clinical purposes. If species identification is required, grow a pure subculture on a suitable nutrient agar or blood agar medium at 37°C and prepare a suspension* for inoculation into the following tests.

7. Test for catalase production (Ch. 8) to distinguish *C. sputorum* (negative) from the *C. fetus* and *C. jejuni* groups (positive).

8. Determine the temperature requirements* to distinguish the *C. jejuni* group, which grow at 37°C and 42°C but not at 25°C from the *C. fetus* group which grow at 25°C and 37°C but not at 42°C (Table 32.2).

9. Test for sensitivity to nalidixic acid* to distinguish *C. jejuni* and *C. coli* (sensitive) from *C. laridis* and *C. fetus* (resistant).

10. Test for the ability to hydrolyse sodium hippurate* and the ability to grow on a nutrient agar medium containing 0.4 g/litre 2,3,5-triphenyltetrazolium chloride (TTC)* to distinguish *C. jejuni* from *C. coli* (Table 32.2).

11. For short-term preservation, grow a culture in cooked meat medium or thioglycollate broth (Ch. 6) for 3 days at 37°C, seal and store at room temperature.

Campylobacter pylori

This species is thought to cause gastritis, duodenitis and peptic ulceration, conditions cured by antibacterial therapy with, e.g. amoxycillin or bismuth salicylate. The curved bacilli are found under the layer of mucus on the epithelium of the gastric antrum in nearly all patients with active chronic gastritis, or gastric or duodenal ulcer. They require protection from the lethal action of the acid gastric secretion by the covering of an intact layer of mucus and, though readily cultivable from biopsies taken from mucus-covered epithelium, are rarely cultivable from acid gastric washings.

The organisms resemble other campylobacters in their general characters, but differ from them in possessing, not one, but four to five polar flagella. They grow well under microaerophilic conditions on blood agar or campylobacter selective medium at 35–37°C, often also at 42°C, but not at 28°C, and form non-pigmented colonies about 1 mm in diameter in 3 days. Marshall & Warren (1984) describe their isolates as being oxidase and catalase positive, glucose and urease negative, sensitive to erythromycin, gentamicin and penicillin, and resistant to nalidixic acid. In contrast, Langenberg et al (1984) and McNulty & Wise (1985) describe their isolates as giving a rapid and strong urease reaction in Christensen's urea broth, within a few minutes when colonial material is emulsified in the broth and within 1–24 h when tissue from a positive biopsy specimen is crushed in the broth and left at room temperature.

Laboratory diagnosis

Specimen. Gastric washings are unsuitable for both microscopical and cultural examination.

A biopsy of mucosa from the gastric antrum should be taken by endoscopy. Place it in a small, e.g. 6 ml, screw-capped bottle containing a small amount, e.g. 0.2 ml, of sterile 0.85% NaCl solution to maintain humidity. Process it as soon as practicable, at least within 2 h.

Gram smear. Smear the specimen on a sterile slide, dry the smear, fix with heat and stain by Gram's method. Examine for the presence of Gram-negative spiral bacteria, which is strongly suggestive of infection with *C. pylori.*

Culture. Crush the specimen and inoculate portions on (1) a blood agar plate, and (2) Skirrow's campylobacter selective medium.* Incubate the plates microaerophilically with 5% O_2 and 10% CO_2 at 37°C and examine after 3, 5 and 7 days. The growth of characteristic oxidase- and catalase-positive colonies consisting of Gram-negative spiral bacteria indicates the presence of *C. pylori.*

Urease test. Emulsify some colonial material in Christensen's urea broth and watch for a colour change after several minutes at room temperature. Also, if some of the biopsy material remains available after inoculation into cultures, crush it into 0.5 ml Christensen's urea broth and incubate aerobically at 37°C.

METHODS FOR VIBRIOS

Alkaline salt transport medium

This non-nutritive fluid helps to maintain the viability of *V. cholerae* in a specimen of faeces and prevent its overgrowth by other bacteria when there may be a delay of more than a few hours in the specimen's transmission to the laboratory.

Boric acid, H_3BO_3	3.1 g
Potassium chloride, KCl	3.7 g
Sodium hydroxide, NaOH, 0.2 mol/litre	133.5 ml
Dried sea salt	20 g
Distilled water	867 ml

Dissolve the boric acid and potassium chloride in 200 ml hot distilled water, cool and make up to 250 ml. Add 133.5 ml of the sodium hydroxide solution and make up with distilled water to 1 litre. Add 20 g of dried sea salt, adjust the pH to 9.2 by the addition of sufficient 5% NaOH or Na_2CO_3 solution and filter through filter paper. Distribute in 10 ml amounts in wide-mouthed 28 ml screw-capped bottles and autoclave at 121°C for 15 min.

A substitute for 20 g sea salt is a mixture of 27 g NaCl, 1 g KCl, 3 g $MgCl_2.6H_2O$ and 1.8 g $MgSO_4.7H_2O$.

Use. Add 1–3 g of the stool to 10 ml transport medium, seal, mix thoroughly and transmit to the laboratory.

Taurocholate peptone transport and enrichment medium

This nutritive selective liquid medium may be used either as a transport (holding) medium to maintain the viability of *V. cholerae* in stool specimens during delay in transmission to the laboratory or as an enrichment medium to promote selective outgrowth of *V. cholerae* from faeces before plating on a selective agar medium.

Peptone, e.g. Trypticase (BBL)	10 g
Sodium chloride, NaCl	10 g
Sodium taurocholate	5 g
Distilled water	1 litre

Dissolve the ingredients, adjust the pH to 9.0 by the addition of sufficient sodium hydroxide solution 1 mol/litre, distribute in 20 ml amounts into 28 ml screw-capped bottles and autoclave at 121°C for 15 min.

To make the medium more selective for vibrios, add sterile potassium tellurite solution to the autoclaved medium to give a final concentration of 1 in 200 000 and use within 2 weeks.

Use. Place about 1 g faeces or a rectal swab in the medium, seal and transmit to the laboratory. In a hot climate, subculture a loopful on to a selective plating medium within 6–8 h at ambient temperature. Also incubate overnight at 37°C and subculture again on a plating medium next day.

Alkaline peptone water

This is an excellent medium for enriching the numbers of *V. cholerae* in a faecal specimen before plating on a selective agar medium.

Peptone	10 g
Sodium chloride, NaCl	10 g
Distilled water	1 litre

Adjust the pH to 8.6, distribute in 10 ml or 20 ml amounts in 28 ml screw-capped bottles and autoclave at 121°C for 15 min.

Use. Inoculate 1 g faeces into 10 ml alkaline peptone water, or about 2 g into 20 ml. Incubate at 37°C for 5 h and then inoculate a loopful from the top of the peptone water on to a selective plating medium. If the incubation is continued for more than 8 h before subculture, the vibrios may be overgrown by other bacteria and it is necessary to perform a second enrichment by inoculating a drop from the top of the peptone water culture into a fresh tube of the medium and incubate the latter for only 5–8 h before plating from it.

Thiosulphate citrate bile sucrose (TCBS)) agar

This is now the most used selective plating medium for vibrios. It was first described by Kobayashi et al (1963). It gives good growth of *V. cholerae*, *V. parahaemolyticus* and other vibrios within 24 h at 37°C (colonies 2–5 mm in diameter) and inhibits most enterobacteria and Gram-positive bacteria, though allowing some strains of proteus, aeromonas and enterococci to form small colonies (1 mm). It resembles deoxycholate citrate agar (DCA) except that it has the high pH value of 8.6 and contains sucrose instead of lactose and indicator dyes that show a change due to acid formation on the alkaline side of neutrality. Sucrose-fermenting vibrios such as *V. cholerae* form yellow colonies and non-sucrose-fermenters such as *V. parahaemolyticus* blue-green ones.

Precautions in the preparation of TCBS agar, e.g. the avoidance of autoclaving certain ingredients, are similar to those for DCA.

Indicator sucrose agar

Yeast extract	5 g
Peptone	10 g
Sodium chloride, kitchen salt	10 g
Sucrose	10 g
Thymol blue 2% solution in 50% ethanol	2 ml
Bromothymol blue 2% solution in 50% ethanol	2 ml
Agar	20 g
Water	800 ml

Dissolve the yeast extract, peptone and sodium chloride in 200 ml water and adjust the pH to 8.6. Dissolve the agar in 600 ml water by steaming at 100°C. Mix the two solutions, add the indicator dyes and the sucrose and mix again. Distribute in accurate 80 ml volumes in screw-capped bottles and autoclave at 115°C for 15 min.

Solution A

Sodium citrate, $Na_3C_6H_5O_7.2H_2O$	10 g
Sodium thiosulphate, $Na_2S_2O_3.5H_2O$	10 g
Ferric citrate	1 g
Water	100 ml

Prepare with sterile precautions, heating at 60°C to facilitate solution.

Solution B

Ox bile, desiccated	8 g
Water	100 ml

Prepare with sterile precautions, heating at 60°C to facilitate solution. Batches of ox bile should be tested for suitability before use.

Complete medium. Melt 80 ml of indicator sucrose agar and, with separate sterile pipettes, add first 10 ml of solution A, mixing well, and then 10 ml of solution B, mixing well again. Pour plates immediately as the medium must not be reheated. Use the plates while they are fresh. If they have to be stored for a day or longer, keep them at 4°C in close-fitting, airtight plastic bags to exclude atmospheric carbon dioxide which lowers the pH.

As the preparation of TCBS agar from its constituents is laborious and complex, it is convenient to use a commercial dried preparation such as Oxoid TCBS Cholera Medium. Dissolve 88 g of this powder in 1 litre of distilled water by heating at 100°C. Do not autoclave. At once pour 20 ml volumes of the melted medium into Petri dishes and dry before use. Any medium not used at once should be discarded; it must not be reheated to melt it again.

Monsur's tellurite taurocholate gelatin agar

This medium (Monsur 1963) is useful for the isolation of cholera and other vibrios from faeces, rectal swabs and other contaminated materials. Classical strains of *V. cholerae* grow more freely on it than on TCBS agar. The high pH and potassium tellurite are inhibitory to most enterobacteria and Gram-positive bacteria, though proteus may form grey-centred colonies without a halo. Vibrios at 24 h show small (1–2 mm) translucent colonies with a grey-black centre and a turbid halo, at 48 h larger (3–4 mm) colonies with a black centre and well defined halo.

Taurocholate gelatin agar

Peptone, e.g. Trypticase (BBL)	10 g
Sodium chloride, NaCl	10 g
Sodium taurocholate	5 g
Sodium carbonate, Na_2CO_3	1 g
Gelatin (Difco)	30 g
Agar	15 g
Distilled water	1 litre

First dissolve the agar and the sodium chloride by heating at 100°C, then add the gelatin and other ingredients, shaking frequently until dissolved. Adjust the pH to 8.5 by the addition of sufficient sodium hydroxide 1 mol/litre solution and distribute in 100 ml volumes into 125 ml screw-capped bottles. Sterilize by autoclaving at 121°C for 15 min. The medium keeps well if stored in a cool place.

Potassium tellurite solution. Prepare a 0.5% solution of potassium tellurite (K_2TeO_3) in water and autoclave at 115°C for 20 min. This solution keeps indefinitely.

Complete medium. With sterile precautions, make a 1 in 10 dilution of the 0.5% potassium tellurite solution. Melt and cool to 50°C a 100 ml volume of the taurocholate gelatin agar and add to it, mixing well, 1 ml of the diluted (0.05%) potassium tellurite solution. While still melted, pour 20 ml volumes into plates. Use the plates soon after setting and drying or, if stored for a few days, keep in closely fitting, airtight plastic bags to exclude atmospheric carbon dioxide. The final pH of the medium should be between 8.5 and 9.2.

Dieudonné's blood alkali agar

Dieudonné's (1909) medium was the classical selective plating medium for the isolation of cholera vibrios from faeces, but has now been surpassed in effectiveness by TCBS and tellurite taurocholate gelatin agars.

Mix equal volumes of defibrinated ox blood and sodium hydroxide 1 mol/litre solution and heat at 100°C for 90 min on each of 8 successive days in a flask large enough to expose a large surface of the fluid to the air. Then allow to stand at ambient temperature for about 10 days, wherein the medium loses ammonia and absorbs carbon dioxide.

Prepare and melt a nutrient agar medium containing 1.5 times the usual concentration of agar, e.g. 2% instead of 1.3%. Cool it to 55°C. Then, to 7 volumes of the melted agar add 3 volumes of the blood-alkali mixture and pour in plates.

Salt requirements

The tolerance or requirement of different concentrations of sodium chloride in the growth medium is a useful distinguishing character of different *Vibrio* species (Table 32.1). The vibrio is tested for its ability to grow in peptone water media with different concentrations of added NaCl. Dried commercial peptones contain mostly between 2% and 10% NaCl, so that 1% peptone water made without any added NaCl may be expected to contain about 0.05% NaCl. This concentration, shown in Table 32.1 as '0% added NaCl', is too low to support the growth of the halophilic vibrios, which give increasing growth with additions of NaCl from 0.5% up to 3% or more.

Prepare a series of 1% peptone waters (pH 7.5) from a low-salt peptone and with the additions of 0%, 0.5%, 3%, 6%, 8% and 10% NaCl. Inoculate each with a loopful of a light suspension of the strain under test in sterile water and incubate at 37°C for 24 h. Recognize growth by the presence of light turbidity in the culture after mixing.

Cholera red reaction

Grow a pure culture in a tube of peptone water for 4 days at 37°C. Add a few drops of concentrated, chemically pure sulphuric or hydrochloric acid. The development of a reddish-pink colour due to the formation of nitroso-indole is characteristic of *V. cholerae* and many other vibrios.

Polymyxin sensitivity

Grow a pure culture of the vibrio in nutrient broth (pH 7.3) for 24 h at 37°C. Spread two or three drops of the culture over a plate of nutrient agar (pH 7.3). After absorption of the inoculum, gently press on to the seeded surface a 6 mm filter paper disk containing 50 units of polymyxin B (Difco). Use of a 300 unit disk has been recommended by von Graevenitz (1983). Keep the plate at 4°C for 1 h and then incubate it at 37°C for 18 h. Resistant bacteria grow right up to the margin of the disk, whilst sensitive ones show a zone of inhibition 1–3 mm wide around it.

Most vibrios, including the classical biovar of *V. cholerae*, are sensitive to polymyxin, but the El Tor biovar and *V. vulnificus* are resistant.

0/129 sensitivity

This test (Shewan et al 1954; Furniss et al 1978) differentiates *Vibrio* species and allied bacteria (Table 32.1). Compound 0/129 as originally used is 2:4 diamino 6,7 diisopropyl pteridine, but a phosphate derivative (BDH Product No. 44169) is now preferred as it is soluble in water. A disk

sensitivity test is done with two 6 mm filter paper disks, one containing 10 μg and the other 150 μg of the compound.

Prepare two solutions of the compound in water, one at a concentration of 500 mg/litre and the other at 7500 mg/litre. Place 0.02 ml drops of these solutions on different 6 mm disks and allow to dry. The disks can be stored at 4°C until required.

Spread a dilute inoculum of the bacterium under test over the surface of a plate of nutrient agar (not a low-salt sensitivity test agar), apply the 10 μg and 150 μg disks at different sites and incubate at 37°C for 24 h. Read the presence of any zone of inhibition as denoting sensitivity to the relevant dose of the compound. *V. cholerae* and other highly sensitive vibrios show sensitivity to the 10 μg as well as the 150 μg disk. Less sensitive vibrios are sensitive only to the 150 μg disk, whilst aeromonads and many other Gram-negative bacilli are resistant to both disks.

Haemagglutination test

El Tor strains of *V. cholerae* agglutinate fowl and sheep red blood cells, whilst classical strains do not cause haemagglutination unless they have aged in the laboratory or been repeatedly passaged in broth.

Prepare a 3% suspension of thrice washed red cells in 0.85% NaCl solution and place a drop of it in the depression on a white porcelain tile or on a clean glass slide. Rub into the drop a small portion of an agar slant culture of the vibrio and mix by tilting the tile to and fro. Haemagglutinating strains cause clumping of the red cells within a few seconds.

H-antigen agglutination

Cholera (O1) and non-cholera (O2–O84) strains of *V. cholerae* share the same H antigen, so that agglutination by an H antiserum identifies a strain as belonging to the species and is useful for the recognition of non-cholera strains.

Grow a pure culture on nutrient agar overnight at 37°C. Suspend portions of it in two separate large drops of phenol saline (1.5%

phenol in 0.85% NaCl) on a glass slide. After 60 s add a loopful of H-antiserum at its test dilution to one drop and a loopful of 0.85% NaCl solution to the other. Mix thoroughly with a loop. With a hand lens look for agglutination within 2 min.

If the culture is autoagglutinating, test another grown at 30°C suspended in 1.5% phenol in distilled water. Cultures should be checked for motility before testing and if poorly motile should be passed through semi-solid agar to obtain a motile line, e.g. by the Craigie tube method (Ch. 29).

METHODS FOR CAMPYLOBACTERS

Skirrow's campylobacter medium

Vancomycin	10 mg
Polymyxin B	2500 IU
Trimethoprim	5 mg
Lysed defibrinated horse blood	50 ml
Nutrient agar	1 litre

Dissolve the antibiotics in a small volume, e.g. 4 ml, of sterile distilled water. Vials of dried antibiotic mixture may be obtained commercially (e.g. Oxoid Campylobacter Selective Supplement). The recommended nutrient agar is Oxoid Blood Agar Base No. 2. Melt it, cool it to 55°C, add sterile saponin-lysed horse blood, mix gently, add the antibiotic mixture, mix again and pour in plates. The plates should be stored away from direct light, which renders blood agar toxic for campylobacters.

Preston campylobacter medium

Cycloheximide ('Actidione')	100 mg
Polymyxin B	5000 IU
Rifampicin	10 mg
Trimethoprim	10 mg
Lysed defibrinated horse blood	50 ml
Nutrient agar	1 litre

Dissolve the antibiotics in a small volume, e.g. 4 ml, of a mixture of equal parts of acetone and sterile distilled water. Vials of dried antibiotic mixture are available commercially (Oxoid). It

is recommended the nutrient agar should not contain yeast extract, in which there are trimethoprim inhibitors not wholly neutralizable by the lysed blood; Oxoid Nutrient Broth No. 2 plus 1.2% New Zealand agar is suitable. Dissolve the agar in the broth at 100°C, sterilize by autoclaving at 121°C for 15 min, cool to 50°C, add sterile saponin-lysed defibrinated horse blood, mix gently, add the antibiotic mixture, mix again and pour in plates.

Preston campylobacter enrichment broth

Cycloheximide ('Actidione')	10 mg
Polymyxin B	5000 IU
Rifampicin	10 mg
Trimethoprim	10 mg
Lysed defibrinated horse blood	50 ml
Nutrient broth	1 litre

Dissolve the antibiotics in acetone/water mixture as described for Preston Campylobacter Medium (above). The recommended nutrient broth is Oxoid Nutrient Broth No. 2. Sterilize it by autoclaving, cool it to 50°C, add sterile saponin-lysed defibrinated horse blood and the antibiotic mixture, and distribute aseptically in 10 ml volumes in test tubes or 5 ml volumes in 6 ml screw-capped bottles. The medium may be stored for up to 7 days at 4°C.

Campylobacter aerotolerance growth supplement

Ferrous sulphate, $FeSO_4.7H_2O$	0.25 g
Sodium metabisulphite	0.25 g
Sodium pyruvate	0.25 g

This supplement (George et al 1978; Hoffman et al 1979) may be added to each 1 litre of campylobacter medium, e.g. Preston Campylobacter Medium or Preston Campylobacter Enrichment Broth, when the microaerophilic incubation atmosphere is procured by an imprecise method, as in a candle jar. Vials of dried mixture are available commercially (e.g. from Oxoid). It should be dissolved in a small volume, e.g. 4 ml, of sterile distilled water and added with sterile precautions to the sterilized and cooled medium.

Inocula for identification tests

Skirrow & Benjamin (1980a) recommend growing the isolate for 24 h at 37°C on a plate of Oxoid Blood Agar Base No. 2 plus 5% defibrinated horse blood and suspending some of the growth in nutrient broth plus the aerotolerance growth supplement to a density matching Brown's opacity standard No. 8 (about 5×10^9 bacilli/ml). Large loopfuls or drops of this suspension may be used to inoculate test media.

Temperature requirements

Campylobacter isolates should be tested for the ability to grow at 25°C, 37°C and 42°C. Preliminary tests may be made on blood agar plates held for 4 days in microaerophilic jars in incubators at the test temperatures. Definitive tests should be made on cultures in deep tubes of Brewer's thioglycollate medium (Ch. 6) incubated for 4 days in waterbaths held at the required temperatures with an accuracy of ± 0.5°C.

Nalidixic acid sensitivity

Perform the test on a nutrient or blood agar plate (e.g. Oxoid Blood Agar Base No. 2). Soak a swab in the dense inoculum suspension described above, press out excess fluid on the side of the tube and then rub the swab over the plate. Apply a 30 μg nalidixic acid test disk and incubate the plate in a microaerophilic atmosphere at 37°C for 42–48 h. Sensitive organisms,

e.g. *C. jejuni*, show a clear zone of inhibition of growth a few mm wide, whilst resistant organisms, e.g. *C. fetus*, grow right up to the disk. Instead of a disk, a strip of heavy filter paper soaked in a 0.06 g/litre solution of nalidixic acid and dried may be applied to the unseeded plate and several isolates tested by inoculating them in streaks at right angles to the strip.

TTC sensitivity

Prepare a plate of nutrient agar (e.g. Oxoid Blood Agar Base No. 2) containing 0.4 g/litre 2,3,5-triphenyltetrazolium chloride. Inoculate suspensions of the isolate under test and, as controls, a TTC-sensitive and a TTC-resistant campylobacter on separate areas of the plate. Incubate in a microaerophilic atmosphere for 42–48 h at 37°C. Read absence of growth as denoting sensitivity.

Hippurate hydrolysis

Grow the isolate under test on blood agar for 18 h at 37°C in a microaerophilic atmosphere. Suspend a 2 mm loopful of the colonial growth in 2 ml distilled water. Add 0.5 ml of a 5% solution of sodium hippurate. Incubate for 2 h in a waterbath at 37°C. Then add 1 ml of a solution of 3.5 g ninhydrin in 100 ml of a mixture of equal parts of acetone and butanol. Leave for 2 h at room temperature. Then read the development of a purple colour as indicating that the isolate has hydrolysed the hippurate to form glycine.

REFERENCES

Agger W A, McCormick J D, Gurwith M J 1985 Clinical and microbiological features of *Aeromonas hydrophila*-associated diarrhoea. Journal of Clinical Microbiology 21: 909–913

Ayres P A, Barrow G I 1978 The distribution of *Vibrio parahaemolyticus* in British coastal waters: report of a collaborative study 1975–6. Journal of Hygiene, Cambridge 80: 281–294

Basu S, Mukerjee S 1968 Bacteriophage typing of *Vibrio eltor*. Experientia 24: 299–300

Basu S, Mukerjee S 1970 A specific phage for pathogenic *Vibrio cholerae*, biotype El Tor (phi-H74–64). World Health Organization Bulletin 43: 509–512

Blaser M J, Hardesty H L, Powers B, Wang W L 1980 Survival of *Campylobacter fetus* subsp. *jejuni* in biological milieus. Journal of Clinical Microbiology 11: 309–313

Blaser M J, Reller L B 1981 Campylobacter enteritis. New England Journal of Medicine 305: 1444–1452

Bolton F J, Coates D, Hinchcliffe P M, Robertson L 1983 Comparison of selective media for isolation of *Campylobacter jejuni/coli*. Journal of Clinical Pathology 36: 78–83

Bolton F J, Robertson L 1982 A selective medium for isolating *Campylobacter jejuni/coli*. Journal of Clinical Pathology 35: 462–467

Buck G E 1984 Recent taxonomic changes in the genus *Campylobacter*. Clinical Microbiology Newsletter 6: 119–120

Butzler J P, Skirrow M B 1979 Campylobacter enteritis. Clinics in Gastroenterology 8: 737–765

Dieudonné A 1909 Blutalkaliagar, ein Elektivnährboden für Choleravibrionen. Zentralblatt für Bakteriologie Abt I Originale 50:107

Ellington E P, Wood J G, Hill E O 1982 Disease caused by a marine vibrio – *Vibrio vulnificus*. New England Journal of Medicine 307:1642

Field M 1971 Intestinal secretion: effect of cyclic AMP and its role in cholera. New England Journal of Medicine 284: 1137–1144

Finkelstein R A, Mukerjee S 1963 A rapid method of differentiating *Vibrio cholerae* and El Tor vibrios. Proceedings of the Society for Experimental Biology, New York 112: 355–359

Furniss A L, Lee J V, Donovan T J 1978 The Vibrios. Public Health Laboratory Service Monograph Series, London, No. 11: 1–58

George H A, Hoffman P S, Smibert R M, Krieg N R 1978 Improved media for growth and aerotolerance of *Campylobacter fetus*. Journal of Clinical Microbiology 8: 35–41

Gilardi G L 1983 Aeromonas and Plesiomonas. Clinical Microbiology Newsletter 5: 49–51

Gracey M, Burke V, Rockhill R C, Suharyong Sunoto 1982 *Aeromonas* species as enteric pathogens. Lancet 1: 223–224

Han G K, Khie T S 1963 A new method for the differentiation of *Vibrio comma* and *Vibrio El Tor*. American Journal of Hygiene 77: 184–186

Hoffman P S, Krieg N R, Smibert R M 1979 Studies of the microaerophilic nature of *Campylobacter fetus* subsp. *jejuni*. I. Physiological aspects of enhanced aerotolerance. Canadian Journal of Microbiology 25: 1–7

Holmgren J, Svennerholm A M, Ouchterlony O 1971 Quantitation of vibriocidal antibodies using agar plaque techniques. Acta Pathologica Microbiologica Scandinavica, Section B, 79: 708–714

Jones D M, Abbott J D, Painter M J, Sutcliffe E M 1984 A comparison of biotypes and serotypes of *Campylobacter* spp. isolated from patients with enteritis and from animal and environmental sources. Journal of Infection 9: 51–58

King E O 1957 Human infections with *Vibrio fetus* and a closely related vibrio. Journal of Infectious Diseases 101: 119–128

King E O 1962 The laboratory recognition of *Vibrio fetus* and a closely related vibrio isolated from cases of human vibriosis. Annals of the New York Academy of Sciences 8: 700–711

Kobayashi T, Enomoto S, Sakazaki R, Kuwahara S 1963 A new selective isolation medium for the Vibrio group, on a modified Nakanishi's medium (TCBS agar medium). Japanese Journal of Bacteriology 18: 387–392

Krieg N R 1981 The genera *Spirillum*, *Aquaspirillum*, and *Oceanospirillum*. In: Starr M P, Stolp H, Trüper H P, Balows A, Schlegel H G (eds) The Prokaryotes. Springer-Verlag, Berlin. ch 52, p 595–596

Langenberg M-L, Tytgat G N, Schipper M E I, Rietra P J G M, Zanen H C 1984 Campylobacter-like organisms in the stomach of patients and healthy individuals. Lancet 1:1348

Lauwers S, De Boeck M, Butzler J P 1978 Campylobacter enteritis in Brussels. Lancet 1: 604–605

Lior H, Woodward D L, Edgar J A, Laroche L J, Gill P 1982 Serotyping of *Campylobacter jejuni* by slide agglutination based on heat-labile factors. Journal of Clinical Microbiology 15: 761–768

McNulty C A M, Gearty J G, Crump B, Davis M, Donovan I A, Melikian V, Lister D M, Wise R 1986 *Campylobacter pyloridis* and associated gastritis: investigator blind, placebo controlled trial of bismuth salicylate and erythromycin ethyl succinate. British Medical Journal 293: 645–649

McNulty C A M, Wise R 1985 Rapid diagnosis of campylobacter associated gastritis. Lancet 1: 1443–1444

Mandal B K, Whale K, Morson B C 1982 Acute colitis due to *Plesiomonas shigelloides*. British Medical Journal 285: 1539–1540

Marshall B J, Warren J R 1984 Unidentified curved bacilli in the stomach of patients with gastritis and peptic ulceration. Lancet 1: 1311–1314

Miyamoto Y, Kato T, Obara Y, Akiyama S, Takizawa K, Yamai S 1969 In vitro hemolytic characteristic of *Vibrio parahaemolyticus*: its close correlation with human pathogenicity. Journal of Bacteriology 100: 1147–1149

Monsur K A 1963 Bacteriological diagnosis of cholera under field conditions. World Health Organization Bulletin 28: 387–389

Moulsdale M T 1983 Isolation of Aeromonas from faeces. Lancet 1:351

Mukerjee S 1961 Diagnostic uses of cholera bacteriophages. Journal of Hygiene, Cambridge 59: 109–115

Owen R J 1983 Nucleic acid in the classification of campylobacters. European Journal of Clinical Microbiology 2: 367–377

Peffers A S R, Bailey J, Barrow G I, Hobbs B C 1973 *Vibrio parahaemolyticus*: gastroenteritis and international air travel. Lancet 1: 143–145

Penner J L, Hennessy J N 1980 Passive haemagglutination techniques for serotyping *Campylobacter fetus* subsp. *jejuni* on the basis of soluble heat-stable antigens. Journal of Clinical Microbiology 12: 732–737

Robinson D A 1981 Infective dose of *Campylobacter jejuni* in milk. British Medical Journal 282:1584

Robinson D A, Jones D M 1981 Milk-borne campylobacter infection. British Medical Journal 282: 1374–1376

Sakazaki R, Balows A 1981 The genera *Vibrio*, *Plesiomonas*, and *Aeromonas*. In: Starr M P, Stolp H, Trüper H P, Balows A, Schlegel H G (eds) The Prokaryotes. Springer-Verlag, Berlin. ch 103, p 1272–1301

Sakazaki R, Tamura K 1971 Somatic antigen variation in *Vibrio cholerae*. Japanese Journal of Medical Science and Biology 24: 93–100

Sakazaki R, Tamura K, Murase M 1971 Determination of the haemolytic activity of *Vibrio cholerae*. Japanese Journal of Medical Science and Biology 24: 83–91

Shewan J M, Hodgkiss W, Liston J 1954 A method for the rapid differentiation of certain non-pathogenic asporogenous bacilli. Nature, London 173: 208–209

Skirrow M B 1977 Campylobacter enteritis: a 'new' disease. British Medical Journal 2: 9–11

Skirrow M B 1982 Campylobacter enteritis – the first 5 years. Journal of Hygiene, Cambridge 89: 175–184

Skirrow M B, Benjamin J 1980a '1001' campylobacters:

cultural characteristics of intestinal campylobacters from man and animals. Journal of Hygiene, Cambridge 85: 427–442

Skirrow M B, Benjamin J 1980b Differentiation of enteropathogenic campylobacter. Journal of Clinical Pathology 33: 1122

Tsukamoto T, Kinoshita Y, Shimada T, Sakazaki R 1978 Two epidemics of diarrhoeal disease possibly caused by *Plesiomonas shigelloides*. Journal of Hygiene, Cambridge 80: 275–280

Von Graevenitz A 1983 Clinical microbiology of *Vibrio* species. Clinical Microbiology Newsletter 5: 49–51

Von Graevenitz A, Bucher C 1983 Evaluation of differential and selective media for isolation of *Aeromonas* and *Plesiomonas* spp. Journal of Clinical Microbiology 17: 16–21

World Health Organization Bacterial Diseases Unit 1974 Guidelines for the laboratory diagnosis of cholera. World Health Organization, Geneva

Brucella

Brucellae are intracellular parasites that infect a wide variety of domestic and free-living animals and may be transmitted to man. There are four species of *Brucella* which can infect man by direct or indirect contact with infected animals. *B. melitensis* is the classical species of the genus and is usually pathogenic for sheep and goats but may also infect cattle. *B. abortus* infects cattle, usually causing abortions in unvaccinated animals; it may also infect a wide variety of other animals including sheep, goats, horses and dogs. *B. suis* infections are reported mainly from North America and Scandinavia; they are primarily infections of pigs. *B. canis* was first isolated in North America from colonies of beagle dogs where it caused outbreaks of abortion and epididymo-orchitis. *B. ovis* and *B. neotomae* do not cause disease in man.

Morphology and staining

Small round or oval cocco-bacilli, about 0.4 μm in diameter, but bacilli 1–2 μm in length may also be seen. Arranged singly; sometimes in pairs, short chains or small clusters. Do not produce capsules, spores or flagella. Fimbriae have not been described. Gram negative; do not usually show bipolar staining; not acid-fast but may resist decolourization by weak solutions of acids or alkalis. A modified Zichl-Neelsen stain is used for screening placentas and other products of abortion.

Cultural characters

Most brucella strains grow poorly on peptone media; growth improved by the addition of serum. Temperature range 20–40°C, optimum 37°C. Brucellae are strictly aerobic organisms but many strains of *B. abortus* require the addition of 5–10% CO_2, especially on primary isolation. On solid culture media colonies may take 2–3 days to develop; they are small, smooth, transparent, low convex with an entire edge.

The isolation of brucellae from milk, dairy products or clinical material usually requires selective agars (described below); comparative trials have shown that these are a satisfactory alternative to guinea-pig inoculation methods.

Viability

Killed after heating at 60°C for 10 min; hence killed in milk by pasteurization. Moderately sensitive to acid and die out in most cheeses involving lactic acid fermentation. Very sensitive to sunlight but may persist in soil or dust for 2–3 months and for longer periods in dead fetal material. Sensitive to many antibiotics including ampicillin, cephalosporins, aminoglycosides, tetracyclines, chloramphenicol, ciprofloxacin, sulphonamides and cotrimoxazole; relatively resistant to vancomycin and polymyxins.

Biochemical reactions

Catalase positive; usually oxidase positive but some strains of *B. abortus* are negative. Urea hydrolysis is variable but often very rapid, especially with strains of *B. suis*. Most strains reduce nitrates to nitrites except *B. ovis*. Brucellae do not ferment carbohydrates in conventional media; oxidative metabolism is the main energy-yielding process.

Table 33.1 Classification into biotypes of *Brucella* species pathogenic to man (see *Methods*).

Species	Biotype	CO$_2$ requirement	H$_2$S production	Thionin a	Thionin b	Thionin c	Basic fuchsin b	Basic fuchsin c	Agglutination A	Agglutination M	Lysis by phage Tb at RTD	Primary host
B. melitensis	1	−	−	−	+	+	+	+	−	+	−	Sheep, goats
	2	−	−	−	+	+	+	+	+	−	−	Sheep, goats
	3	−	−	−	+	+	+	+	+	+	−	Sheep, goats
B. abortus[b]	1	+(−)	+	−	−	−	+	+	+	−	+	Cattle
	2	−(+)	+	−	−	−	−	−	+	−	+	Cattle
	3	+(−)	+	+	+	+	+	+	+	−	+	Cattle
	4	+(−)	+	−	−	−	+	+	−	+	+	Cattle
	5	−	−	−	+	+	+	+	−	+	+	Cattle
	6	−	−(+)	−	+	+	+	+	+	−	+	Cattle
	7	−	+(−)	−	+	+	+	+	+	+	+	Cattle
	9	−	+	−	+	+	+	+	−	+	+	Cattle
B. suis	1	−	++	+	+	+	−	−	+	−	−	Pigs
	2	−	−	−	+	+	−	−	+	−	−	Pigs, hares
	3	−	−	+	+	+	+	+	+	−	−	Pigs
	4	−	−	+	+	+	−	−	+	+	−	Reindeer
B. canis	1	−	−	+	+	+	−	±	−	−	−	Dogs

[a] Dye concentrations: a, 1 in 25 000; b, 1 in 50 000; c, 1 in 100 000.
[b] *B. abortus* biotype 8 is no longer recognized.

Classification of brucellae

Brucellae may be categorized into species and biotypes by the following tests (see Table 33.1): (1) CO$_2$ requirement; (2) H$_2$S production; (3) inhibition by bacteriostatic dyes; (4) agglutination reaction with monospecific sera; (5) lysis by specific bacteriophage.

Most brucella strains isolated during the course of diagnostic procedures or epidemiological investigations can be readily identified as members of the genus *Brucella* by the colonial morphology and Gram stain appearance, agglutination with specific antiserum and lysis by specific phage. Oxidative metabolic tests with manometric techniques may be essential for the satisfactory identification and classification of aberrant brucella strains. These techniques require specialized expertise to perform and interpret and may be particularly hazardous because of the increased risk of accidental infection. Identification and biotyping are best undertaken in a reference laboratory, e.g. the Central Veterinary Laboratory, New Haw, Weybridge, KT15 3NB, for strains isolated in the UK.

Variation

Whilst typical virulent brucellae produce colonies which are smooth and transparent, growth on laboratory media may result in spontaneous dissociation to non-smooth variants. The non-smooth variants include intermediate (I), rough (R) and mucoid (M) variants. Non-smooth variants may show loss of virulence, and R and M strains will not agglutinate with homologous antisera prepared against smooth strains. *B. abortus*, *B. melitensis* and *B. suis* are almost always smooth on primary isolation; *B. canis* is invariably non-smooth but can be agglutinated with antiserum prepared with R strains.

Laboratory diagnosis

Man is usually infected with brucella organisms either by direct contact with infected animals or indirectly by infected dairy products or by accidental exposure to animal vaccines or laboratory isolates. The organism must be handled with particular care and under appropriate containment conditions in the laboratory. Human brucellosis can vary from an acute febrile illness to a chronic, low-grade, ill defined disease.

Culture of brucellae

An attempt should always be made to isolate brucellae from patient's blood during the febrile stages of the disease. Approximately 5 ml of blood should be inoculated into each of 4 blood culture bottles containing serum dextrose (SD) broth*, on 3 successive days. The bottles should be subcultured twice a week for 8 weeks on to SD agar.* The Castaneda blood culture technique may be useful in reducing the risk of contamination during the long incubation period. When *B. abortus* infection is a possibility incubation should be in an atmosphere with added CO_2. Blood cultures should be maintained for at least 8 weeks before they are discarded as negative. In *B. abortus* infections, blood cultures are often negative even when satisfactory blood culture systems have been used. Isolation rates can be markedly improved if material from bone marrow or liver biopsy is also cultured. Brucellae may also be isolated by inoculation into guinea-pigs.*

Serological tests

In the absence of an isolate of the infecting organism from the blood or other clinical material, serological investigation of the patient is of paramount importance for diagnosis of the disease and the future management of the patient.

Brucella antibodies can be detected by a variety of serological tests. The most widely used are the standard agglutination test (SAT)* and the complement fixation test (CFT);* additional information can be obtained from the mercaptoethanol (ME) agglutination* and anti-human globulin (Coombs) tests*. More recently radioimmune assay (RIA) and enzyme-linked immunosorbent assay (ELISA) have been shown to be useful in the diagnosis of brucellosis, but these should be regarded as specialized reference laboratory techniques.

As brucella antibodies may be detectable for many years after acute or subclinical infection, the possibility of residual antibody from a previous infection must be borne in mind when considering the significance of brucella antibodies in a patient's serum. In persons whose symptoms are of recent onset the presence of low titres of brucella antibodies may be significant and in such instances a rising titre may be demonstrated by either the SAT or the CFT and

* Refer to *Methods* at end of this chapter.

can be of considerable help in confirming the clinical diagnosis. It is at this stage of the disease that a significant amount of specific IgM antibody is present; this is indicated by the presence of ME-sensitive agglutinins or can be shown more directly by RIA or ELISA.

Patients with brucellosis may have been ill for many weeks or months before a diagnosis of brucellosis is considered. In these cases the antibody titres are often high, with agglutinating titres exceeding 640 in both SAT and ME agglutination tests, and usually with high CFT titres also. In the chronic stage of the disease brucella antibodies persist for many years after infection; in most cases only ME-sensitive agglutinins persist. Serological findings in the investigation of chronic brucellosis are difficult to interpret as they may be attributable to previous infection and not to chronic infection.

Other tests

Other tests which may be of value although not themselves diagnostic are the *brucellin skin test*, which detects delayed hypersensitivity reaction to brucella antigens, and a *liver biopsy*, which may show the presence of granulomata.

METHODS

Serum dextrose (SD) agar

Base medium

Davies' New Zealand agar	15 g
Bacteriological Peptone (Oxoid)	10 g
Lab-Lemco Extract (Oxoid)	5 g
NaCl	5 g
Distilled water	1 litre

Adjust the pH of the medium to 7.5 and sterilize at 121°C for 20 min. Enrich the base medium with 1% glucose and 5% inactivated horse serum before dispensing into Petri dishes, or into tubes for slants.

SD broth, omitting the agar, may be used as a liquid medium, e.g. for blood culture.

Selective media

Table 33.2 details the composition of five selective media recommended for isolation of

Table 33.2 Composition of selective media for isolation of *Brucella* species.

Selective agent	Concentration of selective agent in basal medium				
	Hartley's digest agar[a]	Serum dextrose agar[b]	5% blood agar[c]	Serum dextrose agar[d]	Tryptone soya broth with 5% horse serum[e]
Bacitracin (units/ml)	—	25	—	25	20
Penicillin (units/ml)	5	—	5	—	—
Vancomycin (μg/ml)	—	—	—	20	20
Ristocetin (μg/ml)	—	—	10	—	—
Polymyxin B (units/ml)	6	4	10	5	5
Nalidixic acid (μg/ml)	—	—	10	5	5
Cetrimide	—	—	1:40 000	—	—
Nystatin (units/ml)	—	—	100	100	100
Amphotericin (μg/ml)	—	10	—	—	4
Cycloheximide (μg/ml)	100	100	150	100	100
Gentian violet (μg/ml)	4	—	—	—	—

[a] Mair (1955)
[b] Leech et al (1964)
[c] Ryan (1967)
[d] Farrell (1969)
[e] Brodie & Sinton (1975).

brucellae. On these media colonies are usually visible after 4–5 days and are 1–2 mm in diameter; on further incubation they increase in size to 4–6 mm. On media that contain gentian violet the colonies are a blue to violet colour with an almost black centre; on SD media without dyes the colonies are translucent, pale yellow colour.

Guinea-pig inoculation

The guinea-pig is the laboratory animal most susceptible to brucellae; the infection is not usually progressive and infected animals may recover spontaneously. A small quantity of prepared biological material is inoculated into the thigh of a guinea-pig. When the animal is killed after 6–8 weeks the lymph nodes in the region of the inoculated site may be enlarged and should be cultured. The spleen should also be cultured by rubbing the cut surface on to the surface of SD agar containing 10 units of bacitracin and 4 units of polymyxin B to suppress contaminants. Blood collected from the jugular vein can be examined for the presence of brucella antibodies.

Tests for identification of brucellae

The tests used for identification and biotyping of *Brucella* species are given in Table 33.1. When identifying unknown strains it is essential to include the WHO prototype strains *B. abortus* 544, *B. melitensis* 16M and *B. suis* 1330. Prepare a suspension of the test strain in 1.5 ml of sterile 0.85% NaCl to give *c*. 10^8 colony-forming units/ml. This is the inoculum for each of the following tests.

1. *CO_2 requirement*. Seed two SD agar plates; incubate both at 37°C, one aerobically and the other in air containing 10% added CO_2. The plates are examined after 4 days incubation and the requirement for CO_2 is recorded.

2. *H_2S production*. Seed an SD agar slope in a tube bearing a lead acetate paper strip held by a loose cap. Incubate the tube in air + 10% CO_2 and examine for the presence of H_2S daily for 4 days. Change the lead acetate strip after each examination, to avoid confusion by the small amounts of H_2S some strains of biotype 5 may produce on the first day.

3. *Dye sensitivity*. Prepare a series of SD agar plates containing thionin at final concentrations of 1 in 25 000, 1 in 50 000 and 1 in 100 000, and another series containing basic fuchsin at 1 in 50 000 and 1 in 100 000. Seed each plate, including a control SD agar plate, with strains to be tested using a cotton-wool swab soaked in the prepared inoculum. The plates are examined after 4 days incubation.

4. *Reaction with monospecific serum*. Antigens

designated A and M (Wilson & Miles 1932) are present in all strains of brucellae but in varying proportions. The predominant antigen in a strain can be determined in a tube agglutination test by testing a killed suspension in mercuric iodide (0.1%) against absorbed monospecific antisera to A and M antigens.

5. *Lysis by bacteriophage.* A standard reference phage, Tbilisi (Tb), is used at RTD (Routine Test Dilution).

Isolation from milk and dairy products

Direct culture

The culture of overnight gravity cream has proved more successful for the isolation of brucellae from cow's milk than culture from centrifuged deposits.

1. Transfer the milk sample to a sterile test tube (180 × 25 mm) and keep at 4°C overnight.

2. Dip a sterile cotton-wool swab into the gravity cream layer and spread it over the surface of well dried selective agar until the fluid has been absorbed.

3. Incubate the plates in air containing 10% CO_2 at 37°C and examine every 2 days for 10 days.

It is advisable to use two selective agars for each specimen; the media of choice are those described by Farrell (1969), Ryan (1967) and Mair (1955; see Table 33.2).

Fluid enrichment

1. Seed each of two or three bottles of 5 ml broth prepared as described by Brodie & Sinton (1975; see Table 33.2) with 0.2 ml of a mixture of the cream layer and deposit from centrifuged milk.

2. Incubate the broths, with the screw caps loose, in air containing 10% CO_2 for 5 days at 37°C.

3. Subculture the broth cultures to a suitable selective agar and incubate in air containing 10% CO_2 for 3 days at 37°C. A more complete account of techniques for the isolation of brucellae from contaminated sources is given by Robertson et al (1980).

Standard agglutination test (SAT)

The procedure is described in detail by Robertson et al (1980). Agglutinins detected in the patient's serum by this test are usually either IgM or IgG. In some sera a blocking factor may interfere with agglutination at low serum dilutions (the prozone phenomenon); this may be due to the presence of IgA (Drutz & Graybill 1976) or other non-agglutinating antibody. False negative results due to this prozone phenomenon can be avoided by testing a series of two-fold dilutions of (uninactivated) serum from 1 in 20 to 1 in 640 in 0.4% phenol saline. Standardized antigen suspension should be used and it is advisable to control each batch of tests with a standardized control serum (e.g. from CPHL, London, or a regional WHO reference centre). The agglutination reactions should be read after 48 h incubation at 37°C. Reactions of partial or complete clearing with agglutination visible with naked eye after gentle agitation of the deposit should be reported as positive; it is important that trace reactions should not be taken as the endpoint of the titration.

Mercaptoethanol (ME) agglutination test

2-mercaptoethanol reduces the disulphide bonds that link IgM molecules to release the subunits. This test estimates the titre of those agglutinins that remain reactive in the presence of ME. The procedure is the same as for the SAT except that the serum dilutions are prepared in 0.85% NaCl containing 0.05 mol/litre ME.

Complement fixation test (CFT)

The test is set up in WHO pattern or similar plastic trays with 80 round-bottomed wells of approximately 1 ml capacity (see Robertson et al 1980). It is a four volume test; a convenient volume is 0.1 ml. Brucella antigen suspensions used for the SAT are suitable if diluted to an optimum concentration as determined by chessboard titrations (see Ch. 49). The long fixation technique at 4°C is recommended with 1.5 haemolytic units of complement when titrated in the presence of antigen and pooled negative serum. A suspension of 2% sensitized sheep red cells is a suitable haemolytic indicator system.

Anti-human globulin (Coombs) test

Serum may contain brucella antibodies which, though combining with receptor sites on the particulate bacterial antigen, do not produce agglutination. These so-called 'incomplete' antibodies can be detected by the addition of rabbit anti-human globulin (Coombs reagent) to antigen coated with such antibodies; the interaction will result in agglutination of the bacterial suspension. The test should be considered positive when there is at least a four-fold difference between it and the SAT titre.

1. Set out a row of seven round-bottomed glass tubes (50 × 9 mm).

2. Into the first tube pipette 0.9 ml sodium barbitone (Veronal) diluent (Oxoid, code BR. 16).

3. Into each of the remaining six tubes pipette 0.5 ml barbitone diluent.

· 4. Into the first tube pipette 0.1 ml of test serum (uninactivated).

5. Prepare two-fold dilutions of serum, discarding the 0.5 ml from the sixth tube; the seventh tube is an antigen control.

6. Prepare the *B. abortus* antigen by diluting the standardized concentrated '0' suspension (Division of microbiological reagents and quality control, CPHL, London) 1 in 5 in barbitone diluent.

7. Into each tube pipette 0.5 ml of diluted *B. abortus* antigen.

8. Incubate the tubes in a covered water bath at 37°C for 24 h.

9. Examine the tubes, record, and discard any showing agglutination.

10. Centrifuge the tubes at 1500 *g* for 20 min.

11. Pour off the supernatant and drain each tube by pressing the rim of the inverted tube against a sheet of filter paper.

12. Add 1 ml of barbitone diluent to each tube and resuspend the deposit with a vortex mixer.

13. Repeat procedures 10, 11 and 12 twice more, and then repeat 10 and 11 once more.

14. Add 0.9 ml of barbitone diluent to each tube. Resuspend the deposit and add 0.1 ml of Coombs reagent diluted so that the final dilution in the tubes is that recommended by the manufacturer.

15. Incubate in a covered water bath at 37°C for 24 h.

The endpoint of the titration is the greatest serum dilution to give partial or complete agglutination. This test is not affected by the prozone phenomenon.

REFERENCES

Brodie J E, Sinton G P 1975 Fluid and solid media for the isolation of *Brucella abortus*. Journal of Hygiene, Cambridge 74: 359–367

Drutz D J, Graybill J R 1976 Infectious diseases. In: Fudenberg H H, Stiles D P, Caldwell J L, Wells J V (eds) Basic and clinical immunology. Lange Medical, Los Altos, USA. p 511

Farrell I D 1969 The development of a new selective medium for the isolation of *Brucella abortus* from contaminated sources. Research in Veterinary Science 16: 280–286

Leech F B, Vessey M P, Macrae W D, Lawson J R, Mackinnon D J, Morgan W J B 1964 Brucellosis in the British dairy herd. Ministry of Agriculture, Fisheries and Food, Animal Disease Surveys Report No 4. HMSO, London

Mair N S 1955 A selective medium for the isolation of *Brucella abortus* from herd samples of milk. Monthly Bulletin of the Ministry of Health and the Public Health Laboratory Service 14: 184–191

Robertson L, Farrell I D, Hinchliffe P M, Quaife R A 1980 Benchbook on *Brucella*. PHLS Monograph Series No 14. HMSO, London

Ryan W J 1967 A selective medium for the isolation of *Brucella abortus* from milk. Monthly Bulletin of the Ministry of Health and the Public Health Laboratory Service 26: 33–38

Wilson G S, Miles A A 1932 The serological differentiation of smooth strains of the brucella group. British Journal of Experimental Pathology 13: 1–13

Yersinia: Pasteurella: Francisella

These three groups of organisms were previously classified together within the genus *Pasteurella*, but some of the species are now considered to be so closely related and to have sufficient distinctive characteristics from the others to warrant their inclusion in a separate genus, *Yersinia*. Thus the plague bacillus, previously known as *P. pestis*, and the causative organism of pseudotuberculosis of guinea-pigs and other animals (*P. pseudotuberculosis*) are now referred to as *Y. pestis* and *Y. pseudotuberculosis* respectively and grouped with *Y. enterocolitica*, an organism that in recent years has been recognized as a cause of enteritis and mesenteric lymphadenitis in man. The bacillus of tularaemia of animals and man now forms a new genus *Francisella* and is known as *F. tularensis*. The genus *Pasteurella* is now restricted to a number of animal pathogens, notably *P. multocida* (*P. septica*), the cause of septicaemic diseases in a variety of animal species. It is of medical importance because it is transmissible to man through contact with infected animals, especially through animal bites. The three genera show differences in the G+C content of DNA, viz. *Yersinia*, 46–47 moles %; *Pasteurella* (except *P. haemolytica*), 37–41 moles %; *Francisella*, 33–36 moles %.

All of these species are small Gram-negative bacilli, some of which show extreme variations in size and shape (involution forms) that are particularly marked in older cultures. When stained with methylene blue, bipolar staining is a characteristic feature. The main distinguishing features of the five species that are of medical importance are shown in Table 34.1.

YERSINIA PESTIS

Y. pestis (*P. pestis*) is the cause of wild, sylvatic plague in many species of wild rodents in various parts of the world. Human plague arises either as a zoonosis through the transfer of infection from rats to man through the bites of infected rat fleas (*Xenopsylla cheopsis*) resulting in bubonic plague, or through droplet infection that gives rise to the highly contagious pneumonic plague that spreads from person to person independently of rats and fleas. Septicaemic plague may also occur either primarily or as a complication of the other two forms.

Morphology and staining

Characteristic morphology is seen best in films made directly from tissues or exudate; short oval coccobacillus with rounded ends, about 1.5 × 0.7 μm, occurring singly or in pairs. On culture, especially in old cultures, pleomorphism is marked, e.g. enlarged, elongated or irregular cells, some of which may be pear-shaped or globular and suggestive of yeast cells. Involution in culture can be hastened by the addition of 3% NaCl and this phenomenon may be used as a means of identification. In fluid culture the bacilli tend to form chains. Capsulate, non-motile, non-sporing, Gram-negative. In smears from the tissues stained with methylene blue the bacilli show characteristic bipolar staining, but in culture the bipolar staining is less obvious and involution forms stain only faintly. In exudates from lesions *Y. pestis* exhibits typical capsules; less obvious in culture although capsules may be

Table 34.1 Criteria for differentiation of *Yersinia*, *Pasteurella* and *Francisella* species.

Species	Growth on routine nutrient medium	Growth on bile-salt medium	Motility at		Acid (no gas) from		Salicin	Indole	Urease	Oxidase	Catalase	ONPG	Ornithine decarboxylase
			22°C	37°C	Maltose	Sucrose							
Y. pestis	+	+	−	−	+	−	+	−	−	−	+	+	−
Y. pseudotuberculosis	+	+	+	−	+	−	+	−	+	−	+	+	−
Y. enterocolitica	+	+	+	−	+ᵃ	+	−	−	+	+/−	+	+	+
P. multocida	+	−	−	−	−	+	−	+	−	+/−	+	−	+
P. pneumotropica	+	−	−	−	+	+	−	+	+	+	+	+	+
P. haemolytica	+	+/−	−	−	−	+	−	−	−	+	+/−	+	+
P. ureae	+	−	−	−	−	+	−	−	+	+	+	−	+
F. tularensis	−	−	−	−	+	−	⋯	−	−	⋯	±	⋯	−

ᵃ Late reaction.

seen in cultures grown at 37°C rather than at the optimum temperature of 27°C.

Cultural characters

Aerobe and facultative anaerobe. Somewhat sensitive to free oxygen and growth may not develop on the surface of an agar plate if the inoculum is small. This inhibition may be avoided by the addition to the medium of blood or 0.025% sodium sulphite or by incubating anaerobically. Temperature range 14–37°C; optimum temperature for primary culture 27°C. Colonies on blood agar are at first very small, transparent, white circular disks, 1 mm or less in diameter but later enlarging to 3 or 4 mm and becoming opaque. In older cultures the mixture of opaque and transparent colonies gives the appearance of a mixed growth.

In broth, growth results in a granular deposit at the bottom and on the sides of the tube. If a drop of oil is allowed to float on the surface of an inoculated flask of broth, a characteristic growth develops, consisting of 'stalactites' hanging down from the oil drop. Like the other yersinias, but unlike *Pasteurella* and *Francisella* species, *Y. pestis* grows on MacConkey medium, but the colonies disappear after 2–3 days probably as a result of autolysis.

Sensitivity

Killed at 55°C in 5 min and by 0.5% phenol in 15 min. Very susceptible to drying but laboratory cultures remain viable for months if kept moist and at low temperature; the risk of laboratory infection from pathological material or cultures is considerable. Sensitive to tetracycline, the drug of choice for bubonic and pneumonic plague, given in large doses (4–6 g daily) during the first 2 days of illness; sensitive to sulphonamides which, however, are not effective for the treatment of pneumonic plague; sensitive to streptomycin; but resistant to penicillin.

Biochemical reactions

Because of poor growth in peptone water, sugar fermentation reactions may take up to 2 weeks to complete. Acid, with no gas, produced in glucose, mannitol, maltose, but not in sucrose, dulcitol or lactose. Other reactions are shown in Table 34.1.

Antigenic structure

It is not possible to distinguish between virulent and avirulent strains of *Y. pestis* serologically; a close antigenic relationship exists with *Y. pseudotuberculosis* through common antigens so that cross-reactions take place in agglutination tests. Two main antigenic complexes, including many antigens, are associated with virulence and immunogenicity. One is somatic and heat stable; it develops at 20°C and 37°C. The other is associated with the capsule (envelope), is heat-labile and develops best at 37°C. The capsular antigen is necessary for efficient vaccine production. It contains the immunogenic fraction F_1 that can be obtained as a non-toxic capsular component from saline extracts of acetone-dried cultures. Fraction F_1 also contributes to the virulence of capsulated organisms because of its antiphagocytic activity. The conditions that determine virulence and immunogenicity vary according to the animal species used. Two other antigens not associated with the capsule, known as V and W, also contribute to the organism's resistance to phagocytosis. For preparation of a killed vaccine effective against plague in man see Meyer (1970) and American Public Health Association (1985).

Laboratory diagnosis of plague

The diagnosis of plague is confirmed by demonstrating *Y. pestis* in stained films from buboes in the case of bubonic plague or in the sputum in pneumonic plague. In septicaemic plague the bacilli may be demonstrated in blood films and isolated in blood cultures, or from the spleen post mortem. The patient's serum may be tested by the complement fixation test or by the haemagglutination test with tanned sheep red cells to which capsular antigen F_1 has been adsorbed. The test may be used for retrospective diagnosis.

Bubonic plague

1. Puncture the bubo with a hypodermic syringe and withdraw the exudate for examination.

2. Prepare films of the exudate and stain by Gram stain and methylene blue. Characteristic Gram-negative coccobacilli and bacilli showing bipolar staining with methylene blue suggest plague bacilli.

3. Culture the exudate on blood agar plates, incubated at 27°C. Pick single colonies and subculture to obtain a pure culture for further identification tests. (a) Demonstrate the ability of the organism to grow on MacConkey medium. (b) Grow on nutrient agar containing 3% NaCl to obtain involution forms. (c) Grow in broth to demonstrate chain formation. (d) Inoculate a flask of broth and allow a drop of oil to float on the surface; examine for the development of 'stalactites' hanging from the oil drop. (e) Carry out biochemical tests and confirm reactions shown in Table 34.1.

4. Inoculate laboratory animals, guinea-pigs or white rats, subcutaneously with exudate from bubo or with 24 h broth culture. Infected animals die in 2–5 days. Post-mortem examination shows a marked local inflammatory condition at the site of inoculation with necrosis and oedema, the regional lymph nodes are enlarged, the spleen is enlarged and congested and may show greyish-white patches in the tissue. Prepare films from the local lesions, lymph nodes, spleen pulp and heart blood; stain and examine for characteristic plague bacilli.

Pneumonic plague

1. Prepare films from the sputum and stain by Gram and methylene blue. Examine stained films microscopically for characteristic Gram negative and bipolar-stained coccobacilli.

2. Culture the sputum and obtain pure culture for identification as with material from bubonic plague. This may be done by inoculating on the simple selective medium of Kniseley et al (1964), which consists of azide blood agar enriched with glucose and calcium.

3. Inoculate sputum into guinea-pigs and/or white rats by applying the material to the nasal mucosa or to a shaved area of skin. This prevents the entry of other virulent micro-organisms that may be present in the sputum. Carry out necropsy on any animals that die as a result of inoculation as for the diagnosis of plague in wild rats (see below).

Diagnosis of plague in wild rats

Before examining rats that may have died as a result of plague, immerse them in disinfectant to kill any infected fleas. It is important to differentiate plague from infection due to Y. pseudo-tuberculosis. In plague, necropsy has the following features: enlargement of the lymphatic nodes with periglandular inflammation and oedema that is most frequent in cervical lymph nodes due to the tendency for the flea to attack the rat's neck region; pleural effusion; enlargement of the spleen which may show small white areas in the pulp; liver congested and mottled; congestion and haemorrhages under the skin and in internal organs.

1. Make films and cultures of heart blood, lymph nodes and spleen.

2. Inoculate material from lesions on to the nasal mucosa of guinea-pigs or white rats as with sputum (see above).

3. Examine stained films and pure cultures for characteristic morphology and biochemical reactions of Y. pestis.

YERSINIA PSEUDOTUBERCULOSIS

Pseudotuberculosis is a zoonosis transmissible from infected animals to man either through skin contact with contaminated water or through the consumption of contaminated vegetables or other foods. It occasionally results in a severe, generalized disease with a high fatality rate. More commonly it gives rise to acute mesenteric adenitis, simulating acute or subacute appendicitis (right iliac fossa syndrome), sometimes with the added complication of erythema nodosum, usually in young males (cf. Y. enterocolitica). Enteritis caused by Y. pseudotuberculosis is rare.

In animals it causes a fatal septicaemia. It attacks wild animals and birds, including rodents, hares and rabbits and also guinea-pigs and other laboratory animals. Subclinical infection may occur. The animal disease must not be confused with so-called pseudotuberculosis of sheep and mice caused by *Corynebacterium ovis* and *C. muris* respectively.

Morphology and motility

A small, oval, non-capsulate, Gram-negative, slightly acid-fast, bipolar-stained bacillus. Differs from *Y. pestis* in being motile at 22°C, readily demonstrated in Craigie tubes (see *Methods*, Ch. 29, but omitting antiserum) incubated at 22°C and at 37°C.

Cultural characters

Aerobe and facultative anaerobe: optimum temperature 29°C. Grows slowly on ordinary nutrient agar; colonies are 1 mm in diameter, raised or umbonate, granular, translucent; non-haemolytic on blood agar; grows poorly on MacConkey medium.

Biochemical reactions

These are shown in Table 34.1. *Y. pseudotuberculosis* strains are biochemically homogenous. They differ from the plague bacillus in their ability to produce urease, and from the *Pasteurella* group in producing β-galactosidase (ONPG positive) (see Ch. 8). Unlike *Y. enterocolitica*, *Y. pseudotuberculosis* does not produce ornithine decarboxylase.

Antigenic structure

The strains of *Y. pseudotuberculosis* are of 6 serological types (serotypes 1–6) based on highly specific somatic antigens, one of which is common to all types, and a thermolabile flagellar antigen (present only in cultures grown at 18–26°C). A rough somatic antigen is shared by all strains and *Y. pestis*. About 90% of human cases of *Y. pseudotuberculosis* infections are due to type 1. An antigenic relationship exists between type 2 and type 4 and certain salmonellas of groups B and D respectively. By means of precipitin and haemagglutination tests the strains of *Y. pseudotuberculosis* have been classified into six O groups (I–VI) on the basis of the O and H antigens so revealed (Thal & Knapp 1971).

Laboratory diagnosis of pseudotuberculosis

The diagnosis is confirmed by isolating the organism from material taken from an excised mesenteric lymph gland and/or by demonstrating antibodies in the patient's serum during the acute phase of the infection.

Culture. Inoculate the excised material on to nutrient agar, blood agar and MacConkey medium and incubate at 37°C for 18 h. Characteristic colonies are granular, translucent with a beaten-copper surface; on blood agar they are non-haemolytic; on MacConkey medium growth is present but poor.

Prepare films of the colonies and stain by Gram, methylene blue and Ziehl-Neelsen stains. The organisms are small ovoid bacilli, bipolar-stained and weakly acid-fast. In broth culture at 22°C they are motile, at 37°C non-motile.

Serology. Carry out tube agglutination tests with smooth suspensions of strains of types 1–6 grown at 22°C, either live or inactivated with ethanol or formaldehyde (Report 1983). The tests are incubated at 52°C and read after 4 and 24 h. In positive sera the H agglutinin titres range from 80–12 800. Antibodies decline rapidly. The majority of cases are due to type 1. Since agglutination of types 2 and 4 may result from coagglutinins due to certain types of *Salmonella*, sera giving these results should be absorbed with salmonellas of groups B and D respectively.

Intradermal test. A skin test similar to the tuberculin and brucellin tests is available to indicate infection by *Y. pseudotuberculosis*. The reaction may be obtained many years after the infection has cleared.

YERSINIA ENTEROCOLITICA

Y. enterocolitica and related species *Y. intermedia*, *Y. frederikseni* and *Y. kristenseni* constitute a heterologous group of organisms, some of which are parasites and potential pathogens of humans and animals, while others are apparently saprophytic and free-living in water, soil and vegetation. *Y. enterocolitica* is becoming increasingly identified as a cause of gastroenteritis in infants and young children and it should be considered in cases of bacillary dysentery or campylobacter-like enterocolitis with abdominal pain and diarrhoea. The incidence is highest during autumn and winter. Occasionally it gives rise to acute terminal ileitis and/or mesenteric lymphadenitis that affects adults of both sexes as well as children. The lesions of this pseudo-appendicular syndrome are more severe than those caused by *Y. pseudotuberculosis*. Septicaemia with a high fatality rate among the elderly also occurs but is rare. There may be immunological complications resulting in erythema nodosum, polyarthritis, Reiter's syndrome, etc. The organism has been isolated from many animal species throughout the world but unlike *Y. pseudotuberculosis*, *Y. enterocolitica* infections are not considered to be true zoonoses. Human infections probably occur from ingestion or contact. Family and other small outbreaks suggest that person to person transmission occurs.

Morphology and motility

Gram-negative coccobacilli showing pleomorphism in older cultures; apparent capsules are seen in vivo but not in culture; motile by means of peritrichous flagella when grown at 22°C, non-motile at 37°C.

Cultural characters

Aerobe and facultative anaerobe. Optimum temperature 22–29°C; multiplies at 4°C (which constitutes a hazard when contaminated food is refrigerated). Grows slowly on artificial media: on blood agar forms non-haemolytic, smooth, translucent colonies, 2–3 mm in diameter in 48 h; grows on MacConkey medium forming pinpoint colonies at 22°C. Selective media or enrichment techniques are necessary for isolation from faecal specimens.

Sensitivity

Like other yersinias, *Y. enterocolitica* is killed by heat at 55°C and by phenol (0.5%) in 15 min. It is susceptible to sulphadiazine, streptomycin, tetracycline and chloramphenicol, but not to penicillin. Antibiotics should be used only for the treatment of severe or generalized infections in adults; cotrimoxazole is effective.

Biochemical reactions

Fermentation of sugars and other biochemical reactions are shown in Table 34.1. *Y. enterocolitica* is more reactive at 28°C than at 37°C. It differs from *Y. pseudotuberculosis* in its ability to ferment sucrose, sorbitol, cellobiose but not salicin, and in being ornithine decarboxylase positive and Voges-Proskauer positive. On the basis of variations in certain biochemical tests *Y. enterocolitica* may be divided into six different biotypes and three new species are now recognized, viz. *Y. intermedia* and *Y. frederikseni* which differ from it in their ability to ferment rhamnose and *Y. kristenseni* which does not ferment sucrose (Report 1983; Mair & Fox, 1986).

Toxin production

Pathogenic serotypes produce a heat-stable enterotoxin similar to that produced by enterotoxigenic *Escherichia coli*. Because the toxin is not produced at temperatures exceeding 30°C it is unlikely that it contributes to the pathogenicity of the infecting strain. However the toxin may be developed by organisms growing in contaminated food stored at low temperatures. This may explain the occurrence of some cases of food poisoning from which no causative organism has been isolated (Francis et al 1980). Toxigenic strains do not ferment rhamnose.

Antigenic structure

Y. enterocolitica is divisible into a large number of serotypes depending on 34 different O antigen factors and 19 H factors. Serotypes 3 and 9 account for the majority of human infections, especially in Europe; in the USA serotype 8 is more common. Other serotypes not associated with human disease have been isolated from healthy individuals and from milk, meat and vegetables. They are probably non-pathogenic. Serotype 9 may cross-react with some *Brucella* species.

For a general review of *Y. enterocolitica* see Swaminathan et al (1982) and Mair & Fox (1986).

Laboratory diagnosis of Y. enterocolitica infections

The diagnosis is confirmed directly by isolation of the organism and indirectly by serological tests on the patient's serum.

Isolation from blood or lymph nodes

Inoculate on to blood agar and MacConkey agar. Incubate plates at 22–29°C for 24 h.

Isolation from faeces, food, soil, etc.

1. Subject heavily contaminated material to preliminary enrichment by mixing with phosphate buffered saline or peptone water, pH 7.6. Maintain at 4°C for 22 days or more.

2. Subculture at weekly intervals on a selective medium (Schiemann CIN Medium, Oxoid) or on MacConkey medium containing a minimum amount of bile salt. Incubate at 22–29°C. Examine plates for colonies of *Y. enterocolitica* which on the selective medium appear like a bullseye, coloured dark red and surrounded by a transparent border. The size varies according to the serotype of the strain. Other organisms that grow produce larger colonies with pinkish centres.

3. Prepare pure cultures; test for motility at 22°C; identify the strain by biochemical tests (see Table 34.1).

4. Determine the serotype of the strain by slide agglutination against rabbit antisera to *Y. enterocolitica* serotypes 3 and 9 using factor O and OH antisera. If serotype 3, subdivide by phage typing (for details, see Bottone 1977).

Serological diagnosis

Use O antigen preparations of serotypes 3 and 9 to test the patient's serum at time of onset of illness and 10 days later by tube agglutination test. A rising titre of 160 and over is significant.

PASTEURELLA MULTOCIDA

P. multocida (*P. septica*) produces a severe fatal haemorrhagic septicaemia in many species of animals and birds. It may also be carried by apparently healthy cattle, sheep, swine, dogs, cats and wild rats. In humans it is the cause of suppurative respiratory tract infections, especially in farmers and other persons living in rural areas in close proximity to animals. It may also lead to septic wounds with involvement of the underlying bone after animal bites or following operations, e.g. for appendicitis (Coghlan 1958). Meningitis may result from infection after head injury. It is thought that the organism may reside as a commensal in the respiratory tract and nasal sinuses from which it passes by way of the blood to damaged tissues where it multiplies.

Morphology and staining

P. multocida is a Gram-negative, non-acid-fast coccobacillus, smaller than *Yersinia* organisms, exhibiting bipolar staining in films made directly from blood and tissues stained with methylene blue: capsulate: non-motile.

Cultural characters

Aerobe and facultative anaerobe; optimum temperature 37°C. Grows on nutrient agar forming circular colonies 0.5–1 mm in diameter in 24 h: does not grow on MacConkey agar: non-haemolytic on blood agar. The colonies may be of three forms – smooth, rough or mucoid.

Sensitivity

Killed quickly by heat at 55°C and by phenol (0.5%) in 15 min. May survive and maintain its virulence in dried or putrified blood for about 3 weeks and in culture or tissue for many months if kept frozen. Sensitive to penicillin, tetracycline, erythromycin, streptomycin and sulphonamides. In osteomyelitis following animal bites, antibiotic treatment must be continued for at least 8 weeks to be effective.

Biochemical reactions

P. multocida differs from other members of the group in certain cultural and biochemical details. Sugars are fermented slowly with acid but no gas production.

Antigenic structure

The species is not antigenically homogeneous. On the basis of capsular and somatic antigens, serological tests have revealed 15 serotypes.

Laboratory diagnosis

Samples from wounds caused by animal bites, CSF in cases of meningitis, or secretions in suppurative conditions of the respiratory tract are cultured on blood agar plates. Identify the organisms that grow by cultural and biochemical tests (Table 34.1).

Other organisms of the Pasteurella genus

Species of *Pasteurella* which differ from *P. multocida* in certain respects include *P. pneumotropica*, occasionally isolated from animal bites; *P. haemolytica* which is pathogenic for sheep, cattle and goats; *P. ureae* sometimes isolated from chronic respiratory tract infections in humans. The pathogenicity of these three species for man has not been proved. *P. haemolytica* differs from *P. multocida* in forming haemolytic colonies on blood agar, in its ability to grow on MacConkey medium and in its greater range of fermentation reactions. For the distinguishing characteristics of the three species see Table 34.1.

FRANCISELLA TULARENSIS

F. tularensis (*P. tularensis*) is the cause of tular-aemia, a plague-like disease of rodents and other small mammals. It is tick-borne among the natural hosts and transmissible to man as a typical zoonosis, either through direct or indirect contact with infected animals, or through handling laboratory cultures without strict safety precautions. The disease is widespread in North America but in Europe it is limited to certain countries and has not yet been identified in the UK. The so-called 'lemming fever' in Norway results from the consumption of water polluted with the carcasses or excreta of infected lemmings or water rats. Water-borne or airborne infections tend to produce influenza-like, pulmonary or typhoid-like illnesses, but in persons such as butchers or trappers who become infected through handling the tissues of animals such as rabbits or hares, there may be ulceroglandular or oculoglandular manifestations.

Morphology

Small coccobacillus which on primary isolation does not exceed $0.7 \times 0.2 \mu m$; in culture pleomorphic, capsulate, non-motile and non-sporing; Gram-negative showing bipolar staining; stains best with dilute (10%) carbol fuchsin as counter-stain. Smears from post-mortem material may require gentle heating to allow penetration of the stain.

Cultural characters

Strict aerobe. Fresh isolates cannot be cultured on ordinary medium but require a complex medium containing blood or tissue extracts and cystine. Optimum temperature 37°C. Minute droplet-like colonies develop in 72 h. Growth in liquid culture medium may be obtained using casein hydrolysate with added thiamine and cystine.

Sensitivity

Killed by moist heat at 55–60°C in 10 min. May remain viable for many years in cultures kept at 10°C and in humid soil and water for 30 and 90 days respectively (Zidon 1966). Very sensitive to chloramphenicol; sensitive to streptomycin. Tetracycline is bacteriostatic and only effective in large doses, 2 g/day for 14 days; it is used for prophylaxis and therapy when the infecting strain is streptomycin resistant (Sawyer et al 1966).

Biochemical reactions

Under suitable conditions acid is formed from glucose and maltose. Indole and urease tests are negative. For other reactions see Table 34.1.

Laboratory diagnosis

Isolate and identify the organism from material taken from the lesions, and demonstrate specific antibodies in the patient's serum.

1. Culture the discharge from local lesions or glands on special medium, e.g. blood agar enriched with 0.1% cystine (see below), or inspissated egg yolk medium. Incubate in air with 10% CO_2 at 37°C for 72 h or more. Small mucoid colonies are characteristic.

2. Inoculate exudates from ulcers and glands into guinea-pigs and mice. Culture the liver and spleen of the infected animals post mortem on special medium.

3. Obtain pure cultures for identification of *F. tularensis*.

4. Perform slide agglutination tests on animal serum and fluorescent antibody tests on spleen imprints.

5. Test patient's serum for specific antibodies

by slide and tube agglutination tests, haemagglutination, complement fixation and anti-human globulin (Coombs) test (see Chs 10 and 33), using antigens prepared from suspensions of *F. tularensis* grown on solid medium (Haug & Pearson 1972). Serum of cases of brucellosis may cross-react with *F. tularensis*. Diagnostic antigens and antisera for use in slide and tube agglutination tests are available from Difco.

Medium for the cultivation of Francisella tularensis

This is a solid medium containing 2.5% glucose and 0.1% cystine hydrochloride.

Glucose cystine solution

Glucose	12.5 g
Cystine hydrochloride	0.5 g
Water	50 ml

Prepare the solution and sterilize it by Seitz filtration.

Preparation of complete medium

Nutrient agar	85 ml
Glucose cystine solution	10 ml
Human blood, fresh	5 ml

Sterilize the agar at 121°C, cool to 50°C and add the remaining ingredients.

REFERENCES

American Public Health Association 1985 Control of communicable diseases in man. Benenson A S (ed) APHA, Washington DC

Bottone E J 1977 *Yersinia enterocolitica*: a panoramic view of a charismatic microorganism. CRC Critical Reviews in Microbiology 5: 211–241

Coghlan J D 1958 Isolation of *Pasteurella multocida* from human peritoneal pus and a study of the relationship to other strains of the same species. Journal of Pathology and Bacteriology 76: 45–53

Francis D W, Spaulding P L, Lovett J 1980 Enterotoxin production and thermal resistance of *Yersinia enterocolitica* in milk. Applied Environmental Microbiology 40: 174–176

Haug R H, Pearson A D 1972 Human infections with *Francisella tularensis* in Norway. Development of a serological screening test. Acta Pathologica Scandinavica, Sect B, 80: 273–280

Kniseley R F, Swaney L M, Friedlander H 1964 Selective media for the isolation of *Pasteurella pestis*. Journal of Bacteriology 88: 491–496

Mair N S, Fox E 1986 Yersiniosis; lab diagnosis, clinical features, epidemiology. Public Health Laboratory Service, London

Meyer K F 1970 Effectiveness of live or killed plague vaccine in man. Bulletin of World Health Organization 42: 653–666

Report 1983 World Health Organization, Yersiniosis. Report on a WHO meeting, Paris, 1981. EURO Reports and Studies 60, Copenhagen

Sawyer W D, Dangerfield H G, Hogg A L, Crozier D 1966 Antibiotic prophylaxis and therapy of airborne tularemia. Bacteriological Reviews 30: 542–548

Swaminathan B, Harmon M C, Mehlman I J 1982 A review of *Yersinia enterocolitica*. Journal of Applied Bacteriology 52: 151–183

Thal E, Knapp W 1971 Antigenic structure of *Yersinia enterocolitica*. In: Topley & Wilson's Principles of bacteriology, virology and immunity, 7th edn. Edward Arnold, London. Ch. 38

Zidon J 1966 Tularaemia. In: van der Hoeden J (ed) Zoonoses. Elsevier, Amsterdam. Ch. 5

Legionellaceae

All members of this family of aerobic Gram-negative rods were originally described as *Legionella* species but some differ sufficiently for it to have been suggested that *L. bozemani*, *L. dumoffi* and *L. gormani* should be placed in a separate genus, *Fluoribacter*, and *L. micdadei* in another genus, *Tatlockia* (Garrity et al 1980). There has been little general usage of these proposed names although they have been accepted by the International Committee on Systematic Bacteriology. In view of common usage, all species will be referred to as *Legionella* in this chapter (see also Brenner 1986).

Members of the Legionellaceae are listed in Table 35.1. *L. pneumophila* is the major pathogen in the group and has often been associated with outbreaks of infection. Most of the other species can occasionally give rise to serious disease, usually in debilitated or immunosuppressed subjects. Some species that have not yet been cultured from man may still prove to be human pathogens, e.g. antibodies to *L. jordanis* and to *L. gormani* have been shown in human sera although the organism has not been isolated from patients. *Legionella* species do not occur as commensal flora in man. Most members of the group have been isolated from aquatic habitats.

These organisms cannot be differentiated microscopically from other Gram-negative rods in clinical specimens, but they stain less well than most other Gram-negative genera. All the Legionellaceae require media enriched with iron and cysteine for primary isolation, e.g. buffered charcoal yeast extract (BCYE) agar. Various species may be distinguished by the characters listed in Table 35.2; in addition they have serologically distinct heat-stable surface somatic antigens, characteristic fatty acid profiles on gas-liquid chromatography (GLC), different isoprenoid quinone content and distinctive DNA (of value in DNA homology studies). On BCYE agar legionellas produce grey-white to pale blue or purple-tinged colonies. On this medium, some legionellas (those designated *Fluoribacter* by Garrity et al 1980, also *L. cherri*, *L. parisiensis*, *L. steigerwalti* plus most strains of *L. anisa*) give a strong blue-white fluorescence under long-wave ultraviolet (UV) light; *L. erythra* and *L. rubrilucens* produce red fluorescence (Brenner 1986; Brenner et al 1985). On Feeley Gorman (FG) agar or other clear tyrosine-containing media, legionellas except *L. micdadei* produce a brown diffusible pigment that fluoresces dull yellow under UV light.

It is difficult to identify these organisms by their colonial appearance alone in mixed culture; Gram-negative rods staining rather poorly with Gram stain and failing to grow on blood agar but growing on BCYE or other supplemented media are examined further. All legionella-like organisms isolated from patient or environmental material should be identified fully, not only so that the full range of infections associated with these organisms and their distribution in the environment is fully documented, but also to differentiate them from nutritionally demanding

---

Note: As explained in the *Preface*, the editors have sought to avoid the use of a double 'i' genitive ending in the specific epithets of species binomials that have been derived from Latinized versions of names. We acknowledge that this is not standard practice for the nomenclature of Legionellaceae; however, for consistency in this volume, the editors have substituted single 'i' forms, e.g. *L. bozemani*, *L. wadsworthi*, in place of the double 'i' forms.

Table 35.1 Members of the family Legionellaceae and their known association with human disease.
Key: Pn = pneumonia; F = Pontiac fever; − = not described; . . . = no information.

Species	Evidence of human infection		Isolated from environment	Disease association in man
	Culture	Serology[a]		
L. anisa	−	−	+	−
L. birminghamensis	+	−	−	?Pn
L. bozemani				
serogroup 1	+	+	+	Pn
serogroup 2	+	+	−	Pn
L. cherri	−	−	+	−
L. dumoffi	+	+	+	Pn
L. erythra	−	−	+	−
L. feelei				
serogroup 1	−	+	+	F
serogroup 2	+	. . .	+	Pn
L. gormani	−	+	+	−
L. hackeliae				
serogroup 1	+	. . .	−	Pn
serogroup 2	+	. . .	−	Pn
L. israelensis	−	−	+	−
L. jamestowniensis	−	−	+	−
L. jordanis	−	+	+	−
L. longbeachae				
serogroup 1	+	+	+	Pn
serogroup 2	+	. . .	−	Pn
L. maceacherni	+	. . .	+	Pn
L. micdadei	+	+	+	Pn
L. oakridgensis	−	−	+	−
L. parisiensis	−	−	+	−
L. pneumophila				
serogroups 1–14	+	+	+	Pn,F
L. rubrilucens	−	−	+	−
L. sainthelensi	−	+	+	Pn
L. santicrucis	−	−	+	−
L. spiritensis	−	−	+	−
L. steigerwalti	−	−	+	−
L. wadsworthi	+	+	−	Pn

[a] Demonstration of antibodies as sole criterion of infection has been validated only for *L. pneumophila* serogroup 1.

thermophilic bacteria that may present similar features.

LEGIONELLA PNEUMOPHILA

This organism gives rise to pneumonia, often serious and sometimes fatal, and also to the brief non-fatal influenza-like illness Pontiac fever. *L. pneumophila* is differentiated from other *Legionella* species by hippurate hydrolysis and by serological tests.

Morphology and staining

Gram-negative rods, 0.3–0.9 × 2–3 μm, with pointed ends and a tendency to filament formation on solid culture medium; smears from infected yolk sac and from clinical material show many shorter forms with rounded ends. Non-sporing; motile with polar flagella; pilated; non-capsulate. In early passage on solid media cells may contain vacuoles which stain with fat stains such as Sudan black.

Cultural characters

Strict aerobe; temperature range 29–40°C; pH optimum 6.9. Requires media supplemented with iron and cysteine for primary isolation. Colonies may take 3–5 days to appear on BCYE agar* at 37°C; strains adapted after animal or agar

* Refer to *Methods* at end of this chapter.

Table 35.2 Some distinguishing characters of the Legionellaceae (see also Brenner et al 1985).
Key: ++, most strains very strong positive; +, most strains moderately strong positive; −, most strains negative; +/−, some strains positive, some negative; ±, most strains weak positive; . . ., not given.

Species	Colony fluorescence (blue/white)	Diffusible pigment (brown)	Pigment fluorescence (dull yellow)	Catalase	Oxidase	Starch hydrolysis	Hippurate hydrolysis	Gelatin liquefaction	β-lactamase
L. pneumophila	−	+	+	±	+/−	+	+	+	+
L. anisa	+/−	+	+	+	+	. . .	−	+	+
L. feelei	−	±	−	+	−	. . .	+	−	−
L. hackeliae	−	+	. . .	±	+	. . .	−	+	+
L. jordanis	−	+	+	+	+	−	−	+	+
L. longbeachae	−	+	+	+	+	−	−	+	+/−
L. oakridgensis	−	+	+	+	−	−	−	+	±
L. sainthelensi	−	+	. . .	+	+	. . .	−	+	+
L. wadsworthi	−	−	−	+	−	−	−	+	+
L. bozemani	+	+	+	++	+/−	+	−	+	±
L. dumoffi	+	+	+	++	−	+	−	+	+
L. gormani	+	+	+	++	−	+	−	+	+
L. micdadei	−	−	−	++	+	−	−	−	−

passage will produce growth in the well of the plate in 24–48 h and individual small colonies in 48–72 h, growing to about 2–3 mm in diameter after 96 h incubation. Colonies circular, low convex, with smooth glistening surface, an entire crenated edge, soft butyrous consistency and a grey or grey-blue appearance. Under the plate microscope a 'cut glass' appearance may be noted, and colonies may also have a lilac colour. On FG agar* colonial growth is poor (other legionellas will not grow on it without adaptation) but a diffusible brown pigment is produced which fluoresces dull yellow under UV light; this may be enhanced by the addition of tyrosine to the medium (Baine & Rasheed 1979). L. pneumophila will produce haemolysis of guinea-pig red cells but this test is not used in identification.

Biochemical reactions

L. pneumophila does not ferment sugars normally used for identification purposes; it does, however, hydrolyse starch, hippurate and gelatin. Catalase positive; oxidase variable. Produces opacity around colonies on an egg yolk medium, with a clearing beyond the zone of opacity; however, tests for lecithinase production are not used for identification. L. pneumophila has a high content of fatty acids and gives rise to a typical profile on GLC; this is an important characteristic in the identification of this species (Moss et al 1977).

Sensitivity to chemical and physical agents

Laboratory cultures survive for months at 4°C or at room temperature. Legionellas may survive for well over a year in unchlorinated tap water. They are readily killed by disinfectants at use-dilution but survive for up to 30 min at pH 2 or at 50°C.

Antibiotic sensitivity

Although L. pneumophila is susceptible to a wide range of antibiotics it is particularly sensitive to erythromycin and rifampicin (Thornsberry et al 1978); these antibiotics have proved effective in vivo, both experimentally and in treatment of patients.

L. pneumophila and most other Legionella species produce a β-lactamase (Thornsberry et al 1978). The enzyme is active on some cephalosporins as well as on benzylpenicillin and ampicillin; its action can only partially be prevented by clavulanic acid and it appears to be different from the β-lactamases found in Enterobacteriaceae and Pseudomonas species.

Serogrouping

To date 14 serogroups of L. pneumophila have been defined, all of which have been implicated in human infection, with most infections being due to serogroup 1. Strains are identified definitively by direct or indirect immunofluorescence with specific antisera, but may also be identified by slide agglutination (Wilkinson & Fikes 1980; Thacker et al 1985). There are serotypes within at least serogroups 1 and 5 of L. pneumophila; strains of serogroup 1 have been placed into provisional types according to their reactions with monoclonal antibodies (Joly et al 1986). Most outbreaks of Legionnaires' disease are caused by one monoclonal antibody type (Tobin et al 1987). Recently subtyping on a genetic basis has been performed by the use of electrophoretic analysis to demonstrate enzyme electromorphs (Selander et al 1985).

Animal pathogenicity

Fresh strains from either human or environmental material are pathogenic for the embryonated hen's egg, which is the most sensitive culture system for legionellas in the absence of other microorganisms. Inoculation into eggs via the yolk sac is lethal in 4–7 days, the organisms being present in the yolk sac in large numbers.

Because of the ability of guinea-pigs to survive intraperitoneal (IP) challenge with grossly contaminated material, together with the animals' susceptibility to legionella infection, guinea-pigs have been used for the attempted isolation of legionellas from patient or environmental material but this technique has now been superseded by the use of selective media. The animal develops fever about 24 h after IP inoculation, the fur becomes ruffled, there is a watery discharge from the eyes and the animal becomes progressively more unwell. Death may not occur, and the animal may recover; thus the guinea-pig should be killed and autopsied when it becomes ill or, in any case, at 4–5 days after inoculation. At autopsy there is a peritoneal exudate or localized abscess which contains large numbers of the organism; the spleen is enlarged and congested and similarly contains many legionellas, usually in pure culture even when the initial inoculum was heavily contaminated with other bacteria. Guinea-pigs may also be infected by the respiratory route and have been used to detect legionellas in air in affected buildings.

Legionellas will infect free-living amoebae of the genera *Acanthamoeba* and *Naegleria* and these organisms have been used experimentally to isolate legionellas from infected material (Rowbotham 1980).

OTHER LEGIONELLA SPECIES

Other *Legionella* species are listed in Table 35.1; at least ten have been isolated from human material and the other 14 only from the environment. *L. feelei* of serogroup 1, although cultured only from coolant used in a car engine plant, was shown to be responsible for an outbreak of Pontiac fever amongst workers at the plant (Herwaldt et al 1984). Antibodies to some species have been demonstrated in man but, in the absence of isolation of these species from man, the specificity of these antibodies is uncertain.

These species have growth requirements similar to those of *L. pneumophila* and are isolated and identified in the same way; they may be distinguished by the features noted in Table 35.2 and by serological examination. Although phenotypically similar to *L. pneumophila* they differ from that species and from each other in DNA content, as shown by DNA homology studies. *L. longbeachae* is similar to *L. pneumophila* in cellular fatty acid content; *L.*

oakridgensis and *L. anisa* also share some components with *L. pneumophila* but differ from it and from each other in a number of details. *L. jordanis*, *L. wadsworthi*, *L. bozemani*, *L. dumoffi*, *L. gormani* and *L. micdadei* form a separate group with similar fatty acid content (Cherry et al 1982; Edelstein et al 1982b). *L. feelei* and *L. sainthelensi* differ from each other in fatty acid content and both differ from other legionellas in some details.

L. oakridgensis differs from other legionellas in that, following original isolation on culture media containing cysteine and iron, they will grow in the absence of cysteine (Orrison et al 1983); other *Legionella* species will grow in the absence of iron but not L-cysteine after adaptation to artificial culture. When grown on BCYE agar with added 0.001% bromocresol purple and 0.001% bromothymol blue, colonies of *L. bozemani*, *L. dumoffi*, *L. gormani* and *L. micdadei* appear blue-grey, whereas *L. pneumophila* colonies are pale green (Vickers et al 1981).

L. feelei, like *L. pneumophila* and *L. spiritensis* but unlike other *Legionella* species, is hippurate positive, and only it and *L. micdadei* do not liquefy gelatin. Its colonies show no autofluorescence. *L. sainthelensi* is biochemically indistinguishable from *L. jordanis*, *L. longbeachae* and *L. wadsworthi*. *L. anisa* resembles *L. bozemani* in biochemical and fatty acid profiles. Most strains of this organism give blue-white fluorescence like *L. bozemani* when colonies are illuminated by UV light, but one strain does not. A new unclassified legionella species isolated from the environment is serologically identical with *L. pneumophila* serogroup 5 but differs when examined by DNA homology (Garrity et al 1982) and by multilocus enzyme electrophoresis (Selander et al 1985). For a more detailed account of *Legionella* species see Bartlett et al (1986).

Laboratory diagnosis of legionella infection

Specimens may be received from patients or from environmental sources. Patient specimens may include sputum, bronchial secretions or biopsy material, lung biopsy or lung taken at post-mortem examination, pleural fluid and blood for culture. Legionellas have also been isolated from other sites including lung abscess, spleen, kidney, small bowel and faeces. Environmental specimens will be swabs from water taps and shower heads, together with rinsings from tap washers, plus centrifuged or filter-concentrated deposits of water from suspect water systems and cooling towers, e.g. in hospitals or hotels where there has been an outbreak.

Legionellas survive well in transit but are not easy to isolate from patient material, especially since their growth may be inhibited by tissue extracts or by other bacteria. Suspect material is cultured directly on selective or unselective media; recent evidence suggests that appropriate selective media may be more sensitive than guinea-pig inoculation (Edelstein et al 1982a). Typical colonies are identified by nutritional requirements followed, where possible, by GLC determination of fatty acid content. Serological analysis is essential, but a negative result does not exclude the diagnosis as the isolate may be of a new serogroup or species. *L. pneumophila* serogroup antigens are excreted in patient's urine and their detection by ELISA or RIA has been used as a rapid diagnostic technique (Kohler & Sathapatayavongs 1983).

In view of the difficulty of culturing these organisms serological diagnostic methods are most commonly used. These are the direct fluorescent antibody test (DFAT) for demonstration of bacterial antigen in tissues, secretions or environmental sources, and the indirect test (IFAT) for demonstration of antibody in patients (Fallon 1981).

Microscopy

1. Examine a Gram stained smear of any specimen of pleural fluid or tissue. The presence of poorly staining Gram-negative rods in a normally sterile site may suggest the presence of legionellas. In any material the presence of other bacterial forms may warn of potential contaminants and that selective media or guinea-pig inoculation may be required for isolation of legionellas.

2. Examine a smear stained by either the DFAT* or IFAT* immunofluorescence method. Positive results should be checked with pre-immune or normal rabbit serum in case the staining is due to naturally acquired antibodies in the rabbit serum. Provided the antisera are specific, the observation of strongly fluorescing short rods may justify the making of a provisional report; with formaldehyde-fixed lung this is the final stage of diagnosis. DFAT with a monoclonal antibody to a common antigen of *L. pneumophila* (Genetic Systems) is effective and specific (Fallon 1986).

Treatment of contaminated specimens

For culture on artificial media, as opposed to guinea-pig inoculation, contaminated specimens may be treated by heat (50°C for 30 min) or with acid before culture on selective medium*, or by simple dilution. The following technique (Greaves 1980), one of a number of variations described, takes advantage of the relative resistance of *L. pneumophila* to acid.

Place a 2 ml sample of homogenized material in a screw-capped bottle with an equal volume of HCl at pH 2 (0.01 mol/l). After 5–15 min at room temperature, neutralize by adding 18 ml of phosphate buffered saline (PBS), pH 7.3, and centrifuge at 1500 g for 20 min. Culture the sediment. An untreated sample of material should also be cultured since the acid reduces the viable count of legionellas by 60–90%. (The heat treatment is less injurious to legionellas.)

Grossly contaminated material may be further treated by suspending the sediment obtained after acid treatment in 2 ml of antibiotic solution containing colistin 15 000 units/litre, vancomycin 50 mg/l, trimethoprim 25 mg/l and amphotericin B 25 mg/l. Transfer 1 ml immediately to 9 ml enrichment broth*; incubate the other 1 ml sample for 2–4 h at 37°C before adding to enrichment broth. Incubate these selective enrichment broths at 37°C for up to 1 week. Inspect daily for turbidity and by Gram stain before subculture to selective and unselective medium. The availability of improved selective media for isolation of legionellas from grossly contaminated material has reduced the need for use of enrichment broth.

Culture of legionellas

The recommended culture medium is BCYE agar*; this has proved more satisfactory than the enriched blood agar media described by Greaves (1980) and Dennis et al (1981), although the latter is useful for antibiotic sensitivity testing of legionellas. Normally sterile material, e.g. pleural fluid, may also be inoculated into the yolk sac of 8–10 day old fertile hens' eggs or into guinea-pigs. Contaminated material may preferably be cultured directly on selective BCYE medium* or inoculated IP into guinea-pigs (at least two animals), preferably test bled before inoculation so that survivors can be examined for development of antibodies. Fluid culture has not been employed commonly for the isolation of *L. pneumophila* but enrichment broth may be used as fluid phase in a Castaneda-type blood culture medium with BCYE as solid phase. Blood cultures should be incubated for at least 1 week.

1. Plate out the specimen, leaving a heavy inoculum in the well of the plate as well as plating to obtain single colonies; seed BCYE agar, both with and without selective antibiotics, and also blood agar, to demonstrate the presence of other organisms. The interfering effects of other organisms can be minimized by diluting the inoculum. Incubate cultures in air or up to 2.5% CO_2 in air, in a container to prevent the plates drying up, for up to 14 days, inspecting daily for likely colonies on specific media and for other organisms on blood agar. On primary isolation colonies may take 3–5 days or more to appear.

2. Examine smears from colonies by Gram stain and the direct fluorescent antibody technique (DFAT)*. Slide agglutination is a rapid technique if high-titre specific sera are available (Wilkinson & Fikes 1980; Thacker et al 1985). Subculture to blood agar; if the organisms are legionellas no growth will occur. Subcultures are made to BCYE agar and also to that medium without added iron and cysteine. Cysteine-dependent legionellas will not grow on this latter medium but will show satellite growth around a filter-paper disk impregnated with a solution of ferric pyrophosphate 12.5 mg/ml and L-cysteine HCl 20 mg/ml (or Oxoid *Legionella* growth supplement SR 110) and then dried and placed in the well of the plate (Smith 1982).

3. Yolk sac material from embryonated eggs that die 3–7 days after inoculation, and peritoneal swabs and spleen smears from dead guinea-pigs or moribund, febrile or well guinea-pigs killed 4–7 days after IP inoculation, should also be examined by microscopy and cultured as described above.

4. Cultures of possible legionellas should be forwarded on a slope of culture medium, in a screw-capped container, to a reference laboratory for serological and GLC examination. Cultures should be checked for growth at 50–55°C before referral, as thermophilic Gram-negative spore-bearing bacilli contaminating culture media may mimic legionellas in cultural requirements (Thacker et al 1981).

Examination of water supplies

Samples (*c.* 5 litres) should be taken from a suspected source of legionella infection. Swabs may also be taken from specific points such as taps (especially hot water taps), tap washers and shower heads. Organisms are concentrated by centrifugation or by filtration through a sterile 142 mm diameter 0.22 μm nylon membrane filter. The filter is removed to a sterile jar and cut into small pieces; 20 ml sterile distilled water (or filtrate) is added. The deposit is removed by shaking or sonication. This deposit or that from centrifugation is examined by DFAT*, by culture on selective and non-selective medium with or without prior holding at pH 2 for 5–15 min or at 50°C for 30 min, and possibly also by IP inoculation of the rest of the suspension into 2–4 guinea-pigs.

Serological diagnosis

This is the way in which most infections with legionellas are diagnosed because of the difficulty of isolating the organisms. The principal technique is the indirect test (IFAT)* although other techniques such as microagglutination (Harrison & Taylor 1982) and ELISA are in use. The microagglutination test is rapid, sensitive and specific but positive results should be confirmed by IFAT (Harrison et al 1987).

Most legionellosis is due to *L. pneumophila* serogroup 1 and antigen made from this organism is available; reference laboratories hold antigens of other serogroups and species that occasionally give rise to infection. Two principal antigens are available for the IFAT, formalin-treated infected yolk sac (Taylor et al 1979) and heat-treated agar-grown cultures (Wilkinson et al 1979). A four-fold rise in titre of antibody in paired sera, from 16 or below to at least 64, or a standing titre of at least 256 in the presence of typical clinical disease, is accepted as evidence of infection. A standing titre of 256 or more in the absence of illness is suggestive of previous infection; antibodies may persist for years in some patients. They may be slow to rise and in some instances seroconversion does not occur until 5–6 weeks after the onset of illness. The specificity of antibody response has not yet been established for species other than *L. pneumophila* serogroup 1.

METHODS

Buffered charcoal yeast extract agar (BCYE)

This medium is recommended for culture of legionellas. Detailed instructions are given below for making BCYE (Pasculle et al 1980, modified by Edelstein 1981; also known as BCYEα medium). A commercial preparation is available, prepared with *Legionella* BCYE supplement (Oxoid SR110) and *Legionella* CYE agar base (Oxoid CM655).

ACES buffer (N-2-acetamido-2-aminoethane sulphonic acid)	10 g
KOH (pellets)	2.8 g
Activated charcoal (Norit A)	1.5 g
Yeast extract (Difco)	10 g
Bacto agar (Difco)	17 g
α-ketoglutarate (mono-potassium salt)	1 g
L-cysteine HCl	0.4 g
Ferric pyrophosphate (soluble)	0.25 g
Distilled water	1 litre

Note: Oxoid yeast extract (L20) may be used instead of Difco, and 12 g Oxoid agar No. 3 (L13) may be used instead of Difco agar.

1. Add ACES buffer to 980 ml distilled water in a flask and stir until dissolved.
2. Add KOH pellets to the solution.
3. Add charcoal, yeast extract, agar and α-ketoglutarate to the solution.
4. Mix well and boil to dissolve agar.
5. Autoclave at 121°C for 15 min and cool to 56°C in a waterbath. The medium must be made fresh each time as reheating the autoclaved base medium reduces its sensitivity.
6. Prepare separate fresh solutions of L-cysteine HCl (0.4 g in 10 ml distilled water) and ferric pyrophosphate (0.25 g in 10 ml distilled water) and sterilize by membrane filtration.
7. Add first L-cysteine solution and then ferric pyrophosphate to the medium.
8. The pH of the medium should be 6.90 ± 0.05; if necessary adjust pH with 1 mol/litre KOH.

Tyrosine BYE medium. This clear medium is the same as BCYE agar but with the omission of charcoal and the addition of 0.45 g L-tyrosine/litre at the same time as the agar.

Selective BCYE agar

BCYE agar may be made more selective for isolation of most legionellas by the addition of antibiotics; however it is important to note that some legionellas e.g. *L. feelei* and *L. anisa*, are inhibited by antibiotics added to culture media. An effective medium is BCYE medium plus ammonium-free glycine 3 g/litre, added to BCYE base before autoclaving. After autoclaving add filter-sterilized polymyxin B 79 200 IU/l, cycloheximide 80 mg/l and vancomycin 5 mg/l (Dennis PJ, personal communication); a lower dose of vancomycin, 1 mg/l may also be used to ensure the growth of less-vancomycin-resistant *Legionella* strains (e.g. *L. anisa*). A similar selective medium containing dyes which aid in the differentiation of *L. bozemani*, *L. gormani*, *L. dumoffi* and *L. micdadei* from most other *Legionella* species has been described and evaluated (Edelstein 1982).

When used to examine potable water specimens no prior acid wash is necessary although heating at 50°C for 30 min is still helpful in eliminating inhibitory organisms.

Feeley Gorman (FG) agar (Feeley et al 1978)

Mueller Hinton agar (BBL)	38 g
L-cysteine HCl	0.4 g
Ferric pyrophosphate (soluble)	0.25 g
Distilled water	1 litre

1. Dissolve the agar in 980 ml distilled water.
2. Autoclave at 121°C for 15 min and cool to 56°C.
3. Add L-cysteine and ferric pyrophosphate solutions as for BCYE medium (above).
4. The final pH should be 6.90 ± 0.05.

Pigment production can be demonstrated in a clear medium such as FG agar and is best seen when the medium is supplemented with 0.45 g L-tyrosine/litre before autoclaving.

Enrichment broth

Yeast extract (Difco)	5 g
Proteose peptone (Difco)	15 g
Liver extract (Panmede, Paines & Byrne)	2.5 g
L-cysteine HCl	0.4 g
Ferric pyrophosphate (soluble)	0.125 g
NaCl	5 g
Distilled water	1 litre

1. Dissolve the ingredients, except L-cysteine and ferric pyrophosphate, in 980 ml hot water and adjust pH to 6.90 ± 0.05.
2. Autoclave at 121°C for 15 min and cool to 56°C.
3. Add L-cysteine and ferric pyrophosphate solutions as for BCYE agar (above).
4. Add 50 ml of sterile defibrinated horse blood.

This medium can also be used as a blood culture medium (Edelstein et al 1979).

Biochemical tests

Hippurate hydrolysis may be demonstrated by the method of Hébert (1981). Make a heavy emulsion of organisms from agar medium in 0.4 ml 1% sodium hippurate (kept in aliquots at −20°C). Incubate at 35°C overnight, then add 0.2 ml of 3.5% ninhydrin in 1:1 acetone:butanol (kept in dark at room temperature) and shake. Incubate at 35°C for 10 min. A positive reaction is when a purple colour develops within the next 20 min.

For *gelatinase* tests, seed the gelatin capsule on an API strip with a heavy saline suspension of agar-grown organisms and incubate for 48–72 h. *Starch hydrolysis* may be demonstrated as described by Weaver (1978). β-lactamase may be detected by the chromogenic cephalosporin test (see Ch. 9).

Direct fluorescent antibody test (DFAT)

The principles underlying the direct immuno-fluorescent antibody test (DFAT) are reviewed in Chapter 10. This technique is suitable for demonstration of bacterial antigen in smears from colonies, and for direct detection of antigen in pleural fluid (centrifuged deposit), sputum, bronchial washings, tracheal aspirates, lung smears, tissues from animals inoculated for isolation studies, formalin-fixed tissues and centrifuged deposits from water samples (because of false positive results DFAT examination of water must always be confirmed by culture). The basic requirements are a suitable fluorescence microscope and antisera to the various sero-groups of *L. pneumophila* and other *Legionella* species. Ideally, the microscope should be equipped for epi-illumination with a × 10 eyepiece and either a × 50 water immersion objective or a × 100 oil immersion objective. Microscopes using transmitted light are generally insufficiently sensitive, although some workers have obtained good results with a quartz halogen source used with darkground condenser, wide aperture objective and an interference filter. The antisera are hyperimmune animal sera or monoclonal antibodies conjugated with fluorescein isothiocyanate for use in a DFAT; however, unlabelled hyperimmune sera may be used in an IFAT.

1. For fluids, make a thin film of the deposit.
2. Fresh tissue is cut with a sterile scalpel blade to give a fresh surface which is pressed and

squeezed with forceps against clean slides to make several imprints. Alternatively, the fresh surface can be scraped with the blade, the debris washed on to a slide with PBS, pH 7.2, and resuspended for spotting on to slides.

3. Dry slides in air. Heat-fix gently, then fix for 10 min by covering with a solution of 10% neutral formalin which should not be allowed to dry. Drain off formalin and dip slides into distilled water before again drying in air.

4. Formalin-fixed lung is cut as above and the fresh surface scraped, the tissue debris smeared on to a slide, dried, and then heat-fixed before washing with distilled water.

5. Place 0.025 ml of fluorescein-labelled antiserum at working dilution on each smear. The serum may be spread lightly with a sterile wire loop. A separate smear is used for antiserum to each legionella serogroup unless polyvalent antiserum pools are available. Dilution of fluorescein-conjugated sera with rhodamine-conjugated normal rabbit serum to working strength reduces background non-specific staining.

Prepare control smears, one with PBS replacing the serum as a negative control, and others with either pre-immune or normal species serum as a serum control. Positive controls should also be included whenever possible.

6. Incubate test and control smears for 30 min at 37°C in a covered chamber to prevent evaporation. Drain off the serum and rinse the smears with a stream of PBS, care being taken not to wash the material off the slide. Negative and positive control smears must be kept separate from test smears. Wash slides in PBS for 5 min.

7. Where the DFAT technique with fluorescein-conjugated antisera has been used, rinse slides briefly in distilled water and allow to dry in air.

8. Where unconjugated antiserum has been used in an IFAT, apply 0.025 ml of the appropriate fluorescein-conjugated anti-species globulin to the smears as above, and to an appropriate control smear for the anti-species globulin. Incubate the slides at 37°C for 30 min in a closed chamber, rinse, wash and finally dry in air as above.

9. For examination, mount smears in buffered glycerol, pH 9.0, or polyvinyl alcohol glycerol medium (Heimer & Taylor 1974). Legionellas appear as short rods or cocco-bacillary forms in contrast to the filamentous forms often seen in smears from cultures. Lung tissue may contain many organisms but sometimes only few. In sputum legionellas are very scanty and smears should be searched as diligently as for tubercle bacilli, e.g. for 20 min. More than five organisms per smear are considered significant. Animal tissues or yolk sac smears usually contain many organisms.

Indirect fluorescent antibody test (IFAT) for legionellosis

This test, used to demonstrate antibody in patient's serum, is based on the reaction of patient's serum with a suspension of legionellas, in which the coating of organisms by the patient's antibody is revealed by staining with fluorescein-conjugated anti-human globulin. Two types of antigen are currently in use. In the UK formalin-killed yolk sac antigen (FYSA) made from embryonated hens' eggs infected with the Pontiac strain of serogroup 1 *L. pneumophila* is available from the Division of Quality Control and Microbiological Reagents, CPHL, London. The other antigen (used widely in the USA and made by the Centers for Disease Control, Atlanta) can be easily prepared by laboratories without egg culture facilities; it is a heat-killed suspension of legionellas mixed with a suspension of normal yolk sac.

IFAT methods using formalinized yolk sac antigens (FYSA)

FYSA consists of infected yolk sacs homogenized with an equal volume of Dulbecco A PBS containing 2% formalin. The antigen issued has been diluted 1 in 50 with PBS containing 0.08% sodium azide for use. Use polytetrafluoroethylene (PTFE)-coated slides with 12 wells such as SMO 10 (Hendley) with 3 mm well.

1. Add 5 μl of FYSA to each well (if 3 mm wells are not used, the volume of antigen must be adjusted). Dry the slides in a 37°C incubator

(20 min) and then fix in acetone at room temperature for 15 min.

2. Make serum dilutions in PBS, pH 7.2, using doubling dilutions starting at 1 in 16. Add 10 μl of serum dilution to each FYSA spot.

3. Incubate the slides in a humid chamber at 37°C for 30 min. Rinse the slides with PBS and then wash in PBS for 15 min with two changes of PBS. Rinse the slides briefly with distilled water, blot and dry at 37°C (10 min).

4. To each FYSA spot add 5 μl of sheep anti-human whole globulin with adequate anti-IgM and anti-IgG activity diluted to working dilution. Incubate the slides in a humid chamber at 37°C for 30 min and wash as above.

5. After drying, mount the preparation in glycerol mounting medium consisting of 1 part buffered saline pH 8.5 and 9 parts neutral glycerol (glycerin). The buffered saline is made as follows. Prepare 0.067 mol/litre K_2HPO_4 by dissolving 1.161 g K_2HPO_4 in 100 ml 0.85% NaCl. Prepare 0.067 mol/l KH_2PO_4 by dissolving 0.907 g KH_2PO_4 in 100 ml 0.85% NaCl. For use, add 10 parts 0.067 mol/l K_2HPO_4 in 0.85% NaCl to 1 part 0.067 mol/l KH_2PO_4 in 0.85% NaCl.

6. Examine the slides by epi-illumination using × 10 eyepieces and a × 100 oil objective. The fluorescence is scored +++, ++, +, ±, −. The endpoint is the last dilution giving + fluorescence, i.e. definite fluorescence and not just dull green colouring of the organisms; the fluorescence must be associated with morphologically recognized organisms.

7. The positive control serum (human) supplied gives + fluorescence at a dilution of 1 in 128 with the system used by the Division of Microbiological Reagents and Quality Control. In order that results are standardized this serum must be used as reference on each occasion. The positive control serum is supplied in measured quantities of 0.2 ml as only small amounts are available at present and it must be used sparingly. Include normal human serum (negative control) in each run; it should give a titre of <16.

8. Sera showing any degree of specific fluorescence at a dilution of 1 in 16 or greater with the FYSA antigen should be forwarded to a reference centre for further study using antigens from strains of other serogroups. Low titres with the serogroup 1 antigen may indicate infection with another serogroup of *L. pneumophila*.

IFAT using heat-killed L. pneumophila

1. Grow *L. pneumophila* on BCYE agar for 3–4 days until there is sufficient growth for it to be scraped off, with a wire loop or a bent glass Pasteur pipette, into PBS, pH 7.2, in a screw-capped container. Place in a boiling waterbath for 15 min. Centrifuge the suspension and suspend the pellet of cells in 2 ml distilled water.

2. Make the working dilution (100–200 cells/high power field) in 0.5% suspension of normal yolk sac in PBS. The yolk sac not only inhibits non-specific background fluorescence seen with culture suspensions in water or PBS, but also increases the sensitivity of the test.

A polyvalent antigen can be made by adding together suspensions of different serogroups or species so as to give 100–200 organisms of each individual serogroup/high power field; a quadrivalent antigen has been shown to work well.

3. Prepare slides as described for FYSA using slides with a 5 mm spot.

4. Make the initial serum dilution of 1 in 16 with 3% suspension of normal yolk sac in PBS. Then make further doubling dilutions in PBS.

5. Add 10 μl of serum dilution to each well. Incubate slides in a humid chamber at 37°C for 30 min, rinse in PBS and wash for 10 min in a PBS bath.

6. Blot slides and add 20 μl fluorescein-conjugated antihuman globulin to each well. Incubate slides, rinse, wash and mount as described above.

7. Examine slides by epi-illumination using a × 6 eyepiece and a × 40 dry objective. Fluorescence is scored as for FYSA, the endpoint being where there is + fluorescence of at least 50% of the bacterial cells present.

8. Prepare a row of six spots with the following controls: a spot using PBS in place of serum, a spot using normal human serum diluted 1 in 32 as a serum control, and dilutions of a known positive serum diluted so that the last of

the remaining four spots on this slide is just beyond endpoint, i.e. shows a ± reaction. The test is read with reference to this serum.

9. Interpretation is as for FYSA. Sera reacting with a polyvalent heat-killed antigen should be titrated against monovalent antigens of available serogroups or forwarded to a reference centre for further examination.

REFERENCES

Baine W B, Rasheed J K 1979 Aromatic substrate specificity of browning by cultures of the Legionnaires' disease bacterium. Annals of Internal Medicine 90: 619–620

Bartlett C L R, Macrae A D, Macfarlane J T 1986 Legionella infections. Arnold, London

Brenner D J 1986 Classification of Legionellaceae. Current status and remaining questions. Israeli Journal of Medical Sciences 22: 620–632

Brenner D J et al 1985 Ten new species of Legionella. International Journal of Systematic Bacteriology 35: 50–59

Cherry W B et al 1982 Legionella jordanis: a new species of Legionella isolated from water and sewage. Journal of Clinical Microbiology 15: 290–297

Dennis P J, Taylor J A, Barrow G I 1981 Phosphate buffered, low sodium chloride blood agar medium for Legionella pneumophila. Lancet 2: 636

Edelstein P H 1981 Improved semiselective medium for isolation of Legionella pneumophila from contaminated clinical and environmental specimens. Journal of Clinical Microbiology 14: 298–303

Edelstein P H 1982 Comparative study of selective media for isolation of Legionella pneumophila from potable water. Journal of Clinical Microbiology 16: 697–699

Edelstein P H, Brenner D J, Moss C W, Steigerwalt A G, Francis E M, George W L 1982b Legionella wadsworthii species nova: a cause of human pneumonia. Annals of Internal Medicine 97: 809–813

Edelstein P H, Meyer R D, Finegold S M 1979 Isolation of Legionella pneumophila from blood. Lancet 1: 750–751

Edelstein P H, Snitzer J B, Finegold S M 1982a Isolation of Legionella pneumophila from hospital potable water specimens: comparison of direct plating with guinea pig inoculation. Journal of Clinical Microbiology 15: 1092–1096

Fallon R J 1981 Laboratory diagnosis of Legionnaires' disease. ACP Broadsheet 99

Fallon R J 1986 Identification of Legionella pneumophila with commercially available immunofluorescence test. Journal of Clinical Pathology 39: 693–694

Feeley J C, Gorman G W, Weaver R E, Mackel D C, Smith H W 1978 Primary isolation media for Legionnaires, disease bacterium. Journal of Clinical Microbiology 8: 320–325

Garrity G M, Brown A, Vickers R M 1980 Tatlockia and Fluoribacter: two new genera of organisms resembling Legionella pneumophila. International Journal of Systematic Bacteriology 30: 609–614

Garrity G M, Elder E M, Davis B, Vickers R M, Brown A 1982 Serological and genotypic diversity among serogroup 5 reacting environmental Legionella isolates. Journal of Clinical Microbiology 15: 646–653

Greaves P W 1980 Methods for the isolation of Legionella pneumophila. Journal of Clinical Pathology 33: 581–584

Harrison T G, Dournon E, Taylor A G 1987 Evaluation of sensitivity of two serological tests for diagnosing pneumonia caused by Legionella pneumophila serogroup 1. Journal of Clinical Pathology 40: 77–82

Harrison T G, Taylor A G 1982 A rapid microagglutination test for the diagnosis of Legionella pneumophila (serogroup 1) infection. Journal of Clinical Pathology 35: 1028–1031

Hébert G A 1981 Hippurate hydrolysis by Legionella pneumophila. Journal of Clinical Microbiology 13: 240–242

Heimer G V, Taylor C E D 1974 Improved mountant for immunofluorescence preparations. Journal of Clinical Pathology 27: 254–256

Herwaldt L A et al 1984 A new Legionella species, Legionella feeleii species nova, causes Pontiac fever in an automobile plant. Annals of Internal Medicine 100: 333–338

Joly J R, McKinney R M, Tobin J O'H, Bibb W F, Watkins I D, Ramsay D 1986 Development of a standardised subgrouping scheme for Legionella pneumophila serogroup 1 using monoclonal antibodies. Journal of Clinical Microbiology 23: 768–771

Kohler R B, Sathapatayavongs B 1983 Recent advances in the diagnosis of serogroup 1 L. pneumophila pneumonia by detection of urinary antigen. Zentralblatt für Bakteriologie Mikrobiologie und Hygiene I. Abt. Orig. A 255: 102–107

Moss C W, Weaver R E, Dees S B, Cherry W B 1977 Cellular fatty acid composition of isolates from Legionnaires' disease. Journal of Clinical Microbiology 6: 140–143

Orrison L H et al 1983 Legionella oakridgensis: unusual new species isolated from cooling tower water. Applied and Environmental Microbiology 45: 536–545

Pasculle A W et al 1980 Pittsburgh pneumonia agent: direct isolation from human lung tissue. Journal of Infection 141: 727–732

Rowbotham T J 1980 Preliminary report on the pathogenicity of Legionella pneumophila for freshwater and soil amoebae. Journal of Clinical Pathology 33: 1179–1183

Selander R K et al 1985 Genetic structure of populations of Legionella pneumophila. Journal of Bacteriology 163: 1021–1037

Smith M G 1982 A simple technique for the presumptive identification of Legionella pneumophila. Journal of Clinical Pathology 35: 1353–1355

Taylor A G, Harrison T G, Dighero M W, Bradstreet C M P 1979 False positive reactions in the indirect fluorescent antibody test for Legionnaires' disease eliminated by use of formalinised yolk-sac antigen. Annals of Internal Medicine 90: 686–689

Thacker L, McKinney R M, Moss C W, Summers H M, Spivack M L, O'Brien T 1981 Thermophilic spore-forming bacilli that mimic fastidious growth characteristics and colonial morphology of legionellae. Journal of Clinical Microbiology 13: 794–797

Thacker W L, Plikaytis B B, Wilkinson H W 1985 Identification of 22 *Legionella* species and 33 serogroups with the slide agglutination test. Journal of Clinical Microbiology 21: 779–782

Thornsberry C, Baker C N, Kirven L A 1978 *In vitro* activity of antimicrobial agents on Legionnaires' disease bacterium. Antimicrobial Agents and Chemotherapy 13: 78–80

Tobin J O'H, McKinney R M, Fallon R J 1987 Subgroups of *Legionella pneumophila* serogroup 1. Lancet 1: 1088–1089

Vickers R M, Brown A, Garrity G M 1981 Dye-containing buffered charcoal yeast extract medium for the differentiation of members of the family *Legionellaceae*. Journal of Clinical Microbiology 13: 380–382

Weaver R E 1978 Cultural and staining characteristics. In: Jones G L, Hébert G A (eds) Legionnaires; the disease, bacteriology and methodology, Centers for Disease Control, Atlanta, Georgia. p 39–43

Wilkinson H W, Fikes B J 1980 Slide agglutination test for serogrouping *Legionella pneumophila* and atypical *Legionella*-like organisms. Journal of Clinical Microbiology 11: 99–101

Wilkinson H W, Fikes B J, Cruce D D 1979 Indirect immunofluorescence test for serodiagnosis of Legionnaires' disease. Evidence for serogroup diversity of Legionnaires' disease bacterial antigens and for multiple specificity of human antibodies. Journal of Clinical Microbiology 9: 379–383

Bacteroides, Fusobacterium and related organisms: anaerobic cocci: identification of anaerobes

This chapter deals with the *Bacteroides/Fusobacterium* group of organisms and, for practical reasons, it embraces *Mobiluncus* and the anaerobic cocci. Many of the principles adopted for laboratory diagnosis and identification of these organisms are also applicable to the clostridia, which are covered in the next two chapters. Some procedures basic to anaerobic technology, such as anaerobic culture methodology, have been detailed in earlier sections of this book (Ch. 7). The first part of this chapter outlines a general approach to the identification of anaerobic bacteria, relevant not only to this chapter but also to the succeeding chapters on clostridia.

General approach to the identification of anaerobic bacteria

Table 36.1 at the end of this chapter outlines the range of tests and media that are of value in characterizing the different groups of strictly anaerobic Gram-positive and Gram-negative bacteria. As it is easy to presume that a demanding aerobe or facultative anaerobe might be an obligate anaerobe, it is most important to subject isolates to a systematic screening procedure as indicated in the first few steps of Table 36.1.

Cell morphology and Gram-stain reaction should be examined in films from blood agar (BA) or cooked meat broth (CMB) cultures incubated for 18–24 h, or longer for anaerobes that grow slowly. Similarly, colonial morphology on BA plates may be examined after 24 h, but prolonged incubation is required for slow growers.

Some organisms, e.g. *Bacteroides melaninogenicus*, produce dark brown or black colonies on blood-containing media, by forming a haem-protein complex. Up to 14 days incubation may be required before this is seen; pigment formation is less delayed if lysed blood is used. Fluorescence of colonies can be detected by exposing BA cultures to long-wave UV light (365 nm) from a Wood's lamp. Colonies of *B. melaninogenicus* fluoresce brick-red, and *Clostridium difficile* colonies fluoresce green. Colonies of fusobacteria fluoresce yellow on media containing cysteine hydrochloride. Note that other clostridia may also fluoresce and that *B. asaccharolyticus* and *B. bivius* colonies on blood agar are pink, red, dark red and purple under UV light at successive stages of growth over 1–4 days.

The further tests indicated in Table 36.1 extend into a range of biochemical and resistance tests that may be of value for determining the individual species within each of the broad groups of organisms. Practical experience with the characterization steps indicated in the subsequent tables in this chapter (or Ch. 37 for clostridia) will allow a bacteriologist to discriminate in the number of tests used for a particular identification, e.g. depending on the nature of a Gram-negative rod isolated, a short-cut approach along the lines set out in Table 36.2 at the end of this chapter might be adopted.

Detection and quantitation of fatty acid end-products of bacterial metabolism by *gas chromatography* (GC) is a useful aid to the identification of anaerobic bacteria. When this information is used in conjunction with details of cell morphology and Gram-stain reaction, it is possible to establish the identity of anaerobes to genus level (as in Table 36.3), and occasionally to species level. The use of GC in characterization of Gram-negative anaerobes is included in the further tables in this chapter, and accounts of GC for identification of the clostridia are given in Chapters 37 and 38. Technical details are given in specialist manuals (or see Deacon et al 1978); a brief account is provided in the *Methods* section of this chapter.

BACTEROIDACEAE

The strictly anaerobic Gram-negative non-sporing rod-shaped bacteria are abundantly represented as commensals in the human gastrointestinal tract, oropharynx and female genital tract and these include many opportunist pathogens. It is increasingly evident that these anaerobes are involved in a very wide range of clinical conditions and that characterization of individual species concerned can be of clinical significance. This section deals with the *Bacteroides, Fusobacterium* and *Leptotrichia* organisms of clinical interest. The description and laboratory guidelines are closely linked with the information given in the associated tables (see end of chapter). Many laboratories find it necessary to restrict the degree of characterization. The information given in Table 36.2 illustrates a short-cut approach in this complex field.

Morphology

Range from short Gram-negative rods to filamentous and fusiform shapes. Pleomorphism is common. All are non-sporing, but some may produce swollen spherical bodies resembling sporing forms when wet films are examined by phase contrast microscopy. Most species of clinical interest are non-motile.

Cultural characters

The nutritional requirements of this heterogeneous group vary. Most of the species of medical interest grow better on enriched media such as freshly prepared or pre-reduced blood agar. Development of visible colonies of some strains may require 48 h or more. Some have special requirements for haemin and vitamin K3 (menadione). The presence of 10% CO_2 in the anaerobic atmosphere often markedly enhances growth. Colonial appearances vary, depending on species and culture media, from tiny translucent colonies to large, grey, circular or irregular colonies at 24–48 h.

Biochemical activities

Active saccharolytic and some non-saccharolytic species are described. Some are proteolytic and a few produce other demonstrable exoenzymes that facilitate their early characterization (see below).

Sensitivity to physical and chemical agents

These organisms vary in their sensitivity to oxygen; in general, colonies on solid media should be picked promptly for subculture. Species variations in sensitivity to dyes, bile and antibiotics can be exploited in simple characterization systems (Table 36.2).

Antibiotic sensitivity

In general, organisms of the *B. fragilis* group are resistant to penicillin and produce potent cephalosporinases and penicillinases. A significant proportion of organisms in the *B. melaninogenicus* group are partially or markedly resistant to penicillin. The fusobacteria are generally sensitive to penicillin. All of these anaerobes are resistant to clinically achievable concentrations of the aminoglycosides. They are often resistant to the tetracyclines. They are generally sensitive to clindamycin, and virtually always sensitive to chloramphenicol and metronidazole.

Serological identification

Several different attempts pioneered by Beerens et al (1971) to develop a serological scheme for identifying *Bacteroides* spp. have been largely empirically based on heated or unheated whole cell antigens and procedures such as agglutination or immunofluorescence. In 1987, when this chapter was written, no serological scheme was widely in use. Two immunofluorescence kits available commercially (Fluoretec F and Fluoretec M; Pfizer) for the identification of the *B. fragilis* group and *B. melaninogenicus* spp. do not differentiate between the likely pathogens and non-pathogens and are still being evaluated. The F kit seems to react with the majority of *B. fragilis* strains but gives variable results with other species in the *B. fragilis* group. The M kit reacts with some *B. bivius* and *B. melaninogenicus* strains, but reactions within this group are not sufficiently specific. As more is understood of the antigens of *Bacteroides* spp., more specific serological schemes will be developed for the identification of these organisms. At present, capsular antigens and outer membrane protein antigens both appear promising for exploitation. The highly heterogeneous LPS antigens have been used in exploratory epidemiological studies.

Other typing methods

Promising results are being obtained with bacteriocin typing, which is simpler than serotyping and may be of diagnostic and epidemiological value (Riley & Mee 1982).

Animal pathogenicity

Animal pathogenicity tests are not performed routinely for any Gram-negative anaerobe. In our limited experience with fusobacteria, *F. necrophorum* is lethal for rabbits when injected intravenously. Various animal models have demonstrated that pathogenic synergy exists between some facultative anaerobes such as *Escherichia coli* and *Bacteroides* spp. (Onderdonk et al 1977; Kelly 1978).

Classification of Bacteroidaceae

The Gram-negative anaerobic non-sporing bacilli of clinical interest are essentially contained within the *Bacteroides/Fusobacterium* group (Bacteroidaceae). A spectrum of Gram-negative rods in this range of organisms extends across many genera, linked by unnamed and, as yet, inadequately characterized groups. There are associated non-anaerobic genera to add to the confusion; recently described genera with characterized species of medical and particular dental interest include the *Eikenella* group which is aerobic and includes capnophilic members, and *Wolinella* which is a group of anaerobic or microaerophilic species. The microaerophilic capnophilic organism formerly known as *Bacteroides ochraceus* is now in the genus *Capnocytophaga* (*C. ochracea*). These 'associated non-anaerobic genera' are not discussed further in this chapter, but there is a note on *Mobiluncus*. *Gardnerella* is described in Chapter 19.

By 1987, there were more than 30 species of *Bacteroides* and 14 species of *Fusobacterium*. Many species occur as normal commensals in man, but some have much greater pathogenic potential than others. *B. fragilis* is accepted as the most commonly encountered pathogenic member of the genus, but other pathogenic associations are increasingly recognized.

Several schemes have been developed for the identification of Gram-negative anaerobic rod-shaped bacteria. Those most widely used are based on publications of the Virginia Polytechnic Institute (Holdeman et al 1977), the Center for Disease Control, Atlanta (Dowell & Hawkins 1976) and the Wadsworth Hospital, Los Angeles (Sutter et al 1975). A shortened, simple and reliable scheme is that of Duerden et al (1980). *Bacteroides* and *Fusobacterium* can be readily separated into major groups by simple tests (Table 36.2) and these groups can be subdivided to species level by further biochemical tests (Tables 36.4–36.7; all at the end of this chapter). The *Bacteroides* organisms can be divided into the *B. fragilis* group, the *B. melaninogenicus/oralis* group, and an asaccharolytic group. In GC tests, the fusobacteria characteristically produce major amounts of butyric acid with varying amounts of other fatty acids but generally excluding iso-butyric and iso-valeric acids. On the other hand, most *Bacteroides* organisms produce major amounts of acetic and succinic acid; the few species that produce butyric acid usually also produce iso-butyric or iso-valeric acid or both of these (see Table 36.3).

Note. In the tables that give differential characteristics of important pathogens in this group of organisms, key reactions are indicated in bold and these provide a short-cut characterization procedure of value to hard-pressed clinical laboratories.

Bacteroides fragilis group

This comprises non-pigmented, strongly saccharolytic and bile tolerant species of *Bacteroides* and includes *B. fragilis, B. vulgatus, B. distasonis, B. thetaiotaomicron, B. ovatus, B. uniformis, B. variabilis, B. eggerthi* and *B. splanchnicus* (see Table 36.4). They are non-motile, non-sporing, small Gram-negative rods 1–4 × 0.4–0.8 μm with rounded ends. Pleomorphism is common and large bizarre rods with round or oval swellings can be seen if fermentable carbohydrate is present. They grow well on freshly prepared blood agar incubated anaerobically with 10% CO_2 at 37°C to produce smooth, circular, convex, opaque, light grey colonies 1–2 mm in diameter at 24 h that are usually non-haemolytic. All members of this group are resistant to penicillin.

Bacteroides fragilis. This organism has the characteristics of the group described above. It is not the most numerous of the commensal bacteroides but it is the most commonly encountered member of the group in a pathogenic role, occurring in postoperative infections associated with abdominal and gynaecological surgery, and in a wide range of other infective situations including cerebral abscess, lung abscess and soft tissue infections, often in concert with other pathogens. The infections are usually endogenous, often assisted by debilitating factors that operate locally or generally in the patient.

It is thought that *B. fragilis* owes its special pathogenic potential to its production of capsular material, but the factor or factors primarily related to the virulence of this organism are still debated. In common with some other pathogenic bacteroides organisms, *B. fragilis* can inhibit the effective phagocytosis and killing of coliform organisms in test mixtures with polymorphs; this

is a likely explanation of the pathogenic synergy exhibited in mixed infections with these organisms. Aggressins produced by *B. fragilis* that may contribute to virulence include a range of proteases, neuraminidase, DNase, heparinase and other enzymes. In addition to this range of biochemical activity against complex substrates, the organism has other activities including the ability to hydrolyse aesculin and to ferment several sugars actively; the latter characteristics are of use in sub-classification (see Table 36.4). *B. fragilis* produces very potent β-lactamases and these preclude the use of antibiotics of the penicillin series and most of the cephalosporin drugs, though cefoxitin has some activity. Some strains are resistant to the lincomycins. All but a very few strains are sensitive to metronidazole which is most often the drug of choice.

Bacteroides melaninogenicus/oralis group

This group (Table 36.5) comprises saccharolytic, bile-sensitive species of *Bacteroides*, some of which produce black-pigmented or brown colonies on blood-containing media. The pigmented species *B. melaninogenicus, B. intermedius, B. corporis* and related organisms not specified here are non-motile, non-sporing, small Gram-negative rods, 0.6–2 × 0.4 μm, often coccobacillary, and sometimes pleomorphic in broth cultures. They grow well on freshly prepared blood agar supplemented with menadione 1 μg/ml incubated anaerobically plus 10% CO_2 at 37°C. At 24 h colonies may be very small; at 48 h they are 1 mm, smooth, circular, convex and opaque. The colour of the colony changes from light grey, through tan and brown, to black. Speed of pigment development is enhanced on lysed blood agar, or by spotting a haemolytic organism on to an inoculated blood agar plate before incubation. Detectable development of pigment by some species may take up to 7 days or more. Colonies of *B. melaninogenicus* on blood agar, and cells of the species in pus or on wound swabs, will fluoresce brickred when subjected to long-wave (365 nm) UV light (Myers et al 1969).

Non-pigmented members of this group include *B. oralis, B. ruminicola, B. bivius* and *B. disiens*. Several new species have recently been proposed.

The cellular and colonial morphology is similar to that of the pigmented members, except that cells are often slightly larger and colonies are light grey to light tan and do not fluoresce brick-red.

B. melaninogenicus and related organisms are associated with periodontal disease, gingivitis, dental abscesses, maxillo-facial sepsis, lung abscess and cerebral abscess. The infections are often mixed. In acute ulcerative gingivitis (Vincent's infection) Bacteroides organisms occur in pathogenic synergy with Vincent's spirochaete and a fusiform organism which may be Fusobacterium nucleatum or Leptotrichia buccalis. The appearances in a Gram smear are diagnostic. Pigmented and non-pigmented members of the melaninogenicus/oralis complex are associated with infections of the female genito-urinary tract. These are assumed to be endogenous as the organisms are encountered frequently (but not invariably) as components of the commensal flora of that site. However, B. fragilis is still regarded as the commonest Gram-negative anaerobic pathogen in female genital tract infections (see Duerden 1980, 1984).

Asaccharolytic bacteroides group

This group (Table 36.6) comprises non-saccharolytic or weakly saccharolytic, usually bile sensitive, species of bacteroides, some of which produce black pigmented colonies on blood-containing media. The pigmented species, B. asaccharolyticus, B. endontalis and B. gingivalis, are non-motile, non-sporing, small Gram-negative rods, $1 \times 0.6\ \mu m$, often cocco-bacillary and pleomorphic. Colonies on freshly prepared blood agar are similar to pigmented members of the melaninogenicus/oralis group.

The non-pigmented asaccharolytic members include a number of species, some of debatable status. Cell and colonial morphology vary among the species. B. praeacutus is motile, and colonies of B. ureolyticus burrow into the surface of agar plates.

Fusobacteria and Leptotrichia

Representative species of fusobacteria are listed in Table 36.7.

These organisms tend to occur in mixed infections such as putrefactive necrotic fusospiro-chaetal conditions with much tissue destruction, as in cancrum oris, other maxillo-facial infections (sometimes following surgical excision for neoplastic disease), septic abortion and lung abscess. Sometimes a fusobacterial infection can be fulminating and can advance with great rapidity from a sore throat syndrome to a necro-tizing pneumonitis. Fusobacteria are commonly involved in dental and periodontal infections, ulcerative gingivitis (see above), liver abscess and cerebral abscess. Fusobacteria and bacter-oides organisms are often involved in concert or separately in necrotizing conditions variously described as anaerobic cellulitis, necrotizing fasciitis and dermal gangrene. The occurrence of these organisms in mixed infections with foul pus is common in infected pilonidal cysts, perianal abscesses, balanitis, and ulcers of the leg and buttocks, including diabetic ulcers and bed sores. Some species of fusobacteria produce long slender Gram-negative rods that are wide at the centre and taper towards the ends (fusiform), but others produce cells that range from cocco-bacilli to long slender rods with parallel sides and these are indistinguishable from other members of the Bacteroidaceae. Isolation is best on blood agar plates containing neomycin and vanco-mycin.* They are strict anaerobes, sensitive to metronidazole, and tolerant of gentian violet. Most are non-motile. After incubation at 37°C for 48 h colonies usually have a raised, irregular or crenated edge, a peaked centre, and may be striate and granular.

Fusobacterium nucleatum is the type species of the genus. It is a slender spindle-shaped Gram-negative rod, $5–10 \times 1\ \mu m$, with tapering pointed ends and often with central or eccentric swellings. After incubation for 48 h on freshly prepared blood agar, colonies are 1–2 mm, irreg-ular, low convex, translucent or opaque, grey and non-haemolytic. The organism is weakly saccharolytic, non-proteolytic and non-motile.

Fusobacterium necrophorum. This Gram-negative anaerobe has a tendency to pleo-morphism and irregular staining. Cells are $1–10 \times 0.5\ \mu m$; long filaments are frequently

_____
* Refer to Methods at end of this chapter.

seen. They are non-motile and non-sporing, but swollen areas sometimes occur. At 48 h, colonies are 1–2 mm, circular, with a flattened edge and raised or convex centre, translucent or opaque, grey and often β-haemolytic. Most strains are lipolytic (see *Methods*, Ch. 37).

Leptotrichia buccalis. This organism is characteristically seen in Gram smears of clinical specimens as long Gram-negative rods of considerable width and with terminal tapering; individual cells may be up to $15 \times 1.5 \mu m$. It is sensitive to metronidazole and tolerant of gentian violet. Colonies on blood agar after incubation for 48 h are 2–3 mm, very irregular and often striate. *Leptotrichia* has been thought of as essentially commensal in the human mouth, but pathogenic associations with other bacteria in the oropharynx are likely to be accepted.

Laboratory diagnosis of bacteroides and fusobacterial infections

The specimens should ideally be of pus, wound exudate, tissue or blood which has been transported to the laboratory in a closed syringe or in a container that has been flushed out with nitrogen. Swabs are not ideal; if they must be used, they should be inoculated on to the media directly, or transported to the laboratory in a reduced transport medium, or thrust into a semi-solid agar medium to avoid desiccation in transit. On receipt, specimens must be processed without delay. Clinical specimens containing fusobacteria or bacteroides can be handled briefly on the open bench and surface plating is suitable, provided that it is expeditious. An anaerobic cabinet (Ch. 7) is not essential, but can be useful if single specimens arrive sporadically or if cultures are to be checked regularly. Freshly poured plates or pre-reduced plates should be used. When seeded with a suitable inoculum, media should be promptly placed in an anaerobic environment with 10% CO_2 and incubated. The steps in a routine investigation are as follows:

1. Make a direct examination of the specimen. Note if it has a foul smell. Observe under a long-wave (365 nm) UV lamp for brick-red fluorescence, which suggests the presence of *B.*

melaninogenicus. Consider preparing an ether extract of the specimen for direct examination by gas chromatography* (Holdeman et al 1977).

2. Prepare films for phase contrast microscopy and Gram stain. Observe characteristic morphology: non-motile, pleomorphic, coccobacillary to fusiform or filamentous, Gram-negative. Consider fluorescent antibody stains for bacteroides, but note cautions (see above).

3. Plate on to two plates each of blood agar (Columbia base containing 4 or 8% whole blood and 1 or 2% freeze-thawed lysed blood and menadione 1 $\mu g/ml^*$) and two selective blood agar plates*. Primary sensitivity tests can be made at this stage by placing disks, e.g. metronidazole 5 μg and penicillin 1 or 2 units, on the first series of streaks. Also seed a tube of pre-reduced cooked meat broth (CMB).

4. Incubate one blood agar plate aerobically and the rest anaerobically with 10% CO_2 at 37°C. Check the CMB, the blood agar and one selective plate after 24 h. Leave the remaining selective plate undisturbed for 48 h.

5. Examine plates for typical colonies. Examine CMB enrichment by microscopy, and subculture as in (3).

6. Pick colonies and subculture into pre-reduced CMB, into PPY medium for subsequent identification by biochemical tests, and into PPY medium containing glucose 1% for gas chromatography,* and also to observe whether or not glucose is fermented.

7. Identification to group level is by observing the tolerance of the organism to bile and gentian violet,* its resistance to a range of antibiotics* and its ability to ferment glucose. Full identification to species level is by selecting the appropriate biochemical tests as indicated in Tables 36.1–7. A more detailed approach is described by Bennett & Duerden (1985).

MOBILUNCUS SPECIES

These are anaerobic or microaerophilic, curved, Gram-negative or Gram-variable rods and they are motile with two or more subterminal flagella. *Mobiluncus* spp. have antibiotic sensitivity profiles that are more typical of Gram-positive organisms, and some features of their cell wall structure are more typical of Gram-positive cells, but this is debated. The organisms may occur in the vagina of apparently healthy women, but seem to have an association with non-specific or bacterial vaginosis. The organisms are fastidious and grow slowly at 33–37°C, producing round, entire, convex, smooth, translucent, colourless colonies, 2–3 mm in diameter, after anaerobic incubation on blood agar medium for 5 days. A suitable selective medium is blood agar supplemented with colistin 10 μg/ml and nalidixic acid 10 μg/ml. Two species are currently recognized, *M. curtisi* and *M. mulieris*. Both accepted species are saccharolytic, but can be differentiated as follows:

M. curtisi is 1.7 × 0.5 μm, Gram-variable, metronidazole resistant, and gives positive results in tests for hippurate and arginine hydrolysis and ONPG. Small amounts of acetic acid and major amounts of succinic acid are produced in glycogen-containing media.

M. mulieris is 2.9 × 0.5 μm, Gram-negative, metronidazole sensitive, and gives negative reactions in tests for hippurate and arginine hydrolysis and ONPG. Major amounts of acetic and succinic acids, and sometimes small amounts of lactic acid are produced in glycogen-containing media.

ANAEROBIC COCCI

Strictly anaerobic Gram-positive cocci have been assigned to the genera *Peptococcus, Peptostreptococcus, Ruminococcus* and *Sarcina*; strictly anaerobic Gram-negative cocci are included in *Veillonella, Megasphera* and *Acidaminococcus*. This brief account is restricted to *Peptococcus, Peptostreptococcus* and *Veillonella*, as these are the genera most commonly associated with clinical infections. Most of the peptococci have now been reclassified as peptostreptococci. *Peptococcus niger* is the only surviving member of the genus *Peptococcus* (see Table 36.8 and Ezaki et al, 1983).

Many species of anaerobic cocci are commonly found as commensals on the human skin, in the female genital tract, in the oropharynx, and in the gastrointestinal tract. These commensal organisms may contaminate clinical specimens. Anaerobic cocci may nevertheless be significant pathogens in intra-abdominal infections, brain abscesses, empyema and aspiration pneumonias, hepatic abscesses, infections of the female genital tract, or infections following maxillofacial surgery in debilitated patients. An association of anaerobic cocci with infected sebaceous cysts is recognized, and anaerobic cocci may also occur in many mixed infections of skin and soft tissues.

The anaerobic cocci are generally sensitive to metronidazole and penicillin, and to a wide range of other antimicrobial drugs including tetracycline, erythromycin, chloramphenicol, clindamycin and the cephalosporins. However, variations in sensitivity make it necessary to check the susceptibilities of isolates in the laboratory. Some cocci that may seem to be anaerobic on primary isolation but are resistant to metronidazole can be shown on subculture to grow aerobically, or microaerophically, or in a CO_2-enriched atmosphere; these isolates are not true anaerobic cocci (Watt & Jack 1977).

Laboratory diagnosis of anaerobic cocci

Table 36.8 indicates some of the representative species and a range of useful tests. Metronidazole sensitivity is used to differentiate true anaerobic cocci from those that may seem to be anaerobic on primary isolation. Vancomycin resistance is typical of Gram-negative anaerobic cocci. The peptococci and some species of peptostreptococci are resistant to novobiocin. Most strains of *Peptostreptococcus anaerobius* are sensitive to sodium polyanetholsulphonate (Liquoid), giving inhibition zones of more than 12 mm diameter with disks containing 100 μg Liquoid/disk; most other anaerobic cocci are resistant in this test. The species noted below merit special attention.

Peptostreptococcus anaerobius. Spherical or lanceolate Gram-positive cocci, diameter 0.8 μm. Short chains with some single and paired cocci are seen in smears from broth culture. Abundant gas produced in broth culture. Colonies on blood agar after anaerobic incubation with 10% CO_2

for 24 h at 37°C are 0.5–1.5 mm in diameter, round, convex, shiny, opaque, grey and non-haemolytic. After further incubation, colonies may become slightly irregular in outline, umbonate, with a light grey centre and darker grey periphery.

Peptostreptococcus magnus. Spherical Gram-positive cocci, diameter 0.8–1 μm. Small and large irregular masses with some single and paired cocci are seen in smears from broth culture. Slight gas production in broth culture. Colonies on blood agar after incubation for 24 h are very small, round, convex, shiny, opaque, grey and non-haemolytic.

Peptostreptococcus asaccharolyticus is similar to *P. magnus*, but colonies on blood agar after incubation for 24 h are usually 0.8–1 mm in diameter. Despite its name, it produces abundant gas in broth culture.

Veillonella parvula. Spherical Gram-negative cocci, diameter 0.3–0.5 μm. Diplococci and single cocci with some clusters are seen in smears from broth culture. Abundant gas is produced in broth culture. Colonies on blood agar after incubation for 24 h are very small, round, convex, shiny, opaque, light grey and non-haemolytic.

METHODS

Growth factors for anaerobes

The inclusion of reducing substances (cooked meat particles, cysteine hydrochloride, sodium thioglycollate, glucose) in culture media improves the growth of anaerobic bacteria. Some anaerobes have a requirement for other growth factors that are not present in the basal media; the addition of haemin and menadione (vitamin K3) enhances the growth of many species of bacteroides. There are claims that the growth of anaerobic cocci is enhanced by Tween 80 (Holdeman et al 1977); the authors could not demonstrate this effect in PPY medium.

Haemin and menadione

Haemin 500 μg/ml. Dissolve 50 mg haematin hydrochloride in 1 ml of 1 mol/litre NaOH solution, and make up to 100 ml with distilled water. Filter sterilize.

Menadione 100 μg/ml. Dissolve 10 mg menadione in 2 ml ethanol, and make up to 100 ml with distilled water. Filter sterilize. Protect from light.

Equal volumes of haemin and menadione solutions can conveniently be mixed before storage. They are added to all media for growth of bacteroides, but can safely be added to all media for growth of anaerobes with no apparent inhibitory effect. The final concentrations in the medium should be haemin 5 μg/ml and menadione 1 μg/ml.

Cysteine HCl 3.75%

Dissolve 3.75 g L-cysteine hydrochloride in 100 ml distilled water. Autoclave at 121°C for 20 min. The final concentration in the medium should be 0.075%.

Sodium carbonate 2%

Dissolve 2 g Na_2CO_3 in 100 ml distilled water. Filter sterilize. The final concentration in the medium should be 0.04%.

Tween 80 10%

Mix 10 ml Tween 80 and 90 ml distilled water. Autoclave at 121°C for 20 min. The final concentration in the medium should be 0.02–0.1%.

Media for anaerobes

Many media in general use are given in Chapter 6. Here we list several media that are specially modified for anaerobic work.

Thioglycollate medium

For fermentation and urease tests use Thioglycollate medium, without glucose or indicator (BBL), supplemented with 0.25% Yeast extract (Oxoid) and 0.25% sodium succinate. Dispense in 5 ml volumes and autoclave at 121°C for 20 min.

Proteose peptone–yeast extract broth (PPY)

Proteose peptone (Oxoid)	2%
Yeast extract (Difco)	1%
NaCl	0.5%

Dissolve the ingredients in distilled water and adjust the pH to 7.4. Dispense in 5 ml volumes and autoclave at 121°C for 20 min. For use, drive off dissolved oxygen by placing in boiling bath for 10 min, then add:

L-cysteine HCl, sterile 3.75% solution	0.1 ml
Na$_2$CO$_3$, sterile 2% solution	0.1 ml

Note: PPY medium with glucose 1% (PPYG medium is used for gas chromatography (see below).

Blood agar for anaerobes

The basic medium is Columbia agar (Oxoid). It is autoclaved at 121°C for 20 min and cooled to about 50°C, when the following are added to give:

Blood agar: 5% defibrinated horse blood.

Lysed blood agar: 5% saponin-lysed horse blood, and menadione to 1 μg/ml.

Combined blood/lysed blood agar: 4% whole blood, 1% freeze-thawed lysed blood and 1 μg/ml menadione. (Use of this medium allows haemolysis to be detected, and speeds up the formation of pigment by pigmented species of bacteroides.)

Selective blood agar

A range of agents can be added to any of the above blood agar media to make them selective for anaerobes as follows (the concentrations given are the final concentrations in the complete medium):

Selective medium for anaerobes. Add gentamicin 20 μg/ml.

Selective medium for bacteroides. Add kanamycin 75 μg/ml and vancomycin 7.5 μg/ml.

Selective medium for fusobacteria. Add neomycin 100 μg/ml and vancomycin 7.5 μg/ml.

Selective medium for clostridia. Add neomycin 70 μg/ml.

Fermentation tests for anaerobes

Dissolve the carbohydrates in distilled water and filter sterilize. Rhamnose, trehalose, melibiose, aesculin, xylan, cellobiose, inositol and mannose are prepared as 10% solutions, and used at a final concentration of 0.5%; the other substrates are prepared as 20% solutions, and used at a final concentration of 1%. Add 0.25 ml amounts of the appropriate test carbohydrate solutions to 5 ml amounts of reduced thioglycollate medium or PPY broth.

After inoculating the test organism, incubate anaerobically with 10% CO$_2$ at 37°C for 24 h, or up to 4 days until reasonable growth occurs. A seeded tube of the test medium without carbohydrate is incubated as a reference control. Read the results, preferably with a pH meter, or by adding a suitable pH indicator solution (e.g. a 0.02 ml drop of a 0.1% aqueous bromothymol blue solution). If a pH meter is used, the test is regarded as positive if the pH falls 0.5 unit below that of the carbohydrate-free reference control culture. If the indicator is used, a yellow colour indicates a positive result, and a green colour indicates a negative result. It is not advisable to incorporate an indicator in the culture medium at the start as indicator dyes may be decolourized, sometimes irreversibly, under anaerobic conditions. When equivocal results are obtained with the indicator solution, they should be verified with a pH meter.

Other tests modified for anaerobes

Urease

Dissolve the urea (10%) in distilled water and filter sterilize. Perform this test in thioglycollate medium or proteose peptone yeast extract (PPY) broth containing 1% urea, and read the results as for the fermentation tests. The test is regarded as positive if the pH rises 0.5 unit above that of the substrate-free reference control culture, or if the indicator turns blue.

Indole production

Extract 5 ml of PPY culture with 0.5 ml toluene. Slowly layer 0.5 ml Ehrlich's indole reagent on to the liquid interface. A red/purple colour indicates a positive result.

Ehrlich's indole reagent. Dissolve 1 g p-dimethyl-aminobenzaldehyde in 95 ml absolute ethanol, then slowly add 20 ml concentrated HCl. Protect from light.

Nitrate reduction

Sterilize a solution of potassium nitrate (KNO$_3$) 2% in distilled water by autoclaving at 121°C for 20 min. Use this to supplement PPY medium with KNO$_3$ 200 μg/ml. To 5 ml of the test culture in this PPY nitrate medium, add 0.25 ml Reagent 1, then 0.25 ml Reagent 2. A red colour indicates the presence of nitrites.

Reagent 1. Add 100 ml distilled water and 30 ml glacial acetic acid to 0.5 g sulphanilic acid and allow to dissolve.

Reagent 2. Dissolve 0.2 g Cleves acid (5-amino-2 naphthalene sulphonic acid) in 120 ml distilled water by warming in a waterbath, then add 30 ml glacial acetic acid.

Gas chromatography (GC) of metabolic products

This procedure can be used with cultures of test organisms, or directly with pus or exudate. Grow cultures for 24 h or longer in 5 ml of PPY medium containing 1% (w/v) glucose (PPYG). After acidification to *c.* pH 2 with 0.1 ml of 50% (v/v) H$_2$SO$_4$, remove the bacteria and insoluble material by centrifugation at 5000 *g* for 15 min. For analysis of volatile fatty acids (VFA) and alcohols, prepare ether extracts by adding 0.2 ml 50% (v/v) H$_2$SO$_4$, 0.4 g NaCl and 1 ml diethyl ether to 1 ml of the prepared culture supernate. After mixing well and centrifuging at 500 *g* for 5 min, carefully pipette the ether layer on to fine-mesh anhydrous CaCl$_2$ to remove water. The CaCl$_2$ should be about one quarter of the total volume, and the mixture should be left for 5 min before use (Holdeman et al 1977). Inject samples (1 μl) into the GC column. It is possible to obtain VFA profiles by injecting samples (1 μl) of acidified culture supernate directly on to some GC columns (Deacon et al 1978) but

these columns become contaminated and the packing must be replaced. Ether extraction is essential for samples of pus or exudate. For non-volatile fatty acids (lactic, succinic and phenyl-acetic), methylate samples by mixing 1 ml of prepared culture supernate, 0.4 ml of 50% (v/v) H$_2$SO$_4$ and 2 ml methanol in a stoppered tube and either leave overnight at room temperature, or heat at 60°C for 1 h. Add 1 ml distilled water and 0.5 ml of chloroform and mix well by inversion. If an emulsion forms, centrifuge at 500 *g* for 5 min. Inject samples (1 μl) of the chloroform layer on to the GC column.

A less hazardous solvent, methyl *tert*-butyl ether, can replace both diethyl ether and chloroform for the extraction of volatile and non-volatile fatty acids (Thomann & Hill 1986).

Following separation of the acids in the column, they are detected and then recorded as a series of peaks on a chart recorder. Identification and quantitation of the substances producing these peaks is done by comparing the retention time and the peak area respectively with peaks produced by standard amounts of known acids.

Useful column packings for analysing metabolic products include; FFAP, SP 1220 (15%) + H$_3$PO$_4$ (1%), or SP 1000 (10%) + H$_3$PO$_4$ (1%) on 100/200 Chromosorb WAW (Supelco), or Chromosorb 101, 100/120 mesh (Supelco, or Phase Sep).

Aesculin hydrolysis

Aesculin cooked meat broth is prepared similarly to CMB, except that aesculin is dissolved in the broth component before autoclaving. Add 0.5 ml of a 1% aqueous ferric ammonium citrate solution to the test culture in CMB containing 1% aesculin, or PPY containing 0.2% aesculin. A black colour indicates a positive result. *Note*: renew the ferric ammonium citrate solution when it changes from green to brown.

Gelatin digestion

Observe a charcoal gelatin disk incubated in a CMB culture of the test organism for up to 2 weeks. Release of charcoal indicates digestion of the gelatin.

Prepare disks by a modification of Kohn's method (1953). Dissolve 12.5 g gelatin (Difco) in 100 ml nutrient broth (Oxoid No. 2). Add 5 g of finely powdered charcoal, pour the mixture into flat dishes to a depth of *c*. 3 mm and allow to solidify at 4°C. Hold the charcoal gelatin in 4% aqueous formaldehyde solution at room temperature for 5 days and then, after rinsing briefly in tap water, cut 1 cm disks. Leave the disks in running tap water for 48 h or longer, until all the formalin is removed. Test this by placing one of the disks on a nutrient agar plate that has been flood-seeded with a 24 h culture of the Oxford strain of *Staphylococcus aureus*. When virtually no zone of inhibition occurs, the disks are considered free from formaldehyde. Place disks in sterile bottles, cover with sterile distilled water and finally pasteurize by heating at 70°C for 20 min. Store at 4°C. Test a random sample of disks for sterility and stability by incubating in CMB at 37°C for at least 14 days.

Tolerance tests

Growth of the test organism is observed in solid media containing the test agent. We recommend separate plates, one containing sodium taurocholate 0.5% and one with gentian violet.

Prepare the media as follows: 0.25% Yeast extract (Oxoid) and 0.25% sodium succinate are added to the Columbia agar base before autoclaving. When cooled to about 50°C, add haemin 5 μg/ml and menadione 1 μg/ml. Then add the inhibitory agents as follows: *bile* medium, 0.5% sodium taurocholate; *gentian violet* medium, Gurr's gentian violet (BDH) to a final concentration of 1 in 100 000. Aqueous stock solutions of the dye are prepared at 100× the final concen-

tration, and the sodium taurocholate at 10× the final concentration, and sterilized by autoclaving at 121°C for 20 min. The control medium has no further additives.

Each medium is seeded with 0.02 ml of starter CMB culture, and this inoculum is spread with a loop over about 1/6 of the area of the plate. After incubation, plates are observed for growth or inhibition. Set up known control organisms on each batch of tolerance plates. Suitable control strains, and the expected results are as follows:

Test organism	Growth on medium		
	Control	with sodium taurocholate	with gentian violet
B. fragilis (NCTC9344)	+	+	−
B. intermedius (NCTC9338)	+	−	−
F. necrogenes (NCTC10723)	+	+	+

Antibiotic resistance tests

These tests are useful in the characterization of some anaerobes. Note that some of the substances are used at levels that could not be safely achieved therapeutically; these tests should not be confused with antibiotic *sensitivity* tests.

Freshly prepared blood agar plates are seeded by spreading 0.02 ml of starter CMB culture on the surface with a glass spreader. The diameters of zones of inhibition are measured after 24 h incubation, or when satisfactory growth occurs. A zone of <15 mm is considered to indicate resistance.

The following antibiotic disks should be used: neomycin, 1000 μg/disk; kanamycin, 1000 μg/disk; benzylpenicillin, 2 units/disk; metronidazole, 5 μg/disk.

Table 36.1 Tests required to identify anaerobic bacteria.

Key: N, necessary; . . ., not necessary; U, use in some cases. For *Methods* see text, Chs 36 and 37. BA, blood agar plate; EYA, egg-yolk agar plate; CMB, cooked meat broth; PPY, proteose peptone-yeast extract broth; TG, thioglycollate medium; SSA, semi-solid agar.

| Test | Test required for identification of | | | | Media employed (see Key) |
	Bacteroides	*Fusobacterium*	*Clostridium*	Anaerobic cocci	
No growth in air	N	N	N	N	BA
No growth in air + 10% CO_2	N	. . .	. . .	N	BA
Gram stain reaction	N	N	N	N	CMB or PPY or BA
Cell morphology	N	N	N	N	CMB or PPY or BA
Spore shape and position	. . .	. . .	N	. . .	CMB
Motility	. . .	. . .	U	. . .	CMB or SSA or BA
Colonial morphology	N	N	N	N	BA
Colony fluorescence at 365 nm	U	. . .	U	. . .	BA
Pigment	N	. . .	. . .	U	Lysed BA or BA
Phospholipase, and neutralization by antisera	. . .	. . .	N	. . .	EYA
Lipase	. . .	U	N	. . .	EYA
Bile and dye tolerance	Sodium taurocholate Gentian violet	. . .	. . .	. . .	Tolerance test agar
Antibiotic resistance	Kanamycin 1000 µg Neomycin 1000 µg Penicillin 2 units Metronidazole 5 µg	. . .		Metronidazole 5 µg Novobiocin 5 µg Vanomycin 5µg Liquoid 100 µg	BA
Indole production	N	N	N	N	PPY
Aesculin hydrolysis	N	N	N	U	CMB + 1% aesculin or PPY + 0.2% aesculin
Gelatin digestion	N	. . .	N	. . .	CMB with charcoal gelatin disk
Meat digestion	. . .	. . .	U	. . .	
Fermentation[a]	Glucose Lactose Sucrose Maltose Rhamnose Trehalose Xylose Xylan	Glucose Lactose Sucrose Mannose Starch Fructose	Glucose Lactose Sucrose Maltose Mannose Mannitol Xylose Melibiose Inositol	Glucose Lactose Sucrose Maltose	PPY or TG
Urease	N	. . .	U	. . .	PPY or TG
Nitrate reduction	U	. . .	. . .	U	PPY with nitrate
Toxin test	. . .	. . .	U	. . .	
Gas chromatography	U	U	U	U	PPY + 1% glucose

[a] The extended range of these useful sugars is not always necessary. The selection depends upon the degree of characterization required (see following tables).

Table 36.2 Typical patterns of results obtained in antibiotic-disk resistance tests and tolerance tests with anaerobic Gram-negative rods.
Key: R, resistant; S, sensitive; S/R, 30–70% of strains give each result; R(S), few species give sensitive result; +, growth; −, inhibited; −(+), few species give positive result; +/−, result varies depending on species.

Test	Pattern of results obtained with strains of				
	B. fragilis group	*B. melaninogenicus/ oralis* group	Asaccharolytic *Bacteroides* group	*Fuso- bacterium*	*Leptotrichia buccalis*
Antibiotic resistance[a]					
Neomycin 1000 μg	R	S	S/R	S	S
Kanamycin 1000 μg	R	R	R(S)	S	S
Penicillin 2 units	R	S/R	S	S	S
Tolerance of:					
Bile salt[b]	+	−	−	+/−	−
Gentian violet[b]	−	−	−(+)	+	+
Fermentation of:					
Glucose	+	+	−	+/−	+

[a] Amount of antibiotic in disk is given.
[b] See *Methods*.

Table 36.3 Identification of anaerobic bacteria to genus level by gas chromatography, cell morphology and Gram-stain reaction.

Gram negative		Gram positive	
Rod-shaped bacilli		*Rod-shaped bacilli*	
a. Peritrichous flagella or non-motile		a. No spores present	
1. Lactic acid only major product	*Leptotrichia*	1. Lactic acid only major product	*Lactobacillus*
2. n-Butyric acid with no (or only trace amounts of) iso-butyric or iso-valeric acid	*Fusobacterium*	2. Lactic and acetic acids in ratio 1: > 1	*Bifidobacterium*
3. Not as (1) or (2) above, and usually acetic and succinic acid produced	*Bacteroides, Capnocytophaga*[a]	3. Acetic and propionic acids as major products	*Propionibacterium*
b. Polar flagella, motile	*Campylobacter*[a]	4. Acetic acid ± formic acid, and lactic or succinic acid or both as major products	*Actinomyces*
c. Spiral cells with axial fibrils	*Treponema, Borrelia*	5. n-Butyric acid + others, or acetic and formic acid, or no major acids produced	*Eubacterium*
		b. Spores present	*Clostridium*
Cocci		*Cocci*	
1. Acetic and propionic acid	*Veillonella*	1. Lactic acid only major product	*Streptococcus*[a]
2. Acetic and butyric acid	*Acidaminococcus*	2. Not as (1)	*Peptococcus, Peptostreptococcus, Ruminococcus*
3. Iso-butyric, butyric, iso-valeric and caproic acid	*Megasphera*		

[a] Although not strict anaerobes, these organisms are included because on primary isolation they may fail to grow aerobically or may grow only anaerobically. They are resistant to metronidazole.

Table 36.4 Differential characters and key for the identification of the *Bacteroides fragilis* group.
Key: +, 95% of strains give a positive result; −, 95% of strains give a negative result; +/−, 30–70% of strains give each result; +(−), 70–95% of strains give the positive result; ..., not tested. For *Methods* see text. Key reactions are printed in bold.

Bile tolerance	Aesculin hydrolysis	Glucose[a]	Lactose[a]	Indole production	Sucrose[a]	Trehalose[a]	Rhamnose[a]	Xylan[a]	Fatty acids[b] produced	Species
+	+	+	+	+	+	+	+	+	A S (p ib iv l)	*B. ovatus*
+	+	+	+	+	+	+	+	−	A S (f p ib iv l)	*B. thetaiotaomicron*
+(−)	+	+	+	+	+	+(−)	−	...	A p S (f ib iv l)	*B. uniformis*
+/−	+	+	+	+	+	−	+	+/−	A p S (iv l)	*B. variabilis*
+(−)	+	+	+	+	+	+(−)	−	...	A p S (f ib iv l)	*B. uniformis*
+	+	+	+	+	−	−	+	+	A p S (ib iv l)	*B. eggerthi*
+	+	+	+	+	−	−	−	...	A p ib b iv S (l)	*B. splanchnicus*
+	+	+	+	−	+	+	+(−)	−	A S (p ib iv l)	*B. distasonis*
+	+/−	+	+	−	+	−	+	−(+)	A p S (ib iv l)	*B. vulgatus*
+	+	+	+	−	+	−	−	−	A p S (f ib iv l)	*B. fragilis*

[a] Fermentation test.
[b] Fatty acids in gas chromatography. Symbols outside brackets, produced by all strains; symbols inside brackets, produced by some strains. The following symbols are used to identify the acids and to indicate the relative amounts produced:

Acid	0.2–10 µmol/ml	>10 µmol/ml
Acetic	a	A
Formic	f	F
Propionic	p	P
Iso-butyric	ib	iB
Butyric	b	B
Iso-valeric	iv	iV
Valeric	v	V
Iso-caproic	ic	iC
Caproic	c	C
Heptanoic	h	H
Lactic	l	L
Succinic	s	S
Phenylacetic	ph	Ph

Table 36.5 Differential characters and key for the identification of the *Bacteriodes melaninogenicus/oralis* group. *Key*: See Table 36.4.

Glucose[a]	Maltose[a]	Xylose[a]	Indole production	Sucrose[a]	Pigment production	Aesculin hydrolysis	Lactose[a]	Fatty acids produced	Species
+	+	+	+	+	-	+	+	A p iv S	B. zoogleoformans
+	+(-)	+	-	+	-	+/-	+	A S (p ib iv l)	B. ruminicola-like[b]
+	+(-)	-	+	+(-)	+	-	-(+)	A iv S (p ib l)	B. intermedius
+	+	-	-	+	+	+/-	+	A S (p ib iv l)	B. melaninogenicus-like[c]
+	+	-	-	+	-	+;/-	+	A S (p ib iv l)	B. oralis-like[d]
+	+	-	-	-	+	-	-	A ib iv S (l)	B. corporis
-(+)	-	-	-	-	-	+	-	a s (pl)	B. capillosus[e]
+	+	-	-	-	-	-	+	A iv S (p ib l)	B. bivius
+	+	-	-	-	-	-	-	A S (p ib iv l)	B. disiens

[a] Fermentation test.
[b] Includes *B. ruminicola*, *B. buccae* and *B. oris*.
[c] Includes *B. melaninogenicus*, *B. loeschi* and *B. denticola*.
[d] Includes *B. oralis*, *B. veroralis* and *B. buccalis*.
[e] Asaccharolytic strains occur; see Table 36.6.

Table 36.6 Differential characters and key for the identification of the asaccharolytic *Bacteroides* group. *Key*: see Table 36.4.

Glucose[a]	Indole production	Motility	Aesculin hydrolysis	Nitrate reduction	Urease production	Pigment production	Phenylacetic acid production	Fatty acids produced	Species
-(+)	-	-	+	-	-	-	-	a s (p l)	B. capillosus
-	-	-	-	+	+	-	-	a s (f p l)	B. ureolyticus
-	+(-)	-	-	-	-	+	+	A p ib B iv ph (l s)	B. gingivalis
-	+(-)	-	-	-	-	+	-	A p ib B iv (l s)	B. asaccharolyticus-like[b]
-	-	+	-	+	-	-	-	A p iB B iv (f l s)	B. praeacutus

[a] Fermentation test.
[b] Includes *B. asaccharolyticus* and *B. endontalis*

Table 36.7 Differential characters and key for the identification of the fusobacteria and *Leptotrichia buccalis*.
Key: see Table 36.4.

Indole production	Aesculin hydrolysis	Mannose[a]	Starch[a]	Sucrose[a]	Fructose[a]	Lipase production	Glucose[a]	Lactose[a]	Butyric acid[b]	Fatty acids produced	Species
+	–	–	–	–	+(–)	–	–	–	+	a p B s (f L)	*F. nucleatum*
+	–	–	–	–	–(+)	+(–)	–(+)	–	+	a p B (f L s)	*F. necrophorum*
+	–	–	–	–	–	–	+(–)	–	+	a p B (f L s)	*F. gonidiaformans*
+	–	–	–	–	–	–	–(+)	–	+	a p B L (f s)	*F. naviforme*
+(–)	–	+	–	–	+	–	+	–	+	A B L (p s)	*F. varium*
–	+	+	–(+)	+/–	+	–	+	+	+	a p B (f iv L s)	*F. mortiferum*
–	+	+	–(+)	+	+	–	+	+	–	L (a f s)	*L. buccalis*
–	+	+	–	–(+)	+	–	+	–	+	a B (f p l s)	*F. necrogenes*
–	+	–	–(+)	–(+)	+(–)	–	+(–)	+(–)	+	B (a f p L s)	*F. prausnitzi*
–	–	–(+)	+	–	–(+)	–	+	–	+	a B L s	*F. plauti*
–	–	+	–	+	+	–	+	–	+	a B L	*F. perfoetans*
+(–)	–	+	–	–	+	–	+	–	+	A B L (p s)	*F. varium*
–	–	–	–	–	–	–	–	–	+	a B (f L s)	*F. russi*

[a] Fermentation test.
[b] Butyric acid is a major product of the fusobacteria.

Table 36.8 Differential characters and key for the identification of the anaerobic cocci. See *Methods* at end of chapter.
Key: S, sensitive; R, resistant; S(R), a few strains give resistant result; See also Table 36.4.

Metronidazole	Vancomycin	Novobiocin	Liquoid	Indole production	Glucose	Lactose	Sucrose	Maltose	Caproic acid	Butyric acid	Fatty acids	Species
S	S	S	R	–	+	+	+	+	–	–	A s (l p)	*Peptostreptococcus productus*
S	S	S	R	–	+	+	–	+	–	–	a L (s)	*Peptostreptococcus parvulus*
S	S	S	S(R)	–	+	–	–	+	–	+/–	A (ib b iv ic l)	*Peptostreptococcus anaerobius*
S	S	S	R	–	–	–	–	–	–	–	A (f l s)	*Peptostreptococcus micros*
S	S	S	R	+	–	–	–	–	–	+	a p b	*Peptostreptococcus indolicus*
S	S	R	R	+	–	–	–	–	–	+	a b	*Peptostreptococcus asaccharolyticus*
S	S	R	R	–	+	–	–	–	–	–	A F	*Peptostreptococcus saccharolyticus*
S	S	R	R	–	–	–	–	–	+	+	ib B iv C (a l s)	*Peptococcus niger*
S	S	R	R	–	–	–	–	–	–	+	A (f l s)	*Peptostreptococcus prevoti*
S	S	R	R	–	–	–	–	–	–	–	a b (f p l s)	*Peptostreptococcus magnus*
S	R	...	...	–	–	–	–	–,	–	–	a p (s)	*Veillonella parvula*[a]

[a] *V. parvula* and related Gram-negative species (see Mays et al 1982).

REFERENCES

Beerens H, Wattre P, Shinjo T, Romond C 1971 Premiers résultats d'un essai de classification sérologique de 131 souches de *Bacteroides* du groupe *fragilis* (Eggerthella). Annales de l'Institut Pasteur, Paris 121: 187–198

Bennett K W, Duerden B I 1985 Identification of fusobacteria in a routine diagnostic laboratory. Journal of Applied Bacteriology 59: 171–181

Deacon A G, Duerden B I, Holbrook W P 1978 Gas-liquid chromatographic analysis of metabolic products in the identification of Bacteroidaceae of clinical interest. Journal of Medical Microbiology 11: 81–99

Dowell V R, Hawkins T M 1976 Laboratory methods in anaerobic bacteriology. CDC Laboratory Manual, CDC, Atlanta

Duerden B I 1980 The isolation and identification of *Bacteroides* spp. from the normal human faecal flora. Journal of Medical Microbiology 13: 69–78

Duerden B I 1984 Infections due to Gram-negative non-sporing anaerobic bacilli. In: Smith G R (ed) Topley & Wilson's Principles of bacteriology, virology and immunity, 7th edn, vol 3 Ch. 62. Edward Arnold, London

Duerden B I, Collee J G, Brown R, Deacon A G, Holbrook W P 1980 A scheme for the identification of Gram-negative bacilli by conventional bacteriological tests. Journal of Medical Microbiology 13: 231–245

Eyaki T, Yamamoto N, Ninomiya K, Suzuki S, Yabuuchi E 1983 Transfer of *Peptococcus indolicus*, *P. asaccharolyticus*, *P. prevotii* and *P. magnus* to the genus *Peptostreptococcus* and proposal of *Peptostreptococcus tetradius* sp. nov. International Journal of Systematic Bacteriology 33: 683–698

Holdeman L V, Cato E P, Moore W E C 1977 Anaerobe laboratory manual, 4th edn. Virginia Polytechnic and State University, Blacksburg, Virginia

Kelly M J 1978 Quantitative and histological demonstration of pathogenic synergy between *Escherichia coli* and *Bacteroides fragilis* in guinea pig wounds. Journal of Medical Microbiology 11: 513–523

Kohn J 1953 A preliminary report of a new gelatin liquefaction method. Journal of Clinical Pathology 6:249

Mays T D, Holdeman L V, Moore W E C, Rogosa M, Johnson J L 1982 Taxonomy of the genus *Veillonella* Prévot. International Journal of Systematic Bacteriology 32: 28–36

Myers M B, Cherry G, Bornside B B, Bornside G H 1969 Ultraviolet red fluorescence of *Bacteroides melaninogenicus*. Applied Microbiology 17: 760–762

Onderdonk A B, Kasper D L, Cisneros R L, Bartlett J G 1977 The capsular polysaccharide of *Bacteroides fragilis* as a virulence factor: comparison of the pathogenic potential of encapsulated and unencapsulated strains. Journal of Infectious Diseases 136: 82–89

Riley T V, Mee B J 1982 A bacteriocin typing scheme for *Bacteroides*. Journal of Medical Microbiology 15: 387–391

Sutter V L, Vargo V L, Finegold S M 1975 Wadsworth anaerobic bacteriology manual, 2nd edn. University of California, Los Angeles

Thomann W R, Hill G B 1986 Modified extraction procedure for gas-liquid chromatography applied to the identification of anaerobic bacteria. Journal of Clinical Microbiology 23: 392–394

Watt B, Jack E P 1977 What are anaerobic cocci? Journal of Medical Microbiology 10: 461–468

Clostridia of wound infection

The genus *Clostridium* is composed of anaerobic large, straight or slightly curved Gram-positive spore-bearing rods, 3–8 × 0.6–1 μm with slightly rounded ends. Gram-variable, Gram-negative and pleomorphic forms are common. A few species can grow poorly aerobically.

General recommendations for anaerobic culture procedures are given in Chapter 7, and principles for the identification of anaerobes are outlined in the first part of Chapter 36, before the systematic treatments of Gram-negative anaerobes and anaerobic cocci. Details of special relevance to the clostridia are given in this chapter and in Chapter 38. For convenience, we deal here with the clostridia that may be involved in wound infections, with brief accounts of the histotoxic group; *Clostridium tetani* and the laboratory diagnosis of tetanus are dealt with separately at the end of this chapter. Enteropathogenic clostridia are discussed in the following chapter.

Identification of clostridia

In practice the routine characterization of pathogenic clostridia is often limited to a few tests that will presumptively indicate the likely species; this simple approach partly explains why many laboratories have experience of a relatively narrow range of clostridial species. Accurate subdivision of the clostridia to species level rests upon morphological criteria, the results of biochemical tests and gas chromatography (GC), together with the identification of some specific toxins (see, e.g. Table 37.1, and see Willis, 1969; Willis, 1977; and Willis & Phillips, 1983). Our approach parallels that adopted in Chapter 36 and is based on a series of simple tests that allow

precise characterization. Initial steps involved in characterization of clostridia and the range of tests of value in detailed identification are given in Chapter 36 (see Tables 36.1 and 36.3). Thereafter, the clostridia can be divided into four groups based on lecithinase production, and lactose and glucose fermentation (see Tables 37.2–37.5, at end of chapter). Whenever possible, the identity of toxigenic species should be confirmed by specific toxin-neutralization tests, although it should be borne in mind that non-toxigenic strains may also occur. Even without GC or animal tests, presumptive identification is often possible. (*Note*: as in Ch. 36, key reactions in the tables that give differential characteristics of important pathogenic species are indicated in bold and these provide a short-cut identification system for the clostridia.)

Many of the techniques used for identification of clostridia are also used for other anaerobes and detailed instructions are given in Chapter 36; tests and procedures of particular relevance to clostridia are included here.

All clostridia produce spores but they vary markedly in their readiness to do so; prolonged incubation of cooked meat broth (CMB) cultures may be required. The spores are most readily demonstrated in wet films examined by phase contrast microscopy. The shape of the spore and its position in the bacillus is of some help in classification. *C. perfringens* and the type species *C. butyricum* produce capsules. Most clostridia are motile, but *C. perfringens* is not. Some motile species do not show active motility under the relatively aerobic conditions of the usual wet film preparations and it may be advantageous to use a semi-solid agar stab (see *Methods* section below). The active motility of species such as *C. septicum* and *C. sporogenes* may be of advantage or of distinct disadvantage in the isolation of pure cultures on solid media (see below).

Biochemical tests are important in the classification of many clostridia. *C. perfringens, C. septicum, C. tertium* and *C. fallax* are predominantly saccharolytic; *C. sporogenes* and *C. histolyticum* are actively proteolytic and *C. tetani* is slightly proteolytic. These activities are reflected in the cultural appearances in CMB (and also in litmus milk medium). The *saccharolytic* clostridia grow rapidly and vigorously in carbohydrate media with production of acid and abundant gas; detailed recommendations for specific sugar fermentation tests are given in the *Methods* section of Chapter 36 (and see Table 36.1). When grown in CMB, saccharolytic clostridia rapidly produce acid and gas but they do not digest the meat; the cultures may have a slightly sour smell and the meat is often reddened. Gas production is not necessarily indicative of sugar fermentation, as proteolysis may be accompanied by evolution of gas bubbles.

The *proteolytic* clostridia digest protein and liquefy gelatin and coagulated serum. Cultures in meat medium produce blackening of the meat, decomposing it and reducing it in volume with the formation of foul-smelling products.

In *litmus milk medium* (Ch. 8), *C. perfringens* produces acid and gas. The acid clots the milk and the gas breaks up the clot, resulting in the 'stormy clot' reaction that is produced by almost all strains of *C. perfringens* but is not specific for this organism as various mixed cultures may mimic the reaction. Litmus milk medium does not support luxurious growth of some clostridia. It is of very limited usefulness in a diagnostic laboratory.

Phospholipase-C (lecithinase) and *lipase* activity can be demonstrated when cultures are grown on egg-yolk media (see *Methods* section below). Zones of opacity produced in egg-yolk agar cultures of phospholipase-producing clostridia can be neutralized by antisera prepared against *C. perfringens* type A and *C. novyi* type A toxins (the Nagler effect). The specificity of this neutralization is valuable in identification of a range of clostridia (see Table 37.2 at the end of this chapter).

Gas chromatography (GC) is also of value in the identification of clostridia. GC used in conjunction with the Gram stain reaction and cell morphology can identify anaerobes to generic level (see Table 36.3). The production of butyric acid by many species of clostridia readily differentiates them from some other genera of anaerobic Gram-positive rods (*Lactobacillus, Bifidobacterium, Actinomyces* and *Propionibacterium*). However, it is necessary to demonstrate spores to differentiate the non-butyric-acid-producing clostridia from these genera, and the butyric-acid-producing clostridia from *Eubacterium* species.

GC, used in conjunction with a suitable range of phenotypic tests, can also help to identify some clostridia to species level. This is especially so when the phenotypic characteristics are similar for more than one species, or when differentiation of the species depends on the results of tests that require prolonged incubation (gelatin liquefaction, spore production), or on tests that give variable results if not done under optimal conditions (motility). Thus, butyric acid production differentiates lecithinase positive strains of *C. subterminale* from *C. limosum*, and *C. butyricum* from *C. clostridiforme*; *C. irregularis, C. cochlearium* and lecithinase negative strains of *C. subterminale* can be differentiated by butyric and isobutyric acid production; isobutyric acid production differentiates *C. difficile* from *C. innocuum* and *C. putrificum* from *C. novyi* type C (see Tables 37.2–37.5, at the end of this chapter). Recommendations for GC technique are given in the *Methods* section of Chapter 36.

CLOSTRIDIUM PERFRINGENS

C. perfringens (*C. welchi*) can be identified as outlined in Table 37.2 (see end of this chapter). Five types (A–E) are distinguished by the different combinations of major lethal toxins that they produce (Table 37.1). *C. perfringens* type A occurs normally in numbers of about 10^4/g wet

Table 37.1 The major lethal toxins and minor lethal or non-lethal factors produced by the various types of *Clostridium perfringens* (after Brooks et al 1957).
Key: +, produced by >95% of strains; +, produced by most strains; (+), produced by some strains; −, not produced.

Type	Occurrence	Major lethal toxins				Minor lethal or non-lethal factors							
		α	β	ε	ι	γ	δ	η	θ	κ	λ	μ	ν
A1	Gas gangrene / Puerperal infection / Septicaemia	+	−	−	−	−	−	(+)	(+)	(+)	−	(+)	(+)
A2	Food poisoning	+	−	−	−	−	−	−	(+)	(+)	−	(+)	+
B	Lamb dysentery	+	+	+	−	+	(+)	−	+	−	+	+	+
C	'Struck' in sheep	+	+	−	−	+	+	−	+	+	−	−	(+)
C	Enteritis in other animals	+	+	−	−	?	−	−	+	+	−	−	(+)
C	Enteritis necroticans in man	+	+	−	−	+	−	−	−	−	−	−	+
D	Enterotoxaemia of sheep and pulpy kidney disease	+	−	+	−	−	−	−	+	+	+	(+)	(+)
E	Doubtful pathogen of sheep and cattle	+	−	−	+	−	−	−	+	+	+	(+)	(+)

weight of faeces in the large intestine of healthy man and animals; this is a median figure and the range is very wide (see Collee 1974). The organism also occurs commonly in soil, water and dust and is particularly associated with manured cultivated soil. The classical *C. perfringens* of gas gangrene belongs to type A1. Note that *C. perfringens* food poisoning is dealt with separately in Chapter 38.

Morphology and staining

A relatively large Gram-positive rod, about 4–6 × 1 μm, with stubby ends, occurring singly or in pairs; often capsulate in tissues. In sugar media the rods are shorter; in protein media they may become filamentous. Non-motile. Spores formed, usually in small numbers and not in the presence of fermentable carbohydrates; typically oval, subterminal or central and not bulging. Spores are produced in special media such as Ellner medium,* but here many bizarre forms occur and sporulation is variable, even with different cultures of the same strain. The improved sporulation media described by Duncan & Strong (1968)* and Phillips (1986)* are now recommended.

* Refer to *Methods* at end of this chapter.

Cultural characters

Anaerobic, but may grow microaerophilically. Optimum temperature range 37–45°C. Grows best on carbohydrate-containing media such as glucose blood agar. Surface colonies large, smooth, regular, convex, slightly opaque disks. On horse blood agar, colonies usually surrounded by a variable zone of complete haemolysis and a wider darker zone of incomplete haemolysis. Other types of colonies include one with a raised opaque centre and a flat radially striate transparent border. Rough flat colonies with an irregular edge resembling a vine leaf may also occur. A variant occasionally produces very mucoid broth cultures and tenacious colonies on blood agar.

Biochemical reactions

Actively saccharolytic. Ferments, with gas production, glucose, lactose, sucrose, maltose, mannose, inositol, starch and (some strains) salicin, glycerol and inulin; mannitol and galactitol (dulcitol) not fermented (see Ch. 36 for *Methods*). Acid and gas produced in litmus milk medium gives the 'stormy clot' reaction; this is produced by almost all strains but is not specific for this organism. The culture has a sour, butyric acid odour. Gelatin liquefied; coagulated serum not usually liquefied. In CMB the meat is reddened but not digested. Hydrogen sulphide is produced; sulphite is actively reduced; most strains reduce nitrates to nitrites.

Viability

Spores generally resist routinely used antiseptics and disinfectants with the exception of formaldehyde and glutaraldehyde. The spores of classical type A1 strains do not survive boiling for more than a few minutes, whereas the spores of type A2 food-poisoning strains and certain type C strains may be markedly heat resistant (see Ch. 38).

Vegetative cells of *C. perfringens* are very sensitive to heat and disinfectants. *C. perfringens* is sensitive to penicillin, erythromycin, many cephalosporins and metronidazole. Generally sensitive to clindamycin. Typically resistant to aminoglycosides.

Toxins

The five types of *C. perfringens* can be differentiated by their production of the four major lethal toxins (Table 37.2). Typing is done by a combination of in-vitro and in-vivo neutralization tests; for details see Volume 2 of the 12th Edition of this book (p 474).

Alpha (α) toxin is produced by all types but notably by type A1 strains; occasional negative strains occur. It is lethal for laboratory animals and necrotizing on intradermal inoculation. The α toxin is a Ca^{2+} or Mg^{2+}-dependent phospholipase, or lecithinase-C (E.C. 3.1.4.3; phosphatidylcholine choline phosphohydrolase). In the presence of free Ca^{2+} or Mg^{2+} it produces opalescence in serum or egg-yolk preparations by splitting phospholipid complexes. The reaction can be inhibited by specific antitoxin; this is the basis of the Nagler test.*

The enzyme is haemolytic for the red cells of most species except the horse and the goat. The clear zones of haemolysis typically seen around colonies of classical type A1 strains grown on horse blood agar are produced by the theta (θ) toxin and not by the α-toxin. With the red cells

of the sheep in particular, the α toxin provides an example of a 'hot-cold' lysin. Activity may be assayed by turbidity tests with egg-yolk emulsion (lecitho-vitellin, LV) or human serum as indicator, or by haemolysis tests incorporating antisera to other haemolytic toxins that may be produced by *C. perfringens*.

Animal pathogenicity

Virulence for guinea-pigs can be demonstrated by subcutaneous or intramuscular injection of 0.5–1 ml of a 24 h culture in CMB into the thigh. A control animal can be protected by an injection of 300–500 units of *C. perfringens* antitoxin given intraperitoneally 24 h before challenge. In the test animal, a spreading inflammatory oedema develops with gelatinous exudate and gas production in the tissue planes; the affected muscles become pink, sodden and necrotic and virtually liquefy at the site of injection. The products of growth in a young culture increase the organism's aggressiveness; washed organisms are practically non-pathogenic. An equal volume of a sterile 5% solution of calcium chloride mixed with the inoculum just before injection increases the pathogenicity of a strain.

CLOSTRIDIUM NOVYI

Four types of *C. novyi* (*C. oedematiens*) types A, B, C and D are specifically differentiated on the basis of the toxins or 'soluble antigens' that they produce; they can be identified as outlined in Tables 37.2 and 37.4 (at the end of this chapter). Type A strains and occasionally type B strains may be associated with a severe form of gas gangrene in man.

Morphology and staining

Large Gram-positive rods (5–8 × 0.8–1 μm) with rounded ends and peritrichous flagella. Spores oval, central or subterminal.

Cultural characters

Type A strains are very strictly anaerobic. Type

B and type C strains are even more exacting, and type D strains are among the most exacting of the strict anaerobes that can be cultured as a routine on solid media. All types may be grown satisfactorily in freshly made CMB. Special solid media are required for reliable surface growth of types B, C and D (see Collee et al 1971); these types are not typically associated with human disease. The following observations relate to type A strains, which will grow on appropriate solid media if the atmosphere is strictly anaerobic; growth is enhanced by 10% CO_2. Surface colonies are raised, opaque, sometimes dome-shaped and circular in very young cultures, but often flattened, large and irregular in older cultures. The colonies tend to fuse and form a spreading, sometimes swarming, growth; tracks produced by motile daughter colonies may be seen. Discrete colonies show two zones of haemolysis on horse blood agar – a narrow inner zone of complete haemolysis, and an outer zone of partial lysis; this is not seen with spreading growth. On egg-yolk media, the organism's gamma (γ) toxin produces a zone of opacity caused by its phospholipase (lecithinase) activity which can be inhibited by specific antitoxin. In addition, the epsilon (ϵ) toxin (a lipase) produces a pearly layer effect that is more restricted and overlies the colonies.*

Biochemical reactions

C. novyi type A is saccharolytic and mildly proteolytic. Ferments glucose with gas production. Some strains ferment maltose and inositol. Various other sugars including lactose, sucrose, fructose and mannose are not fermented. Changes produced in litmus milk medium are slight and indefinite. Gelatin is liquefied, but milk agar, coagulated serum and cooked meat are not digested. Hydrogen sulphide is produced. Nitrates and nitrites reduced. Type A strains do not produce indole or reduce sulphite (Rutter 1970).

Serology

All types seem to share at least one common surface antigen and this is exploited in a direct immunofluorescence procedure for the prompt identification of C. novyi.*

Animal pathogenicity

An intramuscular injection of 0.2–1 ml of an actively growing culture of C. novyi type A in CMB into the thigh muscles of a guinea-pig may cause overwhelming gas gangrene, with minimum gas production but with massive oedema. With some strains there may be difficulty in initiating the infection and the procedure outlined above for C. perfringens should be followed.

CLOSTRIDIUM SEPTICUM

C. septicum and C. chauvoei are very similar (Table 37.3). Both organisms occur widely in the soil and in animals in health and disease, but C. septicum is also well recognized as a pathogen of man. It may be involved in gas gangrene (clostridial myositis) on its own or in association with other clostridia.

Morphology and staining

Moderately large Gram-positive rods with rounded ends, 3–20 × 0.6–1 μm. Pleomorphic; short forms, swollen 'citron bodies' and long curved filaments occur; degenerate Gram-negative forms common. Actively motile with peritrichous flagella. Spores readily formed; oval, central or subterminal and distend the bacillus.

Cultural characters

Obligatory anaerobe but less strict than C. tetani. Optimum temperature 37°C. Grows on ordinary media, but glucose promotes growth. Grows well on blood agar to produce irregular transparent colonies, later becoming greyish and opaque with fairly coarse projecting radiations; often confluent spreading growth. Colonies on horse blood agar may show a narrow zone of haemolysis.

Biochemical reactions

Ferments various sugars including glucose,

lactose, maltose and salicin, but not mannitol or sucrose. Slight acid production in litmus milk medium may cause slow clotting. Liquefies gelatin but not coagulated serum; no proteolytic effect on milk agar. The meat in CMB is reddened but not digested. Hydrogen sulphide is produced but not indole. Nitrates reduced to nitrites. Sulphites reduced. *C. septicum* does not produce a phospholipase or lipase effect on egg-yolk agar.

Antigenic characters

Six groups distinguished on the basis of two somatic antigens (1, 2) and five flagellar (H) antigens (a–e). Marked cross-relationship with *C. chauvoei*, which shares a common spore antigen with *C. septicum*. There are good reasons to consider *C. septicum* and *C. chauvoei* as different types within the same species. However, most *C. chauvoei* strains have a distinct specific antigen and this is exploited in a direct immunofluorescence procedure for the prompt identification of these two species by ultraviolet microscopy.*

Soluble antigens

The α toxin of *C. septicum* is lethal, haemolytic and necrotizing. The β toxin is a deoxyribonuclease. The γ toxin is a hyaluronidase, and the δ toxin is an oxygen-labile haemolysin. A fibrinolysin is produced and the organism also produces a haemagglutinin and a neuraminidase.

Animal pathogenicity

Intramuscular injection of cultures into guinea-pigs produces gas gangrene. The organisms invade the blood and the animal dies within a day or two. Smears from the liver show long, filamentous forms and 'citron bodies'.

CLOSTRIDIUM BIFERMENTANS AND CLOSTRIDIUM SORDELLI

C. bifermentans and *C. sordelli* are closely related, but *C. bifermentans* is non-pathogenic whereas pathogenic strains of *C. sordelli* produce a lethal necrotizing toxin and are occasionally associated with wound infections in man. Their identification is outlined in Table 37.2.

Morphology

Short stubby Gram-positive rods with rounded ends, often occurring in chains and showing large oval central spores that do not typically bulge but seem to make the whole organism look bigger. Chains of these forms in Gram smears or in wet films give the appearances of necklaces set with bright beads.

Cultural characters

Grow readily and are relatively non-exacting anaerobes. Growth on blood agar abundant and may spread. Colonies grey-white, convex, roughly circular with irregularly crenated edges; more irregular colonies common. Colonies on blood agar are often, but not invariably, haemolytic.

Biochemical reactions

The name *bifermentans* refers to the ability to decompose both sugars and proteins, and the *sordelli/bifermentans* group shares this double activity with variations: *C. bifermentans* ferments glucose, maltose, mannose, sorbitol and salicin, whereas *C. sordelli* ferments glucose and maltose but not the other sugars in this list; neither ferments lactose nor sucrose. Both are strongly proteolytic; they liquefy gelatin and decompose milk protein, coagulated serum and cooked meat. *C. bifermentans* does not decompose urea, whereas *C. sordelli* usually produces an active urease. Both produce indole and hydrogen sulphide, and both produce a serologically related phospholipase (lecithinase) that is partially neutralized by *C. perfringens* antitoxin.*

Animal pathogenicity

Experimental inoculation of 0.5–1 ml of an actively growing CMB culture of a pathogenic strain of *C. sordelli* into the thigh of a guinea-pig produces a rapidly lethal oedematous myonecrosis.

CLOSTRIDIUM HISTOLYTICUM

This long slender Gram-positive rod is not a strict anaerobe and can be cultured aerobically. Proteolytic but non-saccharolytic. In meat medium, digestion occurs with the formation of white, crystalline masses of tyrosine. Pathogenic to experimental animals and man. When a culture is injected into the muscle of an animal, in-vivo digestion of the tissues results. Produces a lethal necrotizing exotoxin, an active collagenase, a proteinase, an elastase, an oxygen-labile haemolysin, and various other biologically active products. It may be associated with gas gangrene in man. Its identification is outlined in Table 37.5.

CLOSTRIDIUM TERTIUM

This slender rod is also a non-exacting anaerobe and will grow sub-optimally under aerobic conditions. Weakly motile. Spores oval, terminal. Actively saccharolytic. In litmus milk, acid is formed with gas production and slow clotting. Meat is reddened but not digested. Neither gelatin nor coagulated serum is liquefied. Its pathogenicity is doubtful, but when present in wounds it may give rise to gas production. No exotoxin is produced. See Table 37.3 for an outline of its identification.

CLOSTRIDIUM SPOROGENES

This Gram-positive motile bacillus is very widely distributed. Generally regarded as a harmless saprophyte, but frequently isolated from wound exudates in association with pathogens. Its identification is outlined in Tables 37.2 and 37.4.

Morphology and staining

Usually longer and more slender than *C. perfringens*. Forms abundant oval, central or subterminal spores which may be highly resistant; hence the organism is frequently encountered in mixed cultures in the laboratory, especially after preliminary heating of these cultures to select heat-resistant pathogens. Its spores may survive boiling for periods of 15 min up to 6 h.

Cultural characters

Relatively strict anaerobe. Grows well on simple media, provided that anaerobic conditions are maintained. Surface colonies may present a medusa-head appearance (cf. *Bacillus anthracis*) if the plate is dry. Young colonies small, circular, raised and slightly opaque; soon produce outgrowths and the spreading margin of the colony becomes irregular with coarse feathery projections. On horse blood agar colonies may appear to be haemolytic but this is not caused by a true haemolysin; they are usually irregular and transparent with some central greyish opacity where the colonies are raised. Colonies in shake cultures show as 'woolly' balls of growth. A stab culture develops with lateral spikes like that of *C. tetani*.

Biochemical reactions

Actively proteolytic and saccharolytic; produces amino acids, ammonia, hydrogen sulphide, etc. and cultures have an exceedingly putrid odour. In milk media, casein is precipitated and digested. In CMB, meat is blackened and digested. Gelatin and coagulated serum liquefied. Acid and gas produced from some sugars, including glucose and maltose; lactose and sucrose not fermented.

Laboratory diagnosis of gas gangrene

The bacteriological diagnosis of gas gangrene is usually combined with a general bacteriological examination of the infected wound with which this condition is associated. It is convenient here to give special reference to the recognition of the clostridia, but see also references to bacteroides infections in Chapter 36.

Take exudate from the wound, particularly

from the deeper parts and from parts where the infection seems to be most pronounced. Sterile swabs rubbed over the wound surface and soaked in the exudate are much less satisfactory than pus and excised tissue fragments. If there are sloughs or necrotic tissue or if there is an adequate amount of exudate present in the wound, place good samples of these in sterile screw-capped bottles. If only swabbed specimens are available, ask for at least two or three; one for film preparations, one for aerobic, and one for anaerobic culture. Prompt submission to the laboratory is imperative; desiccation in transit must be avoided. It is good practice to put a swab directly into a screw-capped bottle of CMB at the bedside. The steps in a routine investigation are as follows:

1. Prepare smears for Gram stain. If gas gangrene is present, Gram-positive rods may predominate. Thick, stubby, Gram-positive rods suggest *C. perfringens* or *C. sordelli*; 'citron bodies', boat- or leaf-shaped pleomorphic bacilli with irregular staining, may indicate *C. septicum*; slender rods with round terminal spores suggest *C. tetani*; *C. novyi* occurs as large rods with oval subterminal spores, but these may be relatively scanty in the wound exudate, even in an active infection. The direct immunofluorescence staining procedure of Batty & Walker (1965) is a most useful diagnostic aid for the prompt identification of *C. septicum* and *C. novyi* and some other clostridia, but not *C. perfringens* (see *Methods* section below).

2. In addition to the media routinely used for detection of aerobes, inoculate a tube of pre-reduced cooked meat broth (CMB), a blood agar (BA) plate and two plates of selective BA containing neomycin 70–100 μg/ml (see Ch. 36). Primary sensitivity tests can be made at this stage by placing disks, e.g. metronidazole and penicillin, on the first series of streaks.

Consider also the use of: plates containing increased agar (4–6%) to prevent swarming by some species of clostridia;* a selective egg-yolk agar plate, with or without antitoxins, to detect phospholipase- and lipase-producing clostridia, and to demonstrate any Nagler reaction;* additional tubes of CMB, heated at 70°C for

20 min or at 100°C for 5–20 min, to select sporing forms.

3. Incubate the CMB, BA and selective BA anaerobically with 10% CO_2 at 37°C. Leave one selective BA incubating anaerobically undisturbed for 48 h. Examine the other media after 24 h incubation.

4. Examine plates for typical colonies. Comparison of the aerobic and anaerobic plates affords some indication of the presence of strictly anaerobic organisms, but any suspect anaerobe must later be tested in subculture to ensure that it is unable to grow under aerobic conditions (see Watt & Jack 1977). *C. tertium*, *C. carnis* and *C. histolyticum* can grow to some extent aerobically.

5. Examine CMB enrichment by microscopy, and subculture to plates. In CMB both aerobes and anaerobes flourish; this growth is useful for later subculture should the plate culture fail to yield successful isolation of organisms present in the wound. Film preparations also yield further information on the morphological types of vegetative organisms, and sporing forms that may have developed can be seen.

Note: *C. perfringens* is a common environmental contaminant and, because of its capacity for rapid growth in CMB, it may be present in misleadingly large numbers on secondary plate cultures seeded from primary broth cultures. When it is truly involved in a clostridial myositis (gas gangrene), *C. perfringens* is usually capsulate and can generally be recovered in large numbers on primary plates.

6. Pick suspect colonies and subculture to pre-reduced CMB or PPY medium for subsequent identification by biochemical tests, and to PPY medium containing glucose 1% for gas chromatography (GC; see *Methods*, Ch. 36).

CLOSTRIDIUM TETANI

C. tetani is a common saprophyte occurring in cultivated soils throughout the world. Tetanus occurs in man and animals when a wound is infected with the organism and conditions permit it to multiply and to produce tetanospasmin, which begins to act on the central nervous system between 7–10 days (range 3–30 days) after infection. The voluntary muscles become hyperexcitable; there is increased muscle tonus and exaggerated muscular responses to trivial stimuli. Trismus occurs when the muscles of the jaw are affected; the disease is sometimes called lockjaw because this is quite frequently an early sign of tetanus in man. Tetanus is now uncommon in the developed world as a result of active immunization programmes.

Morphology and staining

Slender Gram-positive rods, 2–5 × 0.4–0.5 μm, with rounded ends; tends to be pleomorphic, sometimes filamentous, with Gram-negative cells most frequently evident. The bacteria are usually sluggishly motile with long peritrichous flagella; some non-motile strains occur. Early in development, spores are subterminal and slightly distend the vegetative cell; the fully developed spore is characteristically terminal and spherical, up to twice the diameter of the vegetative cell, giving the typical drumstick appearance. This morphology may be an artefact of staining; wet films do not show the classical appearance. Strains vary in their tendency to produce spores.

Cultural characters

A strict anaerobe. Temperature range 14–43°C; optimum 37°C. Grows on ordinary nutrient media but more readily grown in CMB or in Fildes peptic blood broth or on fresh blood agar. Colonies on solid media show fine branching projections. After incubation for 48–72 h, the central part of the colony becomes slightly raised and has a ground-glass appearance with a delicately filamentous edge. A fine spreading growth may extend over the entire surface of the medium and may not be apparent on cursory examination. On blood agar, haemolysis is evident under initial confluent growth and may develop below individual colonies, but frequently does not appear below the spreading growth in young cultures. Non-motile variants may produce quite isolated colonies lacking the characteristic feathery processes.

Biochemical reactions

Most strains are asaccharolytic. Most strains can slowly liquefy gelatin, but they are not strongly proteolytic. Indole is formed by almost all strains. (See Ch. 36 for *Methods*.)

Sensitivity to physical and chemical agents

The resistance of spores of *C. tetani* varies. Some are killed by exposure to boiling water for 5–15 min, but rarer more resistant strains require boiling for up to 3 h before being killed. They may resist dry heat at 150°C for 1 h and 5% phenol or 0.1% mercuric chloride for up to 2 weeks or more, but are inactivated by exposure to iodine 1% in watery solution or hydrogen peroxide (10 volumes) within a few hours. Vegetative cells of *C. tetani* are generally sensitive to penicillin and various other antibiotics including clindamycin and metronidazole. The occurrence of *C. tetani* typically in wounds infected with a variety of organisms including penicillinase-producing bacteria must be taken into account in the clinical management of wounds and prevention of tetanus.

Serotyping

Ten types are distinguishable by agglutination tests involving flagellar H antigens; type 6 consists of non-flagellate strains. This serotyping is not done as a routine. All types produce an antigenically identical neurotoxin, and toxigenic and non-toxigenic strains may belong to the same type.

Toxins and animal pathogenicity

The neurotoxin *tetanospasmin* develops in CMB cultures after growth for 2–14 days at 35°C, the optimum time varying with the strain. When crude tetanus toxin is injected into guinea-pigs or mice, the animals die within a day or two with the typical signs of tetanus. In animals, local tetanus spasms may occur in the muscles related to the site of injection.

The mouse is used as a routine for demonstrating the presence of tetanus neurotoxin in culture supernates; a pair of mice is used for each test. Protect one animal by intraperitoneal injection of 500–1500 units (0.5 ml) of tetanus antitoxin 1 h before the test. Inject 0.1 ml of a 48 h CMB culture supernate of the organism intramuscularly into a hind limb of the test and control animals. Signs of ascending tetanus develop in the unprotected animal after several hours; they begin in the inoculated leg and extend to the tail; then the other hind limb is affected and then generalized signs appear. The animal responds to the slightest stimulus with generalized spasms. If large doses of toxin are injected, death may occur in 18–24 h without any of the intermediate symptoms.

Tetanolysin, an oxygen-labile haemolysin, is distinct from the true tetanus toxin.

Laboratory diagnosis of tetanus

The specimen will be wound exudate or tissue removed from the wound.

1. Make a direct smear, Gram stain, and examine for drumstick spore-formers. *Caution*: only a minority of specimens will show these and they are not an invariable index of the presence of *C. tetani*. The use of immunofluorescence staining should be considered here.*

2. Inoculate exudate or homogenized tissue into CMB and on to a BA plate and two selective BA plates (see *Methods* Ch. 36). Incubate anaerobically with 10% CO_2 at 37°C. Consider also seeding an antitoxin-controlled plate for the presumptive identification of *C. tetani*. This involves the use of a freshly prepared BA plate half-smeared with tetanus antitoxin (Lowbury & Lilly 1958). *C. tetani* produces haemolysis which is inhibited by the antiserum. Although there are several objections to this technique, the method is convenient for the provisional screening of large numbers of strains. Confirmation by mouse inoculation is recommended.

3. Leave one selective BA plate undisturbed in the anaerobic atmosphere for 48 h. Check the other plates after 24 h incubation, and daily for up to 4 days. Examine the plates with a hand lens or plate microscope for fine spreading growth. (Note that *C. tetani* type 6 is non-

motile). If present, make a pure subculture from the spreading edge to BA and pre-reduced CMB, and incubate anaerobically for 48 h.

4. Examine the CMB enrichment culture daily by microscopy. If clostridial forms are seen, do the following:

a. Heat part of the culture at 80°C for 10 min and then subculture the heated and unheated samples to BA. Incubate the plates anaerobically. (Note that some *C. tetani* spores are heat sensitive.)

b. Direct immunofluorescence staining.

c. Although it is usual to wait until a pure culture is available, toxicity testing can be done with the supernate from the CMB enrichment culture.

5. Check the subculture in CMB. If it is not pure, subculture from the spreading edge of growth on BA to pre-reduced CMB. If the CMB is pure, set up toxin tests in protected and unprotected mice (see above), set up a range of biochemical tests, and examine the fatty acid profile by GC (see Table 37.5).

METHODS

Identification of clostridia by direct staining with fluorochrome labelled antibody

This procedure (see Batty & Walker 1965) is of use for the identification of *C. septicum*, *C. chauvoei*, *C. novyi*, *C. botulinum* types A, B, F, C, D and E, and *C. tetani*. Conjugated immunoglobulins are commercially available from Wellcome.

An air-dried smear is fixed by immersion of the slide in reagent grade anhydrous acetone for 10 min. A drop of the conjugated immunoglobulin is spread on the smear and left at room temperature for 30 min in a humid atmosphere provided by a wet filter paper in a plastic box.

The excess conjugate is quickly rinsed off the smear with phosphate buffered saline at pH 7.6 (NaCl 8.5 g, Na_2HPO_4 1.28 g, $NaH_2PO_4.2H_2O$ 0.156 g, in 1 litre of distilled water); the smear is held in several changes of this buffer during the following 10–15 min. It is then gently blotted dry and mounted with buffered glycerol at pH 8–9 ($NaHCO_3$ 0.0715 g, Na_2CO_3 0.016 g, water to 10 ml, glycerol to 100 ml) and a glass (not plastic) coverslip for UV microscopy.

Preservation and storage of strains

Strains may be preserved by freeze-drying or by storage in various media. Cooked meat broth containing chalk and minced cooked egg-white is a useful preservation medium (Ch. 6). Germination of spores is sporadic, especially following heat-resistance tests, and this is considered to be partly due to fatty acids in the subculture medium. The inhibitory effect may be reduced by incorporating soluble starch or serum in the medium when subcultures are made from preservation media or from heat-resistance tests.

Media that induce sporulation

Ellner's (1956) medium

This medium is used to induce spore formation in C. perfringens. Anaerobiosis may be ensured by heating at 100°C for 10 min and cooling just prior to inoculation. It is important that the inoculum should be adequate; 0.5 ml of an actively growing 4–12 h meat broth culture should be introduced with a pipette into the bottom of the tube of medium. Incubation is in an anaerobic jar at 37°C.

Peptone (e.g. Proteose peptone, Difco)	10 g
Yeast extract	3 g
Soluble starch	3 g
$MgSO_4$	0.1 g
KH_2PO_4	1.5 g
$Na_2HPO_4.12H_2O$	67 g
Water to	1 litre

Steam briefly at 100°C to dissolve, adjust to pH 7.8 with sodium hydroxide 1 mol/litre, dispense in tubes and autoclave at 121°C for 20 min. Tubes should be half to two-thirds full.

Medium of Duncan & Strong (1968)

This medium should be pre-steamed and then cooled to 37°C just before being seeded with a 10% volume of a 4 h active culture of the strain

of C. perfringens in thioglycollate broth. Addition of activated carbon (1%) may increase the sporulation of some strains. Although high numbers of spores are produced by many test strains, the medium is not invariably successful; this reservation should be applied to all currently developed media for the sporulation of C. perfringens.

Proteose peptone	15 g
Yeast extract	4 g
Soluble starch	4 g
Sodium thioglycollate (mercaptoacetate)	1 g
Disodium hydrogen phosphate $Na_2HPO_4.7H_2O$	1 g
Water to	1 litre

The pH of the medium is about 7.0. Steam at 100°C to dissolve, and dispense into screw-capped bottles which should be at least two-thirds full of medium. Autoclave at 121°C for 15 min. After inoculation and incubation, sporulation should be evident within about 6 h; maximum sporulation is likely to be achieved at 10–16 h.

Medium of Phillips (1986)

A plate of this sporulation medium for Clostridium perfringens should be seeded by rubbing a dry swab charged with a blood agar culture of the organism over the whole surface. Incubate in an atmosphere of nitrogen 80%, CO_2 10% and hydrogen 10% at 37°C for 48 h.

Blood agar base No. 2 (Oxoid CM27)	39.5 g
Desiccated ox bile (Oxoid L50)	10 g
Sodium bicarbonate, $NaHCO_3$	5 g
Quinoline (BDH No. 30012)	0.5 ml
Defibrinated horse blood	50 ml
Distilled water	1 litre

Dissolve the blood agar base, the ox bile and the quinoline in 800 ml of the water and sterilize at 121°C for 15 min. Cool to 50°C. Add the sodium bicarbonate (dissolved in 200 ml of the water and filter sterilized) at 50°C. Then add the horse blood and pour plates. The pH of the medium should be 8.5.

Alkaline egg medium

This medium promotes spore formation by clostridia. Clostridia remain viable in it for years.

Egg yolk	1
Egg whites	2
Sodium hydroxide, NaOH, 1 mol/litre	6 ml
Water to	500 ml

Beat the yolk and whites, add the sodium hydroxide and water. Heat slowly to 95°C for 90 min, filter through cotton wool and distribute. Sterilize by autoclaving at 121°C for 15 min.

Reinforced clostridial agar

This medium is specially enriched with substances that might promote the growth of clostridia. Its preparation involves the heating of cysteine in the absence of any chemical that could protect it substantially against prompt oxidation, but the medium is nevertheless widely used for the culture of various anaerobes in the following form.

Peptone	10 g
Yeast extract	3 g
Meat extract	10 g
Glucose	5 g
Sodium acetate	3 g
Sodium chloride	5 g
L-Cysteine hydrochloride	0.5 g
Soluble starch	1 g
Distilled water to	1 litre

Steam the ingredients in a flask; filter when dissolved. Adjust pH to 7.4. Add agar 10 g and sterilize by autoclaving at 121°C for 20 min.

Cysteine dithiothreitol blood agar

Moore (1968) described the use of the reducing agents cysteine and dithiothreitol to improve solid media for *C. novyi*, particularly of the more fastidious types B and D. Collee et al (1971) modified Moore's medium by increasing the concentrations of cysteine to 1 mg/ml, dithiothreitol to 0.09 mg/ml and of human blood to 33% and later substituted 10% horse blood for the human blood. This latest modification is described here.

Cysteine-dithiothreitol solution

Cysteine	150 mg
Dithiothreitol	13.5 mg
Distilled water	3 ml

Prepare the solution immediately before use and sterilize by membrane filtration.

Preparation of complete medium

Nutrient agar (Oxoid blood agar base, No. 2)	88 ml
Cysteine-dithiothreitol solution	2 ml
Horse blood	10 ml

Melt the nutrient agar, cool to 45–55°C and add the remaining ingredients, mixing carefully before pouring plates. Dry the plates briefly at 60°C for 10 min to protect the reducing agents. Inoculate and incubate immediately.

Motility

Motility may be difficult to demonstrate with some species and it is advantageous to use more than one method.

1. With some species there is active swarming of the culture on the surface of an anaerobic BA plate.

2. Motility may be demonstrated directly by examining freshly made wet films from log-phase CMB cultures, preferably by phase contrast microscopy under a sealed coverslip.

3. A semi-solid agar stab technique can also be used for demonstration of motility (see Ch. 8). Stab cultures in this medium, freshly prepared with added 1% glucose to enhance anaerobiosis, should be examined frequently before excessive gas production invalidates the test. A non-motile species (e.g. *C. perfringens*) may show lateral spikes of growth along faults extending from the stab line, but the appearance is not likely to be confused with the diffuse growth of a truly motile species.

Control of spreading growth on anaerobic plates

Control of the swarming growth of unwanted organisms in plate cultures presents various problems. Pre-treatment of the proposed inoculum by differential heating may be effective, but it carries the risk of killing vegetative cells of likely non-sporing and sporing pathogens. Moreover, the spores of some pathogens are not markedly heat resistant and may be inactivated, or their prompt germination may be inhibited. The use of firm agar containing 3–4% agar is recommended as a general control method (see Ch. 8), but colonial morphology is altered. Alternatively, some workers pay particular attention to drying the surface of agar plates to inhibit swarming; but the availability of nutrients for the initiation of colonial growth on a relatively dry surface may be critically impaired. An 'alcohol' plate is sometimes used; here the surface of the unseeded medium is flooded with ethanol, the excess is removed and the plate is exposed in an incubator to dry it at 37°C. The medium is then seeded in the usual manner. If the pathogen to be isolated can grow on MacConkey agar, it should be noted that *Proteus* and *Pseudomonas* species do not spread on this medium. It is sometimes possible to exclude these spreading species by exposing the seeded plate to chloroform vapour for some minutes prior to anaerobic incubation.

Specific serological control of the swarming growth of *C. tetani* and *C. septicum* is possible (see Willis & Williams 1972). When commercial tetanus antitoxin 40–60 units/ml is incorporated into the agar medium, motile strains of *C. tetani* grow as discrete colonies. Similarly, *C. septicum* does not spread on plates on which 0.2–0.5 ml of a *C. septicum* antiserum prepared against the two serological groups is spread.

Tests for phospholipase and lipase; Nagler's reaction

Several clostridia produce phospholipases that give rise to a zone of opalescence extending beyond the colony or line of growth on human serum or egg-yolk media (see Ch. 8). Proteolytic colonies produce zones of clearing on these media, whilst opalescence restricted to the medium underlying a colony and associated with an overlying iridescent 'pearly layer' indicates lipase activity. The phospholipase reaction produced by *C. perfringens* is specifically neutralized by *C. perfringens* antitoxin (Nagler reaction), but the serologically related phospholipases of *C. bifermentans* and *C. sordelli* and some other clostridia are also inhibited. The phospholipase of *C. novyi* type A can similarly be inhibited by specific *C. novyi* antitoxin (see Table 37.2).

For the presumptive detection of *C. perfringens* in direct plate culture, prepare and dry a plate of good quality digest agar containing egg-yolk 5%. On one half of the plate spread 2–3 drops of *C. perfringens* antitoxin (Wellcome) and allow to dry. Then seed with the test organism or with the exudate under investigation, stroking from the antitoxin-free on to the antitoxin-bearing half, and incubate anaerobically at 37°C. On the section containing no antitoxin, *C. perfringens* colonies show a surrounding zone of opacity, i.e. the Nagler reaction, whereas colonies of the organism on the remainder of the plate do not. Parallel stroke cultures of different strains or isolates may be done on one plate, with a known positive control included, for identification of pure cultures.

Lowbury and Lilly's medium

An indicator medium for *C. perfringens* containing Fildes peptic digest of blood to stimulate the production of lecithinase, human serum or egg-yolk to show lecithinase production and *C. perfringens* antitoxin spread over the surface of half the plate to show neutralization of the lecithinase was devised by Hayward (1943) who named it the Nagler plate. Nagler (1945) observed the lipase in addition to the lecithinase reaction in egg-yolk and proposed an egg-yolk medium as indicator of the lecithinase and lipase of *C. novyi*. Lowbury & Lilly (1955) modified the human serum medium by increasing the concentration of agar to prevent the swarming of *Proteus*, making a double layer medium to allow a clearer demonstration of lecithinase reactions and adding neomycin (100 μg/ml) to inhibit lecithinase-producing aerobic sporing bacilli. However in the description given here the concentration of neomycin is only 70 μg/ml, the maximum that is not markedly inhibitory to many clostridia (Collee & Watt 1971). The neomycin potency of neomycin sulphate is 700 μg/mg. This 70% factor is taken into account in the following recipe.

Agar base

Agar	50 g
Peptone water (Ch. 6)	1 litre

This agar base autoclaved at 121°C for 20 min is used for the lower layer of the medium and as basal medium for the upper layer.

Preparation of complete medium

Agar base	100 ml
Fildes peptic digest of sheep blood	6.5 ml
Human serum, sterile	40 ml
Neomycin sulphate (Upjohn), sterile aqueous solution: 10 000 μg/ml	1.47 ml

The serum may be prepared by treating plasma with 5% of sterile 10% calcium chloride at 37°C. *Note*: Special precautions must be taken when human blood products are used (Chs 7, 15).

Heat the Fildes digest at 55°C for 30 min, melt the agar base and cool it to 56°C. Add the remaining ingredients and pour the medium as the upper layer of double layer plates on a nutrient agar base. Spread 250 international units of *C. perfringens* antitoxin over half of the agar surface.

Willis and Hobbs medium

This medium for the isolation of clostridia (Willis & Hobbs 1959) is a lactose egg-yolk milk agar made selective for various clostridia, particularly *C. perfringens*, by the addition of neomycin. The recommended concentration of 250 μg neomycin sulphate/ml inhibits some clostridia, usually inhibits strains of *Bacillus* and *Staphylococcus*, and greatly reduces the growth of coliform bacilli. As results of culture on Willis & Hobbs medium can be variable and are occasionally confusing, a simpler selective medium such as egg-yolk agar with a good base and neomycin 70 μg/ml is preferred for general use.

Egg yolk suspension. Break eggs with precautions to keep their contents sterile, as described for Löwenstein medium (see Ch. 6), at the same time separating the yolks from the whites. Discard the whites and dilute the yolks with an equal volume of sterile 0.9% sodium chloride solution.

Sterile stock milk. Remove the cream from ordinary milk by centrifuging. Sterilize the skimmed milk by autoclaving at 121°C for 20 min.

Basal medium

Agar	4.8 g
Lactose	4.8 g
Neutral red, 1% solution	1.3 ml
Meat infusion broth, pH 7.0	400 ml
Egg-yolk suspension	15 ml
Milk	60 ml

Dissolve the agar and lactose in the neutral red and broth by steaming, and sterilize at 121°C for 20 min. Cool to 50–55°C and add the egg-yolk and milk. Pour plates.

Possible additions to basal medium

Neomycin sulphate (Upjohn)	250 μg/ml
Sodium thioglycollate	0.1%

Stock sterile solutions of neomycin may be stored in the refrigerator with little loss of potency. The antibiotic is not decomposed by heating at 60°C for 20 min. Thioglycollate may assist the growth of the stricter anaerobes.

Either or both of these reagents may be added at the same time as the egg-yolk and milk.

Table 37.2 Differential characters and key for the identification of the lecithinase-positive clostridia.

Key: +, 95% of strains give a positive result; −, 95% of strains give a negative result; +(−), 70–95% of strains give a positive result; +/−, 30–70% of strains give each result; . ., not tested. Key reactions are indicated in bold.

Species	Fatty acids[c] produced	Iso-butyric acid produced	Gelatin liquefaction	Motility	Maltose[b]	Inositol[b]	Lactose[b]	Glucose[b]	Urease production	Indole production	Lipase production	Inhibition by antitoxin[a]	Lecithinase production
C. novyi type A	a P B (f v l s)	−	+	+	+(−)	+(−)	−	+	−	−	+	+	+
C. sordelli	A ic (F p ib b iv l s)	+/−	+	+	+(−)	−	−	+	+	+	−	+	+
C. bifermentans	A F (p ib b iv ic h l s)	+/−	+	+	+	−	−	+	−	+	−	+	+
C. perfringens	A B L (f p s)	−	+	−	+	+	+	+	−(+)	−	−	+	+(−)
C. sardiniensis	A B (f p L s)	−	+	+	+	−	+	+	−(+)	−	−	+	+
C. absonum	A B L	−	**+**	−	+	−	+	+	. .	−	−	+	+
C. barati	A B L (f p s)	−	**−**	−	+	−	+	+	−	−	−	+	+
C. subterminale	A ib b iv (f p l s)	**+**	+	+	−	−	−	−	−	−	−	+	−(+)
C. limosum	A (f l s)	**−**	+	+	−	−	−	−	−	−	−	+	+
C. botulinum type C	A P B (f v l s)	+	+	+	+(−)	+(−)	−	+	−	+(−)	+	−	−(+)
C. sporogenes	A ib B iv (p v ic s)	+	+	+	+	−	−	+	−(+)	−	+	−	−(+)
C. novyi type B	a P B (f v s)	−	+	+	**+**	+(−)	−	+	−	+(−)	−	−	+
C. novyi type D	A P B (l s)	−	+	+	−	+(−)	−	+	−	+	−	−	+

[a] Observe inhibition of lecithinase by a mixture of *C. perfringens* and *C. novyi* type A antitoxins (see *Methods*).
[b] Fermentation test.
[c] See Table 36.4 for standard key to fatty acid profiles.

Table 37.3 Differential characters and key for the identification of the lecithinase-negative, lactose-positive clostridia.
Key: see Table 37.2.

Species	Fatty acids[c] produced	Butyric acid produced	Motility	Melibiose[a]	Spore position[b]	Xylose[a]	Sucrose[a]	Mannose[a]	Mannitol[a]	Indole production	Aerotolerance	Lactose[a]	Lecithinase production
C. tertium	A b L (f s)	+	+	+	T	+/-	+	+	+	-	+	+	-
C. carnis	A f B l (s)	+	+	-	S	-	+	+	-	-	+	+/-	-
C. sphenoides	A (F l s)	-	+	-(+)	S/T	+/-	-(+)	+	+	+	-	+	-
C. clostridiforme	A (F l s)	-	+	-(+)	S	+	+	+	-	-(+)	-	+/-	-
C. indolis	A F (p b l)	+/-	+	-	T	+(-)	+/-	-	-	+	-	+	-
C. butyricum	A F B (l s)	+	+	+	S	+	+	+	-	-	-	+	-
C. beijerincki	A B (F p l s)	+	+	+/-	S	+	+	+	-	-	-	+	-
C. clostridiforme	A (F l s)	-	+	-(+)	S	+	+	+	-	-(+)	-	+/-	-
C. ramosum	A F L (p s)	-	-	+	T	-	+	+	+(-)	-	-	+	-
C. paraputrificum	A B L (F s)	+	+(-)	-	T	-	+	+	-	-	-	+	-
C. chauvoei	A F B (l s)	+	+	-	S	-	+	+	-	-	-	+	-
C. perfringens	A B L (f p s)	+	-	+/-	S	-	+	+	-	-	-	+	+(-)
C. septicum	A B L (f s)	+	+	-	S/C	-	-	+	-	-	-	+	-

[a] Fermentation test.
[b] T = terminal; S = subterminal; C = central.
[c] See Table 36.4 for key.

Table 37.4 Differential characters and key for the identification of the lecithinase-negative, lactose-negative clostridia.
Key: see Table 37.2.

Species	Fatty acids[d] produced	Iso-butyric acid produced	Motility	Spore position[c]	Toxin test[b]	Indole production	Maltose[a]	Xylose[a]	Sucrose[a]	Mannitol[a]	Aesculin hydrolysis	Lipase production	Aerotolerance	Lactose[a]	Lecithinase production
C. botulinum type A and proteolytic types B and F	A p ib B iV (f ic 1 s)	+	+	S	+	-	+/-	-	-	+	+	+	-	-	-(+)
C. sporogenes	A ib B iv (p v ic s)	+	+	S	-	-	+	-	-	-	+	+	-	-	-(+)
C. botulinum type E and non-proteolytic types B and F	A B (f l s)	-	+	S	+	-	+/-	-	+	-	-	+	-	-	-
C. botulinum types C and D	A P B (f v 1 s)	-	+	S	+	-	+(-)	-	-	-	-	+	-	-	-(+)
C. difficile	A ib b iv v ic (p c)	+	+(-)	S/T	+	-	-	-	+(-)	+	+(-)	-	-	-	-
C. innocuum	A B L (f s)	-	-	T	-	-	-	-	+	+	+	-	-	-	-
C. clostridiforme	A (F l s)	-	+	S	-	-(+)	+	+	+	-	+	-	-	+/-	-
C. glycolicum	A ib iV (f p l s)	+	+	S	-	-	+/-	+	-	-	-(+)	-	-	-	-
C. fallax	A B (L s)	-	+	S	-	-	+	-	-	-	+	-	-	-	-
C. cadaveris	A B (f p s)	-	+	T	-	+	-	-	-	-	-	-	-	-	-
C. putrificum	A ib B iv (f p ic 1 s)	+	+	T	-	-	-	-	-	-	-(+)	-	-	-	-
C. novyi type C	a p B (v)	-	-	S	-	-	-	-	-	-	-	-	-	-	-
C. carnis	A f B 1 (s)	-	+	S	-	-	+	-	+	-	+	-	+	+/-	-

[a] Fermentation test.
[b] Relevant tests indicated in text for different toxins.
[c] S = subterminal; T = terminal.
[d] See Table 36.4 for key.

Table 37.5 Differential characters and key for the identification of the lecithinase-negative, asaccharolytic clostridia. *Key*: See Table 37.2.

Lecithinase production	Glucose[a]	Aerotolerance	Spore position[b]	Indole production	Gelatin liquefaction	Toxin test	Meat digestion	Butyric acid produced	Iso-butyric acid produced	Fatty acids[c] produced	Species
−	−	+	S	−	+	−	+	−	−	A (f l s)	*C. histolyticum*
−	−	−	T	+	−	−	−	+	−	A B (f p l s)	*C. malenominatum*
−	−	−	T	+(−)	+	+	−	+	−	A p b (s)	*C. tetani*
−	−	−	S	−	+	+	−	+	+	A ib b iv l	*C. botulinum* type G
−	−	−	S	−	+	−	+(−)	+	+	A p ib B iv (f ic l s)	*C. hastiforme*
−(+)	−	−	S	−	+	−	−	+	+	A ib b iv (f p l s)	*C. subterminale*
−	−	−	S	−	+	−	−	+	−	A p B (f l s)	*C. cochlearium*
−	−	−	S	−	+	−	−	−	+	A ib iv (f p iC l)	*C. irregularis*

[a] Fermentation test.
[b] S = subterminal; T = terminal.
[c] See Table 36.4 for standard key to fatty acid profiles.

REFERENCES

Batty I, Walker P D 1965 Colonial morphology and fluorescent labelled antibody staining in the identification of species of the genus *Clostridium*. Journal of Applied Bacteriology 28: 112–118

Brooks M E, Sterne M, Warrack G H 1957 A re-assessment of the criteria used for type differentiation of *Cl. perfringens*. Journal of Pathology and Bacteriology 74: 185–195

Collee J G 1974 *Clostridium perfringens* (*Cl. welchii*) in the human gastro-intestinal tract. In: Skinner F A, Carr J G (eds) The normal microbial flora of man. Academic Press, London. p 205–219

Collee J G, Rutter J M, Watt B 1971 The significantly viable particle: a study of the sub-culture of an exacting sporing anaerobe. Journal of Medical Microbiology 4: 271–288

Collee J G, Watt B 1971 Changing approaches to the sporing anaerobes in medical microbiology. In: Barker A N, Gould G W, Wolf J (eds) Spore research 1971. Academic Press, London

Duncan C L, Strong D H 1968 Improved medium for sporulation of *Clostridium perfringens*. Applied Microbiology 16: 82–89

Ellner P D 1956 A medium promoting rapid quantitative sporulation in *Clostridium perfringens*. Journal of Bacteriology 71: 495–496

Hayward N J 1943 The rapid identification of *Cl. welchii* by Nagler tests in plate cultures. Journal of Pathology and Bacteriology 55: 285–293

Lowbury E J L, Lilly H A 1955 A selective plate medium for *Cl. welchii*. Journal of Pathology and Bacteriology 70: 105–109

Lowbury E J L, Lilly H A 1958 Contamination of operating-theatre air with *Clostridium tetani*. British Medical Journal 2: 1334–1336

Moore W B 1968 Solidified media suitable for the cultivation of *Clostridium novyi* type B. Journal of General Microbiology 53: 415–423

Nagler F P O 1945 A cultural reaction for the early diagnosis of *Clostridium oedematiens* infection. Australian Journal of Experimental Biology and Medical Science 23: 59–62

Phillips K D 1986 A new sporulation medium for *Clostridium perfringens*. Letters in Applied Microbiology 3: 77–79

Rutter J M 1970 A study of the carbohydrate fermentation reactions of *Clostridium oedematiens* (*Cl. novyi*). Journal of Medical Microbiology 3: 283–289

Watt B, Jack E P 1977 What are anaerobic cocci? Journal of Medical Microbiology 10: 461–468

Willis A T 1969 Clostridia of wound infection. Butterworth, London

Willis A T 1977 Anaerobic bacteriology. Clinical and laboratory practice, 3rd edn. Butterworth, London

Willis A T, Hobbs G 1959 Some new media for the isolation and identification of clostridia. Journal of Pathology and Bacteriology 77: 511–521

Willis A T, Phillips K D 1983 Anaerobic infections. Public Health Laboratory Service Monograph Series 3, 2nd edn. HMSO, London

Willis A T, Williams K 1972 Prevention of swarming of *Clostridium septicum*. Journal of Medical Microbiology 5: 493–496

Enteropathogenic clostridia and Clostridium botulinum

This chapter deals with the pathogenic clostridia that affect the bowel. Some of the disease associations are definite and dramatic; others are less clearly defined, and some are still debated.

CLOSTRIDIUM PERFRINGENS FOOD POISONING

Food poisoning caused by C. perfringens type A

Strains of *C. perfringens* type A that produce enterotoxin are associated with a mild form of food poisoning (Vol. 1, 13th Edn, Ch. 36). The so-called 'typical food-poisoning strains' (type A2) that are non-haemolytic or feebly haemolytic on horse blood agar plates and have markedly heat-resistant spores are most frequently encountered, but classical (type A1) strains that are β-haemolytic and have relatively heat-sensitive spores can also be involved (see Table 37.1).

Many opportunities arise for spores of *C. perfringens* to contaminate meat and meat products at the abattoir, in transit to shops and market places, and in catering establishments and in the home. As the organism is encountered so frequently and so widely, it is not usual to attempt to trace the ultimate source in an outbreak of food poisoning but rather to determine the circumstances or conditions that allowed the almost inevitable contamination to be boosted during processing of the food concerned. The heat resistance of type A2 spores allows them to survive the whole cooking procedure, whereas type A1 spores are not likely to cause trouble unless they are introduced by faulty catering practice during the period between cooking and serving.

The bacteriological investigation of *C. perfringens* food poisoning must take account of the findings of Collee et al (1961) and Sutton et al (1971). Virtually 100% of the healthy population carries classical β-haemolytic *C. perfringens* in their gut, and 2–30% may be healthy carriers of heat-resistant *C. perfringens*. The faecal counts of *C. perfringens* just after food poisoning caused by this organism are higher than the counts for healthy people, or for people with diarrhoea due to other causes (median counts 8.5×10^6/g; cf. 1.5×10^4/g in normal subjects). However, it should be noted that the range of counts for commensal *C. perfringens* in normal subjects is wide. The spores of heat-resistant strains often require heat treatment before they grow quantitatively. A semi-quantitative procedure for the isolation of *C. perfringens* from food and faeces is outlined in Figure 38.1. Techniques for identification of *C. perfringens* are discussed in Chapter 37.

Samples of suspect foods should be examined if possible but they are often not available by the time the diagnosis is suggested. The organism will be present as vegetative cells in food and the samples should not be heated before culture. Although the organism does not readily sporulate in routine culture media, it does so in the human gut and considerable numbers of spores of *C. perfringens* may occur in faeces of affected persons. Faecal specimens should be examined for vegetative cells and spores of *C. perfringens*. If faecal samples are boiled before culture, heat-resistant strains will be isolated but the spores of many enterotoxin-producing strains will be killed by this treatment. Mild heating is, however, of value in recovery of heat-sensitive *C. perfringens*

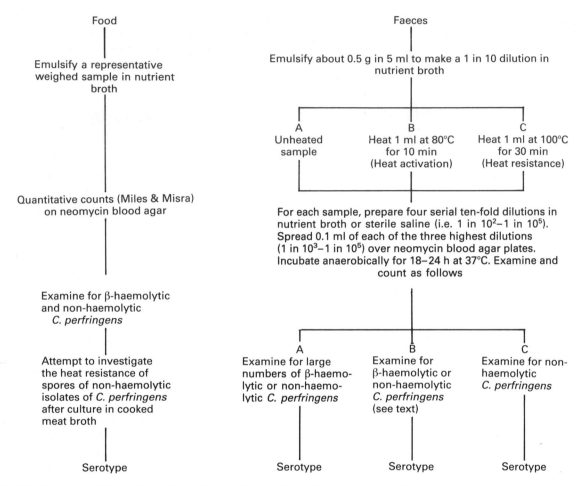

Fig. 38.1 Isolation of *C. perfringens* from food and faeces after a food-poisoning incident.

from faeces as heat shock activates the spores and increases the rate of germination.

The demonstration of *C. perfringens* in the faeces of affected people is of limited value. The qualitative evidence requires to be substantiated by quantitative evidence, because many foods are contaminated with *C. perfringens* and the organism occurs regularly in the faeces of normal people. The count of organisms in remnants of suspect food will depend on the conditions under which the food has been kept and little reliance can be put upon high counts unless the food was held in the refrigerator after serving. Under normal circumstances, counts of the organism do not usually exceed 10^5 per gram of food or faeces, whereas in *C. perfringens* food poisoning

the affected food may contain very high counts of *C. perfringens* (up to 10^9 per gram) and the faeces of affected people may contain *C. perfringens* in counts of $10^5–10^8$ per gram for some days after the food-poisoning incident.

The approach outlined in Figure 38.1 for examination of faeces includes a mild heat activation step as well as a procedure for selecting the very heat-resistant spores of type A2 strains. The yield obtained from sample A (unheated) represents vegetative cells and some of the spores that may germinate, with either type A1 or A2 strains appearing. Sample B (heat activated) will yield colonies, either type A1 or A2, derived purely from spores, as vegetative cells will not withstand heating at 80°C. Colonies of

C. perfringens grown from sample C (boiled) are derived from markedly heat-resistant spores of type A2 strains.

If a faecal sample yields large numbers of type A1 or A2 colonies, this is compatible with a diagnosis of *C. perfringens* food poisoning, but supportive evidence is really needed. If samples from several people involved in an incident yield the same colony type, the evidence is stronger. If the suspected food yields a similar organism in larger numbers, the case is virtually made.

However, the identity of isolates should be finalized by serotyping, so that a relationship can be established between them. The isolation of classical type A1 β-haemolytic *C. perfringens* from food or faeces must be interpreted with caution if this is not possible. Serotyping of food-poisoning strains by slide agglutination tests is done at the Food Hygiene Laboratory, Central Public Health Laboratory, Colindale Avenue, London NW9 5HT. Food-poisoning strains can be assigned to serotypes 1–75 (Stringer et al 1980) but untypable strains also occur quite frequently.

Send several colonies for each specimen, as strains of more than one serotype of *C. perfringens* may be present in the same specimen. If only one single-colony isolate is examined from each specimen, the identity of serotype may not be observed.

A test has been developed for the direct detection of *C. perfringens* enterotoxin in faeces, food, or culture supernates (Bartholomew et al 1985). A reverse passive latex agglutination kit is now available commercially (Oxoid).

C. perfringens enterotoxin-associated colitis

A syndrome differing substantially from that of *C. perfringens* food poisoning has been reported by Borriello et al (1984). Features include abdominal pain and diarrhoea with blood or mucus in the stools. Vomiting sometimes occurs. Patients are usually elderly; an association with current antibiotic therapy is common but not invariable.

Large numbers of *C. perfringens* (10^7–10^{10}/g) are excreted in the stool, predominantly in spore form, along with the enterotoxin which can often be detected in high titre. The enterotoxin produces a cytopathic effect on Vero cells and can be neutralized by specific antiserum raised against it.

Enteritis necroticans: Clostridium perfringens type C

Enteritis necroticans caused by type C strains of *C. perfringens* (originally designated type F) was recognized in Germany in the late 1940s. The form of the disease associated with pork feasting in the highland natives of Papua New Guinea, called 'pig bel', has been studied in detail (Egerton & Walker 1964). There is segmental involvement of small bowel that may be thickened and tender on palpation; loops of dilated intestine with subsequent fibrinopurulent peritonitis and adhesions and intestinal obstruction develop. The disease is a common cause of death in the native children. *C. perfringens* type C (see Table 37.1) produces heat-resistant spores, which are not so markedly heat-resistant as the original type F German strains, but resist 95°C wet heat for some minutes. The organism produces α-toxin, but it is the β-toxin which causes the disease when produced by organisms multiplying and attaching to the villi of the small gut; the toxin is protected from proteolytic digestion by the simultaneous ingestion of a sweet potato vegetable which contains a protease inhibitor. The low protein diet, and the consequent low intestinal protease activity of the natives, further increase vulnerability to the β-toxin. The organism can be demonstrated in the lesions by special immunofluorescence staining and can be cultured from the intestinal content of patients with the disease. It is also present in the stools of healthy carriers and in environmental samples of soil from native cooking areas where 'pig-bel' is endemic.

CLOSTRIDIUM DIFFICILE

Until recently, this organism was regarded as a component of the normal faecal flora of 40–50%

of neonates, but it was rarely isolated from adults. Since 1977 it has been detected with increasing frequency and is now accepted as a cause of pseudomembranous colitis (PMC) and antibiotic-associated colitis (AAC) (Bartlett 1979). The spectrum of disease caused by *C. difficile* is still not fully known, but it appears to range from PMC through AAC to antibiotic-associated diarrhoea (AAD), and may also include exacerbations of chronic inflammatory bowel disease, post-operative diarrhoea and non-antibiotic-associated diarrhoea (British Medical Journal 1981; Brettle et al 1982). Evidence from animal studies and from the observed clustering of some cases favours the view that infection may be exogenous with colonization of a compromised gut.

Morphology and staining

Rod-shaped (4–8 × 0.5–1 μm) with subterminal or terminal non-bulging oval spores. Gram positive, becoming Gram negative in older cultures. In wet films from cooked meat broth (CMB) cultures it exhibits a characteristic oscillating motility. Electron microscopy shows sparse peritrichous flagella.

Cultural characters

A strict anaerobe. Grows well on blood agar (BA) and cefoxitin cycloserine fructose agar (CCFA) at 37°C. On BA, colonies are glossy, greyish, low convex, roughly circular with an irregular edge sometimes becoming spreading; non-haemolytic. On CCFA medium with blood, colonies are similar to those on BA. On CCFA with egg-yolk and neutral red, colonies at 24 h appear large (2–5 mm), flat to low umbonate, yellow, with a ground-glass appearance and a slightly filamentous edge. In films from this growth, organisms may appear much longer, sometimes almost filamentous, and spores are absent; motility is much reduced. Colonies on CCFA are very susceptible to oxygen and must be subcultured without delay. In solid and liquid media, *C. difficile* produces a characteristic farmyard smell which is unlike that of any other *Clostridium* species.

Biochemical reactions

The biochemical reactions of *C. difficile* are summarized in Table 37.4. Most strains ferment glucose, fructose and mannitol, although we have isolated an asaccharolytic strain of *C. difficile*. Aesculin is hydrolysed and some strains produce gelatinase. All are indole negative and lecithinase negative. Gas chromatography (GC; see *Methods*, Ch. 36) of the volatile fatty acid metabolic products after culture in proteose peptone yeast extract glucose (PPYG) medium gives a characteristic profile (Fig. 38.2) which is diagnostic for an organism that can grow on CCFA medium. *C. difficile* produces *p*-cresol from *p*-hydroxyphenyl acetic acid and this is exploited in the indicator medium developed by Phillips & Rogers (1981) for use with GC.

Toxins

A cytotoxin (toxin B) that causes a cytopathic effect on most tissue cell monolayers is neutralized by certain batches of *C. sordelli* antitoxin. An enterotoxin (Sullivan et al 1982), probably produced by all enteropathogenic strains of *C. difficile*, is only weakly cytotoxic but provokes haemorrhagic dilatation when injected into ligated ileal loops of rabbits; this (toxin A) is thought to be the major virulence factor. In 1987, it was not yet practicable to detect the enterotoxin in the diagnostic laboratory. Detection of the cytotoxin is readily performed; although a few enterotoxin positive, cytotoxin negative strains may be missed, it is a worthwhile addition to culture in investigating a possible *C. difficile* infection (see below).

Sensitivity to chemical and physical agents

Vegetative cells of *C. difficile* are sensitive to oxygen. Spores are resistant to oxygen, to heat (75°C for 10–20 min) and to alcohol, which can be used for their selection. Cresols and phenols have been used as selective agents (e.g. 0.2–0.4% *p*-cresol) but this approach is not recommended (see George et al 1979).

Sensitivity to antimicrobial agents

Most strains are sensitive to low concentrations

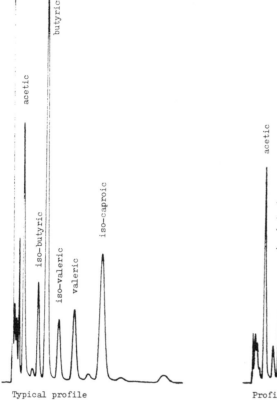

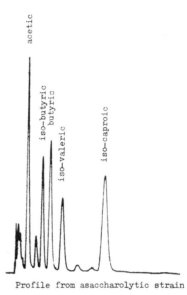

Fig. 38.2 Gas chromatograms of volatile fatty acid metabolic products from 18 h PPYG cultures of a typical and an asaccharolytic strain of *C. difficile* on columns of SP 1220 (see Poxton 1982). *Note*: The small peak between acetic and iso-butyric acids represents propionic acid.

of metronidazole, benzylpenicillin, ampicillin and vancomycin (MIC usually <4 μg/ml, but some up to 32 μg/ml). Most strains are also sensitive to clindamycin, tetracycline and erythromycin, but some are resistant to high levels of these antibiotics. Relatively resistant to aminoglycosides, cephalosporins and cephamycins.

Typing

No generally accepted typing method was available in 1987 when this chapter was written. Various biotypes can be distinguished by a range of simple biochemical tests (Poxton 1982), but this approach is not promising. An immunological fingerprinting method based on visualization of cell surface antigens, after separation on polyacrylamide gel electrophoresis (PAGE), by immunoblot transfer and immunoperoxidase labelling appears more satisfactory (Poxton et al 1984; Sharp & Poxton 1985). A typing method based on PAGE of ^{35}S methionine-labelled proteins has been described by Tabaqchali et al (1986).

Animal pathogenicity

Several investigations of the pathology and epidemiology of *C. difficile* have employed a hamster model. A fatal enterocaecitis can be induced in hamsters if *C. difficile* and antibiotics are given concomitantly. *C. difficile* alone does not usually cause disease but antibiotics alone can result in disease: *C. difficile* is apparently acquired from the environment and then from other animals (Larson et al 1980).

Most strains produce soluble products in broth cultures that are lethal for most laboratory animals. Intramuscular injection of washed live organisms kills mice. Animal tests are not used for diagnostic purposes at present.

Laboratory diagnosis of C. difficile infection

Send a fresh specimen of faeces or diarrhoeal fluid for examination. The vegetative organisms are sensitive to oxygen and are probably unlikely to survive transportation on a swab. Faeces should be investigated for the presence of cyto-toxin*. A direct presumptive diagnostic test (API) based on latex particle agglutination can be applied to a faecal supernate.

The primary assignment is to examine the specimen microscopically and to culture the organism. The introduction of CCFA medium* greatly facilitated the selective isolation of *C. difficile*.

1. Prepare a Gram film and note the presence of any Gram-positive sporing rods. Also prepare a wet film and look for sporing rods showing typical oscillating motility when viewed with phase contrast microscopy. Note the presence of polymorphonuclear leucocytes and red blood cells.

2. Plate out the specimen on fresh CCFA medium, with a large initial inoculum to ensure detection of small numbers of organisms. Incubate the seeded plate anaerobically without delay.

3. Increased yields of *C. difficile* may be obtained by the use of CCFA with reduced concentrations of antibiotics (cefoxitin 8 μg/ml, cycloserine 250 μg/ml) if the sample is previously treated with alcohol to reduce the numbers of non-sporing vegetative commensal species in the inoculum (Borriello & Honour 1981; Levett 1985). The original method used absolute ethanol and homogenized samples were allowed to stand at room temperature for 1 h before plating to selective medium. In our experience, satisfactory results are obtained when a pea-sized sample is homogenized in *c*. 1 ml of industrial methylated spirit; the sample may be plated out within 1–2 min; this makes the method suitable for routine use in the diagnostic laboratory. This procedure gives a significantly higher isolation rate than direct culture on full-strength CCFA.

4. *Enrichment culture.* In addition to primary selective culture, an enrichment procedure may also be employed. Inoculate a portion of the specimen into CMB, or into cycloserine cefoxitin fructose broth (CCFB) which is CCFA medium omitting agar and egg-yolk; O'Farrell et al (1984) recommend including sodium tauro-cholate 1 g/litre in CCFB for enrichment of non-faecal specimens. Incubate anaerobically for 24 h at 37°C and subculture on fresh CCFA as above.

5. Examine plates after anaerobic incubation for 24 h at 37°C. The CCFA medium is highly selective, but an occasional yeast or lactobacillus may grow. On CCFA medium, or on CCFA in which the egg-yolk has been replaced by blood, *C. difficile* colonies show a yellow/green fluor-escence in long wave (365 nm) UV light. Re-incubate plates for a further 24 h before discarding. The use of an anaerobic cabinet for incubation of CCFA plates is particularly valu-able since it allows reincubation of plates after inspection at 24 h without exposure to air.

6. Subculture any suspect colony to BA and incubate anaerobically without delay. Subculture to PPYG medium; after 24 h at 37°C prepare a specimen from the PPYG culture for GC (see Ch. 36, *Methods*). A more rapid GC confir-mation of this organism is done by demon-strating the presence of *p*-cresol and caproic acid in cores of agar beneath suspect colonies on CCFA medium supplemented with *p*-hydroxy-phenyl acetic acid and DL nor-leucine (Phillips & Rogers 1981).

7. If GC is not available, do a range of biochemical tests as indicated in Tables 36.1 and 37.4.

8. Consider a biotyping or serotyping approach if this is available for the investigation of any suspected *C. difficile* outbreak. Isolates may also be assessed for cytotoxin production.

CLOSTRIDIUM BOTULINUM

Botulism is a rare but often fatal intoxication of man and animals. *C. botulinum* spores are widely distributed in nature and botulism is the

---

* Refer to *Methods* at end of this chapter.

result of ingesting food in which *C. botulinum* has multiplied and produced toxin. The disease is characterized by pronounced toxic effects on the peripheral cholinergic nervous system in which the release of acetylcholine at peripheral synapses is irreversibly blocked. After ingestion of the toxin, within 24 h or less, there is progressive paralysis, often initially affecting oculomotor and oropharyngeal muscles. Death usually results from paralysis of the muscles of respiration. *C. botulinum* types A–G are differentiated on the basis of their antigenically distinct but pharmacologically identical toxins. Types A, B and E are most frequently associated with human cases of botulism, but all types can cause disease in man.

Infant botulism is a recently recognized disease in which ingested *C. botulinum* spores multiply in the immature infant gut and produce toxin which is absorbed and produces a spectrum of disease ranging from a mild failure to thrive to paralysis and a sudden infant death syndrome (Arnon 1980).

Wound botulism is an extremely rare disease arising from contamination of a wound or devitalized tissue with *C. botulinum*. The toxin gives rise to neurological symptoms after an incubation period of 4–14 days.

Morphology and staining

Straight or slightly curved rods, 4×1 μm but ranging from 2–10×0.5–2 μm, arranged singly or less commonly in pairs or short chains. Spores oval, subterminal and may slightly distend the cell; some highly toxigenic strains produce few spores. Motile with peritrichous flagella. Gram positive, but become Gram negative when sporulating.

Cultural characters

Strict anaerobe. Grows well on most rich laboratory media. The different toxin types also differ in their cultural characters and there is some variability within each toxin type. Smith (1977) divided the species into four groups

(I–IV, see Table 38.1) based on cultural characters. Optimum temperature 30–37°C, depending on strain. Colonies on solid media after incubation for 48 h are irregularly circular, large (3 mm), smooth, greyish, translucent, with a fibrillar edge that often becomes spreading. Most strains are haemolytic on horse blood agar. Proteolytic strains (A, B, F and G) produce partial clearing on heated blood agar. All types except G produce restricted opalescence and a pearly lipolytic effect on egg-yolk agar (Willis 1977). Recent experience with selective egg-yolk agar containing cycloserine, sulphamethoxazole and trimethoprim indicates that this is very useful for the confirmation of botulism, especially infant botulism (Hatheway & McCroskey 1981).

Biochemical reactions

The groups shown in Table 38.1 show different biochemical reactions. Group I strains ferment glucose and fructose and produce variable or negative results with other sugars; group II strains ferment fructose, glucose, mannose and sucrose; group III strains ferment glucose, mannose and ribose; and group IV (type G) is asaccharolytic. The proteolytic activities of the various types are summarized in Table 38.1. Most strains are indole negative. Tables 37.2, 37.4 and 37.5 indicate other biochemical reactions of interest.

Table 38.1 Cultural groups of *C. botulinum* (after Smith 1977).

Characters of organism	Cultural group			
	I	II	III	IV
Fermentation of glucose	+	+	+	−
Digestion of coagulated protein	+	−	−[a]	+
Hydrolysis of gelatin	+	+	+	+
Major metabolic products[b]	A, P, iB, B, iV	A, B	A, P, B	A, iB, B, iV
Toxin types	A, B, F	B, E, F	C₁, C₂, D	G

[a] Some strains show weak proteolysis.
[b] Volatile fatty acids detected by gas chromatography (GC): A, acetic; P, propionic; iB, iso-butyric; B, butyric; iV, iso-valeric.

C. sporogenes is biochemically indistinguishable from *C. botulinum* group I, and *C. novyi* type A is biochemically indistinguishable from *C. botulinum* group III; differentiation of these organisms depends on specific toxin testing (Smith 1977).

Toxins

There are eight serologically distinct types – A, B, C_1, C_2, D, E, F and G. Slight cross-reactions occur between C_1, C_2 and D, and between E and F. Most but not all of these toxins are synthesized as non-toxic or slightly toxic protoxins. Type A strains and some of the proteolytic type B and F strains produce a protease that activates the toxin; most type E strains and the non-proteolytic B and F strains require an exogenous protease to activate the toxin. Some strains of types C and E produce fully active toxins. All toxins are thermolabile and are inactivated by formaldehyde. Specific phages are involved in the production of toxin by *C. botulinum* types C and D, which can be interconverted; similarly, *C. botulinum* type C and *C. novyi* type A can be interconverted by phages (Eklund & Poysky 1981).

Spores

C. botulinum spores are among the more resistant bacterial spores. There is a descending gradient of heat resistance from the most resistant spores of group I to the less resistant spores of group III. Spores of type A strains can resist boiling at 100°C for some hours. Spores of type E strains are said to be relatively heat sensitive, but this may be misleading; the heated spores of some type E strains do not germinate until they have been treated with lysozyme or a proteinase. Spores of *C. botulinum* are also resistant to radiation, UV light, alcohols, and phenolic and quaternary ammonium compounds. They are relatively susceptible to hypochlorite, ethylene oxide and formaldehyde. The reader is referred to a review by Smith (1977, Ch. 3).

Typing methods

The specific toxin type is determined by toxin/antitoxin neutralization tests in mice. Fluid specimens are mixed with monovalent type-specific antitoxins (Institut Pasteur, 28 Rue du Docteur Roux, 75724 Paris) and injected intraperitoneally into mice. Controls include heated and unheated specimens without antitoxins.

The four groups of *C. botulinum* determined on the basis of cultural and biochemical tests appear to possess group-specific surface antigens. Immunofluorescence procedures with fluorescein-labelled antibodies (FA) can achieve partial typing, but preparations have varied greatly in their usefulness (see Walker & Batty 1964). Three FA reagents available from Wellcome are: anti-type A with activity against A, B and F; anti-type C which reacts with C and D; and anti-type E which reacts specifically with type E. A polyvalent anti-ABF FA reagent is available in the USA. Note that some immunofluorescence reagents cross-react with *C. sporogenes*.

Animal pathogenicity

Intraperitoneal inoculation of culture fluid or culture supernate into mice gives rise to respiratory difficulty in the animals within a few hours. Paralysis of abdominal muscles gives a wasp-waist appearance. A flaccid or generalized paralysis develops; death usually follows within 18–24 h but may take up to 4 days. The internal organs are congested, and thromboses and haemorrhages are seen at autopsy.

Laboratory diagnosis of botulism

Note that *C. botulinum* and materials that may be contaminated with *C. botulinum* must be handled under appropriate containment conditions (Ch. 15). Guidelines for submission of specimens to the Food Hygiene Laboratory, CPHL, London, should be consulted (Report 1979).

Specimens to be investigated may include faeces, food, vomit, gastric fluid, serum, environmental samples and occasionally wound exudate or tissue. The most conclusive proof of botulism is the detection and specific neutralization of toxin in the patient's serum by toxin/antitoxin tests in mice. As direct toxin detection is not always possible, other investigations are added as a routine, and these include culture and identification of the organism from specimens with subsequent detection of toxigenicity. Sometimes the organism may be detected by direct immunofluorescence.

Detection of toxin in serum, food, vomit, faeces or supernates

The following procedure is adapted from that described by Willis (1977).

1. Prepare liquid extracts of solid specimens by homogenization with an equal volume of sterile saline and subsequent centrifugation.

2. As some toxins are activated by trypsin, treat half of the extract with trypsin solution (1% Difco Trypsin 1:250 in distilled water) in the proportions of 9 parts extract to 1 part trypsin solution, held for 1 h at 37°C. The trypsin-treated and untreated samples are again divided into two; heat one portion of each sample to 100°C for 10 min to provide inactivated controls. *Note*: when testing for toxin in serum, trypsin treatment is unnecessary.

3. Add penicillin to each of the four specimens to give a final concentration of 200 units/ml.

4. Challenge three pairs of mice by intraperitoneal inoculation of the untrypsinized material as follows. Protect the first pair with intraperitoneal polyvalent botulinum antitoxin (A, B and E; Institut Pasteur) and challenge with 0.5 ml doses of the unheated material. Challenge the second pair, unprotected, in the same way. Challenge the third pair, also unprotected, with 0.5 ml doses of the heated material.

5. Challenge a further three pairs of mice as above but with the trypsinized material.

Five results are possible: (a) Unprotected mice receiving unheated sample die, while protected mice, and those receiving heated sample survive; this confirms the presence of botulinum toxin. (b) Increased toxicity of some toxins (e.g. type E) by trypsinization may cause death of protected animals – check by diluting sample. (c) If none of the protected animals survives, either toxin C, D or F, or a potent toxin of the other types is present. Repeat with mice protected with C, D and F antisera and use diluted samples. Tetanus intoxication is another possibility – use mice protected with tetanus anti-toxin. (d) All animals die including those receiving heated sample – indicates a non-specific toxic substance. (e) All survive – indicates the absence of botulinum toxin.

Culture of C. botulinum

Direct detection of the organism in the specimen by a fluorescent antibody (FA) procedure is possible, but culture is often necessary and this is generally regarded as technically difficult. See Willis (1977) and Hatheway & McCroskey (1981) for a fuller account.

1. If Gram-positive sporing rods are observed in a specimen, try direct plating, especially in a case of infant botulism. Egg-yolk agar (EYA) has been the medium of choice; a new selective EYA, *C. botulinum* isolation (CBI) medium* will probably supersede it.

2. Attempt enrichment as follows after adding sterile saline to the sample and homogenizing it if necessary. Divide the sample into two. Add an equal volume of absolute ethanol to one half, and leave the other portion untreated. Take 1 ml volumes of ethanol-treated and untreated samples and add these to two sets of three tubes of CMB. Hold one of each set in an 80°C water bath for 10 min, and another pair for 20 min; the final pair is left unheated. This procedure selects for resistant spore-formers but also allows sensitive spores to survive in the untreated cultures.

3. Incubate these cultures anaerobically at 30°C and screen at intervals for toxin production by mouse tests as above; FA tests may be of value as a first screen (see *Methods*, Ch. 37). If no toxin is detected after incubation for 3–5 days, *C. botulinum* should be considered not present.

4. Plate any toxin-positive broth culture on to EYA and CBI medium. An anaerobic chamber should be used, especially if types C or D are suspected. Incubate plates at 30°C for 36–48 h. Colonies showing restricted opalescence and a pearly layer (lipase activity) should be subcultured to CMB and tested for specific toxin in due course. If toxin was detected at the enrichment stage and no opalescence or pearly layer effect is observed on the EYA subcultures, type G may be suspected. FA procedures may

again be useful at this stage for rapid confirmation.

METHODS

Cycloserine cefoxitin fructose agar (CCFA) (George et al 1979)

Basal medium

Proteose peptone No. 2 (Difco)	40 g
Na$_2$HPO$_4$	5 g
KH$_2$PO$_4$	1 g
NaCl	2·g
Anhydrous MgSO$_4$	0.1 g
Fructose	6 g
Agar	20 g
1% ethanolic solution of neutral red	3 ml
Distilled water	1000 ml

Method. Sterilize basal medium at 121°C for 15 min in 100 ml portions. Add to 100 ml melted base at 50°C: D-cycloserine (Sigma) to a final concentration of 500 μg/ml, cefoxitin (MSD) to a final concentration of 16 μg/ml, and 5 ml of 50% Egg-yolk suspension (Oxoid). Alternatively, the egg-yolk may be replaced with 5 ml of whole horse blood to make CCFA with blood.

Note that the concentration of antibiotics can be halved when CCFA is used with an alcohol procedure to select for spores of *C. difficile* (see text).

Assay for C. difficile cytotoxin

The specimen may be a liquid stool, or the homogenate of a solid stool in physiological saline, or the supernate of a 5 day culture of *C. difficile* in BHI/PP broth (Brain heart infusion (Oxoid) 3.7% w/v and Proteose peptone (Difco) 1% w/v). The supernate may be filter-sterilized, but this is unnecessary.

Prepare four-fold serial dilutions of the test liquid in physiological saline and add 10 μl volumes to 90 μl of Eagle's modified maintenance medium (Gibco; Flow) containing penicillin (200 units/ml), streptomycin (200 μg/ml), gentamicin (10 μg/ml) and amphotericin B (20 μg/ml), over monolayers of human embryo fibroblasts (or a wide range of other cell lines) in Microtitre plates (see Ch. 50). The highest dilution of the test fluid that produces complete rounding of more than 50% of the cells after incubation for 24 h at 37°C gives the cytotoxin titre. Neutralization is performed by adding 10 μl of a 25-fold dilution of *C. sordelli* antitoxin (Wellcome) to a duplicate series of wells. A positive control, either a known positive stool extract or a purified *C. difficile* cytotoxin, should be included; we have found no loss in potency if the toxin control is frozen and thawed several times.

Clostridium botulinum isolation (CBI) medium (Dezfulian et al 1981)

Antibacterial supplements. Prepare the following solutions and sterilize by filtration: D-cycloserine, 1% solution in water; sulphamethoxazole, 1.9% solution in water – add 10% NaOH till dissolved; trimethoprim, 0.1% solution in water – add 0.05 mol/litre HCl till dissolved.

Basal medium

Trypticase peptone (BBL)	40 g
Na$_2$HPO$_4$	5 g
NaCl	2 g
MgSO$_4$ 5% aqueous solution	0.2 ml
D-glucose	2 g
Yeast extract (Difco)	5 g
Agar	20 g
Distilled water	900 ml

Method. Adjust to pH 7.4 and autoclave at 121°C for 15 min; cool to 55°C. Add 100 ml of Egg-yolk suspension (50% in saline; Difco) and antibacterial supplements prepared as above: D-cycloserine, 25 ml (250 mg); sulphamethoxazole, 4 ml (76 mg); and trimethoprim, 4 ml (4 mg).

Store plates in an anaerobic chamber for at least 4 h before use.

REFERENCES

Arnon S S 1980 Infant botulism. Annual Review of Medicine 31: 541–560

Bartholomew B A, Stringer M F, Watson G N, Gilbert R J 1985 Development and application of an enzyme linked immunosorbent assay for *Clostridium perfringens* type A enterotoxin. Journal of Clinical Pathology 38: 222–228

Bartlett J G 1979 Antibiotic associated pseudomembranous colitis. Reviews in Infectious Diseases 1: 530–539

Borriello S P, Honour P 1981 Simplified procedure for the routine isolation of *Clostridium difficile* from faeces. Journal of Clinical Pathology 34: 1124–1127

Borriello S P, Larson H E, Welch A R, Barclay F, Stringer M F, Bartholomew B A 1984 Enterotoxigenic *Clostridium perfringens*: a possible cause of antibiotic-associated diarrhoea. Lancet 1: 305–307

Brettle R P, Poxton I R, Murdoch J McC, Brown R, Byrne M D, Collee J G 1982 *Clostridium difficile* in association with sporadic diarrhoea. British Medical Journal 284: 230–233

British Medical Journal 1981 Antibiotic-associated colitis – the continuing saga (leading article). British Medical Journal 282: 1913–1914

Collee J G, Knowlden J A, Hobbs B C 1961 Studies on the growth, sporulation and carriage of *Clostridium welchii* with special reference to food poisoning strains. Journal of Applied Bacteriology 24: 326–339

Dezfulian M, McCroskey L M, Hatheway C L, Dowell V R 1981 Selective medium for isolation of *Clostridium botulinum* from human feces. Journal of Clinical Microbiology 13: 526–531

Egerton J R, Walker P D 1964 The isolation of *Clostridium perfringens* type C from necrotic enteritis in Papua-New Guinea. Journal of Pathology and Bacteriology 88: 275–278

Eklund M W, Poysky F T 1981 Relationship of bacteriophages to the toxigenicity of *Clostridium botulinum* and related organisms. In: Lewis G E (ed) Biomedical aspects of botulism. Academic Press, New York. p 93–107

George W L, Sutter V L, Citron D, Finegold S M 1979 Selective and differential medium for the isolation of *Clostridium difficile*. Journal of Clinical Microbiology 9: 214–219

Hatheway C L, McCroskey L M 1981 Laboratory investigation of human and animal botulism. In: Lewis G E (ed) Biomedical aspects of botulism. Academic Press, New York. p 165–180

Larson H E, Price A B, Borriello S P 1980 Epidemiology of experimental enterocecitis due to *Clostridium difficile*. Journal of Infectious Diseases 142: 408–413

Levett P N 1985 Effect of antibiotic concentration in a selective medium on the isolation of *Clostridium difficile* from faecal specimens. Journal of Clinical Pathology 38: 233–234

O'Farrell S, Wilks M, Nash J Q, Tabaqchali S 1984 A selective enrichment broth for the isolation of *Clostridium difficile*. Journal of Clinical Pathology 37: 98–99

Phillips K D, Rogers P A 1981 Rapid detection and presumptive identification of *Clostridium difficile* by *p*-cresol production on a selective medium. Journal of Clinical Pathology 34: 642–644

Poxton I R 1982 Detection and isolation of *Clostridium difficile*. European Journal of Chemotherapy and Antibiotics 2: 123–128

Poxton I R, Aronsson B, Möllby R, Nord C E, Collee J G 1984 Immunochemical fingerprinting of *Clostridium difficile* strains isolated from an outbreak of antibiotic-associated colitis and diarrhoea. Journal of Medical Microbiology 17: 317–324

Report 1979 Botulism. Communicable Diseases Report, 79/22. Communicable Diseases Surveillance Centre (PHLS) of England, Wales and Ireland

Sharp J, Poxton I R 1985 An immunochemical method for fingerprinting *Clostridium difficile*. Journal of Immunological Methods 83: 241–248

Smith L DS 1977 Botulism: the organism, its toxins, the disease. Thomas, Springfield, Illinois

Stringer M F, Turnbull P C B, Gilbert R J 1980 Application of serological typing to the investigation of outbreaks of *Clostridium perfringens* food poisoning, 1970–1978. Journal of Hygiene, Cambridge 84: 443–456

Sullivan N M, Pellett S, Wilkins D D 1982 Purification and characterization of toxins A and B of *Clostridium difficile*. Infection and Immunity 35: 1032–1040

Sutton R G A, Ghosh A C, Hobbs B C 1971 Isolation and enumeration of *Clostridium welchii* from food and faeces. In: Shapton DA, Board R D (eds) Isolation of anaerobes. The Society for Applied Bacteriology Technical Series 5. Academic Press, London

Tabaqchali S, O'Farrell S, Holland D, Silman R 1986 Method for the typing of *Clostridium difficile* based on polyacrylamide gel electrophoresis of [^{35}S] methionine-labelled proteins. Journal of Clinical Microbiology 23: 197–198

Walker P D, Batty I 1964 Fluorescent studies in the genus *Clostridium*. II. A rapid method for differentiating *Clostridium botulinum* types A, B and F, types C and D, and type E. Journal of Applied Bacteriology 27: 140–142

Willis T 1977 Anaerobic bacteriology: clinical and laboratory practice, 3rd edn. Butterworth, London

Laboratory strategy in the diagnosis of infective syndromes

This chapter outlines laboratory strategy in dealing with the following types of sample or infective syndrome:

1. Blood culture
2. Upper respiratory tract infections, including throat, nose, ear, eye infections
3. Lower respiratory tract infections
4. Wound, skin and deep sepsis
5. Genital tract infections
6. Meningitis
7. Gastrointestinal infections
8. Urinary tract infections
9. Pyrexia of unknown origin.

A major responsibility of the head of a clinical laboratory is to determine the laboratory's policies for dealing with the different kinds of specimens and requests received and the manner of reporting the results of the investigations. The number of specimens submitted to a microbiology laboratory is likely to be very great, e.g. 100 000–200 000 a year, and the majority will need to be examined by staff of different grades applying standardized procedures laid down in a laboratory manual. It will not be possible for senior staff to scrutinize individually each request and specify the particular tests to be performed.

Thus, a policy for procedures must be determined for each major category of specimens and requests, e.g. for blood cultures, throat swabs from pharyngitis, faeces from diarrhoea or gastroenteritis, sputa from suspected lower respiratory tract infections and urines from suspected urinary tract infections. Extra examinations, outwith the standard procedures, may be required if specifically requested by the phys-

ician or if the clinical information provided on the request form suggests that an unusual infection may be present. For example, if throat swabs are not routinely examined for diphtheria bacilli or sputa for tubercle bacilli, the laboratory manual should lay down the clinical indications requiring these extra examinations to be made in particular cases. Moreover, staff must be instructed about the kinds of requests or findings, e.g. those of exotic pathogens, that they should at once bring to the attention of senior staff for a decision on the initial or further procedures to be adopted.

There is a great diversity in the types of tests that may be used to make a particular finding and in the sequences of tests that may be chosen for the investigation of a particular type of specimen. Indeed, almost every laboratory differs from every other in its policies for investigations and reporting. Heads of laboratories take satisfaction in their independent authority to determine their laboratory policies so as best to meet the often conflicting local requirements of special clinical needs, helpfulness to physicians, scientific accuracy, speed of reporting and economy in the use of scarce laboratory staff, finance and other resources. But it is incumbent on them to avoid adhering to outmoded, parochial or deviant policies, and to keep in touch with workers in other laboratories in order to inform themselves about new developments and the advantages and disadvantages of alternative procedures and policies. The continuing rapid advances in medicine and science make it essential for laboratory policies to be subjected to continuous review and development.

Clinical bacteriologists rightly wish to obtain

the fullest pertinent information from the specimens they examine and an adequate confirmation of their findings, but they should avoid obsessively burdening their staff with the requirement of such laborious investigations that the work cannot be done safely and reliably, without haste or the taking of improper shortcuts. An over-ambitious investigative policy is self-defeating, and the procedures should be kept simple enough to be undertaken carefully by the available staff. Thus, it is better for the investigation on an organism isolated from sputum or urine to be confined to showing reliably that it is a coliform bacillus with particular antibiotic sensitivities than for the work to be rushed and made unreliable, and the reporting delayed, in an attempt to identify it as a particular species of *Klebsiella* or *Citrobacter*.

Caution should be exercised before requiring staff to perform additional procedures for research purposes, particularly if only with the vague idea that something interesting may be discovered. Even if the staff have adequate time to perform the extra work carefully, they may not be motivated to do it with the intense interest, attention and precautions necessary for worthwhile research. Moreover, the amount and reliability of the clinical information provided to the laboratory about the patients yielding the specimens, e.g. about their response to antibiotic therapy, are generally insufficient to make the laboratory results useful for research purposes.

There are, however, two kinds of extra investigations that do require to be undertaken in a good clinical laboratory. One is the running of a new type of test in parallel with the existing test to determine the former's advantages and disadvantages under local conditions as a prelude to possibly adopting it in the place of the latter. The other is the examination of unknown specimens provided from an external quality control scheme and the performance of additional tests with known cultures for the purpose of internal quality control. Thus, with each day's batch of tests of a particular kind, extra tests should be set up with stock cultures known to give positive and negative results when the test is properly done. Each batch of enriched or selective medium should be tested for growth or

inhibition of appropriate stock cultures, except perhaps those of media used so commonly that many positive and negative results are regularly obtained from the clinical specimens received.

As the choice of procedures must be determined in light of the special requirements and conditions in each laboratory, the following suggestions for investigative procedures will require to be qualified to meet the local needs.

1. BLOOD CULTURE

Culture of patient's blood is one of the most important investigations in clinical microbiology, for the demonstration of septicaemia or bacteriaemia indicates that there is an immediate threat to the patient's life and an urgent need for appropriate antibiotic therapy. Procedures must be planned to ensure reliability and rapidity in obtaining results, and to this end should, if necessary, be given priority over other work in the allocation of staff labour and material resources. For a review of problems, see Gould & Duerden (1983).

Blood culture is requested mainly in two clinical situations: (1) where the possibility of septicaemia or bacteriaemia is suggested by the presence of fever, shock or other symptoms occurring in association with a known or suspected local infection such as sepsis in a surgical wound, puerperal sepsis, pneumonia, meningitis, osteomyelitis or endocarditis; and (2) where it is one of the procedures required in the investigation of a fever difficult to diagnose because of the absence of signs of a specific infection or local infective lesion, i.e. a pyrexia of unknown origin (PUO). The laboratory diagnosis of PUO is discussed at the end of this chapter and the following discussion is concerned mainly with the former clinical situation.

The isolation of a bacterium from the blood of a patient with a local infection such as wound sepsis or pneumonia is valuable firstly in indicating the urgent need for antibacterial therapy, secondly in revealing the species of bacterium against which therapy should be directed, and thirdly in providing a culture for the performance of in-vitro drug sensitivity tests. Culture of a specimen from a local site of infection, e.g. a wound swab or sputum specimen, often yields a mixture of contaminating commensal bacteria and potential pathogens, the clinical significance of which is unclear, but the demonstration of one of these species in the blood indicates that it at least is an invader of clinical significance. If, for instance, a pneumococcus is cultured from sputum from a patient with suspected pneumonia, it may have been derived from its site of commensal carriage in the throat and not from the lungs, which may instead be infected with an undetected virus or mycoplasma. But if the pneumococcus is cultured from the blood, it may be concluded that it is probably present as a pathogen in the lungs and that the patient certainly requires anti-pneumococcal therapy.

Contamination. A difficulty in interpreting results arises from the liability of the specimen to be contaminated with organisms that are commensals or common contaminants on the skin. Albus staphylococci are the commonest contaminants, but diphtheroid bacilli, coliform bacilli, anthracoid bacilli, *Clostridium perfringens*, candida and other organisms are sometimes present, and the finding of one of these organisms in a blood culture should be viewed with the strong suspicion that it is a contaminant from the skin. But in a patient with debility, immune deficiency, an intravascular line, a prosthetic implant or some other condition favouring an opportunistic infection, the saprophytic or commensal organism isolated may indeed have an important pathogenic role. Consideration must be given to the probability of its having such an opportunistic role in the circumstances of each particular case. To this end, culture should be attempted on several separately collected samples of blood, for the isolation of the same species of organism from repeated specimens suggests that it is probably present as a cause of infection and not merely as a contaminant. This probability is strengthened if it can be shown that the different isolates are identical with one another in their pattern of antibiotic sensitivities, biotype or phage type.

Collection of sample. To minimize difficulty in interpretation, every care must be taken to prevent contamination of the specimen during its collection from the patient and its examination in the laboratory. Those collecting the blood samples should be given advice on the correct aseptic procedures (Ch. 7). They should be instructed how to disinfect the skin over the vein, to use a fresh sterile syringe for the venepuncture and to replace the needle used for the venepuncture with a fresh sterile needle before inoculating the blood into the culture bottles. They should hold the needle by its butt, not shaft, either with sterile forceps or with the fingers covered with a dry sterile rubber glove, and should take care to avoid contaminating themselves or the outside of the culture bottles with potentially infective blood. They should also be warned that contamination is very likely if the sample is collected from an indwelling peripheral venous catheter or a long central venous line instead of from a fresh venepuncture. In some cases such lines themselves become colonized with skin commensal bacteria, which are then seeded into the circulation.

Examination in the laboratory should be planned with a view to minimizing the opportunities for contamination of the specimen or its subcultures with airborne dust or from the bacteriologist's skin or equipment. However it should be noted that despite insistence on aseptic precautions, most laboratories report finding contamination in 1–5% of the blood cultures they examine.

False-negative results. The media and methods used for blood culture should be such as to support growth of nutritionally exacting organisms, and both strict aerobes and strict anaerobes as well as facultative organisms. Even so, a single negative culture should not be taken as proof that a patient does not have a blood infection. In bacteriaemic illnesses the number of bacteria in the blood may vary rapidly between many and few or none as they are introduced intermittently from a local infective focus and removed by the reticuloendothelial tissues. To maximize the chances of isolation when the bacteria may be scanty, a large volume of blood, e.g. 10–20 ml, from each collection should be cultured, and a number of samples should be collected on separate occasions. Thus, in attempting to discover the organism causing a suspected endocarditis, at least six samples collected at intervals of several hours in the course of 3–6 days should be cultured.

Antibiotics in the blood. The blood sample should be diluted between 1 in 5 and 1 in 10 in the culture medium in order to reduce the concentration of natural antibacterial constituents to a sub-effective level. The dilution also reduces the concentration of any therapeutically administered antibiotic. But when an antibiotic is present in the undiluted blood at more than 10 times its minimum inhibitory concentration, it may still, after dilution, prevent the growth of viable bacteria in the specimen.

For this reason, every attempt should be made to ensure that samples of blood are collected *before* the start of antibiotic therapy. If an antibiotic has already been given to the patient, the collection of the blood sample should preferably be delayed until at least 24 h after a dose has last been given. Otherwise, it may be possible to add an antibiotic-inactivating agent to the culture bottle. Para-aminobenzoic acid used to be added routinely to blood culture media to neutralize any sulphonamide administered. If the patient has been treated with a β-lactam antibiotic (a penicillin or cephalosporin), a broad-spectrum β-lactamase should be added to the culture bottle as soon as possible after introduction of the blood, e.g. 0.2 ml of Wellcome penicillinase to a bottle containing 50 ml medium. Special blood culture media are commercially available that contain resins that are said to be capable of inactivating a variety of antibiotics (Marion).

In a study of 2010 blood cultures, 147 (7.3%) of the seeded broths (10 ml blood in 50 ml broth) were found to contain detectable levels of antibiotic and of these 14 (9.5%) grew bacteria (Rodriguez & Lorian 1985). Use of a device to remove the antibiotic did not improve the bacterial recovery rate. Only resistant organisms grew in blood cultures with more than 0.6 μg/ml of a β-lactam antibiotic, 2 μg/ml of aminoglycoside or 4 μg/ml of tetracycline, but sensitive organisms grew in cultures with lower concentrations of the antibiotic. These findings indicate that in patients receiving antibiotics the timing of the collection of a blood sample to just before the next dose is more valuable than the attempt to remove the antibiotic from the sample.

Culture systems. A choice has to be made between the traditional system of examining blood cultures by filming and subculturing after different periods of incubation and an automated system that monitors the culture for an early sign of bacterial growth, such as a change in electrical impedance or the release of radioactive CO_2 or non-radioactive gas. The traditional method will be discussed first. It is the method of choice for laboratories receiving only a small number of requests for blood culture and has the advantages of flexibility and freedom from the need to maintain expensive, complicated equipment.

If the traditional system is to be used, decisions have to be made about (1) the kinds and numbers of culture media to be seeded from each sample of blood, (2) the arrangements for issuing the culture bottles to those who collect the samples, (3) the arrangements for instructing the collectors about the size and method of collection of the samples, (4) the methods of incubation of the culture bottles in the laboratory, (5) the number and times of examinations of the bottles during their incubation, and (6) the methods of examination by filming and subculture.

Culture bottles. It is necessary to culture at least several millilitres of blood diluted 1 in 5 to 1 in 10 in a culture medium. This is conveniently done by inoculating 5–10 ml blood into 50 ml liquid medium in a bottle of 90–125 ml capacity. To maximize the chances of detecting scanty bacteria, a larger volume, e.g. 10–20 ml, of blood should be collected and half of it should be inoculated into each of a 'set' of two such culture bottles. The use of two bottles has several further advantages: they may contain different media or be incubated in different atmospheres, and scanty contaminants are likely to grow in only one of them.

As detailed in Chapter 7, the bottles of sterile medium should be tightly closed with a perforated aluminium or plastic cap over an entire rubber washer, and these should be covered and kept sterile till the moment of inoculation by a metal foil cover. After removal of the foil, the blood is inoculated into the bottle by inserting the syringe needle through the rubber washer, the bottle remaining unopened and unexposed to the entry of airborne dust. Instructions for the collection of the sample and its introduction into the bottle should be given on a printed label attached to the bottle.

Culture media. The chance of detecting scanty or exacting bacteria will be maximized if a variety of rich media are seeded from each sample and different media are used for aerobes and anaerobes. But use of a single, good all-purpose medium will give nearly as many positive results, saves in labour and cost of materials, and reduces the risk of confusion in the issue and use of the culture bottles.

Suitable media are described in Chapters 6 and 7. If a single, all-purpose medium is to be used, it should be richly nutritive and capable of supporting the growth of both strict aerobes and strict anaerobes when incubated sealed and unexposed to an external atmosphere. A good choice is a Robertson-type cooked-meat medium based on brain heart infusion broth and having at its foot a layer of pieces of lean meat about 3 cm deep (Ch. 6). The inoculated blood adds nutrients, including X and V factors, and small amounts of O_2 and CO_2. When the bottle is incubated while still sealed, most anaerobes will find suitable conditions for growth among the pieces of meat and strict aerobes will grow at the surface of the broth where they have access to oxygen in the overlying air. If the bottle has been autoclaved with its cap tightly closed, its original content of air will still be present. If it has been autoclaved with its cap loose, the air expelled during autoclaving will have been replaced by air drawn into it during the

subsequent cooling, unless the washer has been sucked tightly on to its mouth.

If two bottles have been seeded from the sample, their caps may be loosened and one of them incubated in air plus 5–10% CO_2, the other in an anaerobic jar, but the advantages of this procedure over that of incubating both bottles still sealed have not been proven.

When the presence of certain exacting organisms is indicated, specially suitable media and methods of incubation should be used, e.g. Sabouraud broth incubated at 28°C for up to 10 days for yeasts and fungi, and Castaneda's medium incubated at 37°C for up to 6 weeks for brucella.

Examination of blood cultures. Depending on the number of bacteria in the bloodstream and other factors, the first appearance of growth may take place after as little as a few hours or only after a longer period of 1 or a few days, or occasionally 1 or 2 weeks. As it is desired to detect any positive culture as early as possible and yet not miss any late-growing culture, the ideal procedure is to make repeated examinations of the culture bottle at different times during its incubation from 4 h to 2 weeks or longer (Ch. 7). If, however, many requests for blood culture are received each day, the amount of labour required for making more than a few examinations on each bottle may be excessive. Moreover, every opening of a bottle for examination affords an extra opportunity for contamination, and overlapping examinations on successive batches of bottles on the same day increase the chance of confusion and mistakes.

Trials of different schedules suggest that a minimal, reasonably effective procedure is the making of just two examinations on each bottle, the first after incubation at 37°C overnight (i.e. for 12–24 h), the second after 4–7 days. Only very few cultures negative at 4 days become positive on longer incubation. When a report is required urgently on a suspected septicaemia, an additional examination may be made after only 4 h incubation.

Some workers, however, consider that an examination should *always* be made on the day the specimen is received, i.e. after incubation for only 4–8 h. Positive findings at that stage are available for earlier reporting to the clinician and are less likely to be due to the growth of scanty contaminants than those obtained after longer incubation. This course requires that staff should be available in the late evening to examine blood cultures received in the late afternoon. Also, the negative cultures, which constitute the majority of all those received, have to be examined again at 18–24 h and 4–7 days, requiring a total of three examinations. The extra work of the early, first-day examination may be minimized by confining it to the making of subcultures and omitting the more time-consuming examination by Gram film.

It is recommended that on each subsequent occasion of examination, the blood culture should be examined both by a Gram film and by subculturing on two plates of blood agar, the one incubated in air plus 5–10% CO_2, the other anaerobically in nitrogen/hydrogen plus 5–10% CO_2. If the presence of meningococcus or haemophilus seems likely, e.g. in suspected septicaemic meningitis, a heated-blood ('choco-late') agar plate may be substituted for the aerobic plain blood agar plate. Gram filming is particularly valuable when the first examination is made only after overnight incubation, i.e. after 12–24 h, for when bacteria are seen to be present in the film, a preliminary report may be phoned to the physician at once, without the need to wait another day to see growth of the bacteria in the subcultures.

The procedures of filming and subculture must be performed in such a way as to minimize the opportunities for contamination of the blood culture with bacteria from the air, fingers or equipment. The bacteriologist should gently mix the contents of the bottle without wetting the inside of the cap, then remove the cap, withdraw 0.5–1 ml of the culture fluid into a sterile Pasteur pipette, and at once replace the cap. (Contamination of the bottle is less likely to occur during one dip with a pipette than during three with an inoculating loop.) He should then let a large drop of the fluid fall from the pipette on to each subculture plate and finally spread a drop on a slide for Gram staining. Lastly, he should spread the drops on the plates over large 'well' areas and streak them out on the remainder.

Castaneda-type bottles. The difficulties of making many repeated examinations of blood cultures may be avoided by the use of bottles of the Castaneda type, which contain an agar surface above the level of the culture fluid (Ch. 7). Repeated attempts at subculture may be made with a minimum of labour and without ever opening the bottle and exposing it to the risk of contamination. The bottle is momentarily tilted to run some culture fluid over the agar surface and then re-incubated until colonies are seen to appear on the latter. A commercially available kit (Roche) supplies the agar medium in a clear plastic container that is attachable to the mouth of a conventional blood culture bottle on its receipt in the laboratory. Another kit (Gibco) contains the agar slope in a parallel chamber of a double bottle into which some of the seeded broth can be tipped.

Reading of Gram film. The Gram film should be examined as soon as the subcultures have been set up, and positive findings reported at once to the physician so that the morphological type of the organism present may serve as a guide to his initial choice of antibiotic. The finding will also indicate to the bacteriologist what further subcultures and tests should be seeded from the positive bottle. Two extra plates should be seeded confluently and the appropriate antibiotic disks applied to them for sensitivity testing on aerobic and anaerobic incubation. Optochin and bacitracin disks may be used on the subculture plates to identify organisms resembling pneumococci and streptococci. A MacConkey plate may be seeded to assist in the identification of Gram-negative bacilli, a DNase test plate for staphylococci, an aesculin-bile plate for diphtheroid bacilli (to exclude listeria, which is positive), and a Nagler plate for bacilli resembling *Clostridium perfringens*.

A possible cause of error must be borne in mind when reading the Gram film. Some media, particularly some batches of meat pieces incorporated in cooked meat medium, may be contaminated with saprophytic bacteria, which, although they have been killed in the steriliz-ation procedure, may be sufficiently numerous to be seen in the film. If only one morphological type is seen, its presence may lead to the making of a false provisional report, but if a mixture of types is seen, their origin as contaminants will be suspected. The error will be recognized next day when the subcultures will be found to be negative.

Examination of subcultures. The plates should be inspected after incubation for 18–24 h, when any growth should be examined in a Gram film and by the setting up of appropriate identifying and sensitivity tests. Plates showing what is possibly very slight growth and plates seeded from film-positive bottles but still devoid of growth should be re-incubated for up to three more days before being discarded as negative.

Reports. Relevant positive findings should be reported by phone to the physician as soon as is practicable and, if requested, advice should be given on the choice of antibiotic therapy. A written report should be issued when the exam-inations made after the first 12–24 h of incu-bation have been completed. For positive cultures, the species and drug sensitivities should be reported, and for negative cultures, the absence of growth and a note that a further report will be issued if growth appears on longer incubation.

When an albus staphylococcus or a commensal type of diphtheroid bacillus is found and no predisposition to opportunistic infection is known, the report should state that the organism is *probably* a contaminant from the patient's skin and omit the drug sensitivity findings. If, however, the patient has suspected endocarditis, an artificial heart valve, an intravenous catheter or a cerebrospinal fluid shunt, or has had heart surgery, or is immunosuppressed or on cytotoxic drugs, the finding of the organism and its sensi-tivities should be reported, but with the caution that it may *possibly* be a contaminant from the patient's skin.

Automated systems

These systems employ equipment that automati cally detects an early sign of bacterial growth in a special blood culture bottle. The system most used is Bactec (Becton Dickinson). It depends on the release of radioactive carbon dioxide ($^{14}CO_2$) into the atmosphere in the culture bottle by the bacterial degradation of ^{14}C-containing nutrients in a special culture medium. Separate bottles of special medium are supplied for aerobic and anaerobic culture, and bottles of medium containing resins to inactivate any anti-biotics that may be present in the specimen.

Normally 10 ml blood would be collected in a syringe and up to 5 ml injected through their rubber caps into aerobic and anaerobic culture bottles containing 30 ml medium. Up to 60 bottles of the one kind seeded from different patients are loaded into an instrument in which they are incubated, agitated and periodically flushed with an appropriate gas (air + CO_2; or $N_2 + H_2 + CO_2$) through two heat-sterilized needles inserted automatically through the rubber cap. The effluent gas is screened, also automatically, for the presence of β-radiation (low-energy electrons) indicating early bacterial growth, which is often detectable on the same day as the specimen is received in the laboratory. When growth is thus first detected, the bottle is removed and examined in the usual way by filming and subculture. Negatively reacting bottles do not need to be filmed or subcultured at any stage.

The costs of purchasing the special media and hiring the equipment are approximately offset by the saving of culture plates that would otherwise be used on at least two occasions in subculturing the numerous bottles remaining free from growth. These latter generally comprise over 90% of all blood culture specimens received and technical staff welcome being freed from the repetitive and uninteresting, yet onerous and exacting work of examining them by film and subculture. The other major advantage of an automatic system is the earlier detection of heavy septicaemia, which often enables a report to be issued a day earlier than by the traditional system.

Before a change is made from the traditional to an automatic system, consideration should be given to the feasibility of making the necessary supporting arrangements. A regular supply of the special culture bottles and facilities for servicing the equipment must be assured. Adequately trained staff must be available at the appropriate times of day to load the bottles on to the machine, read the results, and unload when finished, and any local requirements for radiation protection must be met. The amount of radioactive material in the bottles is so small that spills should present no hazard to human health and, after sterilization, the spent medium may be discarded via the laboratory drain into the public sewer. Nevertheless, radiation protection officers may require that stocks of bottles issued to users in hospitals and clinics should be kept in secure places and that a balancing inventory should be kept of the number of bottles issued and the number returned. Such difficulties may be avoided by use of the more recent Bactec system which detects the production of non-radioactive CO_2.

Gas capture system. A simple blood culture system recently developed by Oxoid obviates the need for expensive automated equipment, demonstrates both aerobic and anaerobic organisms in a single culture bottle, and permits frequent, easy observation of the onset of growth. The blood culture bottle contains a medium specially formulated to promote gas production on the growth of any aerobic or anaerobic organism and the gas pressure forces medium into a reservoir where it can be observed visually in the course of incubation. In a comparative evaluation the gas capture system gave very similar results to the Bactec radiometric system (King et al 1986).

2. UPPER RESPIRATORY INFECTIONS

The commonest respiratory infections are localized in the oropharynx, nasopharynx and nasal cavity, causing sore throat, nasal discharge and often fever, but the throat pathogens may also

spread to infect the larynx, causing hoarseness, the middle ear, causing otitis media with earache, a paranasal sinus, causing sinusitis with pain in the face or head, and the eye, causing conjunctivitis or keratitis. The upper respiratory tract may also be involved in wider respiratory or generalized infections such as whooping cough, influenza, measles and infectious mononucleosis.

In most cases the primary infection is viral, though the causal virus is generally not demonstrated, and there is often concomitant carriage or secondary infection with one of the potential bacterial pathogens commonly present in the nasopharynx, e.g. pneumococcus, *Haemophilus influenzae*, *Staphylococcus aureus* and *Streptococcus pyogenes*. Drug-resistant coliform bacilli or yeasts may come to dominate the throat flora in patients receiving antibiotics, but their presence is generally of little pathological significance.

Streptococcal pharyngitis

The only common primary bacterial cause of sore throat is *S. pyogenes*, which is found in about 30% of cases of pharyngitis, with or without tonsillitis. Its detection is the main purpose of the bacteriological examination of throat swabs, for it is the only common throat pathogen for which antibiotic therapy is clearly indicated. When it is thought or shown to be present, benzylpenicillin and procaine penicillin should be given by intramuscular injection and followed by phenoxymethyl penicillin given orally for 7–10 days; commonly, the injections are omitted. Erythromycin should be given to patients allergic to the penicillins. Effective therapy should cause rapid amelioration of symptoms, e.g. within 24–48 h, and prevent serious complications such as otitis media and rheumatic fever. Streptococcal pharyngitis cannot be distinguished clinically from viral pharyngitis, so whenever practicable throat swab examinations should be made on patients with sore throat.

In only a few cases in the UK are there clinical indications requiring the examination of throat swabs for other pathogens, such as the diphtheria bacillus, Vincent's organisms, candida or gonococcus, and in the absence of such indications, swabs from pharyngitis should be examined only for *S. pyogenes*. If the presence of commensal nasopharyngeal residents like *H. influenzae*, pneumococcus, *S. aureus* and coliform bacilli is reported to the physician, he may be induced to give inappropriate antibiotic therapy.

Throat swabs. A plain, albumen-coated or charcoal-coated cotton-wool swab should be used to collect as much exudate as possible from the tonsils, posterior pharyngeal wall and any other area that is inflamed or bears exudate. If the patient permits, the swab should be rubbed with rotation over one tonsillar area, then the arch of the soft palate and uvula, the other tonsillar area, and finally the posterior pharyngeal wall. An adequate view of the throat should be ensured by good lighting and the use of a disposable wooden spatula to pull outwards and so depress the tongue. The swab should be replaced in its tube with care not to soil the rim. If it cannot be delivered to the laboratory within about 1 h, it should be placed in a refrigerator at 4°C until delivery or, preferably, it should be submitted in a tube of transport medium (Ch. 6).

In the laboratory the swab should be rubbed, while being rotated, over large 'well' areas, about one-third of the surface on each of two blood agar plates, and the wells should be streaked out with a loop over the remainder of the plate. The plates should be incubated at 37°C for 18–24 h, one in air plus 5–10% CO_2, the other anaerobically in nitrogen or hydrogen plus 5–10% CO_2. It is advantageous, before incubation, to place a 6 mm disk containing 1 unit of benzylpenicillin on the well area of one plate and a disk containing 0.1 units of bacitracin on that of the other.

Next day, colonies of *S. pyogenes* are recognized by their zones of β-haemolysis, larger and clearer on the anaerobic than the aerobic plate, and their sensitivity to both penicillin (zone diameter >16 mm) and bacitracin (zone >12 mm). Haemolytic haemophili, which have streptococcus-like colonies, give stronger haemolysis on the aerobic than the anaerobic plate and

are resistant to penicillin. The results of these primary sensitivity tests make possible the provisional identification of *S. pyogenes*, and its immediate reporting to the physician, even when the streptococci and their haemolysis are confined to the confluent mixed growth in the well of the plate and separate β-haemolytic colonies are not available for testing.

The bacitracin test fails to identify rare strains of *S. pyogenes* that are bacitracin-resistant and misidentifies rare strains of other streptococci that are bacitracin-sensitive. If, therefore, well-separated β-haemolytic colonies are present on the streaked-out area of the plate, they should be picked and their Lancefield group determined by a rapid co-agglutination or precipitation test (see Ch. 17). When separate colonies are not present, it is necessary to replate the confluent β-haemolytic growth to obtain a pure culture for grouping, but a report to the physician should not be delayed until the results of this confirmatory test are available.

Quantitative culture. Note and report the relative abundance of *S. pyogenes* colonies in the primary plate culture, for the organism is more likely to have a pathogenic role when it is numerous (e.g. >100 colonies/plate) than when it is scanty. An appreciable proportion of healthy persons, e.g. 1–10% of adults and up to 20 or 30% of children, carry the streptococcus in the throat, apparently without harm, and the organism will be detected in a throat swab when a carrier develops a sore throat due to some other pathogen, such as an undetected virus. Such a finding could lead to a misdiagnosis, and if the streptococci are scanty the possibility that they are not the cause of the pharyngitis should be borne in mind.

In a study of the value of standardized quantitative culture, Bell & Smith (1976) found large numbers of *S. pyogenes* in throat swabs from 71% of children with streptococcal pharyngitis, but in swabs from only 10% of well children who were throat carriers of the organism. But the numbers of streptococcal colonies on the culture plate are greatly influenced by the efficacy of the procedures of swabbing the throat and transfer to the plate, so that they may not fairly reflect the number of the organisms in vivo. As these procedures cannot be rigidly standardized, account should also be taken of the number of *S. pyogenes* colonies relative to the number of colonies of throat commensal bacteria in the culture. Although a scanty growth of the streptococcus is likely to be due to harmless throat carriage, the uncertainty of the quantitative distinction makes it advisable that in all cases the organism's presence should be reported and antibiotics given to eradicate it.

Reports may be given as 'Many', 'Few' or 'No *S. pyogenes* found in culture'. When none is found, it is advisable to add to the report a statement that 'Other pathogens, including viruses, were not sought'. If a negative result is reported only as 'No pathogens isolated', the physician may think that the swab has been examined for viruses, mycoplasmas, chlamydias, diphtheria bacilli, Vincent's organisms, gonococci and other rarer throat pathogens.

Anti-streptolysin-O (ASO) titre. In cases of suspected streptococcal infection, e.g. acute rheumatic fever, where throat and other cultures have failed to reveal the organism, the patient's blood serum should be tested for its content of antibodies to streptolysin-O. In such infections there is usually a steep rise of ASO titre to values well in excess of 200 Todd units/ml after 2–4 weeks. If the titre is not raised, the patient's illness is unlikely to be rheumatic fever. A reference to a description of the classical method of performing the ASO test is given in Chapter 17. A commercial kit (Rapitex ASL) is available from Behring for rapid testing with a suspension of latex particles sensitized with streptolysin-O.

Other throat infections

Haemolytic streptococci other than *S. pyogenes* are often present in the throat as harmless commensals, but those of groups C and G occasionally, and B rarely, cause pharyngitis. If their presence in large numbers suggests they may have a pathogenic role in the patient, their presence and antibiotic sensitivities should be reported to the physician.

Haemophilus influenzae. As haemophili are carried as commensals in the throat in a large proportion of adults and children, their finding in a throat swab should generally be ignored. There are, however, certain circumstances in which a search should be made for them and their presence regarded as possibly significant. Thus, *H. influenzae* of capsule serotype b is a fairly common pathogen in young children, especially under the age of 4, in whom it may cause pharyngitis, tracheo-laryngo-epiglottitis (croup), bronchopneumonia, bacteriaemia and meningitis, and in such cases it should be sought in throat swab cultures. Moreover, in children with suspected bronchitis or pneumonia, it is often difficult to obtain a satisfactory specimen of sputum, and it may then be helpful to examine a throat swab for the presence of haemophilus and other potential lung pathogens and determine their drug sensitivities. The physician should, however, be warned that though the pathogen in the throat *may* also be present in the lower respiratory tract, it is more probably confined to carriage in the throat. It may be difficult or hazardous to collect a throat swab from a child with croup, in which case an attempt should be made to demonstrate the pathogen in blood culture, as should also be done in suspected pneumonia and meningitis.

When haemophilus is to be sought, the throat swab should be inoculated on to a heated-blood agar or Fildes agar plate as well as on to blood agar, and that plate incubated aerobically. A 2 μg amoxycillin or ampicillin disk may be placed on the well of the plate so that both the presence and sensitivity of the haemophilus may be reported next day. Until the ampicillin sensitivity is known, the drug of choice for the initial treatment of severe haemophilus infections is chloramphenicol, but its prolonged administration may be dangerous.

Diphtheria. In countries where diphtheria is even moderately common, all swabs from sore throats should be cultured on a selective tellurite medium for *Corynebacterium diphtheriae* and *C.*

ulcerans as well as on blood agar for *S. pyogenes*, but in communities where artificial immunization has made diphtheria rare, the chance of making a positive finding may be too low to justify the large expenditure of labour and materials in routinely setting up the extra cultures. In that case, reliance must be placed on the physician to indicate the few cases in which the possibility of diphtheria has been suggested by the presence of membrane in the throat, extreme constitutional upset or nerve paralyses, and which therefore require examination of the swab by the methods described in Chapter 22.

Vincent's infection. A foetid, ulcerative inflammation of the throat (Vincent's angina) or gums (gingivitis) is occasionally caused by a combined infection with Vincent's spirochaetes and anaerobic fusiform bacilli. When the clinical findings suggest the condition, a swab from the affected areas should be examined in a Gram smear. The presence of many Gram-negative spirochaetes and fusiform bacilli, e.g. at least two of each per field well filled with pus cells and debris, may be reported as 'Many Vincent's organisms in film'. Small numbers of such organisms may be present in the healthy mouth and throat, and should be ignored.

Gonococcal pharyngitis. This condition should be suspected in promiscuous persons who engage in oral intercourse and a swab should be examined for gonococcus by culture on selective medium (Ch. 21).

Candidosis (thrush). In newborn babies and debilitated elderly persons, infection with *Candida albicans* may cause an acute inflammation with plaques of soft white exudate in the mouth and throat. In patients with these manifestations, a swab taken from the lesions should be examined for the fungus. An aerobic blood agar plate may show the small opaque white colonies of candida, typically with short pointed 'rootlets' projecting from their margins, but their growth may be slow and incubation at 35–37°C may have to be continued for 48 h before they become recognizable. When an examination for candida is indicated, it is best to inoculate the

swab on to a plate of Sabouraud agar as well as on to blood agar. A 50 unit nystatin disk and a 20 μg amphotericin disk should be placed on the 'well' of the Sabouraud plate. Growth of candida sensitive to the antifungal drugs may then be observed and reported after 24 or 48 h, and later be subjected to confirmatory tests (Ch. 42). The presence of small numbers of yeasts in material from the mouth or throat may reflect selection and opportunistic colonization during antibiotic therapy. In such a case, further antibiotic therapy may be contraindicated.

Viral infections. Several viruses may cause an exudative pharyngitis resembling that caused by *Streptococcus pyogenes*. One that commonly does so is the virus of infectious mononucleosis, a condition which may be diagnosed by the demonstration of a lymphocytosis and atypical lymphocytes in a blood film and that of heterophile antibodies in a Paul-Bunnell test on the patient's serum. Diagnostic tests are usually not attempted for other viral infections of the throat unless the identification is required for epidemiological purposes, when viral culture and serological diagnosis may be attempted (Ch. 48).

Nasal, oral and sinus infections

The organisms infecting the nasal cavity are mainly the same as those infecting the throat and the two regions are often infected simultaneously. A deep nasal swab generally yields the same information as a throat swab, and it is usual to examine only the latter as a nasal swab seldom gives a positive result when the throat swab is negative. Nasal swabs are more often taken to detect healthy carriers than to diagnose infection, deep nasal swabs being taken for *S. pyogenes* and diphtheria bacillus and swabs from the skin of the anterior nares for *S. aureus*. Nasal carriers are a more dangerous source of infection for others than are throat carriers of the same organism, for they disseminate much larger numbers of organisms into the environment than the latter.

Stomatitis. Acute infections of the mouth are commonest in neonates and debilitated elderly persons. They can be caused by Vincent's organisms, *Candida albicans*, and herpes simplex, Coxsackie A and various other viruses. Swabs from the lesions are examined for the first two of these infections as described for throat swabs (see above).

Sinusitis. The paranasal sinuses are normally sterile, but in the course of a nasal infection, a nasopharyngeal bacterium such as *H. influenzae* or pneumococcus may invade a sinus, most commonly the maxillary or frontal sinus, which then becomes filled with pus. Pus aspirated from the sinus, or a saline 'wash-out', should be examined in a Gram film and by culture on aerobic and anaerobic blood agar plates. Preferably the aerobic plate should be of heated blood agar.

Nasopharyngeal swabs. The collection of nasopharyngeal secretion by a *pernasal swab* in charcoal transport medium for the diagnosis of whooping-cough is described in Chapter 20. A suitable pernasal swab kit with Amies charcoal transport medium is produced by Medical Wire. A *postnasal* swab, in which the terminal 2 cm of wire bearing the swab is bent at an angle of 45°, is passed behind the soft palate and rubbed on the posterior wall of the nasopharynx; it may be used for the detection of potential pathogens carried in the nasopharynx of healthy persons, e.g. meningococcus, which generally cannot be recovered from parts of the throat bathed with saliva from the mouth.

Ear infections

Swabs are taken from the external auditory meatus mainly in three suspected conditions, acute otitis media, chronic suppurative otitis media and otitis externa. The provisional clinical diagnosis will indicate the different organisms likely to be present.

Acute otitis media. This infection is usually caused by *S. pyogenes*, pneumococcus, *H. influenzae*, *Branhamella catarrhalis* or, in many cases, one of the respiratory tract viruses. The organism spreads to the middle ear via the Eustachian tube from the nasopharynx, which is the primary site of infection. As long as the eardrum remains intact, none of the infected exudate can be collected on an ear swab, though culture of a throat swab may give a provisional indication of the causal organism. Antibiotic therapy is urgently required to prevent a possible bacterial infection damaging the hearing mechanism, and amoxycillin, erythromycin or cotrimoxazole may be used when the causal organism is unknown. Amoxycillin is the drug of choice unless a β-lactamase-producing variety of *H. influenzae* is the cause, when the absence of a rapid response will indicate the need for a change of drug.

If the eardrum has ruptured spontaneously, or a myringotomy has been performed to relieve pressure, exudate may be collected on a thin swab introduced carefully into the external meatus. It should be examined in a Gram film and by aerobic and anaerobic culture plates of heated blood agar and blood agar.

Chronic suppurative otitis media. When the eardrum has been perforated in an acute attack of otitis media and remains patent, infection with the original pathogens may persist or repeated infections may be caused by secondary invaders such as *S. aureus*, coliform bacilli, pseudomonads and bacteroides. Swabs of the discharge in the external meatus should be cultured to guide the choice of antibiotics for systemic and topical therapy, but it must be borne in mind that such swabs are liable to be contaminated with commensal bacteria from the skin lining the meatus. These contaminants are mainly albus staphylococci, diphtheroid bacilli and saprophytic mycobacteria, which should be ignored, but may include *S. aureus* and coliform bacilli.

Otitis externa. Chronic inflammation of the skin of the external meatus, with irritation and discharge, may be caused by bacteria, particularly *Pseudomonas aeruginosa*, coliform bacilli and *S. aureus*, or fungi, most commonly candida or aspergillus. A swab should be taken from the meatus and cultured aerobically on blood agar and MacConkey plates for the bacteria, on a Sabouraud agar plate with a nystatin 50 unit disk for 48 h at 35–37°C for candida and on a

Sabouraud agar slope for 10 days at 28°C for aspergillus. The results will guide the choice of drug for topical antibacterial or antifungal treatment.

Eye infections

Conjunctivitis and keratitis. The healthy conjunctiva and cornea usually bear a few albus staphylococci and diphtheroid bacilli, mainly derived from the edges of the eyelids. In the newborn, a severe form of acute conjunctivitis, ophthalmia neonatorum, may be caused by the gonococcus in the first 2 or 3 days of life and is liable to damage the cornea unless promptly treated with antibiotics. And a much less dangerous infection, 'sticky eye', may be caused by *S. aureus* during the first week or two. At any age, *Haemophilus aegyptius* may cause acute epidemic conjunctivitis and *H. influenzae*, pneumococcus and meningococcus may cause sporadic cases. *Pseudomonas aeruginosa* may cause serious superficial or deep infections after trauma or surgery to the eye, and *Moraxella lacunata* is found in a rare, subacute or chronic angular conjunctivitis.

Many cases of conjunctivitis are due to viruses of different kinds, e.g. adenovirus type 8 which causes epidemic kerato-conjuctivitis in factories, shipyards and hospitals, whilst herpes simplex virus may cause keratitis. *Chlamydia trachomatis* causes trachoma, a common cause of corneal scarring and blindness in many undeveloped countries, and also a much milder, inclusion conjunctivitis in developed countries, e.g. swimming pool conjunctivitis in older subjects and congenital conjunctivitis within a few days of birth.

The principal difficulty in laboratory diagnosis is that of obtaining an adequate specimen in which the viability of the more delicate pathogens is preserved. It is best to make smears and seed culture plates beside the patient immediately after collecting material from the eye. Because the volume of exudate obtainable is generally small, a dry cotton-wool swab, which would absorb and retain most of the specimen, is unsuitable as a means of collection. The exudate should be picked up with a sterile plati-num loop or on the smoothly rounded tip of a thin glass or plastic rod; otherwise, on the tip of a thin, serum-coated swab. It should be collected from the conjunctiva, e.g. from under an everted eyelid, and contamination from the skin and margin of the eyelid should be avoided. A separate collection should be made for inoculation on to each culture plate and for the making of a smear. The cultures should be on blood agar and heated-blood agar plates incubated in air with 5–10% CO_2. When the specimen material is little, the smear should be confined to a small marked area of the slide, e.g. 5–10 mm in diameter; it should be stained by Gram's method with a strong counterstain.

If it is necessary to dispatch a specimen to the laboratory before inoculation on to culture media, it should be taken on an albumen-coated swab which is placed at once in Stuart's transport medium.

For examination for chlamydia by immunofluorescence or culture in cells, scrapings must be taken from the affected conjunctiva after wiping off the exudate (Ch. 46). For examination for viruses, a swab from the conjunctiva should be submitted in a virus transport medium (Ch. 50).

Infections of orbit and eyeball. These may be caused by any of a variety of aerobic and anaerobic bacteria of the types found in pyogenic and wound infections. Any exudate obtainable should be examined for such organisms and a blood culture should be done. *Iritis* and *choroidoretinitis* may occur in the course of systemic viral infections, e.g. with cytomegalovirus, and toxoplasmosis, for which serological diagnosis should be attempted (Ch. 43). *Styes* are small boils affecting the follicles or the eyelashes on the edges of the eyelids; they are usually caused by *S. aureus* and treated without bacteriological investigation.

3. LOWER RESPIRATORY INFECTIONS

Unlike most regions of the upper respiratory tract, the trachea, bronchi and lungs are normally free from colonization with commensal and potentially pathogenic bacteria, but when their defences are upset they are liable to be invaded by organisms from the throat. They are also susceptible to primary infection with various inhaled pathogens, such as the tubercle and whooping-cough bacilli, and to be involved in generalized infections such as measles and chicken-pox.

The commonest infections are acute tracheo-bronchitis, acute exacerbations of chronic bronchitis, and the pneumonias. In many or most cases the primary infection is caused by a virus, e.g. rhinovirus, myxovirus, adenovirus or respiratory syncytial virus, but there is often a secondary infection with a bacterial pathogen from the nasopharynx, most commonly pneumococcus or *Haemophilus influenzae*. Pneumococcus also appears to be the primary cause of many cases of pneumonia, particularly lobar pneumonia, but often these pneumonic infections are triggered by a preceding viral infection of the upper respiratory tract, such as the common cold. Other secondary invaders of the lower tract include *Staphylococcus aureus*, which may cause fatal pneumonia after influenza, coliform bacilli and *Pseudomonas aeruginosa*, *Branhamella catarrhalis*, *Candida albicans* and *Aspergillus fumigatus*. The staphylococcus, coliforms and candida are found particularly in hospitalized patients treated with antibiotics to which these organisms are resistant.

Other organisms that may cause primary infection in the bronchial tract or lungs are *Mycoplasma pneumoniae*, which is the commonest, *Legionella pneumophila*, *Chlamydia psittaci B* and *Coxiella burneti*. The protozoon *Pneumocystis carini* is liable to cause diffuse infection of the lungs in persons who are immunosuppressed or immunodeficient, e.g. patients infected with human immunodeficiency virus.

Identification of a viral pathogen is attempted only occasionally, as when the information is required for epidemiological purposes or the diagnosis of an obscure infection (but see Ch. 48). Laboratory diagnosis is employed mainly for the identification of other, particularly bacterial pathogens, which may be susceptible to treatment with an antibiotic chosen with the knowledge of their identity.

In suspected pneumonia and other severe infections it is usual to start antibiotic therapy without waiting for the results of laboratory tests, and as pneumococcus and haemophilus are the likeliest bacterial pathogens, the blindly chosen drug is generally ampicillin, amoxycillin, augmentin or cotrimoxazole, though erythromycin or tetracycline should be substituted if failure of response or the clinical features suggest that the infection may be due to a β-lactamase-producing haemophilus, or a mycoplasma or legionella, and flucloxacillin should be added if *S. aureus* may be the cause. As the drugs so chosen may still be inappropriate, laboratory identification of the causal organism should always be attempted at the earliest possible stage. For the best chance of success, specimens of sputum and blood for culture should be collected *before* the start of any antibiotic therapy. In suspected atypical pneumonia an initial blood sample for serology should be taken at the same early stage.

Specimens

Sputum. The material from lower respiratory infections most commonly submitted for bacteriological examination is sputum, a mixture of bronchial secretion and inflammatory exudate coughed up into the mouth and expectorated. There are, however, difficulties both in collecting a suitable sample and in interpreting the results of its culture. In some infections, e.g. those due to mycoplasma or legionella, there is often a lack of secretion and sputum cannot be obtained.

Sputum from a bacterial infection is purulent, containing yellow or green opaque material as well as clear mucoid secretion. Staff collecting specimens should be instructed in how to obtain and recognize the correct material. Many patients tend to swallow their sputum when it is coughed into the throat and, when asked to spit some out, may expectorate mainly saliva. Saliva can be recognized because it is relatively clear and is watery rather than viscous.

Busy or uninstructed staff may send such collections of saliva to the laboratory, but they should not be examined, for the results are likely to be misleading. Thus, the specimen may fail to yield a culture of the pathogen in the lower tract and may give growth of an irrelevant potential pathogen that is being carried in the throat. Any salivary specimen should therefore be discarded and a report sent to the physician stating that the specimen was mainly saliva and thus unsuitable for examination. The regular practice of rejecting unsuitable specimens usually induces staff in wards and clinics to take greater care in the collection procedure.

The decision to reject specimens should not be left to junior staff and clear criteria for rejection should be laid down for general application. Preferably the criteria should be based on a microscopical as well as a naked-eye assessment. Thus, if a Gram-stained smear of a homogenized specimen shows less than 10 polymorphs to every squamous epithelial cell, and the patient is not leucopenic, the material probably consists mainly of saliva.

Instructions for collecting sputum should include the following advice.

1. Make the collection in a disposable, wide-mouthed, screw-capped plastic container of about 100 ml capacity.

2. If possible, collect the sputum before any antibiotic therapy is begun, and when the patient first coughs on waking in the morning.

3. Instruct the patient to wait until he feels material coughed into his throat and then to work it forward into his mouth and spit it directly into the opened container, trying to avoid spilling over the rim. At once tightly screw on the cap of the container. Wipe off any spilled material on its outside with a tissue moistened with disinfectant, but take care not to let any disinfectant enter the container.

4. If the patient has difficulty in coughing sputum into his mouth, ask a physiotherapist to pummel his chest. This exercise often causes exudate to move in the bronchi and stimulate productive coughing.

5. Deliver the specimen to the laboratory as quickly as possible, preferably within 2 h, for delicate pathogens such as pneumococcus and haemophilus may die out during any longer delay.

Bronchial swabs and aspirates. The principal difficulty in sputum examinations arises from the inevitable mixing of the expectorated specimen with throat secretion and saliva. It thus becomes contaminated with hardy mouth commensal bacteria that may overgrow the more delicate lung pathogens, and often also with potential lung pathogens, such as pneumococcus and haemophilus, which are commonly carried in the throat. When found, the latter may be wrongly thought to have been infecting the lower respiratory tract.

This confusing contamination can be avoided if a specimen of bronchial secretion is collected by some means that prevents its contact with the throat and mouth. Such collection may be done by transtracheal puncture and aspiration or by the use of a protected swab passed through a bronchoscope into the bronchi (Brumfitt et al 1957; Lees & McNaught 1959). Direct aspiration of secretion through a bronchoscope, e.g. by bronchial lavage, is unsatisfactory as the inside of the bronchoscope is liable to become soiled with throat secretion.

However transtracheal aspiration and bronchial swabbing require anaesthesia of the patient and the attention of skilled medical staff, and for these reasons are generally not performed. Nevertheless they may be attempted for the diagnosis of unusual or obscure infections.

Blood culture. In all cases of suspected pneumonia a sample of blood should be taken for culture before antibiotics are given. Lung infections are commonly associated with bacteriaemia and it may be possible to culture from the blood a delicate pathogen whose growth is suppressed in cultures of sputum contaminated with salivary organisms. Moreover, the finding of a bacterium in the blood is strong evidence that it has been infecting the lungs and is not merely a throat organism contaminating sputum.

Examination for tuberculosis

A policy must be decided for determining which specimens of sputum are to be examined for tubercle bacilli. Pulmonary tuberculosis is both a threat to the life of the patient and a dangerous source of infection to others. It is therefore essential that cases should be correctly diagnosed at the earliest possible stage and that drug therapy should be based on sensitivity tests made on a culture grown from the patient.

In communities where tuberculosis is moderately or very common, every specimen of sputum received in the laboratory should be screened for tubercle bacilli, regardless of whether the physician requests the examination. At least microscopy of a Ziehl-Neelsen or auramine-stained smear should be done and the positive specimens then cultured (see Ch. 25 for methods).

In communities where tuberculosis is now relatively rare it is generally considered unnecessary to make the laborious tests for tubercle bacilli on all the many sputa received in the laboratory, most of which are from hospital patients with suspected pyogenic pneumonia or an exacerbated bronchitis. If there are good clinical and public health services, reliance may be placed on the physicians to indicate which specimens come from possibly tuberculous patients, and these should be examined for tubercle bacilli by both microscopy and culture (Ch. 25). That this is the laboratory's practice should be made known to family doctors, chest physicians and public health staff, so that these staff are warned always to indicate the possibility of tuberculosis on the request form accompanying the specimen to the laboratory. They should be asked to determine the criteria for deciding which patients require examination for tuberculosis, e.g. all patients with unexplained cough continuing for more than 4–6 weeks, elderly persons with supposed 'smoker's cough', coughing patients with haemoptysis or cachexia, persons who have been in close contact with patients diagnosed as tuberculous, and patients with illnesses that make them specially vulnerable (e.g. AIDS).

Laboratory staff must be protected against the risk of becoming infected from specimens containing tubercle bacilli. If, therefore, there may be cases of pulmonary tuberculosis in the patient population served by the laboratory, *all* specimens of sputum should be regarded as possibly dangerous and the procedures of making smears and seeding cultures should be performed in a safety cabinet (Ch. 15).

Examination for common infections

All sputa should be examined for pneumococcus, haemophilus and the other aerobic pathogens that commonly infect the bronchi and lungs. The recommended procedures are as follows.

1. Note whether the specimen contains opaque green-yellow pus. Do not examine specimens consisting of clear, watery saliva.

2. *Homogenization*. There are advantages in homogenizing the specimen before making films and cultures. Most sputa are inhomogeneous. The purulent material, which contains most of the relevant pathogens, is usually embedded in clear mucoid secretion, and if the specimen is not first homogenized it is difficult to separate out a purulent portion for filming and culture. If the specimen is homogenized, every drop and loopful of it will contain some of the pathogens present. Moreover, the homogenized material is suitable for quantitative examinations.

To homogenize, mix and incubate equal volumes of the sputum and a solution of dithiothreitol (e.g. Sputolysin, Calbiochem) or buffered pancreatin (Oxoid) made up according to the manufacturer's instructions. With dithiothreitol, either mix rapidly on a vortex mixer for 15 s and stand for 15 min at ambient temperature or, preferably, mix gently and continuously on a machine that tilts to and fro placed in an incubator for 30 min at 37°C. With pancreatin, incubate for 30 min at 37°C with continuous or occasional shaking.

3. *Microscopy*. Make a smear of the homogenized sputum, or a purulent portion of the sputum if it is not homogenized. Stain by Gram's method and examine with oil-immersion. First note the presence and relative numbers of polymorphs and squamous epithelial cells. If there are less than 10 polymorphs per squame, the specimen is probably mainly saliva; if more, it is probably derived from an infected site in the lower respiratory tract.

Next note whether there is a wide diversity of bacterial forms, suggesting salivary contamination, or the predominance of one potentially pathogenic form, e.g. Gram-positive diplococci (probably pneumococci), small slender Gram-negative bacilli (probably haemophili), or clustered Gram-positive cocci (probably *Staphylococcus aureus*). Any of the latter three findings warrants the phoning of a provisional report to the physician to guide his initial choice of antibiotics for therapy. The finding of numerous staphylococci is particularly significant, as it indicates that treatment with a β-lactamase-resistant penicillin, such as flucloxacillin, is urgently required.

If fungal infection, e.g. aspergillosis, is suspected, a wet film should be carefully searched for the presence of conidiophores (Ch. 42). The presence of such sporing heads indicates that the fungus is growing in the bronchial tract, whilst the observation of a few colonies growing in a culture of the sputum may reflect only the recent inhalation of spores from the environment.

4. *Culture*. A semi-quantitative method of culture is recommended, so that the presence of a potential pathogen in only small numbers, e.g. less than 10^6/ml sputum, may either be ignored or be reported to the physician as probably representing contamination of the specimen from the throat (Dixon & Miller 1965). If, however, antibiotic treatment had been started before the specimen was taken, or if special considerations apply, as in cystic fibrosis, the presence of a potential pathogen in small numbers should not be ignored.

A satisfactory procedure is to dilute the 1-in-2 homogenized sputum a further 1 in 100 in sterile broth and to inoculate a 0.005 ml loopful of the dilution on to each culture plate. The inoculum should be spread confluently over half of the plate and streaked out over the other half. The growth on the whole area of the plate of 25 or more colonies of the same potential pathogen will then indicate that 10^6 or more of that pathogen were present in each millilitre of the original sputum. The cultures should be incubated at 37°C for 18–24 h in humid air plus 5–10% CO_2, and re-incubated if the colonies are then still small and indistinct. Only if lung abscess or bronchiectasis is suspected, need

additional plates be set up for anaerobic incubation, which should be for 2–4 days. However, a few strains of pneumococci appear to grow in primary cultures only under anaerobic conditions, so it may be best to culture all specimens anaerobically on an extra blood agar plate having a 5 µg optochin disk placed on a confluently seeded area and examine this after 18–24 h.

A plate of good blood agar should suffice to give characteristic growth of the main pathogens, but it is preferable also to seed a plate of either heated-blood ('chocolate') agar, which may give better growth of pneumococcus and haemophilus, or Fildes digest agar, which gives a very distinctive growth of *H. influenzae* and tends to suppress the growth of many salivary commensal bacteria (Ch. 19, *Methods*).

5. *Identification tests*. If, before incubation of the primary cultures, a 5 µg optochin disk and a 1 unit benzylpenicillin disk are placed on the confluently seeded area of the blood plate and a 2 µg amoxycillin disk on that of the Fildes plate, the identity and sensitivities of pneumococcus and haemophilus isolates may be read and reported the day after receipt of the specimen. Further identification and sensitivity tests (Chs 18, 19) may be considered unnecessary, but care should be taken not to overlook β-lactamase production in a haemophilus.

Staphylococcal isolates should be tested by the coagulase or DNase test for identification of *S. aureus* and tested for drug sensitivities, particularly to benzylpenicillin and a β-lactamase-resistant penicillin, such as methicillin (Chs 9, 16). Pseudomonas should be identified by an oxidase test performed on a colony on the primary plate, and tested for sensitivity to antipseudomonas drugs (Chs 9, 31). It is seldom necessary to identify other coliforms, but if one is numerous and thought possibly to be of pathogenic significance, not merely an overgrowing contaminant, its antibiotic sensitivities should be tested. Any numerous neisseria-like colonies should be tested by a rapid method for the fermentation of glucose, maltose and sucrose to identify *Branhamella catarrhalis*, which does not ferment them (Ch. 21).

6. *Fungal cultures*. Candida may be recognized as small opaque cream-coloured colonies with spiky projections on blood agar. These should be subcultured for tests of sensitivity to nystatin and amphotericin and germ tube formation (*C. albicans*, Ch. 42). If, however, the request form indicates that a candidal or fungal infection is suspected, the homogenized sputum should be seeded on to a plate of Sabouraud or malt extract agar with a 50 unit nystatin disk for aerobic incubation at 35–37°C for 2 days for the culture of candida, and a slope of Sabouraud or malt extract agar for aerobic incubation at 28°C for 10 days, or as recommended in Chapter 42, for the culture of aspergillus.

Pneumocystis pneumonia. In an immuno-suppressed or immunodeficient patient with signs of pneumonia or diffuse infiltration of the lungs, infection with *Pneumocystis carini* must be considered and its diagnosis made quickly, for treatment with cotrimoxazole or pentamidine is required for this often fatal condition.

The diagnosis depends on the microscopical demonstration of the Gram-negative tropho-zoites (1–2 μm) or the more easily seen Gram-positive cysts (*c.* 5 μm) of the protozoon. Sputum, or a tracheal or bronchial aspirate rarely gives a positive result. A specimen of lung tissue should be obtained by percutaneous needle aspiration or open lung biopsy (Rosen et al 1975) or one of alveolar fluid by broncho-scopic alveolar lavage (Hopkin et al 1983).

Press the cut surface of tissue on a slide to yield an 'imprint' without smearing. Centrifuge lavage fluid and spread about 0.1 ml of the deposit as a thick film on a slide. Dry the imprint or film and fix with brief heating. Stain the film by the Grocott methenamine silver nitrate method (taking *c.* 3 h), its rapid (5 min) modifi-cation (Smith & Hughes 1972), or the method described in Chapter 43 (*Methods*). The silver stains the thin wall and two internal comma-shaped bodies of the cysts black, and their cyto-plasm a light golden colour, but does not stain the trophozoites. The cysts are commonly seen in clusters embedded in amorphous debris. Care must be taken to distinguish them from yeasts, which usually stain solidly and may show

budding. A second film may be stained by the Gram-Weigert method (Rosen et al 1975), which colours the wall and internal bodies of the cysts purple-black.

Rarer bronchopulmonary infections. When suspected, infections with mycoplasma, legion-ella, chlamydia, coxiella and viruses may be diagnosed as described in the chapters on these organisms. Serological tests can be helpful.

4. WOUND, SKIN AND DEEP SEPSIS

This section deals with the diagnosis of mainly suppurative infections of wounds, burns, the skin, ulcers and sinuses, sites that are open to contamination with more than one of a variety of organisms from the skin, respiratory tract, alimentary tract or the environment; also of closed abscesses and other infections of deep sites, e.g. osteomyelitis and septic arthritis, usually infected by only a single species of pathogen.

Wound infections may be *endogenous* or *exogenous*. Endogenous infections, or auto-infections, are caused by organisms that have been leading a commensal existence elsewhere in the patient's body; for example, an abdominal surgical wound may become infected with organisms from the large bowel after an operation involving incision of the colon. In exogenous infections the source of the infecting organism is outwith the body of the patient who becomes infected; *cross-infection* is a particular example of exogenous infection in which the causal organism is spread from person to person. Infection may occur after accidental or intentional trauma of the skin or other tissue; the latter type is often called 'surgical' or 'postoperative sepsis'.

Infection of a wound is difficult to define and no clear rules can be given to distinguish it from contamination and colonization. Wounds and other open lesions are liable to *contamination* with a multiplicity of organisms from the body surfaces and environment; the contaminating organisms are at first generally present in relat-ively small numbers, as originally introduced, and need not subsequently multiply. *Infection* occurs when one or more of the contaminants evades the clearing effect of the host's defences, replicates in large numbers, and attacks and harms the host's tissues. In the case of a commensal or low-grade pathogen, the multiplication may cause little or no harm to the host and may best be described as *colonization*. Whether harmful infection or harmless colonization occurs is dependent on the virulence of the organisms and the local and general resistance of the host. A knowledge of the patient's general and local condition is therefore important in assessing the significance of bacteriological findings.

Infections of soft tissues are generally associated with the production of pus and the bacteria involved are said to be 'pyogenic' (pus-producing). As there is a wide range of possible causative organisms, a degree of selectivity is inevitable in the choice of examination procedures in the laboratory. The physician has a responsibility to guide the search by noting clues to the nature of the infection in the patient's history and clinical appearance. In many cases the likely cause is fairly obvious. There are well recognized associations of *Staphylococcus aureus* with pustules, boils, carbuncles, stitch abscesses and wound infections. Similarly, *Streptococcus pyogenes* is classically associated with the spreading lesion of erysipelas, which may present as a fulminating infection. However, such associations are not invariable, and vigilance and awareness are essential.

A wide variety of aerobic and anaerobic species of bacteria may be present, either singly or in combination, in infections of wounds and other soft tissues. The commonest pyogenic bacteria are *S. aureus*, *S. pyogenes*, pneumococcus and coliform bacilli such as *Escherichia coli*, *Proteus* species and *Pseudomonas aeruginosa*. Anaerobic organisms, particularly *Clostridium perfringens* and other clostridia, *Bacteroides* species and anaerobic cocci, may be important in infections of wounds, especially abdominal wounds, soiled deep or lacerated wounds, and wherever devitalized tissues provide suitably anaerobic conditions. Preliminary infection with aerobic bacteria, by consuming the available oxygen, may encourage the growth of clostridia and lead to gas-gangrene or tetanus (Ch. 37).

In many cases there is a mixed infection with more than one bacterial species, and in some of these cases a pathogenic synergy may be evident with two or more species acting in concert to cause more damage to the tissues than would be caused by either alone. Mixed infections with Gram-positive cocci and coliform bacilli are not uncommon and polymicrobial infections with anaerobes such as bacteroides and fusiforms, or fuso-spirochaetal associations are well recognized. In Vincent's infection of the gums, for example, and in various other fuso-spirochaetal conditions, the mixture of species may be associated with a fulminating attack.

Special associations of certain pathogens with particular conditions should be borne in mind, e.g. those of bacteroides and anaerobic cocci with dental and cerebral abscesses, capnophilic cocci with dental, cerebral and hepatic abscesses, and anaerobes with pelvic inflammatory disease. Many postoperative abdominal or pelvic wounds have coliform bacilli associated with a moderate exudate during the early healing stage, the infection being often superficial and resolving without specific therapy. But a combination of coliforms with bacteroides may cause a more severe, synergic infection calling for prompt antibacterial therapy.

Among species much less commonly encountered are *Pasteurella multocida* in animal bites, *Corynebacterium diphtheriae* in wound diphtheria, and *Bacillus anthracis* in malignant pustule of the skin. In chronic infections that are slow to heal and in pus showing no other microbes, the possibility of infection with *Mycobacterium tuberculosis*, other mycobacteria, *Actinomyces israeli*, nocardiae or fungi must be considered.

Collection of specimens

Pus or *exudate* is often submitted on a swab for laboratory investigation. The swab is an inefficient sampling device and tends to desiccate the specimen and trap the bacteria, which are then not released on to the culture plate. Whenever possible, pus or exudate should be submitted in a small screw-capped bottle, a firmly stoppered tube or syringe, or a sealed capillary tube. Some workers advocate the sending of pus in oxygen-free, gassed-out vials or in special transport media. We recommend the routine use of transport medium swab kits where delay in transit is likely, as from general practice patients. Appropriate recommendations are made at relevant sections in this book (Chs 6, 7, 36, 37). Fragments of excised tissue removed at wound toilet, or curettings from infected sinuses and other tissues, should be sent in a sterile container without fixative. They are homogenized in a tissue grinder with a little sterile broth and subsequently treated in the same way as exudates. Delay in the transit of specimens to the laboratory must be avoided, especially in the case of swabs, where the exudate may dry into the cotton-wool.

If it is decided to compromise and send a swab, load the swab well with the material. If possible, send two swabs taken from the depths of the wound or lesion, so that one can be used for the preparation of a smear for microscopy and the other for the seeding of cultures. It is difficult to make a good smear from a swab, and quite impossible if the swab is dry; a dry swab must first be moistened with a little sterile broth or saline, and even then the smear may be inadequate. To avoid contamination of the swab before it is used to seed the cultures, either it must be smeared on a sterilized slide or else used to make the smear only after it has been seeded on to all the culture media. The latter procedure is often followed and a poor, unrepresentative smear is usually the result. The submission of duplicate swabs avoids this difficulty. The examination of material on swabs for mycobacteria is almost always unsatisfactory.

If it can be arranged, an extra swab should be placed and broken into a cooked-meat broth immediately it has been taken from the lesion in the ward or at operation, and this broth containing the swab head should be sent to the laboratory in addition to two conventionally packaged swabs. Pathogens sometimes grow in the directly seeded broth, and in subcultures from it, when they cannot be recovered in culture from the conventional swabs.

Physicians should be instructed that when a special investigation is required, they should state this clearly on the request form. Thus the routine investigation is usually confined to a search for the common pyogenic bacteria and anaerobic pathogens and does not include an examination for the tubercle bacillus, other mycobacteria, actinomyces, nocardia, the diphtheria bacillus, the anthrax bacillus or fungi.

Blood culture. If the patient is febrile or in shock, or it seems possible that his local infection is accompanied by a bacteriaemia, a sample of blood should be taken for culture.

Laboratory examination

It is general practice to lay down a basic set of procedures for the examination of all wound swabs and other specimens of pus, exudate or tissue for the commoner pathogens, and the circumstances in which other, special methods of examination should be applied to particular specimens, e.g. when requested by the physician or indicated by clues on the request form to the possible presence of an uncommon pathogen. The basic procedures usually include a naked-eye examination of the specimen, the microscopical examination of a Gram film, and culture on aerobic and anaerobic blood agar plates, on MacConkey agar and in cooked-meat broth. Gas chromatography may be performed directly on liquid specimens to indicate the presence of anaerobes (Ch. 37).

Naked-eye examination

The appearance of a specimen of pus or exudate, and that of any appreciable amount of pus on a swab, should be noted on initial examination. The pus of a staphylococcal lesion is typically creamy and thick in consistency, with pus cells evident on microscopy. That of a *Streptococcus pyogenes* infection is generally straw-coloured and watery, with lysis of pus cells seen on microscopy. That of proteus infection has a fishy smell and that of pseudomonas infection a sweet, musty odour and often a blue pigmentation. Pus containing anaerobic organisms often has an offensive putrid smell, and that of actinomycosis often contains small microcolonies that appear as 'sulphur granules' (Ch. 27). In some fungal infections such as mycetoma, black or brown granules may be present (Ch. 42). The pus of an amoebic abscess is said to resemble anchovy sauce.

Microscopy

Much useful information may be obtained from a smear stained by Gram's method. First note the presence and relative numbers of poly-morphs and bacteria. Pay particular attention to the numbers and variety of different morpho-logical forms of Gram-positive and Gram-negative bacteria. If in a serious infection the appearances suggest the presence of a particular pathogen, a provisional report should be tele-phoned to the physician to guide his initial treat-ment of the patient. Gram-positive cocci in typical clusters or chains may suggest a staphylo-coccal or streptococcal infection, but care should be taken, as the sheared edge of a cluster of cocci may simulate a chain of streptococci and a tangled streptococcal chain may simulate a staphylococcal cluster; mixed staphylococcal and streptococcal infections also occur. The appear-ance of Gram-positive diplococci may be given by either pneumococci or enterococci. Faintly staining Gram-negative rods are sometimes missed if much background debris is heavily counterstained. Gram-variable filaments of actino-myces may appear like chains of cocci and their fragments as diphtheroid bacilli. Many Gram-positive clostridia appear as Gram-negative forms in pus.

Examination of a wet film may reveal the pres-ence of fungi or motile bacteria and fluids aspir-ated from inflamed joints resembling septic arthritis should be examined in a wet film for the presence of uric acid crystals, which may be responsible for the condition in the absence of any infection. Darkground microscopy of a wet film is useful in the diagnosis of primary syphilis.

A smear stained by the Ziehl-Neelsen method should be examined when the clinical circum-stances suggest that the tubercle bacillus, another mycobacterium or a nocardia may be present, e.g. in chronic and neck abscesses (Chs. 25, 26, 27). Immunofluorescent staining allows the prompt identification of pathogens for which specific antisera are available, e.g. some pathogenic clostridia.

Culture

The specimen should be inoculated on to two plates of blood agar, the one for incubation at 37°C aerobically, preferably in air plus 5–10% CO_2, the other for incubation anaerobically in nitrogen/hydrogen plus 5–10% CO_2. It should also be plated for aerobic incubation on MacConkey agar (Ch. 6) or CLED agar (Ch. 28, *Methods*) for the differentiation of coliforms, staphylococci and enterococci, and be inoculated into a tube of cooked-meat broth (Ch. 6) for the enrichment of exacting aerobes and anaerobes. If the specimen is a scantily charged swab, it should be inoculated first on to the blood agar plates, then on to the MacConkey, and finally into the cooked-meat broth, where it should be soaked in the broth and squeezed out on the inside wall of the tube several times.

If there is reason to expect the presence of a spreading organism such as proteus, which might overgrow to obscure and prejudice the isolation of other pathogens, the specimen should also be inoculated on to a plate of a medium that inhibits spreading, e.g. PNPG blood agar containing 0.43 g *p*-nitrophenylglycerol per litre (Ch. 28) or blood agar containing two to three times the usual concentration of agar. If the firm agar is to be used, the bacteriologist should have familiarized himself with the small, often atypical appearance of the colonies of the common path-ogens grown on it. Spreading of proteus is inhi-bited on MacConkey agar, but the use of that medium is insufficient as some common patho-gens, such as *Streptococcus pyogenes*, fail to grow on it.

It is a useful practice to place one or two anti-biotic disks on the 'well' areas of the blood agar plates before incubation, e.g. a 1 unit benzylpenicillin disk and a 10 μg gentamicin disk on the aerobic plate and a 5 μg metronidazole disk and a 50 μg neomycin disk on the anaerobic plate. These 'primary sensitivity tests' may give an early indication of an important aspect of antibiotic sensitivity, assist in the identification of colonies of species with constant sensitivities, and facilitate the isolation of resistant species from mixed cultures by the picking of colonies from the inhibition zones. Thus, strict anaerobes but not aerobes or facultative organisms are inhibited by metronidazole, whilst many anaerobes are resistant to neomycin which inhibits most aerobes. If the appearances in the Gram smear suggest the extra procedures will be worthwhile, a full set of antibiotic disks may be used on a separate plate seeded heavily and confluently from the specimen.

The culture plates are examined after overnight incubation at 37°C for 18–24 h, when the relative numbers and types of the colonies should be noted and any further tests required for their identification and determination of their antibiotic sensitivities done. If there is no growth on the plates, or no growth of a type of organism seen in the Gram film, the aerobic and anaerobic blood agars should be reincubated for another 24 h. If there is still no growth, the plates may be discarded unless there is an indication for longer incubation, as for 7 days when the presence is suspected of a slow-growing pathogen such as *Actinomyces israeli* or some species of bacteroides. If at 24 h or 48 h there is growth in the cooked-meat broth, indicated by turbidity in its supernate, but no growth on the plates, the broth should be filmed and subcultured, both aerobically and anaerobically.

There is a difficulty relating to the culture of slow-growing anaerobes that are highly sensitive to killing by oxygen. Their still invisible growth may be killed by the exposure to air when the anaerobically incubated plate is opened and examined on the bench at 18–24 h, and so not develop further when the plate is reincubated anaerobically. It is important therefore to return the plates to an anaerobic atmosphere as quickly as possible after their opening and examination, but when many specimens are being examined it may be difficult to avoid exposure to air for up to an hour or more. There are thus advantages in continuous anaerobic incubation of primary culture plates (Ch. 7). This may be done by the use of an anaerobic cabinet in which the plates are incubated continuously, but may be inspected at intervals through a window without being removed from the anaerobic atmosphere. Otherwise, the specimen may be inoculated on to two anaerobic plates, the one to be removed for examination after 18–24 h, the other to be left undisturbed in a separate anaerobic atmosphere for later examination after 4–5 days. This second procedure requires the availability of large numbers of anaerobic jars.

If tuberculous or fungal infection is suspected, whether from the clinical circumstances, the appearances in a film, or the absence of growth of bacteria on the ordinary media, the specimen should be cultured by the appropriate methods on the appropriate special media (Chs 25, 42).

Identification of isolates

After the bacteria cultured have been obtained in pure subcultures, any further necessary tests for their identification should be done, e.g. the coagulase test on staphylococci, Lancefield's grouping of β-haemolytic streptococci, and biochemical tests on coliform bacilli and anaerobes. At the same time the pure cultures should be tested for sensitivity to an extended range of antibiotics useful in therapy. When mixed bacteria are grown from a wound or other superficial lesion liable to be contaminated with commensal and saprophytic bacteria, the isolates judged to be such harmless contaminants, e.g. albus (coagulase-negative) staphylococci, diphtheroid bacilli and aerobic spore-formers, need not be fully identified or tested for antibiotic sensitivities.

Interpretation and reporting

A pure growth of a recognized pathogen obtained from a wound or closed abscess is easily interpreted as significant and will be reported to the physician as being so. Difficulties arise in the interpretation of mixed cultures grown from superficial lesions contaminated with commensal and saprophytic organisms. Scanty growths of skin commensals such as albus staphylococci and diphtheroid bacilli are usually disregarded and not reported, and similarly a few colonies of *Escherichia coli* grown from a perineal or other wound liable to be contaminated with faecal bacteria. If a potentially dangerous faecal commensal such as *Clostridium perfringens* is isolated in small numbers under such circumstances, the physician should be made aware of the potential danger while being advised of the probability that the organism is present only as a contaminant. It is particularly in *chronic* superficial lesions, such as varicose ulcers, that the presence of mixed commensal bacteria can confidently be disregarded as insignificant. The result may then be reported on the following lines, 'Many mixed faecal and skin bacteria present', without giving identities or antibiotic sensitivities. But a pure growth of a commensal-type bacterium grown from a specimen aspirated from a deep site not subject to contamination, e.g. joint or pleural fluid, should be reported, together with sensitivities, unless the number of the organisms is so small as to indicate they are contaminants picked up during collection of the specimen or inoculation into the media.

Some indication of the importance of the different bacteria cultured from a lesion may be seen in the number and proportion of their forms in the Gram film and their colonies on the primary plates. In general, a numerous or predominant organism is likely to have pathogenic significance, but the relative numbers of the colonies of the different organisms on a culture plate may not reflect the relative numbers of the organisms in the lesion, for they are subject to many variations such as the relative speed of growth of the different species under the cultural conditions used, antibiotic interactions between species, the presence of traces of antibacterial drugs in the specimen, and the greater tendency of the more delicate pathogens, such as pneumococcus, haemophilus and anaerobes, to die during transport of the specimen to the laboratory. For such reasons, a causal pathogen may be cultured in smaller numbers than a contaminating commensal.

It must be borne in mind that the number of colonies grown in a subculture from a primary enrichment culture of the specimen in cooked-meat broth bears no relation whatever to the number of organisms in the lesion. Even a single bacterium inoculated into the broth may yield a profuse culture in 18 h. When, however, the broth shows growth of an organism not found on the culture plates, it may be concluded that probably only very small numbers of that organism were present in the specimen. Thus, when a growth of *Staphylococcus epidermidis* is obtained in the broth but not on the plates, it is likely the organism was present only as a scanty contaminant of the specimen.

Sometimes the significance of a growth is difficult to assess in the laboratory, but the problem may often be resolved by discussion with the physician and examination of a further carefully taken specimen from the lesion.

Fluid aspirates

Aspirated specimens of joint, pleural, pericardial and peritoneal fluids are examined generally as described above, but if the fluid is relatively clear and its volume sufficient, it should first be centrifuged to deposit the cells and bacteria, and the supernate discarded into disinfectant. As nutritionally exacting pathogens, such as pneumococcus, haemophilus and gonococcus may be present, an extra plate of heated-blood ('chocolate') agar should be seeded for incubation in air plus 5–10% CO_2. Deposits from joint and pleural fluids not yielding other bacteria should be examined for tubercle bacilli by Ziehl-Neelsen film, culture on Löwenstein-Jensen medium and possibly inoculation into guinea-pigs (Ch. 25).

Peritoneal dialysis

Many patients with renal failure are now treated by the procedure of peritoneal dialysis, which exposes them to the risk of bacteria being introduced into the peritoneum and causing a serious peritonitis. Laboratory examination of the effluent fluid is required so that the infection may be recognized at the earliest possible stage and appropriate antibiotic therapy given. When the effluent fluid is turbid to the naked eye, it is obvious that infection has occurred, but examination by cell count, Gram film and culture may reveal the development of the infection at an earlier stage, as well as identifying the infecting organism. Most infections are caused by coagulase-negative staphylococci, usually *Staphylococcus epidermidis* derived from the skin, but a few are caused by coliform bacilli, enterococci, viridans streptococci, *S. aureus*, diphtheroid bacilli, candida and anaerobic bacilli. Until the identity and sensitivities of the causal organism are known, the infection may be treated with antibiotics, e.g. cefuroxime, gentamicin, added to the dialysis fluid.

The whole bag of effluent should be delivered to the laboratory, where there are the skilled staff and facilities to remove a sample without introducing contaminating bacteria. The clip on the spout of the bag should be loosened, a little fluid run to waste, and then about 200 ml fluid collected in four 50 ml lots in sterile bottles suitable for centrifuging. Before centrifugation, a little of the mixed fluid should be taken for a leucocyte count, which is done in a counting chamber as used for cerebrospinal fluid cell counts. In the absence of infection the fluid will contain 10, 20 or 30 leucocytes/ml, but in peritonitis often 500/ml, 1000/ml or more. A count higher than 100/ml should arouse the suspicion of a developing infection. The presence of eosinophilic polymorphs may suggest that the patient's symptoms are due to hypersensitivity to components of the dialysis fluid rather than to infection.

The 200 ml of fluid should then be centrifuged, the supernates discarded and the cellular deposits pooled in about 20 ml of residual fluid. This suspension should be used to make a film for Gram staining and several drops of it should be inoculated on to blood agar plates for aerobic and anaerobic incubation, and a MacConkey plate for aerobic incubation. The remainder of the deposit should be added to a tube of cooked-meat broth. The plates are examined after 18–24 h and again at 48 h. If they show no growth the cooked-meat broth is incubated for up to 3 weeks, or until it becomes turbid, when it should be examined by film and subculture. An alternative approach is to inoculate samples of the dialysis fluid into a standard set of blood culture bottles in the place of the cooked-meat broth; the bottles are then incubated and subcultured by the standard procedures. Any organism isolated is identified and its sensitivities are determined. If the leucocyte count is raised, or if bacteria are seen in the Gram film or in culture, the finding should immediately be telephoned to the physician without waiting for identification of the bacteria.

For a discussion of the diagnosis and management of peritonitis in continuous ambulatory peritoneal dialysis, see Report (1987).

5. GENITAL TRACT INFECTIONS

The laboratory approach to the diagnosis of genital tract infections is best considered in relation to the sex of the patient. Although some of the specific infections, e.g. gonorrhoea, syphilis and chlamydial infection, are common to both sexes, there are usually differences in the presenting symptoms and the sites and methods of collection of specimens in these infections. Moreover, some other infections, e.g. vaginitis and uterine sepsis, are confined to women.

Genital infections in women

These include urethritis, vaginitis, vaginosis, genital ulceration, cervicitis, uterine sepsis, salpingitis, oophoritis and the condition recognized as pelvic inflammatory disease.

Vaginal discharge. Excessive vaginal discharge which is purulent or normal in character is a common complaint, especially in sexually active women, and accounts for a large proportion of specimens submitted for laboratory examination for genital tract infection. A wide range of organisms may be associated with leucorrhoea, but the roles of some are still uncertain. In *acute vaginitis* the squamous epithelial lining of the vaginal wall is invaded and inflamed, causing discomfort, pruritis or pain in addition to discharge. It is most commonly caused by *Trichomonas vaginalis* (Ch. 43) or *Candida albicans* or other yeasts such as *Torulopsis glabrata*

(Ch. 42). Another common condition is *anaerobic vaginosis* (Ch. 19), in which the vaginal epithelium is not invaded or inflamed and the main presenting symptom is the presence of a putrid or fishy-smelling discharge. It appears to be caused by the excessive growth of a mixture of bacteria, including anaerobes, that are commonly present in smaller and harmless numbers in the healthy vagina, e.g. *Gardnerella vaginalis, Bacteroides* species, anaerobic cocci and anaerobic vibrios (mobiluncus). The value of its diagnosis in the laboratory is that it often responds to treatment with metronidazole.

Cervicitis with or without urethritis may be caused by infection with the gonococcus or *Chlamydia trachomatis* and may lead to vaginal discharge. In gonorrhoea there is also often infection of Bartholin's glands, but only rarely infection of the vaginal epithelium. Chlamydial infection may occur with minimal signs and symptoms. Infection of the uterine tubes (salpingitis) with gonococci, streptococci or coliform bacilli may or may not be accompanied by vaginal discharge.

Uterine sepsis, either puerperal or post-abortion, may or may not lead to an increased or abnormal discharge of lochia from the vagina, and the main clue to its diagnosis is the onset of pyrexia. *Streptococcus pyogenes* is the classical cause of puerperal uterine infection, which may lead to fatal septicaemia. Streptococci of other Lancefield groups, anaerobic cocci, *Staphylococcus aureus*, coliform bacilli, bacteroides and clostridia are sometimes involved, either singly or in combination. These organisms may also be involved in postoperative infection of the genital tract, which may proceed to a life-threatening peritonitis or septicaemia.

Genital ulceration may be caused by herpes simplex virus, notably type 2, *Treponema pallidum, Haemophilus ducreyi*, chlamydiae of group A, and *Calymmatobacterium granulomatis*. Pathologists and clinicians recognize abnormal states of the epithelium of the uterine cervix, variously described as cervical ulceration, erosion, metaplasia and dysplasia. There have been debated associations of herpes simplex virus type 2 (HSV2) with these conditions and possible neoplastic change, and more recently a link with certain human papilloma viruses (HPV) or a combined effect of HSV2 and HPV has been suggested. The cervix should be sampled directly when genital herpes is suspected in a pregnant woman.

Tuberculous infection of the uterus and uterine tubes may be caused by *Mycobacterium tuberculosis, M. bovis* or one of the other pathogenic mycobacteria. Actinomycotic infection of the uterus may be associated with the use of an intra-uterine device (Ch. 27). The *toxic shock syndrome* is attributed to the elaboration of a potent exotoxin by staphylococci contaminating and growing on vaginal tampons.

Commensal flora. In relation to the collection of specimens and the interpretation of laboratory findings, it must be borne in mind that the vulva and urethral meatus are contaminated with skin, faecal and vaginal organisms, that the vagina has an indigenous commensal flora, and that the uterus, uterine tubes and ovaries are normally free from microorganisms. It is only for a few days after abortion or childbirth that bacteria from the vagina or environment are likely to pass into the uterus, though gonococci, pneumococci and other organisms occasionally cause ascending infections under other circumstances.

The commensal flora of the vagina varies with age. Before puberty, when the secretion is not acid (pH 6.5–7.5), the flora consists mainly of staphylococci, streptococci other than *S. pyogenes*, diphtheroid bacilli and coliforms. From puberty to the menopause, the secretion is acid (e.g. pH 4.5) and lactobacilli predominate, though various other organisms are present in smaller numbers, e.g. staphylococci, enterococci, streptococci other than *S. pyogenes*, diphtheroid bacilli, coliform bacilli, bacteroides, anaerobic cocci, anaerobic vibrios, yeasts and mycoplasmas. After the menopause the secretion is again non-acid and lactobacilli no longer predominate in the flora.

Collection of specimens

The specimen generally collected for the diagnosis of vaginitis, vaginosis or uterine sepsis is a *high vaginal swab*. The swab is inserted into the upper part of the vagina and rotated there before withdrawing it, so that exudate is collected from the upper as well as the lower vaginal wall. Such a specimen, however, is quite unsuitable for the diagnosis of gonorrhoea, for gonococci derived from the infected cervix tend to die off in the acid vaginal secretion and, if remaining viable, are likely to be overgrown by the vaginal commensal bacteria.

An *endocervical swab* must be collected for examination for gonococci. A vaginal speculum must be used to provide a clear sight of the cervix and the swab is rubbed in and around the introitus of the cervix and withdrawn without contamination from the vaginal wall. Other swabs should also be taken from any exudate discharged from the meatus of the urethra, or a Bartholin's gland. Rectal and pharyngeal swabs should also be considered. There are, clear advantages in referring a patient to a special clinic for these investigations which are fully detailed in Chapter 21.

Swabs for culture should be placed in tubes of Amies' transport medium (Ch. 6) for delivery to the laboratory. If possible, two swabs should be collected and submitted from each site, the one for making films and the other for seeding cultures. Alternatively, and preferably, the physician should use a second swab to make a smear with both thick and thin areas immediately it has been collected and, after drying and heat-fixation, submit the smear to the laboratory along with the first swab in a tube of transport medium. Smears prepared thus directly after collection of the discharge give much better results than smears prepared from swabs that have been transported to the laboratory.

For examination for trichomonas, further, special specimens should be collected from the vagina and cervix, including a swab placed in clear trichomonas transport medium (Ch. 43) for microscopy and possibly culture.

Microscopical examination

Both a wet film and a Gram-stained film should be examined. The wet film, between slide and coverslip, is examined for the presence of motile *Trichomonas vaginalis* as soon as possible after the specimen has been collected from the patient. If enough fluid cannot be expressed from the swab on to the slide, a little sterile saline may be added. If only one swab has been submitted, a sterile slide must be used, for the film must be prepared before the swab is inoculated on to culture media. The film is searched with × 10 and × 40 dry objectives for the presence of rounded or pear-shaped trichomonads showing jerky motility (Ch. 43). The presence of polymorphs or the yeast and hyphal forms of candida should also be noted, though these are generally looked for in the Gram smear.

The Gram-stained smear should be examined particularly for evidence of candidosis (vaginal thrush), anaerobic vaginosis and, if from an endocervical swab, gonococcal infection. *Candidosis* is commonest in pregnancy and diabetes, and after the administration of broad-spectrum antibiotics, steroids or oral contraceptives. The presence of Gram-positive hyphae (pseudomycelium) in addition to numerous Gram-positive yeast forms is diagnostic. In *anaerobic vaginosis* there are very numerous, small Gram-negative or Gram-variable bacilli of diphtheroid morphology (*Gardnerella vaginalis*), squamous epithelial cells covered with many such bacilli ('clue cells'), a variety of other bacterial forms, e.g. Gram-negative bacilli and vibrios, and a relative scarcity of Gram-positive lactobacilli and polymorphs. Direct tests on the foul-smelling secretion will show it contains amines and has a pH of 5 or higher (Ch. 19).

The presence of Gram-negative diplococci intracellularly situated in a limited proportion of polymorph leucocytes, as well as some situated extracellularly, is almost diagnostic of gonorrhoea, but presumptive positive smears must be confirmed by culture, particularly in cases that may involve legal proceedings.

Culture

The specimen should be inoculated on to two plates of a rich blood agar medium, the one for incubation at 35–37°C in a humid atmosphere of air plus 5% CO_2 and the other in an anaerobic atmosphere with CO_2. The plates should be examined after 18–24 h and again after reincubation for another 24 h, as *Gardnerella vaginalis*, anaerobic cocci and bacilli, and candida may show very little growth after 18–24 h. It may be helpful to have placed a 5 μg metronidazole disk and a 50 μg neomycin disk on the 'well' area of the anaerobic plate to assist in the recognition and isolation of anaerobes. Additional media should be seeded when the presence of particular pathogens is expected. Culture of an additional, confluently-seeded aerobic blood agar plate bearing several different antibiotic disks may assist in the separation and provisional identification of the organisms in a mixed flora.

Colonies of *Candida albicans* can often be recognized on the aerobic blood agar plate, either by the appearance of their white colonies with spiky projections or by their growth in the inhibition zones around disks with antibacterial antibiotics. However, if the clinical features or the appearances in the Gram smear suggest that the patient may have candidosis, it is advisable initially also to inoculate the specimen on to a plate of Sabouraud's agar or malt extract agar for aerobic incubation for 48 h at 35–37°C. The placing of a 50 unit nystatin disk and a 20 μg amphotericin disk on the heavily inoculated 'well' area of the Sabouraud plate will assist in the recognition of a candida growth, distinguishing sensitive yeast colonies from resistant staphylococcal and other bacterial colonies, as well as confirming the strain's sensitivity to these therapeutic drugs. In the interpretation of findings, it must be borne in mind that small numbers of candida organisms are commonly present as commensals in the healthy vagina and that the finding of a few colonies in culture is not diagnostic of candidosis. In a true infection the numbers of the organisms will often be sufficiently great for many to be seen in the stained smear.

Gardnerella vaginalis may be recognized by the growth in 48 h of numerous very small colonies on both the aerobic and the anaerobic blood agar plate. But when the clinical features or the appearances in the Gram-stained smear suggest the patient has anaerobic vaginosis, it is

helpful to inoculate the specimen also on to peptone-starch-dextrose agar or one of the selective media described in Chapter 19.

Neisseria gonorrhoeae may grow well enough on the rich moist blood agar incubated in air plus CO_2, but if the clinical features or the appearances in the Gram smear suggest that there may be a gonococcal infection, the specimen should be inoculated additionally on to a plate of moist heated-blood ('chocolate') agar and a plate of the modified New York City selective medium (Ch. 21) for incubation at 35–37°C in air plus 5–10% CO_2.

When *uterine sepsis* is suspected, the specimen should be inoculated on to a MacConkey plate and into a cooked-meat broth as well as on to aerobic and anaerobic blood agar plates, and examined for pyogenic bacteria as described above for wound swabs. When an actinomycotic infection is suspected, anaerobic culture should be continued for 7 days and the specimen should be seeded on to an additional plate of selective medium, e.g. blood agar containing metronidazole 2.5 g/litre (Ch. 27).

Non-specific genital infection (*NSGI*). Non-specific (i.e. non-gonococcal) genital infection in women is generally due to *Chlamydia trachomatis*. The chlamydial infection is primarily a cervicitis, which in over half the patients may be symptomless. It may also cause urethritis, clinical or silent salpingitis leading to infertility, pelvic inflammatory disease or, *post partum*, inclusion conjunctivitis or pneumonitis in the patient's newborn baby.

Laboratory facilities for the demonstration of chlamydia are often unavailable, and diagnosis is based on the clinical features and the laboratory exclusion of gonococcal and trichomonas infection. If facilities are available, scrapings of epithelial cells from the cervix and urethra should be collected on microscope slides for the identification of elementary chlamydial bodies and larger inclusions in the cells' cytoplasm by immunofluorescence with specific, preferably monoclonal antiserum (Alexander et al 1985). Scrapings may otherwise be examined in an enzyme-linked immunosorbent assay (ELISA) test (Caul & Paul 1985) or scrapings collected in antibiotic-free transport medium for culture in irradiated McCoy cells (Ch. 46).

Mycoplasma infection. The role of myco-plasmas in non-specific genital infections is uncertain. T strain mycoplasmas (*Ureaplasma urealyticum*) have been associated with abnormalities of reproduction including infertility, habitual abortion and low birth weight, but the significance of these associations is difficult to evaluate, for vaginal and urethral colonization with ureaplasma is found in a majority of sexually active women. Ureaplasmas can be cultured from cervical or vaginal swabs and the centrifuged deposit from the first 30–40 ml of voided urine. Their isolation and identification is aided by their ability to hydrolyse urea.

Perform quantitative culture by making 10-fold dilutions of the specimen in small (0.9 ml) volumes of liquid medium comprising PPLO broth, horse serum, urea and phenol red indicator (Ch. 45). Express the exudate from the swab into 0.9 ml medium to obtain a 10^1, dilution and prepare further dilutions up to 10^6. Incubate at 37°C and examine for a colour change each day up to 7 days. With colour changes resulting from ureaplasma growth the medium remains clear; any turbidity is a sign of bacterial contamination which invalidates the result.

Syphilis and herpes. Serological tests for syphilis should be performed not only in cases where there is a clinical indication of this infection, but also in cases of other genital and sexually transmissible conditions, for syphilis may be present in addition to a diagnosed gonococcal, trichomonal or chlamydial infection. If an accessible ulcer is present, exudate from it should be examined by darkground microscopy for the presence of treponemes (Ch. 40). In suspected genital herpes, fluid from any vesicle and exudate collected from the base of ulcers should be placed in virus transport medium and submitted for culture for herpes simplex virus (Ch. 50).

Genital infections in men

The infections in men are mostly caused by the same organisms as in women, but are seldom asymptomatic. In practice, urethritis is classified as gonococcal or non-gonococcal (NGU, NSU) depending on whether or not gonococci are found in a Gram film or a culture of the discharge (Ch. 21). Most cases of NGU are caused by *C. trachomatis*, whilst ureaplasmas probably account for about 10% of cases. Prostatitis is rare in sexually active men and when it occurs is usually caused by gonococci or chlamydiae. The subacute or chronic prostatitis found in older men is usually associated with the presence of coliform bacilli or enterococci. The same differences in aetiology between younger and older patients apply also to epididymitis. A tuberculous epididymitis is occasionally found in patients with latent or active tuberculosis.

Balanitis and balano-posthitis often occur as mixed infections of the preputial sac and sulcus associated with inflammation and ulceration; skin and faecal bacteria are usually present and there is often an active bacteroides component. Ulceration of the penis may be caused by herpes simplex virus, usually type 2, the primary chancre of syphilis by *Treponema pallidum*, the soft sore of chancroid by *Haemophilus ducreyi*, lymphogranuloma venereum by chlamydia, and granuloma inguinale by *Calymmatobacterium granulomatis*. Orchitis may be a reaction to mumps.

Collection of specimens

Urethral discharge milked from the urethra may be expressed directly on to slides for examination in Gram-stained films for gonococci. Discharge collected in an inoculating loop should, if possible, be inoculated immediately on to warmed plates of heated-blood agar and selective medium for the culture of gonococci. If specimens have to be transported to the laboratory for the preparation of films and inoculation into culture, as much exudate as possible should be collected on a swab and the swab at once plunged into a tube of Amies' transport medium (Ch. 6). When prostatitis is suspected and there is no spontaneous discharge from the urethra, massage of the prostate *per rectum* may express some exudate for examination. The examination of a chancre requires the careful collection of exudate and its preparation for darkground microscopy (Ch. 40). A specimen of clotted venous blood should be collected for serological examination.

Laboratory examinations

Comparable specimens are examined for pathogens on the same lines as those from infections in women. The interpretation of results is usually easier in male than female infections, for specimens of urethral discharge and exudate from ulcers are less likely to be contaminated with organisms from the perineum. Nevertheless, the distal urethra in men does possess a commensal flora, including diphtheroid bacilli, albus staphylococci, enterococci and coliform bacilli. The presence of these bacteria is unlikely to be related to infection and should be ignored.

Confidentiality. In principle, laboratory reports are confidential to the physician requesting the examination, but many laboratories dispatch batches of reports to hospital wards and medical clinics where they are opened by secretaries, nurses or junior medical staff for distribution into the patients' records. Confidentiality is particularly important in the case of reports, whether positive or negative, on the results of examinations for sexually transmitted infections. Such reports, or at very least the positive ones, should be posted separately and directly to the physician in charge of the patient's case, and the use of code numbers rather than names merits serious consideration.

6. MENINGITIS

There is urgent need for the laboratory diagnosis of suspected meningitis, for bacterial meningitis is life-threatening and requires appropriate antibiotic therapy at the earliest possible moment. An out-of-hours laboratory service should be available so that calls for examinations can be met at any time of the day. Preliminary findings should be telephoned at once to the physician to guide his initial choice of therapy.

The clinical signs of meningeal irritation always suggest infection of the meninges, but they sometimes occur in association with certain other acute infections not involving the meninges (meningismus) and with certain non-infective conditions such as subarachnoid haemorrhage. Infants, moreover, may have meningitis without the usual localizing signs. Laboratory examinations therefore have an important role in establishing whether or not there is meningitis as well as in determining the causal organism in cases of infective meningitis. Every patient suspected of having meningitis should have a specimen of cerebrospinal fluid (CSF) examined in the laboratory.

Most cases of meningitis fall into one of two categories: purulent meningitis and aseptic meningitis. In *purulent meningitis* the CSF is typically turbid due to the presence of large numbers of leucocytes, e.g. from 100 to several thousands per mm^3, most of which are polymorphs. The majority of cases are caused by one or other of three bacteria: meningococcus, pneumococcus and *Haemophilus influenzae*, which generally pass to the meninges from the respiratory tract via the bloodstream. In neonates and infants, coliform bacilli, group B streptococci and, less commonly, pseudomonads, salmonellae and *Listeria monocytogenes* may be the cause. Infections acquired through a carelessly performed lumbar puncture, an accidental wound or an infected neurosurgical wound may be due to pyogenic staphylococci or streptococci, coliform bacilli, anaerobic cocci or bacteroides. In patients with CSF-venous shunts, infection may be caused by *Staphylococcus epidermidis* or some other commensal or saprophytic bacterium. The meninges may become inflamed in reaction to an underlying brain abscess, in which case the CSF may or may not contain large numbers of polymorphs and may or may not yield a culture of the causal organism.

In *aseptic meningitis*, which in Britain is much commoner than purulent meningitis, the CSF is clear or only slightly turbid and contains but moderate numbers of leucocytes, e.g.

10–500/mm³, most of which are lymphocytes, except in the earliest stage. The great majority of cases are due to viruses (viral meningitis), particularly enteroviruses of the echo, coxsackie and polio groups. Mumps virus is a moderately common cause and a few cases are due to herpes simplex, varicella-zoster, measles and adenoviruses. Arboviruses cause cases in countries where these viruses are common.

A few cases with CSF findings resembling those of viral meningitis are caused by leptospires (serovars canicola and icterohaemorrhagiae), fungi (*Cryptococcus neoformans* or *Candida albicans*) and amoebae (*Naegleria* or *Hartmanella*). And an underlying viral encephalitis may give a moderate lymphocytic exudate in the CSF. It should also be noted that when antibiotic therapy is started at an early stage in a bacterial meningitis, the CSF findings may be like those of aseptic meningitis.

Tuberculous meningitis, now rare in Britain, results from a progressive primary infection, usually pulmonary or mesenteric, and is often associated with miliary tuberculosis. It is fatal unless specific anti-tuberculous therapy is given, so its prompt diagnosis is essential. The CSF findings often resemble those of aseptic meningitis, but the cell count is usually slightly higher, e.g. 100–500 leucocytes/mm³, mostly lymphocytes, and a veil clot (fibrin web) often develops when the CSF is allowed to stand undisturbed.

Collection of specimens

The principal specimen to be examined is of CSF collected by lumbar puncture. The procedure should be attempted only by physicians well trained in its performance and rigorous aseptic precautions must be observed to prevent the introduction of infection. Only 3–5 ml of fluid should be collected, for the removal of a larger volume may lead to headache, and the rate of collection should be slow, about 4 or 5 drops a second. When there is increased intracranial pressure, the fluid may tend to spurt out, in which case the withdrawal should be quickly checked, for a large sudden removal of fluid may draw down the cerebellum into the foramen magnum and compress the medulla.

Container for CSF. The laboratory should supply fresh sterile screw-capped containers exclusively for the collection of CSF. These should not be containers that have been cleaned and sterilized after previous use for other purposes. Such re-used containers may contain bacteria from a previous specimen, e.g. urine, or a culture, which, although killed by the sterilization procedure, may be seen in a Gram-stained film of the CSF and lead to the issuing of an erroneous preliminary report based on the findings in the film.

Lumbar puncture. The patient should lie on his side with his back overhanging the edge of a firm couch or bed. His head, flexed forwards, should be on the same level as his sacrum, and his knees should be drawn up. The best site for the puncture is the interspace between the third and fourth lumbar vertebrae, which is at the level of a line joining the highest points of the iliac crests. The skin at this site should be disinfected with, e.g., alcoholic iodine solution, and anaesthetized by the intradermal and subcutaneous injection of a little local anaesthetic. A sterile, hollow lumbar puncture needle containing an occlusive stylet should be used. The operator, wearing sterile gloves, should push the needle deeply between the third and fourth lumbar spines, either in the mid line or slightly to one side of it, so that the tip of the needle, with its bevel downwards, passes slightly headwards into the spinal canal, which it should reach at a depth of 4–6 cm. The stylet should then be withdrawn and, if the needle is correctly placed, the first drops of CSF should appear within a few seconds. If no fluid appears, the stylet should be replaced and the needle pushed a little farther on. If the needle strikes bone, it should be withdrawn a short distance and pressed in again in a different direction. The fluid should be allowed to fall drop by drop into the container until 3–5 ml has been collected. The needle should then be withdrawn, a sterile occlusive dressing applied to the puncture site and the patient left lying down for several hours afterwards.

The specimen must be dispatched to the laboratory as quickly as possible, for delay may result in the death of delicate pathogens, such as meningococci, and the disintegration of leucocytes. It should not be kept in a refrigerator, which tends to kill *H. influenzae*. If delay for a few hours is unavoidable, the specimen is best kept in an incubator at 37°C.

Blood culture. Blood for cultures should be collected at the same time as the CSF, if possible before antibiotics are given. Bacterial meningitis is often associated with a bacteriaemia and the delicate causal organism may sometimes be isolated from the blood when culture of the CSF is negative. *Septic spots* are often present on the skin in cases of meningococcal meningitis and bacteriaemia. One should be scraped and fluid expressed on to a microscope slide for Gram staining, for the cocci may be demonstrated in this material when they cannot be seen in the CSF.

Laboratory examination of CSF

The specimen should be examined with the naked eye for the presence of turbidity and any sign of contamination with blood from the puncture wound. Normal CSF is clear and colourless like water. A yellow colour may result from a previous cerebral haemorrhage. The specimen should then be examined by cell count, Gram film, culture and, if facilities are available, for its glucose and protein contents and the presence of haemophilus, meningococcal or pneumococcal antigens.

Cell count

The leucocytes in the CSF are counted by microscopical observation of well mixed, uncentrifuged fluid in a slide counting chamber. The relative numbers of polymorphs and lymphocytes should be noted, and the number of erythrocytes in specimens contaminated with blood. Normal CSF contains only 0–5 leucocytes/mm^3, mainly lymphocytes, though in neonates up to 30/mm^3, mainly polymorphs. In purulent meningitis there are usually 100–3000 leucocytes/mm^3, mostly polymorphs, though in some cases much higher

numbers. In aseptic meningitis there are usually 10–500 leucocytes/mm^3, mostly lymphocytes, though polymorphs may predominate in the earliest acute stage of the illness. In tuberculous meningitis there are usually 100–500 leucocytes/mm^3, mostly lymphocytes.

If the CSF is heavily blood stained, it is not worthwhile to attempt to make a cell count, for numerous leucocytes derived from the blood will be present. But if there is only slight contamination with blood, the leucocytes and erythrocytes should be counted separately. The finding of leucocytes in numbers greatly in excess of 1 per 1000 erythrocytes, the approximate ratio in blood, will suggest the presence of meningitis.

When examining the wet film of CSF for the cell count, care should be taken not to mistake the rare presence of yeasts or amoebae for leucocytes. A wet film of centrifuged CSF deposit mixed with India ink will, when examined under oil-immersion, demonstrate the characteristic capsulate yeast cells of *Cryptococcus neoformans* and a wet film examined on a warm stage will show the slowly motile trophozoites of *Hartmanella* or *Naegleria*.

Counting chamber. The cell count is usually performed in a modified Fuchs-Rosenthal slide chamber, which has a film depth of 0.2 mm between the counting surface of the slide and the overlying coverslip. The counting surface is marked with triple lines into nine large squares, each 1 mm^3 in area and subdivided into 16 small squares. The volume of fluid in the film overlying five large squares is thus 1 mm^3 and the count of the cells on five large squares is thus the count per mm^3.

Dilution. CSF that is clear or only slightly turbid should be examined undiluted, but when the specimen is highly turbid and its cell count very high, it may be necessary to dilute it 1 in 10 or 1 in 100 before examination. When separate counts are to be made of the leucocytes and erythrocytes, 0.85% NaCl solution should be used as diluent. If, however, the presence of large numbers of erythrocytes makes the recognition and counting of the leucocytes difficult, the dilution should be done with a *counting fluid* which lyses the erythrocytes and stains the nuclei of the leucocytes. A suitable fluid contains acetic acid and crystal violet, e.g.

Glacial acetic acid	1 ml
Propan 1, 2 diol	2.5 ml
Crystal violet 1% in water	1.5 ml
Distilled water	100 ml

Procedure. 1. Make sure the surfaces of the counting chamber and its coverslip are clean and dry. Press the coverslip on to the support areas at the sides of the counting surface until broad bands of rainbow colours (Newton's rings) appear and indicate that close and even contact has been made.

2. Gently but thoroughly mix the diluted or undiluted uncentrifuged CSF. Take up about 0.2 ml in the capillary end of a Pasteur pipette. Carefully apply the tip of the pipette to the counting surface at the edge of the coverslip and allow the fluid to run into the chamber so that it fills the whole chamber without the presence of bubbles of air and yet does not spill over to the support areas on either side. Newton's rings should still be apparent.

3. First inspect the area of the counting grid with the low power of the microscope. Defocus the condenser to make the unstained cells clearly visible. Then count the cells with a × 40 dry objective (magnification × 300 or × 400). Count the cells on five of the large squares. Include in the count any cells that overlap the innermost line of the triple-lined border on the left-hand and distal sides of the square and exclude from the count the cells that overlap the border on the right and proximal sides. Take care not to count erythrocytes as leucocytes.

4. Add together the counts for the five large squares and, in the case of diluted specimens, multiply by the dilution factor to get the count per mm³.

Differential leucocyte count. If there is any difficulty in differentiating polymorphs and lymphocytes in the counting chamber, make a film of the cellular deposit after the specimen has been centrifuged, fix with heat, stain with methylene blue, Leishman or carbol thionine and examine by oil immersion to assess the relative numbers of the two types of leucocytes.

Gram film of CSF

After taking some CSF for the cell count, the remainder should be centrifuged to deposit any cells and bacteria and a film of the deposit should be stained by Gram's method. As cells and bacteria may be scanty, it is generally helpful to make a thick film within an area of about 10 mm diameter encircled by a scratch on the surface of the slide, so that the area to be searched is clearly defined. When the CSF is highly turbid and proteinaceous, part of the film should be thin, for sometimes a wholly thick film, although dried and fixed by heat, becomes washed off the slide in the course of staining.

A very careful search for bacteria should be made particularly in areas of the film where there are plenty of leucocytes, and the search should be continued for at least 10 min before accepting the result as negative. The finding of bacterial forms resembling meningococci, pneumococci, haemophili, coliform bacilli, streptococci or listeriae should at once be reported to the physician, for different antibiotics are preferred for treatment of the different infections: e.g. benzylpenicillin (or chloramphenicol) for meningococcus and pneumococcus; chloramphenicol for haemophilus; chloramphenicol, ampicillin or cotrimoxazole for coliforms; benzylpenicillin or chloramphenicol for group B streptococci; and ampicillin or chloramphenicol for listeria. Benzylpenicillin and chloramphenicol are often given blind to cases of suspected meningitis before laboratory results are available, but it is important to avoid overdosage or prolonged dosage with chloramphenicol in infants, especially neonates, and the earliest indication of the type of bacteria present may be helpful in enabling the physician to change to other drugs.

When a variety of bacterial forms is seen in the film, the probability of the specimen being contaminated with live or dead bacteria should be suspected.

Culture of CSF

Immediately after centrifugation of the CSF and the removal of some of the deposit for the Gram film, the remainder of the deposit should be seeded heavily on to culture media, e.g. a plate of blood agar and a plate of heated-blood ('chocolate') agar for incubation in humid air plus 5–10% CO_2, and a tube of cooked-meat broth. Particularly when there may be a brain abscess, possibly due to bacteroides or anaerobic cocci, a further blood agar plate should be seeded for incubation for 2–5 days in an anaerobic atmosphere with 5–10% CO_2. When organisms are sufficiently numerous to be seen in the film, another blood agar plate should be seeded confluently and antibiotic disks applied, including disks with benzylpenicillin and chloramphenicol, so that sensitivity results may be obtained with minimal delay, but they must be regarded with caution, especially those for *Haemophilus influenzae*.

The cultures should be inspected after overnight incubation. Any growth should be identified and if primary sensitivity results are not available, tests with appropriate antibiotics should be done on the isolate. If no growth is apparent after overnight incubation, the plates should at once be reincubated for another day and then again inspected for growth. If the plate cultures remain free from growth and turbidity develops in the cooked-meat broth, the broth should be filmed and subcultured on to blood agar and heated-blood agar plates, incubated aerobically and anaerobically.

Biochemical tests

The supernate from the centrifuged CSF should be tested for its content of glucose and protein. Normal CSF contains 2.2–4 mmol glucose/litre (about 60% of the plasma glucose value) and 0.15–0.4 g protein/litre (in neonates up to 1.5 g protein/litre). In purulent bacterial meningitis the glucose concentration is reduced (0–2 mmol/litre) and the protein concentration increased (0.5–3 g/litre). In aseptic (viral) meningitis the glucose concentration is normal and the protein concentration raised a little (0.5–1 g/litre).

Bacterial antigens

If appropriate reagents are available, a rapid indication of the type of infection may be obtained by the performance of a coagglutination or counter-immunoelectrophoresis test on the CSF (or blood serum) to demonstrate the presence of the antigens of meningococci of serotype A, B or C, or the capsular antigens of the commoner types of pneumococci or Pittman's type b of *Haemophilus influenzae* (Wasilavskas & Hampton 1982; Chs 19, 21). Convenient kits for the coagglutination test are available commercially (e.g. Wellcome).

Viral meningitis

If the clinical findings and the results of microscopical and biochemical examinations of the CSF suggest the presence of aseptic meningitis, an attempt may be made to isolate the virus from the CSF, a throat swab or a specimen of faeces, and paired sera may be examined for viral antibodies. Some CSF should be kept at −70°C until it can be inoculated into cell cultures, which may yield an echo, coxsackie or herpes virus. A throat swab submitted in viral transport medium may be cultured for these and mumps virus, and faeces may be cultured for echo, coxsackie and polio virus.

Tuberculous meningitis

When a tuberculous infection is suspected, the centrifuged deposit of the CSF should be examined in a Ziehl-Neelsen stained film for acid-fast bacilli and cultured on one or two slopes of Löwenstein-Jensen medium (Ch. 25). The film should be searched for at least 5 min before being accepted as negative. If facilities are available, some of the CSF should be inoculated into a guinea-pig (Ch. 25). As in purulent meningitis, the glucose content of the CSF is reduced and the protein content increased.

Leptospiral meningitis

When the CSF appearances are those of aseptic meningitis and the clinical features, e.g. conjunctivitis, jaundice or nephritis, suggest that the infection may be leptospiral, paired sera should be collected to demonstrate a rising titre of leptospiral antibodies in the serovar-specific microscopical agglutination test or the genus-specific complement-fixation and sensitized erythrocyte tests (Ch. 41). Occasionally, motile leptospires may be seen in the CSF under dark-ground illumination and occasionally leptospires may be cultured from the CSF or blood inoculated into Korthoff's or other leptospiral medium (Ch. 41).

7. GASTROINTESTINAL INFECTIONS

The commonest specimens examined for gastrointestinal infections are those of faeces from patients with diarrhoea, with or without abdominal pain or vomiting. Formed stools may be submitted from patients suspected of having enteric fever, helminthiasis or the subclinical carriage of an intestinal pathogen, and clotted blood may be submitted for serological examination for suspected enteric fever or an intestinal virus infection.

In Britain the commonest infectious causes of diarrhoea in adults and children over 2–3 years old are infections with *Campylobacter* spp. (Ch. 32), *Salmonella typhimurium* and other animal-derived salmonellas (Ch. 29) and *Shigella sonnei* (Ch. 30), and food-poisoning due to these and other bacteria, e.g. *Staphylococcus aureus* (Ch. 16), *Clostridium perfringens* (*C. welchi*) (Chs 37, 38), *Bacillus cereus* (Ch. 24) and *Vibrio parahaemolyticus* (Ch. 32). A moderate number of cases are caused by the protozoon, *Giardia intestinalis* (*G. lamblia*) (Ch. 43) and the fungus, *Cryptosporidium* (Ch. 42), and a few cases by *Shigella flexneri*, *Salmonella typhi*, *Salmonella paratyphi B*, *Aeromonas hydrophila*, *Plesiomonas shigelloides* and *Yersinia enterocolitica*.

In infants under 3 years old, many cases of gastroenteritis are caused by rotaviruses and certain other viruses, and by intestinal pathogenic strains of *Escherichia coli* (Ch. 28). These organisms also cause some infections in adults, e.g. in persons travelling abroad and encountering an enterotoxigenic strain of *E. coli* of a serotype not previously encountered at home ('traveller's diarrhoea').

Various exotic intestinal pathogens may be acquired by persons travelling abroad and cause diarrhoeal illness soon after the traveller has returned to Britain by air. These pathogens include *Vibrio cholerae* (Ch. 32), *Shigella dysenteriae*, *Shigella boydi*, *Salmonella paratyphi A* and *Entamoeba histolytica* (Ch. 43). Physicians should be advised always to inform the laboratory about any recent foreign travel by the patient so that the microbiologist is warned to perform the special examinations required for demonstration of the exotic pathogens.

In patients treated with antibiotics, e.g. for prophylaxis during intestinal surgery, severe enterocolitis may be caused by a drug-resistant strain of *Staphylococcus aureus* and a life-threatening pseudomembranous colitis by *Clostridium difficile* (Ch. 38). Milder, simple diarrhoea often follows prolonged treatment with any of a variety of antibiotics which deranges the bowel flora and predisposes to superinfection with various drug-resistant bacteria, *Candida albicans* or *Cryptosporidium*.

Particularly in childhood, diarrhoea may be caused by infections elsewhere than in the gastrointestinal tract, e.g. by respiratory, urinary and septicaemia infections, and by certain non-infective conditions such as the food allergies.

Collection of specimens

Whenever possible, a specimen of *faeces* should be obtained. A *rectal swab* is unsatisfactory unless it is heavily charged and visibly stained with faeces collected from the rectum, not anus. A swab heavily charged with faeces wiped from toilet paper is usually satisfactory. If enteric fever is suspected, a specimen of venous blood should be collected for *blood culture*. If food-poisoning is suspected because a cluster of cases are related to the eating of a common foodstuff, a sample of the suspect food should be collected (Ch. 11). For serological examinations, paired acute and convalescent samples of clotted blood should be collected at an interval of about 10 days in suspected enteric fever and 2–4 weeks in suspected viral infection.

Faeces. The specimen may be collected from faeces passed into a clean bedpan, unmixed with urine or disinfectant, or from the surface of heavily soiled toilet paper. The container is a 25 ml screw-capped, wide-mouthed glass or plastic bottle with a 'spoon' projecting from the underside of the cap. Collect 1–2 ml of faeces on the spoon and insert it, carried on the spoon, into the bottle. Take care not to soil the rim or outside of the bottle. Apply the cap tightly. Do not collect several spoonfuls or attempt to fill the container. Transmit the specimen quickly to the laboratory. If delay is unavoidable, and particularly when the weather is warm, collect the faeces in a container holding about 6 ml buffered glycerol saline transport medium (Ch. 6).

Examination of faeces

The faecal sample should first be inspected with the naked eye for its consistency, whether formed or fluid, the presence of mucus, pus and blood, indicative of severe dysentery, and the presence of helminths. It is usual then to proceed to culture on media suitable for isolation of the common bacterial pathogens. In Britain it is generally sufficient to culture for campylobacters, salmonellas and shigellas, and to search for other pathogens only when the clinical features or epidemiological circumstances suggest the need to do so, e.g. in infantile or post-antibiotic diarrhoea, in suspected outbreaks of food-poisoning, when the patient has recently returned from travel abroad, and when there has been failure to isolate a common pathogen in a case of persistent diarrhoea. Some bacteriologists, for instance, search for *Clostridium difficile* in all hospital patients, others for cryptosporidium in all young children and immunodeficient patients. In well staffed laboratories it is recommended that all faecal specimens should be examined microscopically for

pus and red cells, protozoa, protozoal and cryptosporidial cysts, helminths and helminthic ova.

A faecal suspension should be prepared for inoculation into the different media. Unless the sample is fluid a portion of it should be suspended to give a 1 in 10 dilution in 2–3 ml of phosphate-buffered (pH 7.3) saline or 0.1% peptone water.

Campylobacter. Inoculate one or two loopfuls of the faecal suspension on a plate of campylobacter selective medium, e.g. the Skirrow or Preston medium (Ch. 32, *Methods*) and incubate for 48 h at 42–43°C under microaerophilic conditions (5–6% O_2, 7–10% CO_2 in H_2 or N_2; see Ch. 32). If the faeces is more than 24 h old, also inoculate one or two loopfuls into a tube of Preston campylobacter enrichment broth (Ch. 32, *Methods*), incubate for 24 h at 42–43°C, and then subculture on to a plate of campylobacter selective medium. Identify *Campylobacter jejuni* and *C. coli* as described in Chapter 32.

Salmonella and Shigella. There is a wide choice of selective and enrichment media for these organisms (Chs 29, 30). A good procedure for routine examinations is to seed a plate of one selective medium, e.g. deoxycholate citrate agar (DCA), and a tube of one enrichment broth, e.g. selenite F broth (Ch. 29, *Methods*). Inoculate one or two loopfuls of the faecal suspension on to the DCA plate, stroking out with care to yield many separate colonies, and one or two drops of the suspension into the selenite F broth, and incubate aerobically for 18–24 h at 37°C. Inspect the plate for pale (non-lactose-fermenting) enterobacterial colonies, pick and prepare a pure subculture (e.g. on a nutrient agar or urea agar slope) from each of any different morphological types of pale colonies, and identify the subcultures as described in Chapters 29 and 30. Streak out a loopful of the selenite culture on DCA, incubate this plate overnight and examine for pale colonies as before. The faeces may contain non-lactose-fermenting commensal bacteria as well as a non-lactose-fermenting pathogen and it is therefore inadvisable to conclude that pathogens are absent from the examination of only a single pale colony. If the only pale colonies are crowded and touching other colonies, pick one as cleanly as possible and plate it out on MacConkey agar to obtain pure, well separated pale colonies the following day. Do not base the identification of a salmonella or shigella on biochemical or serological tests made on a possibly mixed culture.

Xylose lysine deoxycholate (XLD) agar (Ch. 29, *Methods*) has considerable advantages as a primary plating medium for faeces and its use instead of DCA is recommended. It is less inhibitory than DCA to *S. dysenteriae* and *S. flexneri*, and it distinguishes most salmonellas (red colonies with black centres) from shigellas (red colonies without black centres) and most non-pathogenic coliforms (yellow colonies).

The chances of isolating a scanty salmonella or shigella will be increased if additional selective and enrichment media are seeded. There are advantages in seeding a MacConkey agar plate and, for the isolation of salmonellas, a plate of brilliant green MacConkey agar, a plate of Wilson & Blair's brilliant green bismuth sulphite agar (BBSA) and a tube of tetrathionate broth (Ch. 29, *Methods*).

Other food-poisoning bacteria

If the epidemiological circumstances suggest that the patient has been involved in an outbreak of food-poisoning and if the sample of his faeces has been collected within 3 days of the start of his illness, examine the sample for *Clostridium perfringens*, *Staphylococcus aureus*, *Bacillus cereus* and *Vibrio parahaemolyticus* as well as for campylobacter, salmonella and shigella. If possible also obtain a sample of the suspected foodstuff for culture (Ch. 11).

Clostridium perfringens. Food-poisoning may be caused by either heat-sensitive strains (spores killed in 10 min at 80°C) or heat-resistant strains (spores survive for 10 min at 80–100°C) of this organism, though the resistant strains are more likely to be the cause of outbreaks due to well cooked foodstuffs as their spores are more likely to survive the cooking. The mere finding of the organism in the faeces, even if it is heat-resistant, does not indicate that it has a causal role in the illness, for normal subjects commonly have 1000–10 000 bacilli or spores of *C. perfringens* per gram of faeces. Culture should therefore be done by a semi-quantitative method, for faeces collected from patients at the height of the illness commonly contain 1 000 000 or more *C. perfringens* per gram and it is only the finding of such high counts that should be reported as probably significant (see Ch. 38).

The demonstration that strains isolated in large numbers from several patients and the suspected food are of the same serotype provides stronger evidence of their causal role.

It may also be helpful to examine the specimens of faeces for *C. perfringens* enterotoxin, for the finding of this toxin in significant amounts may confirm the diagnosis in an outbreak when the cultural results are equivocal. The examination for toxin may be made in a reference laboratory on faeces transmitted by post, but reversed passive latex agglutination kits are now available commercially (e.g. Oxoid) for testing in the general clinical laboratory.

Staphylococcus aureus. Plate out a few loopfuls of a 1 in 10 saline suspension of the faeces on plates of blood agar, MacConkey agar and a selective medium, e.g. 6% NaCl nutrient agar, mannitol salt agar (Ch. 16) or phenolphthalein phosphate agar (Ch. 16) plus 1250 units polymyxin B/litre. Incubate aerobically for 18–24 h at 37°C and examine for colonies of *S. aureus*. In an outbreak, send subcultures from each patient to a reference laboratory for phage-typing and tests for enterotoxin production.

S. aureus may often be isolated from the faeces of healthy persons, so that its isolation from the faeces of a patient with diarrhoea is not proof of a causal role. Identity of phage-type among the isolates from several patients in an outbreak and from a specimen of suspected foodstuff is fair evidence that the outbreak is due to staphylococcal food-poisoning. Some outbreaks, however, are caused by a foodstuff that has been heated, e.g. pasteurized, at a temperature sufficient to kill the staphylococci though insufficient to inactivate the more thermostable enterotoxin. In such cases the diagnosis requires the demonstration of staphylococcal enterotoxin in the faeces or food. Kits for the detection of staphylococcal enterotoxins A, B, C and D by reversed passive latex agglutination are available commercially (Oxoid).

Bacillus cereus. Particularly when the outbreak is attributed to the eating of a rice dish, inoculate loopfuls of faecal suspension on to plates of blood agar, MacConkey agar and, if available, the selective medium of Holbrook & Anderson (see Ch. 11). After aerobic incubation for 18–24 h at 37°C, look for large rough pale colonies on MacConkey agar and blue colonies surrounded by a precipitate on Holbrook & Anderson's medium. Identify them by their appearance in a Gram film and other tests (Ch. 24).

Vibrio parahaemolyticus. 1. Particularly in outbreaks attributed to raw sea fish and shellfish, plate a few loopfuls of a 1 in 10 suspension of faeces on thiosulphate citrate bile sucrose (TCBS) agar (Ch. 32, *Methods*) and incubate aerobically for 18–24 h at 37°C.

2. Also inoculate a portion of the faecal suspension into an equal volume of double-strength alkaline (pH 8.8) peptone water (Ch. 32), incubate 18–24 h at 25°C, then subculture on to a TCBS plate and incubate for 18–24 h at 37°C.

3. Inspect the plates for large (2–5 mm) blue or green (non-sucrose-fermenting) colonies. Demonstrate they contain vibrios by Gram filming and that they are oxidase positive.

4. Suspend a colony in 3% NaCl solution and inoculate drops of the suspension into media for identifying *V. parahaemolyticus* (Ch. 32), which is motile, ferments glucose but not sucrose with the production of acid but not gas, grows in alkaline peptone water with 8% NaCl but not in peptone water without NaCl or on CLED medium (Ch. 28, *Methods*), and fails to agglutinate with *Vibrio cholerae* O1 antiserum. Send a subculture to a reference laboratory for serotyping.

Infantile gastroenteritis

Most cases appear to be caused by viruses, particularly rotaviruses, which only rarely cause gastroenteritis in children more than a few years old or in adults. As yet, tests are generally not done to demonstrate viruses in the samples of faeces and a viral aetiology is assumed from the failure to demonstrate a bacterial pathogen. When facilities are available a centrifuged concentrate of the faeces may be examined by the electron microscope, which in the acute phase of the illness will show the presence of large numbers of rotaviruses. Rotavirus antigens may also be demonstrated in the faeces by a serological method (e.g. ELISA or latex agglutination), but the use of such tests requires careful and informed laboratory monitoring (see Ch. 48).

Enteropathogenic Escherichia coli. These enteropathogenic strains of *E. coli* (Ch. 28) often cause gastroenteritis in neonates and infants under 3 years old and occasionally also in older subjects. Strains of certain serotypes of the species possess the intestinal pathogenic properties more commonly than strains of other serotypes (Ch. 28). Thus the demonstration that a dominant strain in a patient's faeces belongs to one of the former serotypes *suggests* that it has a pathogenic role, but some strains of these serotypes lack the pathogenic properties. Thus, reliance should not be placed on serotyping as indicative of enteropathogenicity, otherwise *E. coli* may wrongly be judged the cause of a diarrhoeal illness that is due to some other, undetected, e.g. viral, cause.

There is still no test for enteropathogenic properties suitable for routine application to faecal isolates. It is therefore probably wisest not to examine faeces for *E. coli* in sporadic cases of infantile diarrhoea, but only to do so when there is an outbreak among infants and other common intestinal pathogens have not been found.

1. Plate a loopful of faecal suspension on a blood agar plate and a MacConkey plate and incubate 18–24 h at 37°C.

2. Test from 3–10 *E. coli*-like colonies from the blood agar plate for slide agglutination within 1 min with pools of polyvalent sera for enteropathogenic serotypes of *E. coli* (Ch. 28).

3. If any colony gives a strong reaction with one of the pools, inoculate the remainder of it

on to a nutrient agar slope and incubate the slope overnight.

4. Prepare a dense suspension from the slope culture in saline and test it by slide agglutination with monovalent sera to identify the K antigen.

5. Then heat the suspension for 1 h at 100°C, cool it and repeat the slide tests with the monovalent sera to identify the O antigen. Confirm the O serotype by demonstrating tube agglutination to the titre of the serum.

Enterotoxigenic Escherichia coli. Strains of *E. coli* producing heat-stable or heat-labile enterotoxin (Ch. 28) may cause diarrhoea in adults and children who have not previously encountered them and should be sought particularly in cases of 'traveller's diarrhoea'. They may be cultured from faeces on MacConkey and blood agar media and serotyped. Not all strains of commonly toxigenic serotypes produce enterotoxins and cultures may be examined for toxin production in a reference laboratory or for heat-labile enterotoxin with a reversed passive latex agglutination kit (Oxoid).

Microscopy for protozoa, cysts and ova

Usually a faeces sample is not examined microscopically unless the clinical particulars or failure to demonstrate an alternative pathogen suggests that the patient's illness may be due to amoebiasis, giardiasis, balantidiosis, cryptosporidiosis (Ch. 43) or helminthiasis, but if sufficient staff is available, all specimens should be examined microscopically. A wet film of a concentrate of the faeces should be examined for protozoa, protozoal cysts and helminth ova, and a stained film for the oocysts of cryptosporidium. An adhesive, Sellotape-tipped swab should be applied to the perianal skin and examined microscopically for threadworm (enterobius) ova.

Vegetative amoebas and giardias. If possible, obtain a fresh, warm specimen of stool. Select a portion, preferably with mucus or pus, and emulsify it in saline solution or saline containing 0.5% eosin on a slide warmed to 37°C. Apply a coverslip and at once examine the film with a

× 40 dry objective for unstained, motile trophozoites (Ch. 43), pus cells and erythrocytes.

Cysts and ova. Microscopic examination for protozoal cysts and helminthic ova should be done on a film of a concentrate of the faeces (e.g. × 20).

1. Pipette 8 ml of 10% formol (4% formaldehyde) saline into a 28 ml Universal container. Thoroughly emulsify about 1 g faeces in the solution by shaking or by rubbing with a swab stick.

2. Add 2 ml diethyl ether to the suspension, shake vigorously for 1 min, then centrifuge at 650 g (e.g. at c. 1000 rev/min) for exactly 2 min.

3. With a swab stick loosen the debris floating near the surface of the ether. Then discard the debris with the ether and supernatant saline.

4. Withdraw a drop of the centrifuged deposit with a Pasteur pipette, place it on a microscope slide, add a drop of 2% iodine in 4% potassium iodide solution, apply a coverslip and seal the film with Vaseline.

5. Search the film thoroughly with a × 40 dry objective for the cysts of entamoeba and giardia (Ch. 43) and the ova of helminths such as ascaris, schistosoma, trichinella and trichuris. Check the morphology of any such bodies with the × 100 oil-immersion objective.

Identify the bodies seen by comparison with illustrations of their morphology and estimation of their size. As size is a helpful identifying feature, use a graduated eye-piece micrometer (Ch. 2) to measure the diameter of the suspect forms.

Giardiasis. Excretion of the giardia trophozoites and cysts is often intermittent, so microscopical examinations should be made on several separate collections of faeces. A rapid enzyme-linked immunoassay (ELISA) has been described, which is more sensitive and less laborious than microscopical examination (Green et al 1985).

Cryptosporidiosis. When other pathogens have not been found, or in children, travellers or immunodeficient subjects with diarrhoea, examine fresh faeces for the oocysts of cryptosporidium (see Ch. 43). These nearly spherical structures, usually 4–5 μm in diameter, resemble weakly acid-fast organisms in being moderately resistant to both the entry and exit of stains, and this property is exploited to facilitate their recognition in films. A quick and easy method of demonstration is by fluorescence microscopy of a film stained with auramine and counterstained with carbol fuchsin (Casemore et al 1985).

1. Make a thick smear of undiluted faeces with some thin areas. Dry it in air, fix it in absolute methanol for 3 min and again dry it in air.

2. Immerse the fixed smear in auramine-phenol (0.03 g auramine-0, 3 g phenol, 97 ml distilled water (Ch. 3), or as supplied by Infrakem) for 5 min at room temperature. Rinse with tap water.

3. Counterstain for 10 seconds in strong Ziehl-Neelsen carbol fuchsin (Ch. 3) at room temperature. Rinse in tap water and dry in air.

4. View the unmounted film under an incident light fluorescence microscope with a dry objective at a magnification of × 100 or × 200 as for mycobacterium fluorescence microscopy. Oocysts appear as bright yellow-fluorescing spheres with dark centres on a dull red background. Yeasts do not fluoresce. Re-examine positive smears at × 1000 by oil-immersion.

When oocysts are scanty, they may be found more easily in films made from a faecal concentrate. A formol-ether method of concentration adapted for cryptosporidial oocysts is described by Casemore et al (1985).

If a fluorescence microscope is not available, a modified Ziehl-Neelsen stain or, preferably, the safranine-methylene blue stain of Baxby et al (1984) may be used. The latter shows orange ring-shaped oocysts on a blue-stained background.

Microscopy for staphylococcal enterocolitis

When this life-threatening condition is suspected, e.g. in a patient with severe diarrhoea following intestinal surgery and antibiotic treatment, a bacteriological diagnosis is urgently required. Make a Gram-stained film of the faeces and examine it for very numerous Gram-positive cocci largely replacing the normal mixed bacterial flora. At once telephone the finding to the physician. Then culture the faeces as described for staphylococcal food-poisoning (see above) and determine the antibiotic sensitivities of any isolate.

Other intestinal pathogens

Culture of faeces for other intestinal pathogens should be attempted when the circumstances suggest they may be present.

Clostridium difficile. Always examine for this organism in cases in which pseudomembranous colitis is suspected, e.g. where there is severe, often blood-stained diarrhoea and toxaemia in a patient who has been receiving antibiotics, especially clindamycin or lincomycin. The condition poses an immediate danger to life and treatment with an effective antibiotic, e.g. oral vancomycin, is urgently required. The clostridium is also present in many cases of milder antibiotic-associated diarrhoea and should be sought when other pathogens are absent or, as recommended by Brettle & Wallace (1984), routinely in all cases of diarrhoea. The selective cultural procedures are given in detail in Chapter 38. The faeces may be tested directly for cytotoxin (Ch. 38, *Methods*).

Vibrio cholerae. This important pathogen is not indigenous in most countries, but its presence should be sought in patients suffering from diarrhoea just after returning by air from a country in which cholera is known to be present.

1. Culture the faeces in alkaline peptone water, on TCBS agar and on tellurite taurocholate gelatin agar as described in Chapter 32.

2. Identify yellow (sucrose-fermenting) colonies on TCBS agar as *V. cholerae* by demonstrating the organisms are motile Gram-negative vibrios, oxidase positive and capable of growth on CLED and other salt-free media.

3. Identify a classical cholera strain of *V. cholerae* by demonstrating that it reacts with *V. cholerae* O1 antiserum in a slide agglutination test.

4. Recognize non-O1 (non-cholera) strains of *V. cholerae* by their failure to react with the O1 antiserum while giving slide agglutination with *V. cholerae* H antiserum.

5. Send a subculture to a reference laboratory for confirmation of an O1 strain and O serotyping of a non-O1 strain.

Aeromonas hydrophila. This organism can cause severe gastroenteritis, though in most areas the number of reported cases is small. It may grow on MacConkey, deoxycholate and other enteric agars, some strains fermenting lactose and others not, but if it is to be sought a selective agar such as sheep blood agar with 15 mg ampicillin/litre should be used (Agger et al 1985). Incubate cultures on this last medium for 24–48 h at 37°C, flood the plate with 1% sodium dimethyl-*p*-phenylenediamine mono-hydrochloride (oxidase reagent) and recognize the aeromonas colonies by their purple-black colour and surrounding narrow zone of haemolysis. Pick quickly to subculture for identifying tests (Ch. 32).

Plesiomonas shigelloides. This organism causes a few cases of diarrhoea in many countries. It may be detected by its growth on MacConkey and DCA media, usually as pale, but sometimes pink colonies, which may be distinguished from those of shigella and escherichia by their oxidase-positive reaction, and identified as described in Chapter 32.

Yersinia enterocolitica. This organism sometimes causes simple gastroenteritis in Britain. Also examine faeces for it in cases of suspected mesenteric lymphadenitis and consider relevant serological investigation (Ch. 34). It may sometimes be isolated in blood cultures incubated at 22–25°C.

1. Inoculate several drops of a 1 in 10 suspension of the faeces in buffered saline into a tube of selenite F broth (Ch. 29, *Methods*) or phosphate-buffered saline, pH 7.6 (Mair & Fox, 1986) and hold the culture for up to 6 weeks at 4°C.

2. Inoculate a loopful of the faecal suspension, and at weekly intervals thereafter loopfuls of the selenite broth culture, on to plates of DCA (Ch. 29, *Methods*) or CIN medium (Yersinia selective agar base, Oxoid CM 653, plus antibiotic supplement, Oxoid SR109) and incubate for 24 h at 32°C.

3. Inspect the DCA plates for pale (non-lactose-fermenting) colonies and the Yersinia selective agar plates for colonies with dark red centres. Identify the organism as *Y. enterocolitica* by demonstrating it is motile at 22°C, ferments sucrose at 22°C, hydrolyses urea at 35°C, and has the other properties described in Chapter 34. It may also be identified by the API 20E kit.

Reporting

Consideration should be given as to whether antibiotic sensitivities should be reported to the physician along with the finding of a particular pathogen. In simple diarrhoea due to *Salmonella typhimurium* or other animal-derived salmonella, *Shigella sonnei*, *Shigella flexneri* or enteropathogenic *Escherichia coli*, treatment with antibiotics is rarely beneficial and may be harmful in prolonging the illness and the duration of carriage of the pathogen. A report of the finding of such a pathogen with its sensitivities may suggest to an ill-informed physician that he should prescribe antibiotic treatment. A note of the sensitivity results should of course be kept in the laboratory and if the physician enquires about them, the circumstances in which antibiotic therapy may be beneficial rather than harmful may be discussed with him. Antibiotic treatment will be positively required for enteric fever and may be indicated when there is evidence of invasiveness (e.g. septicaemia) with other gut pathogens, or severe dysentery.

Whilst a diagnosis of enterocolitis due to *Clostridium difficile* is a signal to stop any current antibiotic therapy and will demand urgent treatment with, e.g. oral vancomycin, the significance of finding this organism in cases of simple diarrhoea in persons who have not been treated with antibiotics is unclear. *C. difficile* is found in the faeces of many healthy infants and is unlikely to be the cause of diarrhoea in children under 2 years old. Such cases should not be treated with antibiotics.

Negative findings should be reported in terms only of the organisms that were sought and not found, e.g. 'No campylobacter, salmonella or shigella isolated', and not in general terms, e.g. 'No pathogens found', for the latter type of report may suggest that examinations were made for all possible kinds of pathogens, including viruses, protozoa, fungi and helminths.

Any isolation of an infectious enteric pathogen should be notified at once to the local public health authority to prompt the investigation of outbreaks and the institution of preventive measures.

8. URINARY TRACT INFECTIONS

Samples of urine from patients with suspected infections of the urinary tract are the most numerous, e.g. 30–40%, of the different kinds of specimens received in most clinical laboratories. The schedule for their routine examination should therefore be carefully determined with a view to obtaining the necessary diagnostic information with the greatest possible economy of labour and resources.

The examinations generally made are the *microscopical examination* of a wet film of uncentrifuged urine to determine whether polymorphs ('pus cells') are present in numbers indicative of infection in the urinary tract, and the *semi-quantitative culture* of the urine to determine whether it contains a potentially pathogenic bacterium in numbers sufficient to identify it as the causal infecting organism ('significant bacteriuria').

The chemotherapy of a proven infection may be guided by in-vitro sensitivity tests on the pathogen isolated in culture and the outcome of therapy assessed by examination of the urine at the conclusion of treatment. Follow-up examination of patients who have had urinary tract infection is advisable because a relapse may be clinically silent.

The common symptoms of urinary tract infection are urgency and frequency of micturition, with associated discomfort or pain. The commonest condition is cystitis, due to infection of the bladder with a uropathogenic bacterium, which most frequently is *Escherichia coli* but sometimes *Staphylococcus saprophyticus* or, especially in hospital-acquired infections, *Klebsiella*

pneumoniae var. *aerogenes* or *oxytoca*, *Proteus mirabilis*, other coliforms, *Pseudomonas aeruginosa* or *Streptococcus faecalis*. Candida infection may occur in diabetic and immuno-compromised patients. Rarer infecting organisms include *Streptococcus agalactiae*, *Streptococcus milleri*, other streptococci, anaerobic streptococci and *Gardnerella vaginalis* (Collins et al 1986). There has been much debate on the significance of so-called fastidious organisms in urinary tract infection. The argument for the role of these organisms is presented by Maskell (1986) and an opposing case is made by Hamilton-Miller et al (1986).

More serious bacterial infections are acute pyelitis and pyelonephritis, in which the symptoms usually include loin pain and fever and which may be accompanied by a bacteriaemia detectable by *blood culture*. The causative organism may be any of those that cause cystitis, but *Staphylococcus aureus* is responsible for some of the cases.

Patients with signs or symptoms of urinary tract infection sometimes produce samples of urine that show pus cells but do not yield a significant growth of bacteria on routine culture. The explanation may be that the patient has been taking antibiotics prescribed on a previous occasion. Alternatively, he may have an infection with an organism that does not grow on the media normally used for routine investigations. In such cases it is important to consider genito-urinary tuberculosis (Ch. 25) or gonococcal infection (Ch. 21), and infection with nutritionally exacting or anaerobic bacteria (Collins et al 1986). But many patients with frequency and dysuria do not have a bacterial infection of the bladder, nor significant numbers of bacteria in their urine (abacterial pyuria). Their condition is known as non-bacterial urethritis or cystitis, or the urethral syndrome, the cause of which may be urethral or bladder infection with a chlamydia, ureaplasma, trichomonas or virus, which often remains unrecognized (Stamm et al 1980).

Screening out negatives

About 70–80% of the urine specimens received in a clinical laboratory are found on full microscopical and cultural examinations to be free from evidence of infection in the urinary tract. Much labour can therefore be saved by the application of a simple and rapid preliminary screening test that will reliably identify these 'normal' specimens and permit their being reported as showing 'no evidence of infection' without the need for the further, full examinations. A variety of chemical and automated methods have been tried for the detection of the negative specimens, but none has yet been generally accepted as sufficiently reliable for its purpose. Recently, it has been reported by Lowe (1986) that the finding of negative results in all of three chemical tests, for nitrite, blood and protein, performed by a rapid automated dip-strip method (N-Labstix, Ames), predicts the absence of bacteriuria in about half of the culture-negative specimens, which may then be discarded.

Significant bacteriuria

The specimen most easily and therefore most commonly collected is mid-stream urine (MSU). Although the greater part of the urinary tract is devoid of a commensal flora and bladder urine in an uninfected person is free from bacteria, a specimen of spontaneously voided urine is apt to be contaminated with some commensal bacteria from the urethral orifice and perineum, particularly in females, even when the most careful precautions are taken to prevent such contamination. As these contaminating commensals include the very bacteria, such as *E. coli* and *S. saprophyticus*, which are the commonest organisms to infect the urinary tract, the simple demonstration that bacteria of one of these species are present in the sample of urine is not proof that it has been derived from an infection in the urinary tract.

Proof of a urinary tract infection requires the demonstration that the potential pathogen is present in freshly voided urine in numbers greater than those likely to result from contamination from the urethral meatus and its environs. The observations of Kass (1957) suggested that this number, taken to indicate *significant bacteriuria*, is about 100 000/ml. In true infections, in the absence of prior chemotherapy, the number of the infecting bacteria is

likely to be at least as great as this. Accordingly, a quantitative method of culture is adopted to estimate the number of viable bacteria in the specimen.

When properly collected specimens of urine are examined, contamination accounts for less than 10^4 organisms/ml and usually for less than 10^3/ml. Counts due to contamination are variable and the colonies often of diverse species. Specimens from urinary tract infections almost always contain more than 10^4 organisms/ml, usually more than 10^5/ml and often up to 10^8/ml. These high counts, which are fairly constant in serial specimens from the same patient, reflect bacterial multiplication in the urine in vivo and are accepted as indicating significant bacteriuria. The growth obtained in such cases usually represents a single infecting species, though some infections with two species, e.g. *E. coli* and *S. faecalis*, are encountered.

Significant bacteriuria (count $>10^5$/ml in a carefully taken and promptly examined sample) may sometimes occur in the absence of symptoms and pyuria in patients who subsequently develop symptoms of urinary tract infection, e.g. in pregnancy. The detection of such asymptomatic bacteriuria is of value, for there is good evidence of its association with the development of pyelonephritis in some patients.

A rigid adherence to the above guidelines should be avoided and the culture counts should be interpreted in relation to the clinical information about the patient (Maskell 1982). Thus a few specimens from symptomatic patients with a true infection may contain as few as 10^3 viable bacteria/ml and if the occurrence of contamination can be shown to be minimal, their sensitivities should be tested and their presence reported as probably or possibly significant. Indications that the scanty bacteria are not merely contaminants are: (1) the observation that all or almost all the colonies grown from the specimen are of the same species and type, for contaminants are generally of mixed species, and (2) the finding on microscopy of the presence of pus cells but the *absence* of squamous epithelial cells, which would be indicative of contamination from the perineum and vagina.

When, moreover, the specimen has been collected from the bladder by suprapubic aspiration (see below) or a freshly inserted urethral catheter, the absence of contamination may be assumed and the presence of even small numbers of bacteria must be regarded as significant.

Specimen collection

Specimens of urine are generally collected in plastic or glass Universal containers, but mid-stream specimens from females are more conveniently collected in a wide-mouthed container such as a 12 oz (350 ml) honey-pot or a sterile waxed cardboard container.

From male patients, a *mid-stream specimen of urine* (MSU, the middle of the urine flow) is collected. From females, in whom it is more difficult to avoid contamination with organisms from the ano-genital region, a *catheter specimen of urine* (CSU) was commonly collected in the past, but catheterization for this purpose is no longer considered justifiable because it carries a 2–6% risk of introducing and initiating infection. A CSU is nowadays taken only if there are special indications for its requirement or in the course of a cystoscopic investigation. Routinely, therefore, MSU samples are now submitted from women and when carefully taken these compare favourably with catheter specimens. The female patient passes urine with the labia separated and the middle of the stream is collected for examination.

The collection of a clean specimen of urine from children and young infants poses problems. Collection in a bag held with adhesive tape over the genitalia inevitably yields a contaminated, and generally a heavily contaminated specimen. However, a 'negative' finding, when occasionally obtained, may be of value. Otherwise, urine may be aspirated from the bladder into a syringe with a needle introduced aseptically through the skin and abdominal wall just above the pubis (supra-pubic stab). There are understandable reservations about subjecting a child to catheterization or suprapubic aspiration, but the importance of getting a reliable specimen sometimes outweighs these considerations (Maskell 1982).

A non-invasive method of stimulating urine flow in a baby is by tapping just above the pubis

with two fingers at 1 h after a feed; one tap/second is given for 1 min, an interval of 1 min is allowed, then tapping is resumed in this cycle. The method was described by Broomhall et al (1985) and has been favourably appraised by Taylor et al (1986).

If tuberculosis of the urinary tract is suspected, the first urine passed in the day (early morning urine) is the most suitable specimen. Three complete early morning urines should be sent to the laboratory, where they are centrifuged and their deposits examined by microscopical and cultural tests (Ch. 25). The individual specimens should be refrigerated pending processing.

In the investigation of urethritis and prosta-titis, the initial flow of urine, rather than a mid-stream specimen should be examined.

Transport of specimen. Once collected, a specimen of urine must be transported to the laboratory without delay, for urine is an excell-ent culture medium and contaminating bacteria can readily multiply to reach apparently signifi-cant numbers. If a delay of more than 1–2 h is unavoidable, the multiplication of bacteria in the urine should be prevented by storage in a refrigerator at 4°C, or by transport in some form of refrigerated container, or by collection and transport in a container with boric acid at a final, bacteriostatic concentration of 1.8% (Porter & Brodie 1969). When samples of urine not so treated are delayed more than 5 h in transit to the laboratory, the doctor should be informed and the samples discarded, for positive findings may be misleading. Collection and transport on a *dip-slide* (see below) avoids the difficulty of bacterial multiplication before quantitative culture, but does not provide for microscopical examin-ation of the cellular content of the urine.

Microscopy of urine

Microscopical examination of urine is done princ-ipally to detect the presence of increased numbers of polymorphs (pyuria) as an indication of infection in the urinary tract when culture may fail to show significant bacteriuria, either because bacteria are being killed as a result of antibiotic therapy or because the infecting organism is one that is unable to grow on the routinely used media, e.g. the tubercle bacillus, a nutritionally exacting or anaerobic bacterium, a chlamydia or a ureaplasma. Such a finding of sterile, or abacterial pyuria serves as an indication that further, special methods of examination should be used to detect the pathogen.

Microscopical examination is laborious, however, and may yield misleading results if performed cursorily by insufficiently experienced staff. Many bacteriologists, therefore, do not offer it as a routine, e.g. where the routine examinations are made on dip-slides. Instead, they reserve it as a special investigation in selected cases, as when examining repeat specimens from patients with urinary tract symptoms persisting after the failure of an initial culture to demonstrate significant bacteriuria, in suspected pyelonephritis or renal tuberculosis, and in cases where information is urgently required to differentiate a urinary tract infection from appendicitis or some other abdominal condition requiring immediate surgery. It is not unreasonable to omit microscopy and rely on culture for examination of the very numerous specimens of urine submitted from general practice or out-patient clinics from patients with symptoms of simple cystitis or urethral syndrome and those undergoing routine or geriatric or ante-natal assessment. If this is the policy, the clinician must ensure that the specimen is properly taken before antimicrobial treatment and submit information about any previous therapy.

In the past, the microscopical examination was commonly done on a wet film or Gram-stained film of deposit centrifuged from the urine, as the concentration by centrifugation made it easier to detect scanty bacteria or cells. Nowadays centrifugation is not recommended, for the presence of scanty bacteria or polymorphs is unlikely to be significant; the procedure is laborious, and unless it is done in such a way as to give a standard degree of concentration, e.g. $\times 10$ or $\times 20$, a sufficiently reliable estimate of the number of polymorphs cannot be made.

Some polymorphs are usually present in the urine of healthy, uninfected persons, and it is only if their number is clearly greater than the normal values that the finding of 'pus cells' is indicative of urinary tract infection. The normal excretion of leucocytes in the urine varies from only very few up to about $10^6/24$ h, and at times up to a few thousand may be present per ml of uncentrifuged urine. Generally it is accepted that the leucocytes should be found in numbers at least as great as $10^4/ml$ before the presence of pyuria is suggested. Thus the microscopical examination must be done in such a way as to provide a reliable estimate of the leucocyte numbers.

Wet film examination. A leucocyte count sufficiently accurate for general purposes may be obtained from examination of a wet film of uncentrifuged urine, provided that the area of the microscope field is known and the depth of the film is standardized. The film is usually observed with the high power ($\times 40$) dry objective of the microscope and the area of the high power field (HPF) so observed may be calculated from its diameter as measured by the use of a slide micrometer. Thus if the field diameter is 0.44 mm, the area of the HPF is 0.15 mm^2.

The depth of the wet film depends primarily on the volume of the drop of urine placed on the microscope slide and the area of the coverslip applied to it. Mix the urine sample carefully and then transfer 0.05 ml on to the middle of a microscope slide. At once apply a coverslip 22×22 mm in dimensions, avoiding trapped bubbles. The film should show a small excess of fluid along the edges of the coverslip and then be about 0.1 mm in depth. If the area of the HPF is 0.15 mm^2, the volume of urine observed in an HPF will be about 0.015 mm^3. Under these conditions the finding of 1 leucocyte per 7 high power fields corresponds with 10^4 leucocytes per ml and the finding of clearly larger numbers than this indicates significant pyuria.

Two sources of error in leucocyte counts have to be avoided. In cases of pyelonephritis or other kidney disease, care must be taken to avoid confusing tubular epithelial cells with leucocytes. In women, contamination from the vagina may introduce large numbers of leucocytes into a sample of voided urine; the presence of squamous epithelial cells along with pus cells in the sample is evidence that such contamination has taken place and the leucocyte count is then invalidated.

There is little value in microscopical examination of the wet film for bacteria. It may be difficult to recognize bacteria amid amorphous urate particles and it is scarcely possible to distinguish whether bacteria present in significant numbers consist of a single infecting species or a mixture of faecal or vaginal contaminants. Contamination from the vagina may lead to the presence of large numbers of lactobacilli which will not grow on the media used routinely for culture. If in cases where pyuria has been recognized an indication of the type of infecting bacterium is urgently required, a Gram film of centrifuged deposit may be examined, but the findings must be interpreted with caution.

Apart from the presence of leucocytes and bacteria in the wet film, note should be taken of the presence of squamous or tubular epithelial cells, tubular casts, red blood cells and crystals, which may have diagnostic significance in non-infective conditions.

Rant-Shepherd method. If the policy in a laboratory is to subject all specimens of urine to microscopical examination, there are great advantages in the use of a method that economizes in labour by obviating the need to prepare separate wet films of the correct depth for each specimen. The following method devised by Mr J D Rant and Dr W Shepherd, PHLS Microbiology Laboratory, Norwich, UK, can be recommended (Maskell 1982). It requires the use of an inverted binocular microscope with a mechanical stage and clear plastic microtitre trays with flat-bottomed wells. The rigid polystyrene trays M29A with 96 numbered flat wells 8 mm in diameter supplied by Sterilin are suitable. Mix the uncentrifuged sample of urine and with an automatic pipette bearing a disposable, single-use tip deliver a 60 μl volume of it into one of the wells. Deliver similar volumes of other samples up to 95 in number into the other wells in the tray. Register the location of each specimen on the tray on a guide sheet and use a microscopy guide system to ensure that when

each specimen is observed it is correctly identified. Place the charged tray on the stage of the inverted microscope and leave it to stand for a few minutes until the cells in the small volumes of urine have settled on to the flat bottoms of the wells. Then observe microscopically each well in turn and record the number of polymorphs per field. From a knowledge of the area of the field and the depth of urine in the well the number of polymorphs per ml urine can be estimated (in an 8 mm diameter circular flat-bottomed well a 60 μl volume makes a layer 1.2 mm deep). This approach has been incorporated in a semi-automated procedure described by Henrichsen & Moyes (1987) for processing urine samples.

Semi-quantitative culture

To count the viable bacteria in urine by an accurate method such as the pour-plate or Miles & Misra method (Ch. 12) is too laborious for routine use. Quicker, semi-quantitative methods are used instead. The common urinary pathogens grow well on simple and selective media within 24 h of aerobic incubation at 37°C. Nutrient agar, blood agar, MacConkey agar (Ch. 6) and CLED agar (Ch. 28, *Methods*) are the media most often used and laboratories generally limit the range to only one or two of these. CLED and MacConkey media have the advantages of distinguishing lactose- from non-lactose-fermenters and of inhibiting proteus from swarming, and as CLED is the less inhibitory to *Staphylococcus saprophyticus*, its use is most strongly recommended. Blood agar has the advantage of promoting the growth of nutritionally exacting strains, which may additionally require incubation for up to 48 h in air with added 5–10% CO_2 (e.g. see Collins et al 1986), but these and anaerobic pathogens are relatively uncommon in urinary tract infections and their culture should be attempted only in cases of pyuria from which significant numbers of a commoner pathogen have not been grown on the routine media.

Standard loop method

An inoculating loop of standard dimensions is used to take up a small, approximately fixed and known volume of mixed uncentrifuged urine and spread it over a plate of agar culture medium. The plate is incubated, the number of colonies counted or estimated, and this number used to calculate the number of viable bacteria per ml of urine. Thus, if a 0.004 ml loopful of urine yields 400 colonies, the count per ml will be 10^5, or just indicative of significant bacteriuria.

If nichrome or platinum wire of SWG 28 is used to make a circular loop of 3.26 mm internal diameter, it will hold a drop of water or urine of 0.004 ml volume when withdrawn slowly and vertically from the liquid so as to produce a 'flat-sided drop'. It is, however, much simpler to purchase standard, ready made sterile disposable (single-use) plastic loops that will hold a fixed volume in the range 0.001–0.01 ml. When loops holding 0.004 ml or more are used and the loopful is spread uniformly over the whole of a plate, colonies may be so numerous as to be confluent and there may be no single, separate colonies available for picking and the preparation of pure subcultures. Accordingly, it is usual to spread these larger loopfuls over only a sector of the plate and streak out from that sector over other sectors to ensure the production of separate colonies. The approximate number of viable bacteria may then be estimated from the number of colonies on the plate or the weight of confluent or semiconfluent growth on the different sectors according to a prearranged scheme (McGeachie & Kennedy 1963).

A better method, however, is to use a smaller standard loopful and spread it over the whole of a plate with an automatic spreading device. A sterile single-use plastic loop holding 0.001 ml (e.g. as supplied by Elkay or Technical Services) should be used to take up 0.001 ml of mixed uncentrifuged urine and spread it in a diametrical stroke across the middle of a culture plate. The plate may then be spread automatically over its whole surface in a self-sterilizing Autospreader (Denley). The growth of 100 colonies by this method indicates the presence of 10^5 bacteria/ml of urine. If a non-selective nutrient agar or blood agar is used in the plate, the same loop should be streaked out on MacConkey or CLED agar lest a swarming proteus is present.

Filter paper method

This method of semi-quantitative culture (Leigh & Williams 1964) is rapid and very economical in the use of culture medium, but growths are often confluent and, if mixed, require to be plated out to obtain pure subcultures for identifying and sensitivity tests. A standard 6 mm wide strip of absorbent fluffless blotting or filter paper is bent into an L shape with a 12 mm long foot (area 12 × 6 mm) and sterilized at 160°C for 1 h. Dip the whole of the angulated end and foot into the mixed, uncentrifuged sample of urine, withdraw it and wait a few seconds to allow all the excess fluid to be absorbed into the paper. Then press the foot on to the surface of a marked section of a well-dried plate of agar culture medium, ensuring that the whole area of the foot makes contact with the medium. Remove the strip and discard it into disinfectant. Up to 8 or 10 samples can be tested in duplicate on different areas of a 9 cm plate. Incubate the plate and afterwards count the colonies growing on the impression area. Up to 50 colonies may be countable and heavier growths are noted as being semi-confluent (+) or confluent (++).

Estimate the number of viable bacteria per ml of urine from the count of colonies on the impression area or the pattern of semi-confluent or confluent growth. Very approximately, the value of 10^5 bacteria/ml corresponds to a count of 25 colonies of bacilli or 30 colonies of cocci. As, however, the porosity and adsorptive power of the papers obtained from different manufacturers often vary, calibration curves should be prepared from impression counts made in preliminary tests on diluted broth cultures for which viable counts are made in parallel by the Miles & Misra method.

Dip-slide method

The method of semi-quantitative culture on dip-slides or dip-spoons is the least laborious for the laboratory and as the medium is seeded with urine immediately it has been passed, obviates the difficulty of having to prevent bacterial multiplication during transport to the laboratory. It is specially convenient for the routine screening of large numbers of patients, e.g. in ante-natal or geriatric assessments, and for use in clinics and practices remote from the laboratory. Its disadvantages are that it does not provide material for microscopical examination for the cellular content of the urine and that when the bacterial count is high and the growth on the dip-slide confluent, it is difficult to judge whether the growth is pure or mixed and to obtain an unmixed inoculum for identifying and sensitivity tests.

The dip-slide is a small plastic tray carrying a layer of an appropriate agar culture medium. Opposite sides of the tray may carry different media, e.g. CLED agar medium on one side and MacConkey, brain heart infusion or pseudomonas selective agar on the other. The slide is supplied in a Universal-type container, being held on a stalk fastened rigidly to the inside of the screw-cap of the container. Such outfits are available commercially (e.g. from Difco, Gibco, Oxoid and Roche).

A mid-stream specimen of urine is collected in a clean container. The cap of the dip-slide container is unscrewed and held while the dip-slide is withdrawn from the container and briefly immersed in the urine. On its removal, the excess urine is drained off by contact of the bottom of the slide with the wall of the urine vessel and the device is then returned into its container and the cap screwed on tightly. Alternatively an intelligent patient may be instructed to grasp the dip-slide by the cap and hold it in such a way as to immerse the agar tray in the stream of urine while the mid portion is being passed; then to shake off the excess urine and replace the device in its container.

The charged dip-slide in its sealed container is sent to the laboratory, the duration and temperature of transport not being critical. It is then incubated at 37°C overnight and examined for a growth of colonies. (Prolonged culture at 15–18°C often gives comparable results to those obtained by incubation overnight at 37°C.)

Where urine samples are collected in a clinic with the facility for incubation at 37°C, the dip-slide can be incubated there and examined next day by a doctor or nurse who has been familiarized with the appearances of growths. The clinician then gets an early indication of the results and as only the minority of dip-slides that show significant growth need be sent to the laboratory for identification and sensitivity tests, the laboratory is spared from undertaking the large amount of clerical work required for the reception and reporting of the negative specimens.

The count of viable bacteria in the urine is estimated approximately from the number of colonies or the pattern of semi-confluent or confluent growth seen on the medium on the dip-slide. Commercial suppliers of dip-slides provide charts showing representing numbers and patterns by comparison with which the viable count can be read. Otherwise, charts may be prepared in the laboratory from the findings in trials of the dip-slides in diluted broth cultures on which viable counts are obtained by the Miles & Misra method.

Identification and sensitivity tests

If similar colonies are found in numbers suggesting significant bacteriuria, a separate colony or a portion of apparently pure growth should be subcultured for identification and testing of its sensitivity to antibiotics. The appearance of the primary growth on CLED or MacConkey medium will suggest the kind of organism that is present. How much more precisely it should be identified is a matter for consideration. Probably coliform bacilli should be differentiated into *E. coli*, klebsiella, proteus, pseudomonas and other 'coliforms'; *S. saprophyticus* and *S. aureus* should be distinguished from other staphylococci, and enterococci should be distinguished from other streptococci. Detailed characterization and typing of isolates may be done in epidemiological studies of cross-infection and in cases where it is important to distinguish between reinfection of a patient with a new strain and relapse of infection with a strain that was formerly present.

Antibiotic sensitivity tests are best done with an appropriately diluted inoculum of a pure subculture (Ch. 9), but if prior microscopy has indicated that infection may be present, primary sensitivity tests may be set up at the same time as the initial culture by flood-inoculating the urine on to a suitable medium, drying the surface and applying sensitivity test disks. The semi-automated method described by Henrichsen &

Moyes (1987) exploits a multi-point inoculator and combines the advantages of primary sensitivity tests with those of a simple identification system.

As antibiotics are concentrated in urine to higher levels than are found in the tissues, high-content test disks should be used (Ch. 9). If the patient is attending a general practice or out-patient clinic, drugs suitable for oral administration should be tested, e.g. amoxycillin or ampicillin (25 μg disk), cephalexin (30 μg), nalidixic acid (30 μg), ciprofloxacin (5 μg), nitrofurantoin (50 μg), and trimethoprim (2.5 μg). Tests with disks containing amoxycillin (20 μg) with clavulanate (10 μg) marketed as Augmentin (30 μg) may be done as a routine on a separate plate with a β-lactamase producing strain of *E. coli* as control organism, but results should not be issued unless resistance to ampicillin/amoxycillin alone is encountered. Tests with disks containing trimethoprim and sulphamethoxazole in combination are not recommended; if an organism is resistant to trimethoprim alone, the use of cotrimoxazole would be inappropriate.

For patients in hospital, for whom parenteral therapy might be appropriate, sensitivities to cefuroxime (30 μg) and gentamicin (10 μg) should also be tested, and when resistant pseudomonas is present, sensitivity to amikacin, netilmicin, tobramycin, azlocillin, ceftazidime, and ticarcillin may be tested.

It is generally of little value to identify the species in the mixed cultures of faecal-type bacteria that are commonly obtained from patients with indwelling catheters. Antibiotics are of little use in the treatment of such infections. The findings may be reported as 'many mixed bacteria' and the patient's bladder may be treated by irrigation with a mild disinfectant such as Hibitane or Noxythiolin (without specific sensitivity testing).

9. PYREXIA OF UNKNOWN ORIGIN (PUO)

The term PUO is generally applied to any febrile illness lasting more than a few days, the cause of which is obscure due to the absence of obvious specific or localizing signs and symptoms. In these conditions there is thus a special need for a laboratory diagnosis to guide the choice of appropriate therapy. About two-thirds of the more acute cases and one-third of the chronic cases are due to infections of one kind or another and the remainder of cases are due to non-infective causes such as leukaemia, early carcinoma, collagen diseases, sarcoidosis, Crohn's disease and drug reactions.

Many kinds of infections may present as PUO, including many common infections that in some patients fail to show their usual diagnostic features. They include: (1) urinary tract infections; (2) lung, subdiaphragmatic, appendicular and other deep abscesses; (3) septicaemia as, for example, that associated with cryptic abscesses, pneumonia, pyelonephritis, biliary tract infection, infective endocarditis and immunodeficiencies; (4) enteric fever, tuberculosis, brucellosis, syphilis, non-meningitic meningococcal infection, rheumatic fever, leptospirosis without jaundice or meningitis, Q fever and toxoplasmosis; (5) many viral infections, e.g. infectious mononucleosis, rubella and other infectious fevers without their typical rashes; (6) malaria and, less frequently, leishmaniasis, trypanosomiasis and other tropical infections in travellers returned from abroad, and (7) helminthic infestations.

Very careful history taking is an essential preliminary to diagnosis. Enquiry must be made about foreign travel, occupation, contact with cases of infectious diseases and contact with animals. The physician must inform the microbiologist of any such relevant facts.

Laboratory diagnosis of PUO infections

The following procedures should be considered. Tests should first be done for the more likely infections and then, if these are negative, tests for the less likely should be done. For fuller details, refer to the chapters dealing with the specific causal organisms.

1. Blood culture should always be attempted. A first specimen should be collected before antibiotics are given, and several specimens collected on separate occasions should be examined before a negative result is accepted.

2. Specimens of urine, throat secretion, sputum (if present) and faeces should be examined for the common pathogenic bacteria, and

faeces should be examined for protozoa, cysts and helminthic ova.

3. Paired sera should be collected for serological tests for antibody responses to a range of possible pathogens, e.g. cytomegalovirus, hepatitis B virus, influenza virus, infectious mononucleosis virus, chlamydia, coxiella, rickettsia, mycoplasma, brucella, legionella, leptospira, syphilis spirochaete, toxoplasma, aspergillus and other fungi, and entamoeba. The antistreptolysin-O (ASO) test should be done for cryptic *S. pyogenes* infection. The first specimen should be taken as early in the illness as possible and the second 2–4 weeks later.

4. Haematological investigations should be done to detect leucocytosis, suggestive of a cryptic abscess; eosinophilia, suggestive of helminthiasis; and atypical lymphocytes, suggestive of infectious mononucleosis.

5. A tuberculin test and a chest X-ray should be done to detect tuberculosis.

6. Thick and thin blood films should be examined for malaria, leishmaniasis, trypanosomiasis and filariasis in travellers returned from countries in which these infections are present.

REFERENCES

Agger W A, McCormick J D, Gurwith M J 1985 Clinical and microbiological features of *Aeromonas hydrophila*-associated diarrhea. Journal of Clinical Microbiology 21: 909–913

Alexander I, Paul I D, Caul E O 1985 Evaluation of a genus-reactive monoclonal antibody in rapid identification of *Chlamydia trachomatis* by direct immunofluorescence. Genitourinary Medicine 61: 252–254

Baxby D, Blundell N, Hart C A 1984 The development and performance of a simple sensitive method for the detection of *Cryptosporidium* oocysts in faeces. Journal of Hygiene, Cambridge 93: 317–323

Bell S M, Smith D D 1976 Quantitative throat swab culture in the diagnosis of streptococcal pharyngitis in children. Lancet 2: 61–63

Brettle R P, Wallace. E 1984 *Clostridium difficile*-associated diarrhoea. Journal of Infection 8: 123–128

Broomhall J et al 1985 A reliable non-invasive technique for obtaining urine samples from babies. British Medical Journal 290:30

Brumfitt W, Willoughby M L N, Bromley L L 1957 An evaluation of sputum examination in chronic bronchitis. Lancet 2: 1306–1309

Casemore D P, Armstrong M, Sands R L 1985 Laboratory diagnosis of cryptosporidiosis. Journal of Clinical Pathology 38: 1337–1341

Caul E O, Paul I D 1985 Monoclonal antibody based ELISA for detecting *Chlamydia trachomatis*. Lancet 1:279

Collins L E, Clarke R W, Maskell R 1986 Streptococci as urinary pathogens. Lancet 2: 479–481

Dixon J M S, Miller D C 1965 Value of dilute inocula in cultural examination of sputum. Lancet 2: 1046–1048

Gould J C, Duerden B I 1983 Blood culture – current state and future prospects. Journal of Clinical Pathology 36: 963–977

Green E L, Miles M A, Warhurst D C 1985 Immunodiagnostic detection of giardia antigen in faeces by a rapid visual enzyme-linked immunosorbent assay. Lancet 2: 691–693

Hamilton-Miller J M T, Brumfitt W, Smith G W 1986 Are fastidious organisms an important cause of dysuria and frequency? The case against. In: Asscher A W, Brumfitt W (eds) Microbial diseases in nephrology. Wiley, Chichester. Ch 2, p 19–30

Henrichsen C, Moyes A 1987 A semi-automated method for the culture, identification and susceptibility testing of bacteria direct from urine specimens. Medical Laboratory Sciences 44: 50–58

Hopkin J M, Turney J H, Young J A, Adu D, Michael J 1983 Rapid diagnosis of obscure pneumonia in immunosuppressed renal patients by cytology of alveolar lavage fluid. Lancet 2: 299–301

Kass E H 1957 Bacteriuria and the diagnosis of infections of the urinary tract. Archives of Internal Medicine 100: 709–713

King A, Bone G, Phillips I 1986 Comparison of radiometric and gas capture systems for blood cultures. Journal of Clinical Pathology 39: 661–665

Lees A W, McNaught W 1959 Bacteriology of lower-respiratory-tract secretions, sputum and upper-respiratory-tract secretions in 'normals' and chronic bronchitics. Lancet 2: 1112–1115

Leigh D A, Williams J D 1964 Method for the detection of significant bacteriuria in large groups of patients. Journal of Clinical Pathology 17: 498–503

Lowe P A 1986 Chemical screening and prediction of bacteriuria – a new approach. Medical Laboratory Sciences 43: 28–33

McGeachie J, Kennedy A C 1963 Simplified quantitative methods for bacteriuria and pyuria. Journal of Clinical Pathology 16: 32–38

Mair N S, Fox E 1986 Yersiniosis: lab diagnosis, clinical features, epidemiology. Public Health Laboratory Service, London

Maskell R 1982 Diagnosis of urinary tract infection, its causes and consequences. In: Urinary tract infection. Current Topics in Infection Series 3. Edward Arnold, London. p 21–41

Maskell R 1986 Are fastidious organisms an important cause of dysuria and frequency? The case for. In: Asscher A W, Brumfitt W (eds) Microbial disease in nephrology. Wiley, Chichester. Ch 1, p 1–18

Porter I A, Brodie J 1969 Boric acid preservation of urine samples. British Medical Journal 2: 353–355

Report of a Working Party of the British Society for

Antimicrobial Chemotherapy 1987 Diagnosis and management of peritonitis in continuous ambulatory peritoneal dialysis. Lancet 1: 845–849

Rodriguez F, Lorian V 1985 Antibacterial activity in blood cultures. Journal of Clinical Microbiology 21: 262–263

Rosen P P, Martini N, Armstrong D 1975 *Pneumocystis carinii* pneumonia: diagnosis by lung biopsy. American Journal of Medicine 58: 794–802

Smith J W, Hughes W T 1972 A rapid staining technique for *Pneumocystis carinii*. Journal of Clinical Pathology 25: 269–271

Stamm W E, Wagner K F, Amsel R et al 1980 Causes of the acute urethral syndrome in women. New England Journal of Medicine 303: 409–415

Taylor M R H, Dillon M, Keane C T 1986 Reduction of mixed growth rates in urine by using a 'finger tap' method of collection. British Medical Journal 292:990

Wasilavskas B L, Hampton K D 1982 Determination of bacterial meningitis; a retrospective study of 80 cerebrospinal fluid specimens evaluated by four in-vitro methods. Journal of Clinical Microbiology 16: 531–535

Treponema: serological tests for syphilis

The general term spirochaete is often used to embrace *Treponema* species and organisms of similar spiral morphology belonging to the genera *Borrelia* and *Leptospira* (see Ch. 41).

Syphilis is an infectious venereal disease caused by *Treponema pallidum*. A primary lesion or chancre tends to appear on the genitalia at the site of entry of treponemes. The disease is systemic from the onset and the natural course of infection may span several decades (Robertson et al 1988a). *T. pallidum* is the only pathogenic treponeme indigenous to Britain. Other morphologically indistinguishable treponemes that are pathogenic for man include *T. pertenue*, the cause of yaws, a non-venereal but communicable disease found in tropical countries, and *T. carateum*, the cause of pinta, a mild contagious disease similar to yaws but confined to Central and South America.

These pathogenic treponemes cannot be cultured in vitro, either alone or with mammalian cells of various types. In contrast commensal treponemes can be cultured successfully in artificial media. Many commensal species occur in the mouth (e.g. *T. macrodentium* and *T. microdentium*) and on the mucous surfaces of the genitalia (e.g. *T. calligyrum*, *T. genitalis*) where their differentiation from *T. pallidum* is of importance in the diagnosis of primary syphilis.

TREPONEMA PALLIDUM

Morphology and staining

A very delicate, spiral filament 6–14 μm (average 10 μm) by 0.2 μm, with 6–12 coils which are comparatively small, sharp and regular; the length of the coils is about 1 μm and the depth 1–1.5 μm; the ends are pointed and tapering. A capsular or slime layer has been observed occasionally on the surface of *T. pallidum* and may explain the lack of serological reactivity of organisms freshly isolated from animal tissues. A multilayered membrane, referred to as the outer envelope or outer membrane, encloses the cell; the viability of spirochaetes is dependent on an intact outer envelope.

Inside the outer envelope lie the axial filaments or internal flagella (Johnson 1977); these are presumed to be responsible for motility although there is no direct evidence for this. Spirochaetes show rotary corkscrew-like motility and also movements of flexion; angulation, with the organism bending almost to 90° near its centre, is highly characteristic of *T. pallidum*. Its progression is relatively slow compared to that of many motile bacteria.

T. pallidum is feebly refractile and darkground illumination is normally used to visualize the organism. It cannot be seen by ordinary staining methods; special techniques such as silver impregnation may be used to demonstrate the organism, particularly in tissue, but this tends to alter the morphology. Immunofluorescent methods can now be used to detect treponemes in tissues and body fluids.

Cultivation

The Nichols strain of *T. pallidum* was isolated in 1913 from the CSF of a patient with neurosyphilis; it is still virulent for man and is maintained in rabbits by intratesticular inoculation and weekly passage. It divides by binary fission approximately once every 30 h when environmental conditions are favourable. It is generally agreed that pathogenic *T. pallidum* has not been cultivated in artificial media, embryonated eggs or tissue cultures. However, there is now a better understanding of the conditions that permit prolonged survival of treponemes in vitro, with retention of their pathogenicity for animals. Pathogenic treponemes (unlike cultivable non-pathogens) attach themselves to mammalian cells in culture. The discovery that *T. pallidum* is microaerophilic rather than a strict anaerobe has aided the prolonged survival of these microorganisms in vitro.

The genetic relationships between *T. pallidum* and cultivable treponemes have been studied by reassociation assays with ^{125}I-labelled treponemal DNA (Miao & Feldsteel 1978). Three groups were distinguished: virulent Nichols strain of *T. pallidum*; *T. phagedenis* and its biotype Reiter; and *T. refringens*. Features such as the diameter and amplitude of the spiral, the number of axial filaments and the presence of intracytoplasmic microtubules can be used to differentiate between the pathogenic non-cultivable treponemes, which have similar if not identical morphology, and the cultivable treponemes (Hovind-Hougan 1976).

Sensitivity to physical and chemical agents

T. pallidum is so feebly viable outwith its host that syphilis is ordinarily acquired only by sexual intercourse. The organism dies rapidly in water and is very sensitive to drying. However, it can remain viable and maintain its virulence in necropsy material for some time at room temperature, and in serum kept in sealed capillary tubes it remains motile for several days. It is readily killed by heat, e.g. 41.5°C for 1 h. When infected blood is stored at 5°C in citrate anticoagulant, infectivity is lost in 120 h or less. Treponemes survive for only a few days or weeks at −10 to −20°C but remain viable for extended periods at −45°C and for an indefinite period when stored at −78°C. Freezing followed by desiccation (freeze-drying) kills the organism.

Antibiotic sensitivity

Penicillin remains the drug of choice in treating syphilis. Therapeutic regimens for early syphilis should aim to maintain a minimum serum penicillin concentration of 0.03 units/ml for a period of 10–15 days. Tetracycline or erythromycin appear to be effective in patients who are hypersensitive to penicillin but results have not been evaluated as fully as for penicillin.

Although *T. pallidum* is extremely sensitive to penicillin (healing of lesions occurs rapidly and treponemes disappear from early stage lesions), biological cure (i.e. eradication of treponemes) is difficult to prove since *T. pallidum* cannot be cultured in vitro. In a few patients who have been adequately treated with penicillin, residual *T. pallidum* has been detected in CSF, lymph nodes, etc. by electron microscopy; in a very few cases some of these treponemes were inoculated into rabbits and produced typical lesions. In such cases the surviving treponemes remained penicillin sensitive and these patients may be considered to indicate treatment failure, probably due to abnormal penicillin metabolism in the patients ('quick penicillin secretors'), rather than acquired drug resistance.

Animal pathogenicity

Intratesticular injection leads to a syphilitic orchitis in rabbits; intradermal inoculation also produces lesions. Experimentally infected rabbits have been widely used to test various antisyphilitic drugs and to study the immune response to *T. pallidum*. Monkeys and anthropoid apes can also be infected experimentally. At present the only source of *T. pallidum* for preparing antigens and for experimental work is from the testes of infected rabbits. Recently, however, *T. pallidum* antigens have been expressed in *Escherichia coli* after gene cloning (Dallas et al 1987).

Laboratory diagnosis of syphilis

The clinical diagnosis of syphilis is confirmed in the laboratory by (1) demonstrating *T. pallidum* in the exudates from the lesions, or (2) demonstrating antibodies in the serum.

Darkground microscopy

The infectious stages of treponemal infections can usually be diagnosed most quickly and effectively by the demonstration of motile treponemes in wet preparations of serous exudate expressed from suspected primary and secondary lesions. Where topical antibiotics have been used, examination of material obtained by lymph gland puncture may prove useful.

As there is a serious risk of infection it is important to use gloves when obtaining material for darkground microscopy. After cleansing the surface of the lesion with a swab soaked in sterile saline, serum is squeezed by gentle pressure from the depth of the lesion. This serum may be collected directly on a glass coverslip or, if this is difficult, in a glass capillary tube. One end of the capillary is heated to expel fluid neatly on to the centre of a coverslip, which is then positioned on a slide. After firmly pressing the coverslip and slide between pieces of filter paper, the preparation can be examined by darkground illumination using the oil immersion objective.

T. pallidum is recognized by its slender structure, characteristic slow movements and angulation. It must be carefully distinguished from other treponemes that may occur in genital ulcers, but these tend to be surface organisms and are not found in the depth of the lesions. If the initial test is negative the procedure should be repeated daily for at least 3 days; antibiotics should be withheld during this period although sulphadimidine and local saline lavage may be used to reduce local sepsis. Since many commensal treponemes occur in the mouth, darkground microscopy is not suitable for examining oral lesions. Organisms are not easily found in skin lesions of secondary syphilis except those in moist skin areas.

A more definite approach to diagnosis is provided by *immunofluorescence staining*. A smear of the material to be tested is made on a glass slide, fixed and sent to the laboratory. The smear is then stained with fluorescein-labelled antibody specific for *T. pallidum* and examined

by fluorescence microscopy (Daniels & Ferneyhaugh 1977). More recently, fluorescein-labelled pathogen-specific monoclonal antibodies have been used to identify *T. pallidum* in lesions (Lukehart & Baker-Zander 1988).

Serological diagnosis of syphilis

There is no demonstrable immunological difference between the treponemes responsible for syphilis, yaws or pinta. Although this should not often give rise to problems in the UK the possibility should be borne in mind with patients from areas where these diseases are endemic.

The various methods used to measure antibody responses in treponemal infection can be divided into two major categories: (1) tests to measure antibodies produced against non-specific treponemal antigens, i.e. the cardiolipin or lipoidal antigen tests, formerly referred to as 'reagin' tests; and (2) tests to measure antibodies against antigens specific for pathogenic treponemes, i.e. the *T. pallidum* haemagglutination assay (TPHA) and the fluorescent antibody absorbed test (FTA-ABS).

Cardiolipin antigen tests. Cardiolipin, a complex diphospholipid, is widespread in nature and can be isolated from many mammalian tissues as well as from treponemes. Cardiolipin for use as antigen is traditionally prepared from mammalian tissues such as beef heart. Only a few of the numerous tests for detection of antibodies to cardiolipin antigen are still widely used. The classical Wassermann complement fixation test has decreased markedly in popularity as it offers no advantage over the modern flocculation tests, such as the Venereal Diseases Research Laboratory (VDRL) test.* The World Health Organization (1982) now recommends that complement fixation tests should be discontinued; the VDRL test is simpler, quicker and cheaper to perform and should be adopted as standard.

In the rapid plasma reagin (RPR) test,* VDRL antigen is suspended in choline chloride and mixed with finely divided carbon particles,

---

* Refer to *Methods* at end of this chapter.

enabling the test to be performed on unheated serum or plasma and read with the naked eye. A fingerprick blood sample can be tested on plastic or paper cards, making the RPR test particularly suitable for use in field studies in developing countries. The test can also be automated for use in centres where large numbers of specimens must be tested.

Because of their simplicity and accuracy, the cardiolipin antigen tests are used as screening or first-line procedures for both routine diagnosis and mass screening programmes. These tests usually become positive 10–14 days after the appearance of the chancre, the titre gradually increasing. The titre diminishes and the test tends to become negative after treatment. In late or latent syphilis the cardiolipin antigen tests are often negative.

Since these tests detect antibodies against a non-specific antigen shared by treponemes and mammalian tissues a positive result is sometimes obtained with sera from healthy individuals or patients without clinical evidence of syphilis; these reactions are termed Biological False Positives (BFP). Tests using specific *T. pallidum* antigen are required to distinguish between positive cardiolipin antigen tests resulting from BFP reactions and those due to treponemal infection.

T. pallidum haemagglutination assay. The TPHA* is very simple to perform and was the first of the specific tests suitable for routine screening. It is often negative in untreated primary syphilis (possibly owing to variability in the IgM-binding capacity of the TPHA reagent). For all other stages of syphilis, the sensitivity of the TPHA is comparable to that of the FTA-ABS (see below). Occasionally, false positive haemagglutination may result from heterophile antibody in the serum of patients with infectious mononucleosis. (This occurs only if the control cells fail to agglutinate, otherwise a non-specific agglutination reaction would be recorded.) In certain tropical countries a small percentage of BFP reactors have also given apparent false positive TPHA results; because of the sensitivity of the test, these could represent the residue of previous infection with endemic treponematosis.

Fluorescent antibody absorbed test. In the FTA-ABS test*, binding of specific antibody by *T. pallidum* is demonstrated by the indirect immunofluorescence technique. The FTA-ABS is an accepted reference test and is highly specific and sensitive at all stages of syphilitic infection although a small percentage of false positive reactions occur, e.g. in patients with systemic lupus erythematosus and other connective tissue diseases.

Other serological tests. The *T. pallidum immobilization* (TPI) test (Nelson & Mayer 1949) was the first to use specific treponemal antigen but it has been superseded by the TPHA and FTA-ABS tests (Rein et al 1980; Sprott et al 1982). Because the TPI test employs live treponemes it is time-consuming, expensive and technically demanding. A few reference laboratories still perform the TPI test on selected sera for research purposes.

The *Reiter protein complement fixation* (RPCF) test detects antibodies produced against a group-specific treponemal antigen shared by pathogenic and commensal treponemes. Since the Reiter treponeme can be grown in relatively simple media sufficient antigen can readily be obtained for large scale screening. The RPCF test has now been superseded by the TPHA. The role of the enzyme-linked immunosorbent assay (ELISA) in the serological diagnosis of syphilis remains to be evaluated (Veldkamp & Visser 1975; Pope et al 1982).

A more detailed discussion of tests available for diagnosis of syphilis is given by Luger (1988) and Robertson et al (1988b).

Interpretation of serological tests

The pattern of results obtained with the VDRL, TPHA and FTA-ABS tests may give valuable information as to the stage of infection. Table 40.1 provides a guide, but it is important to remember that each case must be interpreted individually in the light of available clinical and epidemiological data. Because of the serious social and medical implications, a diagnosis of syphilis should never be made from the results of a single blood specimen.

Table 40.1 Pattern of results of serological tests in different stages of acquired syphilis.
Key: +, positive; −, negative; −/+, often negative but may be positive at low titre. *Note*: in endemic treponemal diseases such as yaws, bejel or pinta, patterns are similar to syphilis.

VDRL	TPHA	FTA-ABS	Interpretation
+	−	−	False positive reaction; repeat to exclude primary infection
+	−/+	+	Primary infection; dark-ground investigation of lesion may be positive
+	+	+	Untreated (or recently treated); probably beyond primary stage
−	+	+	Treated or partially treated at any stage; untreated latent or late
−	+	−	History of treated syphilis

Quantitative test results may also prove helpful. During the primary stage of infection the VDRL titre rises to 8 or 16. VDRL tests with titres of 16–128 are commonly found in secondary syphilis and active cardiovascular or neurosyphilis. After the secondary stage the VDRL titre declines and eventually becomes negative in *c*. 30% of untreated latent and late cases.

The TPHA test is often negative in early primary syphilis but may become positive at low titre (80–320) towards the end of the primary stage. Titres rise sharply during the secondary stage and commonly reach 5120 or greater. The TPHA titre declines during the latent stage but invariably remains positive at low titre (80–640).

Response to treatment. The cardiolipin antigen tests primarily reflect disease activity. These tests tend to become negative after treatment, particularly in early syphilis. Serial quantitative VDRL testing provides the best means of measuring response to treatment in most stages of treponemal infection.

Differentiation of treated, partially treated and untreated syphilis. The TPHA and FTA-ABS tests usually remain positive for life, even in those who have been fully treated with adequate doses of penicillin. On the premise that detection

of specific anti-treponemal IgM will denote active syphilis, several methods for demonstrating specific IgM antibodies have been investigated.

One of the most widely used methods relies on the detection of anti-treponemal IgM with monospecific fluorescein-labelled anti-human immunoglobulin in the FTA-ABS test. The performance of this test with unfractionated serum (the IgM-FTA-ABS test) is unsatisfactory as false positive and false negative results are common. Reliable results are obtained when 19S (IgM) antibodies are separated from those of the 7S (IgG) class by gel filtration before performing the test; this test is known as the 19S-IgM-FTA. However this is a time-consuming and technically demanding procedure and is normally restricted to research and reference laboratories. Simpler methods of detecting specific IgM by haemagglutination and enzyme-linked immunosorbent assays are being investigated (Luger 1988).

Serological screening

The continuous serological screening of pregnant women, blood donors and 'at risk' groups is helpful in the detection and control of syphilis. When used together, the VDRL and TPHA tests provide a highly efficient screen for the detection or exclusion of treponemal infection; both are simple to perform and can be readily quantitated. Their activity is complementary; the VDRL test is more sensitive than the TPHA in the detection of very early syphilis while the TPHA is more sensitive than the VDRL in the detection of latent and late infection. The FTA-ABS is not suitable for screening large numbers of sera but should be used as a confirmatory test when one of the screening tests is positive. When both screening tests are unequivocally positive further testing is not essential but a confirmatory FTA-ABS test is usually done if available.

Congenital syphilis

Early-stage congenital syphilis is a rarity in the UK and there are few up-to-date serological data available. Since IgM antibodies do not cross the intact placenta a reliable method for demonstrating specific IgM antibodies should indicate active infection of the neonate. Also, antibody titres will rise if a baby has been infected, whereas in the absence of infection, e.g. when the mother has been treated during pregnancy, passively transferred antibody detected by the VDRL will decrease in titre and the test will become negative in approximately 3 months; owing to their greater sensitivity treponemal antigen tests usually take slightly longer to become negative.

Diagnosis of neurosyphilis: examination of CSF

The use of CSF for routine screening tests in patients in whom there is no clinical suspicion of syphilis is unjustified; a negative TPHA test on the blood will virtually exclude active neurosyphilis and is a better screen for the detection of all forms of late syphilis.

However, in cases selected on clinical grounds backed by a positive TPHA test on blood, investigations should be carried out on the CSF to detect early invasion of the central nervous system (CNS). A total volume of 8–10 ml is usually sufficient to carry out the necessary tests; note that contamination of the CSF specimen with even a small amount of blood can give misleading results.

Investigation of the CSF should include a cell count, estimation of total protein and estimation of IgG and IgM. Cell counts exceeding 5 cells/mm^3 (5×10^6/litre) and total protein values above 40 mg/100 ml are signs of inflammation but are non-specific as indicators of syphilitic involvement of the nervous system. Specific tests such as the VDRL, TPHA and FTA-ABS should also be performed.

The VDRL test alone is not a reliable indicator of CNS involvement since it is non-reactive in 30–60% of patients with active neurosyphilis. However, a negative TPHA test in CSF excludes neurosyphilis. A positive TPHA or FTA-ABS test in CSF does not necessarily indicate active disease, since reactivity may be caused by transudation of immunoglobulins from the serum into the CSF. The TPHA index, which relates CSF TPHA titre to the albumin quotient (CSF

albumin concentration $\times$ 10^3/serum albumin concentration), should help exclude errors associated with disturbed function of the blood-brain barrier. The TPHA index and methods for the demonstration of specific IgM antibodies in CSF are being evaluated as indicators of active neurosyphilis (Luger 1988).

Thus, although active neurosyphilis can be excluded reliably and simply by a negative TPHA test result on the CSF, unequivocal serological evidence of CNS involvement is essentially a procedure for a specialized laboratory.

METHODS

The Venereal Diseases Research Laboratory (VDRL) test

This simple flocculation test of high sensitivity can be performed as a tube test but is more widely employed as a micro-slide test. A macroscopic test using carbon antigen is increasing in popularity.

Preparation of the specimen. Transfer a portion of serum from 5–10 ml of clotted blood into a clean tube. Heat in a waterbath at 56°C for 30 min and allow to return to room temperature before testing. Sera that are excessively haemolysed, grossly contaminated with bacteria, or very turbid are unsatisfactory for testing. Specimens to be tested more than 4 h after the original heating period should be reheated at 56°C for 10 min. Sera need not be heated for testing with carbon antigen.

Preparation of the antigen. VDRL antigen is a colourless alcoholic solution containing cardiolipin (0.03%), lecithin (c. 0.2%) and cholesterol (0.9%). The antigen is widely available commercially in a variety of volumes; vials containing 0.5 ml are most convenient for the majority of laboratories. Buffered saline diluent is also available commercially and contains: 37% (w/v) formaldehyde neutral reagent, 0.5 ml; Na_2HPO_4 (anhydrous), 0.037 g; KH_2PO_4, 0.15 g; NaCl, 10 g; distilled water, 1000 ml. The diluent has a pH of 6.0 ± 0.1.

1. Pipette 0.4 ml of buffered saline into a 30 ml round bottle.

2. Add 0.5 ml of antigen (from the lower half of a 1 ml pipette graduated to the tip) directly on to the saline while continuously but gently rotating the bottle on a flat surface; the antigen should be added over a period of approximately 6 s.

3. Blow the last drop of antigen from the pipette without the pipette touching the diluent and continue to rotate for 10 s.

4. Add 4.1 ml of buffered saline from a 5 ml pipette.

5. Replace the top on the bottle and mix well by inverting approximately 30 times in 10 s.

The antigen suspension must be used only on the day that it is prepared; the amount (5 ml) is sufficient for approximately 250 tests. Check each batch of antigen with sera known to give negative, weak positive and positive reactions as defined below.

Carbon antigen (RPR) which requires no prior preparation can be obtained commercially (RPR Card Test Antigen, Gibco). It should be stored at 4°C but it is essential to allow the antigen to reach room temperature before use.

VDRL screening test

Screening tests can be carried out on glass slides (10 × 5 cm), each with six paraffin-ringed or ceramic-ringed areas; slides with concavities, wells, or glass rings are not recommended. Oxford-type pipettes and disposable plastic tips are convenient for measuring volumes.

1. Add 60 μl of serum to a clean glass slide.

2. Add 20 μl of antigen to the serum.

3. Mix with a wooden stick and rotate slide for 4 min; mechanical rotators should be set at about 180 rpm.

4. Read and test microscopically with a × 10 eyepiece and × 10 objective immediately after rotation.

Read the screening test as follows: *negative*, smooth homogeneous particles of antigen; *weak positive*, small clumps of antigen with little or no background clearing; *positive*, large clumps of antigen with marked background clearing. Any specimen giving a weak positive or positive reaction should then be tested quantitatively. Occasionally a test result will be intermediate between negative and weak positive; any serum giving this 'rough' type of reaction should also be tested quantitatively in case of a prozone reaction (Ch. 10).

The test with *carbon antigen* is usually performed on disposable plastic cards (12.5 × 7 cm), each with 10 clearly defined test areas. Volumes of antigen and serum remain the same but the shaking time is extended to 8 min and the test is read macroscopically.

Quantitative VDRL tests

When performing quantitative tests it is a useful check to return to the original blood tube and remove additional serum. This should be heated at 56°C for 30 min as before.

1. Place 100 μl of 0.9% saline in five tubes (7 × 1 cm) for each serum to be tested.

2. Add 100 μl of serum to the first tube and double dilute to give a range of dilutions from 1 in 2 to 1 in 32.

3. Test the serum and dilutions as for the screening test (see above). Any serum giving a positive reaction at a dilution of 1 in 32 should be further diluted and retested to determine the endpoint.

Test results are reported as follows: *borderline reaction*, a weak positive reaction with undiluted serum and a negative reaction with all dilutions; *positive undiluted serum*, a positive reaction with undiluted serum and a weak positive or negative reaction with dilutions; *positive 2, 4, 8*, etc, titre reported as the last serum dilution to give a positive reaction.

The Treponema pallidum haemagglutination (TPHA) test

In this test sheep erythrocytes coated with an extract of *T. pallidum* are agglutinated by antibody from the serum of patients with syphilis. To eliminate non-specific reactions, sera are first absorbed with a special diluent containing soni-cated cell membranes from sheep and ox erythrocytes, normal rabbit testicular extract, sonicated Reiter treponemes, normal rabbit serum, Tween 80 and acacia powder. The following method employs commercial reagents supplied by the Fujizoki Pharmaceutical Company, Tokyo, Japan (distributed in the UK by Mast). Each kit comprises lyophilized test (antigen-coated) and control cells, absorbing diluent and a reactive control serum. (Reagents based on fowl erythrocytes are also available commercially from Whitley and from Wellcome.)

Preparation of the specimen. Prepare heat-inactivated serum as for the VDRL test (the TPHA may be performed without heat inactivation but the pattern of haemagglutination is more distinct with heated serum).

Preparation of the reagents. Kits with different volumes of reagents are available and enable approximately 100–500 screening tests to be carried out.

1. Rehydrate test and control cells with the specified volume of sterile distilled water, mix thoroughly and allow to stand at room temperature for 1 h.

2. Prepare the working dilutions of test and control cells by adding 1 volume of the rehydrated suspension to 5.5 volumes of absorbing diluent.

3. Rehydrate reactive control serum with 1 ml of sterile distilled water.

Reconstituted reagents should be stored at 2–10°C and used within 5 days. Working dilutions of test and control cells should be stored at 2–10°C and used within 1 day.

TPHA screening test

All sera are screened at a 1 in 80 final serum dilution against sensitized (test) cells only. Specimens giving positive or doubtful reactions are then tested quantitatively and also checked for non-specific agglutination with non-sensitized (control) cells. By using only the first 10 wells of alternate rows of a microtitre plate, 40 specimens are conveniently tested on a single plate, leaving sufficient space for appropriate controls.

1. Prepare a 1 in 20 dilution of inactivated serum in a tube by mixing 10 μl serum and 190 μl absorbing diluent. Leave for 30 min at room temperature to absorb.

2. Transfer 20 μl of absorbed serum to the 1st well of a U-type microtitre plate.

3. Transfer 60 μl of test cells to each absorbed serum: the final serum dilution is now 1 in 80.

4. Set up a negative control by treating a known non-reactive serum as above.

5. Determine the titre of the reactive control serum. Place 20 μl of diluent in wells 2–6 of a row. Add 20 μl of reactive control serum to wells 1 and 2. Double dilute from well 2 through to well 6, discarding the last 20 μl. Add 60 μl of test cells to wells 1–6. (Since the positive serum is prediluted to 1 in 80 the final serum dilutions range from 1 in 320 to 1 in 10 240.)

6. Set up a reagent control well containing 20 μl test cells and 60 μl absorbing diluent.

7. Mix the contents of each well by shaking the plate gently. Alternatively place the plate on a Microtiter Microshaker (Denley) for 20 s. Leave plates undisturbed at room temperature for at least 4 h; overnight incubation is often convenient.

Examine individual wells and record the degree of haemagglutination, if any, as follows: +++, smooth mat of agglutinated cells covering more or less the entire bottom of the well; ++, smooth mat of agglutinated cells with a narrow red circle near the perimeter of the agglutination; +, small smooth mat of agglutinated cells with a thicker red circle near the perimeter of the agglutination; ±, a slightly enlarged ring of cells surrounded by a rough margin; −, definite compact button of cells in the centre of the well, with or without a very small 'hole' in the centre. Results for a batch of screening tests are valid only if the negative control serum and the reagent control set up with test cells give a negative reaction and the reactive control serum gives a positive (+) reaction within one doubling dilution of 1 in 2560.

Although specimens giving + to +++ reactions are considered positive they must be tested against control cells to confirm the specific nature of the haemagglutination. This is normally carried out at the same time as the quantitative test. Specimens giving doubtful (±) reactions should also be tested quantitatively.

Quantitative TPHA test

Allow one row of a microtitre plate for each quantitative test.

1. Prepare a 1 in 20 dilution of inactivated serum by mixing 10 μl of serum and 190 μl of absorbing diluent.

2. Add 20 μl of absorbing diluent to wells 2–10, but miss out well 9.

3. Transfer 20 μl of the 1 in 20 diluted serum to wells 1, 2 and 10. Make a series of doubling dilutions from well 2 through to well 8 and discard 20 μl of diluted serum from well 8. Allow to absorb for 30 min at room temperature.

4. Add 60 μl of test cells to wells 1–8 and 60 μl non-sensitized (control) cells to well 10.

5. Set up controls for the sensitized (test) cells and non-sensitized (control) cells by mixing 20 μl of absorbing diluent and 60 μl of cells.

6. Set up a negative control and titrate the positive serum as for the screening test.

7. Allow to stand undisturbed at room temperature for 4 h and examine for haemagglutination.

Results for a batch of quantitative tests are valid only if cell, positive, and negative controls give the expected reactions (as defined for the screening tests). Individual test results are valid only if there is no agglutination of the control cells. Test results are reported as follows: *positive 80, 160, 320*, etc, titre reported as the last serum dilution to give a positive (+) reaction (see above); *negative*, any specimen giving a − or ± reaction at 1 in 80; *borderline reaction*, used for the very occasional specimen that gives a reaction intermediate between ± and +; *non-specific agglutination* (*test invalid*), any specimen causing agglutination of non-sensitized (control) cells.

Fluorescent treponemal antibody absorbed (FTA-ABS) test

In this test the patient's serum is absorbed with an autoclaved supernate from cultures of Reiter treponemes in order to remove group-specific antibody. Binding to *T. pallidum* of antibody specific for pathogenic treponemes is then demonstrated by the indirect immunofluorescence method.

Reagents. The following reagents for this test are widely available commercially (e.g. Wellcome).

1. Phosphate buffered saline (PBS) pH 7.6 (NaCl, 8.5 g; Na_2HPO_4, 1.28 g; $NaH_2PO_4.2H_2O$, 0.156 g; distilled water, 1000 ml).

2. Treponemal antigen (lyophilized suspension of the Nichols strain of *T. pallidum*).

3. Known strongly reactive serum.

4. Known minimally reactive serum.

5. Non-specific serum: a non-syphilitic serum which is reactive when diluted in PBS but negative when diluted in sorbent.

6. Sorbent: a product prepared from cultures of Reiter treponemes.

7. Fluorescent anti-human immunoglobulin reagent.

8. Acetone.

9. Buffered glycerol mounting fluid (1 volume PBS, pH 7.2 + 9 volumes glycerol). A commercial product, Bacto FA Mounting Fluid (Difco), may also be used.

Preparation of antigen smears. PTFE-coated 'multispot' slides with a dark background containing 12 wells, each 3 mm in diameter, are available from Hendley.

1. Place eight slides in a staining dish and cover with absolute alcohol for 1 h to remove grease; pour off alcohol and allow slides to dry.

2. Reconstitute a vial of treponemal antigen with 1 ml sterile distilled water. Break up any clumps in the antigen suspension by repeated aspiration into a syringe fitted with a 25 gauge needle.

3. Transfer 10 μl of antigen suspension to each well of the multispot slides.

4. Allow smears to stand for 5 min at room temperature, remove excess liquid from each well and allow to dry completely for a further 10–15 min.

5. Place slides in a staining dish and fix by covering with acetone for 10 min.

6. Pour off acetone and allow smears to dry in air.

This procedure should give antigen smears with 50–100 evenly distributed treponemes per field when viewed at a magnification of × 400. Slides will keep for at least 6 months if stored at −20°C in airtight containers. Do not thaw and refreeze smears.

Method for the FTA-ABS test

1. Calculate how many antigen wells will be required for tests and controls and remove the appropriate number of slides from the freezer.

2. Inactivate test and control sera at 56°C for 30 min. If sera have already been heat treated, reheat for 10 min at 56°C.

3. Label one test tube to correspond to each serum being tested and place in a rack. Dilute test sera, and control sera known to give strong, weak and negative reactions, 1 in 5 in sorbent (10 μl serum + 40 μl sorbent).

4. Transfer 10 μl of each serum to an antigen well on the multispot slide; specimens can be identified on the slide by writing on the black background with a lead pencil.

5. Incubate at 37°C for 30 min in a humid atmosphere.

6. Place slides in slide carrier and rinse off excess serum with PBS. Wash slides in four changes of PBS for a total of 20 min, rinse in distilled water, blot gently and allow to dry in air.

7. Remove an aliquot of fluorescein-conjugated anti-human globulin from the freezer. Allow to thaw and dilute with PBS to give the predetermined working dilution (see below); add 10 μl to each antigen well.

8. Repeat steps (5) and (6).

9. Add a small drop of buffered glycerol mounting fluid to each well and apply a coverslip.

Results. Examine slides as soon as possible. (If a delay is necessary place slides in a darkened room and read within 4 h.) Locate treponemes using a high-power dry objective and darkground illumination before assessing the degree of fluorescence with a suitable optical system, e.g. a microscope fitted with an HBO 200 W lamp,

BG12 primary filter and OG4 and GG9 secondary filters. Positive reactions are shown by fluorescent treponemes, in contrast to almost invisible non-fluorescent organisms in negative reactions. Results are scored and reported as shown in Table 40.2.

The following additional controls should be set up when testing new batches of reagents (new reagents should be tested in parallel with the existing reagents): (a) *weak positive serum* diluted 1 in 5 in sorbent and 1 in 5 in PBS. These should give equivalent fluorescence, demonstrating the failure of sorbent to remove specific antibody which would give rise to false negative results with weak positive samples. (b) *Non-specific staining controls* comprising antigen + PBS + conjugate, and antigen + sorbent + conjugate. The non-specific serum should give a positive reaction (++) when diluted in PBS but a negative reaction when diluted in sorbent, demonstrating the efficacy of sorbent in inhibiting non-specific staining. Non-specific staining controls should always be negative.

Preparation of the working dilution of conjugate. An economical working dilution of the fluorescent antibody is the highest dilution which will give intense specific staining with negligible background staining. The approximate range of working dilutions of conjugate for use in the FTA-ABS test is stated by the manufacturer. Variations in the optical and test systems used in different laboratories make it desirable to

Table 40.2 Reporting of results in FTA-ABS test for antibody to *T. pallidum*.

Appearance of treponemes	Fluorescence score	Report
Brilliant green fluorescence	+++	Positive
Moderate to bright green fluorescence	++	Positive
Weak but definite uniform green fluorescence, equivalent to weakly reactive control	+	Weak positive
Weak but definite fluorescence, less than weakly reactive control	±	Borderline reaction
No fluorescence, treponemes vaguely visible or completely invisible	−	Negative

confirm the most suitable working dilution by titration under local conditions.

1. Rehydrate the contents of a vial of fluorescein-labelled anti-human globulin with 1 ml sterile distilled water. Mix the contents thoroughly by swirling gently and allow to dissolve slowly; vigorous action is not recommended.

2. Prepare a series of doubling dilutions of conjugate in PBS to cover the range of approximate working dilutions, e.g. 1 in 10 to 1 in 2560.

3. Test each conjugate dilution, and the existing batch of conjugate at its working dilution, with the strong positive, weak positive and negative sera by the standard FTA-ABS procedure.

4. Include a non-specific staining control (antigen + PBS) for each conjugate dilution.

5. Read the slides and determine the endpoint of the titration, i.e. the highest dilution of conjugate giving strong (+++) fluorescence. The working dilution of the new conjugate is one doubling dilution below the endpoint. This dilution should give acceptable fluorescence (+) with the weakly reactive serum. If it does not, repeat the titration with a series of intermediate dilutions, e.g. 1 in 15 to 1 in 1920. The conjugate must not stain non-specifically at 3 doubling dilutions below the working dilution.

6. Aliquot undiluted conjugate in amounts suitable for 1 day's testing when diluted to the working dilution and store at −20°C. Do not refreeze after thawing.

Note: Commercial kits containing all of the necessary reagents and controls, pre-tested and ready for use, are now available.

REFERENCES

Dallas W S et al 1987 Identification and purification of a recombinant *Treponema pallidum* basic membrane protein antigen expressed in *Escherichia coli*. Infection and Immunity 55: 1106–1115

Daniels K C, Ferneyhaugh H S 1977 Specific direct fluorescent antibody detection of *Treponema pallidum*. Health Laboratory Science 14: 164–171

Hovind-Hougan K 1976 Determination by means of electron microscopy of morphological criteria of value for classification of some spirochaetes, in particular treponemes. Acta Pathologica et Microbiologica Scandinavica Sect B Suppl 225: 1–41

Johnson R R 1977 The spirochaetes. Annual Review of Microbiology 31: 89–106

Luger A 1988 Serological diagnosis of syphilis: current methods. In: Young H, McMillan A (eds) Immunological diagnosis of sexually transmitted diseases. Marcel Dekker, New York. p 249–274

Lukehart S A, Baker-Zander S A 1988 Diagnostic potential of monoclonal antibodies against *Treponema pallidum*. In: Young H, McMillan A (eds) Immunological diagnosis of sexually transmitted diseases. Marcel Dekker, New York. p 213–247

Miao R, Feldsteel A H 1978 Genetics of treponema: relationship between *Treponema pallidum* and five cultivable treponemes. Journal of Bacteriology 133: 101–107

Nelson R A, Mayer M M 1949 Immobilization of *Treponema pallidum in vitro* by antibody produced in syphilitic infection. Journal of Experimental Medicine 89: 369–393

Pope V, Hunter E F, Feeley J C 1982 Evaluation of the microenzyme-linked immunosorbent assay with *Treponema pallidum* antigen. Journal of Clinical Microbiology 15: 630–634

Rein M F et al 1980 Failure of the *Treponema pallidum* immobilization test to provide additional diagnostic information about contemporary problem sera. Sexually Transmitted Diseases 7: 101–105

Robertson D H H, McMillan A, Young H 1988a Syphilis: introduction. In: Clinical practice in sexually transmissible diseases. Churchill Livingstone, Edinburgh Ch. 7.

Robertson D H H, McMillan A, Young H 1988b Diagnosis of syphilis. In: Clinical practice in sexually transmissible diseases. Churchill Livingstone, Edinburgh Ch. 8.

Sprott M S, Selkon J B, Turner R H 1982 Evaluation of the role of the *Treponema pallidum* immobilization test in Britain. British Journal of Venereal Diseases 58: 147–148

Veldkamp J, Visser A M 1975 Application of the enzyme-linked immunosorbent assay (ELISA) in the serodiagnosis of syphilis. British Journal of Venereal Diseases 51: 227–231

World Health Organization 1982 Treponemal infections. Technical Report Series 674, WHO, Geneva. p 27

Leptospira: Borrelia

Leptospira and *Borrelia* are two of the genera of medical importance which, along with *Treponema* (Ch. 40), make up the group known as the Spirochaetes.

LEPTOSPIRA

Members of the genus *Leptospira* differ from other spirochaetes morphologically, in their type of motility and in the ease with which they can be cultured. Some leptospires are free-living saprophytes, commonly found in fresh water and occasionally in brackish and even salt water. Others are parasitic and potentially pathogenic organisms that are normally carried by wild vertebrate animals, especially rodents. Under certain conditions they may be transmitted accidentally to man and domestic animals, causing leptospirosis with clinical manifestations of varying degrees of severity. Characteristically the disease in man occurs as a haemorrhagic jaundice, Weil's disease, but a febrile anicteric syndrome is common, sometimes with meningitis as a prominent feature. Subclinical cases are common in certain occupational groups, e.g. agricultural workers, where the risk of infection from animal sources is high.

When working with leptospira standard safety precautions should be observed as indicated in Chapter 15. Care should be taken not to contaminate the skin with leptospiral cultures or with blood or urine of infected animals. Cuts and abrasions should be covered. If accidental contact takes place with the likelihood of infection, a course of penicillin should be started without delay (dose at least 2 g/day for 5 days).

Before treatment, obtain a sample of blood. If fever subsequently develops a second sample should be taken and tested with the first against the relevant serovar. A rise in antibody titre would confirm infection.

Two species of *Leptospira* are recognized, *L. interrogans*, which includes those leptospires that are parasitic and potentially pathogenic, and *L. biflexa*, that comprises all free-living, non-pathogenic strains. The two species are morphologically similar but can be distinguished by the ability of *L. biflexa* to grow at temperatures as low as 13°C and by its resistance to 8-azaguanine (225 μg/ml). Parasitic leptospires do not grow at low temperatures and are usually sensitive to 8-azaguanine.

Morphology and motility

Darkfield microscopy is required in order to see leptospires in the living state. They are recognizable in clinical specimens such as blood, urine and CSF as spiral organisms, 6–20 μm (average 10 μm) in length, 0.1–0.3 μm in diameter and 0.3–0.5 μm in wavelength. They have numerous closely wound primary coils, so closely set together that they are difficult to demonstrate in stained preparations although they are quite obvious in the living state by darkfield microscopy ($\times$ 400). They are fairly rigid organisms with one or both ends hooked. As they move across the field, secondary coils appear and then disappear again, sometimes with a lashing motion. The movement of leptospires is characteristically vigorous, quite unlike the lazy undulating movement of other spirochaetes. In blood films or in semi-solid medium they show sinuous corkscrew-like movement, occasionally bending and straightening again into the characteristically rigid form. This detailed description of the movement of leptospires is important because, unless one is experienced in the work, it is easy to be misled by spiral artefacts that are normally present in blood films and which undulate as a result of Brownian movement. In case of doubt the film should be compared with a film of normal blood and, if possible, with one from a culture of leptospires in semi-solid medium.

Staining

It is not easy to stain leptospires satisfactorily with the usual bacterial stains, but they may be demonstrated by the silver impregnation methods of Levaditi and Fontana (Ch. 3). Faulkener & Lillie's modification of the Warthin-Starry silver impregnation technique is recommended for demonstrating leptospires in sections of infected tissue (Faine 1965).

Cultural characters

Aerobic: optimum temperature for growth 28–32°C: optimum pH 7.2. For routine purposes, liquid or semi-solid media are used; for cloning and research purposes, solid medium is sometimes used.

Liquid medium is used for growing leptospires intended for use as antigens in serological tests. It consists of a buffered salts base with or without peptone, to which is added either rabbit serum, as in Stuart's or Korthof's medium*, or preferably serum derivatives as in Ellinghausen & McCullough's (EM) medium* in which bovine serum albumin (fraction V) and polysorbate (Tween 80) replace whole serum.

Semi-solid medium is prepared by adding 0.2–0.5% (w/v) agar to any suitable liquid medium. Agar appears to favour the multiplication of leptospires and semi-solid medium is used when attempting the isolation of leptospires from blood or urine of patients or from animal

tissues. It has the added advantage that it evaporates less rapidly than liquid medium and helps to maintain the virulence of freshly isolated strains since less frequent subculture is required. It is also used for preparing cultures intended for intravenous inoculation into rabbits for production of hyperimmune serum. A simple semi-solid medium is Fletcher's medium* which consists of nutrient agar and rabbit serum.

Solid culture medium is used for cloning and other specialized purposes. Leptospires produce discrete hemispherical colonies just below the surface of the medium in Petri dishes; they may be difficult to see without oblique light against a dark background. For best results seal the plates to prevent evaporation and incubate at 28–32°C in a moist chamber or in a polythene bag. Keep the plates for at least 6 weeks before discarding them as negative; the colonies are slow to develop (Cox & Larson 1957; Cox 1966).

Survival

Pathogenic leptospires do not multiply readily outside the animal body although they may survive for many days if the external conditions are favourable. They require moisture and since they are particularly sensitive to acid seldom remain viable for long where the pH of the water or soil is less than 6.8. Salt water has a deleterious effect. They die out rapidly in urine, sewage and badly polluted water. They are susceptible to heat; 10 min at 50°C or 10 s at 60°C kills them. Rapidly killed by bile or trypsin, hypochlorite detergents, desiccation, and by exposure to pH values outside the range 6.2–8.0.

They may survive for a time in infected animal tissue at low temperatures. Thus guinea-pig liver has remained infective for up to 26 days at 4°C, and for 100 days at −20°C; leptospires of the pathogenic serovar *canicola* have been cultured from pigs' kidneys on sale in a butcher's shop.

Sensitivity to antibiotics

Leptospires have been shown by culture and animal experiments to be sensitive to penicillin, streptomycin and the tetracyclines. Penicillin has

* Refer to *Methods* at end of this chapter.

Table 41.1 Serogroups and subserogroups of *Leptospira interrogans* with a few of the more important serovars they contain and the reference strains used in the identification of isolates and in the serological diagnosis of leptospirosis of man and animals.

Serogroup	Serovar	Reference strain	Some animals from which the serovar has been isolated
Australis	*australis*	Ballico	Rats, field mice, hedgehogs
	bratislava	Jez Bratislava	Hedgehogs, pigs
Autumnalis	*autumnalis*	Akiyami A	Voles, field mice
Ballum	*ballum*	Mus 127	House mice
	castellonis	Castellon 3	Pigs
	arborea	Arborea	Field mice
Bataviae	*bataviae*	Van Tienen	Rats, voles, field mice, cats
Canicola	*canicola*	Hond Utrecht 1V	Dogs, pigs, jackals
	schuffneri	Vleermuis 90 C	Bats
Celledoni	*celledoni*	Celledoni	Not known
Cynopteri	*cynopteri*	3522 C	Bats
Djasiman	*djasiman*	Djasiman	Rats
Grippotyphosa	*grippotyphosa*	Moskva V	Voles, field mice, cattle
	valbuzzi	Valbuzzi	Not known
Hebdomadis			
a. Hebdomadis	*hebdomadis*	Hebdomadis	Voles, field mice
b. Borincana	*borincana*	HS 622	Not known
Icterohaemorrhagiae	*icterohaemorrhagiae*	RGA	Rats, dogs
	copenhageni	M 20	Rats
Javanica	*javanica*	Veldrat Bataviae 46	Rats, cats
	poi	Poi	Shrews
Louisiana	*louisiana*	LSU 1945	Armadillos
Mini	*mini*	Sari	Rats, voles
	georgia	LT 117	Voles, field mice, raccoons
Panama	*panama*	CZ 214 K	Opossums
Pomona	*pomona*	Pomona	Pigs, cattle
Pyrogenes	*pyrogenes*	Salinem	Rats
Sejroe			
a. Sejroe	*sejroe*	M 84	Field mice
b. Saxkoebing	*saxkoebing*	Mus 24	House mice, field mice
c. Wolffi	*wolffi*	3705	Rats
Shermani	*shermani*	LT 821	Rats, opossums
Tarassovi	*tarassovi*	Perepelicin	Pigs

value as a therapeutic agent for man especially if given in large doses early in the course of the infection.

Serotyping

Within the two species there are many serotypes (now referred to as sero-varieties or serovars) that are distinguished by cross-agglutinin-absorption tests or by antigenic factor analysis (Kmety 1967). Some of the serovars are closely related because of common antigens and form clearly defined serogroups. A list of serovars of medical importance and the groups into which they fall was given by Dikken & Kmety (1978); a shortened and more up-to-date version is given in Table 41.1.

Laboratory diagnosis of leptospirosis

Because of the variability in the signs and symptoms of infection and the frequent absence of jaundice, leptospirosis cannot be diagnosed on clinical grounds alone but should be considered as a possibility in cases of undiagnosed pyrexia (PUO), especially if the patient's living and working conditions allow likely exposure to infection from animal sources, or if the patient has been swimming in or has accidentally fallen into fresh water in areas that harbour rodents and are liable to flooding.

Demonstration of leptospires

1. During the first week of illness the leptospires are present in the blood. They may be seen by darkfield microscopy, especially after differential centrifugation of the blood*. Daily culture of the blood* may result in isolation of the infecting strain. Leptospiraemia is rare after the eighth day. When there is strong evidence of infection, inoculation of laboratory animals* may be used for isolation of leptospires from the blood.

2. Leptospires may be found in the urine during the second week and intermittently for 4–6 weeks or even longer; they are most readily demonstrated during the second and third weeks. Examine the urine immediately after it has been voided; leptospires are sensitive to acid urine and are lysed by antibodies present in the urine. For microscopic examination, centrifuge a portion of freshly voided urine at 3000 rpm for 10 min and examine a drop of the sediment by darkfield microscopy (magnification × 400).

Also attempt urine culture* in semi-solid medium or by animal inoculation.

3. Identify newly isolated strains by immunization of rabbits and serological analysis.* These procedures are lengthy and may be difficult for the average laboratory; strains may be sent for identification to Leptospira Reference Laboratories recognized by the World Health Organization.

Serological diagnosis of leptospirosis

Antibodies are usually detectable in the serum towards the end of the first week after onset but this may be delayed until the second week. The level of antibody increases until the end of the third week and then begins to decline. Residual agglutinating antibody may remain detectable for many years after the patient's recovery. It is advisable to examine a specimen of serum during the early days of the illness and at intervals of 4–5 days thereafter, in order to demonstrate any rise (or fall) in antibody level which may confirm the diagnosis and eliminate the possibility that a single positive reaction reflects residual antibody.

Tests for detection of leptospiral antibodies in sera are of two kinds, genus-specific and serogroup-specific. Genus-specific tests are positive whatever the serovar of the infecting strain. They include complement fixation*; haemagglutination (HA) or haemolysis (HL) tests with sheep or human red cells treated with erythrocyte sensitizing substance (ESS) (Chang & McComb 1954; Sharp 1958); enzyme-linked immunosorbent assay (ELISA) (WHO 1982); and a macroscopic slide agglutination test* against a heated antigen preparation of the saprophytic strain Patoc 1 of serovar *patoc* which appears to contain a large amount of antigen common to all leptospires.

Serogroup-specific tests, on the other hand, are reactive mainly with strains of the same serogroup as the infecting strain. They comprise agglutination tests that are either macroscopic, i.e. read by the naked eye, as with Galton's slide test (Galton et al 1958), or microscopic*, read by darkfield microscopy at low magnification (× 100).

Since agglutinating antibodies of the IgG class remain detectable in the serum for many years after the infection has cleared it is important to demonstrate a rise (or fall) in antibody to confirm the diagnosis of current infection. On the other hand, complement fixing and macroscopically agglutinating antibodies are mainly IgM; they react in the acute stages of infection and decline thereafter. They are not usually detectable for more than a few months after recovery.

The ELISA test is used in some laboratories to detect leptospiral antibodies in human and animal sera. The test can assess separately the levels of specific IgM and IgG, thereby indicating the likely stage of the infection. For details refer to World Health Organization (1982).

BORRELIA

Some of the members of this genus are commensals on the mucous membranes of healthy individuals; others are pathogenic to man. Borrelias that cause relapsing fever are blood parasites that are transmitted among animals of various species and from animals to man by ticks, e.g. *B. duttoni*, or from man to man by the body louse, e.g. *B. recurrentis*. One species, *B. vincenti*, (sometimes classed as *Treponema*), is found in conjunction with a fusiform bacillus, *Fusobacterium fusiforme* and with *Bacteroides* spp. in necrotic areas of the mouth in the ulcerative gingivostomatitis known as Vincent's angina.

A recently described species *B. burgdorferi* (Johnson et al 1984) is now known to be the cause of Lyme disease that was first recognized as an entity in Lyme, Connecticut, in 1975 and is now the most commonly reported tick-borne spirochaetosis in the USA where it is transmitted by ticks of the genus *Ixodes*. Cases have also been diagnosed in Europe and Australia. In the UK it is thought to be spread by the tick *I. ricinus* which is widespread. Lyme disease is characterized in the early stages by a distinctive skin lesion known as erythema chronicum migrans (ECM) and later by cardiac, neurological and arthritic complications that may become chronic.

Morphology

Members of the genus *Borrelia* can be easily distinguished from spirochaetes of the genera *Leptospira* and *Treponema* by their much larger size (10–30 μm in length by 0.3–0.7 μm in width), by their irregular, wide-open, loosely wound primary coils and by the ease with which they can be stained with the usual laboratory aniline dyes; they are Gram-negative. They are actively motile by means of about 10 axial filaments attached at either end of the organism and entwined around the cell within the cytoplasmic membrane (Pl. 38.3, Vol. 1, 13th Edn, p. 395).

Culture and survival

Unlike leptospires, borrelias are not easy to culture in the routine laboratory although some species can be grown in specially devised media (Felsenfeld, 1971). *B. hermsi*, the aetiological agent of tick-borne relapsing fever in the USA, was the first to be successfully cultured through many passages. The medium used was devised by Kelly and subsequently modified to allow the isolation and growth of *B. burgdorferi* from the midgut of infected ticks, with growth from inocula as small as 1–2 organisms. This medium is known as Barbour Stoenner Kelly medium or BSK II* (Barbour 1984). The optimum temperature for growth is 34°C. Some borrelias, including *B. burgdorferi*, are microaerophilic and others, e.g. *B. vincenti*, are strict anaerobes.

B. duttoni may be maintained in ticks for long periods in a sandbox kept at room temperature. The ticks are fed on newborn mice once a year. The ticks remain infective and the borrelias retain their virulence for many years. Borrelias have also been preserved in ticks and lice deep-frozen at -76°C (Felsenfeld 1971).

Sensitivity to antibiotics

Relapsing fever borrelias respond to tetracyclines. *B. burgdorferi* isolated from human CSF has been shown to be sensitive to ceftriaxone, erythromycin, tetracycline and penicillin (Johnson et al 1987) and Lyme disease responds to early treatment. It is suggested that adult patients be treated with tetracycline (250 mg four times daily for 10 days) and children with phenoxymethylpenicillin (50 mg/kg weight daily in divided doses) (Parke 1987).

Classification of borrelias

Antigenic variation readily occurs among relapsing fever borrelias, especially during relapses, and their classification by serological methods is not possible. They are classified as species, some of which are named according to their animal hosts or the vectors that transmit them. Borrelias responsible for Lyme disease on the other hand have been found to be antigenically stable and all isolates so far obtained appear to belong to the single species *B. burgdorferi*. A full description of the genetic and phenotypic characteristics of the species is given by Johnson et al (1984).

Louse-borne borrelias of the species known as *B. recurrentis* (syn. *Spirochaeta obermeieri*) are the cause of epidemic relapsing fever in North Africa, Asia and Europe. Infection is spread from man to man by the body and head louse *Pediculus humanus*. The organisms enter the body probably as a result of scratching the skin and rubbing the body of the louse into the abrasion. The disease occurs in overcrowded communities where the standard of hygiene and nutrition is low.

Tick-borne relapsing fever borrelias infect rodents and other wild animals including porcupines, opossums and armadillos. Pigs, cows and other domestic animals may also be infected. Various species of tick are responsible for transmitting the organism from animal to animal and from animal to man. Human cases of relapsing fever of this nature occur in North and South America, Central and South Africa, Palestine and Iran. They occur endemically as a result of tick-bites or from the coxal fluid after crushing of the tick into a skin abrasion. Species of tick-borne *Borrelia* include *B. duttoni*, the cause of East African relapsing fever, which is spread by the species of tick known as *Ornithodoros moubata*, and *B. persica*, the cause of Asian relapsing fever, spread by *O. tholozani*. *B. turicatae*, *B. parkeri* and *B. hermsi* are responsible for forms of relapsing fever that occur in the USA; they are spread by the ticks *O. turicata*, *O. parkeri* and *O. hermsi* respectively.

Lyme disease spirochaetes identified as *B. burgdorferi* have been isolated from the tick species *Ixodes dammini* and *I. pacificus* in the USA and from *I. ricinus* in Switzerland and other parts of Europe including the UK. Mammalian hosts on which the ticks feed include mice and other rodents and deer.

Borrelias that are found on the mucous membranes of the human mouth and genitalia in healthy and in diseased conditions include *B. buccalis* and *B. vincenti*, both of which are found in normal healthy mouths, but the latter is also present in exudate from the necrotic lesions of the gums in Vincent's angina. *B. refringens* is found on the healthy genital membranes but may also be present in large numbers in cases of vulvo-vaginitis and balanitis.

Laboratory diagnosis of borrelial infection

Relapsing fever

Because of the difficulty of culturing borrelias and the unreliability of serological tests, routine laboratory diagnosis of relapsing fever depends on demonstrating the spirochaetes either in the living state or after staining.

1. During the pyrexial phase of the illness prepare thick and thin films of the patient's blood on microscope slides. Fix by treating with methyl alcohol or acetone for 3 min. Alternatively, for thick blood films, dehaemoglobinize with 0.5% acetic acid. Stain thin films with Giemsa stain or gentian violet and thick films by Leishman's method (Ch. 3; and see Fig. 43.3a).

2. During the pyrexial phase of the illness mount a drop of the patient's blood on a slide with a coverslip and examine for live spirochaetes by darkfield microscopy.

3. If no spirochaetes are seen, inoculate intraperitoneally 1–2 ml blood into six young white mice. Examine drops of blood obtained by clipping the tip of the tail 48 h later and daily thereafter for up to 1 week. Examine by darkfield microscopy for living spirochaetes, or after staining by Giemsa.

4. Inoculate 0.2 ml patient's blood into the chorio-allantoic sac of a chick embryo, 17–18 days old. After the chick has hatched examine the blood for borrelias.

5. Examine films of the stomach contents of ticks caught in the vicinity of the case. In the case of louse-borne relapsing fever, examine body lice taken from the patient. Place the louse in a test tube for 24 h. Remove the louse to a drop of distilled water on a slide. Pierce the body of the louse with a needle to allow the coelomic fluid from the body cavity to mix with the water. Examine microscopically with darkfield illumination and high magnification.

Lyme disease

It is possible to isolate *B. burgdorferi* from the skin lesions, blood, CSF and synovial fluid of patients but its successful cultivation from those sources is rare and laboratory diagnosis usually depends on serological tests.

Apply the indirect immunofluorescent antibody test and/or the ELISA test to the patient's serum. A rise in specific IgM from the 3rd to 6th week after onset of symptoms tends to confirm the clinical diagnosis. IgG antibodies rise more slowly and continue for long periods in patients who develop chronic symptoms. A continued high level of IgM indicates persistent infection (see Craft et al 1984, Steere et al 1986).

In the USA a high recovery rate has been achieved from the tissues of feral rodents and deer on which the ticks feed. This technique may prove to be a suitable method for identifying areas where *B. burgdorferi* is endemic (Anderson et al 1985).

Vincent's angina

The diagnosis of Vincent's angina is normally made by microscopic examination. Prepare smears of exudate from the ulcers and stain with dilute carbol fuchsin. Examine microscopically with a high power objective. The clinical diagnosis is confirmed when large numbers of spirochaetes are seen in conjunction with barred fusiform bacilli and Gram-negative bacilli, together with pus cells that indicate active infection.

In order to exclude other pathogenic bacteria such as haemolytic streptococci or diphtheria bacilli as possible causes of the condition, seed plates of appropriate media with swabs of the lesions. *B. vincenti* may grow in primary culture but, since it is difficult to obtain and maintain a pure culture of the spirochaete, this is not undertaken as a routine in diagnosis of Vincent's infection. When it is desired to culture *B. vincenti*, inoculate into digest broth, e.g. Hartley's Broth (see Ch. 6), enriched with ascitic fluid. Incubate anaerobically (see Ch. 7) at 28–30°C and examine daily for growth.

METHODS

Modified Korthof's medium for leptospires
(Alston & Broom 1958)

All glassware used in preparing culture media for leptospires must be perfectly clean and free from any trace of soap or detergent since these are lethal to the organisms. After cleaning and rinsing, soak for 24 h in phosphate buffered saline (PBS), pH 7.6, and rinse again in distilled water.

Serum. This liquid medium requires the addition of serum. Rabbit serum is generally most satisfactory for culture of leptospires though the serum of some larger animals, e.g. sheep or newborn calf, has been used successfully. Serum from individual rabbits may be inhibitory to leptospires because of agglutinins or other agents. For this reason the sera of several rabbits should be tested individually for agglutinins and suitable animals retained to supply serum as required. Collect the blood from an ear vein or, preferably, by cardiac puncture and allow to clot. Pipette off the serum, inactivate by heating at 56°C for 30 min and sterilize by Seitz filtration.

Haemoglobin solution. To the blood clot after removal of the serum add an equal volume of distilled water and freeze and thaw repeatedly to haemolyse the corpuscles. Sterilize by Seitz filtration.

Peptone salt solution. Different brands of peptone vary in their growth-promoting ability; Difco peptone is recommended.

Peptone (Difco)	0.8 g
NaCl	1.4 g
$NaHCO_3$	0.2 g
KCl	0.04 g
$CaCl_2$	0.04 g
KH_2PO_4	0.24 g
$Na_2HPO_4.2H_2O$	0.88 g
Distilled water	1 litre

Steam the ingredients at 100°C for 20 min and filter through double thickness Whatman No. 1 paper. The pH should be *c.* 7.2. Bottle in 100 ml amounts and autoclave at 115°C for 15 min.

Preparation of complete medium

Peptone salt solution	100 ml
Sterile serum	8 ml
Sterile 'haemoglobin solution'	0.8 ml

Mix the ingredients with sterile precautions. Distribute the medium in 2–3 ml amounts in sterile screw-capped bijou bottles. Test for sterility by incubating at 37°C for 2 days and at 22°C for 3 days.

Solid medium for colonial growth of leptospires (Cox & Larson 1957)

Tryptose-phosphate broth dehydrated (Difco)	0.2 g
Agar (Difco)	1 g
Distilled water	90 ml

Adjust pH to 7.5 and sterilize mixture by autoclaving at 121°C for 15 min. After cooling add 10 ml sterile rabbit serum. Also add 1 ml haemoglobin solution prepared by lysing washed and packed sheep erythrocytes in 20 volumes of cold distilled water; remove stroma by centrifugation and sterilize by Seitz filtration. Heat mixture at 56°C for 30 min and pour into Petri dishes to give a depth of medium of 6–8 mm.

To seed the plates, prepare a series of 10-fold dilutions of a fluid culture and spread 0.1 ml volumes of each dilution evenly over the surface of separate plates to allow the distribution of well spaced individual organisms.

Fletcher's agar for leptospires (Fletcher 1928)

This semi-solid agar is suitable for isolating strains of leptospires and for maintaining them for many months. They multiply within the upper part of the tube forming zones of turbidity at varying depths, known as Dinger's rings.

Peptone	0.3 g
Beef extract	0.2 g
NaCl	0.5 g
Agar	1.5 g
Distilled water (pH 7.4)	920 ml

Mix the above ingredients and bring to boiling point to dissolve. Sterilize by autoclaving at 121°C for 20 min. Cool to 50°C and add 10% (v/v) filter-sterilized rabbit serum warmed to 50°C. Dispense in 8–9 ml volumes in tubes. Heat inactivate at 56°C for 1 h on 2 successive days. Check for sterility by incubating at 37°C and at 30°C for 24 h at each temperature.

Ellinghausen & McCullough (EM) medium for leptospires

A modification of this medium known as EMJH medium (Johnson & Harris 1967) is available commercially from Difco.

For the original EM medium (Ellinghausen & McCullough 1965) prepare the following *stock solutions* and store in refrigerator until required.

a. *Phosphate buffer solution* (conc. × 25)

Na_2HPO_4	16.6 g
KH_2PO_4	2.172 g
Distilled water	1 litre

b. *Salts solution* (conc. × 20)

NaCl	38.5 g
NH_4Cl	5.35 g
$MgCl_2.6H_2O$	3.81 g
Distilled water	1 litre

c. *Copper solution.* $CuSO_4.5H_2O$, 30 mg in 100 ml distilled water.

d. *Zinc solution.* $ZnSO_4.7H_2O$, 80 mg in 200 ml distilled water.

e. *Iron solution.* $FeSO_4.7H_2O$, 500 mg in 200 ml distilled water.

f. *Vitamin B12.* Concentrated stock: 10 mg in 100 ml distilled water. Working stock: 10 ml concentrated stock in 90 ml distilled water.

g. *Thiamine hydrochloride* (stock solution), 200 mg in 100 ml distilled water.

h. *Tween 80.* Dissolve 10 ml Tween 80 in 70 ml distilled water at 60°C, adding it drop by drop. Adjust the volume to 100 ml and then further dilute to 1000 ml. Store this 1% solution at −60°C in convenient amounts.

For special purposes, e.g. for the preparation of protein-free medium, it may be necessary to purify the Tween by charcoal treatment (Bey & Johnson 1978).

i. *Bovine albumin.* Prepare a 5% albumin solution by dissolving 5 g bovine albumin, fraction V (Armour) in 100 ml single strength phosphate buffer (i.e. 40 ml of × 25 conc. stock solution in 960 ml distilled water). Adjust pH to

7.4 by adding 0.4 mol/litre NaOH. Sterilize by membrane filtration (pore size 0.22 μm).

Preparation of medium

1. To 700 ml distilled water add:

Phosphate buffer solution ($\times$ 25 conc.)	40 ml
Salts solution ($\times$ 20 conc.)	50 ml
Copper solution	1 ml
Zinc solution	10 ml
Iron solution	20 ml

Shake the mixture for 5 min.

2. Add L-cystine, 200 mg. Shake the mixture for 3 min (the cystine does not dissolve completely). Filter through double thickness Whatman No. 1 paper.

3. Add: Vitamin B12 (working stock) 20 ml; Thiamine stock solution 0.1 ml; and Tween 80 (1% solution) 120 ml.

Adjust total volume to 1 litre. Dispense this basal mixture in tubes (4 or 8 ml). Autoclave at 121°C for 15 min.

4. Cool and then add sterile bovine albumin solution in proportion of 1 vol. to 4 vols basal medium. Sterilize by filtration through a sandwich of Millipore membrane filters, pore sizes 1.4 μm, 0.45 μm and 0.22 μm.

Differential centrifugation of blood for the detection of leptospires by microscopy (Wolff 1954)

1. Prepare an anticoagulant solution of either 1% sodium oxalate in phosphate buffer, pH 7.5, or 1% 'liquoid' (polyanethol sulphonate – see Ch. 7) in sterile saline. These are preferable to sodium citrate which may be deleterious to leptospires.

2. Add 5 ml blood to 0.5 ml sodium oxalate solution or to 1 ml liquoid solution and centrifuge at *c*. 1000 *g* for 15 min.

3. Examine a drop of the plasma by darkfield microscopy ($\times$ 400).

4. If no leptospires are seen, centrifuge the plasma at 3000–4000 *g* for 20 min. Carefully remove the supernatent and examine a drop of sediment microscopically as above.

Once again it must be emphasized how important it is not to confuse artefacts, such as protoplasmic extrusions from red cells, with leptospires.

Blood culture for leptospires

1. Sample the patient's blood aseptically during the febrile stage of the illness and before treatment with antibiotics.

2. Inoculate a number of bijou bottles containing 3 ml liquid or semi-solid culture medium with varying amounts of blood ranging from 1–4 drops. Alternatively, after differential centrifugation (see above), resuspend the deposit in 2 ml PBS, pH 8.0, and add a few drops of the suspension to each of four bottles of medium.

3. Incubate at 28–30°C and examine periodically for leptospiral growth for up to 6 weeks before discarding as negative.

Daily culture of the blood in either of these ways during the first week of the infection considerably increases the chance of isolating the organisms.

Animal inoculation for isolation of leptospires

Use weanling animals, as older animals tend to be resistant. Guinea-pigs (4 weeks old) or hamsters (3 weeks old) are suitable.

1. Inoculate into the animals intraperitoneally a few drops of patient's blood during the first few days of the illness.

2. Three days later, and daily thereafter, withdraw a drop of peritoneal fluid with a finely drawn Pasteur pipette introduced into the lower quadrant of the abdomen while the animal is held in the upright position with outstretched legs. Discharge the drop on to a slide and examine microscopically.

3. As soon as leptospires are seen in the peritoneal fluid, where they multiply during the early stages of infection in the animal, withdraw blood by cardiac puncture and introduce a few drops into several small bottles of culture medium.

4. Incubate at 28–30°C and examine daily for leptospiral growth.

Culture of urine for leptospires

Leptospires may be present in the patient's urine towards the end of the second week after onset and for several weeks thereafter.

1. Into a number of tubes or bottles containing 5 ml semi-solid culture medium add a disk of neomycin sulphate (content 10 μg) or 5-fluorouracil (final concentration 100 μg/ml) to prevent the growth of contaminants.

2. Serially dilute the urine five or six times in PBS, pH 8.0, and add 1 drop of each dilution to the tubes of culture medium.

3. Incubate at 28–30°C and examine periodically over a period of up to 6 weeks. Contaminants may grow in cultures of undiluted urine and in the first few dilutions, but subsequent dilutions may yield a pure growth of leptospires.

For culture of urine by animal inoculation, inoculate 2 ml urine into young guinea-pigs or hamsters. Culture the animal's blood subsequently as described above.

Identification of newly isolated leptospiral strains: immunization of rabbits

Subculture the isolate over a period of several weeks until the leptospires are sufficiently adapted to laboratory conditions to provide a culture dense enough for serological identification.

1. Prepare a homologous antiserum by immunizing a rabbit against the isolate as follows: Choose a healthy 3–4 kg rabbit and test to ascertain the absence of leptospiral antibodies. Use live or formalin-treated culture of density 2×10^8 orgs/ml. Inject into the marginal vein of the ear 1 ml of culture, followed at 7 day intervals by 4 more injections of 2, 4, 6 and 6 ml. One week after the final injection, test a sample of blood taken from the ear vein and determine the homologous antibody titre. If it is at least 12 800, bleed the rabbit by cardiac puncture 7 days later; if the titre is less than 12 800, inject a further dose of 6 ml. Store the antiserum in 2 ml amounts at 4°C (or freeze-dry).

2. Test the unknown strain by the microscopic agglutination test against a battery of reference antisera representing all known serogroups (or those known to prevail in the locality).

3. Compare the isolate with each of the serovars within the serogroup or serogroups indicated by a positive reaction in the preliminary tests. Use either the technique of agglutinin-absorption or factor analysis (Dikken & Kmety 1978), using reference strains and antisera (available from Leptospira Reference Laboratories) and the homologous antiserum.

Complement fixation test for leptospirosis

This genus-specific test is of value as a screening test for acute leptospirosis. It can be done in laboratories where the procedure is routinely applied to all cases of PUO and other febrile illnesses. The standard technique is used but with an antigen prepared from the saprophytic leptospire Patoc 1.

Complement fixation test antigen. 1. Inoculate 10 ml of an actively growing culture of strain Patoc 1 of *L. biflexa* into 1 litre of EM medium. Allow to grow for *c.* 7 days at room temperature.

2. Treat with merthiolate (final dilution 1 in 10 000) to kill the leptospires.

3. Centrifuge at 10 000 g for 1 h to deposit the leptospires.

4. Discard the supernate and resuspend the deposit in CFT diluent (Oxoid, Code No. BR 16, CFT Diluent Tablets; 1 tablet makes 100 ml buffered saline).

5. Repeat the washing and centrifuging twice more and then resuspend the final deposit of leptospires in 20 ml diluent containing sodium azide (1 in 10 000). The amount of suspension is now 2% of the original volume.

6. Allow the concentrated suspension to stand at 4°C for at least 4 days with periodic shaking.

7. Treat to remove any anticomplementary activity as follows: To 20 ml concentrated antigenic suspension add diluent to make up to 100 ml. Add 5 ml 0.4 mol/litre HCl and mix well. Warm some flat bottles of 50 ml capacity to 60°C and half fill them with the acidified antigen. Place the bottles in a beaker of boiling water, with the caps slightly loosened, for 15 min. Cool the antigen suspension and shake thoroughly to disperse any flocculation. Restore the pH to the original value (7.2) by adding

0.4 mol/litre NaOH. This treatment should ensure that the titre of the complement in the presence of the antigen is near to that with diluent alone.

8. Finally titrate the antigen in the presence of a standard positive rabbit serum and 2 haemolytic units of complement (2 × HD50) to determine the optimum working dilution for use in the complement fixation test.

Slide agglutination test for leptospirosis with heat-treated antigen (Patoc slide test)

This simple test (Mazzonelli et al 1974, modified by Coghlan; see WHO 1982) provides a rapid and reliable means of screening human sera for leptospiral genus-specific antibodies. It allows a provisional diagnosis of acute leptospirosis to be made within a few minutes of receipt of the serum in the laboratory; it is not suitable for retrospective or survey work.

The tests are carried out on a thin glass plate, 15 × 7.5 cm, divided into 3 rows of 2.5 cm squares etched with a diamond cutter. This provides 18 squares/plate, enough for testing 9 sera at a time. It is advisable, but not essential, to have a mechanical rotator (Thomas).

Antigen for Patoc slide test. 1. Inoculate 1 litre of a suitable liquid medium, preferably EM medium, with 5 ml of an actively growing culture of the saprophytic strain Patoc 1. Allow to stand at room temperature. Aeration by means of a mechanical stirrer or magnetic rotator will help to produce a dense culture within 7–10 days.

2. Kill the leptospires by adding neutralized formalin to give a final dilution of 0.5% (0.2% formaldehyde) and allow to stand for at least 2 h at room temperature.

3. Centrifuge at 13 000 g for 30 min. Wash the deposited cells by resuspending them in PBS, pH 7.2, containing sodium azide 1 in 100, and again centrifuge at 13 000 g. Carefully withdraw and discard the supernate from the centrifuge buckets.

4. Add a little PBS to the deposit and by means of a Pasteur pipette or a syringe fitted with a 16–18 gauge needle, mix and transfer to flat screw-capped bottles of 50–60 ml capacity containing some sterile glass beads. Shake periodically over a period of at least 24 h. The suspension should now be of a creamy consistency.

5. Place the bottles in a large beaker of cold water and heat to boiling point. Allow to boil for 30 min.

6. Cool thoroughly and adjust the density of the suspension to twice that of No. 10 on the McFarland scale.

7. Centrifuge lightly to deposit any gross particles or agglutinated leptospires. Decant carefully. Adjust the pH to 7.2.

Although the antigen is now ready for use it improves with time. It should be stored at 4°C and shaken from time to time (but not just before using in the test). If a deposit develops the suspension should be lightly centrifuged and decanted. It is then necessary to readjust the density to McFarland 10 × 2. The sensitivity of each new batch of antigen should be checked against known positive and negative human sera.

Method for Patoc slide test. 1. Dilute the patient's serum 1 in 10 by adding 1 drop to 9 similar drops of PBS in a small test tube.

2. Place 1 drop (0.02 ml) of the 1 in 10 dilution and 1 drop of the undiluted serum side by side in 2 squares of the glass plate. To each drop add 1 drop (0.02 ml) of antigen. Carefully mix the serum and antigen by means of a wooden applicator stick, starting with the mixture containing the diluted serum. Up to 9 sera, 1 of which should be a known positive control, can be accommodated on the plate and tested at the same time.

3. Rotate the plate at 120 rpm for exactly 4 min.

4. Read the reaction by holding the plate against a dark background illuminated from above by a lamp shaded from the eyes.

Record the strength of the reaction as follows: ++++, clearly defined clumps against a cleared background; +++, obvious agglutination but suspension not completely clear; ++ and +, progressively weaker reactions with small clumps, sometimes formed around the periphery of the drop, and with little clearing; a negative (−) result is recorded when the even suspension of the antigen-serum mixture is unchanged. It may be difficult to read the strength of the reaction if the serum is cloudy due to a high lipid content.

Reactions of ++ to ++++ with diluted serum in conjunction with a strong positive reaction with the neat serum indicate present or very recent leptospiral infection. Strong or moderately strong (++++ or +++) reactions with neat serum combined with a negative result with diluted serum suggest the presence of antibodies at an early stage, i.e. within 2–3 days of onset, or they may be residual from a recent infection. When no reaction occurs either with diluted or undiluted serum, it is unlikely that the patient is suffering from leptospirosis. However if the specimen was taken early in the course of the illness and the reaction is negative or weakly positive, it is advisable to test a later specimen which may show a rise in antibody level; this is diagnostic. At the height of infection the reaction with diluted serum may be stronger than with neat serum, due to a prozone effect.

Positive reactions should, if possible, be confirmed by complement fixation and microscopic agglutination tests (see below).

Microscopic agglutination test (MAT) for leptospirosis (Wolff 1954)

Prepare well grown cultures of strains of *L. interrogans* in liquid medium, representing all serogroups known to be prevalent in the locality. Alternatively use cultures of reference strains of serovars that represent all known serogroups (c. 20) to cover all possible types of leptospira infection.

Use living cultures, or cultures killed by the addition of formalin (0.5% w/v) neutralized with magnesium carbonate (traces of formic acid cause non-specific agglutination of leptospires). Add excess $MgCO_3$ to a stock solution of formalin (40% formaldehyde); remove small quantities as required and filter before use. Killed suspensions are more convenient and safer for routine work and they may be stored for a month or longer before use; however if any suspension shows spontaneous agglutination during storage, discard it. Formalinized cultures of several serovars for use as antigens in the MAT are also available commercially (Difco).

1. Dilute the patient's serum serially from 1 in 5 to 1 in 15 000 by the dropping technique, either in tubes or in the wells of polystyrene plates. To 3 drops (0.02 ml) of each dilution add 3 drops of antigen suspension. The procedure is summarized in Table 41.2; this provides a series of dilutions of 1 in 10, 1 in 30, 1 in 100, etc, to 1 in 3000 or more. Alternatively prepare a series of 2-fold dilutions, 1 in 10 to 1 in 5120.

2. If living cultures are used, incubate the mixtures at 32°C (or 37°C) for 3 h and allow to stand at room temperature for 1 h before

Table 41.2 Scheme for preparing a wide range of serum dilutions by a dropping technique in a polystyrene plate for the microscopic agglutination test.
Key: . . . = none added

Reagent	Number of drops of stated reagent added to well no.					
	1	2	3	4	5	6
First row (dilution of serum)						
Saline (drops)	8	9	9	. . .	. . .	. . .
Serum (drops)	2	1[a]	1[b]	. . .	. . .	. . .
Initial serum dilution	5	50	500	. . .	. . .	. . .
Second row (test proper)						
Saline (drops)	. . .	2	. . .	2	. . .	2
Serum 1 in 500 (drops)	. . .	. . .	. . .	. . .	3	1
Serum 1 in 50 (drops)	. . .	. . .	3	1	. . .	. . .
Serum 1 in 5 (drops)	3	1	. . .	. . .	. . .	. . .
Culture (drops)	3	3	3	3	3	3
Final serum dilution	10	30	100	300	1000	3000

[a] Serum diluted 1 in 5 from well no. 1.
[b] Serum diluted 1 in 50 from well no. 2.

reading or, if the specimen is received late in the day, hold the test mixtures at 4°C overnight and read the following morning. If formalinized antigens are used, keep the mixtures at room temperature overnight (covered to prevent evaporation) and read the reactions the following morning. Include a no-serum control with each test whatever the method used, to ensure that the antigens are satisfactory.

3. To read the tests, place a drop of the antigen-serum mixture from each well or tube on a microscope slide (or thin glass plate, c. 12 × 8 cm, prepared for the purpose). Examine the drops with a 16 mm objective (× 100–120) using darkfield illumination. It is not necessary to place a coverslip over the drop and if each drop is quickly examined consecutively, starting with the highest dilution of serum, a large number of readings can be made on the same slide or glass plate. Agglutination of living leptospires appears as lightly refractile, spherical masses. Lysis, which was previously thought to occur, does not take place. With formalinized cultures, agglutination appears as loose irregular cotton-wool-like clumps, quite different from agglutinated living leptospires.

4. Determine the highest dilution of serum which agglutinates 50% or more of leptospires in the drop of suspension. This is judged by the proportion of organisms free between the agglutinated clumps. Compare with the no-serum control. This dilution represents the titre of antibody specific for the particular serovar used.

Interpretation. The test is essentially serogroup-specific but many serovars are related serologically through their minor antigens and there is a certain amount of cross-reaction between the various strains used as antigens, especially in the early stages of the infection, and it may not be possible to obtain a true indication of the serogroup of the infecting strain at that stage. Later specimens however tend to react mainly with the strain that represents the serogroup to which the infecting strain belongs. A

series of specimens of serum taken over a period of several weeks will result in a demonstrable rise in the titre of the homologous antibodies which confirms the diagnosis of present infection. The strain that reacts most strongly with the late specimens indicates the serogroup of the infecting strain.

BSK II medium for Borrelia burgdorferi

The following medium is described by Barbour (1984). After detergent cleaning, all glassware is rinsed thoroughly with glass-distilled water and autoclaved.

Basal medium. Prepare 1 litre working strength CMRL 1066 (a tissue culture medium) by adding 100 ml of ×10 concentrate without glutamate (Gibco) to 900 ml glass-distilled water.

Supplemented medium. Add to the basal medium in the following order:

Neopeptone (Difco)	5 g
Bovine serum albumin, Fraction V (Miles No. 81–003)	50 g
Yeastolate (Difco)	2 g
HEPES (Sigma)	6 g
Glucose	5 g
Sodium citrate	0.7 g
Sodium pyruvate	0.8 g
N-Acetylglucosamine (Sigma)	0.4 g
Sodium bicarbonate	2.2 g

Adjust pH at 20-25°C to 7.6 with NaOH, 1 mol/l. Then add 200 ml of 7% (w/v) gelatin (Difco), previously dissolved in boiling water. Sterilize by Millipore filtration (0.2 μm, nitrocellulose). Store at 4°C.

Preparation of complete medium. Before use add unheated rabbit serum ('trace haemolysed'; Pel-Freez Biologicals Inc., Rogers, AR, USA) to a final concentration of 6% (v/v). Dispense to containers filled 50-90% capacity; cap tightly; incubate at 34-37°C.

REFERENCES

Alston J M, Broom J C 1958 Leptospirosis in man and animals. Livingstone, Edinburgh

Anderson J F, Johnson R C, Magnarelli L A, Hyde F W 1985 Identification of endemic foci of Lyme disease: Isolation of *Borrelia burgdorferi* from feral rodents and ticks. Journal of Clinical Microbiology 22: 36–38

Barbour A G 1984 Isolation and cultivation of Lyme disease spirochaetes. Yale Journal of Biology and Medicine 57: 521–525

Bey R F, Johnson R C 1978 Protein-free and low-protein media for the cultivation of Leptospira. Infection and Immunity 19: 562–569

Chang R S, McComb D E 1954 Erythrocyte sensitizing substances from five strains of leptospirae. American Journal of Tropical Medicine and Hygiene 3: 481–489

Cox C D 1966 Studies on the isolation and growth of leptospirae from surface waters. Annales de la Société Belge de Médicine Tropicale 46: 193–200

Cox C D, Larson A D 1957 Colonial growth of leptospirae. Journal of Bacteriology 73: 587–589

Craft J E, Grodzicki R L, Steere A C 1984 The antibody response in Lyme disease: evaluation of diagnostic tests. Journal of Infectious Diseases 149: 789–795

Dikken H, Kmety E 1978 Serological typing methods of leptospires. In: Bergan T, Norris J R (eds) Methods in microbiology, vol. 11. Academic Press, London. Ch. 8, p 259–307

Ellinghausen H C, McCullough W G 1965 Nutrition of *Leptospira pomona* and growth of 13 other serotypes; fractionation of oleic albumin complex and a medium of bovine albumin and polysorbate 80. American Journal of Veterinary Research 26: 45–51

Faine S 1965 Silver staining of spirochaetes in single tissue sections. Journal of Clinical Pathology 18: 381–382

Felsenfeld O 1971 Borrelia. Strains, vectors, human and animal borreliosis. Warren H Green, St Louis, Missouri, USA

Fletcher W 1928 Recent work on leptospirosis, tsutsugamushi disease and tropical typhus in the Federated Malay States. Transactions of the Royal Society of Tropical Medicine and Hygiene 21: 265–282

Galton M M, Powers D K, Hall A D, Cornell R G 1958 A rapid macroscopic slide screening test for the serodiagnosis of leptospirosis. American Journal of Veterinary Research 19: 505–512

Johnson R C, Harris V G 1967 Differentiation of pathogenic and saprophytic leptospires. 1. Growth at low temperature. Journal of Bacteriology 94: 27–31

Johnson R C, Schmid G P, Hyde F W, Steigerwalt A G, Brenner D J 1984 *Borrelia burgdorferi* sp. nov.: etiologic agent of Lyme disease. International Journal of Systematic Bacteriology 34: 496–497

Johnson R C, Kodner C, Russell M 1987 In vitro and in vivo susceptibility of the Lyme disease spirochaete, *Borrelia burgdorferi*, to four antimicrobial agents. Antimicrobial Agents and Chemotherapy 31: 164–167

Kmety E 1967 Faktorenanalyse von leptospiren der Icterohaemorrhagiae und einiger verwandter serogruppen. Thesis, Slovak Academy of Sciences, Bratislava

Mazzonelli J, Dorta de Mazzonelli G, Mailloux M 1974 Possibilité de diagnostic sérologique macroscopique des leptospires a l'aide d'un antigène unique. Médicine et Maladies Infectieuses 4: 253–254

Parke A 1987 From New to Old England: the progress of Lyme disease. British Medical Journal 294: 525–526

Sharp C F 1958 Laboratory diagnosis of leptospirosis with the sensitized-erythrocyte lysis test. Journal of Pathology and Bacteriology 76: 349–356

Steere A C, Taylor E, Wilson M L, Levine J F, Spielman A 1986 Longitudinal assessment of the clinical and epidemiological features of Lyme disease in a defined population. Journal of Infectious Diseases 154: 295–300

Wolff J W 1954 The laboratory diagnosis of leptospirosis. Thomas, Springfield, Illinois, USA

World Health Organization 1982 Guidelines for the control of leptospirosis. Faine S (ed) WHO Offset Publication No 67, Geneva

Fungi

Many microbiology laboratories are generally inefficient in diagnosing fungal infections. Since mycological investigations require relatively simple technology and equipment, medical microbiologists have an obligation to make amends especially as the introduction of potent chemotherapeutic agents that alter the host's immune response has resulted in a concomitant increase in the incidence of serious fungal infections. It is impossible within the confines of this chapter to raise the level of mycological competence to that already attained in bacteriology. However, it is hoped to acquaint medical microbiologists with basic procedures necessary to establish a provisional diagnosis for some common fungal infections. It may be necessary thereafter to seek the help and advice of an experienced mycologist, whose specialist assistance must also be sought in the diagnosis of other mycoses that may be endemic in some areas of the world. Some fungal diseases with special geographical associations are being more frequently diagnosed elsewhere as a result of modern travel and migration.

The laboratory diagnosis of fungal infections relies largely on direct as opposed to indirect methods. Thus, whilst serology often contributes to the definitive diagnosis of a bacterial or viral infection, it is rarely helpful in diagnostic mycology. One reason is the failure to apply sophisticated serological methods, but a more significant cause is the degree of antigenic cross-reactivity between fungi of different genera. Another consideration is that patients suffering from a systemic mycosis are often immunologically unresponsive as a result of the cytotoxic therapy that made them vulnerable to the infection. In these patients particularly, there is hope that the detection of specific antigenaemia may prove to be a reliable guide in the future.

Diagnosis is almost always based upon the mycological laboratory investigation. Considerable importance should be placed upon direct microscopy in addition to isolation of the organism. In some cases, microscopy is of special importance. For example, the growth of *Aspergillus fumigatus* from sputum culture may represent no more than the trapping of spores from the atmosphere in the bronchial secretions. The presence of the characteristic hyphae in a sputum smear, however, is presumptive evidence of bronchopulmonary aspergillosis. Speciation of bacteria is achieved almost exclusively by performing biochemical tests whereas considerable taxonomic importance is placed upon the greater morphological variation expressed by fungi. This variation is at its most critical in the way fungi reproduce by spore formation; hence direct observation of the sporing apparatus takes precedence over biochemical reactions.

A fact that must influence all mycological investigation from the collection of clinical material to the techniques required for microscopy and culture of the causal organism is that fungi are much less abundant than bacteria in affected clinical material. This is the key to understanding the techniques and methods

As explained in the Preface, the editors have sought to avoid the use of a double 'i' genitive ending in the specific epithets of species binomials which have been derived from Latinized versions of names. We acknowledge that this is not standard practice for the nomenclature of fungi; however, for consistency in this volume, the editors have substituted single 'i' forms for double 'i' forms, e.g. *Microsporum audouini*.

employed in medical mycology. In bacterial skin infections a surface swab is sufficient to provide hundreds of colonies of the pathogen on an agar medium; in order to establish a diagnosis for a dermatophyte infection, however, several samples of the affected tissue taken for investigation may ultimately yield only one colony on culture. Similarly, in bronchopulmonary aspergillosis, a complete 24 h collection of sputum may be required for culture as the number of colony-forming units may be as low as 10/ml and rarely exceed 1000/ml. Thus, in comparison with bacterial pathogens, pathogenic fungi are about one million times less abundant in similar clinical material. Provided that the techniques employed in mycological investigations compensate for the relative scarcity of the causal organism, the bacteriologist need not fear the transition to mycology. Media used for the isolation of fungi are acidic (pH 5.5–5.6) and contain relatively high concentrations of a sugar such as glucose or maltose at *c*. 2% by weight.

In this chapter a practical approach gives some recognition to the genera and their disease manifestations but priority to the types of specimen received in the laboratory and methods applied to their investigation. There are three sections: (1) the isolation and identification of *yeasts*, with methods for the handling and processing of all specimens, except skin; (2) the *superficial mycoses* and the investigation of skin, nail and hair specimens, this section being primarily concerned with the dermatophyte or ringworm fungi, but yeasts and other filamentous fungi may also be significant and their role is discussed; and (3) *Aspergillus* infection is the subject of the final section with special emphasis on bronchopulmonary aspergillosis.

COLLECTION, STORAGE AND TRANSPORT OF SPECIMENS

The proper collection of relevant clinical materials of primary importance. In view of the scarcity of viable fragments in many specimens it is advisable to collect as much material as possible. This is especially true in the diagnosis of cryptococcal meningitis, dermatophyte infections and bronchopulmonary aspergillosis.

Skin, hair and nail samples

Skin scrapings. Grossly contaminated skin or that to which antifungal agents have been applied should be cleaned thoroughly with 70% alcohol.

A curved disposable scalpel blade is preferable for taking samples by scraping across the inflamed margin of the lesion into the apparently healthy tissue. Invading hyphae tend to grow radially from the centre of the lesion which becomes devoid of viable fragments as acquired local immunity develops. The inflamed margin is evidence of a late immunological reaction; actively growing healthy hyphae may be found some centimetres beyond this margin.

If vesicles are present, the tops should be removed with fine scissors and sent for examination.

Skin strippings. An alternative method for the collection of skin specimens is to apply waterproof transparent vinyl adhesive tape (3M type 681) firmly to the affected area and peel it off; the tape, now bearing a thin layer of skin, is then applied to a sterile glass microscope slide for transport to the laboratory. This is a rapid and efficient method of collecting skin samples for the isolation of dermatophytes and yeasts by culture (Milne & Barnetson 1974) but strippings are unsuitable for microscopical examination except in cases of pityriasis versicolor and this is an important consideration if the early presumptive information provided by microscopy is also needed.

Nail. Friable material should be removed from under the nail, or clippings may be taken from the distal border with scissors or nail clippers. In cases of paronychia, i.e. where a yeast infection is suspected, exudate is expressed from the paronychial folds by probing with a flat excavator and collecting on a swab previously moistened with sterile saline.

Hair. Infected hairs should be removed by plucking with epilating forceps and never by cutting which fails to remove the area most likely to harbour the fungus, i.e. the base of the hair shaft around the follicle. The species most frequently associated with scalp ringworm cause the affected hairs to fluoresce under a Wood's lamp and this is a useful means of selecting material.

Storage and transport of skin, nail and hair. All three types of keratinous material should be allowed to dry out to prevent the overgrowth of saprophytic bacteria and fungi that occurs if moisture is retained by holding these specimens in airtight containers such as small glass bottles. Black paper folded to form a packet is most suitable. In such conditions ringworm fungi remain viable for weeks or even months and so specimens may be stored and forwarded with confidence even if the laboratory is remote. Specimens should not be refrigerated as the viability of some species of dermatophyte is affected. Fungi pathogenic to skin survive well as tape strippings stuck to a microscope slide which should be placed in a protective box for transport. Swabs should be sent to the laboratory in a transport medium suitable for yeasts.

Sputum

Since the pathogenic fragments of aspergillus organisms can vary both in numbers and size over a given period, it is advisable to assume difficulty in obtaining positive microscopy and culture; accordingly, total sputum collections should be obtained. To establish or exclude a definitive diagnosis a 3 day collection is often required. Sputum may be collected as three 24 h samples but a convenient system for ward and laboratory handling is for specimens to be batched every 8 h. Whenever possible, sputum should be refrigerated to reduce the saprophytic growth of bacteria and yeasts. Experience has shown that aspergillus hyphae produce little or no growth in sputum even after several days at room temperature and viability is not affected.

Cerebrospinal fluid

Lumbar punctures should be carried out in the same way as for bacteriological sampling, taking precautions to minimize contamination by yeasts colonizing the surface skin. A large volume should be taken if this is clinically permitted whilst taking account of the dangers to the patient if the CSF pressure is increased, i.e. a minimum of 5 ml is recommended, especially where investigations for *Cryptococcus* are requested. Transport the CSF to the laboratory without delay.

Swabs

These should be heavily charged with exudates, pus or other secretions. Where plaques are present such as in the mouth, throat or vagina, the swab should be repeatedly rubbed firmly over these areas. As a general rule, the survival of yeasts on dry swabs is inversely related to time and storage temperature. Delays should be avoided whenever possible. If delay is inevitable, swabs may be held at 4°C and preferably in a suitable transport medium containing antibiotics such as Trichomonas medium (Oxoid).

Other specimens

Tissue biopsies, urine, blood and all materials not mentioned above should be collected, stored and transported in a manner similar to that employed for bacteriology.

1. YEAST INFECTIONS

Yeasts are the most common cause of human fungal infections and, being opportunists, their severity is greatly enhanced in the presence of predisposing factors such as immunosuppressive drug therapy, diabetes, prosthetic devices and drug abuse. Isolation of a yeast is not in itself diagnostic; yeasts occur as part of the commensal flora on the surface of the body and in the gastrointestinal tract. Except in aseptically collected specimens of normally sterile material, interpretation of the mycological results is therefore necessary. Clearly, the clinical signs and symptoms and existence of predisposing factors will be helpful in determining the significance of a yeast isolate but a valuable contribution can often be made by the laboratory. In this respect, helpful information can be obtained by carrying out direct microscopy on the specimen, determining the quantity of yeast present and identifying the isolate fully.

Laboratory diagnosis of yeast infections

Procedures for direct examination of specimens and for culture and identification of yeasts are described below.

Direct examination

Microscopical examination may give an early indication of the presence of yeasts. The finding of yeasts in normally sterile tissue or fluids collected aseptically is significant. In contaminated material such as faeces and sputum the observation is much less conclusive. On a few occasions the presence of hyphae can assist in establishing a differential diagnosis. The observation of a capsule surrounding a yeast cell in CSF provides a presumptive diagnosis of cryptococcosis. The duration and conditions of storage of a specimen should always be taken into account in determining the significance of the microscopical findings as well as those of culture.

Many bacteriologists experience difficulty in differentiating fungal elements from fibrous material and other artefacts, especially in unstained films. Calcofluor white fluorescent staining* is a simple technique that has gained favour recently and overcomes the difficulties and time involved in staining by more conventional means. It also has the advantage of working in the presence of strong concentrations of KOH. When viewed in blue light, fungi possess an inherent weak fluorescence that can be usefully enhanced by the fluor on becoming attached to the chitin and cellulose of the cell wall.

Tissue

The most important factor is to obtain as thin a film as possible by manipulation of a representative portion of the biopsy or post mortem material with a scalpel. Transfer a section 1 mm thick to a drop of 20% potassium hydroxide (KOH) on a microscope slide. Allow to stand for

*Refer to *Methods* section at end of this chapter.

a few minutes, place a coverslip on top and tap gently with a rod. The unstained preparation may be viewed by conventional transmitted light but it is usually beneficial to examine under phase contrast or darkground microscopy. Alternatively, before transferring the tissue to the slide, a drop of 0.1% calcofluor white in 0.05% Evans blue may be added to the 20% KOH. Process as before and view under a fluorescent microscope with a UV light source capable of producing blue light.

Swabs

Prepare a smear from swabs, heat fix and stain by Gram's method. The characteristic budding cells and yeast hyphae are Gram positive and frequently the cell contents have a beaded appearance. Swabs received in transport medium may be handled in a similar manner but usually a wet film is prepared by expressing some of the moisture from the swab, covering with a coverslip and examining the unstained film under suitable illumination as outlined for tissue above. All preparations should be examined thoroughly by traversing several fields since only small numbers of cells may be present. High vaginal and cervical swabs merit special mention as some workers regard the presence of hyphae as a diagnostic criterion in vaginal thrush. This is unwise because (1) hyphae may be scarce and may not be detected, and (2) some species, e.g. *Torulopsis glabrata*, causing yeast vaginitis never produce hyphae.

Cerebrospinal fluid

These specimens must be concentrated before making any attempt to carry out microscopy. A sample of the centrifuged deposit should be Gram stained; then only if budding cells are found should a further preparation be made to examine for capsule formation. To a drop of the resuspended sediment add a similar volume of India ink. Capsules appear as large clear areas surrounding the yeast cell. When present, capsules are presumptive evidence of *Cryptococcus neoformans*.

Urine

Concentration by centrifugation is necessary. A smear should be prepared from the sediment and Gram stained. Care should be taken during collection to minimize contamination especially from the vagina in women. Specimens exposed to prolonged storage at ambient temperature should be discarded.

Isolation

Culture media

Sabouraud's medium* is used worldwide and is generally satisfactory. Some workers prefer malt extract agar* prepared from desiccated malt extract (at 2% by weight of the medium) or from the syrup (4%). It is claimed that in the latter form, malt agar is slightly more inhibitory to bacteria and produces more rapid growth and sporulation of fungi than Sabouraud's medium. In addition it is often possible to distinguish mixed cultures of yeast species by their colony morphology on malt agar. Such media are suitable for the isolation of all the medically important yeasts except, in some instances, for primary isolation of *Cryptococcus neoformans* when a duplicate series of plates containing enriched blood agar should be inoculated.

Blood cultures

Biphasic blood culture bottles with agar and a mycological broth, or simple malt or Sabouraud broth media may be employed*. As most of the generally available blood culture media support the growth of yeasts, these are recommended to avoid confusion in the ward and to reduce the possibility of missing a bacterial pathogen. It is advisable, however, to aerate the cultures periodically by shaking and to subculture routinely rather than to wait until the medium becomes cloudy.

Amongst the pathogenic fungi, the yeasts are most akin to bacteria in terms of numbers present in clinical material, but it is best to assume that the specimen contains few colony

forming units and a good volume of blood should be sampled (see Ch. 39).

Tissue

Biopsy and other tissues should be reduced in size to approximately 1–2 mm in overall dimensions and a few such pieces lightly implanted into the agar medium; the medium should contain antibiotics* if the material is contaminated with bacteria. As an additional safeguard where very small numbers may exist, similar pieces should be inoculated into malt or Sabouraud broth.

Swabs

Heavily seed a well on one quadrant of the agar plate by rotating the swab and sweeping over the surface several times. Secondary and successive dilution strokes should be made with a sterile loop.

Cerebrospinal fluid

A representative loopful of spun deposit should be taken to inoculate the agar media in the usual fashion. Any deposit remaining after samples have been removed for microscopy may be transferred to a suitable mycological broth.

Urine

Spread 0.1 ml of the unconcentrated urine over the surface of malt agar, or an equivalent medium, containing antibiotics. Centrifuge the specimen and remove a loopful of sediment to another agar plate of the same medium and streak out from the well in the normal way.

Incubation

All pathogenic yeasts grow at 37°C but it is advisable to diverge slightly from this general rule for *Cryptococcus neoformans* which merits a duplicate series of plates incubated at 28°C for up to 10 days. With all other specimens (except skin) incubation for 48 h is sufficient for colonies to become visible; it is stressed that 24 h is not sufficient to record no growth of yeasts, particularly from heavily contaminated material.

Identification

The yeasts pathogenic to humans appear as pasty, opaque and usually pale coloured (white, off-white or beige) colonies often with a sweet smell reminiscent of ripe apples. Depending upon the medium used for isolation, it may be possible to distinguish the presence of more than one species. This occurs frequently in specimens originating from the gastrointestinal tract and especially from the mouth. Yeast colonies may be confirmed microscopically by emulsifying a portion of the colony in sterile water or lactophenol cotton blue* and observing the characteristic budding cells. Hyphae may also be present.

Germ tube test

About 90% of yeasts isolated from human material are *Candida albicans* and a rapid method of identification is fortunately available.

The ability of this species to produce a pseudogerm tube in serum is shared only with *C. stellatoidea* which is very much less common. For the 'germ tube' test lightly touch a single colony with a loop or Pasteur pipette; remove excess inoculum and then emulsify the yeast cells in 0.5 ml of horse or other serum in a small test-tube with a loose cotton-wool plug or cap. Failure to achieve a light inoculum inhibits germ tube formation. Incubate at 37°C in a waterbath (for more rapid temperature equilibration) for 2–4 h. Prolonged incubation is not recommended as mycelium production can obscure the germ tubes which are seen as extensions of a typical yeast cell and give a drumstick appearance. Examine carefully to ensure that the parent cell and the germ tube are one continuous cell and that a cell wall does not separate the two as in *C. tropicalis*.

The presumptive identification of *C. albicans* is usually sufficient but where absolute certainty is required, the inability of *C. stellatoidea* to assimilate sucrose (see below) is diagnostic. Identification of germ tube negative yeasts may

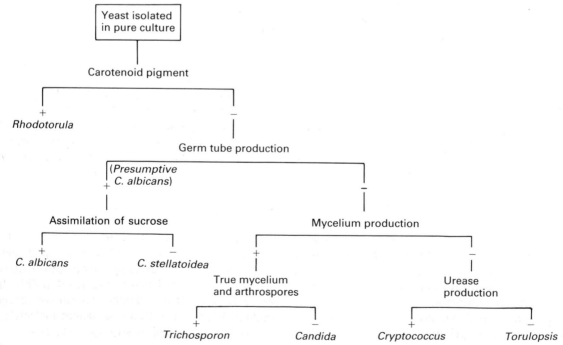

Fig. 42.1 Initial stages in the identification of medically important yeasts.

also be necessary on occasions, especially to determine the role or possible source of the isolate. Commercially prepared systems for the identification of yeasts have become available and these are based upon an auxanogram, i.e. the ability of an isolate to assimilate a series of sugars. A separate test is necessary to determine mycelium production. The series of tests and procedures given below can be used to identify most yeasts from human sources with readily available reagents and equipment.

Steps in the identification of medically important yeasts are outlined in Figure 42.1. Tests for the ability to form a pseudo-germ tube, to form mycelium (Dalmau culture plate) and arthrospores, and various other morphological and metabolic tests are exploited.

1. Dalmau culture plate

This tests the ability of the isolate to form mycelium under optimum conditions. Load a loop with the test organism and form a well at the top of a plate of cornmeal agar.* Make dilution strokes by cutting into the agar with the edge of the sterilized loop. Dip a glass coverslip in alcohol, sterilize it by flaming, and let it cool; then put it on the agar to cover part of the well and some of the dilution strokes. Incubate at 22°C for 48 h and then examine by placing the plate on a microscope from which the slide carrier has been removed. Begin by scanning the area under the coverslip and then, if no filamentous structures are found, carefully focus on the submerged growth that tracks along the incisions in the agar. Further examination of hyphae should be made to distinguish true mycelium from pseudomycelium. A pseudomycelium is composed of cells of varying width with rounded ends (Fig. 42.2) rather like a chain of sausages, whereas a true mycelium has cells of constant width with square ends and has a pattern of intertwining lines of bricks laid end to end (Fig. 42.3a). When a true mycelium is found, individual hyphae should be checked for arthrospore formation (Fig. 42.3b) which identifies the genus *Trichosporon*. Production of pseudomycelium and/or true mycelium in the absence of arthrospores signifies *Candida* species. Round

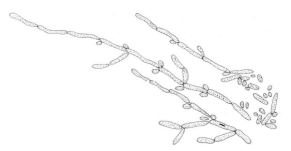

Fig. 42.2 Pseudohyphae showing varying width, rounded ends and blastospore formation.

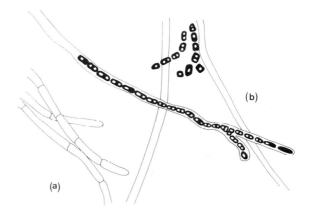

Fig. 42.3 (a) True mycelium formed by hyphae of constant width and end walls at right angles to longitudinal walls. (b) True mycelium of *Trichosporon cutaneum* showing multiple segmentation and ultimately fragmentation into arthrospores.

terminal chlamydospores are formed by *C. albicans* and *C. stellatoidea* and provide confirmatory or alternative evidence for identification. Three genera, *Rhodotorula*, *Cryptococcus* and *Torulopsis*, fail to produce mycelium but one (*Rhodotorula*) is readily identified on primary isolation by the pink colour of its carotenoid pigments. The urease test assists in distinguishing the other two genera.

2. Urease test

Cryptococcus can be reliably differentiated from *Torulopsis* by its ability to produce urease. Seed a slant of Christensen urea agar* and incubate at 30°C for 48 h. Conversion of the phenolphthalein indicator in the medium from yellow to pink or red denotes the alkaline change when urease liberates ammonia from urea. Be particularly vigilant for bacterial contamination as the cause of a false positive result in this test.

Tests 1 and 2 allow identification of the yeast isolate to genus level as shown in Figure 42.1. Speciation can usually be achieved by completing the following two tests, but identification of the genus *Rhodotorula* requires test 5 (nitrate assimilation). If uncertainty persists, confirmation of an identification may be achieved by testing for the ability of the isolate to ferment certain sugars (test 6).

Preparation of inoculum suspension for tests 3, 4, 5 and 6

Before setting up any of the following tests, prepare an inoculum pool by emulsifying a heavily loaded loopful of the strain to be identified in 5 ml of sterile saline.

3. Surface growth

The production and form of surface growth in broth produced by some species is helpful in identification. Put a drop of the inoculum pool suspension into a standard test tube approximately half filled with malt broth or an equivalent medium. Incubate for 48 h at 30°C. Surface growth may be present as a pellicle, a ring around the surface of the tube at the broth interface (e.g. *Candida tropicalis*) or a climbing film on the sides of the glass (presumptive of *C. krusei*).

4. Sugar assimilation test (auxanogram)

Assimilation tests have largely replaced fermentation as a means of species identification in view of equivocal fermentation test results. The method consists essentially of growing a yeast on a basal carbohydrate-free medium supplemented with the test sugar. There are many variations on the number of sugars and the method of their application to the basal medium. The following approach conveniently overcomes some of the practical problems.

a. Prepare Basal medium I or Basal medium II as described in *Methods.** Dispense in 10 ml amounts and autoclave.

b. While the medium is cooling, dispense about 0.5–1 mg of the test sugar into a compartment of a 10 cm square 'Repli dish' (Sterilin) which has 25 divisions. Five sugars that suffice for identification in most instances are glucose (positive control), sucrose, trehalose, lactose and raffinose. Five isolates may be tested on each plate.

c. Allow the agar medium to cool to approximately 45°C; if Basal medium II is used, add a few grains of powdered yeast extract to supply essential vitamins.

d. Seed the medium with 1 ml of the test organism from the prepared inoculum suspension.

e. Use a Pasteur pipette to distribute sufficient of the seeded medium to cover the base of each compartment. A constant depth of medium should be maintained.

f. Incubate at 30°C for 48 h. Growth produces an opacity in the medium and indicates the ability of the isolate to assimilate a sugar. All yeasts assimilate glucose.

The assimilation pattern for individual species is given in Table 42.1. As yeasts can show variation through loss of an enzyme, a wider range of sugars may be tested and/or fermentation tests performed if there is any doubt.

5. Nitrate assimilation

This test assists in the differentiation of the two species of *Rhodotorula* isolated from human sources.

a. Weigh out 1 g of potassium dihydrogen phosphate, 0.5 g magnesium sulphate, 20 g glucose and 25 g agar and steam to dissolve in 1000 ml of distilled water. Dispense in 10 ml amounts and autoclave at 115°C for 15 min.

b. Dispense a few crystals (around 1 mg) of potassium nitrate to one of the compartments of a 'Repli dish', a similar quantity of peptone (dry powder) to another (as positive control) and leave a third compartment free of additives (negative control).

c. Inoculate the test organism from the inoculum suspension into the cooling medium as

Table 42.1 Salient features of the medically important yeasts: ( ) indicates variation, with most likely reaction given within the brackets.

Species	Fermentation of				Assimilation of					Surface growth in broth	Nitrate assimilation	Capsules	Urease	Arthrospores	Pseudo or true mycelium	Germ tubes and/or chlamydospores
	Maltose	Lactose	Sucrose	Glucose	Raffinose	Trehalose	Lactose	Sucrose	Glucose							
Candida albicans	+	−	−	+	−	+	−	+	+	−	−	−	−	−	+	+
C. guilliermondi	−	−	+	+	+	+	−	+	+	−	−	−	−	−	+	−
C. intermedia	+	−	+	+	+	+	+	+	+	+	−	−	−	−	+	−
C. krusei	−	−	−	+	−	−	−	−	+	+	−	−	(+)	−	+	−
C. parapsilosis	−	−	−	+	−	+	+	+	+	−	−	−	−	−	+	−
C. pseudotropicalis	−	+	−	+	+	−	+	+	+	−	−	−	−	−	+	−
C. stellatoidea	−	−	+	+	−	+	−	−	+	−	−	−	−	−	+	+
C. tropicalis	+	−	−	+	−	+	−	+	+	+	−	−	−	−	+	−
C. zeylanoides	+	−	+	(−)	−	+	−	−	+	(+)	−	−	−	−	(−)	−
Cryptococcus neoformans	+	−	−	−	(+)	+	(+)	+	+	(+)	−	+	+	−	−	−
Rhodotorula glutinis	−	−	−	−	+	+	−	+	+	+	+	−	+	−	−	−
R. rubra (R. mucilaginosa)	−	−	(−)	(−)	+	+	−	+	+	(+)	−	−	+	−	−	−
Torulopsis candida	−	−	−	+	+	+	+	+	+	−	−	−	−	−	−	−
T. glabrata	−	−	−	+	−	−	−	−	+	−	−	−	−	−	−	−
Trichosporon capitatum	−	−	−	−	−	−	−	−	+	+	−	−	−	+	+	−
T. cutaneum (T. beigeli)	−	−	−	−	(+)	(+)	+	(+)	+	+	−	−	(+)	+	+	−

in the sugar assimilation test procedure and follow steps c to f in (5) above. Growth must be present in the compartment containing peptone, otherwise the test is invalidated.

6. *Sugar fermentation*

a. Prepare fermentation test media with a suitable range of sugars as described in *Methods* at the end of this chapter.

b. Inoculate the test organism by adding one drop of the inoculum suspension into each tube. A duplicate series should be seeded with the test inoculum as variation can occur.

c. Incubate for 48–72 h at 30°C.

d. The ability to ferment a sugar is shown by the presence of acid (indicator becomes pink) and gas trapped in the Durham tube.

The fermentation patterns of the medically important yeasts are given in Table 42.1. If an isolate does not conform to any of these, consult a specialist text such as Kreger-Van Rij (1984) or forward the strain to a mycology reference laboratory.

Serodiagnosis

Serological tests are of little practical use in the diagnosis of systemic candidosis. Rising titres of precipitins or agglutinins may provide a valid index but all too often there is insufficient time to allow a prognostic diagnosis by such means. Moreover, false positive results are encountered in tests with healthy subjects or with patients suffering from superficial candidosis, and false negatives may occur with immuno-incompetent patients with proven deep-seated yeast infections. A further complication is that cross-reactions may be obtained in patients with tuberculosis and other infections. Considerable efforts are being made to find a practical and reliable method for the detection of candida antigenaemia.

A latex agglutination test for cryptococcal antigen in CSF is commercially available and is of value in the differential diagnosis of meningitis.

2. SUPERFICIAL MYCOSES

Fungal infections of the horny layers of the body surface are common in all countries of the world. The majority are caused by the dermatophyte fungi of the genera *Epidermophyton, Microsporum* and *Trichophyton*. They can all lyse keratin. Some species of the dermatophytes or ringworm fungi have a worldwide distribution whilst others are endemic within clearly defined geographical areas. Their distinct host preferences allow an arbitrary classification: anthropophilic species predominantly infect man; zoophilic species preferentially infect animals; and geophilic species are essentially soil organisms and rarely infect man or animals. Not all superficial mycoses are caused by dermatophytes; the yeasts give rise to intertrigos and infect moist skinfolds. Yeast infections are often associated with predisposing factors such as diabetes, obesity or constant immersion of the hands in water. A very small proportion of superficial infections is caused by filamentous fungi other than dermatophytes. This miscellaneous group almost exclusively parasitizes toenails, frequently following injury. A definitive diagnosis of a fungal infection can only be established by mycological investigation. Although the majority of skin specimens processed in the mycology laboratory yield negative results, exclusion of fungal involvement is of considerable assistance to the dermatologist. The positive identification of a fungus allows a definitive diagnosis, determines the correct treatment, and enables action to be taken on the possible source of the infection and prevention of further spread.

The efficiency with which skin, nail and hair are investigated in the mycology laboratory is largely dependent upon the quantity of material submitted for examination. Attention is drawn to the relevant part of this chapter dealing with collection and storage of specimens (above). It is essential for laboratory workers to familiarize themselves with these procedures in order to instruct clinical colleagues.

Most species of dermatophyte produce two types of asexual conidia (aleuriospores). Microconidia are small and unicellular whereas macroconidia are large and septate and may have thick or thin walls. The latter spores provide differentiation of the dermatophytes into three genera:

Epidermophyton. This genus, of which there is only one species, *E. floccosum*, produces large, smooth, thick walled macroconidia that are usually composed of two to four cells (Fig. 42.4). They are usually abundant and measure from 20–40 μm long by 6–8 μm across and occur in clusters of two or three. Microconidia are not produced.

Microsporum. The macroconidia, which vary in numbers from rare to numerous, are spindle-shaped with thick roughened walls (Fig. 42.5). Each macroconidium may be divided into five to ten cells and can be up to 100 μm long and 6–8 μm wide.

Trichophyton. The macroconidia vary in shape from that of a cigar to a cylinder and measure from 8–50 μm in length and 4–8 μm across (Fig. 42.6). Walls are smooth but may be thick or thin. Unlike macroconidia, microconidia are mostly produced in large numbers.

Identification of a dermatophyte may not be possible on the gross morphology of the colony or by the presence of macro- or microconidia on microscopy. In these cases more detailed examination of the preparation should be carried out under the microscope in order to distinguish other structures that may assist identification. As well as chlamydospores, features such as spiral and racquet hyphae, favic chandeliers and nodular bodies should be noted.

If microscopy fails to place the isolate in a taxon, it is sometimes useful to determine the effect of certain media and growth factors on the development of the colony. Potato dextrose agar* is a reference medium, especially for the production of pigment, as for example in *Trichophyton rubrum*, and it is useful in differentiating this species from anthropophilic *T. mentagrophytes* isolates. Rice grains are used to separate *Microsporum audouini* and *M. canis* as the

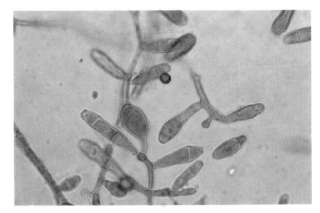

Fig. 42.4 *Epidermophyton floccosum*: mycelium and macroconidia (lactophenol cotton blue × 880).

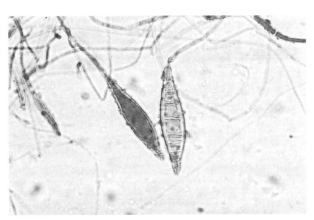

Fig. 42.5 *Microsporum canis*: mycelium and macroconidia (lactophenol cotton blue × 880).

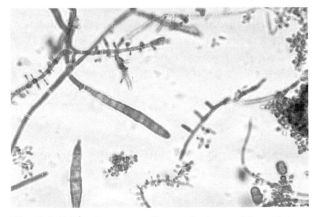

Fig. 42.6 *Trichophyton*: mycelium and microconidia and macroconidia (lactophenol cotton blue × 880).

former grows very poorly on this substrate. A series of agar media (Trichophyton agars, Difco) incorporating growth factors can be helpful in grouping species of *Trichophyton*. Information on the execution of some of these tests and full descriptions of species and their variants is given by Rebell & Taplin (1974).

Characteristics of the common British dermatophytes

Epidermophyton floccosum. On malt peptone agar the colony appears early and enlarges fairly rapidly; surface velvety and powdery and either flat or folded; khaki to tan in colour with tan to dark brown underside. No microconidia produced. Macroconidia usually abundant as described above. Chlamydospores may be produced as the colony ages. This anthropophilic species is isolated almost exclusively from groins and feet; rarely infects nails and never hair.

Microsporum audouini. This species is now rare in Britain where it used to cause epidemic tinea capitis in children. Colony flat and grows slowly with a cream to tan upper surface and a pink or brown underside. Microconidia and macroconidia are rarely formed. When present, the latter are variable in shape but are essentially spindle-shaped with rough or smooth walls. Although anthropophilic, this species rarely infects adults; it is restricted almost entirely to hair in children.

Microsporum canis. Now the most common member of the genus found in Britain. Two forms are recognized on culture. One, fast growing, has white aerial mycelium which becomes tan as the colony ages, bright lemon-yellow to orange on underside. Characteristic spindle-shaped macroconidia are usually present, with rough walls and an asymmetric terminal spiny knob (Fig. 42.5). The second form is termed dysgonic and produces a slowly growing colony with a very irregular colony edge and a mass of submerged mycelium. The aerial part of the colony is shiny and waxy; both surface and undersurface are brown. Isolates from dogs and cats tend to be dysgonic. Human infections usually acquired by contact with infected animals, particularly cats. This zoophilic species can cause tinea capitis in children and tinea corporis in all age groups.

Microsporum gypseum. Granular light to mid-brown colony grows rapidly with an irregularly fringed border and cinnamon undersurface. Numerous spindle-shaped macroconidia formed with up to six cells in each; walls thick and roughened. Geophilic; infection in humans rare and usually as a result of contact with animals such as pet rodents infected from the soil.

Trichophyton mentagrophytes. Two distinct forms recognized. The zoophilic subspecies var. *granulare* produces a fast growing colony with a flat powdery or granular surface, which is an indication of abundant sporulation, and an irregular edge. The anthropophilic subspecies var. *interdigitale* is often indistinguishable from *T. rubrum* on primary isolation since it produces a white fluffy aerial mycelium which may become yellowish or tan with age. The underside of both colony types may be pink, red, yellow or rose brown. Sporulation is much more pronounced in the granular form which also shows the presence of spiral hyphae and macroconidia that are up to six-celled and have smooth thick walls. Macroconidia rare in the anthropophilic form. Both forms produce microconidia either borne along the sides of vegetative hyphae (Fig. 42.6) or in grape-like clusters – especially common in zoophilic isolates.

In practice it may be difficult to differentiate *T. mentagrophytes* var. *interdigitale* from *T. rubrum* on both macroscopic and microscopic characteristics. The isolate should be subcultured to a potato dextrose agar (PDA) plate* and to a slope of Christensen's urea medium supplemented with glucose 10 g/litre*. After incubation at 28°C for 7 days, *T. mentagrophytes* will have degraded the urea sufficiently to change the indicator in the medium to pink. *T. rubrum* requires a longer incubation period of at least a further 7 days to produce a similar pH change. On the PDA medium *T. mentagrophytes* var. *interdigitale* produces a colony similar to that of var. *granulare* on primary isolation, usually with an unpigmented undersurface or rarely a brownish undersurface. A colony of *T. rubrum* on PDA characteristically has a white cottony aerial mycelium, an entire edge and a pink or red underside.

The zoophilic subspecies var. *granulare* commonly causes ringworm of animals especially rodents. In man it tends to form lesions on exposed parts of the body such as forearms and face. All sites of the body but particularly feet, groins and nail, may be infected by *T. mentagrophytes* var. *interdigitale* which has been replaced by *T. rubrum* as the most frequently isolated species in Britain.

Trichophyton rubrum grows more slowly than *T. mentagrophytes* to produce a white colony with a cottony mycelium that may become pink with age. The underside is typically deep red. Many variations have been noted but have not yet been well defined. Tear-shaped microconidia are borne along the sides of undifferentiated vegetative hyphae. The production of macroconidia is variable but usually rare. When present they are long, narrow and cylindrical with rounded ends and can have up to 10 cells with thin smooth walls. *T. rubrum* is the most frequently isolated species of the dermatophytes and can infect all sites of the body, commonly feet, groins and nails, but rarely causes tinea capitis.

Trichophyton tonsurans grows slowly. The colony has a powdery surface which becomes heaped, folded and velvety with age. The surface is usually tan or yellow (var. *sulphureum*) and the underside a deep mahogany or yellow. The microconidia are numerous and transform with maturity into large irregular spores borne in branched clusters or formed on thickened terminal hyphae. Macroconidia are rare in most strains; when present they are cylindrical to club-shaped with five or six cells and often curve towards their apices. This anthropophilic species causes epidemic tinea capitis in the USA. Various skin sites and the nails may be parasitized.

Trichophyton verrucosum grows slowly and almost exclusively on nutrient agar. The colony is white, waxy and heaped. It is unique amongst the dermatophytes by growing more rapidly at 37°C than at 28°C. Macroconidia are almost unknown whereas chlamydospores are common and may occur in chains. Predominantly causes ringworm in cattle. Human infections are acquired by direct contact with infected stock; exposed sites such as face and arms are most at risk.

Trichophyton violaceum. Until recently this anthropophilic species was almost unknown in Britain. Infected immigrants arriving from endemic areas of the world have provided a source from which *T. violaceum* has rapidly spread. Growth is very slow and produces a heaped waxy colony that becomes deep purple at maturity. The mycelium is usually non-sporing, although chlamydospores may be formed. Skin, nail or hair may be infected.

A summary of the characteristics listed above is given in Table 42.2.

Laboratory diagnosis of superficial mycoses

Procedures for direct examination and culture are described below.

Direct examination

Direct microscopy provides an early and reasonably reliable method of diagnosing or excluding a fungal infection. It should be performed on all specimens of skin and nail. Whilst microscopy is equally important in the investigation of hair infections, additional information may be obtained by examination under Wood's light – a source of filtered UV light with maximum emission at 366 nm. When hair is parasitized by *Microsporum audouini* or *M. canis*, a greenish fluorescence is produced at the base of the hair shaft and indicates the most productive area to sample for microscopy and culture. None of the other species commonly associated with hair infections produces fluorescence.

Prepare specimens for microscopy by reducing to thin fragments on a slide and adding a drop of 20% potassium hydroxide dissolved in 40%

Table 42.2 Characteristics of the common British dermatophytes.

Species	Colony Morphology		Microscopy		Host preference	Main sites	Spread of infection
	Surface	Underside	Macroconidia	Microcondia			
Epidermophyton floccosum	Velvety, greenish yellow	Brown	Club shaped. Abundant	Not produced	Anthropophilic	Foot, groin	Man to man through exposure to desquamated skin. e.g. clothing, towels, changing-room floors
Microsporum audouini	Cream to tan	Pink or brown	Spindle shaped. Rare	Rare	Anthropophilic	Scalp	Man to man, (puberty). Sharing of brushes and combs
Microsporum canis	White becoming tan	Lemon-yellow to orange	Spindle shaped. Normally present	Few	Zoophilic	Scalp, body	In children by man to man contact via combs and brushes. Adult skin lesion acquired by contact with infected cats and dogs
Microsporum gypseum	Granular, mid-brown	Cinnamon	Short ovoid to spindle shaped. Abundant	Few	Geophilic	Scalp, body	From soil or infected animal
Trichophyton mentagrophytes var. granulare	Powdery, white to tan	Pink, yellow or rose-brown	Cigar shaped, thick or thin walled. Occasional	Abundant in grape-like clusters	Zoophilic	Beard, head, body	Contact with infected animal, especially rodent
Trichophyton mentagrophytes var. interdigitale	Fluffy, white becoming yellowish or tan	Pink, yellow or rose-brown	Cigar shaped, thick or thin walled. Rare	Commonly borne along sides of hyphae	Anthropophilic	Foot, groin, nails	Man to man. Contact with desquamated skin on floors, towels etc.
Trichophyton rubrum	Fluffy, white becoming pink	Pink or red	Long cylindrical, thin walled. Rare	Borne laterally on vegetative hyphae	Anthropophilic	Foot, groin, body, nails	Man to man. Contact with desquamated skin.
Trichophyton tonsurans	Cream to tan or yellow	Deep red or yellow	Cylindrical with curved tips. Rare	Irregular in size and shape. Numerous	Anthropophilic	Scalp, body, nails	Contagious in schools and other institutions
Trichophyton verrucosum	White waxy on nutrient agar	White or yellow	Variable in shape Almost unknown	Small and thin. Borne on sides of hyphae. Rare	Zoophilic	Head, body	Contact with infected cattle
Trichophyton violaceum	Waxy, deep purplish-red	Deep red to violet	Thin walled, cylindrical. Very rare	Tear shaped. Very rare	Anthropophilic	Head, body, nails	Man to man. Contact with desquamated skin

aqueous dimethyl sulphoxide (KOH/DMSO). This allows rapid penetration and maceration of the tissue without resort to heating before viewing. Apply a coverslip; after a few minutes, tap gently to achieve as thin a preparation as possible. For bright field illumination, the microscope condenser should be racked completely down. Alternatively, when available, phase or darkground illumination greatly facilitates the observation of hyphae which are seen as fine filaments that traverse the tissue unimpeded by the host cell structure (Fig. 42.7).

The calcofluor white fluorescent stain may be used to advantage, especially where the laboratory worker lacks experience. The procedure set out above should be followed except that a drop each of KOH 20% and calcofluor white* is substituted for the KOH/DMSO mixture and the final preparation is viewed by fluorescence microscopy. Fungal hyphae appear bright green against a dark background.

Dermatophyte hyphae, especially in hair, frequently round off with the production of arthrospores. Take care to avoid confusing hyphae and arthrospores with deposits of cholesterol on the surface of the squamous cells. This artefact is often referred to as 'mosaic fungus'.

The bases of hair shafts, particularly those areas that fluoresce or have visible crusted areas, should be selected and closely examined microscopically to determine whether the hyphae and arthrospores form a sheath around the outside (ectothrix) or if they are situated totally within the hair shaft (endothrix). This information is often helpful in identifying the isolate obtained on culture.

The finding of hyphae in a specimen of keratinous material enables a diagnosis of fungal infection to be made. More specific identification of the causal fungus is impossible by simple microscopy, except in the case of pityriasis versicolor (see below). With skin infections, a positive microscopy finding should be the signal for treatment with a broad spectrum antifungal drug; for hair and nail infections, griseofulvin should be prescribed on a 'best guess' basis until the results of culture are known.

Pityriasis versicolor

The definitive diagnosis of pityriasis versicolor by direct microscopy rests on the unique appearance of the causal organism in skin. Adhesive tape strippings provide the simplest means of identification once they have been stained by running a drop of Parker's blue-black Quink ink or methylene blue or lactophenol cotton blue* under the tape. The fungal elements absorb the dye preferentially and appear as abundant short curved hyphae associated with groups of spherical cells giving a 'bananas and grapes' arrangement (Fig. 42.8). It was thought originally that the agent of pityriasis versicolor was an obligate parasite and the name *Malassezia furfur* was applied to its appearance on direct microscopy.

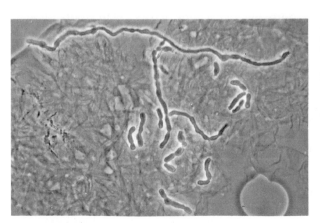

Fig. 42.7 Hyphae of a dermatophytic fungus in skin (KOH preparation, phase contrast × 880).

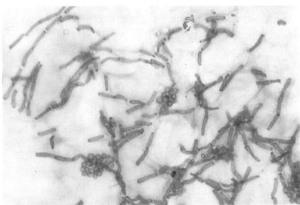

Fig. 42.8 *Malassezia furfur* (*Pityrosporum orbiculare*): yeast and short hyphal forms in the skin from pityriasis versicolor (Parker's Quink ink × 880).

Subsequently, however, it was discovered that the yeast *Pityrosporum orbiculare* could be isolated if the culture medium is overlaid with olive oil to satisfy an absolute requirement for fat. *P. orbiculare* may cause seborrhoeic dermatitis but it may also form part of the commensal flora of skin. The microscopical findings for this condition are diagnostic and the subsequent culture of the causative fungus is accordingly not performed in the routine mycology laboratory.

Isolation

Although methods for isolation of dermatophyte species vary considerably from one laboratory to another, they have several features in common: a typical mycological medium such as malt or Sabouraud's agar is used, with minor modifications such as adjustment of the pH; incubation is at 28–30°C, which is the optimum for all except one of the dermatophytes, for up to 4 weeks. Diseased keratinous tissue harbours a great many organisms and it is necessary to inhibit or reduce the growth of contaminating bacteria and fungi by the addition of selective agents, such as antibacterial antibiotics and the antifungal cycloheximide, to the media. An effective scheme for the isolation of dermatophytes, yeasts and the miscellaneous filamentous fungi causing superficial mycoses is as follows.

Culture media

The basal medium is malt* or Sabouraud's agar* with added peptone or yeast extract respectively. A typical composition is malt extract (syrup) 4%, mycological peptone 0.5% and agar 2% in distilled water.

Table 42.3 lists the range of media employed in the mycological investigation of skin, nail and hair and their effect on the fungi that may be present. This shows that a medium lacking selective agents is necessary for the reliable isolation of yeasts and on those few rare occasions when a filamentous fungus other than a dermatophyte is causative. Cycloheximide (C), also known as actidione, reduces the growth of some yeasts and fungi other than the dermatophytes when it is incorporated at a concentration of 500 mg/litre. Natamycin (N), also known as pimaricin, is more inhibitory towards contaminating fungi and all yeasts at 0.1 g/l but it may also restrict the growth of some strains of *E. floccosum* and *M. canis*. Natamycin unlike cycloheximide may be added prior to autoclaving. Penicillin (P) at a concentration of 20 000 units/l and streptomycin (S) at 40 mg/l should be added to all media after autoclaving. As the causative agent of cattle ringworm, *T. verrucosum*, is a fastidious organism that produces little or no growth on malt agar, a nutrient agar (25 g Oxoid nutrient broth No. 2 and 20 g agar/l) containing cycloheximide, should be prepared. Four media, as shown, are therefore inoculated (see *Methods** for recipes). Occasionally, a yeast and a dermatophyte may be present in the same specimen and since the former rapidly overgrows the latter, the natamycin plate ensures that the dermatophyte has the opportunity to grow.

Inoculum

Skin and nail should be reduced in size to pieces approximately 1 mm across. Hair roots should be selected especially where crusted or fluorescent material is found and cut into similarly sized fragments. Because of the scanty presence of fungi in the tissue, pieces smaller than 1 mm

Table 42.3 The growth of fungi from skin, nail and hair on selective media.
Key: +, growth; −, no growth; ±, some restricted growth; ∓, little or no growth.

Medium[a]	Result of culture on stated medium with			
	Dermatophytes	Yeasts	Contaminants	*Trichophyton verrucosum*
Malt peptone agar	+	+	+	−
Malt peptone agar + P + S + C	+	±	∓	−
Malt peptone agar + P + S + N	+	−	−	−
Nutrient agar + P + S + C	+	∓	∓	+

[a] See *Methods* for details.

are less likely to contain viable hyphae whilst larger fragments may not allow adequate diffusion of nutrients and selective agents into the tissue. Four inocula should be gently implanted into the agar on each plate at well spaced intervals.

Incubation

All dermatophytes have an optimum temperature for growth in culture of 28–30°C with the exception of *T. verrucosum* which grows best at 37°C. Since there is little appreciable difference in the growth rate of this species at the lower temperature and there is less drying out of the media, it is more convenient to incubate all plates containing selective agents at 28°C. The malt peptone agar without additions should be incubated at 37°C and checked for growth of yeasts or other sgnificant fungi for up to 1 week and discarded if it has become overgrown with contaminants. The three other plates should be incubated for 3–4 weeks before recording no growth.

No growth from positive material

Failure to isolate a fungus from a specimen of skin or hair in which hyphae were seen in the microscopy sample can usually be attributed to:

1. Insufficient or incorrectly collected material for culture.

2. Prior treatment of the lesion with an agent possessing antifungal activity.

3. Incorrect storage such as refrigeration, or holding the material in a container that retains moisture.

With nail tissue, failure to isolate a fungus occurs in up to 50% of specimens seen to contain hyphae. This is a well recognized worldwide phenomenon and though it is evident in other fungi causing onychomycosis, the most likely pathogen is a dermatophyte which should respond to griseofulvin therapy. Paradoxically it has been shown (Gentles 1971) that the chances of isolating a dermatophyte from nail tissue actually increase after griseofulvin has been administered for a few months.

Identification

Cultures should be examined at 4 or 5 day intervals from the outset. Growth of a dermatophyte usually occurs within 7–10 days and colonies are recognized as being light coloured, often white and shades thereof, and never blue, black or dark green.

Yeasts

Yeasts grow as typical pasty colonies and are readily recognized. Their significance, however, is less obvious. The clinical information accompanying the specimen is often helpful in determining a yeast isolate's relevance to the disease syndrome but there are no hard and fast rules for interpreting laboratory results. The following factors should be considered when a yeast has been isolated in the absence of a dermatophyte:

1. Hyphae should have been observed on microscopical examination of the tissue and it may have been possible to distinguish pseudomycelium and associated budding cells. The possibility of a yeast pathogen should be considered when the hyphae are abundant, long and thin and less conspicuous than those of a dermatophyte.

2. Growth should be present from the majority of inocula on the medium without selective agents. It is likely that growth, although less extensive, will also be present on the media incorporating cycloheximide.

3. Identification of the yeast (as set out in the previous section) is helpful. For instance, *Candida albicans* or *C. parapsilosis* may be either commensal or pathogenic, whereas *Rhodotorula glutinis* or *Trichosporon cutaneum* are almost exclusively commensal.

Miscellaneous filamentous fungi

True fungi, other than dermatophytes, are seldom pathogenic on skin but on rare occasions they can invade nail tissue – especially traumatized nail tissue of the great toe. They should be considered as potential pathogens only where abnormal hyphae and frequently large chlamydospores are seen on microscopy. Identification of the filamentous fungi is achieved in the conventional manner by reference to appropriate texts such as Barnett & Hunter (1972) and Barron (1968). *Fusarium oxysporum*, *Hendersonula toruloidea* and *Scopulariopsis brevicaulis* are amongst the more commonly isolated species in this rare group.

Dermatophytes

The gross appearance of the colony serves as the first important step in the recognition and identification of a dermatophyte. Colonies that are blue, black or dark green should be regarded as non-dermatophytes. The following characteristics should be noted; the rate of growth of the colony; the texture, colour and shape of the upper thallus; and the production of pigment on the underside. With experience it becomes possible to identify an isolate on those gross morphological characteristics alone.

Precise identification is generally accomplished by examination of a representative section of the sporulating area of the colony under the microscope. The conventional method of making a preparation for microscopy consists of using mounted needles to take a representative sample of the area of the colony that is mature and likely, therefore, to be spore-producing*. The sample is then teased out in a drop of lactophenol cotton blue on a microscope slide and a coverslip applied. This is a time-consuming process and requires considerable skill to separate out the individual hyphae without damage. Spores are readily released from the spore-bearing structures and so the point of greatest significance may be lost. A more rapid method that allows even the completely inexperienced worker to achieve satisfactory preparations is performed thus:

1. Place an elongated drop of lactophenol cotton blue on a clean microscope slide.

2. Take a piece of clear vinyl adhesive tape (e.g. Sellotape or Scotch Tape type 361) 6–7 cm long and hold loosely between the thumb and forefinger of each hand. Allow the centre of the adhesive side of the tape to touch the colony lightly under its own weight.

3. Transfer to the slide, placing the area with adhered mycelium on to the lactophenol cotton blue. Microscopical examination reveals spores and other relevant structures fixed in place by the adhesive.

3. ASPERGILLOSIS

The genus *Aspergillus* consists of hundreds of species, many of which can exploit a variety of substrates and grow and reproduce within a wide range of environmental conditions. *Aspergillus fumigatus* is a ubiquitous example and its airborne spores can cause respiratory allergies directly or give rise after germination to infection of the respiratory tract.

Generally the term aspergillosis is taken to imply an infection caused by *A. fumigatus* in the bronchopulmonary system but it should not be forgotten that other species, such as *A. flavus*, *A. niger* and *A. terreus*, can infect the lungs, and that aspergillus infection may occur at other sites such as the eyes and ears. Kerato-mycosis can be caused by several *Aspergillus* species and mostly follows trauma. *A. niger* is the species predominantly isolated from otitis externa although it is less common in air than *A. fumigatus* and so a degree of specialization or adaptation to the microenvironment of the ears and the respiratory tract is evident. All organs of the body have been recorded as invaded by aspergillus and disseminated aspergillosis is being more widely recognized as advances in medicine enable severely debilitated and immunologically compromised patients to survive.

The inhalation of aspergillus spores can give rise to a hypersensitivity reaction producing symptoms of asthma and rhinitis in atopic individuals (Type I); inhalation in large numbers may induce an allergic alveolitis (Type III) in atopic and non-atopic individuals. Maltworker's lung is an example of the latter and is caused by the inhalation of large numbers of spores of *A. clavatus* released into the atmosphere during the turning of contaminated malting barley.

Bronchopulmonary aspergillosis has been divided into three arbitrary types (Crofton & Douglas 1981) in all of which there is vegetative growth of the fungus within the bronchopulmonary system and the (sometimes spasmodic) expectoration of hyphae in sputum:

1. In *bronchial aspergillosis* with allergic manifestations, reflecting hypersensitivity to antigenic material released from colonization of the bronchial lumen, there is no invasion of lung tissue or of the bronchial wall. The fungus appears to colonize the bronchial secretions. Occasionally, bronchial plugs may be formed consisting mainly of mucus rather than mycelium and these may obstruct the bronchi to cause segmental, lobar or whole lung collapse. Bronchial casts may be coughed up spontaneously, or it may be necessary to remove the plugs at bronchoscopy to allow reinflation of the affected part of the lung. These plugs are ideal specimens for microscopy and culture but it should be emphasized that, contrary to expectations, few hyphae are present in a direct smear and such specimens should be processed as sputum.

2. *Aspergilloma* is the most common form of bronchopulmonary aspergillosis and is produced by the colonization of a lung cavity created by previous disease, typically tuberculosis, but occasionally sarcoidosis, pulmonary infarction, bronchiectasis or invasive aspergillosis. A typical aspergilloma is composed of a cavity wall developed from modified bronchial epithelium enclosing a mass of fungal mycelium and detritus that almost completely fills the cavity leaving a 'halo' of air space that is often visible on X-ray. The mycetoma tends to consist largely of amorphous material with relatively few hyphae.

3. *Invasive* or *necrotizing aspergillosis* occurs in predisposed patients such as those receiving immunosuppressive therapy or the severely debilitated. Active invasion of healthy lung tissue by the fungus usually occurs as a solitary event but it may result in, or from, disseminated aspergillosis. It is imperative to establish a definitive diagnosis quickly as the disease spreads rapidly throughout the lungs causing respiratory failure.

Laboratory diagnosis of aspergillosis

In view of the variable output of fungal fragments in the sputum of patients with aspergillosis, an entire 3 day collection should be made as directed at the beginning of this chapter. This allows a more conclusive investigation and can establish a baseline for future reference, for example to assess the efficacy of treatment.

The laboratory diagnosis of bronchopulmonary aspergillosis has to be made by taking into account, on the one hand, the frequency with which aspergillus spores are present in the atmosphere, and on the other, the relative scarcity of the diagnostic fungal hyphae in sputum. Even quite large numbers of colonies, up to 1000/ml of sputum, can be obtained from spores that have been inhaled and trapped in the bronchial secretions or by contamination of the sputum during collection and processing. Isolation alone is not indicative, therefore, of bronchopulmonary aspergillosis and a definitive diagnosis is only possible by the observation of the characteristic hyphae on microscopy. Conversely, failure to isolate *A. fumigatus* on culture is usually conclusive evidence against aspergillosis and some use can be made of culture in primary screening of sputum from suspected cases.

Primary screening tests for Aspergillus

Screening tests are at their most valuable in invasive aspergillosis since precious time can be saved. Remove the entire sputum specimen (preferably at least 2 ml) with a sterile cotton-wool swab and spread over the surface of a plate containing malt peptone agar to which penicillin and streptomycin have been added*. The swab, having become suitably charged during the process, should be used to seed a second plate of the same medium in the conventional manner. Incubate the entire sputum plate at 45°C and the swab plate at 37°C for 48 h. The higher temperature is selective and prevents the overgrowth of the profuse numbers of bacteria and yeasts present in such a large inoculum whereas *A. fumigatus* grows well although more slowly than at 37°C.

Aspergillus species can be identified by the characteristic sporing head seen on microscopy (Fig. 42.9), strong colour and by the marked colour that it confers on the colony. For example, *A. fumigatus* produces a deep blue-green colony, *A. flavus* light to yellow green, *A. terreus* cinnamon to beige or sandy brown, and

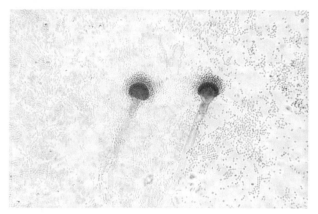

Fig. 42.9 Two conidiophores of *Aspergillus fumigatus* (lactophenol cotton blue × 880).

A. niger dark brown to black. Various morphological features associated with the sporing head allow accurate identification (Thom & Raper 1951).

It is difficult to interpret the results of culture without parallel observations from sputum microscopy. As a general rule, a few aspergillus colonies on the plate incubated at 45°C suggests spore contamination. If colonies are more numerous, further collections should be made and the sputum processed to establish the presence of the diagnostic hyphae by microscopy and to obtain a quantitative count of colony forming units.

Microscopy and culture for Aspergillus

Because of the variable nature of sputum and the small numbers of hyphal fragments that may be present, homogenization and concentration are necessary. Mechanical degradation is inadequate to allow centrifugation and pipetting, and the fungus is unlikely to survive caustic hydrolysis. Chemical agents such as cystine hydrochloride and dithiothreitol appear to yield variable results depending upon the nature of the sputum being processed. Experience has shown that a combination of mechanical agitation and enzymic hydrolysis offers the most satisfactory method.

1. Prepare a 5% suspension of Pancreatin (Grade III, Sigma) in sterile distilled water. Shake vigorously and centrifuge. Remove supernate (which may be stored at −20°C) and dilute 1 in 10 in saline to provide a working strength solution in 10 ml amounts.

2. Transfer the sputum to a squat 60 ml specimen container and add 10 ml of Pancreatin solution for every 5–10 ml of sputum. Shake well for a few minutes (a magnetic stirrer may be used) and transfer to a waterbath at 37°C. Occasional stirring may be necessary for rapid breakdown which is usually complete within 3–4 h.

3. Transfer the digested sputum to a Universal container and centrifuge.

4. Record the volume of the sputum, having removed a volume of supernate equivalent to that of the pancreatic enzyme suspension added at the beginning of the process.

5. Resuspend the sediment in the remaining supernate and remove 0.1 ml and spread over a malt peptone agar plate containing antibiotics. Remove a further 0.1 ml and prepare dilutions at 1 in 10 and 1 in 100 in sterile saline. Use 0.1 ml of each dilution to inoculate on to two further plates. Incubate these plates at 45°C.

6. Centrifuge the digested sputum once more and discard the supernate almost entirely.

7. Emulsify a loopful of sediment *either* in a drop of KOH/DMSO *or* in a drop of KOH 20% and calcofluor white* on a microscope slide and apply a coverslip. Take another loopful and make a heat-fixed smear on a slide.

8. Resuspend the sediment in sufficient supernate or sterile saline for inoculation of the entire homogenate by pipette on to two malt agar plates containing antibiotics.

9. Incubate one plate at 37°C and the other at 45°C for 48 h.

Microscopy

The KOH/DMSO preparation (see above) can be viewed immediately, preferably by phase or darkground rather than bright field illumination. Fluorescence microscopy should be used to examine the preparation stained with calcofluor white which causes the hyphae to fluoresce a bright green colour. The characteristic aspergillus hyphae are scanty and extreme care and patience are required; scan the entire area of the preparation. On occasions aspergillus hyphae may be difficult to differentiate from candida hyphae which are frequently present in sputum and are of little or no pathological significance. Typically, the fragments of *A. fumigatus* are wavy and densely branched, often dichotomous with undeveloped branch initials (Fig. 42.10). An experienced mycologist can suggest the type of aspergillosis that yielded the sputum on the basis of the size, frequency and morphology of the hyphae.

The heat-fixed preparation should be stained with methenamine silver nitrate (Grocott 1955). It may be examined at any time, but it should be retained until the results of culture are known. Fungal elements stain dark brown or black.

Culture

Isolates of *A. fumigatus* are often visible as small, faint, filamentous colonies, with some sporulation after 1 day but it is essential to continue incubation for a further 24 h. Record the number of colonies on the dilution plates and multiply by the appropriate factor to calculate the counts/ml of sputum. The counts on the total sediment plates should correlate with these calculations and they also serve to detect small numbers. On occasion, *A. fumigatus* is present only on the plate incubated at 45°C as growth may be suppressed at 37°C by contaminating yeasts and bacteria. Conversely, some strains of *A. fumigatus* and other species of *Aspergillus*

grow poorly at 45°C and are detected on the 37°C plate alone.

There is no hard and fast rule for the interpretation of the results of culture on their own. In general, the greater the numbers of *A. fumigatus* on culture, the greater is the significance. In exceptional circumstances up to 1000 colonies/ml of sputum may result from inhalation of spores from a heavily contaminated atmosphere. Profuse growth is not diagnostic but should encourage the collection of more sputum for further mycological examination.

The laboratory proof of bronchopulmonary aspergillosis is provided by a positive finding on both microscopy and culture. In very exceptional circumstances false positives may arise in, for example, mechanically ventilated patients where the fungus appears to grow saprophytically in the bronchi. These patients will show an absence of signs and symptoms but the potential risk of such colonization should be related to their general state in any clinical assessment (see Park et al 1982). Morphological variants of *A. fumigatus* (and other species) are sometimes isolated (Milne, unpublished). These tend to grow more slowly and their paler green colour than the wild type is an indication of reduced spore production. Significantly, morphological variants have only been recorded in the sputum obtained from patients with an aspergilloma.

ANTIFUNGAL DRUGS

The range of systemically active antifungal drugs is limited. New antifungals that have been recently introduced have largely been imidazole derivatives for topical use. The imidazoles have the advantage over the polyenes of possessing a broader spectrum and are active against dermatophytes as well as yeasts.

Sensitivity and assay of antifungal drugs

Topical agents

Primary resistance to the topical antifungals is unknown, and resistance does not develop during treatment – possibly because 'overkill'

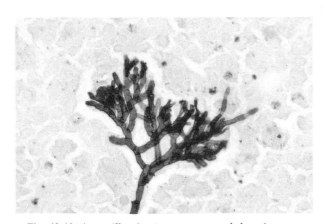

Fig. 42.10 *Aspergillus fumigatus*: wavy and densely branched hyphae in sputum (methenamine silver × 880).

concentrations of the drug are applied. Failure to respond to a course of therapy is likely to be attributable to lack of patient compliance, or to an untreated reservoir of infection or to uncontrolled predisposing factors.

Since topical antifungals are not absorbed to a detectable level, there is no need to determine their presence in body fluids.

Systemically active drugs

There is no standardized method for the sensitivity testing of fungi, because there is such wide variation in growth forms (yeast cells and/or hyphae) of the organisms and in the composition of culture media and culture conditions.

Amphotericin B. The buffered desoxycholate complex of amphotericin has been available for intravenous use for over 20 years and is still the most effective drug for serious and life-threatening infections. There is little or no need for sensitivity testing as all clinical isolates of yeasts and aspergillus are sensitive. Amphotericin can cause a variety of side-effects with renal toxicity related to total dose. As none appears to correlate with the level of amphotericin in serum, drug assay serves no purpose.

Flucytosine. This drug is available for oral and intravenous administration and should be given only in combination with amphotericin except in cases of urinary tract yeast infections. It is essential that sensitivity of the isolate is determined. Regardless of the method employed, extreme care should be exercised in the choice of culture medium as purines and pyrimidines in the medium act as antidotes. For practical guidance on sensitivity testing and the assay of flucytosine in body fluids see the report of the British Society for Mycopathology (1984).

Griseofulvin. Taken orally griseofulvin becomes incorporated into newly synthesized keratin and thus can only affect those fungi, viz. the dermatophytes, that have keratinolytic properties. In-vitro examination against dermatophytes is of no practical significance and unless malabsorption is suspected the determination of serum levels of the drug is not undertaken.

Ketoconazole. This is the first imidazole to yield significant blood levels without a high incidence of side-effects when taken orally. Its main uses are in chronic conditions such as chronic mucocutaneous candidosis and in prophylaxis. Sensitivity testing has limited application since there is poor correlation between attainable serum level, minimum inhibitory concentration and clinical efficacy.

GENERAL MYCOLOGICAL METHODS

Staining of fungi in wet mounts

Transparent self-adhesive tape may be used to transfer fungal elements to a slide for examination either unstained or stained by lactophenol blue (see under *Dermatophytes* above).

Lactophenol cotton blue stain

Phenol crystals	20 g
Lactic acid	20 ml
Glycerol	40 ml
Distilled water	20 ml
Cotton blue (or methyl blue)	0.075 g

Dissolve the phenol crystals in the liquids by gentle warming and then add the dye.

Needle-mount method

1. Place a drop of 95% alcohol on the slide. Gently tease out a fragment of the culture in the alcohol with needles or straight wires. When it is satisfactorily spread, let most of the alcohol evaporate and then add a drop of stain.

2. Apply a coverslip, avoiding bubbles, and exert gentle pressure if the fungus fragments do not lie flat.

3. Remove any excess stain round the coverslip with the edge of a piece of blotting paper. Let the stain penetrate; it may be satisfactory within a few minutes but differentiation may go on improving for up to 24 h. For permanent preparations, seal the edges with nail varnish or cellulose lacquer.

Calcofluor white fluorescent stain

Stock solution A

Calcofluor white (Fluorescent Brightener, Sigma)	1 g
Distilled water	100 ml

Stock solution B

Evans blue (Sigma)	0.05 g
Distilled water	100 ml

Working solution

Solution A	1 ml
Solution B	9 ml

Tissue and sputum (including spun deposit) should be mixed with a drop of the working solution and one of KOH 20%. Note that dimethylsulphoxide (DMSO) should not be employed in order to minimize background fluorescence. Allow a few minutes for maceration/clearing, place a coverslip on top and tap gently to obtain as thin a film as possible. View under a fluorescent microscope with a UV light source or one capable of producing blue light (wavelengths longer than 410 or 450 nm). Fungal cell walls fluoresce a bright green.

Culture media for fungi

Media for the isolation of pathogenic fungi are designed to be inhibitory to bacteria and in certain cases other fungi as well.

Agar is hydrolysed by heat at a low pH and acid media for fungi are not heated above 115°C. After autoclaving, the medium may be allowed to solidify in bulk but it should be remelted only once and then with a minimum of heating. The high concentration of sugar in some media for fungi is another reason for avoiding overheating and repeated heating, because heat tends to char sugar.

Malt peptone agar

Malt extract (syrup)	40 g
Peptone (e.g. Oxoid mycological)	5 g
Agar	15 g
Water	1 litre

Note: 20 g desiccated malt extract such as that produced by Oxoid may be substituted for the syrup.

Steam to dissolve the ingredients and adjust pH to 5.4. Autoclave at 115°C for 15 min. Cool to 50°C and dispense approximately 20 ml amounts into Petri dishes.

Malt peptone agar with antibiotics

Prepare and autoclave medium as above. Allow to cool to 50°C and add the following volumes from stock solutions of antibiotics:

		Final concentration
Malt peptone agar	1 litre	
Streptomycin 10 000 µg/ml)	4 ml	40 µg/ml
Penicillin (10 000 units/ml)	2 ml	20 units/ml

Mix well and dispense 20 ml amounts into Petri dishes as before.

Malt peptone agar with antibiotics and cycloheximide

Prepare malt peptone agar and autoclave as above. Allow to cool to 50°C and add the following.

		Final concentration
Malt peptone agar	1 litre	
Streptomycin (10 000 µg/ml)	4 ml	40 µg/ml
Penicillin (10 000 units/ml)	2 ml	20 units/ml
Cycloheximide (10 000 µg/ml)	50 ml	500 µg/ml

Mix well and dispense 20 ml amounts into Petri dishes.

Note: Prepare the cycloheximide just before use by dissolving 1 g in 100 ml distilled water.

Malt peptone agar with antibiotics and natamycin

Prepare malt peptone agar as above. Allow to

cool to 50°C after autoclaving and add the following:

		Final concentration
Malt peptone agar	1 litre	
Streptomycin (10 000 µg/ml)	4 ml	40 µg/ml
Penicillin (10 000 units/ml)	2 ml	20 units/ml
Natamycin (25 000 µg/ml suspension)	4 ml	100 µg/ml

Mix well and dispense 20 ml amounts into Petri dishes.

Malt broth

Malt extract (desiccated)	20 g
Water	1 litre

Steam to dissolve and adjust pH to 5.4. Autoclave at 115°C for 15 min and dispense 20 ml amounts.

Sabouraud agar

Glucose	20 g
Peptone (e.g. Oxoid mycological)	10 g
Agar	15 g
Water	1 litre

Steam to dissolve and adjust pH to 5.4. Autoclave at 115°C for 15 min and dispense 20 ml amounts into Petri dishes.

Sabouraud agar with antibiotics

Prepare basal medium as indicated above and add penicillin and streptomycin as directed for malt peptone agar with antibiotics.

Sabouraud agar with antibiotics and cycloheximide

Prepare basal medium as indicated above and add selective agents as directed for malt peptone agar with antibiotics and cycloheximide.

Sabouraud agar with antibiotics and natamycin

Prepare basal medium as indicated above and add selective agents as directed for malt peptone agar with antibiotics and natamycin.

Sabouraud broth

Glucose	40 g
Peptone (e.g. Oxoid mycological)	10 g
Water	1 litre

Steam to dissolve and adjust pH to 5.4. Dispense in required amounts and autoclave at 115°C for 15 min.

Sugar assimilation agar

Basal medium I

Yeast nitrogen base (Difco)	6.7 g
Agar	20 g
Water	1 litre

Steam to dissolve and dispense in 10 ml amounts in Universal containers. Autoclave at 115°C for 15 min.

Basal medium II

Ammonium sulphate	5 g
Potassium dihydrogen phosphate	1 g
Magnesium sulphate, $MgSO_4.5H_2O$	0.5 g
Agar	20 g
Water	1 litre

Steam to dissolve ingredients and dispense in 10 ml amounts in Universal containers. Autoclave at 115°C for 15 min.

Appropriate sugars are added as described above (see *Sugar assimilation tests* for identification of yeasts). *Note*: Basal medium II requires the addition of yeast extract as a source of vitamins and trace elements.

Potato dextrose agar

For convenience this potato dextrose agar (PDA) is generally prepared from dehydrated medium (e.g. Oxoid) according to the manufacturer's instructions. Alternatively, this medium may be prepared from raw materials as follows:

Potato	200 g
Dextrose	20 g

Agar	20 g
Water	1 litre

Scrub but do not peel the potatoes and cut into 12 mm cubes. Boil 200 g in 1 litre of water for 60 min. Squeeze as much of the pulp as possible through a fine sieve. Add agar and boil till dissolved. Add dextrose and make up to 1 litre. Dispense in required amounts taking care to keep solids in suspension. Autoclave at 115°C for 30 min. Cool to 50°C and pour approximately 20 ml amounts into Petri dishes.

Cornmeal agar

This medium may be prepared either from commercially available dehydrated ingredients (e.g. Oxoid) according to the manufacturer's instructions or, as indicated below, from basic ingredients.

Cornmeal	40 g
Agar	15 g
Water	1 litre

Boil the cornmeal in 1 litre of water for 60 min. Filter through muslin and add the agar. Steam to dissolve, dispense in required amounts and autoclave at 115°C for 30 min. Allow to cool to 50°C and pour approximately 20 ml amounts into Petri dishes.

Christensen's urea agar containing glucose

Glucose	5 g
Sodium chloride	5 g
Potassium dihydrogen phosphate	2 g
Peptone	1 g
Agar	20 g
Water	1 litre

Steam to dissolve ingredients in 1 litre of water. Add 6 ml phenol red (0.2% in 50% alcohol). Dispense in convenient amounts, e.g. 200 ml. Autoclave at 115°C for 30 min. Steam base to melt, allow to cool to 60°C and add 5 ml of urea (40% aqueous filter sterilized solution) to every 100 ml of medium. Dispense 5 ml amounts of the medium aseptically into test tubes and slope.

Sugar fermentation medium

Peptone (Oxoid)	15 g
Andrade's indicator	10 ml
Sugar to be tested	20 g
Water	1 litre

Andrade's indicator is prepared from 0.5% aqueous acid fuchsin to which sufficient 1 mol/litre sodium hydroxide has been added to turn the colour of the solution yellow.

Dissolve the peptone and Andrade's indicator (Ch. 8) in 1 litre of water and add 20 g of the sugar to be tested; sugars to be tested generally include glucose, sucrose, lactose and maltose. Distribute 3 ml amounts in standard test tubes containing an inverted Durham tube. Sterilize by steaming at 100°C for 30 min on 3 consecutive days.

REFERENCES

Barnett H L, Hunter B B 1972 Illustrated genera of imperfect fungi, 3rd edn. Burgess, Minneapolis
Barron G L 1968 The genera of hyphomycetes from soil. Williams and Wilkins, Baltimore
British Society for Mycopathology 1984 Report of a working group on laboratory methods for flucytosine (5-fluorocytosine). Journal of Antimicrobial Chemotherapy 14: 1–8
Crofton J, Douglas A 1981 Respiratory diseases, 3rd edn. Blackwell Scientific, Oxford
Gentles J C 1971 Laboratory investigations of dermatophyte infections of nails. Sabouraudia 9: 149–152
Grocott R G 1955 A stain for fungi in tissue sections and smears using Gomori's methenamine-silver nitrate technic. American Journal of Clinical Pathology 25: 975–979

Kreger-Van Rij N J W 1984 The yeasts: a taxonomic study, 3rd edn. North-Holland, Amsterdam
Milne L J R, Barnetson R StC 1974 Diagnosis of dermatophytoses using vinyl adhesive tape. Sabouraudia 12: 162–165
Park G R, Drummond G B, Lamb D, Durie T B M, Milne L J R, Lambie A T, Cameron E W J 1982 Disseminated aspergillosis occurring in patients with respiratory, renal and hepatic failure. Lancet 2: 179–183
Rebell G, Taplin D 1974 Dermatophytes: their recognition and identification, 2nd edn. University of Miami Press, Coral Gables, Florida
Thom C, Raper K B 1951 Manual of the aspergilli. Williams and Wilkins, Baltimore

Protozoa

Unicellular eukaryote organisms (Protista) fall into three main groups with organizations akin to multicellular plants, fungi, or animals respectively. The Protozoa belong to the last group. Their modes of living and their life histories are extremely diverse and complex and consequently they display a far wider range of morphology than do bacteria. Many species are parasites or commensals of higher plants and animals. This chapter deals with those of medical importance.

The various functions of the multicellular higher animals are performed in the Protozoa by the differentiation of parts of the single cell into organelles that perform particular functions. Examples are: pseudopodia, flagella, cilia, or undulating membranes, for locomotion; pseudopodia, cytostomes or pinocytotic systems for food ingestion. Thus the microscopical observation of morphology, often after staining, is particularly important in diagnosis.

The classification of the Protozoa, greatly simplified to present only those important as parasites of man, is given in Table 43.1 with the organisms broadly grouped as flagellates, amoebae, sporozoa and ciliates. The distinctions are not absolute, as some organisms are flagellate or amoeboid at different stages of their existences. The flagellates and the amoebae have relatively simple life histories in which binary fission is the main method of reproduction. Both

the sporozoa and the ciliates have conspicuous sexual cycles. To facilitate quick reference the organisms are treated in this chapter in the taxonomic order given in Table 43.1.

Chapter 54 in Volume 1 of the 13th Edition of this work provides summaries of the protozoological, clinical and epidemiological aspects of these medically important Protozoa; for more extensive treatments see Belding (1965), Faust & Russell (1964), Wilcocks & Manson-Bahr (1972) and Kreier (1977, 1978).

Protozoa are mainly important in warm countries as causes of the major health problems of malaria, leishmaniasis, trypanosomiasis and amoebiasis. Other protozoal infections are also of significant importance, such as giardiasis, trichomoniasis and toxoplasmosis. Modern developments which are contributory to an increase in protozoal disease in temperate countries are the tourist industry, which may expose people to insect-transmitted tropical infections such as malaria and trypanosomiasis, alterations in sexual mores, which result in increased person-to-person transmission of conditions such as trichomoniasis and amoebiasis, and immunosuppression, which may allow a normally commensal protozoan such as *Pneumocystis* to become a pathogen.

Many of the protozoal agents described are not special to man and occur also in other mammals. Transmission of some of these zoonoses to man may be an occasional accidental event as with *Balantidium*; for others, it may be an important epidemiological factor providing a reservoir in other animals from which man is more or less frequently infected, as in leishmaniasis and trypanosomiasis. Zoonoses may raise

As explained in the Preface, the editors have sought to avoid the use of a double 'i' genitive ending in the specific epithets of species binomials which have been derived from Latinized versions of names. We acknowledge that this is not standard practice for the nomenclature of protozoa; however, for consistency in this volume, the editors have substituted single 'i' forms for double 'i' forms, e.g. *Pneumocystis carini*, *Toxoplasma gondi*.

Table 43.1 Classification of the medically important protozoa. (Simplified from Baker 1977.)

Phylum Protozoa		
Subphylum I Sarcomastigophora		
Superclass 1 Mastigophora		
Class 2 Zoomastigophorea		
Order Kinetoplastida	*Leishmania, Trypanosoma*	
Order Retortamonadida	*Retortamonas, Enteromonas, Chilomastix*	Flagellates
Order Diplomonadida	*Giardia*	
Order Trichomonadida	*Trichomonas, Dientamoeba*[a]	
Superclass 3 Sarcodina		
Class 1 Rhizopodea		
Order Amoebida	*Entamoeba, Endolimax, Iodamoeba, Naegleria, Acanthamoeba*	Amoebae
Subphylum II Sporozoa		
Class 1 Telosporea		
Subclass 2 Coccidia		
Order Eucoccida		
Suborder Eimeriina	*Isospora, Cryptosporidium, Toxoplasma, Sarcocystis*	Sporozoa
Suborder Haemosporina	*Plasmodium*	
Class 2 Piroplasmea		
Order Piroplasmida	*Babesia*	
Subphylum V Ciliophora		
Class 1 Ciliatea		
Subclass Holotrichia		
Order Trichostomatida	*Balantidium*	Ciliates
Of uncertain taxonomic position	*Pneumocystis*[b]	

[a] Previously placed in the Order Amoebida; transferred on ultrastructural evidence.
[b] A unicellular eukaryote organism, perhaps to be placed in the Sporozoa, perhaps with the *Ascomycetes* yeasts.

problems of organism identification. For example, different 'subspecies' of *Trypanosoma brucei*, all morphologically identical, may be non-infective to man, or cause rapidly or slowly progressive lethal disease. Recently, objective methods, particularly isoenzyme-typing, have been developed for the characterization of such organisms by recognizing genetically different subpopulations within a single 'species' (see Gibson et al 1980). These greatly improve understanding of pathology and epidemiology, but are not yet generally available.

Most protozoal pathogens are readily propagated in culture but a few, e.g. *Giardia*, remain recalcitrant. Many conveniently infect small laboratory animals. All can be preserved for reference, research and diagnostic purposes by cryopreservation, usually in liquid nitrogen (for methods, see Lumsden et al 1973).

Diagnosis by protozoological methods

Direct methods, in which the organisms are sought directly in specimens of tissue or in the contents of a hollow organ, are often helpful. In many protozoal infections, however, the diagnostic problem is mainly due to the paucity of the organisms present. Pathological effects may be due to organisms which are present in extremely small concentrations in the tissues or visceral contents that are readily accessible to sampling. Direct examination methods are thus sometimes only of low efficiency. For instance, in the direct examination of a wet mount of blood for trypanosomes, which being motile are quickly recognized if seen, the recognition threshold is about 250 000 orgs/ml if examination is not to be laboriously protracted. In fixed stained blood films where objects have to be individually visualized and assessed so as to be differentiated from blood constituents the threshold of recognition is probably higher.

Methods to enhance the chance of detecting organisms in such situations include *concentration methods* whereby the protozoal content of a specimen is concentrated into a small volume easily searched by microscopy, and *multiplicative methods*, in which specimens selected as likely to contain organisms are seeded in culture media, or introduced into receptive animals or insects in which they may multiply to produce populations sufficiently numerous for detection and identification by microscopy. Methods of cultivating protozoa in vitro are exhaustively treated by Taylor & Baker (1968, 1978).

Protozoological methods of diagnosis fall into two broad groupings suitable for those organisms that inhabit tissues, including blood, and for those that primarily inhabit the mucous surfaces of hollow viscera communicating with the exterior. Methods of examination for these two groupings are broadly similar in principle but differ in detail.

Tissue protozoa. Direct examination of easily accessible body fluid (blood, CSF), lymph-node or tissue aspirate, and tissue biopsy. Concentration methods involve centrifugation of samples with no, or only small, host cell content, or centrifugation of samples after separation of host cells. Multiplicative methods include cultivation, mostly on blood agar media, animal inoculation, or arranging the ingestion of a blood sample by the insect vector appropriate for multiplication of the organism (xenodiagnosis, as for *Trypanosoma cruzi*, see below).

The conspicuous motility of some of the stages of these protozoa is exploited in wet-mount microscopy. This is used for the direct detection of *Trypanosoma brucei* in specimens of blood, lymph-node aspirate or CSF, or the detection of *Leishmania* and *T. cruzi* in cultures or in animals at appropriate periods after inoculation with suspect materials. Sometimes the wet mount will provide an unequivocal diagnosis, as with *Trypanosoma brucei*, but sometimes fixed stained thin films of deposits from fluids or of tissue or culture smears are required for further morphological studies to confirm diagnosis. Thin films fixed with methanol and stained with Romanowsky stain are most used. Of the Romanowsky stains, Giemsa's is preferred as the simplest and most flexible.

Hollow viscus protozoa. Specimens for diagnosis include faeces, aspirates of intestinal contents, mucous membrane exudates, biopsy sections and impression smears, fluid from ulcers, and abscess aspirates. Unstained wet mounts are used for the direct recognition of motile organisms, and stained with iodine or other stains for visualizing structures within encysted organisms. The observation of nuclear structure and other intracellular organelles necessary for identification may sometimes require special staining methods, such as iron-haematoxylin after fixation in Schaudinn's fluid. Organisms may be concentrated from specimens, e.g. faeces or vaginal exudate, by differential flotation and centrifugation. Multiplicative methods include cultivation on a variety of special media, sometimes containing other living organisms such as *Escherichia coli* for the cultivation of *Entamoeba histolytica*, and sometimes under anaerobic conditions.

Microscopy

Although search for these organisms may be done at lower magnifications, their critical recognition demands high quality, high resolution, oil-immersion objectives. As relative size is often an important diagnostic feature, the microscope used for routine protozoological diagnosis must have a 100-division eye-piece micrometer permanently in place and must bear a permanent label giving the 'per division' calibration in microns of each of its eye-piece and objective combinations. Take care to obtain the most favourable specimens for examination: fresh wet mounts sufficiently thin for the organisms to be easily seen and for the coverslip to be stable; stained preparations with good fixation and consistent staining, with as little as possible extraneous material on the slide, such as deposit from stain.

Diagnosis by immunological methods

Methods for the demonstration of antibodies to protozoa are reviewed in general by Lumsden (1973), and as applied to the diagnosis of protozoal diseases by Kagan & Walls (1981). Practically every serological test known has been investigated but those which have been significantly used for diagnosis are: direct agglutination (DA), tanned cell haemagglutination (TCH), latex agglutination (LA), modification of staining reaction – methylene blue dye test (MBD, for *Toxoplasma* only), indirect immunofluorescence (IF), enzyme-linked immunosorbent assay (ELISA), complement fixation (CF) and double diffusion (DD). Apart from these immunologically specific tests, the simple quantitation of immunoglobulin has been used, as for African trypanosomiasis, in which there is gross elevation of serum IgM early in the disease. Cell-mediated immune responses are sometimes exploited as a diagnostic index, such as the delayed hypersensitivity (DH) skin reaction in leishmaniasis.

Positive immunological results are never considered as indications for treatment of protozoal diseases but are useful in directing the search for a specific protozoal pathogen, or for indicating the extent of tissue invasion by *Entamoeba histolytica* in individual patients, or for epidemiological purposes. For a summary of more recent applications of immunology to protozoal diseases, e.g. for the detection, characterization and location of antigens, which may ultimately alter this statement, see Lumsden (1986).

Since the antigens/antisera necessary for setting up many of the tests will not be available in most clinical microbiological laboratories and are seldom commercially available, except in a few cases as complete kits, attention is directed here to cite the serological tests that are most useful for specific organisms. In the UK specimens can be sent to specialist laboratories equipped to carry out immunological diagnostic tests for protozoal infections at the London School of Hygiene and Tropical Medicine (Keppel Street, London WC1E 7HT; tel. 01–836 8636) or at the Liverpool School of Tropical Medicine (Pembroke Place, Liverpool L3 5QA; tel. 051–708 9393); or in USA to the Centers for Infectious Diseases and for Disease Control (Atlanta 30333, Georgia, USA).

FLAGELLATES

The following organisms are classified as flagellates (Table 43.1) and are discussed below: *Leishmania; Trypanosoma; Retortamonas,* *Enteromonas* and *Chilomastix; Giardia; Trichomonas; Dientamoeba*.

Leishmania

Leishmania occurs in man as intracellular amastigotes in cells of the mononuclear phagocytic system (MPS). In visceral leishmaniasis (VL) the MPS cells affected are mainly in the spleen, liver, bone marrow and lymph nodes. In cutaneous leishmaniasis (CL) the skin is affected mainly, sometimes also the mucous membranes of the nose and pharynx (mucocutaneous leishmaniasis). Although there are differences in size, in the relation of the kinetoplast to the nucleus and in vacuolation, the *Leishmania* spp. in man show practically no serviceable morphological differences either by light or electron microscopy.

The specific names given to *Leishmania* spp. were conferred originally in relation to particular clinical syndromes, geographical distributions and responses to chemotherapy. The following taxonomic arrangement is derived from a comprehensive review by Zuckerman & Lainson (1977).

Leishmania donovani complex. These agents of VL occur in eastern Asia and in the countries bordering the Sahara on the south (*L. donovani*), on the Mediterranean littoral, the Arabian Gulf, southern Russia and north China (*L. infantum*), and in America from Mexico to Argentina (*L. chagasi*). *L. donovani* infects people of all ages, *L. infantum* infects children only, and *L. chagasi* children predominantly. No animal hosts are known for *L. donovani* except in the Sudan where wild rodents and small carnivores may be involved. The animal hosts for *L. infantum* are dogs, and for *L. chagasi*, foxes, dogs and cats.

Leishmania tropica complex. These agents of CL occur in the Mediterranean littoral, the Arabian Gulf, southern Russia, Afghanistan and India, and in the African desert oases (*L. tropica* – 'dry, urban' CL), in southern Russia, in eastern Mediterranean countries and in Africa on the north coast and in the countries bordering the Sahara on its south (*L. major* – 'wet, rural' CL).

Leishmania mexicana complex. These agents of CL occur in the Americas, in Mexico, Belize and Guatemala (*L. m. mexicana* – 'chiclero's ulcer'), in the Amazon basin and Matto Grosso of Brazil and in Trinidad (*L. m. amazonensis* – limited CL), in the Amazon basin and Matto Grosso of Brazil and in Venezuela (*L. m. pifanoi* – diffuse cutaneous leishmaniasis, DCL). The animal hosts are forest rodents and marsupials.

Leishmania braziliensis complex. These agents of CL occur in South America from Venezuela to Paraguay (*L. b. braziliensis* – 'espundia' or muco-CL), in the Guyanas and north Brazil (*L. b. guyanensis* – 'pian bois' CL), in Panama and perhaps adjacent countries (*L. b. panamensis* – single ulcer CL), and in the Peruvian Andes (*L. peruviana* – 'uta' CL). The animal hosts are forest rodents, except for *L. peruviana* which infects dogs.

Visceral leishmaniasis

Roughly in ascending order of diagnostic sensitivity, the tissues to be sampled are blood, lymph node* (inguinal lymph nodes preferred), bone marrow, liver and spleen.* Blood examination is useful only in untreated patients but seeding of cultures with the buffy layer from a sample of the patient's centrifuged citrated blood is often effective (Belding 1965). Failing diagnosis from blood, the other tissues are sampled. Bone marrow aspiration, from the sternum or the iliac crest, is free from hazard but is painful. Splenic aspiration is most sensitive.

Microscopy. Use thin blood films* or smears of the specimen, fixed with methanol and stained with Giemsa's stain as for a thin blood film.* Search for *Leishmania* amastigotes (the Leishman-Donovan or LD bodies) (see Fig. 43.1b, at end of chapter). They are spherical or oval organisms 2–6 μm in length with two internal staining organelles – a larger, spherical, paler staining, nucleus and a smaller, rod-like, more densely staining, kinetoplast. Amastigotes occur mainly within macrophages but sometimes they appear free, released from cells disrupted in making the film. In intracellular amastigotes the organism's cytoplasm may not be differentiated by the

staining from that of the surrounding host cell and so each amastigote may appear as larger paler staining and smaller darker staining dots paired together, i.e the nucleus and the kinetoplast of each.

The promastigotes into which the amastigotes transform in diphasic culture,* are spindle-shaped motile organisms up to *c.* 20 μm long with a single anterior flagellum of about the same length (Fig. 43.1b); the promastigotes occur in rosettes or clumps. The liquid phase of the medium is sampled and examined as a wet mount* for motile organisms, and fixed and stained as for a thin blood film* to confirm morphology.

Culture. Inoculate the specimen into the liquid phase of diphasic blood agar medium.* Incubate at 21–26°C. This temperature favours the development of the organism in the insect vector and amastigotes transform to promastigotes in about 24 h. However, multiplication of the organisms may be slow and promastigote numbers may not reach detectable levels for several weeks. Sample the liquid phase of the medium every few days and do not discard the cultures for at least 3 weeks. Some strains of *L. donovani* are particularly slow to grow. Substitution of tissue culture medium (e.g. 199) enriched with 10% fetal calf serum for the usual liquid phase of the diphasic medium, or the use of a monophasic blood lysate medium ('EPLB'), have been recommended for such strains (Evans 1978).

Animal inoculation. *Cricetulus barbarensis griseus* (Chinese hamster) and *Mesocricetus auratus* (golden hamster) are extremely susceptible to *Leishmania* spp. and are the animals of choice for diagnostic inoculation. Inoculate specimens intraperitoneally. Examine spleen impression smears, stained as for thin blood films, from the animals if they die, or after killing them at 6 months.

Immunological diagnosis. Serological tests such as the Napier formol-gel test (see Lumsden & Sargeaunt 1975), which are mediated by non-specific changes in the immunoglobulin in VL, still have field applications (Zuckerman &

---

* Refer to *Methods* at end of this chapter.

Lainson 1977). Specific serological tests include complement fixation, indirect haemagglutination, fluorescent antibody and passive cutaneous anaphylaxis but Zuckerman & Lainson (1977) comment that antigenic overlapping and group-specific cross-reactivity with different *Leishmania* spp. and with trypanosomes limit their usefulness; in general they are more useful in sero-epidemiological studies than in individual diagnosis. The delayed hypersensitivity skin (DHS) test* (leishmanin or Montenegro test) is more useful. In visceral leishmaniasis it becomes positive usually only after cure of the disease (Zuckerman & Lainson 1977), but see below.

Cutaneous leishmaniasis

CL is a spectrum of disease states rather than a single disease entity, the lesions varying widely depending on the cell-mediated response (CMR) of the person infected (Zuckerman & Lainson 1977). At one end of the spectrum are anergic individuals with defective CMR in whom lesions are widespread and organisms plentiful (diffuse cutaneous leishmaniasis, DCL). At the other end are allergic individuals in whom antibody production is marked, CMR is overdeveloped and organisms are very few (leishmaniasis recidiva – LR).

Obtain a tissue sample by puncture of the periphery of the lesion.* Avoid the centre of the lesion where there is bacterial contamination and organisms tend to be scarce. Make tissue smears and inoculate into cultures as for VL.

Microscopy. The recognition of the organism is as for VL. Amastigotes generally are plentiful in an active lesion but may be scarce in a resolving one, in both the cutaneous and mucocutaneous lesions due to *L. braziliensis* in South America, and in LR.

Culture. As for VL. Most CL species grow readily on the diphasic medium* except for some strains of *L. braziliensis*. With these, the same changes in the medium as recommended for VL can be used, or the substitution of rat for rabbit blood in the solid phase (Taylor & Baker 1968).

Animal inoculation. As for VL except that the animals are inoculated intradermally and any cutaneous lesions appearing are sampled for microscopy.

Immunological diagnosis. For the value of non-specific and specific antibody tests, see under CL above. The delayed hypersensitivity skin (DHS) test is typically positive in *L. tropica* infections, sometimes very soon, even only a few days after infection, but sometimes only after about 6 months. In patients with healed lesions it may remain positive indefinitely. The test is generally weak or negative in patients with New World CL and almost invariably negative in DCL (Zuckerman & Lainson 1977).

Trypanosoma cruzi

The two trypanosomiases that occur in man differ fundamentally and are considered separately. American trypanosomiasis (Chagas disease) is caused by *T. cruzi*, a member of the Section Stercoraria (Hoare 1972) – those trypanosomes transmitted by infective forms occurring in the faeces of the vector insects. African trypanosomiasis (sleeping sickness) is caused by *T. brucei* spp. *gambiense* and *rhodesiense*, which are members of the Section Salivaria – those trypanosomes which are transmitted by infective forms injected by the bite of the vector insects; *T. brucei* is considered in the following section.

American trypanosomiasis (Chagas disease) is widely but sporadically distributed in all the Central and South American states from Mexico to Argentina and Chile. It is transmitted by several genera (*Triatoma, Panstrongylus, Rhodnius*, etc.) of blood-sucking bugs of the Family Reduviidae (assassin or kissing bugs). Animals (dogs, cats, armadillos, opossums, etc.) may be involved as reservoir hosts but most human infections are probably man-derived in poor rural housing infested with the vector bugs. A primary lesion often occurs at site of introduction of the infective faeces of the insect – an indurated inflamed slightly painful oedematous lesion, the 'chagoma', if the infection is via the skin; a unilateral bipalpebral oedema if infection is via the conjunctiva.

Multiplication of the organism is by repeated binary fission of amastigotes within the cells of many tissues but particularly of MPS system and muscles, both cardiac and skeletal. Ultimately, infected cells burst and the released amastigotes transform to trypomastigotes which are carried by the circulation to infect new cells, in which they transform back to amastigotes and set up new cycles of multiplication. Thus in the early acute stage of dissemination of the infection through the host's body, trypomastigotes are often abundant in the peripheral blood; in the later chronic stage, multiplication may be at a low level so that trypomastigotes may be extremely rare in the peripheral blood. Herein lies the main diagnostic difficulty. The trypomastigotes in the blood, as well as infecting new host cells, are also the stages infecting the vector bug. The vector bugs ingest large volumes of blood, sometimes more than 600 μl, and ingested *T. cruzi* trypomastigote forms easily establish in them. This is exploited for diagnostic purposes in the chronic stage (xenodiagnosis, see below).

T. cruzi is classed as a Category 3 pathogen (see Ch. 15), not so much because it is a highly infective agent – barring accidents, ordinary laboratory handling procedures will avoid infection – but because *T. cruzi* infections are often lethal or seriously damaging, and no efficient specific chemotherapy exists. Where *T. cruzi* infection is suspected, therefore, all investigative procedures in the UK will require to be conducted under the conditions laid down for Category 3 pathogens. This will limit investigations to culture of specimens on diphasic blood agar medium and the examination of fixed stained smears from the cultures.

Specimens. In early stage disease, if a chagoma is present, take aspirates of the chagoma tissue* for fixing and staining as for a thin blood film; or sections of a biopsy of the chagoma. Examine blood, thin and thick films*, and lymph node aspirate,* thin films.

In late stage disease blood specimens may be examined as for the early stage of the disease but organism numbers are usually extremely low and they are very rarely found by direct microscopy.

Organisms may be *concentrated* in blood by centrifugation as follows: heparinize about 10 ml of blood; centrifuge minimally so as just to deposit the blood cells; take off the supernatant plasma and centrifuge it to deposit the trypanosomes; examine the second deposit as a wet mount* or fix and stain it as for a thin blood film. Alternatively, agglutinate 10 ml of blood with phytohaemagglutinin; take off the supernate and centrifuge it, and then examine the deposit as above.

Note. The miniature anion-exchange/centrifugation (MAEC) technique for concentrating trypanosomes in blood used for *T. brucei* spp. is not used with *T. cruzi* because the electric charges carried by the blood cells and the organisms are too closely similar.

Microscopy. In smears made from tissue aspirates or biopsies or in biopsy sections, search for nests of intracellular amastigotes in host cells – 'pseudocysts'. *T. cruzi* amastigotes are similar to the amastigotes of *Leishmania* spp., but smaller (about 4 μm long), and infect many types of cells, particularly cardiac and skeletal muscle cells (see Fig. 43.1c, at end of chapter). In the peripheral blood of patients or laboratory animals, *T. cruzi* occurs as trypomastigotes (Fig. 43.1c), 15–20 μm long, often strongly curved, C-shaped, with a large kinetoplast which often appears to transgress the outline of the organism (Fig. 43.1c). In culture and in the faeces of the bugs used for xenodiagnosis all developmental stages occur – amastigotes, epimastigotes and trypomastigotes (Fig. 43.1a).

Culture. Inoculate specimens into diphasic blood agar medium.* Growth may be slow. Sample the liquid overlay by wet mounts and Giemsa-stained thin films weekly for 6 weeks.

Animal inoculation. Mice, rats, guinea-pigs and dogs have been used. Mice are most susceptible though in some individuals the infection disappears spontaneously (Belding 1965). If no *T. cruzi* parasitaemia is detected by microscopy after inoculation, kill the animals at 6 weeks and examine atrial heart muscle sections for intracellular *T. cruzi* amastigotes.

Xenodiagnosis. Laboratory-bred bugs of the species *Triatoma infestans*, *Panstrongylus megistus* or *Rhodnius prolixus*, fed on chickens or pigeons so that they can be known to be free from natural trypanosome infections, are required. Allow 10–20 3rd or 4th instar nymphs to engorge with blood from the suspect patient either directly or, more acceptably, from a lake of defibrinated blood through a membrane. Express the faeces of the bugs into a small drop of saline on a slide and examine wet mounts and Giemsa-stained thin films weekly from 2–8 weeks after the blood meal. Colonies of these reduviid bugs are maintained in the UK at the London School of Hygiene and Tropical Medicine and the Liverpool School of Tropical Medicine (addresses above) and the assistance of these institutions may be enlisted.

Immunological diagnosis. CF is preferred because reactivity usually indicates active clinical disease (Kagan & Walls 1981). DA with trypsinized and formalin-fixed *T. cruzi* epimastigotes from cultures is also used; the sera may need treatment with 2-mercaptoethanol to reduce non-specific agglutination (Kagan & Walls 1981).

Trypanosoma rangeli

This non-pathogenic stercorarian trypanosome must be distinguished from *T. cruzi*. It occurs in man in Central America and in South America as far south as Argentina and Chile. As many as 60% of the population may be infected (Belding 1965). It also is transmitted by reduviid bugs. It may be found by the same kind of examinations as are carried out for *T. cruzi* – in blood films, in diphasic blood agar media or in bugs used for xenodiagnosis. Trypomastigotes in blood are differentiated from those of *T. cruzi* by being 24–34 μm long, slender with tapering ends and with a minute kinetoplast. Hoare (1972) details the characters differentiating the two species in each context, but in general the kinetoplast in *T. rangeli* is minute whereas it is large in *T. cruzi*.

Trypanosoma brucei

African sleeping sickness occurs in a band (15°N to 15°S) across tropical Africa from Senegal and Angola to Kenya, Tanzania, Mozambique and Zimbabwe. It exists, broadly, in two forms; the

T. b. gambiense form is characteristically slowly progressive and lethal only after some years, whereas the *T. b. rhodesiense* disease is more acute and sometimes causes death within a few weeks of infection. *T. brucei* has also a third 'subspecies', *T. b. brucei*, which by definition does not infect man but infects many wild animals, antelopes, etc., and domestic cattle and horses. Although some minor morphological differences are held to occur between different subspecies, these are not sufficient for identification in individual infections. This leads to difficulties in defining epidemiological transmission patterns, since wild animals act also as reservoirs for human-infecting subspecies. Objective methods are now becoming available, mainly from isoenzyme studies (e.g. Gibson et al 1980), for subspecific differentiation. Transmission is, as far as man is concerned, solely by the bite of an infected tsetse fly (*Glossina*), in the *T. b. gambiense* context usually a forest-dwelling species, and in the *T. b. rhodesiense* context usually a savannah, open forest country, species. Since the latter type of country is typical of the African game parks, tourists visiting these are at particular risk of infection.

A primary lesion, the trypanosome chancre, at the site of the infective tsetse bite is more often noted and associated with subsequent pyrexia in the rapidly progressive *T. b. rhodesiense* disease than in *T. b. gambiense* infections. It is an inflamed indurated swelling 5 cm or more in diameter, occurring 7–10 days after the infecting bite. There is local multiplication of the organisms in the tissue fluids at the site of the bite; the blood is soon invaded and multiplication, which is by repeated binary fission of trypomastigote forms, takes place widely in the body, in the blood, lymph and tissue interstitial fluid. There is no intracellular phase. Organisms are usually abundant in the blood and lymph in the early stages of the disease. They are pleomorphic, some individual organisms being long, others short (Fig. 43.1d, at end of chapter). Later, after CNS invasion, organisms are typically scanty in these fluids, but may be found in CSF.*

Specimens. In early stage disease, aspirate a chancre* if present and lymph nodes* if enlarged. Make wet mounts* and thick and thin blood films* for staining with Giemsa's stain. If all these examinations are negative try the MAEC procedure.*

In late stage disease, examine thick and thin blood films repeatedly, on successive days. Try the MAEC procedure. Obtain CSF by lumbar puncture for cell count and protein estimation and search for trypanosomes.*

Concentration. The MAEC test* is the most sensitive (Lumsden et al 1981). Nearly as sensitive is the following microhaematocrit buffy coat microscopy (MBCM) technique. Centrifuge blood samples in heparinized capillary tubes in a microhaematocrit centrifuge and examine the buffy coat and adjacent plasma under the × 40 objective through the wall of the capillary tube (Woo 1970). Centrifugation and microscopy must be done expeditiously, within 20 min, as organisms rapidly lose motility and cannot then be recognized with confidence (Duvallet et al 1979).

Ogbunude & Magaji (1982) have proposed a new method for detection of low parasitaemias. Samples of blood are dispensed into 1.5 ml tapered centrifuge tubes containing 500 μl of a silicone fluid (Siliconöt; Bayer PH300/1000 sp gr 1.075 (-IE 3457)). Centrifugation at 150 g for 5 min deposits the heavier erythrocytes below the silicone leaving a plasma fraction above the silicone containing the lighter leucocytes and any trypanosomes. The trypanosomes can then be searched for in wet mounts.*

Culture is not used practically as an aid to diagnosis of *T. brucei* infection as the organism is much more difficult to culture than *T. cruzi.*

Animal inoculation. This is often effective in *T. b. rhodesiense* infections but less useful in *T. b. gambiense* infections which frequently fail to infect mice or produce only low parasitaemias difficult to detect by microscopy. Inoculate 0.5 ml doses of heparinized blood intraperitoneally into several mice and examine wet mounts* of tail blood daily from 3–20 days.

Microscopy. In wet mounts, in the centrifuge tube of the MAEC method, or in the haemo-cytometer cell, *T. brucei* can be recognized by its form and movement even under the × 40 objective. Scan Giemsa-stained blood films, uncovered, with the × 100 oil-immersion objective for trypomastigotes (Fig. 43.1d). As regards lymphocytes in CSF, 95% of normal adults have counts between 0 and 5.3 cells/μl (Diem & Lentner 1970); 30 or more cells/μl is indicative of cerebral involvement; the presence of morula cells (Fig. 43.1d) is pathognomonic (Wilcocks & Manson-Bahr 1972).

Immunological diagnosis. The serum IgM is raised early in the disease (Mattern et al 1967). The 95% range of total proteins in CSF in normal adults is 123–503 mg/litre (Diem & Lentner 1970); CSF proteins are raised particularly in the IgM fraction if there has been CNS involvement.

Many specific tests have been developed, some particularly for field use. In the laboratory, the indirect fluorescent antibody (IFA) test and ELISA are most extensively used (de Raadt & Seed 1977).

Retortamonas, Enteromonas and Chilomastix

One species of each of these three genera inhabits the human large intestine, *Retortamonas intestinalis*, *Enteromonas hominis* and *Chilomastix mesnili*. All occur as motile trophozoites and resistant cysts. They are found mainly in populations where standards of hygiene are low. Infection is by ingestion of cysts. Although all are considered generally as commensals, *C. mesnili* may be associated with diarrhoea.

Concentration. These organisms and their cysts are not found in concentrates of faecal specimens as they are fragile.

Culture. All the species grow well in Robinson's medium.* Trophozoites are generally seen within 48 h of inoculation of the specimen.

Microscopy. Tables 43.2 and 43.3 and Figure 43.2a (at end of chapter) indicate the specimens to be examined and the microscopical features of the trophozoites and cysts of these protozoa. Trophozoites, and occasionally also cysts, of all species may be seen in saline mounts of fresh faeces.* Trophozoites move rapidly in a jerking fashion. Identification is difficult in unstained preparations, requiring microscopic examinations of iron-haematoxylin stained smears.* Attention should be paid to the position, shape and staining characteristics of the nucleus; the flagella are rarely seen.

Giardia

Giardia lamblia (*G. intestinalis*) is the only human parasite of the genus. The trophozoite inhabits the duodenum and jejunum where encystation also occurs. Although many infected individuals have no symptoms, diarrhoea and steatorrhoea may be presenting features. The organism is found throughout the world and is acquired by drinking water or eating food contaminated with cysts.

Specimens (Table 43.2 at end of chapter). Diarrhoeal stools should be examined for trophozoites within 15 min of their passage or, if this is not possible, collected into polyvinyl alcohol (PVA) fixative.* Cysts, but not trophozoites, may be found in formed stool samples. Microscopic examination of fresh jejunal aspirate, and of Giemsa-stained impression smears of mucosa and of jejunal secretions are the most sensitive procedures.

Concentration. For the detection of light infection with *G. lamblia* use the formol-ether concentration method.*

Culture. Trophozoites of *G. lamblia* in duodenal aspirates have been cultured (Meyer 1976), but only rarely.

Microscopy. The trophozoites of *G. lamblia*, in a saline mount of diarrhoeal stool* or in jejunal aspirate, move rapidly in a tumbling fashion. They are pear-shaped (10–20 × 5–15 μm), rounded anteriorly, pointed posteriorly and convex dorsally (Table 43.3, Fig. 43.2a). On the ventral surface is a large concave adhesive disk. In stained preparations, e.g. in jejunal mucosal impression smears,* two nuclei with prominent karyosomes are seen. Each organism possesses eight flagella which originate in one midline kinetosomal complex; two flagella

emerge anterolaterally, two ventrally, two posterolaterally and two caudally. At the posterior end of the adhesive disk are two median bodies, which stain deeply with haematoxylin. In histological sections of jejunal mucosa, stained with Giemsa, the trophozoites appear as pear- or crescent-shaped structures with two nuclei. However, as serial sections must be examined, this is laborious; microscopy of a stained impression smear is preferred.*

G. lamblia cysts, 8–20 μm in diameter, (Table 43.3, Fig. 43.2a) may be found in both fluid and formed stools. Axonemes of the flagella are seen as a single longitudinal fibre extending from one end of the cyst to the other. Four nuclei and two crescentic structures are visible within cysts stained with iodine.

Immunological diagnosis. Although serum antibodies against *G. lamblia* may be detected by immunofluorescence or by ELISA (Ridley & Ridley 1976; Smith et al 1981) their clinical significance has yet to be determined.

Trichomonas

Two of the three trichomonad species found in man are harmless commensals, *Trichomonas tenax* in the mouth and *Pentatrichomonas hominis* in the caecum. *T. vaginalis* is a common cause of vaginitis. Transmission is sexual but the organism is only rarely pathogenic in the male. Diagnosis is by recognition of the organism in samples of fluid or in scrapings from the genito-urinary system. Diagnosis is generally easier in the female than in the male in whom the organism is typically scanty and difficult to demonstrate.

Specimens. In females, specimens are taken from the posterior vaginal fornix by means of a sterile cotton-wool swab, or preferably, by the polyester sponge method*, and from the urethra by a bacteriological loop or by scraping before the first morning micturition. In males, the urethra is sampled with a cotton-wool or, preferably, polyester swab (Robertson et al 1980).

If the specimen cannot be examined immediately it should be placed in modified Stuart's transport medium (Amies 1967; Robertson et al

1980), although the dilution of the specimen in the transport medium inevitably reduces the chance of visualizing organisms. The duration of survival of *T. vaginalis* in transport medium is fairly limited (see Nielsen 1969).

The organisms die rapidly when dried on a swab and an alternative approach is to place the loaded swab promptly into a tube of trichomonas culture medium, e.g. Oxoid Trichomonas Medium, for transport to the laboratory. The medium should be supplemented with horse serum, penicillin and streptomycin.

Concentration. The deposit obtained by centrifugation with the polyester sponge method is used for microscopy and for inoculation into culture medium. The deposit from centrifugation of a large volume of the first morning specimen of urine can be used in the same way and is particularly useful in males, from whom urethral samples are troublesome to obtain.

Culture. Media for the cultivation of *T. vaginalis* basically provide essential salts, nutrients, reducing agents and antibiotics to inhibit bacterial growth, in the absence, or in low concentrations, of oxygen. The variations on these basic requirements are legion (Taylor & Baker 1968; Honigberg 1978). Media used in the USA commonly include 0.05–0.1% agar to increase viscosity and reduce oxygen diffusion into the medium (Honigberg 1978). Oxoid Trichomonas Medium is commonly used in the UK. The media given below* omit agar for ease of handling; incubation should be anaerobic or in closed containers filled very nearly full. Two media are given; the isotonic medium* is preferred as it is easy to adjust to optimum initial pH (6.1–6.4) by altering the buffer component to compensate for variation in other components, notably the liver digest. An indicator (bromocresol purple) is included to save time in examination; a colour change to yellow indicates cultures in which *T. vaginalis* is likely to be present. Incubate cultures at 37°C for up to 4 days.

Cultivation is a more sensitive diagnostic method than either immediate microscopy of a wet mount or of the centrifuged deposit (see Robertson et al 1969). *T. vaginalis* infection should not be diagnosed unless the characteristic morphology is clearly recognized.

Microscopy. Phase contrast microscopy of a fresh wet mount of the specimen or culture, diluted with a minimum of isotonic saline if necessary, is the method of choice, but bright field or darkground microscopy are also satisfactory. *T. vaginalis* (Fig. 43.2b, at end of this chapter) is recognized as an oval, pyriform or spindle-shaped organism about 15 μm in length, i.e. larger than a neutrophil leucocyte and smaller than an epithelial cell. In fresh specimens the organisms are conspicuously motile, and recognition of the anterior tuft of flagella and the lateral undulating membrane provides a certain identification. Dead and degenerating organisms are difficult to recognize with certainty.

Staining has been advocated by many workers so as to recognize non-motile, dead or degenerating *Trichomonas* in specimens. Dried films fixed with methanol and stained with Giemsa or Papanicalaou stains have been most used. Fixation and staining has the advantage that, if immediate microscopy is not possible, the slide may be sent away for examination. But the examination is laborious and the recognition of the organisms among a profusion of other staining objects is not easy unless organisms are numerous (see Robertson et al 1980). Balsdon et al (1979) have recommended Dip-Quick (Harleco), a haematological stain incorporating arylmethane, xanthene and thiazine dyes, for recognizing *T. vaginalis* in dried films of vaginal discharge.

Immunological diagnosis. Local antibodies to *T. vaginalis* have been demonstrated in vaginal exudate of infected women by Ackers et al (1975) by radioimmune assay. Honigberg (1978) reviews the work on other immunodiagnostic approaches; complement fixation, agglutination, haemagglutination, fluorescent antibody and delayed hypersensitivity test results have all been shown to correlate with protozoological evidence, though results are affected by the antigenic type of the organisms used in the tests. Although these have applications for epidemiological purposes, for tracing contacts or for following treatment, they are not in general use for clinical diagnostic purposes.

Dientamoeba

Only one species, *D. fragilis* from the human colon, is known. Infection may be associated with diarrhoea. Previously grouped with the amoebae, *D. fragilis* has now been shown on ultramicroscopic evidence to be most closely related to the trichomonad flagellates. Its mode of transmission is unknown but does not appear to be directly contaminative and may be via the eggs of intestinal nematode worms.

Concentration. Since trophozoites of this organism are fragile and no cysts are known, concentration methods are not used.

Culture. *D. fragilis* grows readily in Robinson's medium.*

Microscopy. Diagnostic features are summarized in Table 43.3 and Figure 43.2c (see end of chapter). Trophozoites are delicate, disintegrating rapidly so that they are rarely seen in wet mounts of faeces. Movement is by the extrusion of broad, hyaline, pseudopodia with serrated margins. In haematoxylin-stained smears,* two nuclei are usually visible, although uninucleated forms are not uncommon. The nuclei are 2–5 μm diameter and have a large central nucleolus composed of separate chromatin granules, but no peripheral chromatin (Fig. 43.2c).

AMOEBAE

The following amoebic protozoa (Table 43.1, above) are discussed in the next section: *Entamoeba, Endolimax* and *Iodamoeba; Naegleria* and *Acanthamoeba*.

Entamoeba, Endolimax and Iodamoeba

The amoebae occurring in the human large intestine are *Entamoeba histolytica*, *E. coli* and *E. hartmanni*, *Endolimax nana* and *Iodamoeba buetschli*, electron microscope studies indicate that

Dientamoeba fragilis is related more closely to the flagellates than to the amoebae (see above). All five species of amoeba occur in the large intestine as trophozoites reproducing by binary fission and producing resistant cysts by which they are transmitted.

Entamoeba histolytica is the only pathogenic amoeba; the others are only of importance in that they may be confused with *E. histolytica*. Infection with *E. histolytica* can produce dysentery, colitis, hepatic abscesses and cutaneous lesions; however, about 90% of infected individuals have no symptoms. Infection, which is cosmopolitan, is usually acquired by ingesting water or food contaminated by cysts. Sexual transmission plays a significant part in the spread of *E. histolytica* among homosexuals in temperate climates.

Specimens to be examined are indicated in Table 43.2 (at end of chapter). Stool samples should be collected in wide-mouthed chemically clean containers (Sterilin). For the detection of trophozoites the specimen must be examined within 15 min of its passage or, if this is not practicable, should be preserved in PVA fixative.* Formed stool specimens up to 3 days old can be examined for the presence of cysts.

Passage of cysts in the faeces is often intermittent and at least three consecutive specimens should be examined before a diagnosis of amoebiasis is excluded. The administration of kaolin, bismuth, barium sulphate, antimicrobial and antimalarial drugs, liquid paraffin and antidiarrhoeal agents interfere with cyst excretion. In patients with dysentery, rectal exudate and material from the bases of rectal ulcers should be sampled.* Histological sections of rectal mucosa and any overlying exudate should be stained with phosphotungstic acid, haematoxylin or trichrome stain.*

Pus, with the appearance of anchovy sauce, aspirated from a hepatic abscess should be examined for trophozoites. Serological tests are of value in the diagnosis of this complication (see below).

Concentration. As the number of cysts in a stool sample may be small, the routine use of the formol-ether concentration method* is recommended.

Culture. Various media have been used for cultivation of *E. histolytica*. A polyxenic culture medium is useful in diagnosis. For routine purposes, Robinson's medium* has proved valuable. Serum, *Escherichia coli* (whose growth is held in check by erythromycin) and starch are included to provide nutrients and growth factors. Trophozoites of *E. histolytica* usually appear in large numbers within 48 h of inoculation.

The non-pathogenic amoebae, with the exception of *I. buetschli*, also grow in the medium but are distinguished from *E. histolytica* by their appearance in iodine- or trichrome-stained preparations. *Giardia lamblia* does not grow in Robinson's medium but *Retortamonas intestinalis*, *Chilomastix mesnili* and *Enteromonas hominis* do. *Dientamoeba fragilis* grows in Robinson's medium but the trophozoites are difficult to identify.

Microscopy. Table 43.4 and Figure 43.2d (see end of chapter) summarize the microscopic features of the trophozoites and cysts of the amoebae from which *E. histolytica* must be differentiated.

A saline mount* of fresh diarrhoeal stool, rectal exudate or material from a rectal ulcer*, should be examined for the presence of active trophozoites; the use of a warm microscope stage facilitates this but is not essential. The trophozoites of *E. histolytica* (usually 15–25 μm in diameter) move unidirectionally by pushing out finger-like hyaline pseudopodia (lobopodia). The nucleus is not visible but ingested erythrocytes may be seen. Differentiation from non-pathogenic amoebae is of paramount importance. Although a tentative diagnosis of *E. histolytica* infection can be made if trophozoites with these characteristics are seen, definitive diagnosis rests with microscopic examinations of a trichrome- or iron-haematoxylin-stained faecal smear.*

The features diagnostic of vegetative *E. histolytica* in stained smears are: (1) trophozoites, 15 μm in diameter; (2) ingested erythrocytes (*E. coli* rarely ingests erythrocytes); and (3) single nucleus (3–5 μm in diameter) with a small central endosome and a finely beaded ring of peripheral chromatin. However, there is considerable variation in nuclear morphology, especially in organisms from cultures. More than one nucleus may occur.

In rectal biopsies* from patients with acute intestinal amoebic colitis, trophozoites of *E. histolytica* may be seen commonly within the exudate overlying the rectal mucosa, less frequently in the necrotic tissue at the base of rectal ulcers or within the lamina propria (Prathap & Gilman 1970). Histological examination of skin or cervical and vaginal biopsy material from patients with cutaneous, vaginal or cervical amoebiasis shows amoebae within necrotic tissue.

Cysts of *E. histolytica* may be found in both diarrhoeal and formed stool samples and must be distinguished from the cysts of the non-pathogenic amoebae (Table 43.4, Fig. 43.2d). Important features of the iodine-stained cysts are: (1) size – *E. histolytica* cysts are spherical and 10–20 μm in diameter; (2) number of nuclei – *E. histolytica* has usually four but less mature cysts have only one or two nuclei; (3) chromatoidal bodies – *E. histolytica* may have one or more densely staining bars with blunt ends; and (4) young cysts sometimes have an ill-defined glycogen vacuole which stains red-brown with iodine.

Immunological diagnosis. Antibodies reactive with *E. histolytica* may be demonstrated by immunofluorescence in the sera of some patients with amoebiasis (Jeanes 1969). Antibodies are found at a titre of ≥ 64 in the sera of over 95% of individuals with extra-intestinal disease, but only in 75% of patients with acute amoebic colitis. Sera from asymptomatic carriers do not contain antibodies at these titres. Thus the test is of value in the diagnosis of extra-intestinal disease. The efficacy of treatment of extra-intestinal amoebiasis can be assessed by examination of the patient's serum at monthly intervals; usually, the antibody titre falls rapidly, within 2–6 months of therapy (Ambroise-Thomas & Kien Truong 1972). In assessment of prevalence of invasive amoebiasis on an epidemiological scale, an ELISA test has proved useful (Bos et al 1980).

Naegleria and Acanthamoeba

These amoebae, which are normally free-living, occasionally appear as opportunist parasites of man (see Červa 1981). *Naegleria fowleri* is the cause of meningoencephalitis usually associated with a history of intranasal contamination with natural water, e.g. during swimming. Invasion of the CNS is believed to be via the ethmoid cribriform plate and the olfactory tract (primary amoebic meningoencephalitis – PAM). Some 80 cases have been reported (Griffin 1978). The course of the disease is rapid, usually leading to death within a week of exposure. *Acanthamoeba* spp. have been reported, as well as from the CNS, from corneal ulcers, the genitourinary tract and many other sites (Červa 1981). It may be that *Acanthamoeba* is sometimes commensal in the nasopharynx as it is not infrequently found contaminating tissue cultures used for virus isolation from nasal swabs (Griffin 1978). *Naegleria* meningoencephalitis typically occurs in healthy active persons, and *Acanthamoeba* infection in the debilitated or immunologically compromised.

Microscopy. Examine fresh wet films of the CSF. *Naegleria*, about 10 μm long, are distinguished from other cells in the purulent CSF by being slowly motile, 1–2 cell lengths/min, by means of broad pseudopodia alternating from side to side (Fig. 43.1e, at end of chapter). *Acanthamoeba* (20–50 μm) has not been clearly recognized in direct specimens from human disease but shows spiky pseudopodia in culture.

Stain thin films of the CSF with iron-haematoxylin.* Both species have round nuclei with a single large central nucleolus (Fig. 43.1e). Make films from other sites, e.g. corneal ulcers, and stain similarly. In these sites *Acanthamoeba* may be in the cyst form, spherical, about 11 μm in diameter with a scalloped wall (Fig. 43.1e).

Culture. Media incorporating killed *Aerobacter aerogenes* and antibiotics for the isolation and maintenance of these amoebae are described by Taylor & Baker (1968).

SPOROZOA

The following protozoa, classified as sporozoa (Table 43.1, above), are discussed in the next section: *Isospora*, *Cryptosporidium* and *Sarcocystis*; *Toxoplasma*; *Plasmodium*; *Babesia*. *Pneumocystis* is also conveniently included in this group although its taxonomic position is uncertain.

Isospora, Cryptosporidium and Sarcocystis

The species infecting man are: *Isospora belli*, *Cryptosporidium* spp., *Sarcocystis hominis*, *S. suihominis* and *S. lindemanni*. All are essentially parasites of the epithelial cells of the gut of mammals. Ingested sporozoites penetrate the host cells, and develop into schizonts. The schizonts produce merozoites which, after rupture of the host cell, penetrate other host cells setting up new generations of schizonts. After a set number of generations a sexual cycle occurs; the merozoites grow to micro- and macro-gametes and the fertilized macrogametes (zygotes) develop to oocysts which are shed into the intestinal lumen on rupture of the host epithelial cell. In the faeces the oocysts are generally immature ('unsporulated'); they develop ('sporulate') outside the host to contain sporocysts, each containing sporozoites. The numbers of sporocysts and of sporozoites contained in each are characteristic of the genera. *Isospora* and *Sarcocystis* have oocysts containing two sporocysts, each with four sporozoites; *Cryptosporidium* oocysts contain four sporozoites not grouped in sporocysts. Sporozoites from ingested sporulated oocysts begin the cycle in a new host. Transmission of *I. belli* is direct (homoxenous) with only one host species involved, infection being initiated by ingestion of sporozoites. In *Sarcocystis* spp. more than one host species is involved (heteroxenous). The intermediate hosts, herbivores, ingest sporozoites and a generalized infection occurs with encystment of the parasite in muscle and other tissues. The definitive hosts are infected by eating intermediate host tissues containing cysts. Man is the definitive host of *S. hominis* and *suihominis*, the intermediate hosts being cattle and pigs, respectively. Very rarely, man is the intermediate host of *S. lindemanni*, cysts occurring in muscle; the definitive host is not known but may be a carnivore predatory on monkeys. The life cycle of *Cryptosporidium* is incompletely understood. For recent extensive reviews of these coccidia see Dubey (1977) and Tadros & Laarman (1982).

I. belli, *S. suihominis* and *Cryptosporidium* spp. are the infections encountered most frequently in man. Infection may be associated with a self-limiting diarrhoea; more severe intestinal disease (explosive diarrhoea) may be caused in immunocompromised individuals (Meisel et al 1976).

Specimens. Faeces for concentration by Sheather's sucrose flotation method;* faecal smears for staining with carbol fuchsin* or safranin O*; biopsies of jejunal and rectal mucosa for sectioning and staining with Giemsa (*I. belli* and *Cryptosporidium* spp.); biopsies of muscle (*S. lindemanni*).

Microscopy. Oocyst features are given in Table 43.5 (see end of chapter); oocysts do not stain with iodine (cf. yeasts). *I. belli* schizonts, merozoites and gametocytes are illustrated in photomicrographs by Brandborg et al (1970) and in electronmicrographs by Trier et al (1974). Oocysts of *Cryptosporidium* stained by the modified Ziehl-Neelsen method appear as bright red oval structures, sometimes containing a deeply stained dot. Safranin-stained oocysts are bright orange, often surrounded by a clear halo. *Cryptosporidium* spp. appear as ovoid or spherical particles (2–3 μm in diameter), staining densely with Giemsa, in the epithelial cells of duodenal, jejunal, ileal, colonic and rectal biopsies. Although in fact intracellular, the particles appear to be attached to the epithelial cells of the villi and crypts. Photomicrographs and electronmicrographs of *Cryptosporidium* are given by Bird & Smith (1980). *S. lindemanni* cysts occur in muscle cells; they are up to 5 mm long and contain hundreds of rounded, oval or sickle-shaped zoites, $12–16 \times 4–9$ μm (Fig. 43.1f); for illustrations see Jeffrey (1974).

Oocysts of non-human coccidia, ingested with food, may pass through the intestine undigested and be found in the faeces, e.g. *Eimeria sardinae* (Fig. 43.2f) of herrings, sardines, etc. and *Eimeria stiedae* of the rabbit. These oocysts require to be differentiated from those of the coccidia actually infecting man.

Toxoplasma

The definitive hosts of *Toxoplasma gondi* are cats which are infected by ingesting oocysts in feline faeces or by ingesting zoites or cysts in the tissues of intermediate hosts. Domestic animals may be infected with cysts and man can then be infected: (1) by ingesting oocysts in food contaminated with cat faeces, (2) by eating raw meat from animals which have cysts of *T. gondi* in their tissues, acquired by ingesting food contaminated with cat faeces, (3) transplacentally, from acutely or chronically infected mothers. Infection, as indicated by serological results, is widespread but clinical effects are largely confined to situations of low immunocompetence – immunological immaturity or inhibition in fetuses, or immunosuppressive therapy in adults. Transplacental infection may cause neurological disease – epileptic seizures, choroidoretinitis, hydrocephalus and intracerebral calcification. In adults the commonest presentation is lymphadenopathy; encephalitis and generalized dissemination of infection occur in immunocompromised subjects.

Animal inoculation. *T. gondi* has been isolated from a variety of tissues, secretions or biopsies by inoculation. Specimens, most conveniently lymph node aspirate, CSF or tissue biopsy, are inoculated intraperitoneally and intracerebrally into mice. Examine the peritoneal exudate after 6–10 days; or make brain impression smears from moribund mice.

Microscopy. Search sections of biopsies for cysts 200–1000 μm in diameter, packed with many zoites. The cysts stain best with silver methenamine stain.* Search smears of peritoneal exudate from inoculated animals after 6–10 days for *T. gondi* zoites (Dubey 1977), crescent-shaped, $6–7 \times 2–4$ μm (Fig. 43.1f, at end of chapter).

Immunodiagnosis. Serological tests are widely used. The methylene blue dye (MBD) test of Sabin & Feldman (1948) is sensitive and specific but involves risks associated with the use of live organisms. The indirect immunofluorescence (IF) test (Frenkel 1971) is simpler, agrees with MBD test results and so is preferred (Kagan & Walls 1981). ELISA and fluorescent immunoassay (FIAX) tests give results parallel to indirect IF tests (Kagan & Walls 1981) and have advantages: ELISA tests are easy and require no special equipment; FIAX requires special equipment but only a single dilution for quantitative determination (Kagan & Walls 1981). Commercial kits are available for some routine tests, e.g. the ToxHA haemagglutination test kit (Wellcome).

In the diagnosis of acute toxoplasmosis, paired sera taken 14 days apart must be examined to determine if a significant (at least 4-fold) rise in antibody titre has occurred. An IgM-IFA test has been used in the diagnosis of congenital toxoplasmosis in babies (Remington 1969). The presence of specific IgM antibodies in the baby's serum indicates active infection.

Plasmodium

Four species of *Plasmodium*, *P. vivax*, *P. malariae*, *P. ovale*, *P. falciparum*, cause malaria. Malaria is distributed as a natural infection of man in both the Old and the New Worlds between 40°N and 30°S latitudes. Man-infecting species are naturally transmitted by *Anopheles* mosquitoes (Diptera, Nematocera). Bizarre transmission sometimes occurs, by blood transfusion or by contaminated syringes, e.g. in drug addicts. Although certain plasmodial infections in the higher apes are closely similar to those of man, and may indeed once have been transmitted to or from him, transmission is now quite predominantly intra-human and no significant wild animal reservoir is involved. *Plasmodium* spp. occur in man as asexually reproducing organisms in the parenchymal cells of the liver (pre-erythrocytic cycle), and in erythrocytes as asexually reproducing and as gamete-producing organisms, the latter preparatory to a sexual cycle which takes place in *Anopheles*. The liver

stages are inaccessible to detection and so diagnosis depends on the finding of organisms of the asexual cycle or of the pre-sexual cycle (gametocytes) in films of the peripheral blood (Table 43.6, at end of chapter). Identification of the infection and of the *Plasmodium* species involved are essential preliminaries to specific chemotherapy. Vitally important is the quick recognition of *P. falciparum* as this species can cause a highly lethal infection in non-immune subjects if treatment is delayed. The possibility of malaria infection must always be entertained in any pyrexic patient who has visited infected areas. Slides are most likely to show parasites if taken during a pyrexial wave before any chemotherapy. If only early trophozoites ('rings', Table 43.6) are present, slides made after a lapse of some hours may show later stages to assist diagnosis, but it should be emphasized that the schizogony of *P. falciparum* occurs practically entirely in the capillaries of internal viscera; peripheral blood films may contain only ring forms, except in terminal cases. Thick blood films should be examined on at least three different occasions before malaria is excluded as a diagnosis.

Microscopy. Identification of malaria parasites in Giemsa-stained blood films is by examination with the × 100 oil-immersion objective, but the films can be scanned either with a × 50 oil-immersion objective or, after covering the film with a thin layer of immersion oil, with the × 40 dry objective. Malaria parasites are recognized as bodies staining red (nuclear material) and blue (cytoplasm), with black or brown pigment granules in later developmental stages, which occur *within* the erythrocytes. They are identified specifically on morphological differences in the organism and by the changes induced in the host cell. Table 43.6 summarizes microscopical features and Fig. 43.1g–i shows some representative forms. The various stages, their characters and the cell changes induced have been profusely illustrated in many books (see Belding 1965; Garnham 1966; Shute & Maryon 1966). Most important is the recognition of *P. falciparum* (Fig. 43.1i) for which the chief diagnostic characters (Garnham 1966) are:

1. Occurrence of ring forms alone or along with crescentic gametocytes.

2. Common occurrence of multiple infections of single erythrocytes with also accolé forms and rings with double chromatin dots.

3. Presence of Maurer's clefts in erythrocytes containing large rings.

Many details of morphology cannot be seen in thick films. Thus, both thick and thin films* should be made so that if parasites are seen in the thick film they may be more critically studied in the thin film. Multiple infections with more than one *Plasmodium* sp. at the same time are not uncommon.

Field's stain (Lumsden & Sargeaunt 1975) is not suitable for work in which large numbers of blood films have to be stained as each has to be treated separately. When, however, a rapid diagnosis is important, as may happen in individual clinical cases, its use can save half an hour in the staining process.

Immunodiagnosis. Indirect fluorescent antibody (IFA), indirect haemagglutination (IHA) and ELISA tests are most used but are limited to specialized laboratories (see introductory section above for addresses). The IFA test is preferred (Kagan & Walls 1981). The tests have been used for epidemiological studies but do not replace microscopical recognition of the organisms for individual diagnosis. Immunological detection of antigen using an ELISA inhibition test is more promising in this respect (Mackey et al 1982).

Drug sensitivity. Resistance of *P. falciparum* to 4-aminoquinoline drugs is widespread in SE Asia and in South America. A specialized technique, based on estimation of the drug concentration inhibiting schizont maturation in vitro is available to estimate drug sensitivity (Rieckmann et al 1978).

Babesia

Babesia spp. are common parasites of a wide range of mammals. They are important causes of disease in cattle and dogs, and are transmitted by ixodid ticks. Human infections, characterized by fever, jaundice and sometimes myalgia, have been reported (Ristic & Lewis 1977). In most of these, there was a history of exposure to tick-infested environments. Subclinical infections may apparently pass unnoticed. The infection may be dangerous in immunologically compromised individuals; three deaths have occurred, all in splenectomized subjects.

In thin blood films stained with Giemsa, the organisms are round, oval or pyriform bodies 1–4 μm long, occurring singly or in multiples of two within red cells (Fig. 43.1j, at end of chapter). They may resemble *P. falciparum* rings but pigment is not formed.

For animal inoculation, use hamsters. CF, IFA and IHA tests are considered to have been critically evaluated for the serological diagnosis of *Babesia* infection (Mahoney 1977).

Pneumocystis

Pneumocystis carini is widely associated with latent infections in man and many other mammals. Acute infections occur mainly in immunocompromised subjects – in debilitated infants or in adults with malignant disease and in patients treated with corticosteroids. Pneumocystis infection is a major problem in patients with AIDS. Acute infections are characterized by massive consolidation of the lungs, the alveoli being filled with plasma cells and microbial debris. Seed & Aikawa (1977) review *P. carini* infection and Hughes (1975) provides a critical discussion of laboratory diagnosis based on identification of the organism in lung samples.

Specimens. Although the organism may be demonstrable in sputum, tracheal aspirates or bronchial washings, examination of lung tissue is the most sensitive diagnostic procedure. Open lung biopsy is traumatic in the debilitated subjects usually under consideration; trans-bronchoscopic and needle aspiration methods are preferred (Seed & Aikawa 1977).

Culture. Although sometimes claimed, cultivation of the organism has not yet been accomplished (Seed & Aikawa 1977).

Animal inoculation. Many laboratory animals harbour latent infections of *P. carini* which are revealed by immunological suppression, e.g. by treatment with cortisone, so animal inoculation is not used for diagnosis.

Microscopy. P. carini is not seen in haematoxylin-eosin stained lung biopsy sections. Toluidine blue O stained sections (Hughes 1975) may show the cyst walls of the organism, but generally a silver stain is preferred; silver methenamine stain* is suitable. Search 'foamy' patches in alveoli for trophozoites 1.2–5 μm in diameter, of irregular shape, and for cysts (Fig. 43.2g, at end of chapter) 10–12 μm in diameter, which stand out clearly against the greenish background and have a black capsule enclosing two to eight trophozoites (Seed & Aikawa 1977). Yeasts may resemble *P. carini* cysts.

Immunodiagnosis. Antibodies against *P. carini* may be demonstrated by IFA tests (Meuwissen et al 1977) in sera from patients with *P. carini* pneumonia and also in sera from normal control subjects. The antibody titres tend to be higher in the former group (Shepherd et al 1979) but serological tests are obviously of limited value.

CILIATES

The only ciliate protozoon of medical importance is *Balantidium*, discussed below.

Balantidium

Balantidium coli is a common parasite of pigs, from which infections of man are believed to be derived. It is most prevalent in man when association with pigs is close, in South and Central America, SW Asia and some Pacific islands, particularly in New Guinea, where 20% of the human population may be infected. It occurs in the caecum and colon and produces acute diarrhoea with ulceration and tissue penetration similar to that caused by *Entamoeba histolytica*. Transmission is by resistant cysts. For a review see Zaman (1978).

Specimens. Faecal samples as for *E. histolytica.*

Culture. B. coli grows well in Robinson's medium.*

Microscopy. Trophozoites are 30–300 × 30–100 μm (Fig. 43.2h, at end of chapter) and are active ciliated organisms with a funnel-shaped depression (peristome, cytostome, cytopharynx) at the anterior end for ingestion of food material. Internally they have two contractile vacuoles, food vacuoles; trichrome staining shows a kidney-shaped macronucleus with a spherical micronucleus enclosed in its concavity. Cysts (Fig. 43.2h) are spherical or ovoid, 40–60 μm in length with a thick hyaline wall.

METHODS FOR TISSUE AND BLOOD PROTOZOA

Tissue aspirates

Lymph node. 1. Massage the enlarged node with the finger and thumb of the left hand.

2. Insert a hypodermic needle through the ethanol-swabbed skin into the substance of the node and continue massage.

3. Withdraw the needle, attach a dry air-filled syringe and gently blow out the needle contents on to slide.

4. Apply a coverslip and examine immediately as a wet film under the × 40 objective.

5. After examination as a wet film, remove the coverslip and fix and stain as for a thin blood film.

Tissue. 1. Puncture the lesion with a dry hypodermic needle and syringe maintaining negative pressure by withdrawing the piston. Move the needle-point back and forwards in the lesion.

2. Release the pressure just before withdrawing the needle.

3. Detach the syringe, draw a few ml of air into it, reattach it and blow out the contents of the needle on to a slide or into culture medium.

Spleen. Splenic aspiration is acceptably safe providing: (a) the spleen is palpable at least 3 cm below the costal margin on expiration (for smaller spleens or when the spleen is impalpable, use lymph node aspiration), (b) the procedure is quick, and (c) the entry and withdrawal track of the needle are identical, so as to avoid tearing the splenic capsule. After splenic puncture, pulse and blood pressure should be closely watched for 12 h with the patient in bed.

1. Have ready: microscope slides; tubes of culture medium (at room temperature); 5 ml syringe; 32 × 0.9 mm needle; ethanol 75%; swabs.

2. Mark the outline of the spleen on the skin; swab area with 75% ethanol; allow to dry.

3. Push the needle (syringe attached) through the skin 2–4 cm below the costal margin and in the middle of the marked area. Aim the needle upwards at about 45° to the abdominal wall.

4. Retract the syringe piston to about 1 ml and then, continuously maintaining that suction, quickly push the needle into the spleen for its full length and then withdraw it completely.

5. Pull the syringe piston back slowly, to 2–3 ml, insert the needle into the tube of culture medium and expel the needle contents vigorously on to the walls of the tube; repeat with a second tube of culture medium.

6. Make smears by spreading the material remaining on the needle tip, on the syringe nozzle or on the end of the syringe piston. Allow to dry; fix and stain as for a thin blood film.

Wet mounts for tissue or blood protozoa

1. Place a drop of the suspension to be examined, diluted with isotonic NaCl if it is too concentrated, on a slide and cover it immediately with a large coverslip (18 × 18 or 22 × 22 mm).

2. Scan with the × 10 objective and change to the × 40 or × 100 objective to examine suspicious structures, e.g. motile organisms in blood.

The mount should be thin enough for things in it to present more-or-less in a single layer and for the coverslip to be stable, not floating on a deep layer of suspension. For most examinations the above-described wet mount is sufficient. If examination is expected to be very prolonged, seal the coverslip along its four sides with molten paraffin wax or petroleum jelly.

Blood films

Use new slides 75 × 25 mm, freed from grease by washing in 70% ethanol, and dried with a non-fraying grease-free cloth or towel. Two types of film are used. *Thin films* are spread on the slide in a layer mostly one-cell thick, so offering the best conditions for microscopy of cells and of blood-inhabiting protozoa. *Thick films* are spread in layers several cells thick, so that larger volumes of blood can be searched, accepting inferior visualization of the organisms found. Blood is most conveniently obtained by puncturing the bulb of the third finger with a disposable lancet (Steriseal). Films are best stained face-downwards (Fig. 43.3b) to minimize adventitious deposit on the film. Thin and thick films should be made on separate slides to avoid inadvertent fixing of the thick film.

Thin film (Fig. 43.3a). 1. Place a drop of blood about 1.5 mm in diameter in the middle of a slide towards one end.

2. Immediately apply the end of another slide at an angle of about 45° to the first slide so that the drop of blood is in the re-entrant angle.

3. Draw the end of the second slide 'backwards' to contact the blood drop and allow a second or so till the blood drop is seen to spread along most of the line of contact of the second slide on the first.

4. Push the second slide 'forwards' along the first in a continuous movement, thereby pulling the blood out in a band along the slide. Ideally the film should be across the middle of the slide, should not extend to the edges of the slide, and should run out at its end in a fringe of 'tails'. If a drop of blood is too large the amount used for making the film can be reduced by lifting the applying slide and immediately reapplying it slightly further along the slide, separated from the first application.

5. Allow the film to dry.

6. Fix the dry film by placing the slide film upwards, and flooding it with absolute methanol with a Pasteur pipette; leave for 30 s; pour off the methanol, drain the slide on a paper towel and set it up on edge in a rack to dry. It is better to fix in this way rather than by immersion of the whole slide in methanol in a jar; methanol in a

jar, unless set up afresh each day, may not be absolute and may contain debris which can attach to the film.

7. Place the slides to be stained face downwards on the staining tray (Fig. 43.3b) abutting edge to edge.

8. Using a 20 ml plastic syringe with a 38×0.9 mm needle, draw in Giemsa's stain to a measured amount, say 0.5 ml. Draw in diluent (distilled water, or preferably isotonic NaCl buffered to pH 7.2–7.4) to 10 ml. Withdraw the syringe piston a little further to introduce an air bubble. Mix the stain by inverting the syringe several times.

9. Fill the space below the slides with the diluted stain from the syringe and needle.

10. Stain for 30–60 min; pick off the slides singly, flush off the stain quickly with distilled water from a wash bottle, drain on a paper towel and place in a rack to dry.

11. Flush off stain remaining on the tray under a water tap and dry. Do not allow stain to dry on the tray.

Thick film. 1. Place a drop of blood about 3 mm in diameter in the middle of a slide and spread it with the corner of another slide to cover an area about 10 mm diameter.

2. Dry the film rapidly by waving the slide in air.

3. Do not fix. The method depends on the leaching out of the haemoglobin in the erythrocytes, so that the erythrocytes stain minimally and remain transparent, thus allowing stained organisms lying deep in the thick layer of blood cells to be seen. The leaching out takes place at the next stage when the haemoglobin dissolves in the watery solution of stain at the same time as staining goes on.

4. Stain exactly as for thin films (Paras 7 *et seq*, above).

It is important to make the film the optimum thickness. Over-thick films have too many leucocytes in the fields for easy microscopy and over-thin films take little advantage of the facility for searching a larger quantity of blood. At optimum thickness small print is just readable through the unstained film placed over it. Thick films may not adhere to the slide if stained immediately after drying. They are best left at 37°C over-

night. If immediate staining and examination is required, place the slides at 60°C for 5 min.

Miniature anion-exchange/centrifugation (MAEC) method for diagnosis of Trypanosoma brucei parasitaemia (Lumsden et al 1979, 1981)

This method was developed for mass surveys of rural populations in the tropics. It uses small quantities of blood ($c.\ 250\ \mu$l) procured with heparinized capillaries from finger punctures. In principle, sensitivity could be increased by the use of larger volumes of blood, columns, etc.

Materials (Fig. 43.3c). 2 ml plastic syringe barrels, washed in detergent, distilled water and dried.

Cellulose sponge plugs to fit syringe barrels, 14 mm diameter, cut with cork borer from domestic sponge (Spontex).

Reservoirs and centrifuge tubes are made from 150 mm glass Pasteur pipettes. Fit the reservoirs with perforated syringe pistons. Draw the centrifuge tubes so that the terminal lumen is about 200 μm in diameter and the terminal bead small. Insert the terminal part of the centrifuge tube into suitably sized automatic pipette tips for protection.

Phosphate buffered saline with glucose (PBSG; Lanham & Godfrey 1970) as follows:

NaCl	2.125 g
$NaH_2PO_4.2H_2O$	0.39 g
Na_2HPO_4 (anhydrous)	6.74 g
Water to	1 litre
Glucose (added just before use)	1% w/v

DEAE cellulose (Whatman DE52) equilibrated in the above PBSG.

Viewing chambers.

Method. 1. Set up the washed syringe barrels nozzle downwards ('Terry' clips of suitable size screwed to a vertical board are convenient).

2. Insert cellulose plugs in the syringe barrels and push down to the bottom to act as a base for the column.

3. Shake up the equilibrated DEAE cellulose and pour it quickly into the syringe barrels so as to fill them almost full. Allow to drain, dry and refill the syringe barrel with PBSG, twice.

4. Discharge the heparinized blood sample (c. 250 μl) on to the top of the DEAE cellulose and allow it to drain in.

5. Deliver about four drops of PBSG on to the top of the cellulose and immediately plug in and fill the reservoir.

6. Leave until all the PBSG has passed through to the centrifuge tube.

7. Centrifuge the eluate-containing tube at about 500 g for 10 min.

8. Examine the fine tip of the centrifuge tube in the viewing chamber (Fig. 43.3c) by microscope (× 40 objective).

The lumen of the fine tip of the centrifuge tube should be about 200 μm in diameter and trypanosomes if present are easily visualized and recognized by their morphology and movement under the × 40 objective.

Examination of CSF for Trypanosoma brucei

CSF should be examined within 30 min of its withdrawal.

1. Fill the haemocytometer chamber (Improved Neubauer) with the CSF. Allow to settle for 5 min and count the leucocytes in the ruled area (× 40 objective). 95% of adults have less than 5.3 leucocytes/μl (Diem & Lentner 1970). Wilcocks & Manson-Bahr (1972) gave 30 leucocytes/μl as the practical threshold for indicating trypanosomal infection.

2. While counting leucocytes be alert, focusing up-and-down, for motile trypanosomes.

3. Centrifuge the CSF at 1000 g for 5 min; examine the deposit as a wet mount for motile trypanosomes (× 40 objective); remove coverslip, make a thin film of the deposit, fix and stain as for thin blood film. Examine for morula cells ('Mott' cells – degenerating plasma cells with morula inclusions; see Fig. 43.1d).

4. Estimate total protein and IgM in the supernate of the CSF.

Diphasic medium for the cultivation of Leishmania and Trypanosoma cruzi

All the innumerable varieties of diphasic, blood agar and overlay media for the cultivation of Kinetoplastida have been based on the original

NNN medium evolved by Novy & McNeal (1904) and Nicolle (1908) (see Taylor & Baker 1968). Many of the modifications, however, have been for particular research purposes and the following is a formula commonly used for diagnostic work (Evans 1978).

1. Dissolve 40 g Blood Agar Base No. 2 (Oxoid) in 1 litre of distilled water. Dispense 5 ml quantities while molten into screw-capped 30 ml (Universal) bottles and autoclave.

2. Allow to cool to about 45°C, and add aseptically 1 ml fresh rabbit blood; put bottles at a slope to cool so that the agar sets in a slant.

3. Add aseptically to each bottle 1 ml of sterile Locke's solution (containing: NaCl, 8.0; KCl, 0.2; $CaCl_2$, 0.2; KH_2PO_4, 0.3; and glucose, 2.5 g/litre). For possibly bacterially contaminated inocula add to this solution penicillin (200 iu/ml) and streptomycin (2 μg/ml).

For ease of handling, the blood component of the medium can be citrated, or it may be defibrinated (Taylor & Baker 1968), and it is inactivated at 56°C for 30 min. The blood should be fresh, i.e. stored for not longer than 7 days at 4°C. Mostly rabbit blood is used, but blood of other species can be substituted; in descending order of suitability Taylor & Baker (1968) cite man, rabbit, guinea-pig, horse, sheep.

To check the sterility of the blood agar slopes, incubate them at 37°C for 24 h, discarding any showing growth; add the liquid phase to the culture at least 24 h before inoculating the specimen.

Since the danger of bacterial or fungal contamination is greatest at the primary inoculation, it is a good precaution to have the primary culture media put up in screw-capped bottles with centrally perforated rubber-wadded caps, so that the culture can be inoculated with the needle through the cap without opening the bottle (Lumsden et al 1973).

Delayed hypersensitivity skin (DHS) test for Leishmania infection (Montenegro or leishmanin test)

1. Harvest promastigotes of any Leishmania sp. from the diphasic blood agar medium in which they are grown.

2. Wash the promastigotes by repeated centrifugation and resuspension four times in buffered isotonic salts solution (e.g. Solution AB, Lumsden et al 1973).

3. Resuspend in 0.5% phenol saline and adjust the suspension with the same solution to the desired concentration: 100 000 000/ml is recommended for VL and American CL; 100/ml for Old World CL (Wilcocks & Manson-Bahr 1972).

4. Inject 0.2 ml of the suspension intradermally and read the test at 48–72 h. A positive test is an area of erythema and induration 5 mm in diameter or larger which heals (or sometimes ulcerates) in 14–25 days (Belding 1965; Wilcocks & Manson-Bahr 1972).

METHODS FOR HOLLOW VISCUS PROTOZOA

Wet mounts for examination of faeces

1. Collect about 5 mg of faeces on the tip of a wooden applicator stick and mix in a drop (0.05 ml) of saline (8.5 g NaCl/litre of water) on a microscope slide.

2. Cover with a coverslip. The suspension should not be so thick that it appears opaque when viewed against a white background. Scan with a low power objective and then a high power ($\times$ 40) lens to examine suspect objects.

3. Stain with iodine prepared as follows:

Potassium iodide	1 g
Iodine	1.5 g
Distilled water	100 ml

Place a drop of the solution at one edge of the coverslip and draw it into the wet mount by placing a piece of filter paper against the opposite edge.

Preserving faeces in PVA fixative for later microscopy

Polyvinyl alcohol (PVA) fixative (Brooke & Goldman 1949):

Mercuric chloride saturated solution in water: 95% ethanol; 2:1	93.5 ml
Glycerol	1.5 ml
Glacial acetic acid	5 ml
Polyvinyl alcohol (Sigma type II low MW)	5 g

Add the PVA with continuous stirring to the rest of the ingredients heated slowly (to about 75°C); when water-clear, dispense in about 5 ml quantities to wide-mouthed, screw-capped containers; these will remain effective for 6 months stored at room temperatures.

1. With an applicator stick, mix about 1 ml of faeces into the 5 ml of PVA fixative in the container; this preparation will remain satisfactory for microscopy for several months.

2. Pipette a little of the suspension on to a clean paper towel.

3. After a few min, when most of the fluid has been absorbed, use an applicator stick to make smears on slides from the specimen.

4. Dry the smears overnight at 37°C.

5. Stain the smears with iron-haematoxylin (see below), entering the process at stage 3 by placing the slides in iodine/ethanol.

Preparation of faecal smears for staining

1. Charge the distal 2 cm of a wooden applicator stick with faeces; deposit some on the distal 2 cm of a slide by rotating the stick held flat. Spread the sample as evenly as possible along the slide using the middle section of the stick in the same way (Fig. 43.3d).

2. Fix immediately in Schaudinn's fluid; leave in fixative 30 min. Schaudinn's fluid is prepared as follows:

Mercuric chloride, saturated solution in water (c. 70 g/litre)	40 ml
Ethanol, absolute	20 ml
Acetic acid, glacial (added immediately before use)	3 ml

Staining faecal smears with iron-haematoxylin

Process the film, fixed in Schaudinn's fluid, as follows:

1. Ethanol 50%, 5 min.
2. Ethanol 70%, 5 min.

3. Solution of iodine in 70% ethanol (deep brown colour), 5 min.

4. Ethanol 70% (two changes), 10 min each.

5. Ethanol 50%, 5 min.

6. Ethanol 30%, 5 min.

7. Distilled water (two changes), 5 min each.

8. Mordant solution, 4 h. (Ferric ammonium sulphate, 4% w/v solution in distilled water; freshly prepared).

9. Rinse in distilled water.

10. Stain with the following stain, 4 h. (Haematoxylin 5% w/v in absolute ethanol, 10 ml; distilled water, 100 ml. This solution requires to be ripened for 1 month before use by being left in a clear glass stoppered bottle exposed to sunlight).

11. Distilled water, 2 min.

12. Differentiate in 1% ferric ammonium sulphate, repeatedly checking differentiation by microscopy and stopping differentiation, when sufficient, by washing in distilled water.

13. Dehydrate in ascending concentrations of ethanol, clear in xylene, and mount in DPX (Ch. 3).

Staining faecal smears with trichrome stain

Use faecal smears fixed in Schaudinn's fixative as above for at least 30 min. Then treat as follows:

1. Ethanol 70%, 5 min.

2. Ethanol 70% with iodine (deep brown colour), 5 min.

3. Ethanol 70%, twice, 5 min each

4. Stain with Wheatley's rapid light-green stain (1951), 30 min.

Chromotrope 2R	0.6 g
Light green SF	0.3 g
12-tungstophosphoric acid	0.7 g
Acetic acid (glacial)	1 ml
Distilled water	100 ml

Add the acetic acid to the mixture of dry stains; after 30 min, add the distilled water.

5. Rinse in 90% ethanol with 1% glacial acetic acid (v/v), 3 s.

6. Rinse in 100% ethanol.

7. Ethanol 100% (two changes), 5 min each.

8. Xylene (two changes), 3 min each.

9. Mount in DPX.

Staining faecal smears with carbol fuchsin (Henriksen & Pohlenz 1981)

Prepare faecal smears as above and air dry for 5 min. Place in the staining rack of a flat type Coplin staining jar containing a wad of cotton wool saturated in formalin (40% formaldehyde) and incubate at 37°C for 20 min. Then proceed as follows:

1. Flood slides on staining rack with cold carbol fuchsin (Ziehl-Neelsen), 5 min.

2. Rinse in tap water.

3. Flood slides with 10% (v/v) H_2SO_4 until dye ceases to pour out of smear, about 30 s.

4. Rinse in tap water.

5. Stain in aqueous malachite green (5% w/v), 3 min.

6. Rinse in tap water and blot dry with filter paper.

Staining faecal smears with safranin O (Baxby & Blundell 1983)

Prepare faecal smears as above and fix for 3–5 min in 3% (v/v) HCl in methanol contained in a Coplin jar. Air dry and proceed as follows:

1. Flood slide supported in a staining rack with aqueous safranin O (1% w/v) and heat until steam rises from the surface of the stain.

2. Rinse in tap water.

3. Counterstain in aqueous methylene blue (1% w/v), 30 s.

4. Rinse in tap water and blot dry with filter paper.

Robinson's medium for cultivation of intestinal amoebae

Robinson (1968) has described a very sensitive method for the culture of *Entamoeba histolytica*. It involves a defined medium for growing *Escherichia coli*, the bacteria then being the substrate for the growth of amoebae; saline agar slopes; and various solutions, either inhibitory or nutrient, which are added in different combinations during amoebic growth. The preparation of the requirements for this method is described here.

Concentrated stock for growing Escherichia coli is prepared as follows:

NaCl	125 g
Citric acid, $C_6H_8O_7.H_2O$	50 g
KH_2PO_4	12.5 g
$(NH_4)_2SO_4$	25 g
$MgSO_4.7H_2O$	1.25 g
Lactic acid BDH 90.08%	100 ml
Water	2.5 litre

This can be kept without sterilization. It should be more than 4 weeks old to avoid change of pH on autoclaving.

Prepare medium diluted for use as follows:

Concentrated stock	100 ml
NaOH, 40% in water	7.5 ml
Bromothymol blue, 0.04%	2.5 ml
Water	890 ml

Adjust to pH 7.0, dispense in 25 ml volumes in screw-capped 100 ml medical flat bottles and autoclave at 121°C for 20 min.

For use *Escherichia coli* strain B is inoculated into the medium; the bottle is then incubated in the horizontal position at 37°C for 2 days. This medium can be stored at room temperature for 2 months.

Saline agar slopes

NaCl	7 g
Agar	15 g
Water	1 litre

Dissolve, distribute in 2.5 ml aliquots in 7 ml screw-capped bottles, autoclave at 121°C for 15 min and allow to set as slopes. The concentration of agar may require to be increased to 2.5%, depending upon its quality.

Erythromycin solution (0.5%)

Erythromycin base	0.5 g
Ethanol, 70% in water	2.5 ml
Water, sterile	97.5 ml

Suspend the erythromycin in the ethanol in a sterile vessel, allow to stand for 2 h, add the water and store at 4°C.

Phthalate solution, 0.5 mol/l

Potassium phthalate, $C_6H_4(COOK)_2$	204 g
NaOH, 40% in water	100 ml
Water	1.9 litre

Dissolve the salt in the liquids, adjust the pH to 6.3, distribute in 1 ml aliquots and autoclave at 121°C for 10 min. For use, add 9 ml sterile water to give 0.05 mol/l phthalate at pH 6.5.

Sheep serum. Serum from the slaughter house, cleared with paper pulp on a filter, is sterilized by filtration, heated at 56°C on 3 successive days and stored at 4°C. Horse, rabbit, ox or human serum can replace sheep serum.

Bactopeptone solution (20%). This brand of peptone must be used.

Bactopeptone (Difco)	20 g
Water	100 ml

Dissolve the peptone and autoclave in a flask at 121°C for 20 min.

Rice starch powder (BDH).

Method

About 50 mg of faeces is added by wire loop to a saline agar culture bottle, which receives at the same time 4 drops (0.12 ml) of 0.5% erythromycin and 10 mg of starch (judged by eye on a knife blade). Basal amoebic medium (*Escherichia coli* culture prepared as above) is added to fill two-thirds of the bottle. After incubating at 37°C for 24 h, the supernate is pipetted off and replaced by a mixture of 25% basal medium, 25% serum and 50% phthalate solution to the same level. Two drops (0.06 ml) of 20% bactopeptone, two drops (0.06 ml) of 0.5% erythromycin and more starch are added. The culture is again incubated at 37°C.

After 24 h, drops of the culture sediment are examined microscopically in double-strength Lugol's iodine. The culture should be re-examined after a further 48 h incubation. The presence of *Entamoeba histolytica* is suggested in the first place by the abundance and rapidity of its growth. It is distinguished from *Endolimax nana* and *Entamoeba hartmanni* by being larger; with these smaller species a change from the × 20 to the × 40 objective is necessary to observe detail. *E. coli* is distinguished from *E. histolytica* by being less often bunched, being larger, more rounded and more 'glassy' and staining deep red with iodine. The distinctive nuclear pattern of *Dientamoeba fragilis* is shown by iron haematoxylin staining. An eye-piece scale is essential for reading these cultures.

Formol-ether method for the concentration of flagellate and amoebic cysts in faeces (Ridley & Hawgood 1956)

The method (modified) is as follows:

1. With a wooden spatula mix about 5 g of faeces with 10 ml of 10% (v/v) formalin (4% formaldehyde).
2. Strain the suspension through a single layer cotton gauze swab (Vernaid, Vernon-Carus) into a conical centrifuge tube.
3. Add about 3 ml of diethyl ether and shake the tube vigorously about 50 times to extract fat from the sample. (*Note*: diethyl either is highly inflammable and over a period of months of storage forms explosive peroxides. Garcia & Shimizu (1981) found ethyl acetate a satisfactory alternative.)
4. Centrifuge at 600 *g* for 1 min.
5. With a wooden applicator stick loosen the fatty plug at the interface and discard it and the liquid contents of the tube into disinfectant.
6. With a Pasteur pipette mix the sediment with a few drops of iodine solution; make a wet mount of the mixture; cover and examine with the × 40 objective.

Concentration of eimerian coccidian cysts from faeces by Sheather's sucrose flotation method (Sheather 1923)

1. Use a wooden applicator stick to mix about 1 g of stool with 5 ml isotonic saline.
2. Filter the suspension through three layers of cotton gauze swab to give 2 ml in a conical centrifuge tube.
3. Add 8 ml sucrose solution (sucrose, 500 g; phenol, 6.5 g; water, 320 ml).

4. Fill tube up to its rim with sucrose solution.
5. Place a 22 × 22 mm coverslip on the top of the tube, contacting the contained fluid.
6. Centrifuge at 600 *g* for 15 min.
7. Pick off coverslip and apply it to a slide for microscopical examination.

Examination of impression smears of jejunal mucosa (Ament 1972)

1. Remove the tissue from the biopsy capsule and place it on the tip of a gloved finger.
2. Use a blunt probe to arrange the biopsy so that the cut surface rests on the finger.
3. Wipe the mucosal surface successively with two slides; let these dry for 60 min.
4. Fix in methanol (30 min), and then stain in Giemsa stain as for thin blood films.

Examination of rectal ulcer biopsies for Entamoeba histolytica

1. Sample the tissue at the base of the ulcer with rectal biopsy forceps.
2. Remove the sample from the forceps with a needle and smear it on a slide.
3. Fix immediately in Schaudinn's solution and stain with iron haematoxylin (see above).

Polyester sponge method for Trichomonas vaginalis (Robertson et al 1969)

Clinicians are supplied with 10 × 10 × 40 mm pieces of polyester sponge (Campbell Brushes) in 7 ml plastic containers (129A bijou; Sterilin). Use Hartman's 'crocodile' oral forceps (Young) to withdraw the piece of sponge from the container and insert it into the posterior vaginal fornix; after 5 s, return it to the container which is then closed and sent to the laboratory.

1. Add 1 ml isotonic NaCl or buffered isotonic salts solution (pH 5.8) to the container and compress the sponge in the liquid several times with a wooden applicator stick.
2. Attach to the container a Hemming's filter, flat side, with washer but *without* filter pad; attach an empty recipient container to the flanged side of the filter (no washer).

3. Invert the assembly and centrifuge at 700 g for 5 min.

4. Remove and discard the upper sponge-containing container and Hemming's filter into disinfectant; take up the deposit from the centrifugate with a sterile Pasteur pipette and use it to prepare wet mounts and for inoculation into culture medium.

Modified CPLM medium for Trichomonas vaginalis

Johnson & Trussell (1943) recommended CPLM (cysteine-peptone-liver infusion-maltose) medium and the following modification of it (Dr K. Smith, personal communication) has been found satisfactory. Agar has been omitted from this modification because it complicates handling of the medium and of cultures in it. Methylene blue is omitted also. Phosphate as such is not added because there is sufficient of it in other ingredients.

This medium supports growth from a single protozoon under strictly anaerobic conditions. Under aerobic conditions, massive inocula are required. *T. vaginalis* is an anaerobe and contains no catalase.

Basal medium

Peptone	32 g
Maltose	1.6 g
Liver digest (Panmede, Paines & Byrne)	20 g
Cysteine hydrochloride	2.4 g
Ringer's solution, ¼ strength	1 litre
NaOH, 1 mol/litre	$c.$ 9 ml

The brand of peptone is not important. Panmede ox liver digest can be replaced by 32% of any brand of liver infusion made according to the manufacturer's instructions. Cysteine is not essential when cultures are incubated anaerobically but it assists the maintenance of anaerobiosis.

Dissolve the ingredients by shaking. Adjust the pH to 6.0 with NaOH, steam at 100°C for 30 min and filter off the fine grey precipitate with Whatman's No. 1 or coarse paper. Bottle in 90 ml lots and autoclave at 115°C for 10 min. This medium keeps for several weeks.

Penicillin streptomycin solution

Penicillin	0.06 g
Streptomycin	0.1 g
Sterile water	10 ml

Dissolve the antibiotics with sterile precautions. The solution contains 6×10^3 μg penicillin and 10^4 μg streptomycin/ml. It will keep up to 10 days in the refrigerator.

Nystatin solution

Nystatin	5×10^4 units
Sterile water	10 ml

Suspend the antibiotic in the water. The suspension contains 5×10^3 units/ml. It keeps in the refrigerator at less than 10°C but is rapidly destroyed at 37°C.

Preparation of complete medium

Basal medium	90 ml
Sterile inactivated horse serum	10 ml
Penicillin streptomycin solution	1 ml
Nystatin solution	1 ml

Before use, add the serum and antibiotics and distribute in suitable quantities with sterile precautions. Serum from human, calf, ox, sheep or rabbit may be used. The addition of antibiotics is unnecessary for routine subcultures but is essential for clinical diagnostic cultures and for isolating axenic cultures. Nystatin can be omitted unless yeast or fungal contaminants are suspected.

Isotonic Trichomonas medium

All the major constituents of this medium (Lumsden et al 1966) are prepared as solutions that are nearly isotonic with blood plasma. This makes the medium flexible and easily modified if differences, such as in pH, are desired.

Salts solution

NaCl, 0.154 mol/litre	1 litre
KCl, 0.154 mol/l	40 ml
MgCl$_2$, 0.103 mol/l	30 ml
CaCl$_2$, 0.103 mol/l	10 ml

Dissolve and autoclave in a flask at 121°C for 30 min. Store at 4 °C.

Buffer solution pH 7.4

NaH$_2$PO$_4$, 0.154 mol/litre	13.6 ml
Na$_2$HPO$_4$, 0.103 mol/l	86.4 ml
Bromocresol purple	15 mg

Dissolve the indicator in the buffer and autoclave in a flask at 121°C for 20 min. Store at 4°C.

Antibiotic solutions. Benzylpenicillin (Glaxo): 0.6 g dissolved in 5 ml sterile salts solution.
Streptomycin sulphate (Glaxo): 0.5 g dissolved in 2.5 ml sterile salts solution.

Preparation of complete medium

Liver digest (Oxoid), 4% solution	300 ml
Glucose, 5% solution	100 ml
Salts solution	392.5 ml
Buffer solution	100 ml
Benzylpenicillin solution	5 ml
Streptomycin sulphate solution	2.5 ml

Calf serum (Oxoid)	100 ml
Sodium thioglycollate (BDH)	1 g

Mix the ingredients at room temperature. The final pH is 6.1–6.4. Sterilize by filtration and distribute to sterile bottles in amounts that nearly fill them (6 ml to bijou bottles, 15 ml to ½ oz round bottles). Medium can be stored at 4°C for 2 weeks, or longer at −20°C.

Silver methenamine stain for Pneumocystis (Mahan & Sale 1978)

Preparation of stain
1. Add 2 ml of silver nitrate solution in water (1% w/v) to 40 ml of hexamethylenetetramine (methenamine) solution in water (3% w/v).
2. Add 3 ml solution of sodium borate Na$_2$B$_4$O$_7$.10H$_2$O) in water (5% w/v).
3. Make up with water to 80 ml.
4. Heat until solution is deep golden brown immediately before use.

Table 43.2 Specimens for the diagnosis of pathogenic intestinal protozoal infections.

Organism	Specimen(s) required	Comments
Entamoeba histolytica	Faeces Rectal exudate Material from base of rectal ulcers	Preparation of wet mounts and fixation of smears should be immediate[a]
	Rectal biopsy	Trophozoites occasionally seen in histological sections
	Liver abscess aspirate	
	Blood for serological examination	Limited value (see text)
Chilomastix mesnili	Faeces	As for *E. histolytica*
Giardia lamblia	Faeces Jejunal aspirate Jejunal impression smear	Microscopic examination of these specimens is the most sensitive method for diagnosis
	Jejunal biopsy	Trophozoites may be seen in histological preparations
	Blood for serological examination	Limited value (see text)
Dientamoeba fragilis	Faeces	As for *E. histolytica*
Balantidium coli	Faeces Rectal biopsy	As for *E. histolytica*
Isospora belli	Faeces Jejunal biopsy	For oocysts For schizogony stages
Sarcocystis spp.	Faeces Muscle biopsy	For oocysts For cysts of *S. lindemanni*
Cryptosporidium spp.	Faeces Jejunal or rectal biopsy	For oocysts For schizogony stages

[a] Diarrhoeal stools should be examined within 15 min of passing or preserved in PVA fixative (see *Methods*).

Method. Paraffin wax sections of biopsies are treated as follows:

1. Xylene, 3 min.
2. Ethanol 75%, 50%, 25% in distilled water, 5 min each.
3. Chromium trioxide in water (10% w/v), 1 min.
4. Tap water, cold, 5 s.
5. Sodium metabisulphite solution in water (10% w/v), 1 min.
6. Tap water, hot (*c*. 56°C), 1 min.
7. Silver methenamine stain, until sections are golden brown, about 2 min.
8. Rinse in hot tap water.
9. Rinse in cold tap water.
10. Rinse in distilled water.
11. Gold chloride solution in water (1% w/v), 10 s.
12. Rinse in distilled water.
13. Sodium thiosulphate in water (5% w/v), 3 min.
14. Tap water, cold, 10 min
15. Haematoxylin/eosin, stain lightly.
16. Dehydrate, clear in xylene, mount in DPX (Ch. 3).

Table 43.3 Microscopical characters of the intestinal flagellates, and ciliate (see Fig. 43.2).

Protozoon	Shape and size	Nuclear characters (stained smear)	Number and position of flagella	Other features
Trophozoites				
Retortamonas intestinalis	Pear shaped, 4–9 × 3–4 μm	Spherical nucleus at anterior end of organism	1 anterior 1 recurrent in cytostome	Ventral cytostome extending for ½ body length
Enteromonas hominis	Pear shaped, 4–10 × 3–6 μm	Anterior oval nucleus with eccentric endosome	3 anterior 1 longer posterior	No cytostome. Conspicuous fibre (funis) along ⅔ of body length
Chilomastix mesnili	Pear shaped, rounded anteriorly, tail-like posterior projection, 6–20 × 4–7 μm	Round anterior nucleus with several peripheral deeply staining plaques	3 anterior, 1 short recurrent in cytostome	Conspicuous cytostomal groove bordered by cytostomal fibres, one recurved posteriorly
Giardia lamblia	Pear shaped, 10–20 × 5–15 μm	2 nuclei with large endosomes	2 ventral 2 anterolateral 2 posterolateral 2 caudal	—
Dientamoeba fragilis	3.5–22 μm diam.; broad hyaline pseudopodia	Usually 2 nuclei but not uncommonly 1 only; large central endosome; no peripheral chromatin	—	—
Balantidium coli	Elongated or ovoid, 30–300 × 30–300 μm	Kidney-shaped macronucleus enclosing micronucleus	(ciliate)	Peristome/cytostome at anterior end; 2 contractile vacuoles
Cysts				
Retortamonas intestinalis	Thick-walled oval or lemon shaped, 4.5–7 × 3–4.5 μm	Single nucleus	—	Internal flagella and cytostomal fibres seen in iodine-stained cysts
Enteromonas hominis	Oval, 6–8 × 4–6 μm	1–4 nuclei	—	—
Chilomastix mesnili	Pear or lemon shaped with hyaline anterior protuberance, 7–10 × 4.5–6 μm	1 nucleus	—	Cytostomal fibres visible in unstained cysts
Giardia lamblia	Oval or round, 8–20 μm	4 nuclei	—	Longitudinal fibres within iodine-stained cyst
Balantidium coli	Spherical or ovoid, 40–60 μm, cytoplasm hyaline	1 macronucleus	—	—

Table 43.4 Microscopical features of *Entamoeba histolytica* and of the four non-pathogenic intestinal amoebae of man; stained iron-haematoxylin.

Character	Entamoeba histolytica	Entamoeba coli	Entamoeba hartmanni	Endolimax nana	Iodamoeba buetschli
Trophozoites					
Size μm	15–50 (usually 15–20)	15–50 (usually 20–25)	5–12 (usually 8–10)	6–18 (usually 8–10)	8–20 (usually 12–15)
Nucleus					
Peripheral chromatin	Fine granules, beaded	Clumped, unevenly arranged on membrane or as solid ring with no clumps	Similar to *E. histolytica*	Absent	Absent
Endosome	Small, central	Large, often eccentric	Small, compact, often central	Large, irregular, usually central	Large, rounded; surrounded by achromatic granules
Cytoplasm					
Appearance	Granular, ectoplasm and endoplasm clearly differentiated	Granular, no differentiation into ecto- and endoplasm	Fine granular	Granular, vacuolated	Coarse granular, vacuolated
Inclusions	Bacteria, may have erythrocytes	Bacteria, debris	Bacteria	Bacteria	Bacteria, debris
Cysts					
Size (μm)	10–20	10–30	5–9	5–12	6–15
Shape	Spherical	Usually spherical	Spherical	Ovoid	Very irregular, ovoid spherical
Nucleus					
Number	1–4	1–8, seldom 2, occasionally 16	1–4, often 2	1–4	1, rarely 2
Peripheral chromatin	As trophozoite	Coarse, granular, may be clumped on membrane	Fine granules on membrane	Absent	Absent
Endosome	As trophozoite	Large, eccentric	Small, central	Large, central	Large, eccentric
Cytoplasm					
Chromatoidal bodies	Common; blunt ends	Infrequent; splinter-like ends	Common; blunt smooth ends	Absent	Absent
Glycogen (iodine stained)	Ill-defined glycogen vacuole	Well-defined mass lying between nuclei in binucleate cysts	Diffuse or absent	Diffuse, if present	Large, well defined

Table 43.5 Microscopic features of coccidial oocysts.

Species	Shape	Size	Sporulated oocyst
Isospora belli	Ellipsoid, thin walled	20–33 × 10–19 μm	2 ellipsoid sporocysts (9–14 × 7–12 μm), each with 4 crescentic sporozoites; uncommonly seen in fresh faeces
Usually found in faeces as immature oocysts containing a single spherical mass of cytoplasm; released sporocysts rarely seen.			
Sarcocystis hominis, suihominis	Ovoid, thin walled	20–30 × 10–12 μm	2 oval sporocysts (10–16 × 7–12.5 μm), each with 4 sporozoites
Sporulated oocysts rarely seen in faeces; released sporocysts usually found.			
Cryptosporidium spp.	Ovoid or spherical, thin walled	5–6 μm	No sporocyst; 4 sporozoites, small spherical residual body

Table 43.6 Differential diagnosis of *Plasmodium* species of man in Romanowsky-stained thin films of peripheral blood.

	Species and disease			
	P. falciparum Malignant tertian	*P. vivax* Benign tertian	*P. malariae* Quartan	*P. ovale* Ovale tertian
Trophozoites (a) Ring forms	0.15–0.5 of diameter of RBC; RBC normal size Cytoplasm – very fine in young rings; thick irregular in old rings. Marginal (accolé) forms, forms with 2 chromatin dots and multiple infections, common	0.3–0.5 of diameter of RBC which is unaltered in size Cytoplasm – circle, thin	0.3–0.5 of diameter of RBC which is unaltered in size Cytoplasm – circle, thicker	0.3 of diameter of RBC which is unaltered in size Cytoplasm – circle, thicker
(b) Growing forms	RBC unaltered in size, sometimes stippled, pale Parasite compact; pigment dense brown or black mass *Not usually seen in peripheral blood*	RBC enlarged, stippled Parasite amoeboid, vacuolated; pigment fine and scattered, golden brown	RBC unaltered Parasite compact, rounded or band-shaped; dark brown or black pigments, often concentrates in a line along one edge of band	RBC unaltered in size, or slightly enlarged, stippled; may be oval and fimbriated Parasite compact, rounded; pigment fine brown grains
Mature schizonts	RBC unaltered in size, sometimes stippled, pale Parasite about 0.6 of RBC; nuclei or merozoites 8–24; pigment clumped, black *Not usually seen in peripheral blood*	RBC much enlarged, stippled Parasite large, filling enlarged RBC; nuclei or merozoites 12–24, usually 16; pigment a golden brown central loose mass	RBC unaltered Parasite fills RBC completely; nuclei or merozoites 6–12, usually 8, sometimes forming rosette; pigment, brown/black central clump	RBC frequently oval, fimbriated, enlarged, stippled Parasite as for *P. malariae* but does not entirely fill the slightly enlarged RBC; pigment, brown central clump
Gametocytes	RBC distorted Parasite crescentic	RBC enlarged, stippled Parasite large, round filling enlarged RBC	RBC unaltered Parasite small, round filling RBC	RBC slightly enlarged, stippled Parasite round
Stippling	Maurer's clefts	Schüffner's dots	None (Ziemann's dots after prolonged Leishman staining)	James's dots

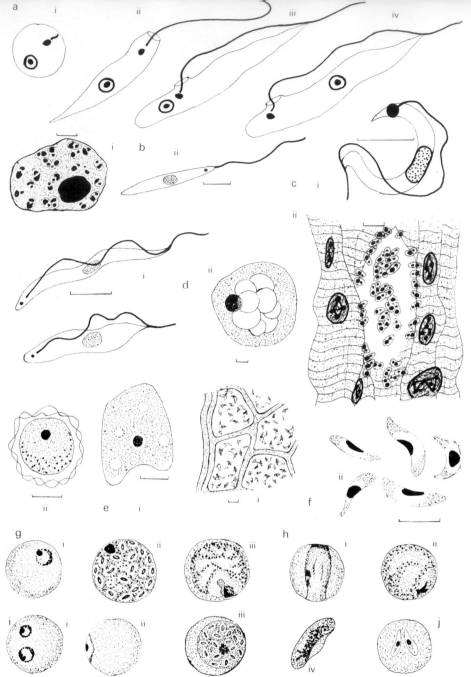

Fig. 43.1 Representative diagrams of the microscopical appearances of stages of the tissue protozoa of man. Romanowsky stain except when stated otherwise. Scale bars are 5 μm.

a. The various developmental stages of the kinetoplastid flagellates (*Leishmania* and *Trypanosoma*): (i) amastigote; (ii) promastigote; (iii) epimastigote; (iv) trypomastigote.

b. *Leishmania*: (i) amastigotes in a macrophage from a tissue aspirate smear; (ii) promastigote form from culture in diphasic medium.

c. *Trypanosoma cruzi*: (i) trypomastigote from thin blood film; (ii) nest of amastigotes in infected muscle cell (pseudocyst).

d. *Trypanosoma brucei rhodesiense*: (i) long slender and short stumpy trypomastigotes in thin blood film of peripheral blood; (ii) Mott or morula cell as seen in CNS tissue sections or in CSF.

e. Soil amoebae: (i) *Naegleria fowleri*, trophozoite from CSF or in culture, iron haematoxylin stain;
(ii) *Acanthamoeba*, cyst from corneal ulcer, unstained.

f. Gut coccidia: (i) *Sarcocystis lindemanni*, zoites in cyst in muscle, haematoxylin and eosin stain; (ii) *Toxoplasma*, zoites from peritoneal fluid or brain smear of mouse.

g. *Plasmodium vivax* in erythrocytes: (i) ring form; (ii) mature schizont; (iii) microgametocyte.

h. *Plasmodium malariae* in erythrocytes: (i) band form trophozoite; (ii) macrogametocyte.

i. *Plasmodium falciparum* in erythrocytes: (i) multiple ring forms in one erythrocyte; (ii) accolé form; (iii) mature schizont; (iv) microgametocyte.

j. *Babesia*, trophozoites in erythrocyte.

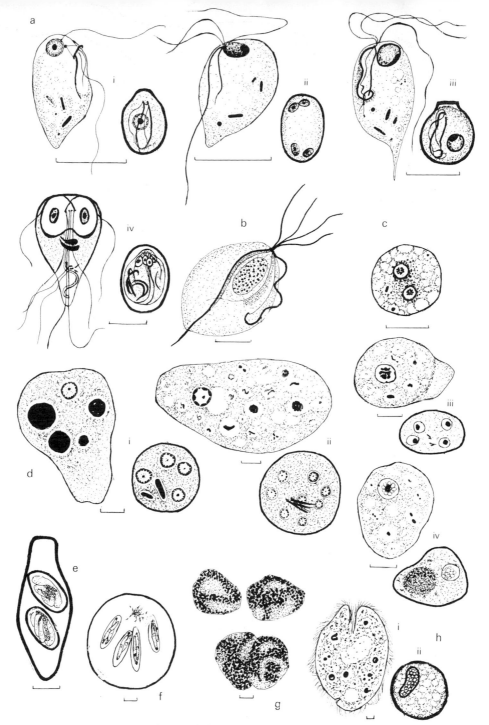

Fig. 43.2 Representative diagrams of the microscopical appearances of stages of the hollow-viscus protozoa of man. Iron-haematoxylin stain except where otherwise stated. Scale bars are 5 μm.

a. Gut flagellates: (i) *Retortamonas intestinalis*, trophozoite and cyst, from faeces; (ii) *Enteromonas hominis*, trophozoite and cyst, from faeces; (iii) *Chilomastix mesnili*, trophozoite and cyst, from faeces; (iv) *Giardia lamblia*, trophozoite and cyst, from duodenal aspirate and faeces, respectively.

b. *Trichomonas vaginalis*, troophozoite, from vaginal exudate, living.

c. *Dientamoeba fragilis*, trophozoite from faeces.

d. Gut amoebae: (i) *Entamoeba histolytica*, trophozoite and cyst, from faeces; (ii) *Entamoeba coli*, trophozoite and cyst, from faeces; (iii) *Endolimax nana*, trophozoite and cyst, from faeces; (iv) *Iodamoeba buetschli*, trophozoite and cyst, from faeces, latter stained iodine.

e. *Isospora belli*, sporulated oocyst, from faeces, unstained.

f. *Eimeria sardinae*, sporulated oocyst, from faeces, unstained.

g. *Pneumocystis carini*, cysts from lung biopsy smear, stained silver methenamine stain.

h. *Balantidium coli*: (i) trophozoite, unstained; (ii) cyst, stained.

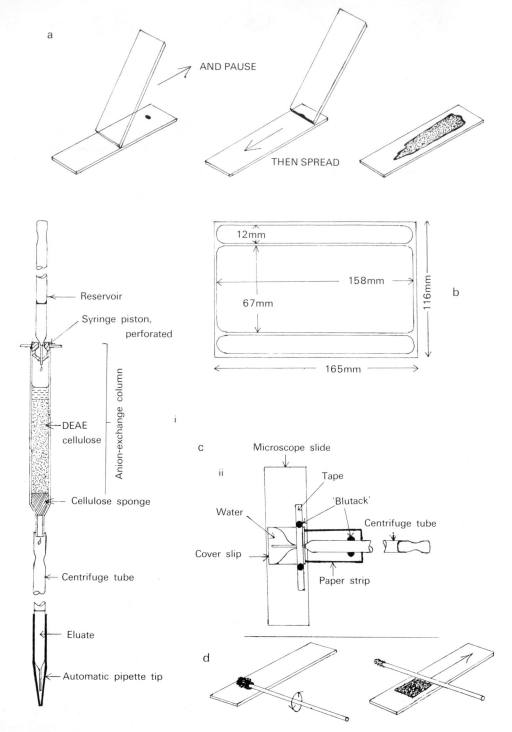

Fig. 43.3 Methods.

a. Method of making a thin blood film.

b. Staining tray machined (1 mm deep) from 6 mm perspex sheet, for staining blood films, tissue smears, etc. with Giemsa stain, face downwards. The tray shown is long enough for 6 slides; the trays can be made longer to accommodate more slides if required.

c. The apparatus for the miniature anion-exchange centrifugation method for the detection of low *Trypanosoma brucei* parasitaemias: (i) the reservoir, anion-exchange column and centrifuge tube assembly; (ii) the viewing chamber for the microscopical examination of the deposit in the centrifuge tube.

d. Preparation of a faecal smear.

REFERENCES

Ackers J P, Lumsden W H R, Catterall R D, Coyle R 1975 Antitrichomonal antibody in the vaginal secretions of women infected with *Trichomonas vaginalis*. British Journal of Venereal Diseases 51: 319–323

Ambroise-Thomas P, Kien Truong T 1972 Fluorescent antibody test in amebiasis. Clinical applications. American Journal of Tropical Medicine and Hygiene 21: 907–912

Ament M E 1972 Diagnosis and treatment of giardiasis. Journal of Pediatrics 80: 633–637

Amies C R 1967 A modified formula for the preparation of Stuart's transport medium. Canadian Journal of Public Health 58: 296–300

Baker J R 1977 Systematics of parasitic protozoa. In: Kreier J P (ed) Parasitic protozoa, vol 1. Academic Press, New York. Ch 4, p 35–56

Balsdon M J, Green N, Andrew C W, Jackson D H 1979 Rapid staining technique for *Trichomonas vaginalis*. Preliminary report. British Journal of Venereal Diseases 55: 289–291

Baxby D, Blundell N 1983 Sensitive rapid simple methods for detecting cryptosporidium in faeces. Lancet 2:1149

Belding D L 1965 Textbook of parasitology, 3rd edn. Appleton-Century-Crofts, New York

Bird R G, Smith M D 1980 Cryptosporidiosis in man: parasite life cycle and fine structural pathology. Journal of Pathology 132: 217–233

Bos H J, Schouten W J, Noordpool H, Makbin M, Oostburg B F J 1980 A seroepidemiological study of amebiasis in Surinam by the enzyme-linked immunosorbent assay (Elisa). American Journal of Tropical Medicine and Hygiene 29: 358–363

Brandborg I L, Goldberg S B, Breidenbach W C 1970 Human coccidiosis – a possible cause of malabsorption. New England Journal of Medicine 283: 1306–1313

Brooke M M, Goldman M 1949 Polyvinyl alcohol fixative as a preservative and adhesive for protozoa in dysenteric stools and other liquid materials. Journal of Laboratory and Clinical Medicine 34: 1554–1560

Červa L 1981 Amebic meningoencephalitis. In: Braude A (ed) Medical microbiology and infectious diseases. Saunders, Philadelphia. Ch 162, p 1281–1287

de Raadt P, Seed J R 1977 Trypanosomes causing disease in man in Africa. In: Kreier J P (ed) Parasitic protozoa, vol 1. Academic Press, New York. Ch 5, p 175–237

Diem K, Lentner C (eds) 1970 Documenta Geigy, 7th edn. J R Geigy S A, Basle. p 635

Dubey J P 1977 Toxoplasma, Hammondia, Besnoitia, Sarcocystis, and other tissue cyst-forming coccidia of man. In: Kreier J P (ed) Parasitic protozoa, vol 3. Academic Press, New York. Ch 4, p 101–237

Duvallet G, Stanghellini A, Saccarin C, Vivant J F 1979 Centrifugation en tubes capillaires: utilisation sur le terrain pour le diagnostic de la trypanosomiase humaine. Nouvelle Presse Medicale 8: 214–215

Evans D A 1978 Kinetoplastida. In: Taylor A R, Baker J R (eds) Methods of cultivating parasites in vitro. Academic Press, London. p 55–88

Faust E C, Russell P F 1964 Clinical parasitology, 7th edn. Lea & Febiger, Philadelphia

Frenkel J K 1971 Toxoplasmosis. Mechanisms of infection, laboratory diagnosis and management. Current Topics in Pathology 54: 29–75

Garcia L S, Shimizu R 1981 Comparison of clinical results for the use of ethyl acetate and diethyl ether in the formalin-ether sedimentation technique performed on polyvinyl alcohol-preserved specimens. Journal of Clinical Microbiology 13: 709–713

Garnham P C C 1966 Malaria parasites and other haemosporidia. Blackwell Scientific, Oxford

Gibson W C, Marshall T F de C, Godfrey D G 1980 Numerical analysis of enzyme polymorphism: a new approach to the epidemiology and taxonomy of trypanosomes of the subgenus Trypanozoon. In: Lumsden W H R, Muller R, Baker J R (eds) Advances in Parasitology 18: 175–244

Griffin J L 1978 Pathogenic free-living amoebae. In: Kreier J P (ed) Parasitic protozoa, vol 2. Academic Press, New York. Ch 4, p 508–549

Henriksen Sr Aa, Pohlenz J F L 1981 Staining of Cryptosporidia by a modified Ziehl-Neelsen technique. Acta Veterinaria Scandinavica 22: 594–596

Hoare C A 1972 The trypanosomes of mammals. Blackwell Scientific, Oxford

Honigberg B M 1978 Trichomonads of importance in human medicine. In: Kreier J P (ed) Parasitic protozoa, vol 2. Academic Press, New York. Ch 4, p 276–454

Hughes W T 1975 Current status of laboratory diagnosis of *Pneumocystis carinii* pneumonitis. CRC Critical Reviews in Clinical Laboratory Sciences 6: 145–170

Jeanes A L 1969 Evaluation in clinical practice of the fluorescent amoebic antibody test. Journal of Clinical Pathology 22: 427–429

Jeffrey H C 1974 Sarcosporidiosis in man. Transactions of the Royal Society of Tropical Medicine and Hygiene 68: 17–29

Johnson G, Trussell R E 1943 Experimental basis for the chemotherapy of *Trichomonas vaginalis* infestations I. Proceedings of the Society of Experimental Biology (New York) 54: 245–249

Kagan I G, Walls K W 1981 Protozoa and helminths. In: Milgrom F, Abeyounis C J, Kano K (eds) Principles of immunological diagnosis in medicine. Lea & Febiger, Philadelphia

Kreier J P (ed) 1977, 1978 Parasitic protozoa. Academic Press, New York

Lanham S M, Godfrey D G 1970 Isolation of salivarian trypanosomes from man and other mammals using DEAE-cellulose. Experimental Parasitology 28: 521–534

Lumsden W H R 1973 Demonstration of antibodies to Protozoa. In: Weir D M (ed) Handbook of experimental immunology, 3rd edn. Blackwell Scientific, Oxford. Ch 42

Lumsden W H R 1986 Application of immunological methods in protozoology. In Weir D M et al (eds) Handbook of experimental immunology, 4th edn. Blackwell Scientific, Oxford. Ch 122

Lumsden W H R, Herbert W J, McNeillage G J C 1973 Techniques with trypanosomes. Churchill Livingstone, Edinburgh

Lumsden W H R, Kimber C D, Dukes P, Haller L, Stanghellini A, Duvallet G 1981 Field diagnosis of sleeping sickness in the Ivory Coast. 1. Comparison of the miniature anion-exchange/centrifugation technique with other protozoological methods. Transactions of the Royal Society of Tropical Medicine and Hygiene 75: 242–250

Lumsden W H R, Kimber C D, Evans D A, Doig S J 1979 *Trypanosoma brucei*: miniature anion-exchange/ centrifugation technique for the detection of low parasitaemias: adaptation for field use. Transactions of the Royal Society of Tropical Medicine and Hygiene 73: 312–317

Lumsden W H R, Robertson D H H, McNeillage G J C 1966 Isolation, cultivation, low temperature preservation and infectivity titration of *Trichomonas vaginalis*. British Journal of Venereal Diseases 42: 145–154

Lumsden W H R, Sargeaunt P G 1975 Protozoa. In: Cruickshank R, Duguid J P, Marmion B P, Swain R H S (eds) Medical microbiology, 12th edn., vol. 2. Churchill Livingstone, Edinburgh. Ch 45, p 544

Mackey L, McGregor I A, Paounova N, Lambert P H 1982 The diagnosis of *Plasmodium falciparum* infection in man by enzyme-linked immunosorbent assay. Bulletin of the World Health Organization 60: 69–75

Mahan C T, Sale G E 1978 Rapid methenamine silver stain for *Pneumocystis* and fungi. Archives of Pathology and Laboratory Medicine 102: 351–352

Mahoney D F 1977 Babesia of domestic animals. In: Kreier J P (ed) Parasitic protozoa, vol 4. Academic Press, New York. Ch 1, p 1–52

Mattern P, Klein F, Radema H, van Furth R 1967 Les γ-macroglobulines réactionnelles et paraproteiniques dans le serum et dans le liquide cephalorachidien humain. Annales de l'Institut Pasteur 113:857

Meisel J L, Perera D R, Meligro C, Rubin C E 1976 Overwhelming watery diarrhea associated with a *Cryptosporidium* in an immunocompromised patient. Gastroenterology 70: 1156–1160

Meuwissen J H E T, Tauber I, Leeuwenberg A D E M, Beckers P J A, Sieben M 1977 Parasitologic and serologic observations of infection with *Pneumocystis* in humans. Journal of Infectious Diseases 136: 43–49

Meyer E 1976 *Giardia lamblia*: isolation and axenic cultivation. Experimental Parasitology 39: 101–105

Nicolle A 1908 Culture du parasite du bouton d'orient. Comptes rendus de l'Académie des Sciences (Paris) 146:842

Nielsen R 1969 *Trichomonas vaginalis*. 1. Survival in solid Stuarts' medium. British Journal of Venereal Diseases 45: 328–331

Novy F G, McNeal W J 1904 On the cultivation of *Trypanosoma brucei*. Journal of Infectious Diseases 1:1

Ogbunude P O J, Magaji Y 1982 A silicone centrifugation method for the detection of low parasitaemias of salivarian trypanosomes. Transactions of the Royal Society of Tropical Medicine and Hygiene 76: 317–318

Prathap K, Gilman R 1970 The histopathology of acute intestinal amoebiasis. American Journal of Pathology 60: 229–239

Remington J S 1969 The present status of the IgM fluorescent antibody technique in the diagnosis of congenital toxoplasmosis. Journal of Pediatrics 75: 1116–1124

Ridley D S, Hawgood B C 1956 The value of formol-ether concentration of faecal cysts and ova. Journal of Clinical Pathology 9: 14–16

Ridley M J, Ridley D S 1976 Serum antibodies and jejunal histology in giardiasis associated with malabsorption. Journal of Clinical Pathology 29: 30–34

Rieckmann K H, Sax L J, Campbell G H, Urema J E 1978 Drug sensitivity of *Plasmodium falciparum*. An in vitro technique. Lancet 1: 22–23

Ristic M, Lewis G E 1977 Babesia in man and wild and laboratory-adapted mammals. In: Kreier J P (ed) Parasitic protozoa, vol 4. Academic Press, New York. ch 2, p 53–76

Robertson D H H, Lumsden W H R, Fraser K F, Hosie D D, Moore D M 1969 Simultaneous isolation of *Trichomonas vaginalis* and collection of vaginal exudate. British Journal of Venereal Diseases 45: 42–43

Robertson D H H, McMillan A, Young H 1980 Clinical practice in sexually transmissible diseases. Pitman Medical, Tunbridge Wells

Robinson G L 1968 The laboratory diagnosis of human parasitic amoebae. Transactions of the Royal Society of Tropical Medicine and Hygiene 62: 285–294

Sabin A B, Feldman H A 1948 Dyes as microchemical indicators of a new immunity phenomenon affecting a protozoan parasite (Toxoplasma). Science 108: 660–663

Seed T M, Aikawa M 1977 Pneumocystis. In: Kreier J P (ed) Parasitic protozoa, vol 4. Academic Press, New York. ch 10, 329–357

Sheather A L 1923 The detection of intestinal Protozoa and mange parasites by a flotation technique. Journal of Comparative Medicine and Therapeutics 36: 266

Shepherd V, Jameson B, Knowles G K 1979 *Pneumocystis carinii* pneumonitis: a serological study. Journal of Clinical Pathology 32: 773–777

Shute P G, Maryon M E 1966 Laboratory technique for the study of malaria, 2nd edn. Churchill, London

Smith P D, Gillin F D, Brown W R, Nash T E 1981 IgG antibody to *Giardia lamblia* detected by enzyme-linked immunosorbent assay. Gastroenterology 80: 1476–1480

Tadros W, Laarman J J 1982 Current concepts on the biology, evolution and taxonomy of tissue cyst-forming eimeriid coccidia. Advances in Parasitology 20: 294–496

Taylor A E R, Baker J R 1968 The cultivation of parasites in vitro. Blackwell Scientific, Oxford

Taylor A E R, Baker J R (eds) 1978 Methods of cultivating parasites in vitro. Academic Press, New York

Trier J S, Moxey P C, Scimmel E L, Robles E 1974 Chronic intestinal coccidiosis in man: intestinal morphology and response to treatment. Gastroenterology 66: 923–935

Wheatley W B 1951 A rapid staining procedure for intestinal amoebae and flagellates. American Journal of Clinical Pathology 67: 300–304

Wilcocks C, Manson-Bahr P E C 1972 Manson's tropical diseases, 17th edn. Baillière Tindall, London

Woo P T K 1970 The haematocrit centrifuge technique for the diagnosis of African trypanosomiasis. Acta Tropica 27: 384–386

Zaman V 1978 *Balantidium coli*. In: Kreier J P (ed) Parasitic protozoa, vol 2. Academic Press, New York. ch 9, 633–653

Zuckerman A, Lainson R 1977 Leishmania. In: Kreier J P (ed) Parasitic protozoa, vol 1. Academic Press, New York. ch 3, p 57–133

Rickettsia: Coxiella

Rickettsial diseases of man may be classified into five major groups – namely typhus fevers, spotted fevers, scrub typhus, Q fever and trench fever. They are caused by various members of the family Rickettsiaceae. Rickettsias are distinguished by their ability to multiply in various arthropods and by their existence in natural reservoirs of one or several warm-blooded animal hosts including man. Rickettsias are for the most part transmitted to human beings by blood-sucking arthropods; the major exception is Q fever which typically is transmitted by aerosol and via the respiratory tract of man and animals.

With the exception of *Rochalimea quintana*, which grows slowly on a modified blood agar medium, rickettsias are obligate intracellular prokaryotes. The individual rickettsial cells are often pleomorphic, rod-like or coccobacillary in shape and occur in chains, pairs or as single cells. In size, members of the spotted fever group are largest (averaging 0.6×1.2 μm); *Coxiella burneti* is the smallest (averaging 0.25×1.0 μm) and representatives of the typhus group fall in between.

Rickettsias vary widely in their resistance to physical and chemical agents. *C. burneti* is the most resistant, in fact more resistant than many non-sporing microorganisms; it can remain infectious for months in milk, tap water, soil or dried blood. Effective disinfection can be achieved with 2% (v/v) formaldehyde, 1% (v/v) Lysol (a mixture of saponified aryl and alkyl derivatives of phenol), ethyl ether and 5% (v/v) hydrogen peroxide. Other common disinfectants should not be relied upon.

Other pathogenic rickettsias such as those of the typhus or spotted fever groups are much less resistant, and may be quickly rendered non-infectious with hypochlorite (available chlorine 50–500 p.p.m.), phenol (1% v/v) or 70% (v/v) ethanol as well as by those disinfectants effective against *C. burneti*.

The clinical presentations and epidemiological features of rickettsial infections and the ecology of the causative organisms are described in Chapter 51, Volume 1 of the 13th Edition of this book. A knowledge of these aspects is pertinent to the laboratory diagnosis of suspected cases of the rickettsial fevers and is summarized in Table 44.1.

Although other species of rickettsias belonging to the typhus group (e.g. *Rickettsia canada*) or the spotted fever group (e.g. *R. slovaca* and *R. rhipicephali*) have been described in recent years, none of them has been shown to be of importance as a source of human disease.

Laboratory diagnosis

In general terms, laboratory confirmation of rickettsial infection may be obtained by isolating and biotyping the rickettsia from the patient, or by demonstrating an antibody response during the disease or, in special circumstances (e.g. biopsy samples from the rash of spotted fever; cardiac vegetations or liver biopsy samples in chronic Q fever) by demonstrating and identifying the organism in the lesions.

The difficulties and dangers of working with live pathogenic rickettsias preclude isolation of the organism as a diagnostic measure in most clinical laboratories. Detailed texts (Lennette & Schmidt 1979; Horsfall & Tamm 1965) should be

Table 44.1 Rickettsial diseases of man.

Disease	Aetiological agent	Geographical distribution	Cycle in nature		Mode of transmission to man
			Arthropod	Mammal	
Spotted fever group					
Rocky Mountain spotted fever	*Rickettsia rickettsi*	Western hemisphere	Ixodid ticks	Rodents, dogs, foxes	Tick bite
Boutonneuse fever	*R. conori*	Mediterranean, Black Sea, Caspian Sea littorals, Middle East, India, Africa	Ixodid ticks	Rodents, dogs	Tick bite
Queensland tick typhus	*R. australis*	Australia	Ixodid ticks	Marsupials	Tick bite
Siberian tick typhus	*R. sibirica*	Central Europe, Armenia, Central Asia, Mongolia, Tadzhikistan	Ixodid ticks	Rodents	Tick bite
Rickettsialpox	*R. akari*	North America, Southern Africa, USSR, Korea	Mites	Mice, other commensal rodents	Mite bite
Typhus group					
Epidemic typhus	*R. prowazeki*	Worldwide	Human body louse, squirrel ectoparasites	Man; flying squirrels	Louse faeces scratched into skin
Brill-Zinsser disease[a]	*R. prowazeki*	Worldwide	· · ·	· · ·	· · ·
Murine typhus	*R. typhi (mooseri)*	Worldwide	Fleas	Rodents	Flea faeces scratched into skin
Scrub typhus	*R. tsutsugamushi*	Asia, India, Australia, Pacific islands	Trombiculid mites	Rodents	Mite bite
Q fever					
Primary Q fever	*Coxiella burneti*	Worldwide	Ixodid ticks	Cattle, sheep, goats rodents	Inhalation of infectious aerosols, tick bite (?)
Chronic granulomatous liver disease[b]	*C. burneti*	Australia, USA	· · ·	· · ·	· · ·
Rickettsial endocarditis[b]	*C. burneti*	Australia, UK, USA, Western Europe	· · ·	· · ·	· · ·
Trench fever	*Rochalimaea quintana*	Europe, Africa, North America	Human body louse	Man	Louse faeces scratched into skin

[a] Recrudescent infection, often many years after primary infection, which may serve as source of infection for body lice and fresh outbreaks of typhus.

[b] Chronic sequelae that may follow soon after a primary attack or after a long latent period; no significance for infection of arthropods.

consulted before such attempts are contemplated. If the isolation and identification of a possible rickettsial agent is crucial, then blood or other samples taken from the patient during the febrile period should be sent to a specialized reference laboratory.

Cultivation of pathogenic rickettsias in animals, eggs or cell cultures should be attempted only in approved containment facilities (Class 3, US Public Health Service 1978; but see also Ch. 15) and then only by workers protected by vaccine or past exposure. Autopsies on fatal cases of Q fever should be conducted only by individuals who have had Q fever vaccine, or who have markers of immunity (antibody or evidence of 'delayed hypersensitivity' to *C. burneti* antigen).

Collection of specimens

In most instances the rôle of the general microbiology laboratory in the diagnosis of suspected clinical cases of rickettsial infection will be restricted to the testing of blood samples for antibody and the aseptic collection of tissues by biopsy or at autopsy for forwarding to a reference laboratory. For serotesting three blood samples should be taken: one as early as possible after onset of disease, one during the second week and one during the fourth week following onset.

Certain points are important to maximize the possibility of isolating a rickettsia, particularly of the typhus or spotted fever group. If isolation attempts in animals are to be made, then ideally they should be injected within 30 min after suspensions of blood or tissue are prepared. Otherwise, the suspect material should be quickly frozen as a layer or 'shell' on the wall of a container rotated in an ethanol/'dry ice' (solid CO_2) bath and stored at $-70°C$. If whole blood is taken for later animal injection, it may also be shell-frozen. If possible, take 10 ml blood samples, allow them to clot, centrifuge immediately and freeze clot and serum separately. The clot may be injected subsequently into the test animals either as a 10% (w/v) suspension in sterile skim milk or in brain heart infusion broth. The use of other common diluents may result in a great and rapid loss of infectivity of the rickettsias present, particularly with members of the typhus and spotted fever groups, but less so with *C. burneti*. Blood specimens taken later than the first week after onset should be separated routinely into cells and serum or plasma because by then the latter may contain significant concentrations of antibodies. Do not add anticoagulants to blood specimens. Never freeze whole blood

specimens to be used for serologic testing. Serum separated from haemolysed specimens may give non-specific reactions.

Frozen specimens *must* be held at a constant $-70°C$ while in storage or transit. It is not sufficient that they merely be kept frozen. They should be shipped to the reference laboratory in a properly insulated container with enough 'dry ice' to maintain the interior temperature at $-70°C$ for at least 24 h longer than the estimated length of time required for shipment. When removed from the shipping carton or $-70°C$ refrigerator, the specimen should be thawed promptly by immersing the container in tepid water, and immediately injected into experimental animals or other culture system. At the time of shipment, the reference laboratory should be notified by telephone of time of departure of the shipment, airline and flight number, and sufficient identification marks to enable the package to be individually recognized and retrieved at the incoming end. Neglect of any of these precautions may result in failure of the very considerable efforts often required to isolate and identify the rickettsial agent.

If ticks or other arthropods collected from the bodies or clothing of patients are to be examined directly for rickettsias, they should be shipped in a tightly stoppered glass receptacle containing a pledget of moist cotton to ensure survival as they are easily killed by desiccation.

Direct microscopic observation of rickettsias

Smears of infected tissue may be examined directly for rickettsias after staining. Stains commonly used are Giménez (Giménez 1964), Macchiavello (Lennette & Schmidt 1979) and Giemsa (for Giemsa staining method see Ch. 46). Except for *R. tsutsugamushi*, rickettsias stain a brilliant red with Giménez stain, red with Macchiavello stain and purple with Giemsa stain. *R. tsutsugamushi* stains reddish-black with a modified Giménez stain. None of these stains will reliably differentiate rickettsias from bacteria. As with the elementary bodies of chlamydia, rickettsias may be fluorochromed with the Hoechst 33258 stain for DNA.

In tissue smears rickettsias are usually seen as

bipolar rods, occurring near cells or free in the cytoplasm. *R. rickettsi* also may be found within the nuclei of infected cells. *C. burneti* grows as a microcolony in a cytoplasmic vacuole with many scores of organisms; individual organisms may be difficult to visualize, the entire contents of the vacuole appearing to be a granular mass which stains red with Giménez or Macchiavello stain.

Infected tissue sections, smears or cells also may be examined directly by immunofluorescence. Specific antisera tagged with fluorescein isothiocyanate (FITC), or the indirect immunofluorescence method may be used successfully to detect and identify pathogenic rickettsias, including those in biopsy material from the early skin lesions in spotted fever (Woodward et al 1976), organisms in ticks or other naturally infected arthropods (Burgdorfer 1970), and *C. burneti* in the vegetations of Q fever endocarditis (Mitchell et al 1966; Lamb et al 1969); the use of guinea-pig or other animal sera containing high levels of antibody against *C. burneti* phase 1 antigen is necessary. The rickettsias may be coated with antibody formed by the patient and pretreatment of the section with a protease may be advantageous. *C. burneti* may be detected in formalin-fixed as well as frozen sections.

Serological diagnosis of rickettsial disease

The natural worldwide distribution of the rickettsial diseases (Table 44.1) has been augmented by worldwide air travel to an extent that the diagnostician should be prepared to identify any of them wherever he may be located.

Except in times of widespread social catastrophe when the typhus fevers often predominate, the most frequently occurring diagnostic problem with a rickettsial disease is probably that of Q fever.

Primary attacks of epidemic typhus or Q fever may result in recovery followed by recrudescent disease. With *R. prowazeki* infections this takes the form of Brill-Zinsser disease which serologically is characterized by an almost pure IgG specific antibody response (Ormsbee et al 1977).

Infection with *C. burneti* may be followed by Q fever endocarditis (Andrews & Marmion 1959; Turck et al 1976), or chronic liver involvement (Peacock et al 1983) or, in women, by placental infection at term (Syrucek et al 1958), a sequel analogous to placental infection of cattle, sheep and goats. Tests for Q fever antibodies should be performed routinely in endocarditis patients with negative blood cultures.

Diagnostic rickettsial antigens and antisera. Rickettsial antigens for diagnostic purposes are in limited supply the world over. Complement-fixing (CF) group antigens and antisera for the typhus and spotted fever groups and for Q fever are available from several sources however. The Commonwealth Serum Labs, Australia, sells Q fever and epidemic typhus antigens for the CF and IF tests. Virion and Behring sell Q fever antigen (Table 49.6). Veterinaria AG, Gruben Str. 40, Zurich, Switzerland, produces Q fever antigen for the capillary agglutination test. The Standards Laboratory, CPHL, Colindale Avenue, London, produces phase 1 and phase 2 Q fever CF antigens which are also satisfactory for microimmunofluorescence tests but distribution is limited.

Finally, the Center for Infectious Diseases, Centers for Disease Control (CDC), Atlanta, GA 30 333, USA, distributes kits for diagnosis by microimmunofluorescence of spotted fever group and typhus group disease. The kits contain antigen, and both reference positive and negative human sera. CF antigens for use in CF, microagglutination and microimmunofluorescence tests for diagnosis of epidemic typhus, murine typhus, spotted fever, boutonneuse fever and Q fever are available in limited amounts from WHO Collaborating Centers for Rickettsial Reference and Research including the Department of Microbiology, University of Maryland School of Medicine, 660 W. Redwood St, Baltimore, Md 21201 USA; the Institute of Virology, Slovak Academy of Sciences, 80 939 Bratislava 9, Czechoslovakia; and the Gamaleya Research Institute of Epidemiology and Microbiology, Moscow, USSR. We know of no commercial source of CF antigens for scrub typhus diagnosis but recent recommendations from a WHO

Consultation on the Diagnosis of Rickettsial Diseases indicates IF antigen for scrub typhus and other rickettsias may become available (contact McDade, CDC).

Antigens of varying reliability for the Weil-Felix test (see below) are available. Particular attention should be given to details of standardization provided by the manufacturer to ensure that the antigens have been tested with sera from patients with rickettsial infections and not simply against sera from experimental animals immunized with the *Proteus* strains.

Rickettsial antigens for use in the CF test are ordinarily made from crude suspensions of heavily infected chick embryo yolk sacs. These are suspended in buffered salt solution containing formaldehyde (10% v/v), ground in a blender and centrifuged to sediment the bulk of the rickettsias. Following resuspension of the pellet in buffered saline, the preparation is shaken with an excess of ethyl ether. This procedure results in a polydisperse preparation of antigen, some of which ('soluble antigen') is not sedimentable by centrifugation at forces up to 18 000 g. Such 'soluble' group-specific CF antigen may be released from members of the typhus, spotted fever and scrub typhus groups but not from *C. burneti*.

Commercially available antigens suitable for the CF test have been made from infected chicken embryo yolk sacs by methods which always include treatment with ether. Such antigen preparations are composed of a mixture of varying proportions of 'soluble' and particulate antigen. Specific and very stable particulate antigen preparations may be produced by first treating the crude yolk sac suspensions of rickettsias with formaldehyde and then purifying them by a high salt process (Ormsbee et al 1977). Antigens prepared by this method can be used interchangeably in CF, microagglutination and microimmunofluorescence tests with highly consistent results.

Antisera for use as positive controls in serological tests for typhus, the spotted fevers or Q fever can be obtained from convalescent human patients or guinea-pigs that have survived infection. Only normal adult animals whose preinfec-

tion sera have been shown to possess no anticomplementary or non-specific activity with human tissues or rickettsial antigens should be used.

Guinea-pigs are inoculated intraperitoneally with infectious spleen and liver suspensions from guinea-pigs, and held for 4–5 weeks. The convalescent animals then are bled from the heart, and the blood is allowed to clot at room temperature in glass tubes. After loosening the clots from the glass of the collection tube, the blood is stored overnight at 4°C and the serum is harvested by pipette. Any remaining erythrocytes are removed by centrifugation. Aqueous merthiolate in a final concentration of 1 in 10 000 is added as a preservative and the antiserum is stored in small aliquots in a freezer. With the possible exception of Q fever antisera the general laboratory would obtain such antisera from a reference laboratory.

Complement fixation test

Human and guinea-pig sera seldom give non-specific reactions although this is not true of sera taken from other animals including sheep, camels, donkeys and some species (*Hemichinus* spp.) of the hedgehog family. Non-specific reactions in human and other serum may often be eliminated by treatment with 'dry ice' (Imam & Alfy 1966). The serum specimen is diluted 1 in 10 with distilled water and a small piece of 'dry ice' added. When the reaction has ceased, 0.1 ml of 8.5% NaCl is added to each 0.9 ml of diluted serum. The serum is then again inactivated by heating to 56°C for 30 min before use in the test.

The micro-CF test described in Chapter 49 may be used for the measurement of rickettsial antibodies; viz, in microtitre plates, a unit volume of 0.025 ml, 3 HD50 of complement, 8 units of antigen and overnight fixation at 4°C.

Commercial rickettsial CF antigens vary significantly with respect to group and species specificity and therefore should be assayed in a 'block' or 'chessboard' antigen-antibody titration with guinea-pig reference sera representing the major species of each group to determine the optimal antigen dose, i.e. that giving the highest serum antibody titre. This value is usually similar in human and guinea-pig antisera but may be substantially different with ovine and bovine sera. Consequently antibody-containing sera from these species should be used to determine the optimal antigen dose when serological surveys of these animals are undertaken.

Finally, because most CF antigen preparations are made from infected chick embryo yolk sacs, a control antigen made from normal yolk sac tissue should be included in each test.

Rickettsial CF antigens should be stored at 4°C. This will not prevent spontaneous loss of species-specificity of typhus and spotted fever antigens however, and commercial ether-extracted antigen may require to be reprocessed and restandardized. Such problems do not arise with Q fever antigens as they are extremely stable if stored at 4°C and *never* frozen. They are particularly susceptible to freezing and thawing, however, which causes spontaneous aggregation and flocculation of the antigen.

Sera are generally tested for rickettsial antibodies in two-fold dilutions from 1 in 10 to 1 in 1280 to bracket the endpoint or, alternatively, 'screened' initially at dilutions of 1 in 10 and 1 in 40 to verify the presence of sera from positive reactors which can subsequently be retitrated to determine the endpoint.

Test antigens for patients suspected of having Q fever, primary typhus or Brill's disease in the United Kingdom (UK) would normally include 'soluble' typhus group and phase 2 CF antigen of *C. burneti*. If hepatic or cardiac disease caused by *C. burneti* is suspected, both phase 1 and phase 2 antigens of *C. burneti* should be included in the test. Although Q fever is certainly the most prevalent rickettsial infection in the UK, others may be not infrequently imported from Western Europe or other areas of the world. For example, boutonneuse fever exists in France and along the entire Mediterranean littoral, and history of recent travel to such areas might prompt inclusion of *R. conori* CF antigen for detection of a spotted fever group infection.

Interpretation of CF test results. Complement-fixing antibodies generally appear in the patient's serum late in the second week of illness, attain peak titres (typically in the range 80–320) within the following 2 weeks and then slowly decline over a period of months. Low levels of antibodies may persist for many years following some primary cases of epidemic typhus or Q fever. The CF antibody response in primary Q fever is essentially to the phase 2 antigen, occasionally accompanied by low level titres (10–40) of phase 1 antibody. Granulomatous hepatitis caused by *C. burneti* exhibits a phase 2 titre of 1280–5120 and usually a phase 1 antibody titre of 20–160 although sometimes higher. Rickettsial endocarditis triggers phase 1 antibody responses that are usually as high or higher (1280–2560) than the concomitant phase 2 response (Andrews & Marmion 1959; Peacock et al 1983; Worswick & Marmion 1985).

Detection of antigen and antibody by immunofluorescence

Antigen detection. Allow a tissue section, tissue smear or impression, or smear of arthropod haemolymph to air dry on a microscope slide. Fix in dehydrated acetone for 10 min. (See also Ch. 48 for discussion of fixation and rehydration of sections.) Cover tissue section or smear with guinea-pig antiserum previously tagged with fluorescein isothiocyanate (FITC) and containing antibodies against the rickettsia suspected to be present. Allow to react for 30 min, in a moist chamber at 37°C. Rinse slide thoroughly, air dry and examine under oil immersion with appropriate fluorescence optics. Indirect immunofluorescence may also be used.

Antibody detection by microimmunofluorescence test. A number of workers (reviewed by Worswick & Marmion 1985) have used immunofluorescence (IF) to distinguish rickettsias of different antigenic composition or to measure antibody. Philip et al (1976) used a microimmunofluorescence method. We describe below a method used for Q fever in our laboratories.

1. *Test for rheumatoid factor (RF).* Sera are first tested for RF. A 50 μl volume of gamma-globulin-coated latex particles in suspension is mixed with an equal volume of patient's serum

on black coated glass slides ('Gonavi slide', Mochida Pharmaceutical Co. Ltd, Tokyo 160, Japan) to check for RF. Those positive are absorbed with latex particles coated with human gammaglobulin (Commonwealth Serum Labs). A volume of 0.25 ml of the coated latex particles is sedimented at 2300 g for 30 min in V-bottomed, polypropylene tubes (45 × 5 mm diameter) and resuspended in 0.25 ml of patient's serum diluted 1 in 5 in phosphate-buffered saline (PBS) pH 7.2. After incubation at room temperature for 1 h or overnight at 4°C, the latex particles are centrifuged out as before and the supernatant fluid is removed and retested for RF. If necessary the absorption procedure is repeated until the serum is clearly RF negative. Sera for immunoglobulin class-specific antibody determinations are absorbed for RF as a routine.

2. *Preparation of slides*. Teflon coated slides are prepared by placing each slide over a cardboard template, on which have been punched 36 equally spaced holes (three rows of 12 holes). A small drop of glycerol is placed on the slide at a spot designated by the template holes underneath the slide. The slide is then sprayed with Teflon. Several slides are stacked laterally in metal racks and the glycerol is removed by immersing the slides in a warm water and detergent solution. After another rinse in running tap water and finally in distilled water they are air-dried. *C. burneti* phase 1 and phase 2 antigens are applied as microdots (100 dots/10 μl) with a microsyringe; the rickettsial concentration is 200 μg dry wt/ml. Phase 1 antigen is added to 18 of the total of 36 wells on the left portion of the slide and phase 2 antigen to the remaining 18 wells on the right half of the slide. The microdots of antigen are dried, fixed in acetone at room temperature for 10 min and stored dry in black, airtight boxes at 4°C up to 3 days before use.

3. *Fluorescent antibody staining*. Serial two-fold dilutions of patient's sera from 1 in 10 to 1 in 320 are prepared in PBS containing normal yolk sac 1% (v/v); each dilution is carefully layered over a microdot of phase 1 and phase 2 antigen set out on each of three slides so as to allow for detection of specific IgG, IgM and IgA antibody. Slides for the detection of IgG and

IgA immunoglobulin class are incubated for 45 min at 37°C whereas slides for the detection of IgM are incubated for 2.5 h at 37°C; these combinations of temperature and time give essentially the same results as overnight incubation at 4°C. Controls include (a) sera positive for IgM, IgG and IgA antibody to phase 1 and phase 2 antigens, and (b) a serum negative for antibody to phase 1 and phase 2 antigens in all three immunoglobulin classes. Normal yolk sac (1% v/v) diluent controls are included in each batch of tests to check for antigen autofluorescence. After incubation, the diluted sera are removed from each slide with a gentle jet of PBS from a wash bottle; slides are then placed in metal racks and washed in two changes of PBS each lasting 10 min. After drying, antigen microdots on each slide are overlaid with an optimal dilution (see below) of the appropriate fluorescein-labelled anti-human IgM, IgG or IgA conjugate and incubated for 30 min at 37°C. They are washed as before, dipped quickly in distilled water, dried, mounted in glycerol 90% in PBS, pH 8.6, and covered with a single large coverslip extending over the whole slide. Slides are examined within 6 h, for example with a Zeiss fluorescent microscope (blue excitation filter BP455/490 and a barrier filter BP520–560) at × 400 magnification with incident illumination or comparable fluorescence optics. Endpoints against each antigen (phase 1 and phase 2) are taken as the highest serum dilution that gives definite fluorescence on the organisms.

4. *Conjugates*. In our laboratories μ-chain-specific rabbit anti-human IgM and Fc-specific goat anti-human fluorescein-labelled conjugates, are obtained from Cappel for the detection of IgM and IgG antibodies respectively. For the IgA test, sheep anti-human IgA fluorescein-labelled globulin is purchased from Wellcome. The appropriate dilution of each conjugate is determined by block or chessboard titration against a positive antiserum and is used at twice the concentration of the optimum dilution.

The indirect IF test has been consistently more sensitive than the CF test in detecting rickettsial antibodies, particularly phase 1 antibodies in Q fever cases. Determination of the immunoglobulin class of the specific antibodies togethe with the ability to detect antibody responses much earlier than by CF has resulted in improved and earlier diagnosis of rickettsial disease (see for example Philip et al 1976; Worswick & Marmion 1985).

Other serological tests

Other tests for detection and measurement of rickettsial antibodies have been developed. They include agglutination (Fiset et al 1969), radio-isotope precipitation (Gerloff et al 1962), hemagglutination (Anacker et al 1979; Shirai et al 1975) and enzyme-linked immunosorbence (Dasch et al 1979) tests. Most of these tests are more sensitive when compared to the CF test. However, most of them require the use of purified antigens which are not available commercially, so the tests remain generally unavailable to diagnostic laboratories.

Weil-Felix (WF) agglutination reaction

This reaction depends on a fortuitous similarity of particular antigenic determinants which occur in most species of pathogenic rickettsias and in the OX-19, OX-2 and OX-K strains of *Proteus vulgaris* and *Proteus mirabilis* (Shaffer & Goldin 1965). The test may be conveniently performed as a microagglutination reaction in microtitre plates with round-bottomed wells, hematoxylin-stained antigen and 0.025 ml unit volumes (Fiset et al 1969). Plates are incubated for 2 h at 37°C followed by overnight incubation at 4°C. The antibody titration may also be run as a tube test (Dreyer tubes or round-bottomed agglutination tubes), in which complete (4+) agglutination is indicated by complete clearing of the supernatant fluid and the formation of white flocculent masses in the bottom of the tube. A serum titre of 80 is the lowest considered 'significant' but four-fold or greater increase of antibody between acute and convalescent sera is considered diagnostic and more reliable than a single reading.

Agglutinins detected by WF reaction appear to be largely in the IgM globulin fraction and appear transiently and early in the course of disease. Thus in typhus patients ultimately shown to have rising antibody titres as deter-

mined by other tests, 55 of 61 patients also were positive by WF test with OX-19 antigen (Ormsbee et al 1977). In contrast, in typhus patients with constant or falling specific antibody titres by other tests, just 18 of 58 were positive by the WF test. Overall, the WF test is less sensitive in detecting rickettsial antibodies than other specific tests with which it has been compared. Table 44.2 summarizes WF reactions found in human rickettsioses.

The WF test is described in this chapter because its antigens and antisera are often more readily available than specific rickettsial antigens. Nevertheless, the use of the WF test has produced more misleading results than any other serological test for the detection of rickettsial antibodies. Commercial antigens are sometimes standardized against sera from rabbits that have been immunized with the homologous strain of *Proteus* spp. Such antisera have little value as controls because they will agglutinate the WF antigen regardless of whether or not it is agglutinated by the cross-reactive rickettsial antibodies. The only valid antigen preparations for the WF test are those which have been standardized against antisera derived from patients infected with rickettsias.

When the proper precautions are taken with respect to standardization of antigen and the inclusion of proper positive serum controls, the WF test can be of help in establishing a presumptive diagnosis of rickettsial disease. It does not distinguish spotted fever group from murine typhus in areas where these diseases co-

Table 44.2 Weil-Felix reactions in rickettsioses.

Disease[a]	Frequency and size of antibody response [b] to *Proteus* type		
	OX-19	OX-2	OX-K
Epidemic typhus	++++	+	−
Murine typhus	++++	+	−
Brill-Zinsser disease	±/−	−	−
Scrub typhus	−	−	+++
Spotted fever group	++++ to +	+ to ++++	−

[a] Q fever, rickettsialpox and trench fever do not produce positive Weil-Felix reactions.
[b] ++++ = frequent and large antibody response; − = no antibody response.

exist, nor is it of any help in detecting antibodies against rickettsialpox, trench fever or Q fever as subjects infected with these organisms do not develop proteus agglutinins. Lastly, it is of little help in the laboratory diagnosis of Brill-Zinsser disease, in which a pure IgG antibody response occurs.

The WF antigens also react with proteus antibodies so that the occurrence of a positive reaction is not, by itself, indicative of the presence of rickettsial antibodies. Positive agglutination reactions in the absence of rickettsial infection have been observed in patients with urinary tract infection with *Proteus* spp., in leptospirosis, in *Borrelia* infections and in severe liver disease.

Demonstration of C. burneti in specimens from infected human beings or animals

The presence of *C. burneti* in specimens such as heparinized blood from a Q fever patient, tissues from suspected cases of rickettsial endocarditis obtained at operation for valve replacement or at autopsy, or milk specimens from infected cattle or goats can be demonstrated by intraperitoneal inoculation of guinea-pigs or hamsters. This appears to be a procedure of low hazard, probably because the number of organisms in an acute stage blood sample from a Q fever patient, or in a contaminated milk sample, is usually small; consequently the likelihood of excretion of many organisms in urine of the infected guinea-pig is also small, as judged by absence of cross-infection among animals held on the same rack of cages or evidence of infection among animal room attendants. This may not apply to infected mice, which excrete the organism more readily. When larger numbers of rickettsias are present as, for example, in an ovine

placenta or a cardiac valve vegetation, accidental infection is more likely. In these circumstances it is best that the processing of specimens and the handling of inoculated animals be done by immune or vaccinated persons.

Mature guinea-pigs (500 g) are anaesthetized and 5 ml of blood is taken by cardiac puncture. The serum is tested by CF for phase 2 antibodies. Several seronegative animals are each inoculated intraperitoneally with 3–5 ml of the sample (milk, blood or blood clot, etc.) without antibiotic. Streptomycin and other antibiotics inhibit rickettsias and penicillin is toxic to guinea-pigs. Place one or more sentinel animals in nearby cages to monitor cross-infection. If the patient has already formed antibody, it is preferable to allow the blood to clot and inject the clot alone after grinding it up in a menstruum of skim milk contained in a screw-topped grinder placed in a hood to minimize the possible escape of infectious aerosols.

Rectal temperatures are taken daily to detect fever ($\geqq 40°C$) in the inoculated animals, if serial passage to other animals or chick embryos is to be attempted. Three and 6 weeks after inoculation the animals should be re-bled. Pre- and post-inoculation sera should be tested with phase 2 *C. burneti* CF antigen (or typhus CF antigen if indicated). A conversion to seropositive (CF titre $\geqq 10$) with negative results from the sentinel animals is decisive evidence for the presence of live *C. burneti* in the original inoculum. Although most rickettsias are quite sensitive to heat and chemical disinfectants, *C. burneti* is not. Material contaminated with this organism should be autoclaved at 115°C for 20 min, or enclosed in two tightly closed plastic bags one within the other and incinerated. Formaldehyde (2% v/v) should be used to disinfect permanent surfaces of benches, hoods, etc.

REFERENCES

Anacker R L, Philip R N, Thomas L A, Casper E A 1979 Indirect hemagglutination test for detection of antibody to *Rickettsia rickettsi* in sera from humans and common laboratory animals. Journal of Clinical Microbiology 10: 677–684

Andrews P S, Marmion B P 1959 Chronic Q fever. 2. Morbid anatomical and bacteriological findings in a

patient with endocarditis. British Medical Journal 2: 983–988

Burgdorfer W 1970 Hemolymph test: a technique for detection of rickettsiae in ticks. American Journal of Tropical Medicine and Hygiene 19: 1010–1014

Dasch G A, Halle H, Bourgeois A L 1979 Sensitive microplate enzyme-linked immunosorbent assay for detection of antibodies against the scrub typhus rickettsia, *Rickettsia tsutsugamushi*. Journal of Clinical Microbiology 9: 38–48

Fiset P, Ormsbee R A, Silberman R, Peacock M, Spielman S H 1969 A microagglutination technique for detection and measurement of rickettsial antibodies. Acta Virologica 13: 60–66

Gerloff R K, Hoyer B H, McLaren L C 1962 Precipitation of radio-labelled poliovirus with specific antibody and anti-globulin. Journal of Immunology 89: 559–570

Giménez D F 1964 Staining rickettsiae in yolk-sac cultures. Stain Technology 39: 135–140

Horsfall F L, Tamm I (eds) 1965 Viral and rickettsial diseases of man, 4th edn. Lippincott, Philadelphia

Imam I Z E, Alfy L 1966 The elimination of the anticomplementary reactions of the sera by CO_2. Journal of the Egyptian Public Health Association 41: 33–36

Lamb R, Boyd J F, Grist N R 1969 Q fever endocarditis. Scottish Medical Journal 14: 10–16

Lennette E H, Schmidt N J (eds) 1979 Diagnostic procedures for viral, rickettsial and chlamydial infections, 5th edn. American Public Health Association, New York. chs 2 and 33

Mitchell R, Grist N R, Bazaz C, Kenmuir A C F 1966 Pathological, rickettsiological and immunofluorescence studies of a case of Q fever endocarditis. Journal of Pathology and Bacteriology 91:317

Ormsbee R, Peacock M, Philip R, Casper E, Plorde J, Gabre-Kidan T, Wright L 1977 Serologic diagnosis of epidemic typhus fever. American Journal of Epidemiology 105: 261–271

Peacock M G, Philip R N, Williams J C, Faulkner R S

1983 Serological evaluation of Q fever in man: enhanced Phase 1 titers of IgG and IgA are diagnostic for Q fever endocarditis. Infection and Immunity 41:1089

Philip R N, Casper E A, Ormsbee R A, Peacock M G, Burgdorfer W 1976 Microimmunofluorescence test for the serological study of Rocky Mountain spotted fever and typhus. Journal of Clinical Microbiology 3: 51–61

Shaffer J G, Goldin M 1965 Serodiagnostic test in diseases other than syphilis. In: Davisohn I, Wells B B (eds) Clinical diagnosis by laboratory methods, 13th edn. Saunders, Philadelphia. ch 24, p 889–890

Shirai A, Dietel J W, Osterman J V 1975 Indirect hemagglutination test for human antibody to typhus and spotted fever group rickettsiae. Journal of Clinical Microbiology 2: 430–437

Syrucek L, Sobeslavsky O, Gutwirth I 1958 Isolation of *Coxiella burneti* from human placentas. Journal of Hygiene and Epidemiology 2: 29–35

Turck E P G, Howitt G, Turnberg L A et al 1976 Chronic Q fever. Quarterly Journal of Medicine 45: 193–217

US Public Health Service 1978 NIH Laboratory safety monograph. Office of Research Safety, National Cancer Institute, Bethesda, Md USA

Woodward T E, Pedersen C E Jr, Oster C N, Bagley L R, Romberger J, Snyder M J 1976 Prompt confirmation of Rocky Mountain spotted fever: identification of rickettsiae in skin tissues. Journal of Infectious Diseases 134: 297–301

Worswick D, Marmion B P 1985 Antibody responses in acute and chronic Q fever and in subjects vaccinated against Q fever. Journal of Medical Microbiology 19: 281–296

Mycoplasma: Acholeplasma: Ureaplasma

These three groups of organisms, previously described under the general title of pleuro-pneumonia-like organisms (PPLO), are small prokaryotic cells (200–250 nm diameter; taxonomy reviewed by Freundt & Edward 1979). They resemble larger prokaryotic cells (e.g. bacteria) in their ability to grow in cell-free media although some are exacting in their growth requirements and grow slowly. Their genome is a single circular double stranded DNA molecule (5×10^8 daltons for mycoplasmas: 1×10^9 for acholeplasmas) in an unbounded nucleus and dense arrays of bacterial type ribosomes. They have no rigid cell wall. There is a trilaminar cytoplasmic membrane, but unlike that of bacteria, it contains cholesterol or carotenol in addition to the usual neutral and phospholipids. The mycoplasmas cannot synthesize their own cholesterol and require it as a growth factor in the culture medium. The acholeplasmas synthesize carotenol as a substitute for cholesterol, but will incorporate cholesterol if it is provided. The absence of a rigid cell wall is reflected in branched and other unusual morphological forms of the mycoplasma cell. Cells of some species have a coccobacillary morphology, others are filamentous; some have specialized processes for attachment to host cells that are probably also related to the capacity for gliding motion. In line with absence of a cell wall the organisms are not inhibited by members of the penicillin family, bacitracin, or polymyxin B; in general they are sensitive in vivo to tetracycline, erythromycin, kanamycin, chloramphenicol, streptomycin, tylosin and to other antibiotics that act at ribosome level; they are also sensitive to arsenical compounds and sodium aurothiomalate.

The ureaplasmas (*Ureaplasma urealyticum*) were previously known as T mycoplasmas; T for *tiny* colony – a reference to the size difference (15–30 μm versus 200–500 μm) of their colonies compared with those of the mycoplasmas and acholeplasmas. As the name implies, they have the ability to split urea to ammonia, unlike the mycoplasmas. Except for the ureaplasmas and *Mycoplasma genitalium*, mycoplasmas are more resistant to the inhibitory action of thallium salts than bacteria, a difference exploited in selective media. Despite some colonial similarities, mycoplasmas are quite distinct from L-phase variants of bacteria and do not revert to bacteria when cultured in media free of inhibitors of bacterial cell wall synthesis or other L-phase inducers (see Hijmans et al 1969 for a discussion of the properties of, and terminology for L-phase/L-form variants of bacteria; also that of spheroplasts and protoplasts).

Mycoplasma cells stain poorly by the Gram method but are negative. Consequently various special staining techniques are used – overnight Giemsa, Dienes' stain, cresyl-fast violet, orcein or fluorochroming with nucleic acid stains such as acridine orange or the Hoechst 33258 dye. The cells from fluid culture may also be visualized by darkground or phase-contrast methods in the light microscope, or in the electron microscope by negative contrast staining or in thin sections; some species have surface projections which resemble those of myxoviruses. The irregular shape in negative contrast preparations may present difficulties in identification (Wolanski &

Maramorosch 1970). Examination of thin sections allows the recognition within the cell of the nuclear area, ribosome arrays and the trilaminar cytoplasmic membrane.

Mycoplasmas are grown in soft agar medium with a high (10–20% v/v) concentration of serum or other protein such as ascitic fluid. The function of the serum or other protein is to provide a source of cholesterol, fatty acids, or urea in the case of the ureaplasmas, and to regulate their availability to the organisms. Yeast extract, nucleic acid mixtures, tissue extracts, coenzymes and other supplements may be required according to species. Some mycoplasma species are aerobes or facultative anaerobes, others grow better in hydrogen or nitrogen with 10% (v/v) CO_2. Initially the mycoplasma cells multiply within the agar to form a ball-shaped colony that grows up to the surface of the agar and spreads along it, giving a halo of delicate growth. When viewed from above such a colony presents a 'fried egg' appearance (13th Edn, Vol. 1, Plate 52.2) with an agar-embedded centre. Colony size varies from 200–500 μm for the 'large colony' mycoplasmas to 15–30 μm for the ureaplasmas; larger colonies of the latter with 'fried egg' morphology may be obtained with specially supplemented media with control of pH. Mycoplasmas also grow in broth, or in semi-solid agar or diphasic broth-agar culture, with serum and other supplements. Many species grow readily in cultures of human or animal cells where they adhere to the cell surface and are also found in the fluid phase of the cultures. Isolation of mycoplasmas in laboratory animals does not play an important part in laboratory diagnosis although M. pneumoniae was first cultivated in hamsters and cotton rats and then in chick embryos.

The established human mycoplasma flora comprises M. hominis, M. pneumoniae, M. salivarium, M. orale, M. buccale, M. faucium (formerly known as M. orale serotypes 1, 2 and 3), M. fermentans, M. genitalium and numerous serotypes of ureaplasmas.

M. genitalium is a recent addition. Taylor-Robinson et al (1981) and Tully et al (1981) observed that darkground microscopy of fresh urethral exudates from non-gonococcal urethritis revealed mobile spiral forms and on the supposition that they might be spiroplasmas, cultured them in SP4 medium (Tully et al 1977); two strains of M. genitalium were isolated. The pathogenic significance for man is under investigation; so far experiments with marmosets suggest that it may be a urogenital pathogen (Taylor-Robinson et al 1982).

Other occasional isolates from human sources include M. lipophilum (Del Guidice & Carski 1968), M. primatum, primarily a simian mycoplasma but originally designated the 'Navel' strain, and the saprophyte, Acholeplasma laidlawi.

Of the mycoplasmas isolated from man, M. pneumoniae is the predominant pathogen; M. hominis, M. fermentans, M. genitalium and U. urealyticum have a variable importance (reviewed by Cassell & Cole 1981). The remaining members of the flora appear to be saprophytic except in unusual circumstances, e.g. M. salivarium and arthritis in hypogammaglobulinaemia (So et al 1983).

Clinical associations are:

1. M. pneumoniae with pharyngitis, sinusitis, febrile bronchitis or pneumonia, accompanied in a proportion of patients by formation of cold haemagglutinins, Streptococcus MG agglutinins, biological false positive WR, or anti-tissue antibodies. In recent years extrapulmonary manifestations such as arthritis, hepatitis and central nervous system involvement (meningoencephalitis, cerebellar ataxia, transverse myelitis, Guillain-Barré syndrome) have been reported. A proportion of patients with erythema multiforme, erythema nodosum or the Stevens-Johnson syndrome may show evidence of infection. Volunteer experiments suggested that myringitis might be a manifestation of M. pneumoniae infection but although otitis media and myringitis have been observed in natural infection, involvement of the ear is not common (Clyde 1979).

2. M. hominis, M. fermentans or U. urealyticum with some cases of salpingitis, tubo-ovarian abscess, pelvic abscess, septic abortion and puerperal infection and fever.

3. An association of U. urealyticum (and perhaps now M. genitalium) with non-gonococcal (NGU) or postgonococcal urethritis

or cervicitis. The pathogenetic significance of these associations has proved difficult to assess. The lower urinary and genital tract of both sexes are commonly colonized by ureaplasmas or *M. hominis*. In a number of studies ureaplasmas have been isolated more frequently from NGU, vaginitis or cervicitis than from controls of variable comparability. NGU has been reproduced in a small number of human volunteers by the instillation of a culture of *U. urealyticum* into the urethra (Taylor-Robinson et al 1977) and in chimpanzees (Taylor-Robinson et al 1978). Nevertheless *Chlamydia trachomatis* appears to be responsible for 30–50% of NGU, and cervicitis. The concurrent presence of both chlamydias and mycoplasmas in some patients clouds the issue. Treatment of NGU with antibiotics with differing actions on chlamydias and mycoplasmas has indicated that a proportion of the non-chlamydial cases are probably due to ureaplasmas (Bowie et al 1976; Coufalik et al 1979). Account has also to be taken of the fact that there are numerous serotypes of *U. urealyticum* and some may be more pathogenic than others; also the numbers of organisms present may be significant (cf. *Escherichia coli* and urinary tract infection). Ureaplasmas have also been associated with male and female infertility and abortion; also with low birth weight in the newborn. They may also play a part in renal infection (reviews: Gnarpe & Friberg 1973; Taylor-Robinson & McCormack 1979; Taylor-Robinson et al 1981).

In practical terms, for the microbiological diagnostic laboratory, it may be concluded that while these detailed research investigations have been useful in establishing the rôle of ureaplasmas and other genital mycoplasmas in infections of the reproductive tract and the neonate, the mere isolation of the organism from clinical samples will frequently serve little purpose in diagnosis and case management. This is a position that differs markedly from the diagnosis of *M. pneumoniae* infection in respiratory disease (see below).

General information on the cell biology of mycoplasmas and accounts of clinical aspects of infection with mycoplasmas may be found in the first two volumes of 'The Mycoplasmas' (Barile

et al 1979). Unusual clinical presentations of *M. pneumoniae* infection are described by Fleming et al (1967), Hodges et al (1972) and Smith & Sangster (1972). Some references to immuno-pathological and heterogenetic serological reactions with *M. pneumoniae* and their effects are Marmion et al (1967); Plackett et al (1969); Biberfeld (1970, 1971); Clyde (1971) and Costea et al (1972).

METHODS FOR THE HANDLING OF MYCOPLASMA CULTURES

Media

The formulae and methods of preparation of solid, semi-solid and liquid media for 'large colony' mycoplasmas and ureaplasmas are described in detail at the end of this chapter.* Attention to the following points is important.

Serum. There is sometimes a difference in growth-promoting properties between sera from different horses and it is advisable to test bleed a series of animals and obtain a large volume of serum from those that are satisfactory and to store it at −20°C or below. Alternatively, tested serum may be available from commercial sources. Serum is used without heat inactivation. Pooled human serum is sometimes used instead of horse serum but may contain antibody to mycoplasmas. Some human mycoplasmas will grow on swine serum but the growth of *M. pneumoniae* is significantly less than on horse serum. The growth-promoting properties of serum from various animal species is related to their cholesterol content. Thus, when it is desired to grow strains of mycoplasma for immunization of rabbits, and to avoid the use of a heterologous serum in the medium, it is necessary to add cholesterol to the rabbit serum in the medium (Taylor-Robinson et al 1963).

Yeast extract. The source and method of preparation of yeast extracts is important. Not all commercially prepared extracts will support the growth of *M. pneumoniae*; that described under

* Refer to *Methods* at end of this chapter.

*Methods** involves low temperature extraction. The pH of the extract and of the final medium should be adjusted to pH 7.0. (Note that the pH of the final medium for ureaplasmas is 6.0).

Growth factors. Much effort has been expended in the search for growth-promoting or inhibitor-neutralizing factors e.g. nucleic acids, coenzymes, extracts of boiled erythrocytes, bovine lung or staphylococci. These substances may be of use in attempts to isolate exacting mycoplasmas and are described by Klieneberger-Nobel (1962), Lemcke (1965) and Rylance et al (1979). Complex tissue culture media (Jensen et al 1965; Quinlan et al 1972) with yeast extract and lipid may be valuable as substitutes for serum-containing medium in antigen preparation or for increasing uptake of isotope-labelled precursors from the medium. The ingredients of tissue culture media have also proved to be valuable supplements to standard mycoplasma media for the growth of *M. genitalium* and *M. pneumoniae* (see SP-4 medium*; also Tully et al 1977; 1979; 1981).

Other requirements. Mycoplasmas are inhibited by some metal ions so it is important to use analytical grade chemicals and double distilled or ion-exchanged water in media preparation. Variation in batches of agar may make it necessary to vary concentration by trial and error; for optimal growth mycoplasmas must have a soft agar. The diphasic and solid media described below* should grow all members of the human flora, but may not be satisfactory for some avian or animal mycoplasmas. Formulae and supplements for some of these species are described by Lemcke (1965). The semi-solid and diphasic versions of the standard medium are valuable in providing a soft yet supporting framework for mycoplasma growth.

Growth of glycolytic species, such as *M. pneumoniae*, in broth may be enhanced by addition of glucose and by shaking or rolling the container. Diphasic medium may be made selective for *M. pneumoniae* by incorporation of 0.001% methylene blue. This inhibits other members of the human flora; if glucose and a pH indicator are also added the medium may be monitored for the growth of *M. pneumoniae* by the change of pH to acid. Subculture on to solid medium must then be done to verify the presence of the mycoplasma.

Ureaplasma media. Solid and fluid media for ureaplasmas described in *Methods** are based on media developed by Shepard and alternative formulae are given in Shepard (1969). The media contain serum (a source of urea), yeast extract and added urea. Growth in both solid and liquid medium is rapid and is conveniently monitored by the change of colour of the indicator to alkaline as the result of formation of ammonia from the urea. The alkaline shift is accompanied by a loss of viability and media with HEPES buffer may be used to counteract this and improve growth and colony size (Manchee & Taylor-Robinson 1969).

Culture

Mycoplasma medium is expensive and it is economical to hold it in small plastic disposable Petri dishes, 50×13 mm, e.g. from Sterilin, Falcon, etc. A vent may be cut in the edge of the dish with a hot wire to allow gaseous exchange. These dishes have good optical properties and the colonies at the surface of the medium should be visualized without opening the dish by placing it, lid down, on the stage of a microscope without stage clamps and equipped with $\times 10$ and $\times 4$ objectives and $\times 10$ oculars. This combination of lenses is optimal for the range (20–500 μm) of mycoplasma colonies. The larger ones may, of course, be visualized with a plate microscope. Examination without opening the plate is important because incubation has frequently to continue for 2 to 3 weeks and contamination, particularly with moulds, may be a problem.

Plates may be labelled with white adhesive tape and an indelible pen (e.g. laundry marker). The small size of the plates and the moist atmosphere in which they are held makes labelling with ordinary ball-point or felt-tip pens or grease pencils unsatisfactory. While the plates are being examined it is advisable to hold them upon a tray lined with filter paper soaked in 70% (v/v) ethanol or methylated spirit and also to wipe the microscope stage with the spirit from time to time to reduce the load of contaminants on the outside of the plates. Mould may grow over the edge of the lid, into the water of condensation on the inside of the lid and finally on to the medium itself.

Plates are incubated aerobically in plastic lunch boxes or in glass jars with sealed lids (fruit preserving jars) with a roll of cotton-wool soaked in water to maintain humidity. It is important to clean, disinfect or autoclave these containers regularly so as to prevent a build-up of fungal contaminants. Anaerobic incubation is effected in a McIntosh & Fildes jar with e.g. GasPak (BBL) or microaerophilic incubation by flushing the jar with 90% nitrogen and 10% CO_2 mixture.

Subculture. The technique of subculturing strains of mycoplasmas differs from the standard 'picking' method with bacteria because of the embedded nature of the colony. Small blocks of agar medium, bearing one or more colonies, are cut from the medium and placed colony-side down on fresh medium. A small stainless steel spatula, or scalpel with detachable blades, may be used for this purpose and is held in boiling water and burned off with spirit between transfers. The block is moved an inch or so across the plate so that mycoplasma cells will rub off on to the new medium. When mycoplasmas are first established on solid media of a different composition to that on which they have been carried, it may be found that growth occurs mainly under the block. Periodic movement of the block around the surface of the medium during incubation may establish growth satisfactorily.

Cloning. The colonial morphology of various species of mycoplasmas is often not distinctive and cross-contamination of strains and colonies made up of sectors of different mycoplasmas is a hazard. For this reason it is important to clone stock strains and isolates by serial subculture from one colony. The culture is grown in broth, filtered (220 nm APD), and two or three ten-fold serial dilutions prepared from it and plated on solid media to give a plate with well dispersed colonies. A small block with one colony is aspir-ated with a wide bore Pasteur pipette. The colony-bearing block is expelled into semi-solid agar, incubated and then subcultured on to solid media. This procedure may be repeated several times to ensure that the strain is pure.

Storage and shipment of mycoplasmas. Lyophilized cultures may be recovered by inoculating the material from the ampoule in 'stab' fashion into the centre of a bijou bottle of semi-solid medium and later subculturing on to solid media. The initial incubation in semi-solid agar may help to establish small numbers of organisms in a medium to which they are unaccustomed. Stock strains or isolates may be preserved by lyophilization, or by placing small amounts of a heavy culture in semi-solid agar medium at $-70°C$. Strains may be transmitted by mail on sealed plates or, more conveniently, as an agar block with colonies in semi-solid agar in a bijou bottle, or as lyophilized cultures.

Identification of isolates

Mycoplasma colonies are differentiated from small bacterial colonies and pseudocolonies by staining methods. They are differentiated from unstable L-phase variants by cultivation on the standard medium without penicillin and thallium acetate to allow the latter to revert to bacteria. Mycoplasmas are further identified by biochemical reactions, by certain biological reactions such as haemolysin production and haemadsorption and, above all, with the large colony mycoplasmas, by serological differentiation into species. Although serological identification is the primary method for the clinical laboratory, speciation of initial or novel isolates can be achieved by a variety of other (research) techniques. These include DNA/DNA or DNA/RNA hybridization between isolates and prototype strains or between mycoplasmas (suspected to be L-phase variants) and the presumptive bacterial parent (see Stanbridge & Raff 1979).

Differentiation of species by sequence homology generally gives clear-cut results. However, ribosomal RNA genes have some sequences that are conserved between mycoplasma species and cross homology may be observed with probes representing ribosomal genes and extracts of mycoplasma cells (see below). Some workers have used electrophoretic analysis of mycoplasma and L-phase variant extracts on polyacrylamide gels; this gives excellent species differentiation and facilitates identification of L-phase variants with bacterial parents (Theodore et al 1971).

In practical terms in the general bacteriological laboratory colony size provides a primary differentiation between mycoplasmas and the much smaller ureaplasmas. The former are identified by biochemical, biological and serological means (Table 45.1). The latter are identified by their ability to split urea, their inhibition by erythromycin and their resistance to lincomycin; they are also inhibited by 5'-iodo-2'-deoxyuridine and hydroxyurea (Shepard 1969). Serological identification of ureaplasmas is complicated by the existence of numerous antigenic subtypes (Lin et al 1972). Simple typing by growth inhibition, which is of such value with the mycoplasmas (Clyde 1964), is possible and has been used by various workers (see Black 1973; Cracea et al 1982). However standardized antisera for the various antigenic subtypes or the prototype strains are not readily available.

Selected laboratory methods are now outlined in principle.

Stains for mycoplasmas

The most generally used stain is that of Dienes* (Dienes 1939; Madoff 1959). Other useful stains are the Giemsa method* and cresyl-fast violet* (Shepard 1967). The former gives a purple-violet staining of both large and small colony mycoplasmas with some definition of the cellular structure of the colony. The latter stains both large and small colonies a red-purple colour. Mycoplasmas may also be detected by fluorochromes for nucleic acid, such as Hoechst 33258 for DNA (see section on *Detection of mycoplasmas in cell culture* below).

Distinction of mycoplasma colonies and artefacts (pseudocolonies)

Although well developed mycoplasma colonies are distinctive enough there may be difficulties in differentiating young or poorly growing colonies from the artefacts known as pseudocolonies (Brown et al 1940) or from the nuclei of tissue cells from cell cultures or clinical specimens. Pseudocolonies are precipitates arising from the high concentration of serum in mycoplasma media. Although they are not biological entities, they may appear to subculture when a block containing them is pushed over the surface of uninoculated medium because fresh collections of 'colonies' appear in the inoculated area, apparently as a result of stress changes in the medium surface or the provision of foci on which precipitates can increase. The agar-embedded centre of a mycoplasma colony is slightly granular and extends through several focal planes whereas a pseudocolony may have a central knob but is a superficial structure found in the focal plane of the medium surface. Mycoplasma colonies and pseudocolonies differ in their staining reactions with Dienes' stain, cresyl-fast violet or Giemsa, which reveal the collections of mycoplasma cells making up the colony. In addition pseudocolonies are not, of course, inhibited by broad spectrum antibiotics, antisera, UV or X irradiation, and do not incorporate thymidine or uridine into their structure.

Biochemical and biological tests

Fermentation of carbohydrates

A 1% (w/v) concentration of the carbohydrate under test is incorporated into an agar slope, or in semi-solid or fluid preparation of the standard medium together with phenol red (0.002% w/v). The range of sugars fermented is limited and is not of great differential importance. For most purposes it is sufficient to test for acid production from glucose. If other sugars are used it is important to remember that a maltase and a diastase in unheated horse serum may lead to false positive reactions. Fermentation may be weak and small changes of pH may be more accurately detected with a microelectrode than by colour change of the indicator; if semi-solid or fluid media are used, growth should be confirmed in negative tubes by subculture. Lemcke (1965) may be consulted for details of other biochemical tests.

Table 45.1 Biological and biochemical reactions of members of the human mycoplasma flora.
Key: . . ., results not available; β = complete haemolysis of erythrocytes (β haemolysis); – or x = no or partial haemolysis.

| Species | Requirement for yeast extract | Inhibition of growth by | | | | Haemolysis | Haemadsorption | Acid from glucose | Ammonia from | | Aerobic reduction of tetrazolium |
		Thallium acetate (0.01% w/v)	Methylene blue (0.001% w/v)	Erythromycin (100 µg/ml)	Lincomycin (200 µg/ml)				Arginine	Urea	
M. pneumoniae	+	–	–	+	–	β	+	+	–	–	+
M. fermentans	–	–	+	+	+	–	–	+	+	–	–
M. hominis	–	–	+	–	+	– or x	–	–	+	–	–
M. orale 1 (*M. orale*)	+	–	+	–	+	–	+[a]	–	+	–	–
M. orale 2 (*M. buccale*)	–	–	+	–	–	–	–	–	+	–	–
M. orale 3 (*M. faucium*)	+	–	+	–	–	–	+[a]	–	+	–	–
M. salivarium	–	–	+	–	–	–	–	–	+	–	–
M. genitalium	+	+	. . .	. . .	. . .	. . .	+	+	–	–	±
Ureaplasma urealyticum	+	+	–	+	–	β	–	–	–	+	–

[a] With chicken erythrocytes, not guinea-pig or human, but see Purcell & Chanock (1969).

Tests for other enzyme pathways

Media and tests for arginine deaminase,* urease* and reduction of tetrazolium* are described under *Methods* (below).

Haemolysis and haemadsorption

Isolates of mycoplasmas are inoculated onto standard medium to give well dispersed colonies and incubated until colonies are well grown (5–8 days). The plate is then overlaid with a thin layer of saline-agar containing 1% (v/v) sheep or guinea-pig erythrocytes and reincubated aerobically overnight.

M. pneumoniae produces a complete clearing, resembling β-haemolysis, of guinea-pig erythrocytes but test conditions are critical. Other mycoplasmas may produce a greenish clearing of the overlay. Haemolysis depends on production of hydrogen peroxide; a simple test for this is described by Lind (1970).

Haemadsorption may be tested by flooding the culture plate, or a block excised from it, with a 1% (v/v) suspension of sheep erythrocytes in saline and leaving them in contact for 30 min. The erythrocyte suspension is then aspirated and the colonies gently washed with saline and then inspected under the microscope. Positive colonies are seen to be plastered with erythrocytes. Spermatozoa and tissue culture cells may also adsorb to colonies (Taylor-Robinson & Manchee 1967a,b); the spectrum of activity is not precisely the same as that of haemadsorption but in each instance pretreatment of the colonies with antiserum to the mycoplasma inhibits the reaction.

Serological identification of mycoplasmas

Serological methods are the most important means of identifying and classifying mycoplasmas. Almost all the known serological techniques, e.g. agglutination, complement fixation, gel diffusion, inhibition of haemadsorption, indirect haemagglutination, immunofluorescence, metabolic inhibition, complement-mediated mycoplasmacidal antibody, radioimmunoassay, etc., have been used either to classify strains or to measure antibody in sera from convalescent patients or hyperimmunized animals

(see Purcell et al 1969). Some of these techniques recognize intratypic differences and are more relevant for a reference, than for the general laboratory. Details are given of two simple methods – growth inhibition on agar and immunofluorescence on colonies transferred to glass slides – that will allow identification of most mycoplasma isolates in a general laboratory.

Growth inhibition on agar

The method follows those developed by Huijsmans-Evers & Ruys (1956) and Clyde (1964). After cloning the isolate, seed a mycoplasma broth with a small (5–10 mm²) block containing colonies and incubate for 3–7 days depending on the strain. Dry plates of standard mycoplasma medium at 37°C and seed by placing a small quantity of the broth on the plate and distributing it evenly with a spreader. Place filter paper disks containing mycoplasma antisera on the seeded plates. The antisera are prepared by hyperimmunization of animals with representative strains of each of the human mycoplasma species. Up to four disks may be placed on each plate; one disk should contain no serum. The disks may be prepared by soaking sterile filter paper disks, 5 mm diameter, and either holding them frozen at −20°C or drying them and storing at 4°C. Alternatively a single multiarmed set of disks may be used, with a different serum on each arm (Stanbridge & Hayflick 1967). Suitable antisera have to be prepared in the laboratory by immunization of rabbits as unfortunately commercial sources of mycoplasma antisera have declined sharply in recent years. Small quantities of reference antisera may be available for calibration of locally produced antisera from the Mycoplasma Section (Dr J. G. Tully), Laboratory of Molecular Biology, NIAID, Building 550, Frederick Cancer Research Facility, Frederick, MD 21701, USA. The plates are incubated, aerobically or anaerobically, depending on the nature of the isolate, and inspected macroscopically and microscopically for a zone of inhibition of growth around the disks (illustrated in 13th Edn, Vol. 1, Plate 52.4). The method is highly specific and shows little of the cross-reactions between species revealed by more sensitive methods such as complement fixation. It may be necessary to seed a smaller dose of organisms if there is evidence of partial inhibition around the disks with 'break-through' of colonies.

Identification of mycoplasmas (not ureaplasmas) by immunofluorescence on slides

Colonies are transferred to microscope slides by placing a 5–10 mm² block with well dispersed colonies face down on an area marked out by glass diamond. The slides should have been chemically cleaned (e.g. chromic acid) and held in ethanol before use. The slide and agar block is lowered into a beaker of water at 85°C. It helps to have a simple platform and handle in light metal to support the slide during this operation. Once in the water the block turns opaque and finally melts over the surface of the slide. At this point a quick swirling motion will dislodge the agar and leave the mycoplasma colonies heat-fixed to the slide. The slide is then removed from the beaker, rinsed briefly in another beaker of water at 85°C to free the preparation of the last traces of agar, then dried and inspected under the low power of the microscope to confirm that colonies have, in fact, been transferred.

The mycoplasma antisera, usually made in rabbit, goat or horse, and the appropriate fluorescein-conjugated antiglobulin, are absorbed with a mixture of packed, washed yeast cells and horse liver powder. This is done to cut down possible heterologous reactions between the antisera, the conjugate and residual traces of medium components (yeast extract or horse serum) on the slide. Sera and absorbents are mixed in a ratio of approximately 0.5 g to 2 ml of serum and held for 1 h at room temperature with periodic shaking, then centrifuged and the supernatant fluid passed through a syringe membrane filter to remove fine particles.

The conjugate and mycoplasma antisera have first to be titrated on known strains to determine the dilution for use in the test with unknown colonies. Mycoplasma antisera may be used at a concentration of 10–20 antibody units. A conjugate will usually have a titration endpoint of 20–40 on antibody coated colonies and may be used at a dilution of one in 5–10. Concentrations stronger than 5 are liable to give non-specific staining.

In the first stage of staining the unknown colonies, a drop of diluted, absorbed, antiserum is spread over the colony-bearing area of the slide with a toothpick or bacteriological loop so as to ensure even dispersion. The slide is placed in a closed, humid chamber for 30 min at 37°C. Next the slide is washed by placing it in a container of phosphate-buffered saline pH 7.0 with a magnetic stirrer for 30 min at room temperature. The excess buffer is then drained from the slide and it is carefully mopped dry with a cellulose wipe without touching the area with colonies. A drop of conjugate is then spread over the colony area and the slide returned to the moist chamber for 30 min at 37°C. The slide is then washed again with fresh buffer and quickly rinsed with distilled water, mopped dry, and the colony area covered with mounting fluid (e.g. buffer pH 8.5 one part, analytical grade glycerol nine parts; or one of the permanent fluorescence-free mountants) and a coverslip; its edges may be sealed with colourless nail varnish. The preparation is viewed in the fluorescence microscope with a darkground condenser or incident optics. Colonies with attached antibody show a bright green speckled fluorescence; negative colonies autofluoresce blue or silver-grey depending on the wavelength of the exciting light (13th Edn, Vol. 1, Plate 7). Controls should include preparations with buffer as the 'middle layer' rather than antiserum and also some with buffer instead of conjugate. There should also be a control preparation of a known strain of mycoplasma and its homologous antiserum to check that the diluted absorbed conjugate is still active.

In general this method gives clear-cut differentiation between mycoplasma species when care is taken to use the antisera at a standard unitage. It is also possible to detect mixtures of mycoplasmas by looking for stained and unstained colonies or parts of colonies with the same preparation.

Antibody in human (or animal) convalescent-phase sera may be titrated on colonies but both this method and growth inhibition are of low sensitivity compared with antibody measurement by metabolic inhibition, indirect haemagglutination, or radioimmunoassay. Del Guidice et al (1967) have developed a method for fluor-staining of colonies directly on agar and detection with the incident illuminator of the microscope.

LABORATORY DIAGNOSIS OF MYCOPLASMA INFECTIONS

M. pneumoniae infection of the respiratory tract

Patients with bronchiolitis or pneumonia may harbour *M. pneumoniae* in the nasopharynx or respiratory secretions for substantial periods of time, even after antibiotic therapy and clinical recovery. Nevertheless there are marked variations in the ease with which the organism is grown by different laboratories. Experience during recent prevalences of *M. pneumoniae* infection shows that a substantial proportion of patients present to the doctor 10–14 or more days from the onset of illness. At this stage, diagnosis may most easily be made by detection of specific IgM antibody*; often complement-fixing antibody will also be present but may not increase in titre. Serodiagnosis may be supported by demonstration of antigen (Kok et al 1988a) or specific nucleotide sequences in the respiratory exudate, or by culture of the organism on solid, diphasic or SP-4 media*, or in the cell-sheet system (see below). A method for the direct detection of antigen* is described under *Methods*; kits for the detection of the specific ribosomal sequences of *M. pneumoniae* may be obtained from Gen Probe. Recent studies (Kok et al 1988a) indicate that antigen detection and nucleic acid probe detection are a convenient substitute for culture of the organism. There are, however, significant numbers of patients whose respiratory secretions are negative for antigen or specific ribosomal sequences who have good serological evidence of current infection.

Collection of specimens

1. *Throat and nose swabs* are taken and the heads broken off into 2 ml of a transport medium in a bijou bottle; the standard myco-

plasma fluid medium will do for this purpose or a mixture of basal broth, bovine serum albumin (1% v/v), gelatin (0.3% w/v) and penicillin (1000 units/ml) may be employed.

2. *Nasopharyngeal aspirates* as collected for virus culture (Ch. 48) are good starting material for isolation of *M. pneumoniae*. Virus transport medium, which contains gentamicin, must not be used to wash the aspirated mucus into the specimen trap; either the broth-albumin mixture described above or modified virus transport medium containing cefotaxime (50 μg/ml) or ampicillin (200 μg/ml) may be used.

Fluid expelled from the swabs, or cells centrifuged from the nasopharyngeal aspirate, are inoculated in a volume of 0.5–1.5 ml into a bottle of diphasic medium* containing glucose and methylene blue, a bottle of SP4 medium*, and one or two drops are plated on to the standard solid mycoplasma medium*.

3. *Sputum* is mixed with an equal volume of mycoplasma broth and lightly homogenized (e.g. in a Nelson blender) and is then inoculated into diphasic medium and onto solid mycoplasma medium. Particularly viscous specimens may be liquefied by digestion with pancreatic dornase or 'sputolysin'. Isolation rates may be improved by inoculation of 10–15 ml volumes of sputum extract into diphasic or SP-4 medium* in small medical 'flats'. Pleural fluid, aspirates from otitis media, cerebrospinal fluid and other miscellaneous specimens for *M. pneumoniae* are also inoculated into diphasic or SP-4 medium*.

4. *Tissue specimens* from the lungs of fatal cases of atypical pneumonia, or from animals inoculated experimentally, may require special treatment to offset the mycoplasmacidal effects of tissue enzymes released on grinding the tissue (Kaklamanis et al 1969). Diphasic or SP-4 medium* should be inoculated with several ten-fold dilutions of the tissue extract as well as with the concentrated material.

Culture

In general, plates and diphasic medium are

incubated aerobically (at 35.5–36.0°C) and the latter is inspected each day for acid production and subcultured on to a plate of solid medium if this occurs. The primary plate seeded with the swab eluates or sputum is inspected at 3–5 day intervals and all media are held for up to 3 weeks before discard. At that stage, apparently negative plates may be flooded with a saline suspension of human or sheep erythrocytes to detect inconspicuous colonies by haemadsorption. Suspect colonies on the primary plate, or from the subcultures from diphasic medium, are subcultured and identified by the biochemical and serological tests already described.

Disadvantages of these standard methods for the culture of *M. pneumoniae* are low sensitivity and the time taken to obtain and identify a positive culture. As an additional approach nasopharyngeal aspirates and other respiratory specimens may be inoculated into mycoplasma-free sheets of HeLa 229 cells, inhibited with cycloheximide and with mycoplasma broth containing thallium acetate as the fluid phase. After 4 days the sheets are stained by immunofluorescence with absorbed polyclonal or monoclonal antibody to *M. pneumoniae*. Positive cell cultures are subcultured on to solid agar for colony identification (Kok et al 1988b).

Infections of the genital tract

Clinical specimens for isolation of mycoplasmas or ureaplasmas from the genital tract may include high vaginal or cervical swabs, urethral swabs or urine after massage of prostate and paraurethral glands, specimens of purulent aspirate from 'non-bacterial' salpingitis, tissue or swabs from membranes or fetus in cases of abortion or prematurity, or semen collected as part of an investigation of infertility. In addition, blood may be taken for culture in puerperal fever. Swabs may be taken into Stuart's transport medium or into mycoplasma broth *without* inhibitors such as thallium acetate or methylene blue. Ampicillin may be added to control bacterial overgrowth.

Swabs are spread on plates of standard ureaplasma media*; eluates from the swabs may also be inoculated into diphasic medium without methylene blue and into liquid ureaplasma

medium. Urine is centrifuged and the deposit inoculated on to plates and into fluid medium. Tissue and pus may be blended with mycoplasma broth, without inhibitors, and the supernatant fluid from a lightly centrifuged suspension inoculated into mycoplasma and ureaplasma media. Blood for culture should be taken into diphasic medium without glucose or methylene blue in a fashion analogous to the Castaneda blood culture bottle and also into ureaplasma broth; both types of media are subcultured at intervals on to the appropriate solid media. Semen should be lightly blended with ureaplasma broth and seeded on to solid and into liquid media.

Incubation of all plates, both for *M. hominis* and *M. fermentans* and for ureaplasmas, should be under microaerophilic or anaerobic conditions. Suspect colonies are subcultured and identified as already described.

Note: These methods are described for completeness but it should be emphasized again (see above) that the mere isolation of mycoplasma or ureaplasma from the genital tract is not necessarily evidence that it is causally related to any disease that is present.

SEROLOGICAL DIAGNOSIS OF MYCOPLASMA PNEUMONIAE INFECTION

The development of antibody to *M. pneumoniae* by infected subjects may be measured by a range of techniques of widely differing sensitivity. The technique commonly used in the general bacteriological laboratory is complement-fixation with whole cell or lipid extracts of the organism, but this is not sensitive enough to detect all cases and some other methods are required.

In addition, about half the patients infected with *M. pneumoniae* develop cold haemagglutinins to their own or group 'O' erythrocytes and a smaller proportion, agglutinins to *Streptococcus* MG. These heterogenetic reactions probably depend on fortuitous similarities between glycolipid haptens in the mycoplasma membrane and carbohydrate determinants in the streptococcal cell (Marmion et al 1967; Plackett et al 1969) or in the 'I' antigen of the erythrocyte (Costea et al 1972). As cold haemagglutinins develop rapidly it may be of value to estimate them as well as testing for complement-fixing or other antibody to *M. pneumoniae*.

Complement-fixation (CF) tests for M. pneumoniae infection

Complement-fixing antigens may be obtained from commercial sources and so their preparation will not be described in detail here (see 12th Edn, Vol. 2, Ch. 43 for details). Lipid extract antigen is supplied by the Commonwealth Serum Laboratories and by Behring.

Whole cell or suspended lipid antigen is titrated in 'chessboard' fashion in the CF test against human and rabbit antisera to determine the optimum antigen concentration, i.e. that dilution giving the highest serum titre, for routine tests (see Ch. 49). The whole cell antigen and the lipid antigen used with acute and convalescent sera from atypical pneumonia patients both detect about the same proportion of the total *M. pneumoniae* infections. As the lipid antigen is free from anticomplementary activity it can be used at high unitage to detect the poor CF antibody responses that occur in a minority of patients. However, the chloroform methanol extraction also makes accessible cardiolipin-like phosphatides so that the antigen will react with WR-positive sera from syphilitics. Paradoxical or conflicting results should therefore be investigated by testing the sera for specific antitreponemal antibody by the TPHA or other techniques (Ch. 40).

Metabolic inhibition (MI) test for measurement of antibody to M. pneumoniae.

This technique is described in detail in the 12th Edition (Vol. 2, Ch. 49) and by Taylor-Robinson et al (1966) and Purcell et al (1969). It is a very sensitive way of measuring antibody to *M. pneumoniae* but complicated by the fact that sera from patients may often contain broad spectrum antibiotics that will interfere with the assay. This can be circumvented to some extent by using an erythromycin resistant strain of *M. pneumoniae*

(Niitu et al 1974). Because of the limitations of the CF and MI tests, we describe two methods of measuring immunoglobulin class-specific antibody, particularly IgM, which are useful adjuncts to the CF test.

Detection of M. pneumoniae IgM antibodies

A useful marker of current or recent infection is to measure the IgM specific antibody. This can be tested by using enzyme immunoassay (Busolo et al 1983; Dussaix et al 1983) or radioimmunoassays (Hu et al 1983; Price 1983) on microtitre plates coated with *M. pneumoniae* antigen. Alternatively, the haemagglutination (HA) reaction with tanned erythrocytes coated with *M. pneumoniae* antigen can be modified as an IgM 'capture' test for the measurement of specific IgM antibody. A direct enzyme immunoassay* and modified HA test* are described in detail in *Methods* below. Specific IgM antibody increases in titre more rapidly than CF antibody, and declines to low levels within a year after infection. Its detection is particularly valuable when unchanging, intermediate levels of CF antibody (e.g. titres of 40–80) are observed in sera taken in the middle and late stages of the illness and when it is uncertain whether the antibody is related to the current or past infection. The use of CF and IgM antibody tests as a part of a general 'screen' test in a patient with respiratory infection is illustrated by the report form in Figure 47.3.

DETECTION OF MYCOPLASMAS IN CELL CULTURE

The frequency with which various species of mycoplasma are found in cell cultures varies from country to country and reflects local practice in handling cells, local commercial arrangements for supply of cells, or private exchange of cultures (see reviews by Hayflick 1965; MacPherson 1968; Stanbridge 1971). Although initially mycoplasmas may have been introduced into cell cultures from the nasopharynx of handlers, or from medium components such as bovine or swine serum, trypsin, chick embryo extract and the like, the prevalence of a single, or limited number of species in many different cell lines indicates that cross-infection between cultures is an important, and too often unrecognized mode of infection. Species reported include *M. hominis, M. orale, M. hyorhinis, M. arginini*, and from time to time, *M. fermentans, M. gallisepticum, M. pulmonis, A. laidlawi* and *A. granularum*.

Mycoplasmas in cell cultures may be detected by light or phase contrast microscopy of cell sheets stained by Giemsa, orcein (Fogh & Fogh 1964), or fluorochromed with acridine orange (Ebke & Kuwert 1972) or Hoechst 33258 dye (Hilwig & Gropp 1972). Cell sheets may also be examined by immunofluorescence with single or pooled antisera to the mycoplasma species likely to be found as cell culture contaminants. Mycoplasmas may be visualized in the electron microscope in thin sections of cell sheets or, much less reliably, in negative contrast preparations of cell lysates (Wolanski & Maramorosch 1970).

Other methods involve detection of enzymes characteristic of mycoplasmas and not of their host cells, e.g. arginine deaminase (Schimke & Barile 1963); such methods have the attraction of speed but suffer from the limitations that not all mycoplasmas have the arginine deaminase pathway and that simple culture of the cells for mycoplasma is more sensitive if somewhat slower. Other workers (Horoszewicz & Grace 1964; Levine 1972) have taken advantage of the fact that mycoplasma-infected cell cultures exhibit abnormal levels of thymidine and uridine phosphorylase; thus estimation of the uracil split from radioisotope tagged uridine can be used as an index of contamination. Tagged thymidine and uridine is incorporated into, respectively, the DNA and RNA of the mycoplasmas and the labelled organisms can be located by the increase of silver grains over the cytoplasm of cells in autoradiographs (Studzinski et al 1973); however, experience again suggests that the method is less sensitive than culture. Mycoplasmas incorporate both uridine and uracil into their RNA, whereas eukaryotic cells incorporate only uridine; this differential activity has been utilized to detect contamination (Schneider et al 1974) but does not always correlate well with the results of other methods.

Todaro et al (1971) have developed an ingenious method in which cell cultures are exposed to thymidine and uridine with different radioisotopic labels, the fluid phase or cell eluates are concentrated and centrifuged on a sucrose gradient, and the fractions examined for double labelling at a characteristic buoyant density (1.20–1.24 g/cm^3). This method would be advantageous for detection of mycoplasmas that grow poorly in cell-free media; some mycoplasmas become highly adapted to life at the cell surface and have a low plating efficiency in cell-free media.

Finally, it has been observed that there is a highly conserved nucleotide sequence among the ribosomal RNA genes of different mycoplasma species (Razin et al 1984); nucleic acid probes have been constructed by cloning the rRNA genes into a plasmid/*E. coli* system and these probes have been used to detect contaminant mycoplasmas in cell culture.

A kit marketed by Gen Probe uses a probe to the common sequences of ribosomal RNA and will detect a variety of mycoplasmas, acholeplasmas and spiroplasmas in the short time of two hours. (This kit should not be confused with the probe for the specific ribosomal sequences of *M. pneumoniae* marketed by the same manufacturer.)

Two simple methods – fluorochroming with Hoechst 33258, and culture – of use in the general bacteriological laboratory are described in greater detail.

Fluorochrome detection of mycoplasmas (after Hessling et al 1980)

The cells are grown at 37°C in air with 5% CO_2. At 2 and 4 days after the cells have been seeded, coverslips are selected upon which the cells are approximately 80–90% confluent. Without removing the medium, 2 ml of Carnoy's fixative (3 parts 100% methanol, 1 part glacial acetic acid) is added gently to the dish containing the coverslip and incubated at room temperature for 2 min. The medium is aspirated and, without allowing the coverslip to dry, fresh fixative is added for an additional 5 min. This step is repeated once. The fixative is then aspirated, and the coverslip allowed to dry. A stock solution of the Hoechst 33258 stain is made at a concentration of 0.05 mg/ml in Hanks' balanced salt solution (see *Methods* Ch. 50), without phenol red, pH 7.0. For the test, a stock solution less than 1 week old is diluted to a concentration of 0.05 μg/ml in Hanks' solution. Approximately 1 ml of the diluted stain is incubated on each dried coverslip for 10 min. The coverslips are then washed three times with distilled water and mounted in 0.1 mol/litre acetate buffer, pH 5.5, on a microscope slide. When almost dry, the slides are sealed and examined at $\times$ 540 magnification with a fluorescence microscope.

Mycoplasmas may also be detected by immunofluorescence and this procedure was described in detail in the 12th Edition, Volume 2, Chapter 43.

Detection of mycoplasmas in cells by culture

Replace the standard culture medium over the cell monolayer or in the flask with lymphoblastoid cells with liquid mycoplasma culture medium and incubate for 4–7 days before subculture on to agar plates or semi-solid medium. This increases the number of the contaminating mycoplasmas present in the culture vessel and hence increases the growth on subculture, particularly with mycoplasmas that are tightly cell-associated or the exacting 'non-cultivable' strains (Hopps et al 1973).

At the same time it is of value to inoculate into glucose broth without inhibitor to detect low grade infection of the cells with bacteria or yeasts. One mycoplasma plate is incubated aerobically and the other anaerobically or in nitrogen and CO_2. It is particularly important to use anaerobic conditions to detect *M. orale* in cell culture. The semi-solid agar is subcultured at 3, 7 and 14 days and the primary plates and the subcultures are examined at the same intervals. Suspected colonies are stained by Dienes' method* or with cresyl-fast violet* and the isolates identified by immunofluorescence and by

subculture and growth inhibition. The presence of L-phase variants simulating mycoplasmas is investigated by subculture on standard medium without inhibitors.

Treatment of contaminated cells

This is a matter of some difficulty as the antibiotic sensitivity of different mycoplasma species varies. Basic policy should include buying in mycoplasma-free cells (and checking them at time of purchase), growing them up and storing clean stocks in liquid nitrogen or at −70°C. Contaminated sublines are rigorously discarded as infection is liable to spread to other cell lines. Separate hoods must be used for contaminated and clean lines along with separate cell culture media, pipette cans, etc. Hoods should be cleaned between handling different cell lines. Cells which cannot be discarded may be treated with tetracycline, kanamycin, tylosin or other broad spectrum antibiotics to which the organism is demonstrably sensitive (see Cross et al 1967; Fogh & Fogh 1969; Stanbridge 1971). Sodium aurothiomalate is effective against some species but disappointing with *M. orale*. Other methods advocated but less effective outside the laboratory of origin are heating cultures at 41°C, or treatment with antiserum to the mycoplasma concerned (see Stanbridge 1971). It must be remembered that even if stock cell lines are mycoplasma-free, many virus stocks will be contaminated and will serve as a source of further laboratory outbreaks of contamination. Treatment of virus-infected cell cultures with antibiotics and gold salts, or gamma irradiation of virus seeds (Polley & Fanok 1973) may overcome the problem.

METHODS

Stains for mycoplasmas and ureaplasmas

Dienes' stain

Azure II	0.25 g
Methylene blue	0.5 g
Maltose	2 g
Na_2CO_3	0.05 g

Benzoic acid	0.04 g
Distilled water	20 ml

Method. (a) Flood the plate, or a portion of the plate containing suspected mycoplasma colonies, with Dienes' stain diluted 1 in 10 in distilled water. Examine the plate microscopically using a low power objective ($\times$ 4 or $\times$ 10).

(b) Alternatively, smear clean coverslips with the 'neat' stain and allow to dry. Cut out a block of agar (5–10 mm square $\times$ 1–2 mm thick) from the plate and place colony-side down on the dry stain. Attach a brass ring (15–20 mm diameter $\times$ 3–4 mm thick) to a microscope slide by warming the ring in a Bunsen flame, dipping in Vaseline and pressing the ring on to a slide. Place the coverslip, agar block side down, on the ring and view the stained preparation microscopically using a low power objective ($\times$ 4 or $\times$ 10).

Colonies of mycoplasma retain the stain for at least 2 days while those of nearly all bacterial colonies lose the colour in half an hour. Mycoplasmas stain an intense royal blue, ureaplasmas stain reddish or greenish-blue. Colonies which have been transferred to slides by the hot water transfer method may be stained by overnight exposure to Dienes' stain or a mixture of Dienes' and Giemsa in equal proportions. By this method the stained preparation may be viewed microscopically with the oil immersion objective.

Cresyl-fast violet stain (Shepard 1967)

Stock solution. Adjust distilled water to pH 3.7 with glacial acetic acid (1–5 drops/100 ml). Dissolve 1 g cresyl-fast violet in 100 ml distilled water, pH 3.7. Allow solution to ripen for 48 h.

Working solution (prepared daily)

Stock solution	20 ml
NaCl	0.05 g
Agitate 1 min, filter and add	
maltose	7 g

Method. The stain may be applied by any of the methods mentioned above although difficulty may be experienced in coating coverslips. If this is so, the block should be stained before applying

a coverslip. Colonies of mycoplasma, both large and ureaplasmas, stain red-purple.

Giemsa stain

Blocks of agar with colonies should be inverted on to microscope slides and immersed in Bouin's fixative overnight. The block is then removed and the slide rinsed in tap water for 1 h. The slide is placed colony-side down on two supports in a Petri dish to which is added Giemsa stain (Ch. 46) diluted 1 in 20 in distilled water. Staining is allowed to take place overnight, before rinsing and microscopic examination.

Hoechst 33258 stain

See also use of Hoechst 33258 stain under *Detection of mycoplasmas in cell culture* (above).

Media for the cultivation of Mycoplasma pneumoniae and other mycoplasmas

For details of the following media, see Lemcke (1965), Marmion (1967) and Shepard (1969). *Note*: Media for mycoplasmas contain horse serum. Some batches may contain inhibitors and each batch should be tested for inhibitory activity before use. Wellcome Horse Serum No. 3 (not inactivated) is suitable.

Standard solid medium

Yeast extract

Baker's yeast	1 kg
Deionized water	1 litre
Hydrochloric acid, HCl, analytical	
grade	c. 6.5 ml

Add the yeast to 500 ml water at 50°C, in a large beaker. Mix and knead well (this is particularly important). Add the remaining water, warm to 80°C and add acid until the pH reaches 4.5, checked with pH papers. Mix well and heat at 80°C for 20 min. Allow the yeast cells to settle and clarify by centrifugation. Filter the supernatant through a hardened filter paper (38.5 cm diameter) and then through a Seitz EK filter or other bacterium-tight grade. Check for sterility by adding 5 ml filtrate to 10 ml nutrient broth, incubating 24 h and subculturing on blood agar. Dispense in convenient amounts and store at −20 or −40°C. Adjust the pH to 7.0 immediately before use.

Preparation of complete medium

PPLO agar base without crystal violet (Difco) pH 7.8	70 ml
Yeast extract, pH 7.0	10 ml
Horse serum (unheated)	20 ml
Sodium deoxyribonucleate (calf thymus) solution, 0.2% (w/v)	1.0 ml
Thallous acetate solution, $TlC_2H_3O_2$, 1 in 80 (w/v)	1.0 ml
Dipotassium hydrogen phosphate solution, K_2HPO_4, 1 mol/l	2.0 ml
Penicillin solution, 50 000 units/ml	0.2 ml

The solutions are sterilized by filtration. The agar is dissolved, sterilized and cooled to 48°C before adding the remaining ingredients which should be at room temperature. The final pH should be 7.8. It is convenient to dispense 10 ml amounts in disposable 5 cm Petri dishes (Sterilin, Falcon, etc.). The poured plates are stored in closed containers at 4°C. Plates should not be used if more than one week old, as mycoplasmas require a soft agar for growth.

Liquid medium

This medium, with or without glucose, may be used for primary isolation of mycoplasmas but it is not so good as diphasic medium. It can be used for antigen production.

PPLO broth without crystal violet (Difco) pH 7.8	70 ml
Yeast extract, pH 7.0, see above	10 ml
Horse serum (unheated)	20 ml
Glucose solution, 10% (w/v)	10 ml
Sodium deoxyribonucleate (calf thymus) solution, 0.2% (w/v)	1.0 ml
Thallous acetate solution, $TlC_2H_3O_2$, 1 in 80 (w/v)	1.0 ml

Dipotassium hydrogen phosphate solution, K_2HPO_4, 1 mol/l	2.0 ml
Pencillin solution, 50 000 units/ml	0.2 ml
Phenol red solution, 0.2% (w/v)	1.0 ml
Methylene blue solution, 0.1% (w/v)	1.0 ml

Methylene blue is omitted unless the examination is only for *M. pneumoniae*. It inhibits the growth of human commensal mycoplasmas. Sometimes it contains inhibitors for *M. pneumoniae* and each batch should be tested for inhibitory activity before use.

Sterilize the solution by filtration and add them to the sterile broth. Dispense, with sterile precautions.

Diphasic medium

For the primary isolation of mycoplasmas.

Solid phase. Standard solid medium, above.

Liquid phase. Liquid medium, above.

Preparation of complete medium. Dispense the solid phase in approximately 5 ml quantities in sterile screw-capped bottles and allow it to set. Overlay with 10 ml of the liquid phase.

Sloppy agar medium

This medium is useful for primary isolation of mycoplasmas.

PPLO broth without crystal violet (Difco) pH 7.8	70 ml
PPLO agar base without crystal violet (Difco) pH 7.8	10 ml
Yeast extract, pH 7.0, see above	10 ml
Horse serum (unheated)	20 ml
Sodium deoxyribonucleate (calf thymus) solution, 0.2% (w/v)	1.0 ml
Thallous acetate solution, $TlC_2H_3O_2$, 1 in 80 (w/v)	1.0 ml
Dipotassium hydrogen phosphate solution, K_2HPO_4, 1 mol/l	2.0 ml
Penicillin solution, 50 000 units/ml	0.2 ml

Sterilize the solutions by filtration and add them

to the sterile broth. Add the 10 ml molten agar base. Mix gently. Dispense aseptically in 4 ml amounts in small screw-capped bottles (bijoux).

SP-4 medium (after Tully et al 1977; 1979; 1981)

The medium consists of a base resembling that used in the standard mycoplasma medium described above together with various supplements, in particular a complex tissue or cell culture medium, CMRL 1066. The latter is a modification of the Healy, Fischer and Parker cell culture medium 858 and contains 21 amino acids, 13 vitamins, nucleic acid precursors and enzyme cofactors. The 10× concentrate of CMRL 1066 contains levels of cholesterol suitable for mycoplasma growth.

The medium may be used in the liquid form without agar and with phenol red, or as a diphasic medium, or in the form of plates. In our experience, the inoculation of specimens into the liquid or diphasic medium with subculture on to plates of the standard mycoplasma medium, rather than plates of SP-4 medium, gives optimal results. The reason why this is so is unclear. Thallium acetate may be added for the culture of *M. pneumoniae*, but must be omitted when culturing *M. genitalium*.

Basal medium

Mycoplasma broth base (BBL)	3.5 g
Tryptone (Difco)	10.0 g
Peptone (Difco)	5.3 g
Glucose	5.0 g
Deionized water	615 ml

Supplements

CMRL 1066 medium, 10× concentrate with glutamine (Gibco 154)	50 ml
Fresh yeast extract, 25% solution (MA Bioproducts)	35 ml
Yeastolate, 2% solution, sterile (Difco)	100 ml
Fetal bovine serum, heated at 56°C for 1 h (Flow)	170 ml
Penicillin, 100 000 units/ml	10 ml
Phenol red solution, 0.1% (w/v)	20 ml

Preparation of complete medium

The quantities shown above are sufficient to make 1 litre of SP-4 medium; the osmolality is 332 mmol/kg; pH 7.0–7.4. Basal medium is prepared and adjusted to pH 7.5 and then autoclaved at 121°C for 15 min. Complete medium is prepared by the addition of each of the sterile supplements. Agar plates are prepared, generally with 200 ml amounts of the complete medium, by the addition of 3.5% (w/v) of Noble agar (Difco) to the basal medium before sterilization. After autoclaving, the basal medium is equilibrated at 56°C, sterile supplements added aseptically (except for the phenol red solution), and plates poured. The agar medium is to be used no later than 7 days after preparation.

Ureaplasma medium

PPLO broth or PPLO agar without crystal violet (Difco) pH 6.0	70 ml
Yeast extract, pH 7.0, (see *standard solid medium* above)	10 ml
Horse serum (unheated)	20 ml
Urea solution, 20% (w/v)	5 ml
Phenol red solution, 0.2% (w/v)	1.0 ml
Penicillin solution, 200 000 units/ml	0.25 ml

The solutions are sterilized by filtration and added to the sterile broth or agar. The pH of the medium is adjusted to 6.0 before dispensing it with sterile precautions.

Media for enzyme tests

Test media for arginine deaminase, urease, and tetrazolium reduction are described below.

Arginine deaminase

The standard liquid medium is supplemented with 1% (w/v) L-arginine HCl and 0.002% phenol red and adjusted to pH 7.0. Production of ammonia is indicated by a change to a deep red colour. Note that the horse serum in the medium contains urea and that an organism with urease may also produce ammonia.

Urease (Shepard & Lunceford 1970; Shepard 1973)

Urease activity may be determined (1) in a liquid medium (Shepard's U9 medium) or (2) by plate tests.

1. Urease colour test liquid medium

   Basal broth
   Tryptic digest broth powder
      (BBL or Difco)   0.75 g
   Sodium chloride, NaCl   0.5 g
   Potassium dihydrogen phosphate
      KH_2PO_4 0.02 g
   Deionized water   100 ml

Note: Not all batches of tryptic digest broth powder are satisfactory and tests with known ureaplasmas are advisable.

The ingredients are dissolved, pH adjusted to 5.5 with HCl 2 mol/l and the basal broth sterilized in the autoclave at 121°C for 15 min.

   Complete medium

   Sterile basal broth   95 ml
   Unheated normal horse serum   4 ml
   10% w/v urea, stock solution   0.5 ml
   0.2% w/v phenol red, stock
      solution   1 ml
   Benzylpenicillin 100 000 units/ml   1 ml

Analytical grade urea is used and sterilized by filtration.

Adjust to pH 6.0. The complete medium is dispensed in 1.5–2 ml volumes in 7 ml screw-capped bottles. Preparations should not be kept longer than 1 week. The medium may also be used for isolation of ureaplasmas from clinical specimens and for this purpose may be supplemented by 2.5 μg/ml of amphotericin B to suppress yeasts and filamentous fungi that give a positive urease test.

2. Plate spot tests for urease and differential media.

A solution containing 1% (w/v) analytical grade urea and 0.8% (w/v) manganous chloride is applied to suspected ureaplasma colonies which must be less than 48 h old. The liberation of ammonia from the urea reacts with the divalent cation indicator – manganous chloride – to give a golden brown precipitate around the colony. Alternatively, 0.03% (w/v) manganous sulphate may be incorporated in the ureaplasma solid medium thus giving a differential medium on which ureaplasmas have a golden precipitate around them while 'large colony' mycoplasmas do not change the medium.

Tetrazolium reduction (Kraybill & Crawford 1965).

Plates of standard mycoplasma agar are prepared with the addition of 2 ml of 1% (w/v) stock solution of 2–3–5 triphenyltetrazolium chloride per 100 ml of medium. The stock solution is sterilized in the autoclave. A block of agar containing numerous colonies is placed, colony-side down, on the tetrazolium plate and the plate reincubated aerobically. In 3–6 days the colony-containing block becomes pink in colour if *M. pneumoniae* is present. It should be noted that under anaerobic conditions many mycoplasmas give a positive tetrazolium reaction and that members of the non-human mycoplasma flora, e.g. *M. gallisepticum, A. laidlawi*, give positive aerobic reduction of tetrazolium. An overlay method has also been described for *M. pneumoniae* (Woods & Smith 1972).

Method for direct detection of M. pneumoniae antigen in respiratory exudates

The principle of the method is described above; plates for the test are prepared as follows:

Antiserum for 'antigen capture'. A rabbit antiserum against *M. pneumoniae* with a titre of

≥2560 in the indirect haemagglutination test (see below) is precipitated three times in 35% (w/v) saturated ammonium sulphate. The precipitated globulin is redissolved in the same volume of PBS pH 7.0 as the original serum and dialysed extensively at 4°C. The globulin fraction is then absorbed with normal human lung homogenate and glutaraldehyde-fixed human serum (Avrameas & Ternynck 1969) – a range of absorbants covering those antigen determinants likely to be present in a sample of human respiratory secretions.

Coating of plates. Duplicate flat-bottomed microtitre wells (Nunc Cat. No. 439454) are coated with antibody diluted in 0.05 mol/l sodium bicarbonate buffer pH 9.6, either at 37°C for 1 h or at room temperature overnight. The dilution of antibody for coating is determined by previous titration in chessboard fashion with a whole-cell *M. pneumoniae* CF antigen. That dilution of antibody which detects antigen at its endpoint ('antigen titre') but is free from non-specific reactions in the absence of antigen, is chosen for coating the wells. In the *M. pneumoniae* system this is about 10 antibody units (i.e. a 1 in 200 dilution of a serum with a titre of 2000), or around 25 μg/ml of protein.

After coating, the unadsorbed antibodies are removed with five washes in PBS pH 7.0 with 0.05% (v/v) Tween 20 (PSB/T). The plates can then be stored for several weeks either at 4°C or −70°C before use.

Test proper. The specimen (a clarified, sonicated sample of nasopharyngeal aspirate) is diluted with an equal volume of diluent buffer (2.5% w/v skim milk in PBS/T) before addition to the wells coated with antibody or pre-immunization serum. After incubation for 2 h at 37°C or overnight at room temperature (or after prior testing for optimal conditions), the unreacted materials are removed by five washes with PBS/T over 10 min.

In a direct enzyme immunoassay (EIA), the enzyme-labelled antibody (diluted in diluent buffer) is then added and incubated at 37°C for 1 h or a predetermined optimal set of conditions.

Before the addition of the substrate, the unreacted labelled antibodies are removed by five washes over 10 min. The enzyme substrate reaction is allowed to proceed at room temperature for 15 min before stopping the reaction with 1 mol/l H_2SO_4. In the indirect EIA, a second antibody (of different animal origin to the primary capture antibody) is reacted with the captured antigen for 1 h at 37°C before addition of an enzyme-labelled antiglobulin.

The colour reaction can be read in an automated spectrophotometer designed for plate reading, and at a wavelength of 490 nm if the enzyme used is horseradish peroxidase or at 405 nm if alkaline phosphatase is used.

The absorbance values may be determined in an automated spectrophotometer designed for plate reading. An absorbance value of 2 is the maximum obtainable in the linear part of the response curve of the instrument.

The amount of antigen 'captured' may be quantitated either in terms of the optical density absorbance measurements (as shown in Fig. 48.7) or expressed as the specific binding % (SB%) from the formula

$$SB\% = \frac{AS \text{ minus } AN}{2} \times 100$$

where AS is the average absorbance value for wells coated with specific antibody and AN is the average absorbance value for wells coated with the negative control serum.

The 'cut-off' value for the SB% that designates a positive or negative test can be determined in various ways. One is to determine that SB% values for a large number (100 plus) of specimens negative on other criteria, such as culture of the organism or serological testing of the patients providing the samples, then to calculate the mean and standard deviation (SD) and take as a 'cut-off' level the mean plus 3 SD.

The system should be calibrated by titration of dilutions of a culture of the mycoplasma to define the sensitivity of the system. Figure 48.7 shows, as an illustration, the curves for relationship between colony-forming units and antigen of *M. pneumoniae* (as well as similar calibrations for an antigen capture system for herpes simplex virus).

Methods for measurement of specific IgM antibody to M. pneumoniae

Detection of M. pneumoniae specific IgM antibody by an indirect solid-phase enzyme immunoassay

For the laboratory equipped with an automated spectrophotometer, the presence of IgM specific antibodies can be detected by coating microtitre wells (preferably those with uniform high binding capacity) with sonicated *M. pneumoniae* whole cell antigen in bicarbonate buffer (pH 9.6) for 2 h at 37°C or overnight at room temperature. The reaction volumes for this assay are 100 μl/well and the washing buffer is PBS with 0.05% Tween 20 (PBS/T). After coating, any unbound sites are blocked with 10% bovine serum albumin-PBS/T at 37°C for 1 h. The wells are washed and the test sera added. The sera are diluted 1 in 200 in 2.5% BSA-PBS/T before addition to the reaction wells. It is preferable to remove any rheumatoid factor in the sera before testing. The test sera are incubated for 1 h at 37°C and then washed at least five times. The appropriate dilution (in 2.5% BSA-PBS/T) of urease-conjugated sheep antihuman IgM (Commonwealth Serum Labs) is then added and incubated for 30 min at 37°C. Before addition of the urea substrate (Commonwealth Serum Labs) the reaction wells are washed three times with washing buffer followed by three washes with distilled water. The distilled water is used to remove the metallic ions which can interfere with the substrate reaction and give spurious results. A purple colour reaction indicates the presence of IgM specific antibody and a yellow colour (unreacted substrate) a negative result. An objective result can be read from an automated spectrophotometer at 588 nm.

Indirect haemagglutination for M. pneumoniae specific IgM antibody

An alternative IgM assay is an antibody capture modification of the indirect haemagglutination (IHA). This indirect haemagglutination assay requires antigen-sensitized sheep erythrocytes and will measure total antibody, i.e. in all immunoglobulin classes, as well as measuring IgG, IgM and IgA specific antibody to *M. pneumoniae*.

Preparation of sheep erythrocytes sensitized with M. pneumoniae antigen. Erythrocytes sensitized with *M. pneumoniae* antigen may be obtained as a kit (Serodia myco kit from Fujirebio Inc., Shirjuku-Ku, Tokyo 161, Japan) or prepared in the laboratory as follows.

The technique was developed with *M. pneumoniae* organisms supplied for the CFT by Wellcome. However, the recent withdrawal of this product means that laboratories will now have to prepare suspensions, preferably by growing the organism on a glass surface (Somerson et al 1967), so as to decrease contamination with serum protein from the growth medium. The organisms are resuspended in 2 ml PBS and sonicated at 4°C in a Branson Sonifier for 10 min with two 1 min cooling intervals. This sonicate is then used at a predetermined dilution (usually 1 in 10) to sensitize tanned sheep red blood cells (SRBC) in the indirect haemagglutination test.

The procedures for fixation, tanning and sensitization for the sheep erythrocytes are essentially those described by Hog & Das (1970). Fresh SRBC are washed 3 times with phosphate-buffered saline (PBS; 0.01 mol/litre, pH 7.2). A 2% (v/v) cell suspension is then made in 1% (v/v) glutaraldehyde. This fixation process is then allowed to proceed by gentle stirring at room temperature for 30 min. The SRBC are then washed 3 times and stored at 4°C until required for tanning. Such fixed SRBC could be stored for up to 6 months, with 0.1% (w/v) sodium azide.

For tanning, a 2% suspension of fixed SRBC is then mixed with an equal volume of freshly prepared tannic acid. The dilution of tannic acid is previously determined by a 'chessboard' titration so as to use the lowest dilution that will not give autoagglutination of the sensitized cells. For most batches of tannic acid, this is usually 1 in 40 000. The mixture is then incubated at 56°C for

30 min with occasional mixing. After tanning, the cells are washed 3 times with PBS.

Sensitization of the tanned cells is then carried out immediately. To a volume of 2% tanned cells is added an equal volume of *M. pneumoniae* sonicate. This is then incubated in a roller drum at 37°C for 1 h. After sensitization the cells are washed 3 times with PBS and a 4% cell suspension is prepared in 2.5% fetal calf serum in PBS (diluent buffer). After 2 days the cells are resuspended in a fresh volume of diluent buffer and then used in the IHA test. Such sensitized cells will store for up to 2 months at 4°C without loss of activity. Before use each time the cells are resuspended in fresh diluent buffer.

Indirect haemagglutination test (IHA). A series of two-fold dilutions of the test sera are made in microtitre trays (25 μl/well) from a starting dilution of 1 in 10. To each well is then added an equal volume of 0.4% *M. pneumoniae* sensitized SRBC (SRBC-Mp). Hence, the final concentration of cells in each well is 0.2% and the first dilution of the serum is then 1 in 20. The plate is read after 2–3 h at ambient temperature or after overnight incubation at 4°C. The latter generally gives a result one doubling dilution higher than that at ambient temperature. An agglutinated mat of cells indicates the presence of specific antibodies; a button of cells at the bottom of the well indicates a negative result. Sera showing a titre of $\geq$ 160 are considered to be serologically positive for *M. pneumoniae*.

Modified IHA test for IgM specific antibodies. To each well of a polystyrene microtitre tray (Linbro, Nunc or Cooke) is added 100 μl of rabbit anti-human μ chain (Dakopatts). The optimal dilution of coating antibody to use is previously titrated. The microtray is then airdried at 37°C and immersed in cold methanol for 10 seconds. The methanol used is previously dried with molecular sieves (Sigma, 3Å) at −20°C as this has been found to give a better fixation of the capture antibody. Two-fold falling dilutions of the patients' sera are then made in the coated cups using diluent buffer. After overnight incubation at 4°C, the tray is then washed three times with PBS, excess fluid drained on a paper towel and to each well is then added 50 μl of 0.2% SRBC-Mp. The plate is left at ambient temperature and read after 1 h. Positive and negative results are read as with the IHA test. With this modified IHA test, it is preferable to use SRBC-Mp cells that were prepared within 2 weeks.

Rheumatoid factor (RF) test. Sera that are positive for IgM specific antibodies to *M. pneumoniae* are also checked for the presence of IgM antibodies (rheumatoid factor) specific for human IgG. The presence of RF is indicated by the agglutination of latex beads coated with human IgG (Commonwealth Serum Labs). Such sera are then absorbed with fixed normal human sera (Avrameas & Ternynck 1969) and then retested for IgM specific antibodies to *M. pneumoniae*.

REFERENCES

Avrameas S, Ternynck T 1969 The cross linking of proteins with glutaraldehyde and its use for the preparation of immunoadsorbents. Immunochemistry 6: 53–66
Barile M F, Razin S, Tully J G, Whitcomb R F (eds) 1979 The Mycoplasmas, vols 1, 2, 3. Academic Press, New York
Biberfeld G 1970 Antibodies to tissue antigens in cases of *Mycoplasma pneumoniae* infection. Acta Pathologica et Microbiologica Scandinavica (B) 78:266
Biberfeld G 1971 Antibodies to brain and other tissues in cases of *Mycoplasma pneumoniae* infection. Clinical Experimental Immunology 8: 319–333
Black F T 1973 Modification of the growth inhibition test and application to human T-mycoplasmas. Applied Microbiology 25: 528–533

Bowie W R, Alexander E R, Floyd J F, Holmes J, Miller Y, Holmes K K 1976 Differential response of chlamydial and ureaplasma associated urethritis to sulphafurazole (sulfisoxazole) and aminocyclitols. Lancet 2: 1276–1278
Brown T M, Swift H F, Watson R F 1940 Pseudocolonies simulating those of pleuropneumonialike microorganisms. Journal of Bacteriology 40: 857–864
Busolo F, Tonin E, Meloni G A 1983 Enzyme-linked immunosorbent assay for serodiagnosis of *Mycoplasma pneumoniae* infections. Journal of Clinical Microbiology 18: 432–435
Cassell G H, Cole B C 1981 Mycoplasmas as agents of human disease. New England Journal of Medicine 304: 80–89

Clyde W A 1964 Mycoplasma species identification based on growth inhibition by specific antisera. Journal of Immunology 92: 958–65

Clyde W A 1971 Immunopathology of experimental *Mycoplasma pneumoniae* disease. Infection and Immunity 4: 757–763

Clyde W A 1979 *Mycoplasma pneumoniae* infections of man. In: Tully J G, Whitcomb R F (eds) The Mycoplasmas, vol II, Human and animal mycoplasmas. Academic Press, New York. p 275–306

Costea N, Yakulis V J, Heller P 1972 Inhibition of cold agglutinins (anti-I) by *Mycoplasma pneumoniae* antigens. Proceedings of the Society of Experimental Biology 139: 476–479

Coufalik E D, Taylor-Robinson D, Csonka G V 1979 Treatment of nongonococcal urethritis with rifampicin as a means of defining the rôle of *Ureaplasma urealyticum*. British Journal of Venereal Disease 55: 36–43

Cracea, E, Botez D, Constantinescu E, Georgescu-Braila M 1982 *Ureaplasma urealyticum* serotypes isolated from cases of female sterility. Zentralblatt für Bakteriologie, Microbiologie und Hygiene 1 AO 252: 535–539

Cross G F, Goodman M R, Shaw E F 1967 Detection and treatment of contaminating mycoplasmas in cell culture. Australian Journal of Experimental Biology and Medical Sciences 45: 201–212

Del Guidice R A, Carski T R 1968 Characterization of a new Mycoplasma species of human origin. Bacteriological Proceedings. p 67

Del Guidice R A, Robillard N F, Carski T R 1967 Immunofluorescence identification of Mycoplasma on agar by use of incident illumination. Journal of Bacteriology 93: 1205–1209

Dienes L 1939 L organism of Klieneberger and *Streptobacillus moniliformis* and other bacteria. Journal of Infectious Diseases 65: 24–42

Dussaix E, Slim A, Tournier P 1983 Comparison of enzyme-linked immunosorbent assay (ELISA) and complement fixation test for detection of *Mycoplasma pneumoniae* antibodies. Journal of Clinical Pathology 36: 228–232

Ebke J, Kuwert E 1972 Detection of *Mycoplasma orale* type 1 in tissue cultures by means of acridine orange stain. Zentrablatt für Bakteriologie Microbiologie und Hygiene 1 AO: 221, 87–93

Fleming P, Krieger E, Watty E I, Quinn P A, Bannatyne R M 1967 Febrile mucocutaneous syndrome with respiratory involvement associated with isolation of *M. pneumoniae*. Canadian Medical Association Journal 93: 1458–1459

Fogh J, Fogh H 1964 A method for direct demonstration of pleuropneumonialike organisms in cultured cells. Proceedings of the Society of Experimental Biology 117: 899–901

Fogh J, Fogh H 1969 Procedures for control of mycoplasma contamination of tissue cultures. Annals of the New York Academy of Sciences 172: 15–30

Freundt E A, Edward D G ff 1979 Classification and taxonomy. In: Barile M F, Razin S (eds) The Mycoplasmas, vol. 1, Cell biology. Academic Press, New York. p 1–41

Gnarpe H, Friberg J 1973 T-mycoplasmas as a possible cause of reproductive failure. Nature 242: 120–121

Hayflick L 1965 Tissue cultures and mycoplasmas. Texas Reports on Biology and Medicine 23: 285–303

Hessling J J, Miller S E, Levy N L 1980 A direct comparision of procedures for the detection of mycoplasma in tissue culture. Journal of Immunological Methods 38: 315–324

Hijmans W, Van Boven C P A, Clasener H A L 1969 Fundamental biology of the L-phase of bacteria. In: Hayflick L (ed) The Mycoplasmatales and the L-phase of bacteria. North-Holland, Amsterdam. p 67–143

Hilwig I, Gropp A 1972 Staining of constitutive heterochromatin in mammalian chromosomes with a new fluorochrome. Experimental Cell Research 75: 122–126

Hodges G R, Fass R J, Saslaws S 1972 Central nervous system disease associated with M. pneumoniae infection. Archives of Internal Medicine 130: 277–282

Hog M S, Das P C 1970 Preparation of human cells for assay of serum fibrinogen degradation products using haemagglutination inhibition. Scandinavian Journal of Haematology Suppl. 13: 10l–106

Hopps H E, Meyer B C, Barile M F, Del Guidice R A 1973 Problems concerning non-cultivable mycoplasma contamination in tissue cultures. Annals of the New York Academy of Sciences 225: 265–276

Horoszewicz J S, Grace J T 1964 PPLO. Detection in cell culture by thymidine cleavage. Bacteriological Proceedings. p 131

Hu P C, Powell D A, Albright F, Gardner D E, Collier A M, Clyde W A 1983 A solid-phase radioimmunoassay for detection of antibodies against *Mycoplasma pneumoniae*. Journal of Clinical and Laboratory Immunology 11: 209–213

Huijsmans-Evers A G, Ruys A C 1956 Microorganisms of the pleuropneumonia group (family of Mycoplasmataceae) in man. II. Serological identification and discussion of pathogenicity. Antonie van Leeuwenhoek 22: 377–384

Jensen K E, Senterfit L B, Chanock R M, Smith C B, Purcell R H 1965 An inactivated *Mycoplasma pneumoniae* vaccine. Journal of American Medical Association 194: 248–252

Kaklamanis E, Thomas L, Stavropoulos K, Borman I, Boshwitz C 1969 Mycoplasmacidal activity of normal tissue extracts. Nature 221: 860–861

Klieneberger-Nobel E 1962 Pleuropneumonialike organisms (PPLO): Mycoplasmataceae. Academic Press, New York

Kok T W, Marmion B P, Vakarnis G, Martin J 1988a Culture of *Mycoplasma pneumoniae* from respiratory exudates on cell monolayers. In preparation

Kok T W, Vakarnis G, Marmion B P, Martin J, Esterman A 1988b Laboratory diagnosis of *Mycoplasma pneumoniae* infection. 1. Direct detection of antigen in respiratory exudates by enzyme immunoassay. In preparation.

Kraybill W H, Crawford Y E 1965 A selective medium and colour test for *Mycoplasma pneumoniae*. Proceedings of the Society of Experimental Biology, New York 118: 965–970

Lemcke R M 1965 Media for the Mycoplasmataceae. Laboratory Practice 14: 712–716

Levine E M 1972 Mycoplasma contamination of animal cell cultures: a simple, rapid detection method. Experimental Cell Research 74: 99–109

Lin J S L, Kendrick M I, Kass E H 1972 Serological typing of human genital T-mycoplasmas by a complement dependent mycoplasmacidal test. Journal of Infectious Diseases 126:658

Lind K 1970 A simple test for peroxide secretion by mycoplasma. Acta Pathologica et Microbiologica Scandinavica (B) 78:256

MacPherson I 1968 Mycoplasmas in tissue culture. Journal of Cell Sciences 1: 145–168

Madoff S 1959 Isolation and identification of PPLO. Annals of the New York Academy of Sciences 79: 383–392

Manchee R J, Taylor-Robinson D 1969 Enhanced growth of T-strain mycoplasmas with N-2-hydroxethylpiperazine-N'-2 ethane sulfonic acid buffer. Journal of Bacteriology 100: 78–85

Marmion B P 1967 The mycoplasmas: new information on their properties and their pathogenecity for man. In: Waterson AP (ed) Recent advances in medical microbiology. Churchill, London

Marmion B P, Plackett P, Lemcke R M 1967 Immunochemical analysis of Mycoplasma pneumoniae. 1. Methods of extraction and reactions of fractions from M. pneumoniae and from M. mycoides with homologous antisera and antisera against Streptococcus MG. Australian Journal of Experimental Biology and Medical Science 45: 163–187

Niitu Y, Hasegawa S, Kubota H 1974 Usefulness of an erythromycin resistant strain of Mycoplasma pneumoniae for the fermentation-inhibition test. Antimicrobial Agents and Chemotherapy 5: 111–113

Plackett P, Marmion B P, Shaw E J, Lemcke R M 1969 Immunochemical analysis of Mycoplasma pneumoniae. 3. Separation and identification of serologically active lipids. Australian Journal of Experimental Biology and Medical Science 47: 171–195

Polley J R, Fanok A G 1973 Inactivation of mycoplasma in seed virus stocks using gamma radiation. Canadian Journal of Microbiology 19: 709–714

Price P C 1983 Direct radioimmunoassay for the detection of IgM antibodies against Mycoplasma pneumoniae. Journal of Immunological Methods 32: 261–273

Purcell R H, Chanock R M 1969 Mycoplasmas of human origin. In: Lennette E H, Schmidt N J (eds) Diagnostic procedures for viral and rickettsial infections, 4th edn. American Public Health Association, New York. ch 23. p 786–825

Purcell R H, Chanock R M, Taylor-Robinson D 1969 Serology of the mycoplasmas of man. In: Hayflick L (ed) The Mycoplasmatales and L-phase of bacteria. North-Holland, Amsterdam. p 221–264

Quinlan D C, Liss A, Maniloff J 1972 Eagles basal medium for Mycoplasma studies. Microbios 6: 179–185

Razin S, Gross M, Wormser M, Pollack Y, Glaser G 1984 Detection of Mycoplasmas infecting cell cultures by DNA hybridization. In Vitro 20: 404–408

Rylance H J, Marr W, Malcolm M G, Stewart S M, Marmion B P 1979 Growth factors for Mycoplasma pneumoniae in yeast and tissue extracts. Journal of Applied Bacteriology 47: 341–345

Schimke R T, Barile M F 1963 Arginine breakdown in mammalian cell cultures contaminated with pleuropneumonialike organisms (PPLO). Experimental Cell Research 30: 593–590

Schneider E L, Stanbridge E J, Epstein C J 1974 Incorporation of 3H-uridine and 3H-uracil into RNA: a simple technique for the detection of mycoplasma contamination of cultured cells. Experimental Cell Research 84: 311–318

Shepard M C 1967 Cultivation and properties of T-strains of mycoplasma associated with nongonococcal urethritis. Annals of the New York Academy of Sciences 143: 505–514

Shepard M C 1969 Fundamental biology of the T-strains. In: Hayflick L (ed) The Mycoplasmatales and L-phase of bacteria. North-Holland, Amsterdam. p 49–65

Shepard M C 1973 Differential method for identification of T-mycoplasmas based on demonstration of urease. Journal of Infectious Diseases 127: Suppl. p 22

Shepard M C, Lunceford C D 1970 Differential agar medium for identification of T-mycoplasmas in primary culture. Bacteriological Proceedings 70:83

Smith C, Sangster G 1972 Mycoplasma pneumoniae meningoencephalitis. Scandinavian Journal of Infectious Diseases 4:69

So A K L, Furr P M, Taylor-Robinson D, Webster A D B 1983 Arthritis caused by Mycoplasma salivarium in hypogammaglobulinaemia. British Medical Journal (Clin Res) 286: 762–763

Somerson N L, James W D, Walls B E, Chanock R M 1967 Growth of Mycoplasma pneumoniae on a glass surface. Annals of the New York Academy of Sciences 143: 384–389

Stanbridge E J 1971 Mycoplasmas and cell cultures. Bacteriological Reviews 35: 206–227

Stanbridge E J, Hayflick L 1967 Growth inhibition test for identification of mycoplasma species utilizing dried antiserum impregnated paper discs. Journal of Bacteriology 93: 1392–1396

Stanbridge E J, Raff M E 1979 The molecular biology of mycoplasmas. In: Barile M F, Razin S (eds) The Mycoplasmas, vol. I, Cell biology. Academic Press, New York. p 157–185

Studzinski G P, Gierthy J F, Cholon J T 1973 An autoradiographic screening test for mycoplasmal contamination of mammalian cell cultures. In Vitro 8: 466–472

Taylor-Robinson D, Csonka G W, Prentice M J 1977 Human intraurethral inoculation of ureaplasmas. Quarterly Journal of Medicine 46: 309–326

Taylor-Robinson D, Furr P M, Hetheringham C M 1982 The pathogenicity of a newly discovered human mycoplasma (strain G37) for the genital tract of marmosets. Journal of Hygiene, Cambridge 89: 449–455

Taylor-Robinson D, McCormack W M 1979 Mycoplasmas in human genitourinary infections. In: Tully J G, Whitcomb R G (eds) The Mycoplasmas. Vol II. Human and animal mycoplasmas Academic Press, New York. p 307–366

Taylor-Robinson D, Manchee R J 1967a Spermadsorption and spermagglutination by mycoplasma. Nature 215: 484–487

Taylor-Robinson D, Manchee R J 1967b Novel approach to studying relationships between mycoplasmas and tissue culture cells. Nature 216: 1306–1307

Taylor-Robinson D, Purcell R H, London W T, Sly D L 1978 Urethral infection of chimpanzees by Ureaplasma urealyticum. Journal of Medical Microbiology 11: 197–201

Taylor-Robinson D, Purcell R H, Wong D C, Chanock R M 1966 A colour test for measurement of antibody to certain mycoplasma species based on the inhibition of acid production. Journal of Hygiene, Cambridge 64: 91–104

Taylor-Robinson D, Somerson N L, Turner H C, Chanock R M 1963 Serological relationships among human mycoplasmas as shown by complement fixation and gel diffusion. Journal of Bacteriology 85: 1261–1273

Taylor-Robinson D, Tully J G, Furr P M, Cole R M, Rose D L, Hanna N F 1981 Urogenital mycoplasma infections of man: a review with observations on a recently discovered mycoplasma. Israel Journal of Medical Science 17: 524–530

Theodore T, Tully J G, Cole R M 1971 Polyacrylamide gel identification of bacterial L forms and mycoplasma species of human origin. Applied Microbiology 21:272

Todaro G J, Aaronson S A, Rands E 1971 Rapid detection of mycoplasma-infected cell cultures. Experimental Cell Research 65: 256–257

Tully J G, Rose D L, Whitcomb R F, Wenzel R P 1979 Enhanced isolation of *Mycoplasma pneumoniae* from throat washings with a newly modified culture medium. Journal of Infectious Diseases 139: 478–482

Tully J G, Taylor-Robinson D, Cole R M, Rose D L 1981 A newly discovered mycoplasma in the human urogenital tract. Lancet 1: 1288–1291

Tully J G, Whitcomb R F, Clark H F, Williamson D L 1977 Pathogenic mycoplasmas: cultivation and vertebrate pathogenicity of a new spiroplasma. Science 195: 892–894

Wolanski B, Maramorosch K 1970 Negatively stained mycoplasmas; fact or artefact? Virology 42: 319–327

Woods L L, Smith T F 1972 Tetrazolium agar overlay in test for *Mycoplasma pneumoniae*. Applied Microbiology 24: 148–149

Chlamydia

Chlamydias are small, obligate intracellular microorganisms; they have a unique growth cycle and their cell walls lack peptidoglycan. They are currently classified with the Gram-negative bacteria within the kingdom Procaryotae, division (phylum) *Gracilicutes*, class *Scotobacteria*, but within their own order *Chlamydiales*, family 1 *Chlamydiaceae*, with one genus, *Chlamydia* and two species: *Chlamydia trachomatis* and *C. psittaci* (Moulder et al 1984). However, the sequences of the 16S rRNA of these 2 species are closely related but are so different from all other Eubacteria that it has been recommended that the chlamydias be placed alone in a new division, as yet unnamed and not fully defined (Weisburg et al 1986; Woese 1987). They stain poorly with the Gram stain, but readily by the Giemsa, Castaneda, Giménez (Giménez 1964) or Macchiavello methods. They have a double stranded DNA genome, prokaryotic type RNA and synthesize their own proteins during their developmental cycle in membrane-bounded vacuoles in the cytoplasm of host cells. However, their synthetic processes are dependent on energy (ATP) and metabolites from the host cell pool.

Two forms of the organism are seen in infected cells. The elementary body (250–300 nm diameter) is the infectious form; the initial or reticulate body (800–1200 nm diameter), with a higher content of RNA, is the metabolically active, non-infectious, fragile form into which the elementary body develops during the multiplication cycle. The reticulate body undergoes a series of divisions by binary fission yielding progeny that are smaller. This culminates in condensation of internal elements, formation of elementary bodies, and their release from the host cell by a phenomenon similar to exocytosis (Todd & Caldwell 1985). The cell wall of the elementary body is somewhat similar to that of Gram-negative bacteria, but contrary to previous reports neither muramic acid (Garrett et al 1974), nor a peptidoglycan layer (Caldwell et al 1981) are present. However, penicillin-binding proteins are present (Barbour et al 1982).

The rigidity of the cell wall of elementary bodies is facilitated and maintained by extensive disulphide cross-linking of the major outer membrane protein (Bavoil et al 1984), which is rich in cysteine, and probably by 3 other cysteine-rich proteins of MW 12, 59 and 62 kilodaltons (Hatch et al 1984). These S-S linkages are not detected in cell walls of reticulate bodies.

There is a major heat-stable complement fixing, genus-specific antigen, extractable from the organism with organic solvents, e.g. ether. This is composed of typical lipopolysaccharide (LPS) components – D-glucosamine, long-chain 3-hydroxy fatty acids, 2-keto-3-deoxyoctanoic acid and phosphate – and resembles enterobacterial LPS of the Re chemotype of *Salmonella* species. It also contains the compound 3-hydroxydocosanoic acid (3-OH C22:0) not previously described in LPS (Nurminen et al 1985).

Chlamydial LPS shares at least two antigenic determinants with the LPS of certain Gram-negative bacteria, e.g. *Acinetobacter calcoaceticus* var. *anitratum*, and Re mutants of *Salmonella* and has at least one immunodominant epitope unique to chlamydias, as demonstrated by reactivity with monoclonal antibodies (Caldwell

& Hitchcock 1984) and in other serological tests (Brade et al 1985). Free chlamydial lipid A has cross reactivity with free enterobacterial lipid A; in the organism both are in the cryptic form, but may be unmasked by acid hydrolysis.

Chlamydias are sensitive to some antibiotics, notably tetracyclines and erythromycin; *C. trachomatis* is sensitive to sulphonamides, but *C. psittaci*, with a few exceptions, is not. Penicillin is chlamydistatic in vitro but is not generally of value in the treatment of human or animal infections.

The two species also differ in structure of the cytoplasmic inclusions, DNA homology, antigenic structure, and most recently, in their 4.4 megadalton plasmid (Peterson & de la Maza 1983).

These organisms cause a wide range of human diseases (see Schachter 1978; and 13th Edn, Vol. 1, Ch. 50).

C. trachomatis causes ocular, respiratory, genital tract, and probably aural infections, lymphogranuloma venereum (LGV), and some cases of endocarditis, and perihepatitis.

Ocular infections take the form of inclusion conjunctivitis in adults or neonates, or trachoma (a more severe condition potentiated by repeated reinfection and probably by secondary infection with bacteria). Genital infections include non-gonococcal or post-gonococcal urethritis, clinical or subclinical cervicitis, epididymitis and salpingitis. A chronic pneumonitis in the newborn has been described (Beem & Saxon 1977).

Species, subspecies and serovar specific antigens have been delineated among *C. trachomatis* strains with the aid of monoclonal antibodies (Stephens et al 1982a), and have been shown to be predominantly associated with the major outer membrane protein which clearly differs between chlamydial species.

Within *C. trachomatis* there are three biovars: (1) Biovar I with 3 serovars, L_1, L_2 and L_3, which cause LGV; (2) Biovar II with 12 serovars A–K, including Ba, which cause ocular, genital and associated infections (Grayston & Wang 1975); and (3) Biovar III which comprises the aetiological agent of mouse pneumonitis, the only animal pathogen classified within this species.

C. psittaci causes psittacosis, and occasionally conjunctivitis and myocarditis in man, and infections associated with abortion, arthritis, conjunctivitis, encephalomyelitis, enteritis and pneumonitis as well as latent infections in many species of animals and in birds (Meyer 1967). Recently, a new group of *C. psittaci* (called TWAR strains) has been isolated from cases of mild pneumonia in man (Saikku et al 1985; Grayston et al 1986); no avian or animal reservoir has yet been identified.

Strains of *C. psittaci* have proved more difficult to divide satisfactorily than have strains of *C. trachomatis*. However, to date, eight biotypes have been identified by the morphology of the inclusions in cell culture, and by the effect of diethylaminoethyl-dextran (DEAE-D) and cycloheximide in facilitating cellular infection (Spears & Storz 1979). These biotypes correlated well with serotypes delineated recently by the indirect micro-immunofluorescence test (Perez-Martinez & Storz 1985).

Both species grow in the yolk sac of the chick embryo. Avian *C. psittaci* and LGV strains grow readily in several cell lines. Other *C. psittaci* and *C. trachomatis* strains require centrifugation with or without metabolic inhibition of cells to facilitate growth. *C. trachomatis* strains form inclusions in a few cell lines only. TWAR strains grow poorly in both yolk sac and cells.

SPECIMENS FOR LABORATORY DIAGNOSIS

For microscopy. Smears from the conjunctiva, nasopharynx, endocervix, urethra or middle ear of patients with suspected *C. trachomatis* infections are prepared on clean microscope slides; material should be evenly spread over an area no greater than 1 cm diameter. Cells for smears from eye infections may be obtained by scraping or vigorous swabbing, with or without local anaesthetic, of the upper (in trachoma) or lower conjunctiva (in inclusion conjunctivitis) and fornices.

For culture. Swabs or scrapings from the appropriate mucosal surface taken as above are placed in transport medium – namely 0.5 ml sucrose phosphate saline (2SP; Gordon et al

1969; 0.2 mol/l sucrose in 0.02 mol/l phosphate buffer pH 7.2) or sucrose potassium glutamate (SPG; Bovarnick et al 1950; 0.218 mol/l sucrose; 0.038 mol/l KH_2PO_4; 0.0072 mol/l K_2HPO_4; 0.049 mol/l potassium glutamate, pH 7.0). To these transport media may be added antibiotics – gentamicin (20 μg/ml), vancomycin (100 μg/ml), amphotericin B (50 μg/ml). Other variants include 5% fetal calf serum (FCS) or bovine serum or bovine serum albumin fraction V, with/without 0.05 mol HEPES (N-2-hydroxyethyl-piperazine-N-2-ethanesulfonic acid) buffer and 2–3 glass beads (2–3 mm diameter). Cotton-tipped aluminium (Medical Wire) and rayon-tipped wooden swabs are more satisfactory – less inhibitory to chlamydias and less toxic to cells – than calcium alginate-tipped aluminium and cotton-tipped wooden swabs (Mårdh & Zeeberg 1981).

Other specimens include blood and sputum from human cases of psittacosis, biopsy or autopsy tissues from avian or other mammalian species infected with *C. psittaci*, bubo pus, biopsied lymph nodes and genital tract specimens from LGV cases (Schachter & Dawson 1979). Note that specimens must not be put into viral or mycoplasmal transport medium which contains penicillin.

Specimens should be inoculated immediately into cell cultures (Ngeow et al 1981) or kept at 4°C if sent to the laboratory within 24 h. If longer storage is needed, this should be at −60°C or in liquid nitrogen (−196°C); the material is taken down to −60°C at a slow rate of one to three degrees C per min.

For antibody studies. Paired sera, or eye or genital tract secretions collected with cellulose sponges or swabs, or nasopharyngeal aspirates or swabs collected 2 weeks apart may be stored at or below −20°C until titrated for antibody.

LABORATORY PROCESSING OF SPECIMENS

Smears for microscopy

Smears should be air dried, fixed appropriately according to the stain to be used, then stained by the Giemsa, Iodine or Hoechst 33258 methods (Salari & Ward 1979) or by immunofluorescence (IF) or immunoperoxidase (IP). Specific antigens in inclusions, or elementary bodies may be demonstrated by IF (Nichols et al 1963; Lewis et al 1972) or inclusions by IP (Woodland et al 1978); in either instance use can be made of polyclonal (Nichols et al 1963) or monoclonal antibodies (Tam et al 1982, 1984). The preparations are then examined for chlamydial inclusions within epithelial cells (Colour plates 13–15, Vol. 1, 13th Edn, facing p. 538); note that only at certain stages of the developmental cycle do inclusions of *C. trachomatis* stain with iodine.

Giemsa staining

For optimal results with the Giemsa method it is important that batches of stain are tested against positive material before use. The air dried smear is fixed in absolute methanol for 5–10 min then placed into Gurrs R66 Improved (BDH) or other tested batch of Giemsa stain which is appropriately diluted in Sorenson's buffer, pH 6.8 (508 ml 0.07 mol/l KH_2PO_4 plus 492 ml 0.07 mol/l Na_2HPO_4). Details of a method for preparation of Giemsa stain are given at the end of the chapter.*

The slide can be inverted on the stain in a Petri dish or placed vertically in a staining jar to avoid stain precipitate on the smear. After staining (time determined according to thickness of smear) the slide is rinsed in buffer then quickly in methanol to remove excess stain and differentiate the preparation, then returned to buffer, dried and examined microscopically.

Attention is paid to the type of cell in the exudate. Chlamydial infections, particularly adult inclusion conjunctivitis, give a mixed cellular exudate containing mononuclear and polymorphonuclear leucocytes as well as the epithelial cells which contain cytoplasmic chlamydial inclusions. If inclusions are not found, smears containing less than 100 epithelial cells are considered 'unsatisfactory' (Nichols et al 1963). The exudate of a chlamydial infection differs from that of an adenovirus or herpes virus

---

* Refer to *Methods* at end of this chapter.

conjunctivitis in which the cells are predominantly mononuclear, and also from that of allergic conjunctivitis or vernal catarrh in which eosinophils may be seen. In trachoma, in addition to the polymorphonuclear leucocytes, lymphocytes, mature plasma cells and macrophages may be present; Leber cells or large macrophages with phagocytosed debris may also be seen. The examination of Giemsa smears from suspected ocular infections is both time-consuming – 30 min per smear – and insensitive (Nichols et al 1963). Detection of inclusions in scrapings from urethra or cervix by Giemsa staining is even less satisfactory.

Immunofluorescence (IF) staining

Alternative methods rely on detection of inclusions by IF with polyclonal antiserum from hyperimmunized animals (Nichols et al 1963), or inclusions and elementary bodies with monoclonal antibodies (Tam et al 1984). Several commercial kits are now available and have proved rapid, sensitive methods for the diagnosis of these infections – elementary bodies appear as small, solid, round, green-yellow particles. These kits utilize monoclonal antibodies against either species or genus-specific antigens, e.g. MicroTrak, Syva; Imagen, Boots-Celltech; Chlamyset, Orion (Krech et al 1985; Francis & Abbas 1985; Parkinson 1985). Care must be taken however in the interpretation of these tests in that false positive reactions may arise from the binding of Protein A of many *Staphylococcus aureus* strains to the Fc piece of the monoclonal antibody, or by cross reactions with certain Gram-negative bacteria. This non-specific binding can be blocked with normal human serum (Krech et al 1985).

Iodine staining of glycogen in C. trachomatis inclusions

This technique is rapid and effective with heavily infected material, e.g. smears from neonatal inclusion conjunctivitis. However, it is not satisfactory with material from the genital tract. It may also be used to detect inclusions in cell cultures (see below) although some cells such as HeLa 229 may have accumulations of glycogen that lead to problems of interpretation. Cell monolayers or air dried smears are fixed in absolute methanol or in 10% (v/v) formalin (4% formaldehyde) saline and stained in 5% iodine in 10% potassium iodide for 5 min (Gordon et al 1969). A coverslip is placed over the slide which is examined as a wet mount.

Antigen detection on solid phase

Chlamydial antigen may be detected using solid-phase antigen capture methods. Specific polyclonal (Jones et al 1984) or monoclonal antibody (Hambling & Kurtz 1985) is adsorbed to wells in a plastic plate or to polystyrene beads and a detector system of anti-*C. trachomatis* antibody coupled to an enzyme such as horseradish peroxidase or urease (see Chs 10 and 48) used to detect specific binding to *C. trachomatis* elementary bodies or antigens. These tests appear to be of similar sensitivity and specificity to culture of the organism in cells, provided precautions to monitor non-specific reactions, 'false positives', are employed (Hambling & Kurtz 1985). They also appear to be equivalent to detection of elementary bodies by direct monoclonal IF (Caul & Paul 1985). Commercial kits employing this approach are available, e.g. Chlamydiazyme, Abbott; IDEIA Chlamydia test, Boots Celltech.

Culture of the organism

Chlamydias are highly infectious human pathogens and laboratory infections are not uncommon. Therefore, attempts at their isolation, especially *C. psittaci*, should only be undertaken in laboratories with suitable isolation/containment facilities (see Ch. 15). Although *C. trachomatis* strains are less infectious, laboratory infections have occurred. Furthermore cross-contamination of specimens during attempts at culture of the organism has given rise to considerable confusion.

Aseptic technique is required throughout all isolation procedures and suitable disinfection procedures must be followed.

Specimens collected by swab should be shaken

for approximately 1 min on a Vortex mixer, or sonicated (Gordon et al 1969). Tissues taken at autopsy, or sputum, should be homogenized or shaken with glass beads in sucrose potassium glutamate (SPG; see above) containing 20 μg/ml gentamicin, and centrifuged at 500 g for 5 min to remove cellular debris, then stored at $-60°$C until tested.

Cell cultures are the most sensitive and convenient host cells for the isolation of chlamydias; mice and the yolk sac of embryonated eggs may be useful for the isolation of *C. psittaci* and LGV strains. The yolk sac is particularly useful when large quantities of organisms are required, e.g. for seed stock for inoculation of cells, preparation of antigens for serological tests or immunization of animals for antisera.

Method A: Cell cultures

Mycoplasma-free, untreated, irradiated or metabolically inhibited McCoy cells (Gordon et al 1972; Schachter et al 1978; Evans & Taylor-Robinson 1979; La Scolea & Keddell 1981; Yoder et al 1981), HeLa 229 cells (Croy et al 1975), BHK cells (Taverne & Blyth 1971; McComb & Puzniak 1974) or 'Buffalo' green monkey (BGM) cells (Hobson et al 1982) may be used for isolation of *C. trachomatis*. For the isolation of *C. psittaci* McCoy cells (Hobson et al 1977), L929 or BGM cells are satisfactory (Hobson et al 1982; Grice & Brown 1985). In fact, most continuous lines of epithelial cells are probably able to support the growth of *C. psittaci*. Centrifugation of the inoculum on to culture monolayers is essential to achieve maximum infectivity especially with *C. trachomatis* serotypes A–K (Gordon & Quan 1965a; Darougar et al 1974) and generally with non-avian *C. psittaci* strains (Storz 1971). The addition of non-essential amino acids to Eagles minimum essential medium (MEMNE) as basic medium for growth (GM) and maintenance (MM) of cells obviates the need for additional treatment (e.g. with DEAE-dextran, etc.) of McCoy and HeLa 229 cells. Cycloheximide 0.5–2 μg/ml in MM prevents continued multiplication of host cells, and allows maximum multiplication of elementary bodies and therefore ease of identi-

fication of chlamydial inclusions (Ripa & Mårdh 1977) but is inhibitory to certain biotypes of *C. psittaci* (Spears & Storz 1979; Grice & Brown 1985); 5–8% fetal calf serum (FCS) in MM allows development of increased numbers of elementary bodies per inclusion; temperature (35–37°C depending on the strain), and pH must be maintained at optimal levels (Rota & Nichols 1973).

Preparation of untreated cell culture monolayers. 1. Inoculate flat-sided flask or bottle with cells in GM – Eagles MEMNE (Cat. No. F15, Grand Island Biological Company, Grand Island, New York, USA) containing 8% FCS, and either no antibiotics or 20 μg/ml gentamicin. Incubate at 37°C.

2. If confluent monolayer has not developed within 5 days, change GM 2 days before monolayer is required.

3. Remove cells with mixture of 0.05% (w/v) trypsin and 0.02% (w/v) versene (disodium ethylene-diamine-tetra-acetic acid, EDTA) in calcium- and magnesium-free phosphate buffered saline, 10–15 min at 37°C. Resuspend cells in GM, then dilute to 4 × 10^5 cells/ml.

4. Dispense in 0.5 ml volumes per 5 ml flat-bottomed polystyrene vial or bijou bottle (Sterilin) containing 12–13 mm glass coverslip.

5. Incubate at 37°C for 18–30 h to allow cells to adhere to glass and to form monolayers.

Basic method for inoculation of cell cultures.
1. Decant GM from vials, replace with 0.25 ml GM.

2. Add 0.2–0.3 ml specimen to each of two vials.

3. Centrifuge horizontally for 1 h at 35°C in a Sorvall RC-3 centrifuge at 3700 g or at higher g if available and breakage of vials, bottles or coverslips does not occur (Darougar et al 1974).

4. Incubate at 35°C for 1–2 h to equilibrate, then remove and discard the medium above the cells.

5. Add 1 ml fresh MM (MEMNE containing 5–8% FCS, glucose 0.03 mol/l, 0.5 μg cycloheximide, 100 μg vancomycin, 20 μg gentamicin and 50 μg amphotericin B per ml).

6. Incubate at 35°C for 48–72 h.

7. Stain coverslip from one vial.

Note: Appropriate changes to this technique can adapt it for use with microtitre plates (Yoder et al 1981).

Staining of infected monolayers, and identification of chlamydias. Cells can be stained by iodine (for *C. trachomatis* inclusions only, but in HeLa 229 cells they can be confused with glycogen granules), Giemsa, Giménez, Hoechst 33258, IF or IP techniques. The use of monoclonal antibodies in IF stains increases the sensitivity of detection of inclusions (Stephens et al 1982b).

Recently a rapid staining method using the nuclear staining part of the three part blood staining kit, 'Diff-Quik' (Harleco), has been described (Hardy & Nell 1985).

Inclusions appear as dense collections of small, round, deeply stained particles within a defined area in the cytoplasm – deep brown/black when stained by iodine, deep purple under brightfield and bright yellow under darkfield illumination when stained by Giemsa, deep red by Giménez, bright green/yellow by IF, brown/yellow by IP, green/blue by Hoechst stain and bright yellow under darkfield illumination by 'Diff-Quik'. Care must be taken to distinguish inclusions from non-chlamydial material that can appear as broken inclusions especially in monolayers seeded with genital tract specimens when stained by Giemsa. By incorporating Evans' Blue into the final wash during IF staining non-specific fluorescence can be reduced.

The species of the new isolate can be determined in cell cultures by the appearance of inclusions (Gordon & Quan 1965b) and confirmed by IF with monoclonal antibodies which recognize the species-specific major outer membrane protein antigen of *C. trachomatis* (Stephens et al 1982b). *C. trachomatis* species can be subdivided into 15 serotypes by micro-IF with standard polyclonal type specific (Wang et al 1973; Grayston & Wang 1975) or monoclonal antisera (Wang et al 1985). To date, no standardized system has been defined for subdividing *C. psittaci* strains, although bovine and ovine strains can be separated into type 1 and type 2 by plaque reduction tests (Schachter et al 1975),

and eight biotypes delineated by inclusion morphology and response to diethylaminoethyl-dextran (DEAE-D) and cycloheximide (Spears & Storz 1979). These latter correlate well with groups delineated recently by micro-IF (Perez-Martinez & Storz 1985).

Establishment of a new strain. If the first vial is positive, remove MM from the second, add 0.3 ml SPG, several 2–3 mm diameter glass beads and shake to disrupt and remove cells from coverslip. Dilute at least 1 in 2 in GM and inoculate on to monolayers as previously or place at −60°C until others are available – do not snap freeze. When required thaw quickly at 37°C. If first coverslip is negative, incubate second for a total of 72 h, then pass as described above; a few additional positive cultures will be detected after this 'blind' passage.

Method B: 6–8 day developing chick embryos

1. Inoculate 0.2–0.5 ml suspension of specimen treated with 500 μg/ml gentamicin and 100 units/ml nystatin into the yolk sac of each of six embryos and incubate at 35°C.

2. Candle eggs daily; discard any which die within 48 h.

3. Harvest yolk sacs from embryos which die subsequent to day 2 on the day of death and from those alive 13 days post-inoculation.

4. Make impression smears of yolk sac taken from near the stalk.

5. Fix and stain by Macchiavello, Castaneda, Giemsa* or Giménez methods, IF or with Hoechst 33258.

6. Examine for elementary bodies. The distinction between elementary bodies and yolk sac granules requires substantial experience. A differential staining method is useful, e.g. Macchiavello's stain or its Giménez (1964) modification. Hoeschst 33258 fluorochrome also gives sharp differentiation with an 'empty' background as the yolk sac granules do not contain DNA (Salari & Ward 1979).

7. If the yolk sac is negative homogenize in Tenbroeck grinder or shake vigorously with glass beads. Add SPG containing 500 μg/ml gentamicin equal to the volume of the yolk sac, and

reinoculate at further 1 in 2 and 1 in 20 dilutions into a fresh batch of embryos; attention is drawn to the hazards of cross contamination between batches of embryos in this blind passage procedure.

8. If yolk sacs are positive grind or homogenize, with equal volume SPG, then centrifuge at 500 g for 5 min. Remove middle layer which contains the chlamydias and store at −60°C.

Method C: Mice

1. For the isolation of *C. psittaci* inoculate suspensions in volumes of 0.5 ml intraperitoneally, 0.1 ml intranasally or 0.03 ml intracerebrally, into three 5-week mice. For isolation of LGV, inoculate suspensions in the same volumes intracerebrally into 3-week mice, or intranasally into 5-week mice. (*Note*: For both these routes of inoculation mice must be anaesthetized; see Ch. 14).

2. Check mice daily. At necropsy make an impression smear from the spleens, lungs and brains of mice that die and those killed 7–14 days after inoculation. Appropriate tissues are collected into 2SP or SPG, processed and stored for further passage.

3. Fix and stain smear by Giemsa, Giménez or IF. Examine for presence of inclusions and elementary bodies.

4. Inoculate negative tissues into mice and/or cell cultures (Schachter & Dawson 1979). Examine as above.

SERODIAGNOSIS OF CHLAMYDIAL INFECTIONS

Paired sera from *C. psittaci* infections or LGV may be titrated for antibody by complement fixation (CF) (Schachter & Dawson 1979); note that an indirect CF must be used for avian sera (Karrer et al 1950). Paired sera, secretions and aspirates from patients with any of the chlamydial infections may be titrated for total or class-specific immunoglobulins by micro-IF (Jones & Treharne 1974; Wang et al 1975; Mhyre & Mårdh 1982), inclusion-IF (Collier et al 1972; Richmond & Caul 1975), enzyme-linked immunosorbent assay (ELISA) (Lewis et al 1977; Levy & McCormack 1982), radioisotope precipitation (Gerloff & Watson 1967) or solid-phase radioimmunoassay (RIA) (Meurman et al 1982). Micro-IF, inclusion-IF and ELISA are the most frequently used tests for titration of antibody to *C. trachomatis*. The latter two measure genus-specific antibody. Therefore to test for antibody against *C. trachomatis* the serovar-specific micro-IF test should be used (Forsey et al 1986). This is particularly important since the finding of the TWAR strains of *C. psittaci* which are thought to have a human reservoir, and against which a considerable percentage of some populations has antibody (Saikku et al 1985; Grayston et al 1986). The serotype of antibody against *C. trachomatis* can be determined with micro-IF and RIA.

Note: While the finding of antibodies to *C. trachomatis* in a single serum sample and/or secretions may indicate current infection in certain individuals, such antibodies, in the absence of isolation of *C. trachomatis* are generally of little diagnostic value, because of the widespread presence of these antibodies in many populations. However the finding of specific antibody in the IgM class is probably of greater predictive value for infection than that in IgG (Treharne & Forsey 1983). Very high titres of IgG or IgM antibody against *C. trachomatis* in single nasopharyngeal aspirates or serum of infants may be indicative of *C. trachomatis* pneumonitis (Beem & Saxon 1977).

Immunofluorescence tests for antibody titration

Microimmunofluorescence test (micro-IF)

In this test elementary bodies of the standard serotypes, in pools or singly, are used for titration of antibodies and for the demonstration of type-specific antibody responses (Wang et al 1973), while reticulate bodies can be used as genus-specific antigens (Young et al 1979). Both types of particles are suspended in 3–5% normal yolk sac (Wang et al 1973) or egg-albumin-glycerol (Nisbet et al 1979). Antigens are spotted with fine pen nibs on to clean glass microscope slides, in order and close together. Normal yolk sac 5% is spotted as control to assist in localization of antigen spots during microscopy. Slides are air dried, then fixed in reagent grade dehydrated acetone, 10 min at room temperature.

10 μl of serum/secretions diluted in phosphate buffered saline (FAPBS) pH 7.4,* are placed over each group of antigens. The slides are placed in a humidified box for 30 min at 37°C, washed in FAPBS for 5–10 min, air dried, then an optimal dilution of fluorescein-isothiocyanate (FITC) conjugated anti-species immunoglobulin is placed over each spot, for 30 min at 37°C. Slides are then washed as above. Evans Blue (0.02%) or rhodamine/bovine serum albumin may be added to the last wash as a counterstain. Slides are then air dried, and covered with glycerol-based mounting fluid, pH 8.9,* and a coverslip. Fluorescence is read by UV microscopy and titres taken as the highest dilution giving positive fluorescence.

Inclusion immunofluorescence test (inclusion-IF)

This test utilizes infected cells grown on polytetrafluoroethylene coated slides (Richmond & Caul 1975), and can detect both genus-specific and type-specific antibodies to *C. trachomatis* serotypes.

METHODS
Giemsa stain

Giemsa powder 0.6 g; methanol (acetone free, neutral) 50 ml; glycerine (neutral, freshly opened bottle) 50 ml. Grind powder in mortar before weighing, weigh, grind again with part of the measured glycerine in a clean mortar, pour off the top third into a clean 500 or 1000 ml flask, and add more glycerine, grind again.

Repeat until most of the powder has been mixed and poured into the flask to give a thin layer of stain. Stopper flask with cotton-wool plug, cover with heavy paper and bind with rubber band. Place flask into waterbath at 55–60°C for 2 h. Ensure flask stays upright and level of stain remains under water and shake every 30 min. Use part of the measured methanol to wash last bit of stain from mortar. Pour washings into small airtight bottle, with remainder of methanol. Remove stain from waterbath and allow to come to room temperature. Add methanol and shake well. Store in dark bottle away from light. Stain may be used immediately but it is preferably left 2 weeks with intermittent shaking. Filter through Whatman No. 1 filter paper before use. For use dilute appropriately in buffer pH 6.8 (Sorenson's; see *Giemsa staining* above).

Phosphate buffered saline for immunofluorescence tests (FAPBS)

Prepare stock solutions:

(i) 8.5% (w/v) NaCl, by dissolving 85 g NaCl in 1 litre distilled water;
(ii) 0.67 mol/l KH_2PO_4, by dissolving 90.7 g KH_2PO_4 in 1 litre distilled water;
(iii) 0.67 mol/l K_2HPO_4, by dissolving 116.2 g K_2HPO_4 in 1 litre distilled water.

To prepare 1 litre working solution, mix together: 100 ml stock solution (i); 2.33 ml stock solution (ii); and 11.67 ml stock solution (iii); with 886 ml distilled water. Check that pH is 7.4.

Mounting fluid for immunofluorescence

Mix 0.0715 g $NaHCO_3$ and 0.016 g Na_2CO_3 with 10 ml distilled water, then add glycerol to make a total volume of 100 ml. Check that pH is 8.9.

REFERENCES

Barbour A G, Amano K-L, Hackstadt T, Perry L, Caldwell H 1982 *Chlamydia trachomatis* has penicillin-binding proteins but not detectable muramic acid. Journal of Bacteriology 151: 420–428
Bavoil P, Ohlin A, Schachter J 1984 Role of disulphide bonding in outer membrane structure and permeability in *Chlamydia trachomatis*. Infection and Immunity 44: 479–485
Beem M O, Saxon E M 1977 Respiratory-tract colonization and a distinctive pneumonia syndrome in infants infected with *Chlamydia trachomatis*. New England Journal of Medicine 296: 306–310

Bovarnick M R, Miller J C, Snyder J C 1950 The influence of certain salts, amino acids, sugars and proteins on the stability of rickettsiae. Journal of Bacteriology 59: 509–522

Brade L, Nurminen M, Mäkelä P H, Brade H 1985 Antigenic properties of *Chlamydia trachomatis* lipopolysaccharide. Infection and Immunity 48: 569–572

Caldwell H D, Hitchcock P J 1984 Monoclonal antibody against a genus-specific antigen of Chlamydial species: location of the epitope on Chlamydial lipopolysaccharide. Infection and Immunity 44: 306–314

Caldwell H D, Kromhout J, Schachter J 1981 Purification and partial characterization of the major outer membrane protein of *Chlamydia trachomatis*. Infection and Immunity 31: 1161–1176

Caul E O, Paul I D 1985 Monoclonal antibody based ELISA for detecting *Chlamydia trachomatis*. Lancet 2:279

Collier L H, Sowa J, Sowa S 1972 The serum and conjunctival antibody response to trachoma in Gambian children. Journal of Hygiene, Cambridge 70: 727–740

Croy T R, Kuo C-C, Wang S-P 1975 Comparative susceptibility of 11 mammalian cell lines to infection with trachoma organisms. Journal of Clinical Microbiology 1: 434–439

Darougar S, Cubitt S, Jones B R 1974 Effect of high speed centrifugation on the sensitivity of irradiated McCoy cell culture for the isolation of chlamydia. British Journal of Venereal Diseases 50: 308–312

Evans R T, Taylor-Robinson D 1979 Comparison of various McCoy cell treatment procedures used for detection of *Chlamydia trachomatis*. Journal of Clinical Microbiology 10: 198–201

Forsey T, Stainsby K, Hoger P H, Ridgway G L, Darougar S, Fischer-Brugge U 1986 Comparison of two immunofluorescence tests for detecting antibodies to *C. trachomatis*. European Journal of Epidemiology 2: 163–164

Francis R A, Abbas A H A 1985 Fluorescein-conjugated monoclonal antibodies to detect *Chlamydia trachomatis* in smears. Lancet 2:222

Garrett A J, Harrison M J, Manire G P 1974 A search for the bacterial mucopeptide component muramic acid in Chlamydia. Journal of General Microbiology 80: 315–318

Gerloff R K, Watson R O 1967 The radioisotope precipitation test for psittacosis group antibody. American Journal of Ophthalmology 63: 1492–1498

Giménez D F 1964 Staining rickettsiae in yolk sac cultures. Stain Technology 39: 135–140

Gordon F B, Dressler H R, Quan A, McQuilkin W T, Thomas T I 1972 Effect of ionising irradiation on susceptibility of McCoy cell cultures to *Chlamydia trachomatis*. Applied Microbiology 23: 123–129

Gordon F B, Harper I A, Quan A L, Treharne J D, Dwyer R StC, Garland J A 1969 Detection of Chlamydia (Bedsonia) in certain infections of man. 1. Laboratory procedures: comparison of yolk sac and cell culture for detection and isolation. Journal of Infectious Diseases 120: 451–462

Gordon F B, Quan A L 1965a Isolation of the trachoma agent in cell culture. Proceedings of the Society for Experimental Biology and Medicine 118: 354–359

Gordon F B, Quan A L 1965b Occurrence of glycogen in inclusions of the psittacosis-lymphogranuloma venereum-trachoma agents. Journal of Infectious Diseases 115: 186–196

Grayston J T, Wang S-P 1975 New knowledge of chlamydiae and the diseases they cause. Journal of Infectious Diseases 132: 87–105

Grayston J T, Kuo C-C, Wang S-P, Altman J 1986 A new *Chlamydia psittaci* strain, TWAR, isolated in acute respiratory tract infections. New England Journal of Medicine 315: 161–168

Grice R G, Brown A S 1985 A tissue culture procedure for the isolation of *Chlamydia psittaci* from koalas (Phascolarctos cinereus). Australian Journal of Experimental Biology and Medical Science 63: 283–286

Hambling M H, Kurtz A E 1985 Preliminary evaluation of an enzyme immunoassay test for the detection of *Chlamydia trachomatis*. Lancet 1:53

Hardy P H, Nell E E 1985 A rapid, simple stain for *Chlamydia trachomatis* inclusions. Abstracts. Annual Meeting of American Society for Microbiology C373

Hatch T P, Allan I, Pearce J H 1984 Structural and polypeptide differences between envelopes of infective and reproductive life forms of Chlamydia spp. Journal of Bacteriology 157: 13–20

Hobson D, Lee N, Quayle E, Beckett E E 1982 Growth of *Chlamydia trachomatis* in Buffalo green monkey cells. Lancet 2: 872–873

Hobson D, Johnson F W A, Byng R E 1977 The growth of the ewe abortion chlamydia agent in McCoy cell culture. Journal of Comparative Pathology 87: 155–159

Jones B R, Treharne J D 1974 Micro-immunofluorescence type-specific serological tests for chlamydial infection applied to psittacosis, ornithosis, lymphogranuloma venereum, trachoma, paratrachoma and 'non-specific' urethritis. Proceedings of the Royal Society of Medicine 67: 735–736

Jones M F, Smith T F, Houglum A L, Herrmann J E 1984 Detection of *Chlamydia trachomatis* in genital specimens by the Chlamydiazyme test. Journal of Clinical Microbiology 20: 465–467

Karrer H, Meyer K F, Eddie B 1950 The complement fixation inhibition test and its application to the diagnosis of ornithosis in chickens and in ducks. Principles and technique of the test. Journal of Infectious Diseases 87: 13–23

Krech T, Gerhard-Fsadni D, Hofmann N, Miller S M 1985 Interference of *Staphylococcus aureus* in the detection of *Chlamydia trachomatis* by monoclonal antibody. Lancet 1: 1161–1162

La Scolea L J, Keddell J E 1981 Efficacy of various cell culture procedures for detection of *Chlamydia trachomatis* and applicability to diagnosis of pediatric infections. Journal of Clinical Microbiology 13: 705–708

Levy N J, McCormack W H 1982 Detection of serum antibody to Chlamydia with ELISA. In: Mårdh P-A, Holmes K K, Oriel J D, Piot P, Schachter J (eds) Chlamydial infections. Fernström Foundation Series 2. Elsevier Biomedical, Amsterdam. p 341–344

Lewis V J, Thacker W L, Cacciapuoti A F 1972 Detection of *Chlamydia psittaci* by immunofluorescence. Applied Microbiology 24: 8–12

Lewis V J, Thacker W L, Mitchell S H 1977 Enzyme-linked immunosorbent assay for chlamydial antibodies. Journal of Clinical Microbiology 6: 507–510

McComb D E, Puzniak C I 1974 Micro cell culture method for isolation of *Chlamydia trachomatis*. Applied Microbiology 28: 727–729

Mårdh P-A, Zeeberg B 1981 Toxic effect of sampling

swabs and transportation test tubes on the formation of intracytoplasmic inclusions of *Chlamydia trachomatis* in McCoy cell cultures. British Journal of Venereal Diseases 57: 268–272

Meurman O, Terho P, Sonck C E 1982 Type specific IgG and IgA antibodies in old lymphogranuloma venereum determined by solid-phase radioimmunoassay. Medical Microbiology and Immunology (Berlin) 170: 279–286

Meyer K F 1967 The host spectrum of psittacosis-lymphogranuloma venereum (PL) agents. American Journal of Ophthalmology. Series 3, 63: 1225/199–1246/220

Mhyre E B, Mårdh P-A 1982 Antibody response in psittacosis. In: Mårdh P-A, Holmes K K, Oriel J D, Piot P, Schachter J (eds) Chlamydial infections. Fernström Foundation Series 2. Elsevier Biomedical, Amsterdam. p 345–348

Moulder J W, Hatch T P, Kuo C-C, Schachter J, Storz J 1984 Genus Chlamydia. In: Krieg N R (ed) Bergey's manual of systematic bacteriology Vol 1. Williams and Wilkins, Baltimore USA. Series 2, p 729–739

Ngeow Y F, Munday P E, Evans R T, Taylor-Robinson D 1981 Taking cell cultures to the patient in an attempt to improve chlamydial isolation. British Journal of Venereal Diseases 57:44–46

Nichols R L, McComb D E, Haddad N, Murray E S 1963 Studies on trachoma. II. Comparison of fluorescent antibody, Giemsa, and egg isolation methods for detection of trachoma virus in human conjunctival scrapings. American Journal of Tropical Medicine and Hygiene 12:223–229

Nisbet I T, Graham D M, Ng K, Lunt R A 1979 Preparation of antigens for microimmunofluorescence testing for antichlamydial antibodies. Lancet 2:859

Nurminen M, Rietschel E T, Brade H 1985 Chemical characterization of *Chlamydia trachomatis* lipopolysaccharide. Infection and Immunity 48: 573–575

Parkinson S T 1985 Fluorescein-conjugated monoclonal antibodies to detect *Chlamydia trachomatis* in smears. Lancet 2: 222–223

Perez-Martinez J A, Storz J 1985 Antigenic diversity of *Chlamydia psittaci* of mammalian origin determined by microimmunofluorescence. Infection and Immunity 50: 905–910

Peterson E M, de la Maza L M 1983 Characterization of chlamydia DNA by restriction endonuclease cleavage. Infection and Immunity 41: 604–608

Richmond S J, Caul E O 1975 Fluorescent antibody studies in chlamydial infections. Journal of Clinical Microbiology 1: 345–352

Ripa K T, Mårdh P-A 1977 Cultivation of *Chlamydia trachomatis* in cycloheximide treated McCoy cells. Journal of Clinical Microbiology 6: 328–331

Rota T R, Nichols R L 1973 *Chlamydia trachomatis* in cell culture. 1. Comparison of efficiencies of infection in several chemically defined media, at various pH and temperature values, and after exposure to diethylaminoethyl-dextran. Applied Microbiology 26: 560–565

Saikku P, Wang S-P, Kleemola M, Brander E, Rusanen E, Grayston J T 1985 An epidemic of mild pneumonia due to an unusual strain of *Chlamydia psittaci*. Journal of Infectious Diseases 151: 832–839

Salari S H, Ward M E 1979 Early detection of *Chlamydia*

trachomatis using fluorescent, DNA binding dyes. Journal of Clinical Pathology 32: 1155–1162

Schachter J 1978 Chlamydia infections. New England Journal of Medicine 298: 428–435, 490–495, 540–549

Schachter J, Banks J, Sugg N, Sung M, Storz J, Meyer K F 1975 Serotyping of *Chlamydia*: isolates of bovine origin. Infection and Immunity 11: 904–907

Schachter J, Dawson C R 1979 Psittacosis-lymphogranuloma venereum agents/TRIC agents. In: Lennette E H, Schmidt N J (eds) Diagnostic procedures for viral, rickettsial and chlamydial infections, 5th edn. American Public Health Association Incorporated, Washington, DC. ch 32, p 1021–1059

Schachter J, Dawson C R, Hoshiwara I, Daghfous T, Banks J 1978 The use of cycloheximide-treated cells for isolating trachoma agents under field conditions. Bulletin of the World Health Organization 56:629–632

Spears P, Storz J 1979 Biotyping of *Chlamydia psittaci* based on inclusion morphology and response to diethylaminoethyl-dextran and cycloheximide. Infection and Immunity 24: 224–232

Stephens R S, Tam M R, Kuo C-C, Nowinski R C 1982a Monoclonal antibodies to *Chlamydia trachomatis*: antibody specificities and antigen characterization. Journal of Immunology 128: 1083–1089

Stephens R S, Kuo C-C, Tam M R 1982b Sensitivity of immunofluorescence with monoclonal antibodies for detection of *Chlamydia trachomatis* inclusions in cell culture. Journal of Clinical Microbiology 16: 4–7

Storz J 1971 Cultivation of chlamydial agents in different host media.Chlamydia and chlamydia-induced diseases. Thomas, Springfield, Illinois, USA. p 71–88

Tam M R, Stamm W E, Handsfield H H, Stephens R, Kuo C-C, Holmes K K, Ditzenberger K, Krieger M, Nowinski R G 1984 Culture-independent diagnosis of *Chlamydia trachomatis* using monoclonal antibodies. New England Journal of Medicine 310: 1146–1150

Tam M R, Stephens R S, Kuo C-C, Holmes K K, Stamm W E, Nowinski R C 1982 Use of monoclonal antibodies to *Chlamydia trachomatis* in immunodiagnostic reagents. In: Mårdh P-A, Holmes K K, Oriel J D, Piot P, Schachter J (eds) Chlamydial infections. Fernström Foundation Series 2. Elsevier Biomedical, Amsterdam. p 317–320

Taverne J, Blyth W A 1971 Interactions between trachoma organisms and macrophages. In: Nichols R L (ed) Trachoma and related disorders caused by chlamydial agents. Excerpta Medica, Amsterdam. p 88–107

Todd W J, Caldwell H D 1985 The interaction of *Chlamydia trachomatis* with host cells: ultrastructural studies of the mechanism of release of a biovar II strain from HeLa 229 cells. Journal of Infectious Diseases 151: 1037–1044

Treharne J D, Forsey B J 1983 Chlamydial serology. British Medical Bulletin 39: 194–200

Wang S-P, Grayston J T, Alexander E R, Holmes K K 1975 Simplified microimmunofluorescence test with trachoma-lymphogranuloma venereum (*Chlamydia trachomatis*) antigens for use as a screening test for antibody. Journal of Clinical Microbiology 1: 250–255

Wang S-P, Kuo C-C, Barnes R C, Stephens R S, Grayston J T 1985 Immunotyping of *Chlamydia trachomatis* with monoclonal antibodies. Journal of Infectious Diseases 152: 791–800

Wang S-P, Kuo C-C, Grayston J T 1973 A simplified
method for immunological typing of trachoma-inclusion
conjunctivitis-lymphogranuloma venereum organisms.
Infection and Immunity 7: 356–360

Weisburg W G, Hatch T P, Woese C R 1986 Eubacterial
origin of *Chlamydia*. Journal of Bacteriology
167: 570–574

Woese C R 1987 Bacterial evolution. Microbiological
Reviews 51: 221–271

Woodland P M, El-Sheikh H, Darougar S, Squires S 1978
Sensitivity of immunoperoxidase and immunofluorescence
staining for detecting chlamydia in conjunctival scrapings
and cell culture. Journal of Clinical Pathology
31: 1073–1077

Yoder B L, Stamm W E, Koester C M, Alexander E R
1981 Microtest procedure for isolation of *Chlamydia
trachomatis*. Journal of Clinical Microbiology 13:
1036–1039

Young E C, Chinn J S, Caldwell H D, Kuo C-C 1979
Reticulate bodies as single antigen in *Chlamydia
trachomatis* serology with microimmunofluorescence.
Journal of Clinical Microbiology 10: 351–356

Virology testing in the clinical microbiology laboratory

In the 12th edition of this practical textbook on medical microbiology, then subtitled 'The practice of medical microbiology', there were two chapters on technical aspects of virology – namely 'Cell, tissue and organ culture' and 'Isolation and identification of viruses' – and two chapters giving synoptic accounts of the properties of various groups of DNA and RNA viruses. This treatment was clearly inadequate from the point of view of clinical or medical diagnostic virology as a well developed and rapidly expanding discipline in its own right. However, attempts to update and expand the treatment of virology for the present text soon served to bring home the near impossibility of condensing into half a dozen chapters not only information about a wide range of techniques for viruses ranging from cell and organ culture, small animal and chick embryo inoculation, centrifugation, protein and nucleic acid chemistry, viral immunology, etc., but also that of giving useful information about the systematics and pathogenic properties of the six groups of DNA and 14 groups of RNA viruses that are now recognized to infect man (see Tables 47.1 and 47.2 below). The full treatment of the latter would give a text comparable in length to that dealing with the groups of bacteria in the present volume.

Further, it could be anticipated that even if achieved, a condensed version of the practical aspects of medical virology would be of limited value to the staff of a full-time virus laboratory or virus reference laboratory who are already well served by detailed practical handbooks such

Table 47.1 Characteristics of major DNA viruses. *Key*: . . ., not stated; icosa = icosahedral shape (no. of capsomers); ds, double stranded; ss, single stranded.

Family	Genus	Important human pathogens	Virion			Genome	
			Shape	Size (nm)	Envelope	MW (×10⁶)ᵃ	Configuration
Adenoviridae	Adenovirus	Human adenovirus	Icosa (252)	~80	No	~22	ds, linear
Hepadnaviridae	None established	Hepatitis B virus	Spherical	42	No	1.8	ds, circular
Herpesviridae Subfamilies:							
Alphaherpesvirinae	Simplexvirus Varicellavirus	Herpes simplex virus Varicella zoster virus	Icosa (162)	120–300	Yes	96 100 145 114	ds, linear
Betaherpesvirinae	Cytomegalovirus	Cytomegalovirus					
Gammaherpesvirinae	Lymphocryptovirus	Epstein Barr virus					
Papovaviridae	Papillomavirus	Human papilloma virus	Icosa (72)	55	No	5	ds, circular
Parvoviridae	Parvovirus	Human parvovirus	Icosa (32)	20	No	1.5–2.0	ss, linear
Poxviridae	Orthopoxvirus	Variola (smallpox) Vaccinia	Brick	250 × 200	Yes	110–140	ds, linear
	Parapoxvirus	Contagious pustular dermatitis virus (orf) Milker's node	Oval	260 × 160	Yes	85	
	Unclassified	Molluscum contagiosum	Oval	250 × 200	Yes	. . .	

ᵃ Molecular wt of nucleic acid in daltons

Table 47.2 Characteristics of major RNA viruses. *Key*: icosa, icosahedral shape (no. of capsomers); ds, double stranded; ss, single stranded

Family	Genus	Important human pathogens	Virion Shape	Virion Size (nm)	Virion Envelope	Genome MW ($\times 10^6$)[a]	Genome Configuration
Arenaviridae	Arenavirus	Lassa virus	Spherical	~120	Yes	3–5	ss, circular 2 molecules Negative stranded[b]
Bunyaviridae	Bunyavirus Phlebovirus Nairovirus	Bunyamwera virus Rift Valley fever virus Crimean Congo haemorrhagic fever virus	Spherical	~100	Yes	4–7	ss, circular 3 molecules Negative stranded
	Hantavirus (proposed genus)	Hantaan virus					
Caliciviridae	Calicivirus	Norwalk (probable member of genus)	Icosa (32 cup-like depressions)	35–39	No	2.6	ss, linear 1 molecule Positive stranded
Picornaviridae	Enterovirus	Poliovirus 1–3 Coxsackie virus A1–22, 24; B1–6 Echovirus 1–9, 11–27, 29–34 Human enterovirus 68–71 Hepatitis A virus (entero 72)	Icosa (32)	22–30	No	2.5	ss, linear 1 molecule Positive stranded
	Rhinovirus	Human rhinovirus 1–113					
Coronaviridae	Coronavirus	Human coronaviruses	Spherical	100	Yes	6	ss, linear 1 molecule Positive stranded
Flaviviridae	Flavivirus	Yellow fever virus Dengue virus 1–4 St Louis encephalitis virus Australian encephalitis virus	Icosa	40–50	Yes	4	ss, linear 1 molecule Positive stranded
Togaviridae	Alphavirus	Chikungunya virus O'Nyong-Nyong virus Ross River virus Sindbis virus Eastern, Western, Venezuelan encephalitis viruses	Spherical	60–70	Yes	4	ss, linear 1 molecule Positive stranded
	Rubivirus	Rubella virus	Spherical	50–70	Yes	2.5–3	
Orthomyxoviridae	Orthomyxovirus	Influenza virus A–C	Spherical or filamentous	~120	Yes	5	ss, linear 8 molecules Negative stranded
Paramyxoviridae	Morbillivirus	Measles virus		100–250	Yes	5–7	ss, linear 1 molecule Negative stranded
	Paramyxovirus	Mumps virus Parainfluenza virus 1–4	Spherical	100–600 150–200			
	Pneumovirus	Respiratory syncytial virus		150–300			
Retroviridae	Oncovirus	Human T cell leukaemia virus, I, II	Spherical	~100	Yes	4–6	ss, linear diploid Positive stranded
	Lentivirus	Human immunodeficiency virus	Spherical	100–140	Yes	4	
Reoviridae	Rotavirus	Human rotavirus	Spherical Icosa	60–80	No	12–15	ss, linear 11 molecules
Rhabdoviridae	Lyssavirus	Rabies virus	Bullet-shaped	75 × 180	Yes	4	ss, linear 1 molecule Negative stranded
Filoviridae (proposed family)		Ebola virus Marburg virus	Filaments	80 × 14 000 (max)	No	4	ss, linear 1 molecule
Not established	Not established	Delta agent	Spherical	36	No	0.5	ss, circular 1 molecule

[a] Molecular wt of nucleic acid in daltons
[b] i.e. sense of strand relative to messenger RNA

as that of Grist et al (1983), Lennette & Schmidt (1979), or the series on Methods in virology by Maramorosch & Koprowski (1967–84) supplemented by exhaustive summaries of the properties of vertebrate virus groups such as that prepared by Andrewes et al (1978), Belshe (1984) or Fields (1985).

To whom, therefore, should a few chapters on virology in a textbook of practical bacteriology be directed and what should they cover? Clearly, the target is not the specialist virus laboratory. In determining content, it is perhaps worth considering the present practices and policies of medium-sized state or private microbiological laboratories in respect of virological testing and the division of work between them and the local virus reference laboratory. A historical perspective on the evolution of virus testing in the microbiology laboratory may assist. In the earliest days of diagnostic virology, tests were confined to the isolation of a limited number of viruses in experimental animals and to performing serological tests – mostly complement fixation tests (CFT) – with a limited range of antigens. Work with experimental animals was costly and laborious and the problems of antigen preparation from the organs of infected animals were substantial, particularly the anticomplementary effects from the local antibody response in the animal. These diagnostic approaches had little impact on the microbiology laboratory or the ward and remained the province of the research or virus reference laboratory.

In the 1940s and 1950s, after some pioneer work in the the 1930s, the scope of diagnostic virology was increased by the wider use of the chick embryo (CE) for virus propagation; more virus groups could be grown and, as importantly, potent antigens, free from anticomplementary activity, became available for the serodiagnosis of diseases such as influenza, herpes simplex, smallpox, some arboviruses and so on. The mainstay of the virus diagnostic laboratory then became CE culture and serodiagnosis on serial samples of serum from the patient. During this period also, inoculation of suckling mice for the isolation of Coxsackie A and B viruses was added to the techniques deployed.

However, these advances were still not of great interest to the general microbiological laboratory, as they remained costly and laborious, even though in some instances, e.g. with herpes simplex virus, they could yield a result in time to influence case management.

In the late 1950s, cell or tissue culture was introduced – or reintroduced – for virus culture and resulted in the recognition of many new groups of viruses and the intensive development of viral molecular biology and viral immunology. Specialist medical virology laboratories changed the direction of their diagnostic approach at this point. Reliance was placed primarily on the culture of viruses in cells with specimens taken during the acute illness and less, or secondary, attention was paid to serodiagnosis; nevertheless the latter remained a valuable discriminatory measure to distinguish virus-related disease from a transient carriage of virus; it was also a necessary quality control of the efficiency of cell culture in detecting a high proportion of cases of infection. In some instances, e.g. with poliovirus from faeces, or herpes simplex virus from a skin lesion or brain biopsy, the speed of cell culture and provisional identification was comparable to or even faster than the culture of common bacterial pathogens on agar plates.

Microbiology laboratories began to be involved at this stage, and some undertook cell culture with a continuous cell line such as HeLa for the isolation of certain enteroviruses, adenovirus or herpes simplex virus; however, the workflow of virological tests in the bacteriological laboratory did not approach that of agar plate culture for bacterial pathogens. Some microbiological laboratories also started to test for viral antibody, often in relation to a special hospital requirement, e.g. screening for cytomegalovirus antibody in renal patients or rubella antibody testing in the maternity hospital. These developments were much assisted by the emergence of firms set up initially to provide viruses and antisera to research institutes, and subsequently able to supply the general microbiology laboratory with reagents of a type previously prepared 'in house' by the specialist virology laboratory.

However, it was not until the late 1960s and early 1970s that technical advances took place that significantly involved the general microbiological laboratory in virus diagnostic testing. The first of these was the recognition of hepatitis B surface antigen in the serum of acute and chronic cases of hepatitis B. Antigen was detected first by gel diffusion and later by radio-immunoassay(RIA); techniques that gave an answer within hours or a day and were of clear value in case management. It is true, of course, that smallpox and chickenpox had been diagnosed in the laboratory by gel diffusion techniques some years previously, but these were specialized applications of less interest to the microbiology laboratory. The clinical advantages of the rapid detection of antigen as a diagnostic measure, as exemplified by hepatitis B, also served to emphasize the importance of the pioneer work of Gardner & his colleagues (see Gardner & McQuillin 1980) in the direct virus diagnosis (DVD) of respiratory and other virus infections by antigen detection with immuno-fluorescence (IF) techniques. The commercial availability of potent, specific IF conjugates and viral antisera enabled this approach to be adopted by the microbiology, as well as virology, laboratory. These approaches with IF tests have been supplemented with antigen detection by enzyme immunoassay (EIA) and may eventually be supplanted by the latter.

A second development was the detection by electron microscopy (EM) of rotavirus virions in the stools of children with gastroenteritis, another direct test providing information of immediate clinical relevance. Again, the electron microscope had been used previously to detect smallpox and vaccinia virions in skin lesions or even respiratory viruses in the nasopharynx. However, the detection of rotavirus had a wider clinical appeal. The use of EM with simple negative contrast staining was soon extended to detect adenovirus, Norwalk agent and other viruses in faeces, and to the detection of those of herpes, molluscum contagiosum, orf, cowpox and milker's nodes in skin lesions.

A third development was the recognition that the (usual but not invariable) rapid rise and fall of specific IgM antibody during a virus infection could in many instances be exploited to speed up serodiagnosis and to provide presumptive evidence of a current virus infection by the examination of a single serum specimen, rather than the 'paired' sera used previously. Complement fixation tests for viral antibodies, which mostly measure IgG antibody, become positive later in the disease. In circumstances when only a convalescent phase serum is available, it may be difficult to distinguish specific IgG antibody from a recent or a past infection. After the application of EIA to the measurement of IgM antibodies to hepatitis A virus there has been a steady expansion of the availability of EIA-based direct or μ-chain capture kits to measure specific IgM antibody to various virus antigens.

Thus, at the end of this evolutionary process, we arrive at a repertoire of virological tests from which medium-sized hospital, state or private laboratories may implement those most suited to their needs. The full repertoire comprises three categories, namely (1) direct detection of infectious agents – usually as antigen – in specimens taken from a variety of sites; (2) serodiagnosis either by examination of paired sera or by the detection of specific IgM antibody in a single sample, and finally (3) diagnosis by virus culture.

Direct detection methods are commonly applied to hepatitis B virus, rotavirus, respiratory syncytial virus and other upper respiratory viruses, herpes simplex virus and some non-bacterial pathogens such as chlamydia and *Mycoplasma pneumoniae*, using commonly available kits or reagents. Hepatitis B testing can usually be restricted to surface antigen detection, leaving antibody, other antigen and DNA tests to the specialist virus laboratory. The complement fixation test is still the most frequently employed serodiagnostic method, making use of readily available commercial antigens. However, for specific applications other tests may be performed, such as haemagglutination-inhibition or single radial haemolysis for the detection of rubella antibodies. Commercially available EIA kits may also be utilized for the detection of specific IgM or IgG antibodies to a limited range of viruses such as hepatitis A, cytomegalovirus and rubella. With regard to virus culture, a suitable continuous cell line such as HeLa, Hep-2 or Vero may be chosen, with the specific intention of detecting commonly isolated pathogens such as herpes simplex virus and respiratory syncytial virus, and perhaps some enteroviruses (e.g. poliovirus). From time to time, the culture system may be supplemented by primary monkey kidney cells or primary human fibroblasts from commercial sources, in order to extend the range of viruses detected.

Those tests which are required infrequently, or those which need more specialized technology, fall outside the scope of the general microbiology laboratory, and requests for these are diverted to a specialist virus laboratory. Examples of such tests are the culture of fastidious viruses such as rubella or the human retroviruses, the isolation and identification of a full range of respiratory viruses, enteroviruses or arboviruses, the serodiagnosis of less commonly sought pathogens, and tests involving nucleic acid hybridization such as probing for human papilloma viruses in biopsy material. Confirmatory tests are also the province of the full-time virus laboratory.

Whether serological screening for human immunodeficiency virus (HIV) infection is performed by the virus section of a regional microbiology laboratory, or by a reference centre, depends largely on the view taken by the nation's health authorities. When centralization of testing is not required, as in the UK, it may be appropriate for a general microbiology laboratory to provide this service using one of the various readily available EIA kits. However, HIV antibody positive samples should be forwarded to a reference virus laboratory for confirmation of the result.

It is important to realize that a limited approach to laboratory diagnosis of virus infections has potential pitfalls. For example, if the diagnosis of herpes simplex infection is based solely on antigen detection without the inoculation of cell cultures, there will be no quality control of the efficiency of the antigen detection method (which typically might be expected to detect about 85% of specimens that are culture positive). Low rates of efficiency may arise, for example, from poor specimen collection or manufacturing failures with kits. It is therefore necessary to make periodic comparisons of the results of direct testing with the 'gold standard' of either culture of the virus, when feasible, or

the serological response of the patient, or both. Most antigen detection systems require between 10^4 and 10^6 infective particles per ml to give a positive result (see Ch. 48) whereas 1–10 particles will infect a cell culture. In practice, direct detection methods work well because the number of virions or amount of free unpackaged antigen in the inflammatory exudate is frequently high. Nevertheless, the microbiology laboratory should make arrangements with the local virus reference laboratory for periodic testing of specimens in parallel by various techniques to gain the requisite quality assurance for their antigen detection methods.

Against this background, the chapters on virological testing that follow have been restricted to consideration of (1) *direct virus diagnosis* (DVD), (2) *serological testing*, with a guide to reagents and kits available from commercial sources and (3) some notes on the handling of *continuous cell lines*.

The remainder of this introductory chapter is concerned with diagnostic approaches in virology, with the choice, recording, processing and storage of specimens and their reporting, and finally with the general organization of the virology section of the microbiology laboratory.

LABORATORY DIAGNOSIS OF VIRUS INFECTIONS

The diagnosis of a virus infection can be established in several ways, often used together, namely:

1. Direct methods such as (a) the cytological or histological examination of cells from the site of the infection in those viral infections in which a characteristic viral cytopathic effect (CPE) is produced (Ch. 48); and (b) the direct detection of virus particles, viral antigen or viral nucleic acid in specimens taken from the appropriate site (Ch. 48).

2. The demonstration of the presence of the virus in appropriate specimens by culture in cells, animals or chick embryos.

3. By serological tests to demonstrate an antibody response to one of a range of known viral

antigens during the course of the patient's illness (Ch. 49). Less frequently, in special circumstances, the development of a cell-mediated immune response to a particular virus rather than antibody may be measured by lymphocyte proliferative response, inhibition of macrophage migration, or by skin test reactions to viral antigen.

The effective use of these laboratory diagnostic approaches is heavily dependent on knowledge of the pathogenesis of viral or non-bacterial infections. It is especially important to be aware of the changing locations and amounts of virus at different stages of the illness and of the patterns of antibody response in the various immunoglobulin classes.

For example, in some acute respiratory infections such as influenza, parainfluenza or respiratory syncytial virus infection, virus is present in the respiratory tract – and in particular in the nasopharynx, the source of most clinical specimens – for only 2–5 days around the onset of illness, although antigen may be demonstrable for a few days longer. Consequently, sampling must be undertaken as soon as possible after onset of illness if culture is to have much chance of success. In contrast, with acute adenovirus infections, while early sampling of the nasopharynx is still desirable, virus may be isolated from the faeces for a longer period than from the nasopharynx; so both faecal and upper respiratory samples should be collected. In this type of acute infection at a mucosal surface, antibody mostly develops some 8–12 days after onset of illness; the documentation and spacing of serial specimens of sera must take account of this pattern. However, during some infections, such as the systemic disease Q fever, CF antibody, predominantly in the IgG class, may rise more slowly and not be detected until 20–30 days after onset. Immunofluorescence (IF) tests for specific IgM antibody to *C.burneti* (Ch. 44) may give a positive result at an earlier stage than the CF, 10–15 days after onset; a knowledge of these differences is critical in planning the investigation of the patient.

Many systemic virus infections have a different pathogenesis that in sequence involves entry of the virus at a body surface, some local replication of virus, then viraemic spread to an internal 'target' organ; viral cytopathic or immunologically mediated damage to the latter signals the onset of clinical disease. These diseases have a longer incubation period and by the time the patient presents to the doctor the virus may have been cleared from the portal of entry and from the blood and be limited to an inaccessible internal organ. In addition, the antibody response may have reached a plateau so that sequential serum samples reveal an unchanging level. This result may be construed as evidence of exposure to the virus concerned, but does not distinguish between a current or a past infection. In some cases, virus-specific IgM tests may be available to help resolve this dilemma.

Two illustrations of the interrelation of pathogenesis and sample collection may be given. The first is *hepatitis A*. The virus (provisionally classed as enterovirus 72) enters the body through the oropharynx or gut. After a viraemic phase in the second part of the incubation period – demonstrated in the early experiments with human volunteers – it reaches the liver cells. Experiments performed in a chimpanzee model show that virus multiplies in the liver without producing disease until the cells are damaged by the emerging immune response to virus antigens expressed on the cell surface. Despite its enterovirus-like properties, evidence that it multiplies in the cells of the intestine is lacking, although virions are present in the faeces and are presumably excreted from the liver into the gut through the bile.

The incubation period of the disease is about a month and the acute onset of general symptoms and hepatitis marks the start of the immunologically mediated damage. At this stage, when the patient presents to the doctor, the laboratory diagnostic approaches are based on the pattern of events just described. Although the faeces may be examined for virus (virions by EM; antigen by EIA), at this stage the number of virions in the faeces is declining rapidly. A direct approach to detection of virus in liver biopsy specimens is limited by the immune clearance of antigen from the liver and, more importantly, by the dangers of liver biopsy in acute hepatitis. Fortunately, serodiagnosis is an effective option and hepatitis A is a good example of a virus disease in which serological tests offer a quicker and more sensitive diagnostic strategy than DVD or virus culture. At the time when hepatitis or jaundice is clinically evident, specific IgM antibody has developed in the majority of patients; this can be detected by EIA or RIA, and lasts for some months after the illness before declining. Specific IgG antibody develops more slowly and an increase in antibody titre can in fact be demonstrated by CFT or other complement-based tests such as immune adherence. The latter tests are of less clinical value than the detection of specific IgM antibody; measurement of specific IgG antibody is however of value as an indicator of past infection and consequent immunity.

A second example with some variations on the theme is that of *poliomyelitis*. Here again, the virus enters by the oropharynx and gut and probably multiplies in the gut-associated lymphoid tissue and reaches the blood stream via the draining lymphatic nodes or thoracic duct. The viraemia occurs during the incubation period of the clinical disease (c. 2 weeks) and is of no diagnostic use to the virus laboratory. In a small minority of patients the blood-borne virus infects the anterior horn cells of the spinal cord and the cells of the motor cortex; cytopathic action in these cells gives rise to the onset of clinical disease (poliomyelitis). Minor, abortive forms of poliovirus infection may take the form of a 'flu-like' illness or aseptic meningitis.

The approach to laboratory diagnosis of paralytic poliomyelitis can only be direct (i.e. examination of the target organ) in fatal cases of the disease or in circumstances in which brain biopsy has been done for other reasons. Polio-virus can be isolated from brain or spinal cord, albeit with difficulty (perhaps the result of masking of virus by antibody); curiously, it is rare to isolate poliovirus from lumbar CSF, in contrast to other enterovirus infections. In fact, the best source of virus is the faeces; excretion of virus, unlike that of hepatitis A, is prolonged and may last for a fortnight or more from the onset of illness. However, polioviruses, particularly live vaccine strains (oral poliovirus vaccine), are found from time to time in the

faeces of healthy persons or those with clearly unrelated diseases. Thus, the coincidence of atypical or equivocal paresis and an unrelated transient gut carriage of virus may give rise to substantial problems of clinical interpretation (see Melnick et al 1979 on the problems of association of enteroviruses with disease). In other words, the conclusion that a poliomyelitis-like illness is caused by poliovirus, because the latter has been isolated from the faeces, is not one of absolute certainty.

Nor may serological examinations resolve this problem. Rising CF or neutralizing antibody titres may be found in children experiencing a first and severe infection. However, in older patients who already have antibody to one or other of the serotypes of poliovirus or to other enteroviruses, the heterotypic CF antibody response may be boosted and be high or unchanging at the time of serum sampling; it may therefore be difficult to obtain clear evidence of a current infection with the prevalent virus or that isolated from the patient's gut.

It is hoped that these examples of the wide variation in host-virus relationships that have such an important bearing on strategies for virus laboratory diagnosis will stimulate the reader to make a systematic survey of this aspect. Excellent accounts of the pathogenesis and pathology of human virus infections are given in the latest edition of the textbook by White & Fenner (1986) as well as in the text by Mims & White (1984).

Choice of specimens for laboratory diagnosis of virus infections

From the foregoing, it should be clear that the principles for the optimal selection of specimens for virus diagnosis are fairly simple and are apparent as answers to 4 questions, namely: (1) Where is the virus at this stage of the disease; is the site accessible without invasive measures or is it necessary to sample some secondary site? (2) Can virions, antigens or specific nucleotide sequences be detected at the lesion site? (3) Can the virus be grown readily in cell culture (e.g. herpes simplex virus or enterovirus), or is it slow growing (e.g. varicella-zoster virus), or not presently cultivable (e.g. hepatitis B virus)? (4) What are the kinetics of the antibody response in the suspected disease and is it necessary to collect 'paired' sera or will measurement of specific IgM antibody in a single sample suffice? The answers to these questions differ from one virus group to another.

Some of the important human viruses, together with their characteristics, have been listed in Tables 47.1 and 47.2 because there have been a number of important changes in virus classification since the appearance of Volume 1, 13th Edition in 1978. In Tables 47.3 and 47.4, an attempt has been made to list some of the

clinical associations of these viruses, and to indicate the optimal diagnostic methods for each. The information contained in these tables is not intended to be exhaustive, and only the most commonly used tests for a particular agent are included. The diagnostic tests for many of the viruses listed are normally performed only by the specialist virus laboratory, but nevertheless, they have been included for completeness. Bold print type has been used to mark first line tests. Those particularly suitable for deployment in the general microbiology laboratory are marked with an asterisk.

In practice, patients rarely present with clinical

Table 47.3 DNA viruses causing disease in man and outline of their laboratory diagnosis. *Key*: Ag, antigen detection; EM, electronmicroscopy; NA, nucleic acid probe; . . ., not in routine use; *, suitable for use in a general microbiology laboratory. First line tests are indicated in bold.

Virus	Disease in man	Laboratory diagnosis		
		Direct	Cell or other culture	Serology
Human adenovirus	Acute respiratory disease Conjunctivitis Gastroenteritis (40,41) Cystitis, urethritis (11,21,37)	**Ag, EM**	**Many cell types***	**Paired sera***
Hepatitis B virus	Hepatitis Chronic liver disease Hepatocellular carcinoma	**Ag*, NA** (HBV DNA)	None	**Paired sera (HBsAg) Specific IgM (HBcAg)**
Herpes simplex virus	Herpes simplex	**Ag*, EM**	**Many cell types***	Limited use
Varicella zoster virus	Chicken pox	**EM, Ag**	**Human fibroblasts**	Limited use
Cytomegalovirus	Cytomegalic inclusion disease	. . .	**Human fibroblasts**	**Paired sera**
	CMV mononucleosis	. . .		**Specific IgM**
Epstein Barr virus	Infectious mononucleosis	. . .	. . .	**Paired sera – Paul Bunnell***
	Burkitt's lymphoma	Ag	Lymphocyte transformation assay	
	Nasopharyngeal carcinoma	Ag		**Specific IgM (VCA)**
	Lymphoproliferative disease	. . .		**Specific IgA (VCA)**
Human papilloma virus	Warts Cervical carcinoma in situ?	NA, EM, Ag Histology	None	Limited use
Human parvovirus	Aplastic crisis	Ag		
	'Fifth' disease	Ag	None	**Specific IgM**
	Abortion?	**NA, Ag** (fetal tissue)		
Variola (smallpox), vaccinia virus (*Note*: Variola – group 4 pathogen)	Smallpox, vaccinia	**EM, Ag**	**Many cell types Chick embryo Chorioallantoic membrane**	Paired sera
Contagious pustular dermatitis virus (orf)	Orf	**EM**	. . .	Paired sera
Molluscum contagiosum	Molluscum contagiosum	**EM**	. . .	. . .

Table 47.4 RNA viruses causing disease in man and outline of their laboratory diagnosis. See *Key* to Table 47.3

Virus	Disease in man	Laboratory diagnosis		
		Direct	Cell or other culture	Serology
Lassa fever virus	Fever, myalgia, hepatitis, shock	Ag	**Vero cells**	Paired sera and specific IgM
Bunyamwera virus	Fever, myalgia and rash	. . .	Many cells especially Vero	**Paired sera**
Rift valley fever virus	Fever and myalgia	. . .	Many cells especially Vero	**Paired sera and specific IgM**
Crimean congo haemorrhagic fever virus	Haemorrhagic fever	. . .	Newborn mice	**Paired sera and specific IgM**
Hantaan virus *Note*: above are Group 3 or 4 pathogens	Rodent-borne nephropathy	. . .	Not routinely practicable	**Paired sera and specific IgM**
Norwalk	Gastroenteritis	**EM**, Ag	None	Paired sera
Polioviruses	Paralysis, meningitis, febrile illness	. . .	**Many cell types**	Paired sera
Coxsackie A viruses	Herpangina, hand foot and mouth disease, meningitis, haemorrhagic conjunctivitis (A24), exanthem, paralysis	. . .	**Suckling mice Rhabdomyosarcoma cells**	Paired sera
Coxsackie B viruses	Pleurodynia, meningitis, severe systemic disease (neonates), pericarditis, myocarditis, exanthem, febrile illness	. . .	**African green monkey kidney cells**	Paired sera and specific IgM
Echoviruses	Meningitis, paralysis, exanthem, myalgia, myocarditis, severe systemic disease (neonates)	. . .	**Human fibroblasts**	Paired sera
Enteroviruses 68–71	Pneumonia (68), haemorrhagic conjunctivitis (70), paralysis (70,71), hand foot and mouth disease (71)	. . .	**Human fibroblasts**	Paired sera
Hepatitis A	Infectious hepatitis	. . .	Not routinely practicable	**Specific IgM***
Rhinoviruses	Common cold	. . .	**Human fibroblasts**	
Coronavirus	Common cold	**Ag**	Not routinely practicable	Paired sera
Yellow fever virus	Fever Hepatic and renal failure	. . .	Specialized cells, mice	**Paired sera and specific IgM**
Dengue virus	Fever, myalgia, rash ± haemorrhage	Ag		
Australian encephalitis virus	Encephalitis	. . .		
Alphaviruses *Note*: many of above are Group 3 pathogens	Fever, arthritis, encephalitis	. . .	Suckling mice, many cells including insect cells	**Paired sera and specific IgM**

Rubella virus	German measles, arthritis, congenital malformation, progressive panencephalitis	. . .	RK13 cells	**Paired sera* Specific IgM antibody**[a]
Influenza viruses	Influenza, pneumonitis	**Ag**	**Primary monkey kidney cell Madin-Darby canine kidney Chick embryo**	**Paired sera***
Measles	Measles, giant-cell pneumonia, encephalitis, SSPE	**Ag**	Primary monkey kidney Primary human kidney	**Paired sera***
Mumps	Parotitis, epidydimo-orchitis, meningitis, encephalitis	. . .	Primary monkey kidney	**Paired sera***
Parainfluenza 1–3	Croup (types 1 and 2), bronchitis in infants (type 3), coryza, pharyngitis	**Ag***	**Monkey kidney cells**	**Paired sera***
Respiratory syncytial virus	Bronchiolitis in infants, rhinitis, pharyngitis	**Ag***	**Many cells especially Hep-2*, HeLa**	Paired sera
HIV	AIDS and related syndromes	Ag	Specialized, peripheral blood lymphocytes	**Presence of antibody is used to indicate exposure***
Rotavirus	Infantile gastroenteritis	**Ag*, EM**	None	**Paired sera**
Rabies virus *Note*: Group 3 pathogen	Rabies	**Ag, Histology**	Many cell types	. . .
Ebola, Marburg *Note*: Group 4 pathogens	Haemorrhagic fever	**Ag, EM (liver)**	**Vero cells**	**Paired sera and specific IgM**
Delta agent	Hepatitis when co-infecting or superinfecting HBV	**Ag, NA**	None	**Paired sera**

[a] Specific IgM antibody for rubella should be determined in reference laboratory.

symptoms and signs that point unequivocally to a single causative virus. More commonly they exhibit a syndrome which may be due to one of several different infective agents. For example 'influenza' or acute respiratory disease may result from infection with not only influenza virus but also adenovirus, parainfluenza virus, respiratory syncytial virus, coronavirus, rhinovirus and a number of other pathogens, including bacteria, although it is conceded that there may be fine points of difference in the clinical presentation or the epidemiological circumstance that will point to the involvement of one particular agent. It follows therefore that a broad approach is necessary and samples should be collected for DVD, cell culture and for serological tests in most instances. Even if the

virology section of the microbiology laboratory does not intend to culture for virus, the specimen can be retained frozen or refrigerated (cf. RSV) for onward transmission to the virus laboratory if DVD yields equivocal results.

In general, specimens collected for these purposes take the form of (1) swabbings of lesion sites (e.g. skin, throat) with swab heads transferred to viral transport medium, (2) scrapings of lesions to obtain infected cells (e.g. base of vesicles, corneal ulcers), (3) aspirates of secretions or exudates (e.g. from posterior nasopharynx, conjunctiva, cervix), (4) excreta such as urine or faeces and (5) biopsy specimens obtained by needle aspiration, open exploration or endoscopy from liver, kidney, heart, lung, brain or intestine. Details of the choice and collection of these specimens are given in the Chapter on DVD (Ch. 48). A portion of the specimen can be put aside for virus culture and processed as described in the notes on cell and virus culture techniques for the microbiological laboratory (Ch. 50).

Serum samples are obtained by collection of 10 ml of blood into a dry sterile container. If virus isolation is to be attempted from peripheral blood leucocytes, heparinized blood is collected and the cells are separated as described in Chapter 48.

The collection and transportation of virological specimens is also described by Madeley (1977).

DOCUMENTATION OF REQUESTS AND RECEPTION OF SPECIMENS

Request forms

Certain basic information is required on the request form in order to ensure unequivocal identification of the patient (viz., surname, given name, sex, date of birth and record number for hospital inpatients), and of the sender or so-called 'requester' (viz., printed name, practice address or hospital and ward, telephone number and signature). In addition, space is provided for a description of the specimen (e.g. clotted blood, urine, etc.), the date of request, the date and time of collection and finally brief clinical information and provisional diagnosis. Of special importance in the interpretation of many virology tests is the date of onset of the illness; a separate box should be provided for this information. A space is normally reserved for a laboratory number stamped, entered with a stamping machine or preprinted on a label; if the request form is to be used as a worksheet, a space is normally reserved for 'laboratory use only' – not infrequently on the reverse of the form.

Figure 47.1 shows one possible example of a request form; it has been designed to aid the requester not only to choose the appropriate

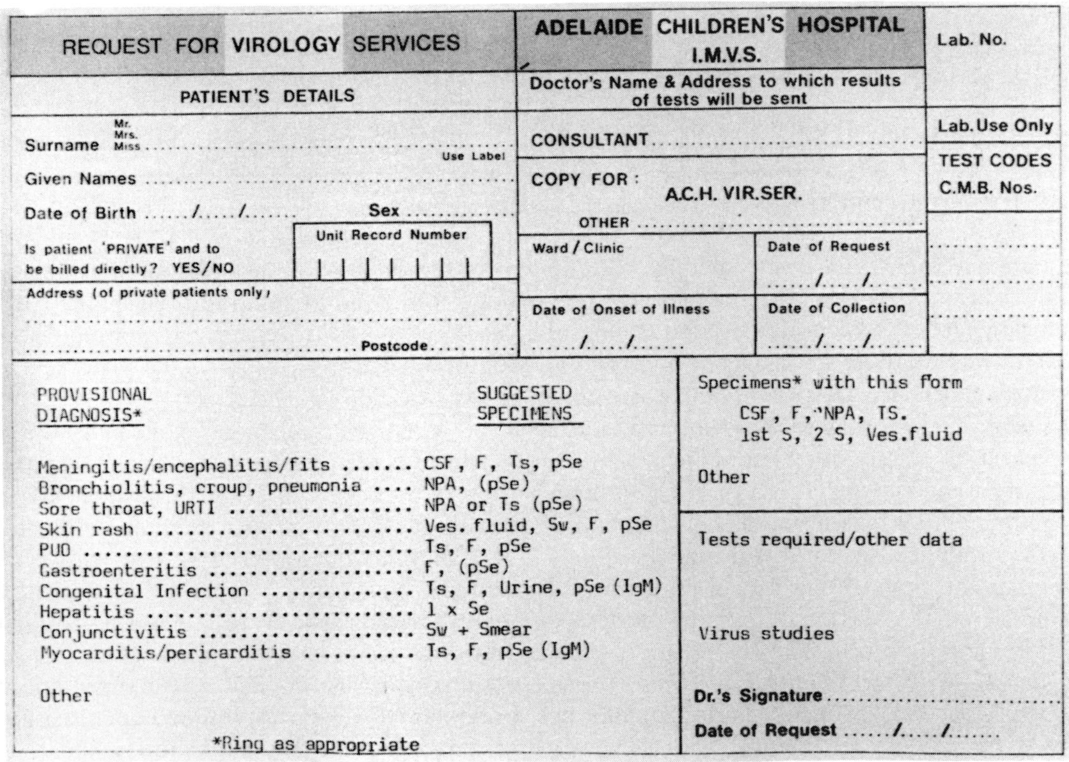
REQUEST FOR VIROLOGY SERVICES

ADELAIDE CHILDREN'S HOSPITAL
I.M.V.S.

Lab. No.

PATIENT'S DETAILS

Surname Mr. Mrs. Miss ....
Use Label
Given Names ....
Date of Birth ....../....../...... Sex ....
Is patient 'PRIVATE' and to be billed directly? YES/NO
Unit Record Number
Address (of private patients only)
....
.... Postcode..........

Doctor's Name & Address to which results of tests will be sent
CONSULTANT..........
COPY FOR: A.C.H. VIR.SER.
OTHER ....
Ward / Clinic
Date of Request ....../....../......
Date of Onset of Illness ....../....../......
Date of Collection ....../....../......

Lab. Use Only
TEST CODES
C.M.B. Nos.

PROVISIONAL DIAGNOSIS* — SUGGESTED SPECIMENS

Meningitis/encephalitis/fits .... CSF, F, Ts, pSe
Bronchiolitis, croup, pneumonia .... NPA, (pSe)
Sore throat, URTI .... NPA or Ts (pSe)
Skin rash .... Ves. fluid, Sw, F, pSe
PUO .... Ts, F, pSe
Gastroenteritis .... F, (pSe)
Congenital Infection .... Ts, F, Urine, pSe (IgM)
Hepatitis .... 1 x Se
Conjunctivitis .... Sw + Smear
Myocarditis/pericarditis .... Ts, F, pSe (IgM)

Other

*Ring as appropriate

Specimens* with this form
CSF, F, NPA, TS.
1st S, 2 S, Ves.fluid
Other

Tests required/other data

Virus studies

Dr.'s Signature..........
Date of Request ....../....../......

Fig. 47.1 Possible request form for virology services.

specimens for investigation, but also to reduce the writing required by a format of 'ring' or 'delete' entries. Other examples of request forms are given by Grist et al (1983).

It is sad to record that the collection of specimens and the completion of request forms by medical or nursing staff often leaves much to be desired; indeed the date of onset of illness is one of the most closely guarded secrets! Our experience shows that better samples are obtained if a specially trained sister or laboratory worker visits the wards, collects the specimens – or is present when the doctor collects a sample requiring special invasive techniques (e.g. liver biopsy) – and documents them according to agreed procedures. A specimen collector is also invaluable in obtaining blood samples from children (constant practice is important) and in ensuring that samples are transmitted promptly to the laboratory in the hospital or via the courier service if the laboratory is at a distance.

Reception of specimens

In the context of the present discussion, it is assumed that the area for reception of specimens will serve for both bacteriological and virological samples.

For safety reasons a separate room or a partitioned area is used for the reception of specimens. This room should be located at the entrance to the department in order to avoid unnecessary traffic through or past test areas. The main function of the reception area is to unpack and record the arrival of specimens. It is often found useful to record on the original request form both the day and time of arrival of the sample, and an automatic 'clock' stamp is frequently used to simplify this task.

On arrival at the laboratory, each specimen is allocated a unique laboratory accession number, most conveniently by utilizing a pad of self-adhesive labels preprinted with numbers in replicate; a stamp machine capable of repeating the same number several times may also be used. Labels with the number are attached to the sample, to the original request form and, if a daybook is kept, one is placed alongside the patient's name or code number and date of birth

in the book. Additional labels with the unique number are required for any other containers, such as serum bottles, into which all or part of the specimen may be transferred. Note however, that while containers labelled in this way are satisfactory for the immediate period of testing when the containers are held at 4°C or at room temperature, they are less satisfactory for long-term storage of virus culture specimens or sera at −20°C or lower temperatures. For the latter purpose, typed labels on white zinc oxide tape which do not come away from the container during freezing and thawing may be used; the typed number remains legible when moist. The strips of tape may be placed on cleared X-ray film for insertion into the typewriter and can be cut to size on the film (but note dangers of sharp points). The need to store samples in the frozen state is a special requirement of virological testing; not only is it necessary to store sera so that acute and convalescent samples can be tested in the same test run, but samples for culture may need to be re-examined if there is a question of laboratory contamination from another sample. Practice in this regard differs from that in the bacteriological or clinical chemistry laboratory which are geared to 'test and discard'.

Many laboratories now use micro or mainframe computers to file patient data and for reporting and billing. Typically, the name, date of birth, sex and hospital record number (or other unique identification) are entered together with the name of the person submitting the sample for examination. The address and telephone number of the requester may be entered or a preformed file may, for example, hold the names, addresses and telephone numbers of all private or general practitioners. Data regarding the specimen include the laboratory accession number, the type of specimen (e.g. blood, swab, cervical smear, etc.), the date of collection and the date of arrival at the laboratory. The date of onset of illness is a valuable additional item. These items need to be entered into the computer file as soon as possible after the specimen arrives, particularly if the computer is also used to generate worksheets.

In our opinion, data entry is best performed

by properly trained clerks, rather than by technical or scientific staff. The location of the computer terminal should be adjacent to, but not in the same room as, the reception area. A convenient system is to provide a hatch through which unpacked forms, with the laboratory accession number allotted, can be passed for registration. After registration, the forms are usually sorted into baskets corresponding to the laboratory section which will perform the test, and either taken to that section along with the specimens, or immediately filed if the computer is used for all further data recording.

Safe handling of virus specimens in the reception area

Specimens are frequently received which are inadequately labelled, so as to make the identification of the source unreliable. Reception staff should be instructed to inform the sender (if identified) that an unlabelled specimen appears to be associated with their request, and that the sample will be discarded. Exceptions to this rule should be made only if the specimen is difficult to replace (e.g. CSF or bone marrow). If such specimens are processed, a clear statement should accompany the report, indicating the possibility of misidentification of the patient.

Whole blood specimens require centrifugation and transfer of serum into a separate container. This may or may not be performed in the reception area, according to the number of specimens processed by the laboratory each day and the facilities available. When the throughput is high, it is often preferred that reception is kept as a 'clean' area; in other words, specimens are unpacked but never opened, and serum separation is performed in the individual sections of the laboratory. Whether blood is centrifuged in the reception area or not, a suitable sealed-bucket centrifuge must be used to guard against accidental breakage of a container; after spinning, many virology laboratories now transfer the serum from the original bottle into new containers inside a safety hood.

Workers in the reception area are the first laboratory staff to handle incoming material. Unless such staff are properly trained in appro-

priate safety precautions, they are at risk of acquiring an infection during the course of their work, particularly from broken or leaking specimen containers or sharp points (needles) or blades contaminated from specimens. It is a general principle in virology laboratories that all specimens are regarded as potential sources of infection; it is prudent for reception staff to wear light plastic gloves (disposable) when handling specimens. Gloves must be removed and discarded if the staff member leaves the reception area, and also before handling the telephone or stationery.

Laboratory outbreaks of hepatitis B, and more recently the world pandemic of AIDS, have stimulated renewed interest in safety in all types of pathology laboratories because, although the infectivity of the majority of specimens from hepatitis and AIDS patients is probably low, the consequences of infection are grave. Blood is one of the body fluids in which hepatitis, HIV and other infectious agents are found, and is also the most likely type of specimen to arrive having leaked from its container. A large proportion of virology tests are performed on blood samples, and in view of the importance of preventing laboratory acquired infection of any kind, it is vital that reception staff are given clear instructions on how to deal with a leaking specimen.

Most hospitals and laboratories have issued instructions about the secure bagging of specimens and request forms, and the use of biohazard stickers.

In general, those specimens which have leaked into the plastic bag surrounding the container should be discarded, and the sender should be informed and asked to send another sample. As with unlabelled specimens, exceptions may be made, at the discretion of senior laboratory staff, to accept specimens which are difficult to replace. In this situation, special arrangements with staff in the relevant laboratory section must be made, in order to ensure that the sample is retrieved while the contaminated container and bag are disposed of in a safe manner.

If the leak is not confined to the plastic bag, or if a leaking specimen was not placed in a bag initially, then reception staff are required to decontaminate, safely, areas of spillage. Again, a clear protocol is required, and all new reception staff should be shown how to deal with a contaminated surface. A 'spillage kit' must be at hand, containing an absorbent cloth and a wash bottle filled with a disinfectant suitable for all kinds of surface. Two commonly used disinfectants are 70% (v/v) ethanol and 2% (v/v) glutaraldehyde, both of which rapidly inactivate a wide range of bacteria and viruses, including HIV. Hypochlorite solution (5000 p.p.m. available chlorine) may also be used, except on metal. All disinfectants, particularly relatively unstable ones like glutaraldehyde, should be replaced regularly.

In order to register the arrival of a leaking specimen and inform the sender of its disposal, the information supplied on the request form is required. If the form has become soiled, a common procedure is to place it, using gloved hands or forceps, inside a clear plastic bag and photocopy it, before throwing it into the infected waste container.

The transport from a single point of origin of a large number of specimens inside a single plastic bag should be strongly discouraged. In this situation, a single leaking container can lead to wastage of all the specimens in the bag. The leak may also not be apparent until the bag has been opened, unnecessarily exposing the staff to a potential source of infection.

When a particular sender initiates a large number of requests, the most satisfactory transport system is to provide racks to keep the blood bottles upright, and to stow the racks inside a sturdy insulated container provided with a carrying handle.

Safety in the virus laboratory is discussed at length, with references to working party reports and codes of practice, by Grist et al (1983), by Pike & Richardson (1979) and by Flewett (1980); see also the discussion of safety in the microbiology laboratory in Chapter 15. Attention is also drawn to the need for collection and storage of a serum from each new member of staff as a 'base line' for subsequent exposure to infection and to the need for vaccination against hepatitis B, poliomyelitis and rubella.

REPORTING VIROLOGY RESULTS

The format of reports prepared by the virology section of a clinical microbiology laboratory will probably adhere as far as possible to that used for microbiology. There are certain differences, particularly relating to the need with serological tests to retrieve results obtained with earlier specimens of serum and reprint them along with those from current tests. Recording systems may either be manual – results are held on worksheets and transferred by typing or photocopying to preprinted report forms (examples shown in Grist et al 1983) – or the collation of results and printing of the report forms can be done through the computer utilizing a commercial data base or programmes generated 'in house'. Computerization of reporting has many advantages, after the inevitable teething problems have been overcome. Test results can be matched up with patient data entered at the time of receipt of the specimen; the file with records of all results can be called up for interpretation while answering telephone enquiries.

Results can either be entered into the computer by laboratory staff as they are generated by test runs or they can be placed on a computer assembly form (Fig. 47.2) which is passed to the data entry staff along with the original request form. The two forms are eventually filed together. The computer assembly form has not only the test values entered on it; it also has references to a set of standard interpretive comments held on computer file, and identified by codes of numbers or combinations of letters (so-called mnemonics). The laboratory staff circle the most appropriate code on the assembly form and the data entry staff have merely to key in the chosen code to have the comment printed on the report form. The code is also printed on the report form so that, if required, the input data on the assembly can be rapidly checked with the report by first scanning the test values and then second checking that the code on the assembly form and the report correspond.

Figure 47.3 shows, as examples, the results of tests on paired sera for CF antibody to various

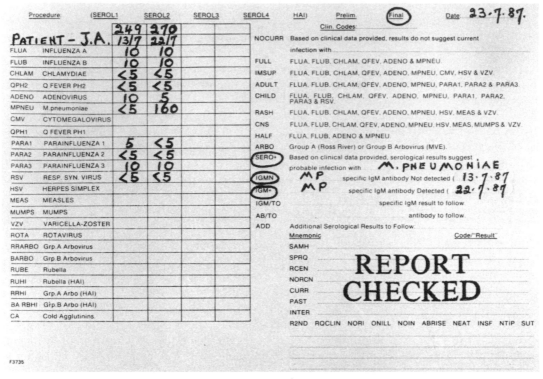

Fig. 47.2 Example of an assembly form for entry of serological tests for certain virus infections into the computer. The form contains both the test results and a signal to use an interpretive comment, held on computer file, and printed as part of the report. After use, the forms are attached to the request form and filed as 'back up' for the information held on computer file. The form above has been completed with the results of tests on paired sera from a patient with respiratory illness caused by *Mycoplasma pneumoniae*. As the illness might have been due to any one of a number of agents, the sera have been tested with a range of viral and nonbacterial antigens.

virus antigens and the format of a report based on these results.

Pre-coded comments generally cover around 90% of reporting situations; obviously 'inspired' comments will be required from time to time and may be generated by the senior technical or the medical staff. Experience shows, however, that complete reliance on inspired comments for every test entry is not only time-consuming but also there are frequently transcription errors at the time of entry of the data into the computer.

OTHER ASPECTS OF THE ORGANIZATION OF A VIROLOGY SECTION IN THE CLINICAL MICROBIOLOGY LABORATORY

Workflow and space

Depending on specimen load, virus work of the scope envisaged above will mostly require two medium-sized laboratories (40 square metres each) with attached offices for maintenance of laboratory records and paper work, reference books, telephone and computer terminal for entry of results and generation of work sheets. These functions should be separated from specimens, test kits and the working bench surface as far as possible.

The flow of work is divided into (1) DVD and simple cell culture in one laboratory and (2) virus serological testing in the other. There is of course some overlap between functions and the division is not absolute. DVD involves antigen detection by IF or EIA; virus serology may involve antibody measurement by the same techniques. Nevertheless antibody testing by any technique requires the same background equipment of refrigerators ($-20°C$ to $-40°C$) to hold serum collections, medium-speed shielded centri-

```
INSTITUTE OF MEDICAL AND VETERINARY SCIENCE
                        DR G.W.
Patient Details                                              Collection Date and Time
J.A.                    TORRENSVILLE          5031   22/07/87
   ref: 001531                                       Lab No: E 270
Birth                                                SEROL2
Date 12/04/1953   Sex M   Ref. on 22/07/87


      Specimen         : BLOOD
      Specimen Received : 23/07/87
      Date onset illness : 7.7.87

      Final Report

      Sera Tested in Parallel

                        Specimen of    13/7/87      22/7/87
      Influenza A                         10           10
      Influenza B                         10           10
      Chlamydiae                          <5           <5
      Q Fever Phase 2                     <5           <5
      Adenovirus                          10            5
      Mycoplasma pneumoniae               <5          160
      Parainfluenza 1                      5           <5
      Parainfluenza 2                     <5           <5
      Parainfluenza 3                     10           10
      Respiratory Syncytial Virus         <5           <5

      Mycoplasma pneumoniae specific IgM antibody NOT detected.
      Specimen of 13/7/87.
      Mycoplasma pneumoniae specific IgM antibody DETECTED.
      Specimen of 22/7/87.


      Lab Use Only:IGMN MPNEU IGM+ MPNEU


   printed 17/09 12:35  for enquiries phone 228 7543
   VIRAL SEROLOGY                              coll-22/07/87
```

Fig. 47.3 Example of a computer-generated virological report from the data supplied on the input form shown in Figure 47.2. The rise in antibody titre to *Mycoplasma pneumoniae* CF antigen from <5 in the first sample of serum to 160 in the second sample should be noted; also the presence of specific IgM antibody in the latter. Antibody titres to the other antigens used showed no significant change between the first and second serum samples.

fuges for serum separation, semi-automated or automated dilution equipment, waterbaths or incubators for incubation of antigen-serum mixtures, plate readers , etc., so that segregation in one laboratory is a functional decision. Similarly, DVD and cell culture have common requirements of refrigerated centrifuges, low temperature (−70°C) freezers or liquid nitrogen containers, stationary rack or rolling drum incubators to hold cell cultures (used both for virus culture and for preparation of positive controls for antigen detection tests), low and high power microscopes, including UV microscopes, etc. (lists of laboratory equipment are given by Hawkes 1979).

There are two policy decisions to be taken. The first concerns the desirability of combining serological testing for bacteriological infections with that for viruses. There are elements in common, e.g. IF for *Legionella pneumophila* antibody. On the other hand, virological testing makes extensive use of complement fixation tests, not commonly used in microbiology. A final decision will depend on the work load; as numbers increase, virological serum testing is probably best done separately.

The second decision concerns testing for hepatitis B immune markers and HIV antibody. Hepatitis B testing may be combined with other serological testing for viral antibody, but given the need for protection of staff (see above), both test procedures are best handled in a separate laboratory if resources permit. It is particularly important that work with these 'high risk' specimens is carried out in an uncluttered area without the pressure associated with multiple serotesting of the serology section.

Staffing and management

Staff numbers will obviously be related to the number of requests handled each year. Each of the two sections of the laboratory would probably have, in a line management capacity, a senior medical laboratory scientist, supported by one or two more junior staff. The seniors would have had a minimum of 5 years experience in virology, preferably including initial training and experience in bacteriology, together with a formal qualification such as Fellowship of the Institute of Medical Laboratory Scientists or a BSc (Hons) or MSc in Microbiology. The senior in charge of the section is responsible to the chief hospital scientist or chief technician in the microbiology laboratory, and through him or her to the medical director or consultant in charge of the laboratory as a whole.

REFERENCES

Andrewes C H, Pereira H G, Wildy P 1978 Viruses of vertebrates, 4th edn. Bailliere, London
Belshe R B 1984 Textbook of human virology. PSG Littletons, Massachussetts
Fields B N 1985 Virology. Raven Press, New York
Flewett T H 1980 Safety in the virology laboratory. In: Waterson A P (ed) Recent advances in clinical virology 2: 169–187
Gardner P S, McQuillin J 1980 Rapid virus diagnosis: Application of immunofluorescence, 2nd edn. Butterworth, London
Grist N R, Bell E J, Follet E A, Urquhart G E D 1983 Diagnostic methods in clinical virology, 4th edn. Blackwell, Oxford
Hawkes R A 1979 Equipping the virus laboratory. In: Lennette E H, Schmidt N J (eds) Diagnostic procedures of viral and rickettsial infections, 5th edn. American Public Health Association, New York p 11–14
Lennette E H, Schmidt N J 1979 Diagnostic procedures of viral and rickettsial infections, 5th edn. American Public Health Association, New York

Madeley C R 1977 Guide to the collection and transport of virological specimens. World Health Organization, Geneva
Maramorosch K, Koprowski H 1967–1984 (eds) Methods in virology. Academic Press, New York
Melnick J L, Wenner H A, Phillips C A 1979 Association of enteroviruses with disease. In: Lennette E H, Schmidt N J (eds) Diagnostic procedures of viral and rickettsial infections, 5th edn. American Public Health Association, New York, p 526–7
Mims C A, White D O 1984 Viral pathogenesis and immunology. Blackwell, Oxford
Pike R M, Richardson J H 1979 Prevention of laboratory infections. In: Lennette E H, Schmidt N J (eds) Diagnostic procedures of viral and rickettsial infections 5th edn. American Public Health Association, New York p 49–63
White D O, Fenner F 1986 Pathogenesis and pathology of virus infections. In: Medical virology, 3rd edn. Academic Press, New York. p 119–145

Direct virus diagnosis

Direct virus diagnosis (DVD) depends on the detection of virus particles, viral antigen or viral nucleic acid in specimens taken from the site of infection (see Table 48.1 at the end of this chapter). The term DVD is preferred to 'rapid virus diagnosis' because (1) the economical operation of the laboratory may require that direct tests are done in batches over a period of 24 h, and (2) in some virus infections, culture of the virus or serodiagnosis by detection of specific IgM antibody may be as quick as a direct detection method.

The methods that may be used for DVD are:

1. Examination of cells from the inflammatory exudate for viral inclusions, or free virus particles (larger viruses only) by standard histological or special histochemical techniques.

2. Demonstration of virions by electron microscopy (EM): mainly by simple negative contrast staining but also by immunoelectron microscopy (IEM).

3. Demonstration of viral antigens, either in cells from the exudate, or in cells from short-term cell cultures (24–48 h) into which the exudate has been inoculated.

4. Demonstration of specific viral DNA or RNA sequences in cells or semi-purified extracts of nucleic acid from the lesion or exudate by a variety of hybridization techniques, mainly on solid supports.

These approaches may be supplemented by measurement of specific IgA antibody at the lesion site, or specific IgM antibody in the patient's serum. As the latter antibody rises and falls away rapidly, its presence suggests a current infection; it may be detected in advance of changing levels of antibody detected by CF or other reactions (see Chs. 47 and 49).

The subject of DVD is covered by Gardner & McQuillin (1980) with particular reference to immunofluorescence, by McIntosh et al (1978, 1980), by Halonen et al (1984), by Richman et al (1984), by Flewett (1985) in a general fashion, and in the general and specific chapters of Lennette & Schmidt (1979).

The methods listed above are now considered in greater detail.

Cytological and histological methods in direct diagnosis

The virions of most viruses are beyond the limits of resolution of the light microscope, but those of the poxviruses can be seen in stained smears from lesions caused by the genus *Orthopoxvirus* (e.g. vaccinia, smallpox, cowpox, monkey pox), or by *Parapoxvirus* (e.g. orf, milker's nodule) or molluscum contagiosum (an unclassified poxvirus). Two stains – Gutstein and the Moroson silver stain – are described by Downie & Kempe (1969); alternatively overnight Giemsa staining of slides pre-treated with weak potassium permanganate may be used (Marmion & Goodburn 1961).

Inclusion bodies, e.g. herpesviruses or paramyxoviruses, in the nuclei or cytoplasm of exfoliated cells (or cells from infected cell cultures) may be fixed in Bouin's solution (Ch. 3) and stained by haematoxylin and eosin, or fixed in 95% (v/v) ethanol and stained with the Papanicolaou stain. A fluorochrome such as acridine orange or coriphosphine gives striking results with viral nucleic acid; use 1 in 2000 to 1 in 4000 (optimum dilution to be determined by trial) in acetate buffer pH 3.0 on smears for 10 min in acetic acid 25% (v/v) in methanol, wash and mount in pH 3.0 buffer. Examine in ultra-violet or blue light in the fluorescence microscope.

For example, with these fluorochromes, the virions of the poxviruses give the orange-green fluorescence of double-stranded nucleic acid (in this instance DNA), both as free virions and as cytoplasmic 'factories' in the cell. Again, the cytoplasmic inclusions of the double-stranded RNA reoviruses appear as a green fluorescing ring around the nuclei of infected cells. Nuclear inclusion bodies of herpesviruses, papilloma viruses or parvoviruses may fluoresce a different shade of green, or show a different intensity of fluorescence that contrasts with the green-yellow of the marginated nuclear chromatin. Hoechst stain No. 33258 (Ch. 45), which stains DNA only and which is effective in revealing cell-dependent prokaryotes such as mycoplasmas, chlamydias or rickettsias, might also be used for the larger DNA viruses.

Several of the microscope manufacturing firms put out useful handbooks dealing with fluorescence microscopy and fluorochromes; one such has been compiled by Holz for Zeiss, West Germany, ('Worthwhile facts about fluorescence microscopy') and lists the wide range of fluorochromes available and their applications.

Standard histological methods for cell and tissue fixation are considered by Hopwood (1985), and methods for staining inclusion bodies in tissue sections or cell sheets are described by Malherbe & Strickland-Chomley (1980).

Detection of virions by negative contrast electron microscopy

Direct method. Vesicular exudates are frequently rich in the virions of, for example, the herpesvirus or the poxvirus groups; they may simply be spun on to an EM grid at 20 000 *g* for 10 min and stained with a mixture of the salts of heavy metals (see Madeley 1972). Serum may be examined for the virions of hepatitis B virus or parvovirus. Faecal extracts may contain large numbers of rotavirus virions in gastroenteritis, usually detectable without any need for concentration. A drop of the faecal suspension may be placed directly on an EM grid and stained with a drop of negative contrast stain mixture, blotted dry, and is then ready for examination. An alternative, sensitive method is to clarify the faecal suspension by light centrifugation (3000 *g* for 10 min) and then spin the supernatant fluid at 20 000 *g* for 10 min on to an EM grid held at the bottom of the centrifuge tube. The initial clarification reduces the amount of bacteria and small debris and facilitates the detection and identification of the virions in EM.

In immunoelecral microscopy (IEM), anti-serum is added to a small volume of the specimen to aggregate virus particles (incubate for 1–2 h at 37°C, then spin at 20 000 *g* for 10 min on to the grid). This method has the advantage that the aggregated virions are easier to see and also that they are concentrated on the grid so that the method is more sensitive than the direct method outlined in the previous paragraph. Alternatively, the grid may be coated with the antiserum, then floated on the surface of the sample for 30–60 min at room temperature. This is particularly useful when the virus suspected to be present is of a single serotype (e.g. varicella-zoster virus). In the latter variant of the method, pre-existing antibody from the host adsorbed to the virus may block attachment to antibody on the grid, thereby reducing sensitivity.

IEM is less valuable with virus groups with numerous serotypes (e.g. enteroviruses); nevertheless, when one particular serotype of virus is circulating in the community, IEM may be used to detect or serotype the prevalent strain in specimens or in new isolates from cell culture. Advantage may also be taken of the prevalence of antibodies to many viruses in pools of sera from human adults. Addition of 1% (v/v) pooled human serum may clump and concentrate virions in the specimen extract; it does not of course provide a specific serological identification.

A general discussion of EM diagnosis is given by Field (1982). An atlas of virus particles stained by negative contrast has been compiled by Madeley (1972) and by McLean & Wong

(1984). The latter text illustrates more clearly the difficulties of detecting virions in partly processed clinical samples as contrasted with the examination of highly purified concentrated virion suspensions.

Detection of antigens by immunofluorescence, antigen capture and other techniques

Historically, the *immunofluorescence* (IF) detection of viral antigens in cells from exudates was the first method to make a substantial impact on the provision of rapid or direct viral diagnosis (see Gardner & McQuillin 1980), although IF detection of antigen in clinical samples or infected cell cultures had been described as long ago as the middle 1950s (Cohen et al 1955, Liu 1956, Goldwasser & Kissling 1958, Koen et al 1958, Biegeleisen et al 1959). Even earlier, as a diagnostic measure for smallpox in the 1940s and 1950s, antigen had been detected in extracts of lesion material using either gel diffusion or 'reversed' complement fixation (see Dumbell & Nizamuddin 1959).

The principle of diagnosis by detection of free antigen was greatly extended by the discovery that hepatitis B surface antigen could be demonstrated in the blood of acute cases and carriers, at first by insensitive techniques such as gel diffusion or immunoelectrophoresis, and later by radioimmunoassay or enzyme immunoassay using competition or '*antigen capture*' techniques capable of detecting antigen at the 1 ng level or lower. This success led in turn to the application of the method to the detection of other viral antigens in exudates and lesion extracts; the approach is now supplanting the labour-intensive method of antigen detection by immunofluorescence, although the latter remains a sensitive and useful technique for examination of cells in inflammatory exudates, as well as being of particular value as an intermediate step in the work-up of new antigen capture tests. It certainly should not be assumed that EIA antigen capture will necessarily be superior in sensitivity to carefully conducted IF examination (see, for example, Hornsleth et al 1982).

Figure 48.1 sets out in general terms the principles of antigen detection by immunofluor-

escence or antigen capture. The two approaches have been illustrated in the same figure because there are evident similarities between them. For convenience, in the discussions that follow, we deal first with the detection of virus antigens in the cell or cell membrane, mainly by immunofluorescence but also by immunoenzyme methods in cells, and second, with the detection of extracellular antigen, mainly by antigen capture techniques but also some others involving the agglutination of inert particles coated with antibody when mixed with viral antigens.

Detection of cell-associated viral antigens

The approaches in Figure 48.1a and b involve layering a known antiserum on the infected cells. If the antiserum is already labelled with a fluorescent, radioisotope or enzyme marker when the antiserum is applied to the cells, the test is said to be '*direct*' (Fig. 48.1a). If a second labelled antibody (antiglobulin) directed against the unlabelled immunoglobulins of the first antiserum is used, then the test is said to be '*indirect*' (Fig. 48.1b). With directly labelled antisera, reactivity must be directed solely to the viral antigen and the antiserum must be shown to be non-reactive with cell antigens or with serum or other proteins in the specimen or the transport media employed. With indirect tests, both the unlabelled 'middle layer' serum and the labelled antiglobulin must be shown to be free of this so-called 'non-specific' (i.e. unwanted) reactivity, or be rendered so by absorption (see below).

The specific detection of antigens present in cells rests primarily on the specificity of the antisera, e.g. absence of reactivity with uninfected cells and high activity. However, the accuracy and validity of the examination of cells for antigen – either by immunofluorescence or histological immunoenzyme techniques – rests on the finding that the antigen is in the correct location (nuclear or cytoplasmic); also on the pattern (punctate or globular) of the antigen masses seen in the cell. Thus, herpes simplex virus type 2 antigen presents as a uniform mass located in the nucleus, whereas respiratory syncytial virus (RSV) antigen presents as a speckled globular inclusion in the cytoplasm.

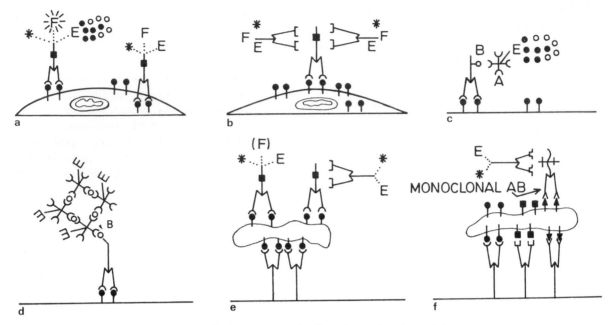

Fig. 48.1 Methods for detection of antigen in tissues, cultured cells or free antigen in exudates.
(a) Direct detection of surface or intracellular antigen with antibody tagged with fluorescein (F), enzyme (E) or radiolabel
(*). Fluorescein emits green light on illumination with blue-violet light in direct or epi-illumination. Enzymes split
non-coloured substrates (○) to coloured products (●). For cellular studies insoluble split products are required.
(b) Indirect detection of antigens with tagged antiglobulin used as a second reactant. Since it attaches at several sites greater
amplification of signal is obtained.
(c) Direct detection of antigen with biotin-tagged antibody (B = biotin) and enzyme-tagged avidin (A). (d) The use of
preformed complexes of biotin and enzyme tagged avidin increases sensitivity.
(e) Direct and indirect antigen-capture methods as used in enzyme immunoassay and radioimmunoassay methods to detect
soluble virions and antigens, using polyclonal antivirus for capture and detection. Fluorescence is less frequently used in this
type of assay although systems are available (see text).
(f) Mixed direct antigen-capture system using a polyclonal antibody to capture several epitopes of an antigen and a
monoclonal antibody to detect any one of these epitopes. Procedure may provide opportunity to use a polyclonal group-
specific capture antibody and a series of monoclonal antibodies to other serotypes or to different epitopes. The
conjugation of enzymes or radiolabels to monoclonal antibodies may be ineffective and thus binding is often detected with
an anti-mouse globulin conjugate.

Detection of extracellular viral antigens by antigen capture techniques

Extracellular antigen is first 'captured' with an antibody bound to a surface, such as a cup in a plastic plate or a polystyrene bead; the presence of the antigen is detected by a tagged antibody of the same species as the capture antibody, in a *direct* system, or by an antibody raised in a different animal species with the corresponding tagged antiglobulin, in an *indirect* system (Fig. 48.1e, and Yolken 1982).

At present, polyclonal antisera against whole virions, or other virus proteins not packaged into the virion, are preferred. This is certainly so for antisera which are to be adsorbed to solid surfaces (beads; wells in plastic plates) with the intention of capturing antigen free in the fluid phase of a clinical specimen (Fig. 48.1e). The place of monoclonal antibodies raised in hybrid-oma culture in these systems is of considerable interest, but still under assessment. Monoclonal antibodies may be highly active – in terms of titre – but of unsatisfactory avidity or unstable when conjugated with dyes or enzymes. A single monoclonal antibody, even of high avidity, may not perform effectively as a 'capture' antibody – given the difficulty of holding a captured antigen by a single species of epitope in the face of thermal agitation and washing. 'Cocktails' of several monoclonal antibodies that recognize different epitopes may be used in attempts to avoid this difficulty. Thus, the Ortho RSV kit uses two monoclonal antibodies directed to different respiratory syncytial virus epitopes and a polyclonal anti-RSV serum conjugated to peroxidase as the detector. Other workers have used a polyclonal anti-mouse globulin antibody to coat the surface of the cup or bead and to hold the cocktail of specific monoclonal antibodies to capture the antigen. In a limited sense, this becomes equivalent to using a polyclonal antiserum; consequently the approach has to be justified by the demonstration of a greater specific activity, and less background non-specificity than can be obtained with a polyclonal antiserum. It is probable that monoclonal antibodies will find a greater application in the direct or indirect detection of antigen in cells by immunofluorescence, or on the 'detector' side of an antigen capture system (as in Fig. 48.1f).

The limits of sensitivity of an antigen capture system are usually in the range of 10^4–10^6 tissue culture infective doses (TCID50) of virus/ml of specimen, or, to take another example, about 10^4 colony-forming units of *Mycoplasma pneumoniae* (see *Methods*, Ch. 45). In practice, around 80% of samples found to be positive on culture of virus in cells will have been positive in antigen capture. The efficiency of the method probably rests on the facts that (1) virus antigen is liberated from cells along with the virions detected by cell culture, and (2) antigen may persist at the lesion site after infective virus has declined.

Efforts to improve or 'fine tune' the sensitivity of an antigen capture system can be directed, logically, to each of the component stages. The evidence that a cocktail of monoclonal antibodies is superior to a potent ('high titre') well adsorbed polyclonal antiserum as a capture antibody is not decisive. Many viral and prokaryotic antigens are quite distinct from the tissue antigen background in the clinical specimen and the unique discriminatory power of a monoclonal antibody is not required.

The use (Fig. 48.1b) of an indirect method with an antiglobulin in the detector system offers some amplification over a direct method (see Ch. 45). The combination of a monoclonal antibody with a mouse antiglobulin with an enzyme tag combines this increased sensitivity with specificity. But it has to be reiterated that heterogenetic antibody interactions may occur between the different species of serum in the different layers of the system and suitable cross-absorptions may be required. Probably most scope for increasing sensitivity resides in improvements to the 'label' attached to the first or second antibody in the detector system. Several ingenious strategies are available.

The number of enzyme molecules anchored to each specific antibody bound to the captured antigen can be increased by exposing the bound antibody to a preformed complex of monoclonal antibody and enzyme (e.g. peroxidase or alkaline phosphatase) and linking with a polyclonal mouse antiglobulin (Fig. 48.2).

An alternative method rests on coupling the small molecule biotin to the first or second anti-

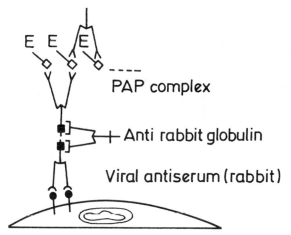

Fig. 48.2 P.A.P. is rabbit anti horseradish peroxidase, formed initially as an insoluble complex, but finally stabilized in solution in slight antigen (i.e. enzyme) excess in acid conditions. It is indicated here as PAP complex.

It is usually present as a pentameric complex of two immunoglobulin molecules with three enzyme molecules, thus allowing a greater output of coloured reaction product.

Because the primary antibody is not covalently linked with a label, its reactivity with viral antigens remains high.

The principle illustrated can be extended to avidin–biotin systems as described in the illustrated text 'The biotin–streptavidin system' available from Amersham.

body (antiglobulin) in the detection system and in turn detecting the biotin-tagged antibody with avidin (chicken avidin or streptavidin) linked to an enzyme, e.g. peroxidase or phosphatase, which then liberate a coloured end-product from a substrate (Fig. 48.1c), as with enzyme immunoassay.

The binding of biotin and avidin is essentially irreversible and the system has a higher binding coefficient than that of antigen and antibody. Avidin has four receptors for biotin and it is possible to couple several enzyme molecules per molecule of avidin without steric interference with these sites. Indeed it is possible to preform complexes of avidin-enzyme linked with biotin which, when bound to the biotinylated antibody, amplify the reaction (Hsu et al 1981, Kendall et al 1983, Yolken et al 1983, Hsu & Raine 1984, Fig. 48.1d).

There are some problems with the system despite its theoretical advantages. Biotin and other groupings present in tissues and exudates may bind the avidin-enzyme complex and give high non-specific background readings. Chicken avidin, a positively charged glycoprotein, is said to bind more readily to cell surface antigens and lectins than streptavidin, which is a protein with a neutral isoelectric point at physiological pH. Consequently, the use of streptavidin-biotin systems may offer advantages over the chicken avidin-biotin system.

There are a number of commercial sources of avidin or streptavidin-phosphatase or peroxidase reagents, and some are listed at the end of this chapter. An interesting variant, offered by Kirkegaard & Perry, links biotin to antibody with a 7 atom spacer, and detects with streptavidin peroxidase; a combination claimed to give higher sensitivity in EIA and immunoblots, and less problems with steric hindrance between antibody and streptavidin.

There are numerous variations in the enzymes used, methods of coupling antibody and the substrates for enzyme action (see Farr & Nakane 1981). The commonly used alkaline phosphatase from calf intestine is coupled to antibody with glutaraldehyde (Avrameas & Ternynck 1971); on addition of substrates such as p-nitrophenyl phosphate, the phosphatase gives a coloured split product. The sensitivity of the phosphatase

system may be increased by using 4-methyl-umbelliferyl phosphate or fluorescein phosphate; enzyme action yields bases that fluoresce brilliantly at short wavelengths of light. Similarly, a combination of umbelliferyl-β-galactoside and β-galactosidase may be used to generate fluorescent end-products (Whitehead et al 1979).

Another commonly used enzyme, peroxidase, has a smaller molecular weight than phosphatase; unbound conjugates are more easily washed out, reducing background. The use of 2,2'-azino-di [3-ethyl-benzthiazoline sulphonate] (ABTS, Boehringer) as a substrate for peroxidase, gives a blue-green colour at 417 nm and generates about 10 times more colour per unit time than phosphatase generates with p-nitrophenyl phosphate.

In further improvements to sensitivity, amplification of enzyme action has been obtained by using the products of one enzyme-substrate interaction to activate, in cascade, a second enzyme-substrate system, which in turn gives a coloured end-product. Thus, Self (1985) has described an enzyme amplification system in which alkaline phosphatase dephosphorylates NADP to NAD. The NAD is then reduced to NADH by alcohol dehydrogenase and then oxidized by a diaphorase, reducing in the transfer a tetrazolium salt to give a coloured formazan which can be detected spectrophotometrically. This system has been used, under licence, by Wellcome to produce a number of viral antigen capture assays starting with hepatitis B surface antigen.

A label of a different kind, the element europium, has been attached to antiglobulin in a system named time-resolved fluorimmunoassay (Soini & Hemmila 1979, Halonen et al 1984). The label is activated by a laser pulse to give out light, and the fluorescence is measured.

Detection of extracellular viral antigens by precipitation and agglutination techniques

Methods of detection of free viral antigen in the fluid phase of clinical specimens may in a sense be considered to have evolved from the simple gel diffusion or counter immunoelectrophoresis – of low sensitivity for antigen detection – via techniques of intermediate sensitivity in which antibody was bound to the surface of particles such as tanned erythrocytes, 'latex' (polystyrene) particles or even bacteria, which agglutinated when exposed to antigen. Finally, these techniques were replaced by the sensitive antigen capture techniques just described.

The agglutination techniques still have a place as rapid screening methods when a very rapid answer is required, e.g. to test a new admission to a renal unit or children's ward at a time when the main laboratory is closed. When used, however, this (provisional) result must be confirmed as soon as practicable by a more sensitive method.

Various test formats are available. Erythrocytes or latex particles coated with antibody to hepatitis B surface antigen (HBsAg) have been used to detect or confirm the presence of HBsAg in serum. Simple agglutination kits with antibody-coated latex particles, though of lower sensitivity that other methods, are supplied by several manufacturers (see below). The techniques may be quite versatile; for example, a faecal extract from a patient with viral enteritis, when mixed with latex particles of different colours, coated either with antiserum to adenovirus or to rotavirus, gives aggregates of different colours, depending on the particular virus present.

Choice of methods for antigen detection

Decisions about the method finally chosen for antigen detection – immunofluorescence (IF) examination of cells, or antigen capture with enzyme immunoassay (EIA) or radioimmunoassay (RIA) – are determined not only by the type of specimen but also the workload and level of equipment in the laboratory. The virological section of a microbiological laboratory dealing with small numbers of specimens from respiratory tract, skin or genital tract will probably opt for IF on separated cells using a simple fluorescence microscope and the high quality antiviral antibodies available commercially. It may combine IF with the use of commercial EIA-based kits for detection of hepatitis B surface antigen, rotavirus antigen in faeces or herpes simplex antigen in skin or other lesions.

Larger specialist virus laboratories are now moving to EIA or RIA-based antigen capture across the whole range respiratory virus pathogens, for rotaviruses and the adenoviruses associated with enteritis, as well as for hepatitis B and herpes simplex testing. The various commercial kits, or 'in house' versions of them, offer the attraction of batch processing and automated printed readout free from the time-consuming processes and skilled interpretations required with immunofluorescence. This approach requires equipment such as automated plate or bead washers and plate readers for EIA and gamma counters for RIA.

In the remainder of this chapter, details are given (1) of the choice and methods of collection of specimens for direct virus diagnosis; (2) of immunofluorescence methods for the detection of viruses in cells from exudates from respiratory infections, in cells from lesions in skin or mucous membranes, and in samples from the central nervous system; and (3) references to 3 and 4 layer antigen capture method based on ELISA technique (EIA). Tabular detail is provided on some of the commercial sources of viral antisera, antiglobulins and other reagents for detection systems and of the kits for a number of viral antigens (see Table 48.2–4 at end of this chapter). Finally, (4) a general illustrative account is given of some developmental directions in the use of nucleic acid probes in direct diagnosis.

COLLECTION AND INITIAL PROCESSING OF SPECIMENS

Specimens should be delivered promptly to the laboratory so that no deterioration in the quality of cells occurs. For patients admitted in the evening, specimens should be collected just before the arrival of laboratory staff the following morning. Attention to detail in taking the specimens will be rewarded by cleaner preparations with less non-specific background.

Skin lesions and vesicle fluids

Vesicle fluids should be taken from lesions with clear contents, indicating a recent eruption. As some of the fluid will be needed for virus culture, the skin should not be swabbed with disinfectants that might leave a residual activity; it may be cleaned with isopropyl alcohol. Separate heparin-treated sterile glass capillary tubes are used to draw up fluids – either by capillary attraction or by gentle aspiration with a rubber teat – from several vesicles after these have been opened with the tip of a hypodermic needle. If the fluids are not readily aspirated, a larger opening may be needed, or a sterile cotton swab may be used to compress the vesicle laterally to expel the contents. The capillaries for EM and EIA studies are left in a labelled Petri dish, while those for virus culture are washed out into a small volume of viral transport medium (Ch. 50) in a bijou bottle or small vial.

Material for virus culture may also be obtained by removing the top of the vesicle, swabbing the exposed base, and then breaking off the head of the swab in a container of virus transport medium. Scrapings may also be taken from the base or side of the lesion with a small curetting spoon or fine scalpel; the harvested cells are smeared on slides for IF examination and the spoon is agitated in virus transport medium to provide a sample for culture. The epithelial cells most likely to contain inclusions and antigens are those taken from the advancing edge of the lesion.

Other methods of making cell spreads from a lesion include collection with a cotton swab followed by 'rolling' the head of the swab on to a microscopy slide; alternatively a sterile microscopy slide may be applied to the lesion, and by a combined squeezing and twisting action, material can be expressed on to a premarked area of the slide.

If specimens contain visible fragments of skin or tissue, it may be more convenient to process them further in the laboratory; small fragments should be covered with a drop of saline during transit. On arrival at the bench, these fragments may be teased out with needles for the production of replicate slides before air drying and fixation.

Suspected *herpetic whitlows* may present some difficulty. The indurated area may give the appearance of containing fluid but incision does not yield fluid or pus. If the lesion has already been incised under the mistaken impression that there is a bacterial infection, then a swab should be dipped in viral transport medium and the wound area swabbed. If the lesion is intact, the skin may be anaesthetized with a cold spray and the centre of the lesion gently penetrated with a fine hypodermic needle to yield at least some tissue fluid and the area then swabbed. Virus culture may be easier than antigen detection in this particular instance.

The *skin nodules* of molluscum contagiosum or orf require a small incision with a scalpel and a squeeze to release the hard molluscum body or internal contents of the lesion. The harvested material may then be dispersed with needles or by squashing between one slide and another in readiness for acridine orange staining for nucleic acids and for electron microscopy to detect the characteristic virions of molluscum or orf. Skin biopsy is less often called for, but if required, can be done with a punch such as that described by Oldig-Stenkvist & Grandien (1976).

Biopsy specimens

Biopsy specimens may be requested by the virologist or reach the laboratory indirectly via the histopathologist. These commonly include samples of tissue from brain, lung, liver, kidney or lymph nodes, although samples may be taken from any level of the gastrointestinal tract or even heart muscle.

Brain biopsy. These specimens, e.g. from suspected herpes encephalitis, are particularly critical samples for case management, and examination is a team effort. The laboratory should be notified well in advance by the neurosurgeon that a biopsy sample is to be taken; its examination should be coordinated with the neuropathologist. A member of the laboratory staff should wait in the outer room of the operating theatre and receive the sample of tissue which should be placed by the surgeon in a dry sterile container. The sample is brought back to the laboratory at once and divided in consultation with the neuropathologist. Part is fixed for histological examination, and part is used for frozen sections, cut either by the neuropathologist or the virus laboratory. The residual material is emulsified in a Ten Brock or other grinder with broth (if bacteriological examinations are also required) or with virus transport medium.

The emulsified suspension can be used for electron microscopy, inoculation of cell cultures and for tests for herpes simplex antigen by antigen capture EIA. The frozen sections are examined at once by IF and perhaps later by immunoperoxidase staining for herpes simplex antigen. It should be appreciated that only a small proportion of presumptive cases of herpes encephalitis eventually prove to be so.

Consequently, the division of the biopsy sample, and the planning for serial serological sampling of the patient, need to take account of 'allergic' encephalitis (histological examination) as a response to viral infection or agents such as *Mycoplasma pneumoniae*; infection with pathogenic amoebae; and bacterial infection partly suppressed by antibiotic treatment. The neurosurgeon may also be able to obtain a sample of CSF from the ventricle at the time of taking the brain biopsy. This may yield cells containing virus or antigen when these are not present in samples of lumbar CSF.

Lung tissue may be obtained by open biopsy or an aspirate by lung puncture with a syringe and needle. Frozen sections of tissue, or cell smears from the aspirates, are prepared. The aspirated or emulsified lung tissue is also used for culture. As with brain biopsy, a team approach is required to ensure that histological examination is performed (viral inclusions and *Pneumocystis carini*); that the clinical microbiologists are involved (*Legionella pneumophila*), and that mycoplasma culture is performed. In addition, IF examination of sections or impression smears and cell culture for viruses, particularly the herpesvirus group (CMV and herpes simplex), should be done. According to the patient's history and age group, consideration should also be given to preparing the specimen for examination for chlamydia antigen or for culture of the organism (see Ch. 46).

Liver tissue. Here again, a broad approach – histological, microbiological and virological – is required as dictated by the clinical history. Many

liver biopsies will have been collected with the object of confirming acute or chronic infection with hepatitis B virus; processing needs to cover histological examination and examination of frozen sections for HBsAg, HBcAg and HBV DNA.

Although HBsAg and HBcAg may be detected in fixed tissues, it is necessary to use frozen tissue sections for maximum sensitivity. Liver biopsies should be snap-frozen and kept frozen to avoid ice crystal damage. This is most conveniently performed by embedding the biopsy specimen in a large drop of OCT embedding compound (Miles) mounted on a 2 mm thick, 1 cm diameter piece of cork. The cork is then held with forceps immediately above the surface of liquid nitrogen until the OCT is three quarters frozen and then plunged into the nitrogen for not less than 1 min. The cork-mounted sample may then be wrapped in precooled aluminium foil for long-term storage at $-70°C$, or attached to or removed from a cryostat specimen holder several times without thawing.

In other circumstances (e.g. investigation of pyrexia of undetermined origin), fixed histological and frozen sections should be prepared and culture strategies must take into account not only viruses such as CMV, rubella and adenovirus, but also agents such as *Coxiella burneti* (Ch. 44) and *Mycobacterium tuberculosis* (Ch. 25). Consequently, rapid transport in a dry sterile bottle and, after decisions about testing have been taken, the use of antibiotic-free transport medium is a wise precaution.

Lymph node biopsy. In addition to planning with other departments for specialized histological examination to exclude, depending on clinical history, infection with mycobacteria, fungi and the organism of cat scratch fever, impression smears are prepared for IF examination with antisera to adenovirus, herpesviruses, and possibly Epstein Barr (EB) virus. Virus culture should include inoculation of tissue homogenate into culture as well as dicing the tissue to make suspended cell fragments which are placed on feeder layers of cells. At the present time, infection with EB virus, hepatitis

B and HIV is probably best excluded by a serological test on the patient rather than by attempts to grow virus or detect viral nucleic acid. Nevertheless, nucleic acid probes for EBV, CMV and HBV are available, and examination by 'cell blot' or in-situ hybridization may eventually become part of direct viral diagnosis with lymph-node and other organ biopsies.

Kidney biopsy. Depending on the clinical history, provision is made for histological examination and culture for fastidious bacteria, e.g. leptospira, as well as for rubella, measles, adenovirus, certain enteroviruses and cytomegalovirus.

Urine

Urine can be a useful source of infected exfoliated cells bearing inclusion bodies of CMV, measles or other viruses. Freshly voided samples of urine are collected in sterile containers with an antibiotic solution (100 μg/ml gentamicin, 100 μg/ml mycostatin) and transferred at once to the laboratory where they are held at 4°C and not frozen. After light centrifugation (500 g for 15 min), the supernatant fluid may be used for inoculation of cell culture. Deposits from the urine may be mixed with an equal volume of 95% (v/v) ethanol and either filtered through a 0.45 μm Millipore filter, from which smears are made on microscopy slides, or deposited on slides with a cytocentrifuge. Smears are covered with a few drops of Parlodion (1 g Parlodion mixed with 200 ml of 95% (v/v) ethanol and anhydrous ether) and then stained with Papanicolaou, Giemsa or haematoxylin and eosin (Fetterman 1952, Margileth 1955, Schumann et al 1977).

Cells separated from urine, or in a similar way from milk, saliva, cervical secretions, or in impression smears from biopsy specimens, may also be fixed for IF examination for CMV and other antigens (see below, and Reynolds et al 1979).

Faeces

Specimens should be obtained in 1–5 g portions or as fluid stools, depending on the circum-stances. The former are resuspended by vortexing in phosphate buffered saline to an approximate 20% (w/v) suspension. Samples are centrifuged at medium speed to remove debris and some bacteria and stored at −20°C.

Nasopharyngeal secretions

Nasopharyngeal secretions are the preferred source of specimens for virus culture and direct diagnosis of respiratory infections in paediatric groups. Collection of post-nasal swabs from young children is not easy and may even be hazardous to the operator whose eyes are in close proximity to the patient. Excellent specimens are obtained, with little trauma, by aspirating secretions from the nasopharynx with a fine feeding catheter, size 8, attached to a plastic mucus extractor (see Fig. 48.3 and Gardner & McQuillin 1980). Several portable suction machines are available commercially; the ward suction lines may be used, or aspiration may be done with a 20 ml syringe.

The tip of the catheter is passed along the floor of the nose for about 7 cm, suction is applied and the aspirated material in the catheter is washed into the mucus trap with virus transport medium; if culture for *Mycoplasma pneumoniae* is also contemplated, a transport medium containing penicillin or ampicillin without aminoglycosides is required.

Nursing staff and virology specimen collectors become very quick and adept in performing the aspiration, and infants find the procedure inoffensive and it is well tolerated; it is less likely to provoke spasmodic coughing than swabbing of the throat. Occasionally, larger size catheters or rough ended catheters lead to minor bleeding; the contaminating erythrocytes may interfere with antigen detection in IF tests, and the problem should be rectified.

Samples from acute infections of the eye

The yield of viruses or chlamydias, and the quality of diagnosis, is heavily dependent on the skill with which samples are collected from the eye. Swabs or scrapings from the tarsal surface of the conjunctiva may be collected in the

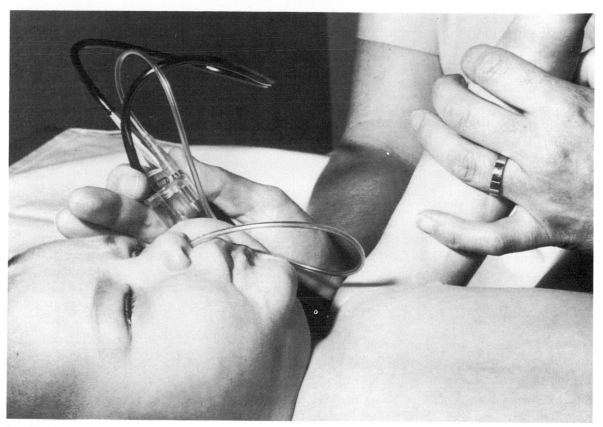

Fig. 48.3 Collection of a nasopharyngeal aspirate from a child with respiratory infection.

patient room attached to the virus laboratory or by staff in the wards. However, we are of the opinion that for examination and sampling of the cornea, regular arrangements should be made with the ophthalmology outpatient department for ambulant patients to be inspected and sampled by a trained ophthalmologist, who can anaesthetize the cornea, examine it with fluorescein and a slit lamp, and collect adequate samples (by swab debridement or impression smears prepared by touching the edge of any corneal ulcer with the flat surface of a small plastic spatula and transferring the cells to a microscope slide). Such procedures as inspection of the eyelids for small vesicles (in herpetic infection), recognition of molluscum bodies, expression of the contents of follicles on the tarsal conjunctiva, all require experience. The samples submitted should include: at least three smears of cells on microscopy slides for Giemsa staining and immunofluorescence for viral and chlamydial

antigens; a swab from cornea or conjunctiva, the head of which is broken off into viral transport medium for virus culture; and swabs for chlamydia culture in the appropriate transport medium (see Ch. 46).

EXAMINATION OF FROZEN SECTIONS OF TISSUE, CELLS FROM EXUDATES AND SECRETIONS, AND CELLS FROM CULTURE FOR VIRAL ANTIGENS

The successful application of antigen detection by immunofluorescence (IF) depends on the availability of high-titre, specific antisera that react with the viral antigen and not with cell antigens or other host proteins in the clinical sample. The increasing number of commercial sources supplying well tested, antigen-affinity purified, fractionated antisera has greatly simplified the task of the DVD laboratory.

Table 48.1 (at the end of this chapter) summarizes the diseases in which DVD by IF may be used. With some virus groups such as the enteroviruses and rhinoviruses which have numerous serotypes, or in which viral antigen is retained in the cell only for short periods, detection of antigen by IF has been less successful, although the IF typing of isolates in cell culture has been exploited to some extent.

An additional 'rapid' method, not strictly speaking DVD, involves inoculation of the specimen into cell culture and the examination, 24–48 h later, of the cell sheet by IF for early or capsid antigens of the virus concerned, or demonstration of antigen in cell homogenate by antigen capture methods. This method has been employed with CMV and varicella-zoster viruses which take many days to produce CPE in cell sheets.

Examination of cells from nasopharyngeal aspirates, sputum, throat washings, bronchial washings and lung puncture or lung aspirates

The specimen is inspected to determine the degree of viscosity due to mucus that might impede the separation of cells from the sample. Specimens that are fluid and clearly non-viscous, such as throat or bronchial washings, are simply centrifuged at 800 g for 10 min to deposit the cells. Semi-fluid samples, such as those obtained by nasopharyngeal aspiration, may be diluted further with viral transport medium to render them rather more fluid and then mixed on a vortex agitator, and the cells deposited by centrifugation. Highly viscous samples such as sputum may be treated with Sputolysin (Calbiochem) or N-acetylcysteine at room temperature for 15 min, followed by vortex mixing and centrifugation. Alternatively, the sputum may be homogenized by repeated aspiration through a small bore pipette, and the cells then deposited from the homogenate. The cell pellet obtained by any of these methods is harvested and given one more cycle of resuspension in phosphate buffered saline (PBS) pH 7.0 and centrifugation, and then suspended in a small volume of PBS with 1–2% fetal calf serum or 0.05% (w/v) gelatin. Volumes of 20–40 μl of the cell suspension are dispensed into each of the 8 wells of a Teflon-coated slide (see Fig. 48.4; available from Wellcome). The preparation is then dried in a stream of cool air from a small fan heater. Once dry, the slide is fixed in reagent grade acetone for 5 min at 4°C. Note that a range of fixatives have been used successfully in immunofluorescence procedures. These include dry methanol or ethanol, carbon tetrachloride, weak concentrations of formalin (0.1–1%) or paraformaldehyde (2% w/v). For formalin fixation the cell sheets are dried and fixed in the formalin at 4°C for 30 min, washed in PBS, dried again and finally hydrated before the antiserum is applied. Stronger concentrations of formalin (around 1% v/v) reveal intracellular antigens; weaker concentrations reveal membrane antigens. For instance, hepatitis B surface antigen in a liver biopsy is well fixed for immunofluorescence with the use of carbon tetrachloride or formaldehyde. The advantages and disadvantages of these fixatives are further discussed by Nairn (1976) and Hopwood (1985).

Some viral antigens, however, may be inactivated by these fixatives; the best all-round fixative appears to be acetone. This may be used in the manner described, or the slides may be fixed in acetone at −20°C overnight. It is important to fix in a fresh batch of acetone each time as the reagent may absorb moisture from the atmosphere and become less effective. Note also that acetone does not necessarily inactivate viral infectivity and that the specimen remains potentially infectious. After acetone fixation the slides may be stored in moisture-tight boxes at −20°C. However, as they are normally to be examined at once, they are first rehydrated by placing in a moist chamber at room temperature for 15–30 min before staining. This step cuts down the non-specific staining in the specimen. The test is then set up by placing an optimal dilution (see below for determination) of a particular antiserum over one of the wells; a whole battery of antisera being deployed over the 8 wells on the slide. The range of antisera used for respiratory tract specimens would usually be influenza A and B (antibody against the internal nucleoprotein or 'soluble' antigen), adenovirus (antiserum against a broadly reacting strain

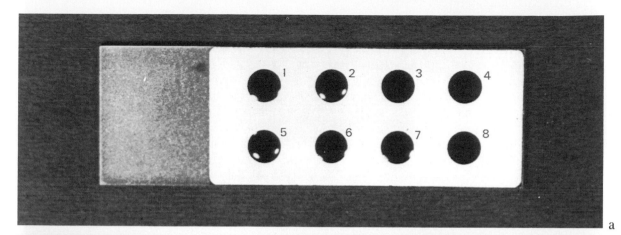

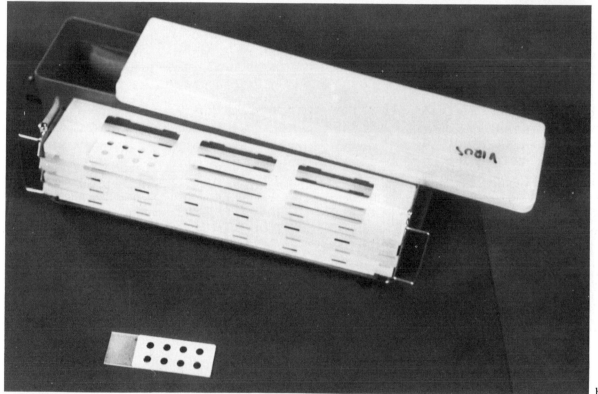

Fig. 48.4 Multi-well slides (teflon coated) as used for an indirect test. Cells from the patient's respiratory tract are first dried onto each well and fixed. See text for details. Antisera are added as described.
(a) Layout: 7 wells with 7 specific rabbit sera to relevant respiratory viruses; one well with plain rabbit serum. After a first incubation period washed slides are blotted dry and all wells reacted with tagged anti-rabbit globulins.
(b) Incubation box keeps reagents from drying out during incubation at 37°C.

representing antibody to the hexon antigen), parainfluenza 1, 2 and 3 and respiratory syncytial virus. Other clinical diagnoses (e.g. chronic pneumonitis in the newborn, post-transfusion pneumonitis, material from an immuno-suppressed patient) may require that antisera to cytomegalovirus, herpes simplex, varicella-zoster, measles or chlamydia be added to the battery of antisera.

The treated multiwell slide with its antisera is

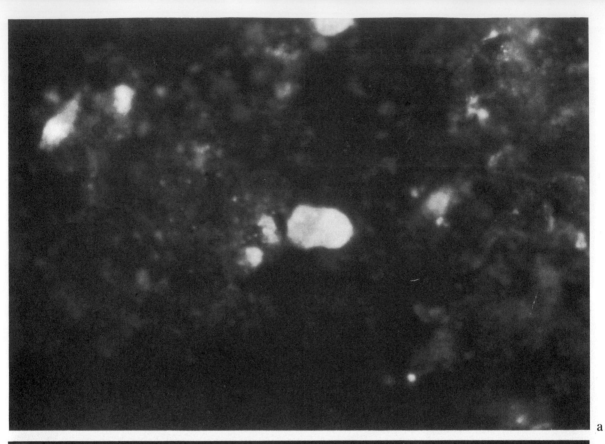

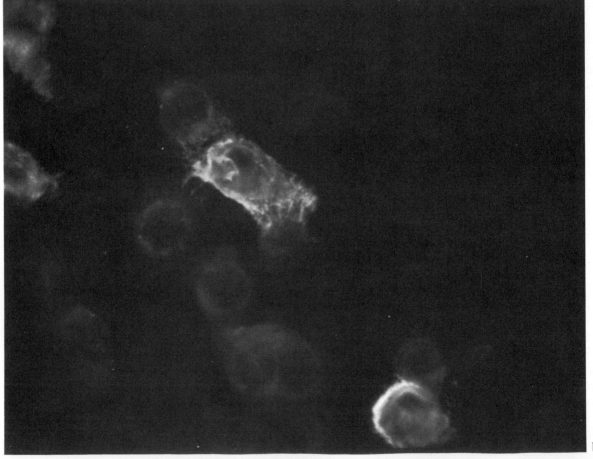

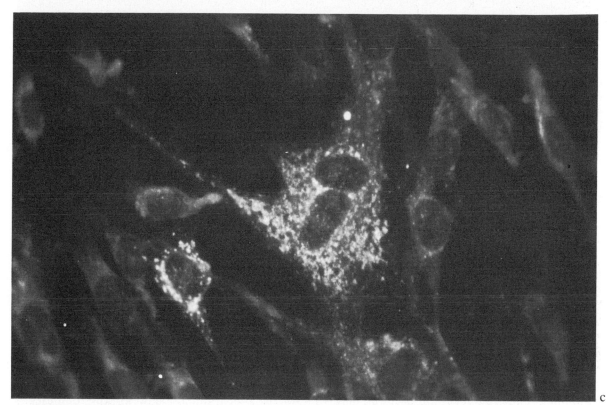

c

Fig. 48.5 Immunofluorescence of cells infected with respiratory syncytial virus and stained by the indirect method with rabbit anti-RSV followed by fluorescein tagged goat anti-rabbit globulins.
(a) cells and debris from nasopharyngeal aspirate; poor morphology, but cells are specifically stained.
(b) HeLa cells grown on a coverslip
(c) Human fibroblast cells grown on coverslip
Minor differences in distribution of antigens are seen between cell lines but only the infected cells show green fluorescence whilst background cells take up a counterstain (Evans Blue). Cells of this type are used to determine the optimal working dilutions of newly prepared sera.

held in a moist chamber at 37°C for 30 min. It is then washed twice with PBS. If a direct test is being used, the slide is mounted for examination at this stage. If an indirect test is used, then it is overlaid with a fluorescein or rhodamine conjugated antiglobulin, and incubated for a further 30 min at room temperature in the moist chamber. After two further washes to remove unbound conjugated antiglobulins, the slide is turned on its edge and gently tapped on a facial tissue or filter paper to drain as much of the PBS off the surface as possible; the tissue (or dry cotton swab) is gently used to dry the surface without touching the contents of the wells. Optional further steps in the staining procedure are (1) to counterstain with Evans blue 0.01% (w/v) in PBS for 10 min with a 10 min PBS wash;

the dye fluoresces red and blankets non-specific cell staining by the fluorescein conjugate, and (2) incorporation of η-propyl-gallate into the mountant as a stabilizer to prevent photobleaching (Giloh & Sedat 1982). The slide is then overlaid with glycerol buffer pH 8.6 and a large coverslip placed over the whole surface and sealed into position with colourless nail varnish round the edges. Alternatively, permanent mounts such as Eukitt (quick hardening mounting medium for microscopy specimens, Zeiss) or Elvanol (Heimer & Taylor 1974) may be used instead of the buffered glycerol. This makes for a stable preparation as the coverslip is firmly anchored, and also permits re-examination of the specimen at a later date if there is doubt about the findings, particularly when the results of virus culture on the same specimen need to be compared with the results of direct diagnosis. The slides are then examined in a fluorescence microscope with transmitted or incident illumination. Figure 48.5 shows the results obtained with an antiserum to respiratory syncytial virus and cells from a nasopharyngeal aspirate of an infant with bronchiolitis.

The control of specificity in this particular test format is determined by the fact that only one of the battery of antisera should react with the cells in the specimen – or at most two if there happens to be more than one virus present. A reaction of the cells with most of the test antisera suggests a non-specific effect. Second, the antigen detected is usually in the form of one or more inclusion bodies in the cytoplasm of the cells, or nuclear staining with herpes simplex virus; this greatly facilitates interpretation of the findings. Extracellular antigen is more difficult to interpret, although with potent monoclonal anti-bodies the individual elementary bodies of organisms such as chlamydia or the larger viruses of the pox group may be seen. Specimens containing large numbers of bacteria may be unsatisfactory; they may adsorb serum proteins non-specifically and fluoresce. Care must also be taken to ensure that each of the wells contains sufficient numbers of cells to ensure that an examination is valid; ≥ 100 cells per well is desirable, < 10 is not acceptable. Moreover, the cells should have come from the respiratory tract; buccal squames are not acceptable.

Immunofluorescence detection of infected cells is a sensitive method but efficiency is highly dependent on the time spent in searching the slide. As a working rule, it would be expected that IF with an antiserum to respiratory syncytial virus and cells from nasopharyngeal aspirates of infants with bronchiolitis or pneumonia would detect at least 85% and preferably over 90% of specimens positive in cell culture.

Determination of working dilutions of viral antisera and 'in test' controls for potency

Suitable test substrates for titration of viral anti-sera and, subsequently, for routine positive controls may be made from mixtures of infected and uninfected cells from cell culture, roughly in the ratio of 1:3. Cell cultures are inoculated with the homologous virus and harvested by trypsin dispersion at the time when CPE first appears in part of the cell sheet. The infected cells are mixed with uninfected cells and dispensed into well slides. Dilutions of the viral antiserum and, separately, the preinoculation sample from the animal immunized, or a negative serum from the same species, are placed in the wells and the staining process completed as described. The endpoint is that dilution of serum that gives a reaction on the infected cells with many nega-tives interspersed. The preparation may be counterstained with 0.01% (w/v) Evans blue to provide a contrast with the positive cells.

The uninfected cells in the mixture serve to detect the development of non-specific staining which may result if the fluorescein or rhodamine dissociates from the antibody and then acts as a simple histological stain. When this occurs, or when the specific staining properties of the diluted serum start to diminish, it is an indication for the preparation of new working dilutions of antiserum or absorption of the working dilution with tissue powder, centrifugation and filtration through a 0.4 μm Millipore syringe filter. Working dilutions of serum may become contaminated with bacteria or precipitated protein; both give rise to undesirable clumps of fluorescent material on the preparation; again these have to be removed either by making up fresh batches of diluted antiserum, or by filtration. Sodium azide (0.1% w/v) may be added to inhibit bacterial contamination.

Examination of cells from conjunctiva or cornea

Preparations are fixed with acetone and stained for chlamydia (Ch. 46), adenovirus and herpes simplex virus type 1 and 2. The procedure of staining, washing and examination is that just described above. The adenovirus antiserum should contain antibody against the group-reactive hexon antigen and should have been shown to react with adenoviruses types 8, 11 and 19, which may be associated with epidemic keratoconjunctivitis. Presumably, keratoconjunctivitis caused by ECHO virus serotype 71 could also be diagnosed by IF/DVD, given potent antiserum, but we have no reports on the matter.

Urine

Details of the process of collection and separation of cells were described above. After acetone fixation, they may be stained with antisera to cytomegalovirus, measles or adenovirus. Standard indirect immunofluorescence may be employed or use may be made of the anti-complement immunofluorescence test in the case of cytomegalovirus.

Biopsy specimens

Frozen sections are cut on a cryostat at 4–6 μm, and mounted on previously acid-washed, gelatin-coated slides (gelatin, 1% w/v in distilled water, melted and slides dipped and drained), air dried and then fixed in dehydrated acetone for 10 min at 4°C. Sections of liver biopsies may be fixed in carbon tetrachloride or in formalin 1% v/v (see above). Punch biopsies from skin lesions suspected to be due to herpes simplex or varicella-zoster viruses may be sectioned in the same way and fixed with dehydrated acetone before staining with the requisite antisera. The examination of brain biopsy specimens from patients with suspected herpes simplex encephalitis is a particularly important application of the IF method. The use of potent type-specific herpes simplex virus antisera and control, antibody-negative serum from the same animal species is imperative. These sera must be shown not to react with uninfected human brain tissue – the negative control. Sections from a known herpes-infected brain must be included in the test run.

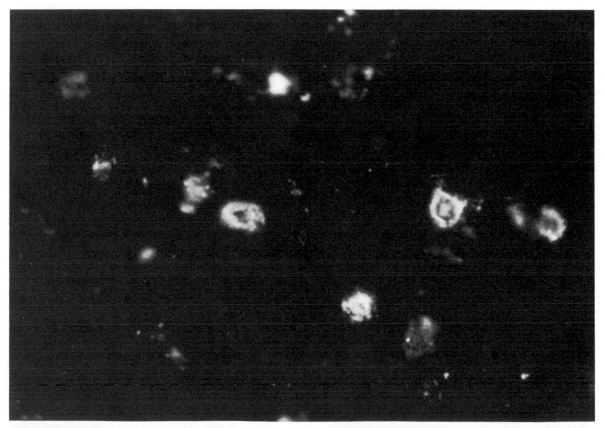

Fig. 48.6 Section from brain biopsy of a patient with herpes encephalitis stained by immunofluorescence with herpes simplex type 1 antiserum.

When a CNS specimen is obtained from a proven case of herpes encephalitis it is prudent to prepare a large number of frozen sections, to fix and store them in an air-tight box at −20°C for use as controls in subsequent tests. Failing this, as second best, control sections may be obtained by inoculating mice intracerebrally with herpes simplex virus and harvesting the brain. However, the lesion in mouse brain tends to be an abscess with extensive antigen deposits in its wall rather than an infection of neurones extending in a network through the brain tissue as in the human being. Figure 48.6 illustrates a positive result with a brain biopsy from a herpes simplex encephalitis stained by IF with herpes simplex virus type 1 antiserum.

DETECTION OF VIRAL ANTIGENS IN HISTOLOGICAL SECTIONS FROM FIXED, EMBEDDED SPECIMENS

Examination of frozen sections of brain or liver biopsies may be complemented or substituted by the use of specimens that have been formalin-fixed, dehydrated, wax-embedded and sectioned by standard techniques. Sections mounted on slides are dewaxed and brought to water. They may then be stained for the presence of viral antigens by using the avidin-biotin complex (ABC) (Hsu et al 1981).

Sections are treated with a protease – protease K or trypsin – a step that will remove any bound antibody from the viral antigens and generally cuts down non-specific background fluorescence. The first antibody (to the virus suspected to be present) is usually reacted with the section overnight at 4°C or room temperature. However, recent studies (Leong & Milios 1986) have shown that microwave irradiation can replace this step and thus shorten considerably the usually long incubation period with the primary antibody. An added advantage claimed for this method is the better retention of cell morphology. The microwave irradiation is usually for about 30 s at the defrost setting. After this, the section is washed over 10 min with three changes of PBS. The second antibody (biotin-labelled) is then reacted for 30 min at room temperature.

The unreacted antibody is washed away over 10 min with two changes of PBS. A preformed avidin-biotin peroxidase complex is then applied for 1 h at room temperature. After washing with two changes of PBS over 10 min the substrate (3, 3-diaminobenzidine tetrahydrochloride – 1 mg/2 ml in buffered saline at pH 7.6 and 1 μl 30% H_2O_2 per ml of working solution) is added and the colour is allowed to develop over 10–15 min at room temperature. After a further wash in PBS, the tissue section may be counterstained with haematoxylin and eosin, and examined under the light microscope.

ANTIGEN CAPTURE METHODS FOR DIRECT VIRUS DIAGNOSIS

Various methods for antigen capture are outlined in Figure 48.1. The simplest 'direct' system (Fig. 48.1e) is one in which a high-titre polyclonal antiserum is prepared by immunizing an animal (e.g. rabbit or goat) with the viral or non-bacterial antigen to be detected. After fractionation of the serum to obtain the antibody globulin and absorption with tissue powders or homogenates to remove so-called 'natural' antibodies (ones that cross-react between animal species) that might react with tissue antigens in the clinical specimens, the antibody is coated on to the surface of a polystyrene bead or a well in a plastic plate. The same polyclonal antibody, conjugated with an enzyme or with a radiolabel, is used to detect antigen 'captured' from the clinical specimen by the antibody on the plastic surface. Other beads or wells are coated with a comparable fraction from the preinoculation serum from the animal providing the antiserum to act as negative controls.

Applications of this direct technique, or the equivalent indirect technique, have been described with influenza A, respiratory syncytial virus, parainfluenza type 2 virus and adenovirus (see, for example, Sarkkinen et al 1981a, b).

It is probable that the virological section of the bacteriological laboratory will make most use of the antigen capture technique using one of the commercial kits for herpes simplex virus. The format of these test kits can be obtained from

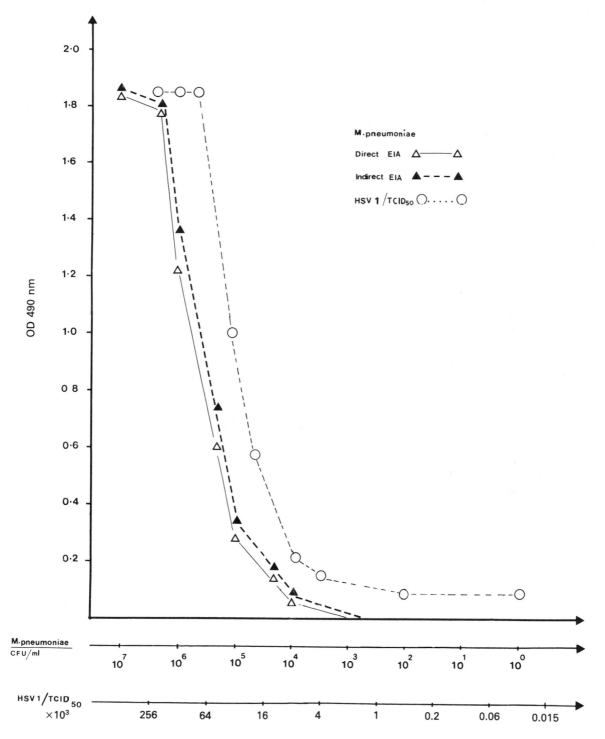

Fig. 48.7 Illustration of dose response curves showing relation between % binding in antigen capture EIA and numbers of colony forming units (cfu) of *M. pneumoniae* or tissue culture infective doses (TCID50) of herpes simplex virus.

the product leaflets. However, the reader may consult the *Methods* section of Chapter 45 for an account of a comparable antigen capture method applied to the detection of *Mycoplasma pneumoniae* antigen in nasopharyngeal secretions and sputum.

Figure 48.7 illustrates dose response curves in antigen capture assays for (1) herpes simplex virus antigen, and (2) *M. pneumoniae* antigen, plotted in the same graph. The left hand axis shows the optical density readings obtained with the coloured 'split product' liberated by the enzyme (peroxidase in this instance) from the test substrate. Inspection of the curves suggests that between 10^4 and 10^5 cfu of *M. pneumoniae* and about 10^6 TCID50 of herpes simplex virus are required to give a 'positive' result. As explained in Chapter 45, the 'cut off' value between 'positive' and 'negative' is ascertained by testing a large number of specimens negative for the viral or non-bacterial antigens on other grounds (e.g. culture; serotesting of patients) and taking a value 3 standard deviations above the mean value as the boundary between positive and negative. It may also be noted that the use of the indirect test format yielded only a small, though consistent increase in sensitivity of antigen detection. It is recommended that any antigen capture kit introduced into the laboratory is calibrated in terms of dose response curve and that a standard positive control antigen at a dilution near detection endpoint is included in each test run.

SEROLOGICAL REAGENTS FOR IMMUNOFLUORESCENCE, ENZYME IMMUNOASSAY OR RADIOIMMUNOASSAY

The virological section of the bacteriological laboratory, for whom this chapter is written, will probably find it more cost-effective to purchase viral antisera and the corresponding detection systems whenever possible, rather than to prepare such reagents in their own laboratory. Comparative costings of 'in-house' preparation and of purchase from commercial sources should take into account not only the cost of the labour

in preparing and purifying antigens, and that of the purchase, housing, bleeding and immunization of animals, but also the costs of the subsequent purification, titration and specificity checks on the antisera thus obtained.

Antisera from commercial sources not only have the advantage of a standardized method of preparation on a large scale, with consequent batch reliability, but in addition they have frequently been purified both by fractionation of the specific globulins and affinity chromatography purification against the antigen for which they are to be used in IF or EIA tests. There are many commercial sources of such excellent reagents. These do not need to be accepted uncritically; the laboratory is obliged in any case to titrate the reagents with known positive and negative control specimens so as to determine the working dilutions of antiserum to be used under their own circumstances and also to check that the dilution nominated by the manufacturer is in fact suitable. Additionally, new batches of the reagents from the same supplier will need to be checked to see if they correspond in potency and specificity to previous batches. Table 48.2 (at the end of this chapter) lists some sources of viral antisera and corresponding detection systems. This list does not claim to be exhaustive and certainly does not imply that any product not mentioned is inadequate. The list is merely intended as an introduction to a wide field of supply which will enable a laboratory undertaking DVD to plan its operations. A more comprehensive guide to laboratory reagents (Linscotts Directory 1986–87) may be consulted for other sources of reagents.

There are however, circumstances in which antisera to particular virus groups may not be available (e.g. adenovirus serotype 40/41) and it is necessary to prepare the antisera in the laboratory.

In planning the immunization schedule several points have to be decided. First, whether a *post-infection* serum from a laboratory animal (e.g. antibody to parainfluenza 2, *Coxiella burneti* or, say, herpes simplex virus in a guinea-pig) will contain antibody at a level and specificity that will do the job. A post-infection serum represents the animal's immune response to replicating virus or other agent uncomplicated by an unwanted hyperimmune antibody response to foreign protein in the inoculum or to contaminants such as mycoplasmas.

Second, if a post-infection serum is not adequate and hyperimmunization of the animal with antigen is unavoidable, then careful consideration must be given to reducing, as far as possible, the number of extraneous antigens in the inocula so that the antibody response of the animal is directed as completely as possible to the viral antigen under study.

Unwanted heterospecific or cross-reacting antibodies may arise during the course of hyperimmunization in several ways:

1. Antibodies may be stimulated by antigens of the cells in which the viral inoculum has been grown. For example, an enterovirus grown in HeLa cells maintained with fetal calf serum will stimulate antibody to human and bovine antigens as well as to the enterovirus. Whenever possible, the virus for immunization should be grown in the same species of cell as the animal to be immunized and with the same species of serum in the cell culture maintenance medium. Thus adenovirus can be grown in RK13 cells with rabbit serum for immunization of rabbits.

When the cell in which the virus is grown and the animal immunized have to be of different species, then the viral harvest should be purified by sucrose density centrifugation or other methods to concentrate the antigen and to reduce the load of contaminating host cell antigen. This may be effective with unenveloped viruses but enveloped ones may acquire cell-surface antigen markers with host specificity as part of their envelope as they bud from the cell.

2. Contaminating mycoplasmas, of human or animal origin, may be present in apparently normal cell culture and in large numbers in the stock virus seeds used to inoculate cell cultures. The same contaminant species of mycoplasma may be present by chance in different lines of virus used to prepare inocula for antiserum production and may well lead to unexplained cross-reactions between the resulting antisera. The virus seed, and the cells, should be cultured or checked for contaminating mycoplasmas and the size of the population of mycoplasmas should

be reduced or eliminated by treatment with antibiotic such as tiamulin, or fresh mycoplasma-free virus and cells should be used (Ch. 45).

3. Animal viruses generically related to those in human beings and sharing antigens with them may be present in the laboratory animal to be immunized and this may alter or even diminish the specific response obtained. For example, rotaviruses are common in many animal species and it may be difficult to find an animal free of cross-reacting antibody before immunization. The immunization course may boost the antibody response against shared viral antigens rather than to the predominant antigen against which it is hoped to raise the antiserum.

4. Finally, in preparing viral inocula for animal immunization, consideration has to be given to the desired spectrum of reactivity of the antiserum in relation to the purpose for which it is to be used. With a virus species of a single serotype, e.g. measles, the use of an inoculum containing the virus-coded envelope proteins and the internal nucleoprotein antigen would be an acceptable strategy; the antiserum would react with membrane antigens and free antigen inside the cell. On the other hand, an antiserum to a single serotype of influenza A, with haemagglutinin and neuraminidase antigens unrelated to currently prevalent strains, and with a low content of antibody to the group-reactive internal nucleoprotein ('soluble') antigen might be of limited value in the IF examination of nasopharyngeal cells from patients with suspected influenza.

When points (1) to (4) have been taken into account, it is probable that semi-purified virus, with some residual contaminating cell protein, will be mixed with complete or incomplete Freund's adjuvant and injected into the animal at several sites and followed by a series of booster injections of the same preparation intravenously or intraperitoneally (Ch. 14).

Once test bleedings of the rabbit or other animal show a satisfactory specific antibody level, attention can be given to removing unwanted specificities from the newly prepared antiserum. The major one will be antibodies directed against the antigens of the cells in which the virus was grown, if this was not autologous.

The serum is first absorbed with a substantial bulk of a lightly homogenized and washed suspension of tissue from an organ of the species from which the host cell was derived, e.g. human liver or kidney when HeLa or other human epithelial cell was used for viral propagation. The tissue homogenate is deposited by centrifugation; a volume of heat-inactivated serum, about 10 times that of the pellet, is added and the mixture resuspended with a Pasteur pipette or by vortex mixing. The mixture is held for 2 h at 20°C followed by 18 h incubation at 4°C with periodic mixing. The tissue suspension is then removed by centrifugation; a final absorption may be done by overlaying the antiserum on a formalin-fixed sheet of the host cell (e.g. HeLa) used to propagate the virus inoculum, with periodic rocking of the serum overlay. After a further period of 10–18 h at 4°C the serum is removed, centrifuged, filtered and tested on virus-infected and control uninfected cells by IF to determine its virus-specific and host-cell antibody levels.

Reactions with the cell culture medium components – usually fetal calf serum – can be removed by heat-coagulated or glutaraldehyde cross-linked serum, which will take out reactivities against serum proteins (Avrameas & Ternynck 1969); these may be different from those on cells of the same species and both absorption steps will probably be necessary.

It should also be noted that the use of Freund's complete adjuvant may lead to the generation of antibodies to cell wall or other components of the mycobacteria used in the mixture. These antibodies may react, for example, with *Mycobacterium tuberculosis* or other mycobacteria in infected tissue (brain biopsy samples, lymph node, liver, etc.), giving misleading results.

Other approaches to avoid anti-host specificities in antiviral antisera may be employed. For example, in difficult cases, an antiserum may be prepared against the cell in which the virus is to be grown, in the same species of animal to be immunized with the virus. This anti-cell serum is mixed with the virus grown in the same cell and used to immunize the animal. The intention is to 'blanket' host-cell specificitis with an antibody that will be recognized as 'self' by the laboratory animal being immunized.

This approach to the preparation of antisera against low potency immunogens that need to be 'recognized' against a distracting background of numerous cellular antigens has been supplemented or supplanted by the preparation of monoclonal antibody to the desired epitope (Gafré & Milstein 1981, Yolken 1983).

Finally, the specificity of viral antisera may be improved by adsorption and elution of the specific antibody to the antigen bound to a solid support (affinity chromatography). This has a number of advantages. The specific antibody is separated from other (unknown) antibody globulins present in the animal's serum and also from non-globulin proteins which may be non-specifically 'sticky'. The affinity-purified antibody has clearly reacted avidly with the antigen and retains its polyclonal character of reacting with a range of epitopes on the virus. Lastly, there is a substantial saving of enzyme or radiolabel in preparing the conjugate. A number of firms offer affinity-purified antibody – Kirkegaard & Perry have a wide range of labelled and unlabelled antiglobulins and Sera-Lab have a kit (Insolmer) for batch affinity purification of soluble protein antigens. The principles of affinity chromatography, including the coupling of proteins in soluble supports, are dealt with in the Pharmacia handbook, Affinity Chromatography, Principles and Methods, (obtainable from Pharmacia Fine Chemicals).

The absorbed sera may then be titrated by immunofluorescence on mixtures of infected or uninfected cells as previously described, or on infected 'flying coverslip' cultures. A dose of virus is used, which at 24–48 h of incubation, shows 50% of the cells with CPE. Cells will be at various stages of virus replication, thus presenting a range of early and late virus antigens, unassembled and assembled, comparable with the range likely to be seen in exfoliated cells taken during an acute infection. An adequate antiserum is considered to be one that can be used in IF tests at a dilution of at least 1 in 100. Similarly, the antisera may be titrated in EIA, and working dilutions for coating of plates, etc., determined as already outlined.

Labelled antisera and antiglobulin conjugates. Similar considerations apply to the procurement and use of these reagents as to the viral antisera described above, i.e. it is quicker and cheaper to buy them than to prepare them, particularly given that the required range of second antibodies or conjugates is much less than that of viral antisera.

Table 48.3 (at the end of this Chapter) details some sources of conjugated sera both for fluorescein and tetramethyl rhodamine labelled reagents. It also gives details of sources of peroxidase, phosphatase and urease detection systems for use on sections or in EIA antigen capture systems.

For those who wish to prepare their own fluorescent conjugates, particularly for direct labelling of viral antisera, reference to the detailed methods may be made to Nairn (1976), Kawamura (1977) and Riggs (1979).

DIRECT VIRUS DIAGNOSIS BY DETECTION OF VIRAL NUCLEIC ACIDS IN CLINICAL SAMPLES

The major part of this chapter has been directed to describing methods whereby viral antigens – virion components or non-virion antigens – may be detected in cells or exudates from lesions for direct diagnosis. Virally infected cells also contain large amounts of viral nucleic acid (DNA or RNA), frequently well in excess of the amounts packaged in virions and exported from the cell.

For many years virologists have quantified and compared viral DNA and RNA by hybridization methods, either as a means of determining relationship among viruses ('speciation'), or as part of analyses of the kinetics and sequence of events in the replication of the viral genome and formation of viral messenger RNAs that code for viral structural proteins and replicative enzymes.

More recently, considerable interest has been generated in the possibility of detecting, as a diagnostic measure, viral nucleic acid sequences in infected cells or free virions in exudates from infected lesions. The nucleotide sequences of a particular virus or group of related viruses are unique, so their detection offers a highly *specific* test for the presence of the virus(es). However, such approaches have also to be as *sensitive* and as *rapid* as detection of viral protein antigens, and to compare favourably with culture of the virus.

Current efforts are directed at assessing all these attributes of viral nucleic acid detection in comparison with antigen detection and culture.

Obviously in those special instances such as infection with viroids, in which a capsid protein is not coded and culture systems are inefficient, the detection of the viral nucleic acid offers clear advantages. Again, with vertebrate viruses that do not grow, or grow poorly in cell culture, such as hepatitis B virus, the parvovirus of erythema infectiosum, or the human papilloma viruses, the detection of viral sequences may offer a viable diagnostic measure, although in the first two of the examples quoted viral antigen can also be detected with high efficiency.

The principles involved in this newly developed variant of DVD follow well-established lines; the molecular biological background is simply and clearly described in the books by Watson et al (1983) and Davis et al (1986) on recombinant DNA technology, as well as in reviews by Meinkoth & Wahl (1984) or the cloning manual by Maniatis et al (1982). Clinical applications are reviewed by Kulski & Norval (1985) and in a published symposium (Wie-Shing Lee 1985).

As is well known, double-stranded DNA consists of a double helix of two nucleotide chains with matched or complementary bases that pair with one another – guanine with cytosine and adenine with thymine. This base pairing may be broken and the two strands of DNA separated by heat or alkali. On removal of the denaturing conditions the strands with sequences of complementary bases will reanneal in a highly specific manner. If DNA is denatured in solution and another species of DNA or RNA is mixed with it, then when the conditions permitting reannealing are re-established, 'mixed' hybrids or duplexes may form between the nucleotide chains of the first and second DNAs, or DNA-RNA heteroduplexes may form. At the same time, of course, some complementary chains of the original DNA will also reassociate and reanneal; a process that will compete with the formation of 'mixed' duplexes.

The extent of hybridization will depend on the amount of base pairing between the two species of DNA, i.e. on the degree of relatedness of the sequences (homology) between the two DNAs. By adjusting the temperature, and concentration of salt and formamide (a denaturing agent), the amount of mismatching that is permitted may be varied.

A large 'mismatch' will be tolerated under conditions of low stringency (low temperature, high salt, low formamide concentrations), but will remain unstable. Such hybrids will be easily disrupted in buffers of higher temperature and low ionic strength. Lesser degrees of mismatch will be permitted as the hybridization temperature is increased, the salt concentration decreased or the formamide concentration increased. These hybrids will be more stable when washed at high temperature or in low salt buffers.

The formation of duplexes between a nucleotide chain of known viral origin ('the probe') and chains of high or complete sequence homology in lesion material – the basis of the nucleic acid probe detection technique – can be demonstrated in various ways. That most commonly used is to denature double-stranded DNA, e.g. by boiling for 5 min or treating with 0.5 mol/litre sodium hydroxide, quickly neutralizing with 0.5 mol/l hydrochloric acid in 1.5 mol/l sodium chloride, and then 'spotting' or filtering the sample on to a nitrocellulose membrane before reannealling can occur. Single-stranded DNA binds to nitrocellulose membranes and the separated complementary strands can then be fixed in position by baking (e.g. at 80°C for 2 h). Such 'target' DNA can then be conveniently handled for hybridization with one or a number of known probes. To do this, the membrane is immersed in a hybridization solution containing complementary DNA (probe) identified with a radio-isotopic label or other tag, in a single-stranded state and held at a predetermined temperature; hybrids readily form. Unstable, mismatched hybrids may then be removed by washing in buffers of varying temperatures and ionic strength depending on the degree of

homology between target and probe that is sought. Hybridization under low stringency conditions and washing under low stringency conditions will enable detection of distantly related DNA, whereas the use of higher temperatures (i.e. more stringent conditions) will detect only closely related DNA. The DNA targets in these 'dot blot' hybridization tests may be purified before they are applied to the nitrocellulose filter or they may be clinical samples without further processing, or the cells extracted from such samples spotted on the membrane samples ('cell blots'). Efforts have been made to improve the specificity of tests with unpurified clinical samples by using a 'sandwich' assay in which a 'capture' strand of DNA anchored to the membrane hybridizes to part of the 'target' and a labelled probe attaches to a contiguous sequence (Fig. 48.8, Ranki et al 1983, Virtanen et al 1983).

Hybridization may also be effected in solution and the duplexes separated from the unhybridized single-stranded nucleic acid by batch or column treatment on hydroxyapatite, which selectively binds duplexes. Another variant of the technique is to hybridize probe to denatured nucleic acid targets in cells in tissue sections or cell monolayers on microscope slides (in-situ cytohybridization) with subsequent location of the bound radioactive probe by autoradiography.

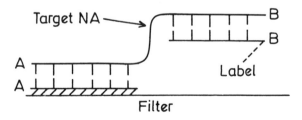

Fig. 48.8 Principle of sandwich hybridization on filters. The target viral nucleic acid (NA) contains contiguous but non-overlapping sequences A and B. A single stranded unlabelled probe for A is attached to the filter and 'captures' the target. A labelled probe (B) for the other sequence is mixed with the denatured viral nucleic acid in solution and applied to the filter during reassociation of the NA. After stringent washing an appropriate detection system for the label is added. This may be an enzyme substrate if probe B is directly labelled with enzyme. Or it may be avidin and enzyme if the probe is labelled with biotin. Or finally, the membrane may be counted if the label is ^{32}P, ^{125}I or other radiolabel.

Probes are prepared in various ways. The DNA sequence of interest – in the case of DVD, part of the viral genome of a DNA virus or a complementary DNA (cDNA) copy of an RNA virus – is cloned in a vector both to produce high yields of probe DNA and a reproducible product representing a particular part of the viral genome, e.g. a conserved portion common to a number of closely related viruses in the group. The commonly used system for propagation of viral nucleic acid is *Escherichia coli* containing the plasmid pBR322 which has antibiotic resistance genes for ampicillin and tetracycline. DNA sequences cloned into a restriction enzyme site in one of the antibiotic resistance genes will interrupt its expression and provide a means of identifying and selecting the colonies of *E. coli* with the plasmid containing the inserted DNA or cDNA (see Watson et al 1983).

The *E. coli* containing the plasmid with insert is grown in broth culture containing the selective antibiotic; the plasmid with insert is extracted from the bacteria and either the whole construct is used as a probe, or the cloned insert may be excised and purified for use as a probe.

Apart from pBR322, many other plasmids and some bacteriophages may be used as vectors. Phage DNA is larger than plasmid DNA and will tolerate the insertion of larger fragments. Phages replicate within a bacterial cell many thousand fold, and are liberated to infect surrounding cells, thus resulting in numerous phage particles and so large probe yields. A synthetic hybrid between plasmid and phage (so called 'cosmid') will carry even larger inserts.

Single-stranded DNA probes may be produced by subcloning into the double-stranded replicative intermediate of the single-stranded bacteriophage M13; yet again other systems (e.g. the SP6 system) have been constructed that have the necessary 'signal boxes' to lead to the production of an RNA transcript from the region of the inserted gene. These single-stranded RNA probes have certain advantages over double-stranded DNA probes in that DNA-RNA hybrids can be formed and remain stable at temperatures over 70°C at which the competing DNA-DNA reassociations are lessened.

Finally, once the base sequence of a viral (or other) gene has been established, it is possible to produce a synthetic DNA probe to key sequences of 25–50 bases. Such 'made to order' probes are still uncommon and most laboratories use an *E. coli*-plasmid or a bacteriophage system.

Labelling of probes

The probe hybridizing with the 'target' nucleic acid has to be detected by a label, commonly a radio-isotope, although efforts are being made to use enzymes directly or indirectly linked to the DNA probe as tags. The isotopes used are ^{32}P ($T_{\frac{1}{2}} = 14$ days), or longer half-life isotopes ^{35}S or ^{125}I; tritium-labelled probes have a use with in-situ cytohybridization.

The radiolabelling is commonly done by enzymic substitution of radiolabelled nucleotides for unlabelled ones – 'nick translation' – or enzymatically extending the ends of the probe fragment with additional radiolabelled nucleotides. In the case of RNA transcripts, radiolabelled nucleotides are supplied in the reaction mix and are incorporated during transcription.

Nick translation uses *E. coli* DNA polymerase I enzyme to simultaneously remove nucleotides from the 5′ phosphoryl-terminus and add nucleotides to the 3′ hydroxyl-terminus of a nick created in the dsDNA by a DNase I enzyme. Conditions may be changed to produce various size fragments with differing degrees of incorporation of radiolabel (specific activity). Radiolabelled probe binding to target DNA on a solid support may then be detected either by scintillation counting or exposure to an X-ray film (autoradiography) in the 'dot' or 'cell blot' techniques or by dipping in photographic emulsion or the stripping film technique with slides in the in-situ cytohybridization technique.

Enzyme labels can be attached to nucleic acids via biotin and chicken avidin or streptavidin with phosphatase or peroxidase, as with the antibody systems described earlier in this chapter. Biotinylated nucleotides can be incorporated into probes by nick translation (Mannelidis et al 1982, Leary et al 1983, Burns et al 1985) or attached by a highly reactive azide group activated by ultraviolet irradiation (Forster et al

1986). Despite initial enthusiasm for biotinylated probes the experience of many workers has been that they are not as sensitive as ^{32}P labelled probes. Biotin or other immunogen attached to DNA could also be detected with specific antibody linked with preformed avidin or antibody complex – as in EIA – in order to increase sensitivity, and the developments with EIA may improve non-radio-isotopic tracing with nucleic acid probes. Liquid hybridization techniques with hydroxyapatite separation employ ^{3}H or ^{125}I labelled probes in a rapid and sensitive fashion, giving a result within a matter of hours.

Specimens

The variety of specimens suitable for DNA hybridization is almost endless. DNA has been extracted from Egyptian mummies and used for hybridization. Less exotically, forensic pathologists have described DNA extraction from blood or semen traces up to many years old. However, most attention in the microbiology/virology laboratory has focused on its application to rapid diagnosis of pathogens difficult or slow to grow in culture, or for which appropriate antigen detection methods have not been developed.

Any tissue or body fluid containing the pathogen or its nucleic acid is suitable. Specimens may be processed either to extract and purify the DNA as a target, or to denature it while still in the tissues, and to probe for it in the presence of cellular debris.

DNA extraction

Briefly, samples are digested with proteinase K plus SDS, the protein is removed by phenol-chloroform extraction and the DNA precipitated in 70% ethanol. The precipitated, denatured DNA may then be filtered under suction on to nitrocellulose membrane. The use of a manifold, e.g. Bio-Dot apparatus (Bio-Rad), enables multiple specimens to be processed in one run. Alternatively, DNA is treated with restriction enzymes, electrophoresed on a gel, then denatured and transferred to a membrane and probed for fragments of specific sizes – Southern blot (see Watson et al 1983).

In-situ hybridization

Filter in situ. In this method, whole cells suspected to contain virus or viral nucleic acid are filtered on to a membrane, lysed with 0.5 mol/l NaOH, neutralized and baked. DNA hybridization is successful despite the presence of extraneous cellular material, e.g. papillomavirus DNA in exfoliated cervical cells.

In-situ cytohybridization. This is, strictly speaking, not a rapid virus diagnostic technique, as the process of exposing tissue sections to probes, particularly those labelled with ^{3}H, and subsequent detection of hybridized probe by autoradiography will take at least several days, and when the targets are present in low copy number, may take several weeks. Details of the techniques employed may be found in papers dealing with the detection of hepatitis B virus DNA in hepatocytes and other tissues (Burrell 1984). The method has also been employed with papillomavirus in cells from cervical smears.

Current status of DVD by nucleic acid hybridization: papilloma virus as illustration

The development of DNA hybridization as a diagnostic tool has been rapid although it is still in its infancy. This is well illustrated by developments with papillomavirus (Schneider et al 1985). In the period mid-1970s to 1986, 46 biotypes or subspecies of human papilloma virus have been described. Human papillomaviruses (HPV) cannot be grown in cell culture, nor can they be divided into biotypes by serological reactions. Their diversity remained unknown until cloning of HPV DNA and cross-hybridization with clinical samples from skin warts, cervical cells and cancers and materials from other sites.

The screening of cell or tissue samples with a library of probes at high and low stringency revealed distantly or closely related HPV sequences in an increasing range of tissues. Further, certain HPV biotypes have been related to specific diseases, e.g. HPV 16 and 18 DNA can be found in 80% of cervical carcinomas (distantly related HPV types probably make up the rest) while HPV 6 and 11 DNA are found in almost all genital warts (Gissman et al 1984, Syrjänen 1986). Dysplastic lesions of the cervix may contain any combination of the four types, but progression to carcinoma in situ occurs more frequently if types 16 and 18 are present (Campion et al 1986).

As an example, Figure 48.9 presents the hybridization patterns of DNA extracted from genital tissue and other cells. Specimens 1, 2, 3 and 4 were genital warts; specimen 5, HeLa cells; and specimen 6 from Bowenoid papulosis of the vulva. Briefly, $c.$ 50 mg of tissue was digested overnight in proteinase K/SDS, extracted with phenol/chloroform and ethanol-precipitated. Following RNAse treatment,

reextraction and precipitation, DNA was quantified by spectrophotometry, 1 μg and 100 ng of DNA were boiled to denature the DNA and applied to nitrocellulose (BA 85).

Plasmids containing HPV 6, 11, 16 and 18 were obtained from Professor L. Gissman (Deutches Krebsforschungszentrom, Heidelburg, West Germany). HPV 6, 11 and 16 were cloned into the Bam Hl site of pBR322 and HPV 18 into the Eco Rl site of pBR322. *E. coli* transformants with these plasmids exhibit the phenotypes ampicillin resistant, tetracycline sensitive for HPV 6, 11 and 16, and ampicillin and tetracycline resistant for HPV 18.

After growth in minimal medium (LB Broth; Maniatis et al 1982), plasmids were extruded by

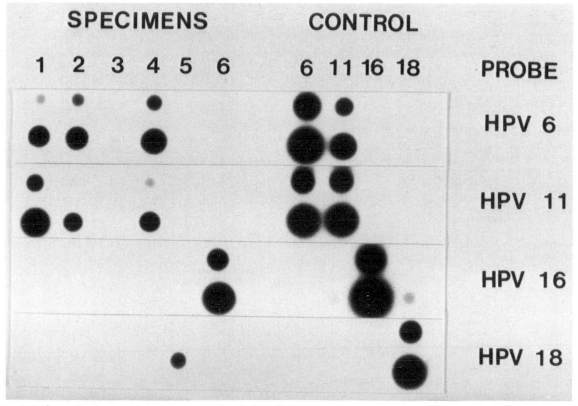

Fig. 48.9 Autoradiograph of Schleicher and Schuell nitrocellulose membrane on which extracted DNA (100 ng and 1000 ng) from genital warts (specimens 1, 2, 3 and 4), HeLa cells (5), and Bowenoid papulosis (6) was applied. 100 pg and 1000 pg of purified insert DNA of HPV 6, 11, 16 and 18 was applied as a control. Replicate filters were hybridized for 16 hours under conditions of high stringency with HPV 6, 11, 16 and 18 labelled by nick translation, then washed and autoradiographed overnight. Extensive cross-reaction between HPV 6 and HPV 11 can be seen in both the controls, and in specimens 1, 2 and 4; the relative intensity of the reactions of these specimens with the probes, suggests that specimen 1 contains HPV 11, and specimens 2 and 4 contain HPV 6. On the other hand, there is relatively little cross-reaction between HPV 16 and 18, as exemplified by the controls, and specimens 5 and 6.

Table 48.1 Methods for direct virus diagnosis in various diseases. *Key*: †, test not available or not applicable; ±, test possible but of low sensitivity; + to ++, test useful to highly effective; *, detection theoretically possible or demonstrated on a pilot scale but not generally in use; . . ., no information.

Organ system and disease	Virus group	Specimen	Microscopy		Antigen detection			Probe for viral nucleic acid
			Bright field	EM	IF	EIA	RIA	
Skin/mucous membranes								
Herpes simplex	Herpesvirus	Vesicle fluid; cells scraped from base of lesion	Cytology for inclusion bodies:	+/+++†	++	++	++	++
Herpes zoster								
Varicella			Giemsa/H and E	+/++	++	++	. . .	*†
			Papanicolaou (Pap)	+/++	++	++	. . .	*
Vaccinia	Poxvirus	Vesicle fluid; cells scraped from base of lesion	Cytology-Gutstein for EBs	++		gel diffusion/CF		
Orf				++				
Paravaccinia			Cytology-acridine orange (AO)	++	−†	−	. . .	. . .
Molluscum contagiosum				++	−	−	. . .	. . .
Warts – Plantar warts –	Papilloma	Cell scrapes Biopsy	Cytology – AO/Pap	++	+	+	+	++
Genital warts (Cervical atypia or neoplasia)		Swab or brushing	Cytology-AO/Pap	−	±	±	±	++
Erythema infectiosum	Parvovirus	Plasma Lesion biopsy	−†		++	−	−	++	++
Respiratory tract								
Influenza	Influenza virus	Mucoid exudate and cells, nasopharyngeal aspirate (NPA)	−		−	++	+	−	*
Croup	Parainfluenza virus		−		−	++	*	−	*
Bronchiolitis	Respiratory syncytial virus		−		−	++	++	++	*
Pneumonia	Respiratory syncytial virus		−		−	++	++	++	*
	Adenovirus		−		−	++	++	++	*
	Cytomegalovirus (CMV)		Cytology, AO/Pap	−	++	++	++	++
	Measles		Cytology, AO/Pap	−	++	++	*	*
URTI – 'colds'	Rhinovirus		−		−	(culture or seroconversion only)			
	Coronavirus		−		−	(culture or seroconversion only)			
Nasopharyngeal carcinoma	Epstein Barr virus	Cells obtained by NPA	−		−	++	−	−	++
Measles	Measles	Urine	Cytology, H and E	−	+	*	*	−
Gastro-intestinal tract								
Enteritis	Rotavirus	Faeces	−		+	−	++	*	+
	Adenovirus		−		+	−	++	*	*
	'Coronavirus'		−		++	−	−	−	−
	'Small round virus'		−		++	−	−	−	−
Hepatitis	Hepatitis A	Faeces	−		++	−	*	*	*
		Serum	−		−	(specific IgM Ab detection)			
	Hepatitis B	Serum	−		++	−	++	++	++
		Liver biopsy	++		±	++	++	*	++
						(HBsAg: HBcAg)		
	Non-A, non-B hepatitis	(Serum)	−		−	(serological diagnosis by exclusion)			
		Liver biopsy	+		−				
	CMV/Epstein Barr virus	(Serum)	−		−	(serological diagnosis)			
Central nervous system								
'Poliomyelitis'	Poliovirus	Faeces	−		±	culture and seroconversion			
	Enterovirus	Faeces	−		±	culture and seroconversion			
		NPA	−		±	culture and seroconversion			
Meningitis	Mumps	Gargle, urine	−		−	culture and seroconversion			
	Enterovirus	Faeces	−		−	culture and seroconversion			

Organ system and disease	Virus group	Specimen	Microscopy		Antigen detection			Probe for viral nucleic acid
			Bright field	EM	IF	EIA	RIA	
Encephalitis	Herpes simplex	Biopsy	H and E, Pap	+	++	++	++	*
	Arthropod borne	Serum	−		(culture and seroconversion)			
Measles Encephalitis	Measles virus	Biopsy	H and E	−	−	−	−	. . .
SSPE	Measles virus	Biopsy (serum/CSF)	H and E, AO	+	++	++	++	−
					(serodiagnosis)			
Rubella SSPE	Rubella	Biopsy (serum/CSF)	. . .		. . .			
					(culture: serodiagnosis)			
Creutzfeldt-Jakob disease	Group unknown	Biopsy	Histology, H and E	+				
					(animal inoculation)			
Progressive multifocal leukoencephalopathy	Polyomavirus (JC)	Biopsy Urine	Histology, H and E	‖	++	. . .	. . .	*
					(culture: human fetal glial cells)			
Eye and uveal tract Keratoconjunctivitis	Herpes simplex	Cell scrapes	Cytology AO/Pap	+	++	++	*	*
	Adenovirus	Cell scrapes	Cytology AO/Pap	+	++	++	*	*
	Enterovirus 71	Swab	−		−			−
	Molluscum contagiosum	Cell scrapes	Cytology		(cell culture)			
	Chlamydia	Cell scrapes	Giemsa	+	++	*	. . .	*
Intra-uterine and perinatal	Rubella	Serum	−		−			
					(serological tests: IgM)			
	CMV	Serum	−		−			
		Urine	Cytology, H and E		(serological tests: IgM)			
					−			
	Herpes simplex	Throat swab,	−		+	+	*	+
		liver biopsy, serum	−		(cell culture)			
					−			
					(serological tests: IgM)			
Miscellaneous Burkitt's lymphoma	Epstein Barr virus	Biopsy	−		−			
					++	−	−	++
Aplastic crisis in anaemias	Parvovirus	Serum	−		+			
					−	−	++	++
AIDS, pre-AIDS	HIV	Serum	−		−			
					(serological tests)			

alkaline lysis and purified. With the appropriate restriction enzyme, the cloned DNA was excised from vector DNA, separated on an agarose gel and purified.

For control, 100 pg and 1000 pg (1 ng) of purified cloned DNA was denatured by heating and applied to the nitrocellulose.

A 100 ng sample of insert was labelled with [^{32}P] dATP and [^{32}P] dCTP by nick translation. After removal of unincorporated nucleotide by separation on a Sepharose G50 column, the probe was used at 10 ng/ml (*c.* 5×10^{6} counts/ml). Hybridization was performed in 50% formamide containing 0.75 mol/l NaCl and 0.075 mol/l Na citrate at 42°C for 16 h. Then filters were washed in 0.3 mol/l NaCl, 0.03 mol/l Na citrate, 0.1% SDS at 68°C for 90 min and exposed overnight to X-ray film (X OMAT RP, Kodak).

Three of the genital warts (Fig. 48.9) contained large amounts of HPV DNA hybridizing to the closely related HPV 6 and 11 probes. A fourth, specimen 3, was too weakly reactive with HPV 6 to show in this plate. HeLa cells are known to contain an incomplete HPV 18 genome DNA. Bowenoid papulosis lesions (which are similar in appearance to squamous cell carcinoma in situ) usually contain HPV 16 DNA.

Cloned viral nucleic acid probes have been described for a number of viruses, and may be

Table 48.2 Serological reagents and some sources of supply: viral antisera.

Antiserum	Antibody	Supplier[a]
Influenza A, B	Polyclonal (chicken/bovine)	Boots-Celltech
Respiratory syncytial virus	(bovine)	Flow
Parainfluenza 1 and 3	(chicken)	Micro Assoc
Respiratory syncytial virus	Monoclonal	Ortho Wellcome Dakopatts Carter-Wallace Sera-Lab
Herpes simplex 1 and 2	Polyclonal (rabbit)	Dakopatts Wellcome MA Bioproducts Sera-Lab
Varicella-zoster	Monoclonal	Ortho MA Bioproducts Sera-Lab
Cytomegalovirus	Polyclonal (goat) Monoclonal	BioGenex MA Bioproducts
Measles	Polyclonal (bovine) Monoclonal	Wellcome Sera-Lab
Rotavirus	Polyclonal (rabbit) (chicken)	Dakopatts Wellcome
Mumps	Polyclonal	Flow
Rubella	Polyclonal	Wellcome Ortho
Coronavirus	Polyclonal	NIAID
Rabies	Polyclonal	Webster
Hepatitis A	Polyclonal	NIAID
Hepatitis B anti HBs anti HBc	Polyclonal	Ortho Hoechst Abbott Behring NIAID Connaught

[a] For addresses of suppliers, see *Appendix 3*.

available for use, e.g. CMV (Spector & Spector 1985), adenoviruses (Gomes et al 1985, Hypiä 1985), herpes simplex viruses (Fung et al 1985), rotavirus (Dimitrov et al 1985).

Commercial kits are increasingly available and currently include biotin-labelled cloned DNA probes for HSV, EBV and CMV (Enzo Biochem) or synthetic oligonucleotide probes labelled with alkaline phosphatase, e.g. for HSV

1 and 2 (Snap:- synthetic *n*ucleic *a*cid *p*robe; Dupont).

General comment on nucleic acid hybridization and DVD

The limitations of nucleic acid hybridization as a viable method in DVD are (1) the need to use radioisotopes to attain sufficient sensitivity –

Table 48.3 Serological reagents and sources of supply: detection systems for immunofluorescence and enzyme-radioimmunoassay. *Key*: . . ., no information.

Reagent	Antibody	Supplier[a]
Fluorescein-labelled antiglobulins (anti-immunoglobulin class: many species: anti-mouse immunoglobulin for monoclonal antibody)	Polyclonal or Monoclonal	Miles Wellcome Orion Silenus Dakopatts Cappell Caltag Kirkegaard & Perry
Peroxidase conjugates	Polyclonal	Sigma Dakopatts Cappell Silenus Miles Caltag Kirkegaard & Perry
Alkaline phosphatase conjugate	Polyclonal	Sigma Dakopatts Cappell Silenus Miles Caltag Kirkegaard & Perry
Urease conjugate	Polyclonal	Commonwealth Serum Labs
Biotin conjugates	Polyclonal	Sigma Amersham Pacific Caltag Kirkegaard & Perry
Avidin-alkaline phosphatase Avidin-peroxidase	. . .	Sigma
^{125}I-antiglobulin	Polyclonal	Amersham
^{125}I-staphylococcal A protein	. . .	Amersham

[a] For addresses of suppliers, see *Appendix 3*.

Table 48.4 Some commercial test kits for detection of virus antigens.

Name	Antigen	Type of assay	Supplier[a]
Abbott RSV EIA	Respiratory syncytial virus	Enzyme immunoassay	Abbott
Imagen	Respiratory syncytial virus	Immunofluorescence	Boots-Celltech
Ortho RSV	Respiratory syncytial virus	Enzyme immunoassay	Ortho
HSV ELISA	Herpes simplex	Enzyme immunoassay	Dakopatts
Ortho HSV	Herpes simplex	Enzyme immunoassay	Ortho
MicroTrak HSV	Herpes simplex	Immunofluorescence	Syva
Rotavirus ELISA	Rotavirus	Enzyme immunoassay	Dakopatts
Wellcozyme	Rotavirus	Enzyme immunoassay	Wellcome
Rotazyme	Rotavirus	Enzyme immunoassay	Abbott
Wellcogen	Rotavirus	Latex agglutination	Wellcome
Slidex	Rotavirus	Latex agglutination	API
Rotalex	Rotavirus	Latex agglutination	Orion
Rotascreen	Rotavirus	Latex agglutination	Mercia
Auszyme	Hepatitis B surface antigen	Enzyme immunoassay	Abbott
HBe EIA	Hepatitis B e antigen	Enzyme immunoassay	Abbott

[a] For addresses of suppliers, see *Appendix 3*.

enzyme tagging is suboptimal at present, and (2) the length of the period needed to complete the test and expose the autoradiographs, often 1–3 days.

The use of high concentrations of probe – perhaps particularly of short synthetic probes – may shorten both the incubation and the autoradiography steps. For example, a recent paper (Gomes et al 1985) described a 2 h procedure for identifying adenovirus in nasopharyngeal ex-

foliated cells by DNA hybridization. Its sensitivity in comparison with IF and EIA remains to be determined.

The recent development of a test utilizing cDNA probes to specific and group mycoplasma ribosomal RNA sequences, which can be done in fluid media with separation on hydroxyapatite and completed in a matter of hours, indicates that the time factor can be reduced, although radiolabels were required (Gen Probe).

REFERENCES

Avrameas S, Ternynck T 1969 The cross-linking of proteins with glutaraldehyde and its use for the preparation of immunoadsorbents. Immunochemistry 6: 53–66

Avrameas S, Ternynck T 1971 Peroxidase labelled antibody and Fab conjugates with enhanced intracellular penetration. Immunochemistry 8: 1175–1179

Biegeleisen J Z, Scott L V, Lewis V Jr 1959 Rapid diagnosis of herpes simplex virus infections with fluorescent antibody. Science 129: 640–641

Burns J, Chan V T W, Jonasson J A, Fleming K A, Taylor S, McGee J O'D 1985 Sensitive system for visualising biotinylated DNA probes hybridised in situ: rapid sex determination of intact cells. Journal of Clinical Pathology 38: 1085–1092

Burrell C J 1984 Cell-virus relationships in persistent hepatitis B infection in man; implications from in situ hybridisation studies. In: Chisari F V (ed) Advances in hepatitis research. Masson, New York, p 62–68

Campion M J, McCance D, Cuzick J, Singer A 1986 Progressive potential of mild cervical atypia: prospective cytological, colposcopic, and virological study. Lancet 2: 273–240

Cohen S M, Gordon I, Rapp F, Macaulay J C, Buckley S M 1955 Fluorescent antibody and complement-fixation tests of agents isolated in tissue culture from measles patients. Proceedings of the Society for Experimental Biology and Medicine 90: 118–122

Davis L G, Debner M D, Battery J F 1986 Basic methods in molecular biology. Elsevier, New York

Dimitrov D H, Graham D Y, Estes M K 1985 Detection of rotaviruses by nucleic acid hybridization with cloned DNA of simian rotavirus SAII genes. Journal of Infectious Diseases 152: 293–300

Downie A W, Kempe C H 1969 Poxviruses. In: Lennette E H, Schmidt N J (eds) Diagnostic procedures for viral and rickettsial infections, 4th edn. American Public Health Association, New York, p 281–320

Dumbell K R, Nizamuddin M D 1959 An agar precipitation test for the laboratory diagnosis of small pox. Lancet 1: 916–917

Farr A G, Nakane P K 1981 Immunohistochemistry with enzyme labelled antibodies: a brief review. Journal of Immunological Methods 47: 129–144

Fetterman G H 1952 A new laboratory aid in the clinical diagnosis of inclusion disease of infancy. American Journal of Clinical Pathology 22: 424–425

Field A M 1982 Diagnostic virology using

electronmicroscopic techniques. Advances in Virus Research 27: 1–69

Flewett T H 1985 Rapid diagnosis of virus diseases. In: Tyrrell D A J, Oxford J S (eds) Antiviral chemotherapy and interferon. British Medical Bulletin 41: 307–403

Forster A C, McInnes J L, Skingle D C, Symons R H 1985 Non-radioactive hybridization probes prepared by the chemical labelling of DNA and RNA with a novel reagent, photobiotin. Nucleic Acid Research 13: 745–761

Fung J C, Shanley J, Tilton R C 1985 Comparison of the detection of herpes simplex virus with specific DNA probes and monoclonal antibodies. Journal of Clinical Microbiology 22: 748–753

Galfré G, Milstein C 1981 Preparation of monoclonal antibodies; strategies and procedures. In: Langone J J, van Vunzkis H (eds) Methods in enzymology 73: 1–46 Academic Press, New York

Gardner P S, McQuillin J 1980 Rapid virus diagnosis: application of immunofluorescence, 2nd edn. Butterworth, London

Giloh H, Sedat J W 1982 Fluorescence microscopy: reduced photobleaching of rhodamine and fluorescein protein by η prophyl gallate. Science 217: 1252–1255

Gissman L, Boshart M, Durst M, Ikenberg H, Wagner D, zur Hausen H 1984 Presence of human papillomavirus in genital tumours. Journal of Investigative Dermatology 63: 265–285

Goldwasser R A, Kissling R E 1958 Fluorescent antibody staining of street and fixed rabies virus antigens in mouse brains. Proceedings of the Society for Experimental Biology and Medicine 98: 219–223

Gomes S A, Nascimento J P, Siqueira M M, Krawczuk M M, Pereira H G, Russell W C 1985 In situ hybridization with biotinylated DNA probes: a rapid diagnostic test for adenovirus upper respiratory infections. Journal of Virological Methods 12: 105–110

Halonen P, Meurman O, Peterson U G, Ranki M, Lövgren T N-E 1984 New developments in the diagnosis of virus infection. In: Kurstak E, Marusyk R G (eds) Control of virus diseases. Dekker, New York, p 501–520

Heimer G V, Taylor C E D 1974 Improved mountant for immunofluorescence preparations. Journal of Clinical Pathology 27: 254–256

Hopwood D 1985 Cell and tissue fixation, 1972–1982. Histochemical Journal 17: 380–442

Hornsleth A, Friis B, Andersen P, Brenoe E 1982 Detection of respiratory syncytial virus in nasopharyngeal secretions by ELISA: comparison with fluorescent antibody technique. Journal of Medical Virology 10: 273–281

Hsu S, Raine L 1984 The use of avidin-biotin-peroxidase complex (ABC) in diagnostic and research pathology. In: DeLellis R A (ed) Advances in immunohistochemistry 2:31. Masson, New York

Hsu S, Raine L, Fanger H 1981 A comparative study of the peroxidase anti-peroxidase method and an avidin-biotin complex method for studying polypeptide hormones with radioimmunoassay antibodies. American Journal of Clinical Pathology 75: 736–738

Hypiä T 1985 Detection of adenovirus in nasopharyngeal specimens by radioactive and nonradioactive DNA probes. Journal of Clinical Microbiology 21: 730–733

Kawamura A Jr 1977 Fluorescent antibody techniques and their applications. University Park Press, Baltimore

Kendall C, Ionescu-Matiu I, Dreesman G R 1983 Utilisation of the biotin-avidin system to amplify the sensitivity of the enzyme-linked immunosorbent assay (ELISA). Journal of Immunological Methods 56: 329–339

Koen S M, Gordon I, Rapp F, Macaulay J C, Buckley S M 1958 Fluorescein antibody and complement fixation tests of agents isolated in tissue culture from measles patients. Proceedings of the Society for Experimental Biology and Medicine 98: 219–223

Kulski J K, Norval M 1985 Nucleic acid probes in diagnosis of viral diseases of man: brief review. Archives of Virology 83: 3–15

Leary J J, Brigote D J, Ward D C 1983 Rapid and sensitive colorimetric method for visualising biotin-labelled DNA probes hybridised to DNA or RNA immobilised on nitrocellulose-bioblots. Proceedings of the National Academy of Sciences, USA 80: 4045–4049

Lennette E H, Schmidt N J 1979 Diagnostic procedures for viral, rickettsial and chlamydial infections, 5th edn. American Public Health Association, New York

Leong A S-Y, Milios J 1986 Rapid immunoperoxidase staining of lymphocyte antigens using microwave irradiation. Journal of Pathology 148: 183–187

Linscotts Directory of immunological and biological reagents 1986–1987, 4th edn. Linscotts, East Grinstead

Liu C 1956 Rapid diagnosis of human influenza infection from nasal smears by means of fluorescein-labelled antibody. Proceedings of the Society for Experimental Biology and Medicine 92: 883–887

McIntosh K, Wilfert C, Chernesky M, Plotkin S, Mattheis M J 1978 Summary of a workshop on new and useful techniques in rapid virus diagnosis. Journal of Infectious Diseases 138: 414–419

McIntosh K, Wilfert C, Chernesky M, Plotkin S, Mattheis M J 1980 Summary of a workshop on new and useful techniques in rapid virus diagnosis. Journal of Infectious Diseases 142: 793–802

McLean D M, Wong K K 1984 Same day diagnosis of human virus infections. CRC Press, Boca Raton, Florida

Madeley C R 1972 Virus morphology. Churchill Livingstone, Edinburgh

Malherbe H H, Strickland-Cholmley 1980 Viral cytopathology. CRC Press, Boca Raton, Florida

Maniatis T, Fritsch E F, Sambrook J 1982 Molecular cloning: A laboratory manual. Cold Spring Harbor Laboratory, Cold Spring Harbor

Mannelidis L, Langer-Safer P R E, Ward D C 1982 High resolution mapping of satellite DNA using biotin-labelled DNA probes. Journal of Cellular Biology 95: 619–625

Margileth A M 1955 The diagnosis and treatment of generalised inclusion disease of the new born. Pediatrics 15: 270–283

Marmion B P, Goodburn G M 1961 Effect of an organic gold salt on Eaton's primary atypical pneumonia organism and other observations. Nature 189: 247–248

Meinkoth J, Wahl G 1984 Hybridization of nucleic acids immobilized on solid supports. Analytical Biochemistry 138: 267–284

Nairn R C 1976 Fluorescent protein tracing, 4th edn. Churchill Livingstone, Edinburgh

Oldig-Stenkvist E, Grandien M 1976 Early diagnosis of virus-caused vesicular rashes by immunofluorescence on skin biopsies. 1. Varicella zoster and herpes simplex. Scandinavian Journal of Infectious Diseases 8: 27–35

Ranki M, Palva A, Virtanen M, Laaksonen M, Soderlund H 1983 Sandwich hybridization as a convenient method for the detection of nucleic acids in crude samples. Gene 21: 77–85

Reynolds D W, Stagno S, Alford C A 1979 Laboratory diagnosis of cytomegalovirus infections. In: Lennette E H, Schmidt N J (eds) Diagnostic procedures for viral, rickettsial and chlamydial infections, 5th edn. American Public Health Association, Washington, p 399 439

Richman D, Schmidt N, Plotkin S et al 1984 Summary of a workshop on new and useful methods in rapid viral diagnosis. Journal of Infectious Diseases 150: 941–951

Riggs J L 1979 Immunofluorescent staining. In: Lennette E H, Schmidt N J (eds) Diagnostic procedures for viral, rickettsial and chlamydial infections, 5th edn. American Public Health Association, Washington, p 141–151

Sarkkinen H K, Halonen P E, Salmi A A 1981a Detection of influenza A virus by radioimmunoassay and enzyme immunoassay from nasopharyngeal specimens. Journal of Medical Virology 7: 213–220

Sarkkinen H K, Halonen P E, Arstila P P, Salmi A A 1981b Detection of respiratory syncytial, parainfluenza type 2 and adenovirus antigens by radioimmunoassay and enzyme immunoassay on nasopharyngeal specimens from children with acute respiratory disease. Journal of Clinical Microbiology 13: 258–265

Schneider A, Kraus H, Schuhmann R, Gissman N L 1985 Papillomavirus infection of the lower genital tract: detection of viral DNA in gynaecological swabs. International Journal of Cancer 35: 443–448

Schumann G B, Berring S, Hill R B 1977 Use of cytocentrifuge for the detection of cytomegalovirus inclusions in the urine of renal allograft patients. Acta Cytologica 21: 168–172

Self C H 1985 Enzyme amplification – a general method applied to provide an immunoassisted assay for placental alkaline phosphatase. Journal of Immunological Methods 76: 389–393

Soini E, Hemmila I 1979 Fluorimmunoassay: present status and key problems. Clinical Chemistry 25: 353–361

Spector S A, Spector D H 1985 The use of DNA probes in studies of human cytomegalovirus. Clinical Chemistry 31: 1514–1520

Syrjänen K J 1986 Human papillomavirus (HPV) infections of the female genital tract and their associations with intraepithelial neoplasia and squamous cell carcinoma. In: Sommers S C, Rosen P P, Fechner R (eds) Pathology annual. Appleton-Century-Crofts, Norwalk, Connecticut, Pt 1, p 53–89

Virtanen M, Palva A, Laaksonen M, Halonen P, Söderlund H, Ranki M 1983 Novel test for rapid virus diagnosis: detection of adenovirus in nasopharyngeal mucus aspirates by means of nucleic-acid sandwich hybridisation. Lancet 1: 381–383

Watson J D, Tooze J, Kurtz D T 1983 Recombinant DNA. Scientific American Books, Freeman, New York

Whitehead T P, Kricka L J, Carter T J N, Thorpe G H C 1979 Analytical luminescence: its potential in the clinical laboratory. Clinical Chemistry 25: 1531–1546

Wie-Shing Lee 1985 (ed) Symposium on nucleic acid probes and monoclonal antibodies in the diagnosis of infectious diseases. Clinics in laboratory medicine. Saunders Philadelphia, 5, No 3

Yolken R H 1982 Enzyme immunoassays for the detection of infectious antigens in body fluids: current limitations and future prospects. Reviews in Infectious Diseases 4: 35–68

Yolken R H 1983 Use of monoclonal antibodies for viral diagnosis. Current Topics in Microbiology and Immunology 104: 177–195

Yolken R H, Leister F J, Whitcomb L S, Santosham M 1983 Enzyme immunoassays for the detection of bacterial antigens utilizing biotin-labelled antibody and peroxidase biotin-avidin complex. Journal of Immunological Methods 56: 319–327

Serodiagnosis of virus infections

The serodiagnosis of virus infections (or of non-bacterial infections caused by agents such as chlamydia, rickettsia or *Mycoplasma pneumoniae* that are often the province of the virus laboratory) depends on the measurement of significant changes in the levels of total antibody, or that in certain immunoglobulin classes during the course of the infection, as outlined in Chapter 47.

In principle, the presence of antibody to a virus in a patient's serum is evidence that the latter's immune system has been exposed and responded to novel virus-specific antigens. This may result either from a symptomatic or an asymptomatic infection with a virus, or one of a group of viruses sharing common antigens, or from vaccination with a live, or killed virus vaccine.

Broadly, therefore, the detection of viral antibody may be used to indicate a current or recent infection, or a past infection with resulting immunity, or to provide epidemiological information about virus exposure and potential immunity in population surveys.

A very wide range of serological techniques can be used in clinical practice to detect virus-specific antibody. Criteria affecting the choice of method include:

1. *The level of test sensitivity required.* With the majority of acute symptomatic virus infections, the antibody response during the course of infection is usually sufficiently great for a method of only moderate sensitivity, e.g. complement fixation, to be perfectly adequate.

When detection of IgM antibody in a single serum sample is the goal, tests of greater absolute sensitivity such as immunofluorescence (IF), enzyme immunoassay (EIA) or radio-immunoassay (RIA) may be advantageous. Similarly, when the intention is to detect – as markers of immunity – low levels of antibody that may persist years after infection or appear in response to vaccination, these more sensitive techniques will often detect many more than an insensitive assay such as the CF test.

2. *The intensity of the antibody response in various immunoglobulin classes during the course of infection.* Some methods are equally suitable for detecting specific IgM and IgG antibody, e.g. haemagglutination-inhibition (HAI), whereas others are poor for detection of viral IgM antibody, e.g. CF, single radial haemolysis (SRH). Thus, after rubella infection, antibody may not be detectable by CF or SRH until 1–2 weeks after the appearance of HA antibody.

3. *A need to batch tests in the laboratory.* It is a common serodiagnostic practice to test a patient's serum for antibody to a number of virus antigens in parallel when the clinical history does not allow a reliable prediction of the particular agent involved, e.g. in respiratory infections. A test procedure that can be easily duplicated to test for multiple agents, e.g. CF, has distinct advantages over those that become more labour intensive with each new viral antigen added to the panel.

4. *The experience and preferences of the testing laboratory.* Despite the qualifications just made, it may nevertheless be desirable in a laboratory that has extensive experience with one method, e.g. IF, EIA or RIA, to use this method more widely than in a laboratory without this experience.

Quantitation of viral antibody: dilutions and titres

In serodiagnosis it is often necessary to determine the *amount* of a specific antibody in the patient's blood serum in order to distinguish between the presence of a large or increasing amount of antibody produced in response to a current infection and the presence of a small amount of antibody, perhaps the result of a previous infection or exposure to a cross-reacting antigen, but not produced in response to the patient's current illness. In routine tests it is impracticable to isolate the specific antibody and measure its mass. Instead, the amount of the antibody is estimated by determining the greatest degree to which the serum can be diluted without losing the power to give an observable primary or secondary reaction when mixed with the specific antigen. Increasing dilutions of the serum are mixed with constant amounts of antigen; the greatest reacting dilution gives a measure of the content of antibody and a value for the *titre* of antibody in the undiluted serum.

The notation for expression of this endpoint dilution or titre is considered at length in Chapter 10; as indicated there, titres should be expressed by the *integers* representing the endpoint of greatest reacting dilutions; e.g. if the greatest reacting dilution of the serum is one in 8, then the *titre* is 8. The term 'reciprocal titre' is incorrect and based on the mistaken use of a fraction to express the endpoint dilution; it should therefore be avoided. It is also recalled that titres reported from tests for bacterial antibody normally indicate the final dilution of the serum in the reaction mixture after all the other reagents have been added – e.g. bacterial suspension and saline diluent – over and above initial dilution of the serum. On the other hand, most serum antibody titres reported from the virological laboratory indicate either the (starting) dilution of the serum in the primary reaction mixture with virus or haemagglutinin, or the initial dilution of the serum without adjustment for the further dilution with the added reactants. In the latter instance the value has absolute meaning only in the context of knowledge of the volumes of the reactants added to each mixture and, more important, diagnostic information is gained from the relative increase or decrease in titre between the samples taken at various stages of the disease. Usually, two-fold differences in titre between serum samples tested in the same assay run are considered to be within the range of chance variations in the serological test, whereas a four-fold or greater difference in titre is taken as 'significant'. The 'four-fold or greater' rule is equally applicable to bacteriological and virological serological tests but bacteriologists tend to place more emphasis on absolute titres.

CHOICE OF SEROLOGICAL TESTS FOR DIAGNOSIS OF VIRUS AND NON-BACTERIAL INFECTIONS

The choice of techniques employed by the virus section of the bacteriological laboratory will mainly be influenced by the properties of the virus groups likely to be involved in a particular disease or syndrome, and to a lesser extent by familiarity with a particular technique or historical circumstances in the 'work up' of the techniques.

Complement fixation tests are widely used, particularly for the orthomyxoviruses (influenza A and B), the paramyxoviruses (parainfluenza 1,2,3, measles, mumps, respiratory syncytial virus), herpes viruses (herpes simplex, varicella zoster and cytomegalovirus), adenovirus and rotavirus. Good quality CF antigens representing these viruses are available from a number of commercial sources.

In circumstances in which the CF test is not sensitive enough or, in particular, when it is necessary to measure a strain-specific or type-specific antibody response to a virus, haemagglutination-inhibition or neutralization of infectivity may be used. For example, CF antibody to rubella virus can be detected during acute rubella, but a more sensitive test such as haemagglutination-inhibition or single radial haemolysis has to be used for assay of immune state in vaccinees or pregnant women. Again, although an enterovirus antigen with group reactivity or a common poliovirus antigen can be used in the CF test for the serodiagnostic confirmation of a suspected enterovirus infection, virus neutralization tests will generally be required for precise information on the infecting agent.

In virus infections, the complement fixation test mostly (but not invariably) measures antibody in the IgG class (Cowan 1973), and consequently its use is quite restricted in the analysis of immunoglobulin class response in infection. The use of the CF test for such analysis would require a preliminary separation of IgG and IgM fractions as a sucrose density gradient, or chromatographically, or perhaps by absorption of some IgG subclasses with staphylococcal protein A. At the end of the process the separated fractions may be anti-complementary. Consequently, the measurement of class-specific antibody responses is more easily accomplished by IF with immunoglobulin-class-specific conjugates and virus infected cells, or by EIA, RIA or adaptations of the haemagglutination-inhibition test. IF, EIA or RIA may also be preferred over CF either in circumstances in which potent antigens are not available or in particular those in which the cost of producing concentrated antigens for the CF test would be prohibitive.

Finally, it can be mentioned that although at the present time most laboratories use CF as their basic technique for antibody detection in the major groups of viruses, continuing improvements are occurring in the range, quality, price and potential for automation of routine EIA tests for this purpose. A laboratory newly setting up would be advised to assess both techniques carefully in the light of their own requirements and the range of tests to be offered.

Tables 49.1, 49.2 and 49.3 set out the possible and optimal tests for use with serum samples from various virus infections of the respiratory tract, central nervous system, and skin. In addition to the virus infections tabulated here, attention is drawn to the involvement of viruses in infections of the *eye*: namely, adenovirus, measles virus, enterovirus 70, Coxsackie A24, herpes simplex and varicella zoster virus in conjunctivitis or keratoconjunctivitis; rubella virus in cataracts and retinopathy in the congenital rubella syndrome, and cytomegalovirus in chorioretinitis. Also to the involvement of EBV, CMV, HSV, rubella virus and hepatitis A, B and non-A non-B viruses in *hepatitis*. Many of these infections can be diagnosed by detection of antigen or antibody.

A comprehensive account of the causes of viral syndromes is given by White & Fenner

Table 49.1 Patterns of involvement of various viruses in acute respiratory disease. Antigens and serological tests for investigation of these syndromes.

Viruses, antigens and serological test[a]	Acute respiratory disease/syndrome				
	Rhinitis	Pharyngitis	Bronchiolitis	Croup	Pneumonia
Rhinovirus*	+++[b]	++[b]	+[b]	−[b]	−
Coxsackie/enteroviruses*	+	++	+	+	−
Coronavirus (EIA)	+++	++	+	−	−
Influenza A (CF, HAI)	+	++	+	++	++
Influenza B (CF, HAI)	+	++	+	+	++
Adenovirus (CF)	+	++		−	++
Respiratory syncytial virus (CF)	+	+	++ (infants)	+	++ (infants)
Parainfluenza 1–3 (CF)	+	+	+	++	++
Measles (CF)	++	++	−	−	++
Herpes simplex (CF, EIA)	−	++	−	−	−
Varicella zoster (CF, EIA)	−	−	−	−	+
Cytomegalovirus (CF, EIA-M)	−	−	−	−	+
Epstein Barr virus (Paul Bunnell, IF-M)	−	++	−	−	−

* = Serological tests of less utility than culture – collect samples for Virus Reference Lab.
[a] = EIA and EIA-M: enzyme immunoassay for total antibody (EIA) or specific IgM antibody (EIA-M).
   CF, HAI, IF-M: antibody detection by complement fixation, haemagglutination inhibition or immunofluorescence for specific IgM antibody. Tests in italic print are those preferred for routine diagnosis.
[b] = − to ++++: indication of the (increasing) frequency with which the virus group is involved in the disease syndrome.

Table 49.2 Patterns of involvement of various viruses in acute infections of the central nervous system. Antigens and serological tests for investigation of these syndromes.

Viruses, antigens and serological tests[a]	Acute CNS disease					
	Meningitis	Encephalitis	Paralysis	Post-infection encephalomyelitis	SSPE	Reye's syndrome
Enteroviruses*	++[b]	+[b]	+[b]	−[b]	−	−
Mumps (CF, HAI)	+++	++	−	−	−	−
Measles (CF)	−	−	−	++	+++	−
Adenovirus (CF)	−	+	−	−	−	−
Influenza A, B (CF, HAI)	−	−	−	+	−	++
Herpes simplex (CF,EIA)	+	++	+	−	−	−
Varicella zoster (CF, EIA)	+	+	+	+	−	++
Epstein Barr virus (Paul Bunnel, IF-M)	+	−	−	++	−	−
Rubella (CF, HAI, EIA-M)	−	−	−	+	+	−
Arboviruses (CF,HAI)	+	+	+	−	−	−
Lymphocytic choriomeningitis(CF)	+	+	−	−	−	−

*,[a,b] See notes to Table 49.1.

Table 49.3 Patterns of involvement of various viruses in skin rashes. Antigens and serological tests for investigation of these syndromes

Viruses, antigens and serological tests[a]	Skin rash		
	Maculopapular	Vesicular	Wart-like or nodular
Enteroviruses*	++[b]	+[b]	−[b]
Arbovirus (CF, HAI)	++	−	−
Rubella (CF, HAI, EIA-M)	++	−	−
Measles (CF)	++	−	−
Herpes simplex (CF, EIA)*	−	++	−
Varicella-zoster (CF)*	−	++	−
Cytomegalovirus (CF, EIA- M)	++	−	−
Epstein Barr virus (Paul Bunnell, IF-M)	++	−	−
Vaccinia (CF)*	+	++	−
Papillomavirus[c]	−	−	++
Molluscum contagiosum[c]	−	−	++
Orf[c]	−	−	++

*,[a,b] See notes to Table 49.1.
[c] Direct diagnosis techniques required, see Chapter 48.

(1986). The possible contribution of non-bacterial agents such as chlamydias (e.g. pneumonitis, conjunctivitis and keratoconjunctivitis); *Mycoplasma pneumoniae* (e.g. pneumonitis, encephalitis, Guillain-Barré syndrome) and *Coxiella burneti* (e.g. hepatitis, pneumonitis, encephalitis) to these syndromes should not be overlooked; the appropriate antigens (Chs. 44, 45, 46) should be included in the panel of antigens used to screen or test the sera.

In summary, the clusters of tests employed by the virus serology laboratory are as follows:

1. *Acute respiratory infection in an adult.* First test for antibody to influenza viruses A and B,

adenovirus, chlamydia group antigen, *C. burneti* Phase 2 antigen, *Mycoplasma pneumoniae*; optional additions are parainfluenza viruses 1, 2 and 3, RSV and measles virus; also cytomegalovirus in an immunocompromised patient or recipient of a recent blood transfusion.

2. *Acute respiratory infection in a child.* Influenza viruses A and B, parainfluenza viruses 1, 2 and 3, RSV, measles virus, adenovirus and *M. pneumoniae*; optional additions, depending on epidemiological circumstances are chlamydia group antigen and *C. burneti* Phase 2 antigen.

3. *Acute CNS disease or peripheral neur-*

opathy. Influenza viruses A and B, adenovirus, chlamydia group antigen, *M. pneumoniae, C. burneti* Phase 2 antigen, mumps, measles and herpes simplex viruses. Coxsackie, echo and polio viruses are covered by culture of throat and faecal samples.

4. *Skin rashes.* Adenovirus, *M. pneumoniae,* measles, herpes simplex, varicella zoster and rubella viruses, cytomegalovirus and local arboviruses. As above, enteroviruses are covered by culture.

5. *Congenital abnormalities.* Rubella virus, cytomegalovirus. Serology for toxoplasma infection is also required (Ch. 43). Maternal serum must be tested in parallel to account for transplacentally acquired antibody. Virus culture from appropriate specimens is also required.

6. *Perinatal infections.* Cytomegalovirus although rarely symptomatic, HIV (when indicated), hepatitis B. Maternal serum must be tested in parallel to account for transplacentally acquired antibody. In addition, culture is necessary to cover herpes simplex virus, RSV and enteroviruses. Perinatal rotavirus infection is diagnosed by EM or antigen detection.

7. *Myocarditis/pericarditis.* Influenza A and B, adenovirus, *M. pneumoniae,* chlamydia group antigen. Tests for Coxsackie B 1–6 antibody by neutralization, IF or other techniques are required.

8. *Pyrexia of undetermined origin.* As for respiratory infections, plus Epstein Barr and cytomegaloviruses and local arboviruses. Enteroviruses have to be covered by culture.

9. *Acute hepatitis.* Hepatitis A and B, cytomegalovirus, rubella, Epstein Barr virus, *C. burneti.* Enteroviruses by culture.

10. *Therapeutically or naturally immunocompromised patients.* Herpes simplex and Epstein Barr viruses, cytomegalovirus, varicella zoster virus, hepatitis B virus and HIV (depending on mode of presentation).

The principles of the techniques are now considered in more detail and the technical details are given under *Methods* at the end of the chapter.

COMPLEMENT FIXATION TESTS

The fact that antibody, once it combines with antigen, is able to activate the complement system is used as a way of showing the presence of a particular antibody in a serum, or, conversely, when used with a known antiserum, to detect viral antigens in inflammatory exudates or in infected cell cultures.

The complement system consists of some 20 plasma proteins arranged in nine interacting groups in the serum of healthy persons. The complement of most species will react with antibody derived from other species; fresh guinea-pig serum is a common laboratory source of complement. The complement in fresh human serum has to be inactivated by heat before the serum is tested for complement-fixing antibody. Some of the components of complement are heat labile and are destroyed by heating at 56°C for 20–30 min. The individual components of the complement system are taken up by an antigen-antibody complex in a particular order; destruction of the heat-labile components – which are taken up early in the cascade reaction – prevents the remaining components from taking part.

For most antigens the reaction of the complement system with the antigen-antibody complex causes in itself no visible effect and it is necessary to use an indicator system, which commonly consists of sheep red cells coated with anti-sheep red cell antibody (see Ch. 10 and Fig. 10.13; also immune adherence and single radial haemolysis below). Complement has the ability to lyse the antibody-coated cells, probably by virtue of the esterase activity of one of the end-products of complement activation on the red cell membrane. In a test for viral antibody, the patient's serum, complement and antigen are first mixed together and after a period of incubation the indicator system, antibody-coated sheep erythrocytes, is added. The complement initially added to the system will, however, have been taken up ('fixed') during the incubation stage by the original antibody-antigen complex (if specific antibody was present) and will not be available to lyse the antibody-sensitized erythrocytes. Thus, a positive complement fixation test is indicated by absence of lysis of the erythrocytes while a negative test, with unused complement, is shown by lysis of the red cells (Fig. 10.13).

Fresh or specially preserved serum from healthy adult (250–300 g) guinea-pigs which have been starved for 24 h before being bled is used as a source of complement. It contains an active haemolytic complement for sheep erythrocytes sensitized with the homologous haemolytic antibody. When fresh serum is used, the blood is obtained by cardiac puncture 12–18 h before the test. It is allowed to clot and stand overnight in the refrigerator. The complement in serum too recently withdrawn is apt to be excessively 'fixable', and in consequence is unsuitable for the CF test.

When possible, the pooled serum of several guinea-pigs should be used. Guinea-pigs may suffer from infections with paramyxoviruses or chlamydias; antibody may be present in their sera and give rise to artefactual reactions when such sera are used as a complement source in the CFT proper. Small portions of the guinea-pig serum harvested for complement should be inactivated and tested with mumps and parainfluenza antigen and with chlamydial group CF antigen before the harvests are pooled for use as a complement source.

Complement is unstable and deteriorates on keeping at ordinary temperatures. It is advisable to keep the guinea-pig serum, particularly when diluted, on ice during the course of setting up CF tests. If storage at −30°C is available the fresh serum may be divided into small portions and kept frozen for a few weeks.

Specially preserved serum (see below) can be kept for several months, and it is now a general practice to use such a preparation made from the pooled blood of a number of animals. This should be absorbed with packed sheep erythrocytes (0.1 ml cells/ml guinea-pig serum for 30 min at 4°C).

Preservation of complement. For the preservation of complement two principles have been applied: (1) rapid drying of the serum from the frozen state in vacuo ('freeze drying') and the reconstitution of the serum when required by dissolving the dried material in the appropriate amount of distilled water; i.e. Rayner's method for the preservation of bacterial cultures and serum (Rayner 1943); (2) addition to the liquid serum of hypertonic sodium chloride or other salts, exemplified by Richardson's method* (Richardson 1941). Preservation of the complement-serum in the liquid state constitutes a simple and convenient procedure, and such preparations are available commercially (e.g. Wellcome), either in liquid form which will keep for a few months at 4°C or in the freeze-dried state. Once the freeze-dried reagent is reconstituted it should be stored at 4°C and used within 1 week as the gradual loss of CO_2 from the serum leads to pH changes and loss of activity.

Complement fixation tests for measurement of viral antibody

Details, including appropriate controls, are given under *Methods**. In principle, serial dilutions of heat-inactivated test sera, preferably paired, acute and convalescent phase samples, are prepared in a buffered CF diluent rich in Mg and Ca ions (co-factors for complement activation). The dilutions are generally made in microtitre plates, using a 0.025 ml unit volume. One volume of complement containing three 50% haemolytic doses (3HD50) is added to each of the serum dilutions, followed by an optimal dose of viral antigen.

Each serum has to be tested with several antigens and the test may be set out so that the serial dilutions of different sera take up the rows on a single plate and the same antigen is added to all wells on the same plate.

When all three reagents have been added and mixed, the plates are incubated, usually at 4°C overnight, to allow fixation of complement. A unit volume of sensitized cells is then added to each well in the plate. After a short incubation at 37°C, reading of the plates is facilitated by settling of the cells so that degrees of haemolysis

---

* Refer to *Methods* at end of this chapter.

may be assessed in the supernatant fluid in the wells; this may be achieved in a plate centrifuge or by gravity on the bench. Wells containing antibody show unlysed cells collected in the bottom (Fig. 49.1a, Plates 11.1 and 11.2, 12th Edn. Vol. 2, p. 259–260). The endpoint (titre) is taken as that dilution fixing 75–100% of complement and is expressed in terms of the starting dilution of the serum.

An alternative test format is to 'screen' sera, particularly the convalescent phase serum, at a standard dilution of, say, one in 40 against each of the viral antigens and then, in a second test run, to titrate both the acute and convalescent serum against those antigens giving a positive result in the initial screen test. While this may be more economical of reagents, reporting is delayed by a day and more labour is required. It is a matter for individual laboratory decision in relation to work patterns and reporting pressures.

ASSAYS FOR VIRAL NEUTRALIZING ANTIBODY

Neutralizing antibodies react with their homologous virus by attaching to certain critical epitopes in the capsid or envelope. This renders the virus incapable of initiating infection in susceptible host cells. The intimate mechanism of neutralization is unclear. In some instances, the critical epitopes appear to be ones related to proteins or other determinants reacting with viral receptors on the cell surface. However, except in strong concentrations of antibody, it is unlikely that the explanation is merely interference with adsorption to receptors. In many cases, the antibody may interfere with the uncoating of the virus in the cell cytoplasm, rendering it liable to destruction in the phagolysosomes. It is clear that the antibody does not invariably destroy the virus, as infective virus can in some cases be dissociated apparently unaltered from the virus-serum complexes by dilution or by lowering the pH of the reaction mixture. The formation of a virus-antibody complex is time-, temperature- and concentration-dependent and the sensitivity of a neutralization test will be governed by these factors and the indicator system. Neutralization

may be enhanced by the presence of complement or IgM rheumatoid factor. Note that not all antiviral antibody is neutralizing.

When carrying out neutralization tests it is necessary to include a virus-diluent control which is treated in exactly the same manner as the virus-serum mixture, since some viruses are thermolabile and their infectivity titre may decrease during the reaction. The interaction of the virus-diluent control with the indicator system (cells in culture, animals etc.) is used as the standard against which the test sample suspected to contain virus-specific antibody is compared.

Titration of neutralizing antibody can be applied to any virus provided there is a suitable indicator system for the presence of unneutralized virus. Neutralization tests are sensitive and often strain-specific, but tend to be costly and labour-intensive. Consequently, measurement of antibody in acute viral infections generally makes use of simpler and cheaper methods, such as the CFT. However, as the spectrum of antibody response to a virus is wide and includes antibody to internal as well as surface antigens, and as not all antibodies neutralize infectivity, there are particular circumstances – e.g. assessment of immune response to vaccine – in which it is necessary to measure neutralizing antibody.

The indicator system for unneutralized virus may be an animal, chick embryo or a cell culture. In all systems quantitation of infectivity of the stock virus preparation is a necessary first step in order to determine the size of inoculum to use in the test. In cell cultures, virus may be quantified as the amount that will infect a certain proportion of tubes of cell cultures (quantal response), or the number of cytopathic or other foci in a cell sheet (focal or plaque assay), or that amount which will inhibit the metabolism of a cell suspension.

Quantal response

In this method, the infectivity of the virus is assessed by the 'units' or 'quanta' of response produced in groups of experimental hosts challenged by inoculation of dilutions of the suspension; it may be measured in animals, chick embryos or in cell culture monolayers. The response may be the death of the animal or chick embryo, or the production of paralysis, or a certain degree of pneumonia, or seroconversion – any marker of infection that can be used to give a 'yes/no' or digital response.

In cell culture monolayers, a unit response in which more than two-thirds of the sheet is destroyed by CPE may be scored as positive or 'dead', or those sheets with less CPE as 'survived' – according to the convention of the laboratory. A dilution of inoculum at which 100% of hosts respond is sometimes used as an end-point, but is subject to greater variability than one at which 50% of the hosts respond. The 50% endpoints obtained thereby are variously described; e.g. when based on mortality, as the 50% lethal dose (LD50); when based on an indication of infection, as the infective dose (ID50); or when based on infection of cell cultures (so-called tissue cultures) as the TCID50, and so on. Determination of the 50% endpoint requires, in strict statistical terms, the use of a large number of animals or other viral substrates inoculated with closely spaced dilutions of virus around the expected 50% endpoint. Such titrations may not be economical in terms of time or animals, chick embryos or cell cultures. Consequently Reed & Muench (1938) devised a treatment of the data that takes into account the experience of the total group of susceptible hosts in the titration, not just the groups near the 50% endpoint.

Some of these points are discussed in Chapter 13; an illustrative virological example is given in Table 49.4. Ten-fold dilutions of virus were inoculated into groups of six cell culture tubes and those showing CPE several days later were scored 'positive' or 'negative'. A table of cumu-

lative values is drawn up in which the positive to negative CPE ratios are determined for each virus dilution by summing the 'positives' from the most dilute virus suspension to the most concentrated, and vice-versa for the 'negatives'. By inspection of the table, it will be seen that the 50% endpoint lies between dilutions of one in 10^3 (87.5%) and 10^4 (28.6%). A more precise estimate of its position between these two values is made using the following formula:

proportionate distance =
$$\frac{(\% \text{ positive at dilution above } 50\%) - 50\%}{(\% \text{ pos. at dilution } >50\%) - (\% \text{ pos. at dilution } <50\%)}$$

In the example given in Table 49.4 this would be:

$$\frac{87.5 - 50}{87.5 - 28.6} = \frac{37.5}{58.9} = 0.64$$

so that in this titration in which the incremental step is 10-fold, the TCID50 is a dilution of $10^{3.64}$.

Karber (1931) described a slightly different method that uses the observed mortality ratios at each of the dilutions of the virus suspension, rather than cumulative mortality and survivor ratios. The end results are quite close to those obtained by the Reed & Muench method. In all statistical methods for estimating a 50% endpoint, it is essential that the range of virus dilution is sufficiently wide to produce infection of all cell cultures at one end of the spectrum and none at the other.

When the value for the TCID50 has been established, neutralizing antibody in a test serum can be estimated either by titrating a range of

Table 49.4 Arrangements for calculating the 50% infective dose in titration of virus in groups of cell cultures by the Reed–Muench method. (For explanation, see text.)

Virus concentration	Effect in cell culture			Cumulative totals of effects		Ratio: positive/ total	Percentage number positive
	CPE positive	CPE negative	Positives total	Positive	Negative		
10^{-1}	6	0	6/6	19	0	19/19	100
10^{-2}	6	0	6/6	13	0	13/13	100
10^{-3}	5	1	5/6	7	1	7/8	87.5
10^{-4}	2	4	2/6	2	5	2/7	28.6
10^{-5}	0	6	0/6	0	11	0/11	0

serum dilutions from, say, 1 in 10 to 1 in 320 against 100 TCID50 of virus, or by testing a single, low dilution of serum against 100, 1000 and 10 000 TCID50 of virus. Details of the former type of neutralizing antibody test are given in Chapter 50. The virus section of a bacteriological laboratory may wish to make use of this type of neutralizing antibody titration, e.g. for the examination of sera for antibody to Coxsackie B virus in patients with carditis, or for antibody to enteroviruses isolated from faeces in order to obtain additional evidence relating the viral isolate to the disease.

Focal response – viral plaque assays

In this method viral suspensions near the infectivity endpoint are absorbed on to cell monolayers and overlayed with a medium that reduces the spread of progeny virus (released from the cells first infected). In this way, virus spreads only to cells adjacent to those infected by the inoculum and thus small foci of infection or plaques are formed, the number of which reflects the number of infectious particles added to the culture. After a suitable incubation period the plaques may be counted and the infectivity of the original inoculum expressed as plaque-forming units per ml (pfu/ml) of the suspension. The containment medium may include (1) an antiserum to the virus – this will prevent spread of released virus through the medium, so only closely adjacent cells will be infected, or (2) agar or agarose – this overlay is useful for small viruses such as polioviruses but has the disadvantage that if it is too hot it will kill the cells, and if too cold it cannot be pipetted; (3) methyl cellulose – this is incorporated in the medium at a final concentration of 0.75%; this overlay is more easily handled but is only sufficiently viscid to inhibit the diffusion of large viruses such as the herpes and pox viruses; (4) substances such as starch or tragacanth gum or combinations of agar and antibody may be used.

Production of plaques. This can be done using either preformed monolayers or by infecting cells in suspension. The details of preparation, in-

fection and enumeration of plaques is described in Chapter 50.

Detection of plaques. Viral plaques may be detected in a number of ways. With cytopathic viruses the vital stain neutral red is commonly employed; on the addition of the stain to the cell monolayer foci of dead cells (CPE) are seen as unstained areas against the sheet of viable cells which take up the stain. The stain may be incorporated into the nutrient overlay (designed to limit virus diffusion) but neutral red is toxic to some viruses; also it damages cells by photodynamic action when the cultures are handled in the light (cultures are incubated in the dark) and thus the number of cells able to support viral replication may be reduced. Consequently the dye is sometimes added as a second overlay at the end of the incubation period of the culture. Note that certain viruses (e.g. cytomegalovirus) which do not kill cells rapidly may enhance the uptake of neutral red producing a reversal of the effect just described.

Plaques produced by actively cytopathic viruses can also be detected by staining the cell monolayers with formol crystal violet, Giemsa stain or carbol fuschin. This treatment kills both cells and virus and does not allow subculture of the plaques to obtain cloned material. It is however very useful in providing a permanent preparation for easy counting of plaques and storage as a record.

Plaques produced by haemadsorbing viruses (myxo- and paramyxovirus, rubella) may be detected by removing the overlay (which has to be fluid enough to be removed cleanly by suction) and placing the appropriate erythocyte suspension on the sheet, incubating, washing and examining for haemadsorbing foci.

Viral plaques in cells sheets may also be demonstrated by immunofluorescence (IF) or immunoperoxidase (IP) staining. For IF staining the cell sheets have to be arranged so that they can be scanned with low and intermediate power objectives in the UV microscope. The cultures are stained and examined for fluorescent foci at a time when only one cycle of replication has taken place and before secondary foci have formed by viral spread to cells elsewhere in the sheet. Both IF and IP staining are particularly effective for those slow-growing viruses which spread from cell-to-cell, such as varicella-zoster virus (Gerna & Chambers 1976) and cytomegalovirus.

Of these techniques for the quantitation of plaque-forming units (pfu) of virus, those depending on a cytopathic effect in the cells are most probably the easiest to adapt to measurement of antibody. In principle, a small dose, say 1000 pfu of virus, is mixed with the test serum, incubated, and then plated as described. The reduction in the number of plaques after incubation of the plates gives a measure of the neutralizing power of the serum. That serum dilution giving a plaque reduction of 50–90% is usually taken as the endpoint.

Measurement of antibody by metabolic inhibition test

This is a useful colorimetric test to simplify the reading of viral CPE in neutralization tests. It is based on the fact that cells that are respiring normally produce acid and change the colour of the medium (which contains phenol red indicator) from orange-red to yellow. If the virus is cytocidal, destruction of the cells reduces the respiration of the culture and there is a rise of pH indicated by a change of colour of the indicator to a dark red or purple colour. Neutralization of the virus with specific antiserum will allow the cells to continue to respire normally and the medium will turn yellow.

Titration of virus and antibody by viral plaque assays or metabolic inhibition tests is normally the province of the virus reference laboratory. However, a general description of the latter techniques are given by Schmidt (1979) which should be consulted for details of all three types of neutralization test.

OTHER SEROLOGICAL TESTS FOR MEASUREMENT OF VIRAL ANTIBODY

In addition to the widely used complement fixation test, and the virus neutralization test,

virtually every other serological technique for measurement of antigen-antibody union has been put into service for measurement of viral antibody. For example, antibody may be measured by (1) *immunofluorescence* or *immunoperoxidase* staining on virus-infected cells grown on coverslips or harvested and spun on to slides; (2) by inhibition of the viral agglutination of erythrocytes (*haemagglutination-inhibition*) or their haemadsorption to infected cell sheets (*haemadsorption-inhibition*); (3) agglutination of viral antigen-coated erythrocytes or latex particles; (4) variants of the complement fixation reaction such as *immune adherence* haemagglutination in which antigen-antibody complexes activate the C3 complement component which adheres erythrocytes and *single radial haemolysis* (see below); (5) *immune electron microscopy*; (6) *immunodiffusion* in which antigen-antibody complexes give precipitation lines in gels.

Two sensitive tests in increasing routine use are *enzyme immunoassay* (EIA) and *radioimmunoassay* (RIA). These techniques may be used to measure the total specific antibody content of a serum, or the specific antibody in a particular immunoglobulin class.

Some of these techniques, e.g. immunodiffusion, immune electron microscopy, are insensitive methods of measuring antibody, labour-intensive or require uneconomical amounts of antigen; further discussion in this chapter is limited to immunofluorescence (IF), haemagglutination-inhibition (HAI), EIA, RIA and single radial haemolysis (SRH).

Measurement of viral antibody by immunofluorescence (IF)

The principle of this test is described in Chapter 10 and the direct and indirect methods are illustrated in Figure 10.14. The union of antibody to antigen may also be detected by treating the preparation with guinea-pig complement and detecting the bound complement with a fluorescent conjugate directed against it. Commercial sources of anti-viral antisera, the preparation of control antisera, and the preparation of virus-infected cell sheets are described in Chapter 50.

The indirect method is used for the titration

of viral antibody. Two-fold serial dilutions of the test sera are made, starting from an initial dilution of 1 in 10. For the anti-complement IF test, the initial dilution should be heat-inactivated (56°C for 30 min) before proceeding. The antigen preparation may take the form of virus-infected cells grown on 'flying coverslips', or cells grown or placed in wells on a Teflon-coated microscope slide (Ch. 48). Serum dilutions are layered on to the cells, slides are incubated in a moist chamber at 37°C for 30 min, washed, and blotted dry. A predetermined dilution of an anti-human globulin conjugated with fluorescein isothiocyanate is then added and the slides or coverslips are incubated at 37°C for a further 30 min. After washing, the preparation is mounted in buffered glycerol pH 8.0, or a permanent mountant (Ch. 48) and examined under the ultra-violet light microscope. The use of mixtures of infected and non-infected cells (Ch. 48) provides an in-built control for non-specific staining of the cells, caused by anti-nuclear factor or other anti-tissue antibodies in the serum under test. In circumstances in which staining is uniform and suspected to be due to anti-tissue antibody, the starting dilution of serum should be absorbed, first with a tissue suspension of the same species as the cell, then with an uninfected cell suspension. The removal of the anti-tissue or cell antibodies may reveal anti-viral antibody previously masked by the general staining.

By convention, the degree of immunofluorescence is expressed on a scale from + to ++++ (maximum). The titre of the serum may be taken as that dilution showing a ++ staining reaction.

The indirect IF may be adapted to measure specific antibody of a particular Ig class by use of fluorescein-conjugated antiglobulins to μ chain, γ chain or α chain. Measurement of specific IgM antibody must take into account the misleading results that may arise from the presence of IgM rheumatoid factor. Sera should be tested and if necessary absorbed with Ig-coated 'latex' beads (see also Meurman 1983).

Details of the preparation of fluorescent conjugates are given in Chapter 10, and sources of antiglobulin conjugates in Chapter 48. Kits for the measurement of specific IgM antibody to Epstein Barr virus and herpes simplex virus may be obtained from Gull Labs.

Although the commonest version of the IF technique uses microscope slide preparations and the visual assessment of fluorescence in the UV microscope, attempts have been made to remove the subjectivity involved in the latter by measurement of the degree of fluorescence in a fluorimeter. One system Fiax (MA Bioproducts) employs a small paddle-shaped sampler with test antigen bound to one surface and a control antigen on the reverse. This sampler is placed successively in the test serum and a fluorescent conjugate, with appropriate washing, and read in a fluorimeter which compares the emission from the two sides of the sampler. The Track XI Diagnostic System (MA Bioproducts) comprises a test 'track' or strip with wells containing a thick film of a gel of polymeric microbeads which provide 3 dimensional binding sites for antigens or antibodies. The gels in the wells of the 'Track', are saturated with various antigens and dried. For use, the test serum is placed in the wells, incubated for a short time, washed, treated with a fluorescent conjugate, washed again and then read in the fluorescence reader. This system has been used to screen rodent colonies for evidence of virus or mycoplasma infection but is obviously of wider applicability.

Haemagglutination-inhibition test (HAI test)

A number of viruses possess surface molecules that bind to receptors on the outer membrane of red blood cells from a species of animal or bird appropriate for the particular virus. This reaction can be visualized macroscopically as an irregular 'carpet' of red cells on the bottom of microtitre plate wells, in contrast to the central 'button' of cells seen when haemagglutination has not occurred. Virus-specific antibody reacting with viral surface antigens can be measured by the ability to block this reaction (Fig. 10.10). Sera may contain low levels of 'non-specific inhibitors' (not antibody) that will also block the reaction without signifying the presence of specific virus antibody. Various methods are available to remove or inactivate non-specific inhibitors from

Table 49.5 Conditions for the haemagglutination-inhibition test

Virus	Optimal type of red cell (and concentration V/V%)	pH	Temperature of incubation	Time of incubation (for reaction of virus and serum)	Diluent[a]	Treatment of serum to remove non-specific inhibitors and agglutinins
Adenovirus	Monkey, rat (0.75%) stabilized with rabbit serum	7.2	37°C	1 h	Saline	Kaolin and red cells
Togavirus Flavivirus	Goose (0.3%)	5.7–7.4[c]	4°C	Overnight	Borate saline solution pH 8–9, according to virus strain	Kaolin pH 9 and red cells
Enteroviruses	Human 'O' (0.75%)	5.8 or 7.4	4°C or 37°C	1 h	PBS pH 5.8 or 7.4	Kaolin. Animal sera have to be absorbed with red cells.
Influenza A (in O phase)	Human 'O' (0.75%) Guinea-pig (0.5%)					
(in D phase)	Fowl (0.5%)		22°C			
Influenza B	Human 'O' (0.5%) Guinea-pig (0.5%) Fowl (0.5%)	7.2		30 min–1 h	CFT diluent	Heat, RDE[d] or trypsin/periodate
Influenza C	Human 'O' (0.5%) Guinea-pig (0.5%) Fowl (0.5%)		0–4°C			
Measles	Monkey (0.5%)	7.2	37°C	30 min–1 h	PBS pH 7.2	Heat. Absorb with monkey red cells overnight at 4°C
Mumps Parainfluenza 1,2,3	Chicken (1.0 to 0.5%) Human 'O' (0.75%) Guinea-pig (0.5%)	7.2	4°C then 37°C	30 min–1 h	PBS pH 7.2	As influenza A
Reovirus	Human 'O' (0.75%)	7.2	22°C	1 h	Saline	Kaolin
Rubella	Day-old chick cells (0.25%)	7.3	RT[b]	1 h	DGV	Kaolin
	Pigeon (0.25%)	6.2	RT	1 h	HSAG	Heparin MnCl$_2$

[a] – PBS = phosphate buffered saline, pH as indicated; for DGV and HSAG diluents see *Methods*.
[b] – RT = room temperature.
[c] Conditions and diluents vary for each virus group. See Clarke & Casals (1958).
[d] RDE = receptor destroying enzyme.

sera prior to the test (see Table 49.5). In practice, routine virus laboratories make much use of HAI tests for rubella antibody testing; less frequently strain-specific antibody responses to influenza virus and arbovirus antigen may be measured by this technique. The other examples of HAI tests listed in Table 49.5 are of limited application and restricted to more specialized laboratories. Conditions for HAI tests are critical and differ between viruses; however, once a particular system is standardized it is a satisfactorily robust test. Details of techniques for influenza and rubella are given under *Methods**.

Enzyme immunoassay (EIA)

The principle of the method is described briefly (as ELISA) in Chapter 10 and its application to the detection of *Mycoplasma pneumoniae* antigen and antibody is found in Chapter 45.

There are two main approaches for the detection of antibody by EIA. In the first, the antigen – sonicated virus particles or extracted antigens – is adsorbed to the wells of a plastic microtitre plate and fixed there. Remaining active adsorption sites on the plastic are blocked with bovine serum albumin or skim milk. The coated well is overlaid with the test serum, incubated, washed to remove unbound serum components and then a detector system of an antiglobulin conjugated with an enzyme (peroxidase, phosphatase or urease) followed by substrate is used to detect antibody bound to the antigen. The antiglobulin may be broadly reactive or it may be specific for one Ig class (IgM, IgG or IgA).

In the second, or 'antibody capture' method, a potent and highly specific anti-immuno-globulin-class reagent, anti-μ, anti-γ or anti-α chain, is adsorbed and fixed to the wells of the plastic plate. Dilutions of the test serum are placed in the antibody-coated wells, incubated, and the unbound antibody and serum components washed away. Bound ('captured') antibody is then detected by first incubating with a viral antigen, and after washing, detecting the complex of bound antigen and captured antibody with an enzyme-conjugated antiserum to the viral antigen.

As explained in Chapter 48, great care must be taken to prevent hetcrogenetic antibody cross-reactions between the sera making up the various 'layers' in this test system. For example, if a rabbit antiserum to human μ chain is used as the capture antibody on the plate, and a guinea-pig antiserum to the virus is used in the detection side of the system, 'natural' antibodies in the two different species of sera may interact and give false positive readings and high backgrounds. It may be necessary to absorb each animal serum with glutaraldehyde cross-linked human serum, and the rabbit serum with insolubilized guinea-pig serum, and vice versa, in order to remove the cross-reactivity.

A second difficulty arises from the presence of IgM rheumatoid factor (RF) in some of the human sera that will be tested. Complexes of IgM RF and specific IgG antibody will be bound to the antigen on the plate or captured by the anti-μ chain serum, and such complexes will then appear to be specific IgM antibody. Sera should therefore be tested for RF before any EIA test for the measurement of IgM antibody and be absorbed with latex particles coated with denatured human globulin until they cease to give a positive RF reaction. (It is presumed that in this absorption the IgM RF-specific IgG antibody complexes are dissociated in favour of IgM RF-IgG latex combinations.) However, with critical specimens (e.g. determination of rubella specific IgM antibody in a pregnant woman) it may be necessary to dissociate and separate the IgM RF-specific IgG antibody complexes in acid sucrose density gradients.

It is probable that the virus section of a bacteriological laboratory will make the most use of EIA for measurement of total and specific IgM antibody in serum by purchasing kits rather than by preparing thcm 'in house'. Kits from commercial sources include ones for the measurement of hepatitis A IgM, hepatitis B core IgG and IgM, and hepatitis B surface antibody (available from a number of manufacturers), rubella IgM (Rubazyme M, Abbott) and for cytomegalovirus IgM (Behring). There are also EIA kits for detection of antibody to human immunodeficiency virus from Abbott, Dupont, Electronucleonics, Organon, Wellcome and others. The list is not exhaustive and docs not constitute an endorsement relative to kits that are not mentioned; it is simply an introductory guide. The hepatitis and HIV areas in particular are highly competitive; the quality of kits in these fields is generally high and under further development. For those laboratories that wish to make up their own test systems, the essential stcps in the preparation of viral antigens are described by Burrell (1986), and the coating of plates and standardization of the system are illustrated by the technique for direct estimation of specific IgM antibody to *Mycoplasma pneumoniae* described in *Methods* in Chapter 45.

Kits based on microtitre trays or the bead systems used by Abbott lend themselves to automation in serum dilution and the reading of results. Abbott have devised and supply their own apparatus. Other automated diluters, plate washers and plate readers are available for the standard microtitre tray system.

Radioimmunoassay (RIA), including radioimmunoprecipitation tests

These methods which offer the advantages of specificity, precision and high sensitivity, have evolved mainly from tests devised to quantitate polypeptide hormones although radioimmuno-precipitation was used to measure antibody to *Coxiella burneti* in the 1950s. They may be used to measure either antibody or antigen. Radioimmunoassay for measurement of antibody may be undertaken in solution (i.e. radioimmunoprecipitation) or with one of the ligands bound to a solid phase such as a well in a microtitre plate, a glass or polystyrene bead, or an insoluble support such as cellulose. In the radioimmuno-precipitation test, radiolabelled antigen is reacted with the test serum in which antibody is to be detected, and the antigen/antibody complex is precipitated and separated from the unbound labelled antigen by treatment either with an antiglobulin, or by ammonium sulphate precipitation (if the antigen is soluble in ammonium sulphate), or by treatment with staphylococcal protein A followed by centrifugation or chromatography to deposit or separate the complexes. A comparison is then made of the radioactivity in the deposit with that in the supernatant and the ratio between the two measurements reflects the amount of antibody present in the test serum. Competition radioprecipitation assays may be used for antigen detection, in which labelled antigen competes with unlabelled antigen in the test sample for a limiting amount of antibody reagent. When complexes are precipitated by one of the above methods, precipitation of labelled antigen is inhibited to an extent reflecting the amount of unlabelled antigen in the test sample. Competition assays for the measurement of antibody generally require the antigen to be bound to a solid phase.

Solid-phase radioimmunoassay offers the advantage that separation of antigen/antibody complexes is more easily achieved. The principle of the method is identical to that of enzyme immunoassay (Ch. 10, Fig. 10.14), except that radiolabelled rather than enzyme-labelled anti-globulins are used. Instead of the addition of substrate, gamma or scintillation counting is required to quantitate the bound antiglobulin. Direct, competition and antibody capture techniques are all applicable to solid phase RIA. As in EIA, rheumatoid factor may interfere with IgM tests.

The most commonly used radionuclide is ^{125}I, which can be linked to antigen or antibody with little damage to their immunological specificity. A disadvantage of radioimmunoassay is that ^{125}I-labelled reagents in common use have a limited shelf-life (commonly 3–6 weeks), owing to the half-life of the isotope (60 days for ^{125}I) and to radiation-induced damage to the ligand on storage. In addition, there is the potential hazard of using radio-isotopes, particularly during the process of labelling antigen and antibody when the largest quantity of ^{125}I is used. There is also the requirement for expensive equipment for counting.

It is probable that the virus section of the bacteriological laboratory will not require to make up solid-phase radioimmunoassays or radioimmunoprecipitation assays, although they may use assays from commercial sources. Consequently, details are not given under Methods. However, further general information may be gained from Bolton & Hunter (1986). An example of the detection of antibody to hepatitis B surface antigen is given by Burrell et al (1978).

Measurement of antibody by single radial haemolysis (SRH)

In this technique, the test sera are placed in wells in an agarose gel containing antigen-coated erythrocytes and complement. As the antibody in each of the test sera diffuses through the agarose, it combines with the antigen on the erythrocytes; complement is bound to the antigen-antibody complex and activated. When the plates are incubated overnight at 37°C, a circular zone of haemolysis develops around the well. The diameter of the zone is proportional to the concentration of antibody in the test serum.

The antigen can be bound to the erythrocyte in various ways; the requirement is to ensure that the complex of antigen-antibody and activated complement is in close proximity to the erythrocyte membrane in order for lysis to occur. The method has particular application to the measurement of antibody to haemagglutinating viruses; its common use is with rubella and influenza viruses (Russell et al 1975). Antibody of the IgG class is measured effectively; IgM and IgA antibodies may react less effectively. An advantage is that the reaction is not affected by non-specific inhibitors of haemagglutination as in the HAI tests with rubella and influenza; sera have only to be heat-inactivated to destroy complement and the test requires only small volumes. As an illustration of the technique, a single radial haemolysis test for rubella antibody* is given below.

METHODS

Antigens for viral serodiagnosis

Table 49.6 lists the range of CF antigens available from 4 commercial sources. As elsewhere, the point is made that the list is introductory and does not constitute an endorsement of the products or imply that these are the only sources. Sources of viral antisera, for use as controls with these antigens, are described in Chapter 48, Table 48.2.

If resources permit, the purchase of standardized antigens offers a considerable saving in time and labour. If antigens are to be prepared in the laboratory, consideration has to be given to the following points: (1) the optimal system for growing the virus to produce high-titre antigen

– this may involve using cells, chick embryos or animals; (2) the efficiency of extracting virions or non-virion antigens from the substrate cells and the complications, if any, that failure to separate cell or tissue proteins from the antigen will impose on the serological technique in which the antigen is to be used; (3) the stability of the antigens during the extraction process. These parameters will differ from virus to virus. Consequently, the relevant chapters of Lennette & Schmidt (1979) should be consulted along with those in Maramorosch & Koprowski (1967), Fraenkel-Conrat & Wagner (1974–1983), and Fields (1985).

Complement fixation tests for antibody and antigen

Patient's serum

A specimen of blood is obtained by venepuncture as for blood culture. The blood is then placed in a sterile stoppered test-tube or screw-capped bottle and allowed to coagulate. It is advisable to obtain at least 5 ml of blood. The serum is pipetted off after separation; some is diluted to the starting dilution for the test and heated in a waterbath at 56°C for 30 min. Heating reduces non-specific fixation effects which may occur with normal unheated sera plus the antigen; it also inactivates its complement.

Reagents

Complement fixation test diluent. (Veronal-NaCl diluent, obtainable in tablet form: Oxoid).

Preserved complement, Richardson's method. Preservation of liquid complement-serum in hypertonic salt solution is effective provided the pH is adjusted to 6.0–6.4. A convenient method (Richardson 1941) employing borate-buffer-sorbitol for control of pH, is described below.

Two stock solutions, which keep indefinitely, are used:

Solution A: boric acid (H_3BO_3) 0.93 g, borax ($Na_2B_4O_7.10H_2O$) 2.29 g, and sorbitol ($C_6H_{14}O_6.\frac{1}{2}H_2O$) 11.74 g are dissolved in and

Table 49.6 Some commercially available antigens for complement fixation tests as at 1987.

Antigen	Source[a]			
	Virion	*MA Bio-products*	Wellcome	Behring
Influenza A	A	A	A	—
Influenza B	A	A	A	—
Influenza C	—	A	—	—
Chlamydial group[b]	A	A	A	A
Adenovirus	A	A	—	A
Mycoplasma pneumoniae[b]	A	—	—	A
Parainfluenza 1	A	A	—	A
Parainfluenza 2	A	A	—	—
Parainfluenza 3	A	A	—	A
Respiratory syncytial virus	A	A	—	A
Cytomegalovirus	A	A	—	A
Herpes simplex	A	A	—	A
Measles	A	A	A	A
Mumps	A	A	—	A
Varicella zoster	A	A	—	A
Rubella	—	A	A	A
Lymphocytic choriomeningitis	A	A	—	A
Coxsackie B1 to B6 inc.	A	A	—	—
Poliovirus types 1,2,3	A	A	—	—
Reovirus	—	A	—	—
Coxiella burneti[b]	A	—	—	A
Rotavirus	A	—	—	A
Epstein Barr virus	A	—	—	—

[a] For addresses of suppliers, see *Appendix 3*; A = available; — = not known to be available.
[b] Also available from the Commonwealth Serum Laboratories, Australia

made up to 100 ml with saturated NaCl solution. The resulting molar concentrations are: 0.27 mol/l boric acid, 0.12 mol/l sodium borate, 0.6 mol/l sorbitol in saturated sodium chloride.

Solution B: borax 0.57 g and sodium azide (NaN$_3$) 0.81 g are dissolved and made up to 100 ml with saturated NaCl solution. The resulting molar concentrations are: 0.03 mol/l boric acid, 0.03 mol/l sodium borate, 0.125 mol/l sodium azide in saturated sodium chloride.

To preserve complement, mix 8 parts of serum with 1 part of solution B, followed by 1 part of solution A. This treated serum keeps very well even at room temperature. At 0–3°C, loss of titre is not noticeable until after 6–9 months. The final concentrations in the mixture are 0.03 mol/l boric acid, 0.015 mol/l sodium borate, 0.06 mol/l sorbitol, and 0.0125 mol/l sodium azide.

For use as a 1 in 10 dilution of complement, 1 part of preserved serum is diluted with 7 parts of distilled water. Any further dilution from this 1 in 10 mixture is made with saline or the Veronal-sodium chloride CFT diluent. The diluted complement preparation should not be kept more than an hour or two and should be kept on ice, or at 4°C when not required on the bench.

Viral antigens. These may be bought commercially (Table 49.6 shows some sources) or made in the laboratory.

Sheep erythrocytes (Oxoid). Either defibrinated or in Alsever's solution. Wash in saline at least three times, until the supernate is colourless. Resuspend the red cells in physiological saline and estimate their concentration in a haematocrit tube by centrifuging at 3000 rpm for 20 min. A concentration of 4% (v/v) in CFT diluent is required for sensitization with antibody.

Rabbit or horse anti-sheep red cell serum (Wellcome). This should have a high haemolytic titre but a low haemagglutinating titre. It is often referred to as haemolysin, immune body (IB)

(Darter 1953), or haemolytic immune body (HIB).

Summary of test procedure

Serum samples to be tested are diluted to an appropriate starting level, e.g. 1 in 5, heat-inactivated, placed in wells at one edge of a microtitre plate and serial two-fold dilutions are prepared in corresponding rows. Complement and virus antigen at the appropriate dilution (see below) are added to all test wells in that order. The plates are then incubated, usually overnight at 4°C, but sometimes at 37°C for 1–2 h to allow antigen-antibody interaction with consumption of complement if antibody is present. Overnight incubation in the cold gives a more sensitive test and better fits the working pattern of the laboratory. On the first day sera are diluted and the test set up. On the second day, the haemolytic system is added, the test read and reported. Reagents standardized for an overnight test must not be used in a short-fixation test, and vice versa.

When the indicator system is added, *inhibition* of cell lysis (i.e. a cell button) indicates absence of free complement; therefore presence of virus-specific antibody. Essential controls included with every test are (1) serum control (the serum under test, at highest concentration used, with complement, but without antigen) to detect naturally occurring anti-complementary activity in the test serum; (2) antigen control (virus antigen and complement, without added test serum) to check for any anti-complementary activity in the virus antigen; (3) a complement titration made by adding successive dilutions of complement to a row of wells, starting with complement at working strength, in order to check the number of complement units in the test; (4) cell control (sensitized cells without added serum, antigen or complement) to detect any spontaneous cell lysis; (5) positive serum control in which a standard known positive anti-serum is titrated to its end-point with the corresponding antigen at the dilution used in the test to check its potency; and (6) a normal yolk sac (for egg-grown antigens) or uninfected cell culture control, or both as appropriate, in order to ensure that the patient's serum does not interact with non-specific components of the antigen preparation.

Complement fixation – detailed procedure

The method described is based on that of Bradstreet & Taylor (1962) but has been modified for use in microtitre plates. All the serum titres quoted are initial dilutions before the addition of the test system.

Apparatus

1. Cooke microtitre disposable 'U' plates (rigid styrene) or permanent lucite 'U' plates (Flow); these plates have 12 × 8 wells.
2. Permanent or disposable 0.025 ml pipettes (Flow) with filters.
3. Microdiluters 0.025 ml (Flow).
4. Go-no-Go sheets to test volume delivered by pipettes and microdiluters (Flow).
5. Automatic syringe (1 ml to deliver 0.1 ml; Turner), for antigen dilutions in chessboard.
6. 1 ml rubber teat.

Titration of complement and anti-sheep cell haemolytic serum

1. Prepare dilutions of the complement in 20% steps as follows. If Richardson's preserved complement is being employed it should be prepared by adding 7 volumes of distilled water to 1 volume of complement. This will give a dilution equivalent to 1 in 10, which can subsequently be diluted with buffer. When using the microtitre plates, only a very small volume of the complement dilutions is required. The quantities suggested are shown in Table 49.7.

2. With the micropipette put 2 drops (0.05 ml) of CFT diluent in each of 70 wells (10 × 7) of a microtitre plate (Table 49.8). These 2 drops replace the antibody and antigen in the test proper.

3. Beginning with column ten, add 1 drop of buffer to each of the 7 wells, then 1 drop of the 1 in 179 dilution of complement to each of the 7 wells of column 9 and work backwards till all the wells contain a total of 3 drops.

4. Cover the plate and incubate overnight at 4°C to mimic the actual test in which the virus-antibody reaction typically requires 18 h to reach completion.

5. Next day, prepare 1 ml amounts of doubling dilutions of the haemolytic antiserum from 1 in 25 to 1 in 800, in 7 tubes. To an equal volume of 4% sheep red cells add these dilutions of haemolytic antiserum. *NB*: Always add haemolytic antiserum to the red cells. As a control, to ensure that the cells do not also lyse in the absence of the haemolytic antiserum, add 1 ml buffer to 1 ml RBC. Place the tubes in a waterbath for 10 min at 37°C, or at room temperature for 30 min to sensitize the red blood cells.

6. After overnight incubation, remove the plate from the refrigerator and place in a 37°C incubator for 30 min (for cells sensitized at 37°C in step 5) or stand at room temperature for 30 min (for cells sensitized at room temperature).

7. Beginning with the tube without any haemolytic antiserum, add 1 drop of the cells to each well of row seven. Then continue to add the

Table 49.7 Dilution series for titration of complement.

Reagent	Volumes of reagents in tube numbers								
	1	2	3	4	5	6	7	8	9
Complement	0.2 ml	—[a]	—	—	—	—	—	—	—
Distilled water	1.4 ml	—	—	—	—	—	—	—	—
CFT diluent	3.2 ml	0.5 ml	0.5 ml	0.5 ml	0.5 ml	0.5 ml	0.5 ml	0.5 ml	0.5 ml
		2 ml	2 ml	2 ml	2 ml	2 ml	2 ml	2 ml	2 ml
Resulting dilution	1 in 30	1 in 38	1 in 47	1 in 59	1 in 73	1 in 92	1 in 114	1 in 143	1 in 179

[a] – = none added.

Table 49.8 Determination of complement dose and optimal concentration of anti sheep cell haemolysin. The titration is set out in a 96 well microtiter plate as shown in Figure 49.1, but the orientation of the plate is different; the dilutions of complement extend across ten cups in the greatest width of the plate so as to accommodate the closely spaced dilutions of complement required in the titration.

		1	2	3	4	5	6	7	8	9	10	11	12	Dilutions of haemolysin (one in)
							Columns							
R	A	0	0	0	2	4	4	4	4	4	4	..	..	25
o	B	0	0	0	0	0	1	3	4	4	4	..	..	50
w	C	0	0	0	0	0	0	1	2	4	4	..	..	100
s	D	0	0	0	0	1	2	4	4	4	4	..	..	200
	E	0	0	0	1	3	4	4	4	4	4	..	..	400
	F	1	3	4	4	4	4	4	4	4	4	..	..	800
	G	4	4	4	4	4	4	4	4	4	4	..	..	0
	H	..	..	..	..	..	..	..	..	..	..	..	..	..
		30	38	47	59	73	92	114	143	179	0			

Dilutions of complement (one in)

0 = complete lysis of erythrocytes.
4 = unlysed cells.
3,2,1 = varying degrees of cell lysis.
. . = unused cup in microtitre plate.

sensitized red cells row by row finishing with the mixture containing the 1 in 25 haemolytic antiserum.

8. Tap plate gently to keep cells in suspension and incubate for 30 min at 37°C. The plate should be shaken at 10 min intervals.

9. Place at 4°C to allow unlysed cells to settle. The degree of haemolysis in each well is then scored as a scale from 0–4 as follows:

$$0 = 100\% \text{ lysis}$$
$$1 = 75\% \text{ lysis}$$
$$2 = 50\% \text{ lysis}$$
$$3 = 25\% \text{ lysis}$$
$$4 = 0\% \text{ lysis.}$$

In addition, trace (tr) is used to denote a few unlysed cells (i.e. between 0 and 1).

The optimal sensitizing concentration (OSC) of the haemolytic serum is that dilution which gives most haemolysis with the highest dilution of complement. In the example shown in Table 49.8, it would be 1 in 100. The 50% haemolytic dose of complement (HD50) is that dose of complement at which lysis of 50% of the cells occurs in the presence of the OSC of haemolytic

serum. In the above example the HD50 would be a 1 in 143 dilution. In the test proper, a satisfactory compromise between sensitivity and specificity is obtained by using 3HD50.

Standardization of antigen and antisera. This is done by a 'chessboard' titration of a series of dilutions of the test antigen against dilutions of a reference antiserum (Table 49.9).

1. Prepare doubling dilutions of the heat-inactivated serum from 1 in 5 to 1 in 640 (8 wells) or to the desired level. This may be done either in tubes followed by transfer of the serum dilutions to the plate, or in the plate itself by the use of the microdiluters. For the latter method, 1 drop of buffer is added to 56 wells (8 × 7) beginning with the second column; 1 drop of serum diluted to 1 in 5 is added to all the wells of the first and second columns. One diluter loop is then placed in each of the wells of the second column, rotated and transferred to the wells of the third column. This is continued until the eighth column is reached when the remaining 0.025 ml is discarded.

2. Add 1 drop of 3HD50 complement to all the wells of the test. The following are also required: (a) a cell control to check for the

Table 49.9 'Chessboard' titration of an antigen and antiserum showing *peak* optimal antigen titre.

			Antiserum dilutions (one in)								Complement controls			
			5	10	20	40	80	160	320	640	3	1.5 HD50	0.75	
			*1	2	3	4	5	6	7	8	9	10	11	12
												With antigen		
Antigen	5	A*	4	4	4	3	0	0	0	0	0	0		4
dilutions	10	B	4	4	4	4	3	0	0	0	0	0		4
(one in)	20	C	4	4	4	4	3 ←	0	0	0	0	0		4
	40	D	4	4	4	3	1	0	0	0	0	0		4
	80	E	4	4	2	0	0	0	0	0	0	0		4
	160	F	2	0	0	0	0	0	0	0	0	0 \		4
											No antigen, complement only			Cell control
	Serum only	G	tr	0	0	0	0	0	0	0	0	0	4	4

* designations of columns and rows of cups in a microtiter plate; see Table 49.8 and Figure 49.1.

absence of spontaneous lysis of the sensitized erythrocytes in the absence of complement (1 well with 3 drops of buffer and no complement); (b) a complement control to check the amount of complement actually used in the test (3 wells with 2 drops of buffer and 1 drop of either 3, 1.5 or 0.75 HD50 complement); (c) antigen controls to test for anti-complementary activity dispensed as in Tables 49.9 and 49.10, containing antigen at each dilution, decreasing amounts of complement and 1 unit volume of buffer in place of serum.

3. Prepare 6 doubling dilutions of antigen (from 1 in 5 to 1 in 160) in test-tubes remembering to change pipettes at each dilution to avoid carry-over of antigen. Beginning with the bottom row, add 1 drop of buffer to all the wells of that row (serum control) and continue up the concentrations of antigen allowing 1 row per dilution.

4. Incubate the plate overnight at 4°C.

5. The following day, prepare and sensitize the sheep red blood cells using OSC of haemolysin. Remember that the diluted haemolysin and the 4% erythrocyte suspension have to be very well mixed. Using 2 flasks, the diluted haemolysin is poured into the erythrocyte suspension, swirling continuously.

6. Warm plate at 37°C or room temperature (as for complement titration) for 30 min.

7. Add 1 drop of sensitized cells to all wells; incubate as for complement titration.

Most antigen-antibody 'chessboards' give one or other of two main patterns: (1) that with a *peak* optimal antigen dilution (Table 49.9); or (2) that with a *plateau* of optimal antigen dilution (Table 49.10). An antigen showing a peak pattern should be used at the optimal peak dilution (OPD). With an antigen showing a plateau pattern, 1 unit of antigen may be taken as the highest dilution of antigen giving a score of 2 or more fixation with the highest dilution of serum; the antigen should be used at 2 or 4 units (preferably 4 units if not anti-complementary). A plateau pattern may indicate anti-complementary activity at low antigen dilutions sometimes detected with 1.5HD50 but not with 3HD50 (Table 49.10). In the example shown, the 1 in 5 and 1 in 10 dilutions of antigen are slightly anti-complementary as judged by the complement titration at the right end of the table.

The titre of the serum is the highest dilution of serum that gives a reading of 2 or more with the antigen. Fixation end-points are marked ← in Tables 49.9 and 49.10. The antigens in both samples would be used at 1 in 20 i.e. OPD in Table 49.9; twice end-point in Table 49.10. The titre of each serum is 80.

Test proper for serological diagnosis

1. Heat 1 in 5 serum dilutions (0.2 ml serum, 0.8 ml CF buffer) at 56° for 30 min to inactivate complement.

2. Put 1 volume (0.025 ml) diluent as indi-

Table 49.10 'Chessboard' titration of an antigen and antiserum showing *plateau* optimal antigen titre.

		Antiserum dilutions (one in)								Complement controls			
		5	10	20	40	80	160	320	640	3	1.5 HD50	0.75	
		*1	2	3	4	5	6	7	8	9	10	11	12
											With antigen		
	5	A*	4	4	4	4	2	0	0	0	2	4	4
Antigen	10	B	4	4	4	4	2	0	0	0	0	2	4
dilutions	20	C	4	4	4	4	2	0	0	0	0	0	4
(one in)	40	D	4	4	4	4	2←	0	0	0	0	0	4
	80	E	4	4	2	1	0	0	0	0	0	0	4
	160	F	4	1	4	0	0	0	0	0	0	0	4

										No antigen, complement only			Cell control
Serum only	G	0	0	0	0	0	0	0	0	0	0	4	4

* designations of columns and rows of cups in a microtiter plate; see Table 49.8 and Figure 49.1.

cated (Fig. 49.1) into wells G–A for each test serum and for the positive serum control.

3. Add 1 volume of diluent to 6 complement control wells (H–C) or complement titration (3, 1.5, 0.75 HD50 with and without specific antigen).

4. Add 3 volumes buffer to a cell control well (well 1A).

5. Using a separate pipette for each serum, put 50 μl of each heated, diluted serum into well H to provide the starting 1 in 5 dilution, and put 25 μl of each heated, diluted serum into well A for serum control.

6. Make doubling dilutions (0.025 ml) by transferring the diluters from wells H–G and so on to well B; mix well at each transfer by rotating the diluters 4 times. Blot diluters dry.

7. Add 1 volume complement 3 HD50 to all rows, wells H–A, and to wells H and E in the complement titration row (step 3). Add 1 volume complement 1.5 HD50, and 1 volume 0.75 HD50 to wells G and D, and wells F and C respectively, in the complement titration row.

8. Add 1 volume of antigen at the OPD or 2–4 units to wells H–B for each test serum and positive control serum row, and to wells H–F in the complement titration row. Add 1 volume buffer to wells E–C in the complement titration row to take the place of antigen.

9. Stack and cover plates and stand overnight at 4°C.

10. Next morning sensitize washed 4% sheep RBC in a conical flask by slow addition with thorough mixing of an equal volume of haemolysin (final mixture 2% cells with optimal sensitizing dilution of haemolytic antiserum. Always add the serum to the cells as addition of the cells to the serum may result in uneven sensitization. Incubate in waterbath at 37°C for 10 min or at room temperature for at least 30 min.

11. Remove plates from refrigerator and warm for 30 min at 37°C or room temperature. Add 0.025 ml of 2% sensitized sheep cells to each well. Cover plates with sealing tape.

12. Reincubate for 30 min to allow lysis, shaking at 10, 20 and 30 min to resuspend cells using a microshaker.

13. Deposit cells by centrifugation in the plate centrifuge, or placing plates in refrigerator overnight, or by standing them at room temperature for several hours until the cells have settled.

The highest dilution of serum giving a fixation value of 4 or 3 is taken as its titre. For routine testing of large numbers of sera, one may put the antigen and serum controls and the known positive control antiserum titration, on separate plates, allowing 12 test sera per plate. If any serum should be anti-complementary, i.e. fixes complement in the absence of antigen, it should be treated by incubating it overnight at 4°C with fresh guinea-pig serum (4 volumes of patient's serum to 1 volume guinea-pig serum). After

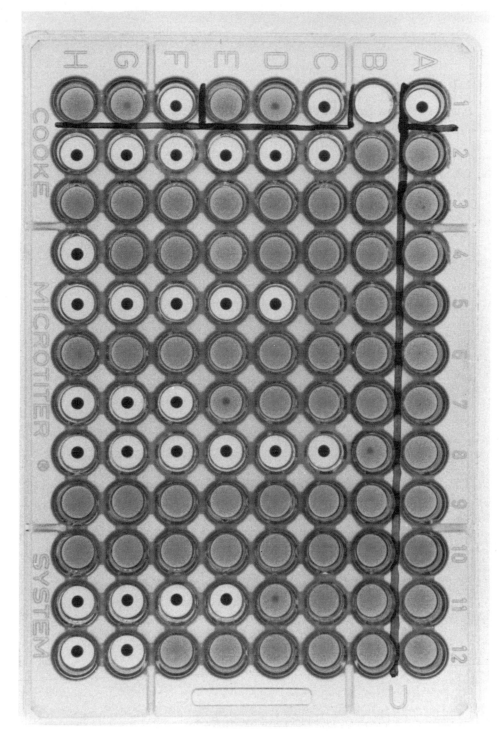

Fig. 49.1 Suggested layout for the complement fixation test in which ten serum specimen (rows 3 to 12) and a positive control antiserum (row 2) are titrated against an optimal dose of one antigen. The starting dilution (1 in 5) of the sera are in the cups on the left hand side of the plate (column H) and dilutions extend across the plate to an end dilution of 1 in 320 in column B. Serum controls at a dilution of 1 in 5 are in the rows under column A. Abbreviated complement titrations (3, 1.5 and 0.75 HD50) with the working dilution of antigen (cups H, G and F) and one without antigen (cups E, D and C) are located at the top of the plate (see also text). Complete fixation of complement is indicated by a clear well with a central button of cells. The titre of the positive control serum is 160.

heating for 30 min at 37°C dilute with buffer to give a 1 in 5 dilution and inactivate any free complement by heating for 30 min at 60°C.

For testing antigens. For virus identification, straight line titrations of antigen from undiluted to 1 in 160 or higher are tested against (1) specific animal antiserum at 4 times titre, (2) negative control serum at same dilution as specific antiserum, and (3) Veronal-NaCl diluent (antigen controls). Specific reagent controls are also included.

Haemagglutination and haemagglutination-inhibition test

Apparatus (Sever 1962)

1. Permanent lucite 'U' or 'V' plates or disposable (Rigid Styrene) 'U' plates.
2. Microtitre droppers 0.025 ml.
3. Microtitre diluters 0.025 ml.

Reagents

1. Diluent – see Table 49.5 for details. Complement fixation test diluent is suitable for influenza as it contains Ca^{2+} and Mg^{2+} ions. See below for recipes for HSAG and DGV diluents.
2. Viral antigen (haemagglutinin).
3. Serum heated to 56°C for 30 min and suitably treated to remove non-specific inhibitors (see below and Table 49.5).
4. Red cells of the optimum species and concentration (Table 49.5).

Titration of virus (haemagglutinin)

1. Place 1 drop of diluent in each of, say, 10 wells of the microtitre plate and in 1 more well to act as a cell control.
2. Place 1 drop of virus in first well giving a 1 in 2 dilution and using a microdiluter prepare doubling dilutions of the virus discarding the last 0.025 ml.
3. Add 1 drop of diluent to each well used, in place of the serum which is added in the haemagglutination-inhibition test.
4. Add 1 drop of red cells to each well including the cell control.

5. Incubate at the appropriate temperature (see Table 49.5) until the control cells have settled to a discrete button.
6. Read the titre of the virus as the highest dilution that gives haemagglutination (1 haemagglutinating unit : HAU).

Haemagglutination-inhibition test

1. Place 1 drop (0.025 ml) of diluent in the second and each of the remaining, say, 10 wells for the serum dilutions and to a control well for each serum.
2. Place 1 drop (0.025 ml) of serum dilution in the first and second well and in each serum control well. The starting dilution depends on the method used for pretreatment of the serum (see below). Also add 1 drop of diluent to each of 4 haemagglutinin control wells, and 2 drops to a single cell control well.
3. Make doubling dilutions of the serum using a microdiluter loop. Ensure that 0.025 ml is discarded from the final well.
4. Add 1 drop 4 HAU virus to each of the test wells and to 1 of the haemagglutinin control wells. Add 2, 1 and ½ HAU to the other three haemagglutinin control wells.
5. Incubate to allow serum and virus to interact for 1 h at room temperature.
6. Add 1 volume of red cells to all the wells.
7. Incubate as when titrating the haemagglutinin.
8. Read the result, when the cell and serum controls are discrete buttons and the haemagglutinin titration shows a diminishing amount of haemagglutination. The titre of the serum is the highest dilution that causes *complete* inhibition of haemagglutination.

Removal of non-specific inhibitors and agglutinins from serum

Heat. By holding the sera at 56°C for 30 min the Chu inhibitors are destroyed.

Receptor destroying enzyme (RDE) obtainable from Wellcome removes the Francis' inhibitor or mucoid inhibitor. Mix 4 parts of RDE with 1 part serum. Incubate overnight at 37°C and follow by incubation for 1 h at 56°C to destroy any remaining RDE. The serum has been diluted 1 in 5. This method depends on the potency of the RDE so if it was not purchased commercially, it needs to be standardized by titration against normal rabbit serum.

Trypsin and periodate will also remove the Francis' inhibitor or mucoid inhibitors.

Reagents: Trypsin 1:250 dissolved in 0.1 mol/litre phosphate buffer pH 8.2 at a concentration of 4 μg/ml; this solution should be clear and requires prolonged shaking. Potassium periodate, 0.011 mol/l

1. Mix 1 volume serum and 1 volume trypsin.
2. Place immediately for 30 min in 56°C waterbath.
3. Cool to room temperature.
4. Add 3 volumes of 0.011 mol/l potassium periodate.
5. Incubate for at least 15 min.
6. Add 3 volume of 1% glycerol-saline solution. This gives a 1 in 8 dilution of the serum.

Kaolin for removal of non-specific inhibitors for rubella HI tests.

Reagents: physiological saline (0.85% NaCl); 25% acid-washed kaolin.

1. Make a 1 in 5 dilution of serum in saline.
2. Add an equal volume of washed kaolin; the serum is now diluted 1 in 10.
3. Allow to stand 20 min at room temperature.
4. Deposit the kaolin by centrifugation.

Heparin MnCl$_2$ for absorbing non-specific inhibitors for rubella HI tests.

Reagents: sodium heparin – 5000 iu/ml; $MnCl_2 4H_2O$ – prepare 1 mol/litre $MnCl_2$ stock solution.

1. Sterilize $MnCl_2$ stock solution by filtration through the millipore membrane, 0.22 μm pore size.
2. Mix equal parts heparin and 1.0 mol/l $MnCl_2$ solution.
3. Store at 4°C (can be used for up to 2 weeks).

4. Add 0.2 ml serum to 0.3 ml HSAG diluent (see below).
5. Add 0.2 ml of Heparin-$MnCl_2$ and mix gently.
6. Hold for 15 min at 4°C.
7. Add 0.4 ml of 50% red cells and shake gently to mix.
8. Add 0.7 ml HSAG diluent to tube and mix gently.
9. Centrifuge for 20 min at 4°C at 900 *g*.
10. Recover supernate – final dilution of serum is 1 in 8.

Red blood cells of the appropriate species, for removal of agglutinins from serum.

Reagent: packed erythrocytes (e.g. day-old chick cells for rubella tests).

1. Add 0.1 ml packed cells to 1.0 ml of a 1 in 10 dilution of serum.
2. Incubate for 1 h at 4°C.
3. Remove the red cells by centrifugation at 4°C.
4. Test the serum for residual agglutinins at 37°C.
5. If any remain repeat steps 1–4.

HSAG diluent

Solution A: HEPES saline (×5 concentration solution)

HEPES	29.8 g
NaCl	40.95 g
CaCl$_2$2H$_2$O	0.74 g
Distilled water to	1000 ml

Dissolve in approximately 900 ml distilled water. Adjust the pH to 6.2 by adding 1 mol/litre NaOH. Add distilled water to 1000 ml. Sterilize by filtration through a 0.22 μm membrane and store at 4°C in convenient amounts.

Solution B: bovine serum albumin (×2 concentrated solution)

Bovine albumin powder	20 g
Distilled water to	1000 ml

Dissolve albumin; sterilize and store as above.

Solution C: gelatin (×10 concentrated solution)

Gelatin	0.025 g
Distilled water to	1000 ml

Dissolve gelatin and sterilize by autoclaving for 15 min at 121°C. Store at 4°C in convenient amounts.

Method. To make 1000 ml of complete HSAG diluent combine:
  200 ml of solution A
  500 ml of solution B
  100 ml of solution C
  200 ml of sterile distilled water
At 25°C the pH of the HSAG diluent should be 6.2. It can be stored at 4°C for several months if kept sterile.

Dextrose-gelatin-Veronal buffer (DGV)

As used in the rubella haemagglutination-inhibition test.

Solution A

Veronal (barbitone, diethylbarbituric acid)	0.58 g
Gelatin	0.60 g

Dissolve Veronal and gelatin in 125 ml deionized water by gentle heating.

Solution B

Sodium Veronal (sod. barbitone, sod. barbiturate)	0.38 g
Calcium chloride (anhydrous)	0.02 g
Magnesium sulphate	0.12 g
Sodium chloride	8.5 g
Dextrose	10.0 g
De-ionized water	875 ml

Method. Combine Solution A with Solution B. Sterilize by autoclaving at 115°C for 10 min (pH 7.3).

Single radial haemolysis for rubella antibody

Apparatus
1. Centrifuge for 25–30 ml screw-capped bottles (Universal container).
2. Waterbath 0–60°C.
3. Square plastic dishes (Sterilin code no. 109).
4. Well punch, 2.5–3.0 mm with suction.
5. 10 × 10 cm square template for cutting wells with well-to-well spacing of 13 mm.
6. Oxford or MLA micropipettes to deliver 5–10 μl.

Red cells. Sheep cells. Fresh or preserved in Alsever's solution (not formalinized). Allow fresh cells to age 1 day before washing 3 times in barbitone buffered saline (BABS) complement fixation buffer containing 0.08% sodium azide. Make up sheep RBC to 15% suspension in BABS (TCS).

Agarose. 1% agarose in BABS + 0.8% sodium azide. (Indubiose 37; Sigma type 11; Koch Light; Miles).

Complement. Reconstituted Richardson's preserved complement (see above).

Rubella haemagglutinin. From Division of microbiological reagents and quality control, Central Public Health Laboratory (CPHL), London, in the UK; and from Behring; Flow; Wellcome. Minimum HA titre must be 128.

Diluent. Complement-fixation buffer tablets Oxoid BR16 (BABS + 0.08% sodium azide).

Control serum. Standardized serum containing 15 International Units (15 IU) of rubella antibody. (Division of microbiological reagents and quality control, CPHL, London; Statens Seruminstitut, Copenhagen, Denmark; or Wellcome). 'In house' standards, assessed against the reference serum, should be included.

Method

Preparation of plates

Test and control gel plates are prepared as described in the box. Leave the gel plates to set for a minimum of 10 min, then store at 4°C for 30 min – 5 days before use.

Preparation of gel plates for SRH test for rubella antibody

Test	*Control*
1. Melt 15 ml 1% agarose in BABS. Hold in 43°C waterbath.	Melt 15 ml 1% agarose in BABS. Hold in 43°C waterbath.
2. Pipette 0.3 ml of 15% sheep RBC into a Universal container. Mark 'test'.	Pipette 0.3 ml of 15% sheep RBC into a Universal container. Mark 'control'.
3. Add 0.3 ml of rubella haemagglutinin (titre $\geq$ 128) to the sheep RBC. Mix. Leave 30 min at room temperature.	Add 0.3 ml of BABS to the sheep RBC. Mix. Leave 30 min at room temperature.
4. Fill universal with BABS. Centrifuge to pellet RBC.	Fill universal with BABS. Centrifuge to pellet RBC.
5. Discard supernatant, resuspend pellet in 0.5 ml of azide barbitone buffer.	Discard supernatant, resuspend pellet in 0.5 ml of azide barbitone buffer.
6. Add 0.5 ml undiluted Richardson's preserved complement to cell suspension in universal.	Add 0.5 ml undiluted Richardson's preserved complement to cell suspension in universal.
7. Place cell suspension into 43°C waterbath for 10 s then add the 15 ml of 1% agarose. Mix and pour contents into 10 × 10 cm square Petri dish on a level surface.	Place cell suspension into 43°C waterbath for 10 s then add the 15 ml of 1% agarose. Mix and pour contents into 10 × 10 cm square Petri dish on a level surface.

Test procedure

1. Heat inactivate 0.1 ml of undiluted test and control serum (15 IU/ml) in test-tubes immersed in a 60°C water bath for 20 min.

2. Place gel plates over template and cut wells with 2.5–3.0 mm tubular well punch attached to a vacuum line and trap (well volume 8–11 μl).

3. Add each serum to its corresponding 'test' and 'control' gel using an Oxford or MLA pipette. Use the template under each plate as a numerical guide. For orientation, mark the top left hand corner of the Petri-dish (not the lid) with an indelible marker pen.

4. The loaded plates are placed in a humidified box and incubated at 37°C overnight.

5. Measure zones of haemolysis next day using trans-illumination against a black background.

Interpretation of results

1. Test zone $\geq$ zone of 15 IU/ml control serum and larger than the zone in the corresponding position on the control plate: rubella antibody present ($\geq$15 IU/ml). Regard as immune.

2. Test zone $<$ zone of 15 IU/ml control serum but larger than the zone in the corresponding position on the control plate: low amount of rubella antibody ($<$15 IU/ml). Regard as non-immune.

3. No test zone or a test zone equal to or less than that of the zone in the corresponding position on the control plate: rubella antibody not detected. Regard as susceptible.

REFERENCES

Bolton A E, Hunter W M 1986 Radioimmunoassay and related methods. In: Weir D M et al (eds) Handbook of experimental immunology, 4th edn. Blackwell, Oxford, ch 26

Bradstreet C M P, Taylor C E D 1962 Technique of complement fixation test applicable to the diagnosis of virus diseases. Monthly Bulletin of the Ministry of Health Laboratory Service 21:96

Burrell C J 1986 Preparation of viral antigens. In: Weir D M et al (eds) Handbook of experimental immunology, 4th edn. Blackwell, Oxford, ch 5

Burrell C J, Leadbetter G, Black S H, Hunter W M 1978 Rapid detection of hepatitis B surface antigen by double antibody radioimmunoassay. Journal of Medical Virology 3: 19–26

Clarke D H, Casals J 1958 Techniques for hemagglutination and hemagglutination-inhibition with arthropod-borne viruses. American Journal of Tropical Medicine and Hygiene 7: 561–573

Cowan K M 1973 Antibody response to viral antigens. Advances in Immunology 17: 195–253

Darter L A 1953 Procedure for production of antisheep haemolysin. Journal of Laboratory and Clinical Medicine 41:653

Fields B N 1985 Virology. Raven Press, New York

Fraenkel-Conrat H, Wagner R R 1974–1983 Comprehensive virology (18 vols). Plenum Press, New York

Gerna G, Chambers R W 1976 Varicella-zoster plaque assay and plaque reduction neutralisation test by the immunoperoxidase technique. Journal of Clinical Microbiology 4: 437–442

Karber G 1931 cited in Schmidt N J 1979 In: Lennette E H, Schmidt N J (eds) Diagnostic procedures for viral, rickettsial and chlamydial infections, 5th edn. American Public Health Association, Washington

Lennette E H, Schmidt N J 1979 Diagnostic procedures for viral, rickettsial and chlamydial infections, 5th edn. American Public Health Association, Washington

Maromorosch K, Koprowski H 1967 Methods in virology, vol II. Academic Press, New York

Meurman O 1983 Detection of antiviral IgM antibodies and its problems – a review. Current Topics in Microbiology and Immunology 104:101

Rayner A G 1943 A simple method for the preservation of cultures and sera by drying. Journal of Pathology and Bacteriology 55:373

Reed L J, Muench H 1938 A simple method for estimating 50% endpoints. American Journal of Hygiene 27:493

Richardson G M 1941 The preservation of liquid complement serum. Lancet 2:696

Russell S M, McCahon D, Beare A S 1975 A single radial haemolysis test for measurement of influenza antibody. Journal of General Virology 27:1

Schmidt N J 1979 Cell culture techniques for diagnostic virology. In: Lennette E H, Schmidt N J (eds) Diagnostic procedures for viral, rickettsial and chlamydial infections, 5th edn. American Public Health Association, Washington, p 65–139

Sever J L 1962 Application of a microtechnique to viral serological investigation. Journal of Immunology 88:320

White D O, Fenner F J 1986 Medical Virology, 3rd edn. Academic Press, Orlando, Florida

Cell and virus culture in the clinical microbiology laboratory

The proposition was advanced in Chapter 47 that a general microbiology laboratory would probably choose to refer many specimens for routine virus isolation to a specialist virus diagnostic laboratory. Nevertheless, the microbiology laboratory may need to use some cell culture methods, for applications such as (1) culture from clinical specimens of rapidly growing viruses such as herpes simplex virus, respiratory syncytial virus, and some enteroviruses (e.g. poliovirus, Coxsackie B viruses); (2) the preparation of virus-infected cell monolayers, dispersed cells, or cell sonicates for use as positive controls in antigen detection tests (Ch. 48), or as sources of antigen for the titration of antibody by immunofluorescence, complement fixation or enzyme immunoassay (Ch. 49); (3) the measurement of neutralizing antibody (Ch. 49); and (4) the detection of bacterial toxins such as that of *Clostridium difficile* (see Ch. 38).

The notes on cell culture techniques that follow are directed to the above applications. Additional information concerning cell culture methods may be obtained from Paul (1970), Kruse & Patterson (1973), Moffat (1973), Jakoby & Pastan (1979), Schmidt (1972, 1979) and Freshney (1983).

Cell culture systems

Monolayer cultures

Cell monolayers are most commonly used for the culture of viruses. There are three categories, namely (1) primary, (2) semi-continuous, and (3) continuous cell cultures (Moffat 1973).

Primary cultures. Viable cell suspensions may be obtained by the dispersion of cells in animal tissues or organs, e.g. monkey kidney or human amnion, by treatment with trypsin, collagenase or other enzymes. When placed in culture vessels with nutrient media, viable cells adhere to the wall of the vessel and begin to multiply. Multiplication ceases when neighbouring cells touch (contact inhibition), resulting in the formation of a sheet of cells, one cell deep (a monolayer). Because metabolic activity in such a culture is low, the accumulation of acid in the medium is slow, which in turn means that the cells are easily maintained. The cells in primary cultures generally possess a diploid complement of chromosomes characteristic of the tissue cells of the donor animal.

Although particularly useful for the isolation of viruses such as the echoviruses or orthomyxoviruses, primary culture techniques have disadvantages for the virus section of the microbiological laboratory. Cultures have to be prepared de novo from fresh tissue samples which may either be difficult to obtain or may require special care in preparation. The presence of contaminating or endogenous viruses, latent in the animal host, may give difficulties with cell growth and virus isolation. Finally, primary cultures established from the organs of different individuals of the same animal species may vary in their ability to support replication of the same virus.

Semi-continuous cell cultures (cell strains). Semi-continuous cell cultures are established with the successful subculture of primary cell monolayers. With methods currently available to the diagnostic laboratory, these cultures mostly consist of spindle-shaped fibroblastoid cells. When established from human embryonic tissues or neonatal foreskin, these semi-continuous cell cultures may undergo up to 50–100 population doublings before senescence and death of the culture. Cultures are maintained by creating a bank of frozen cells (in liquid nitrogen) from early passage harvests, from which samples are periodically revived to initiate cultures that may be used for up to 8–10 passages before a change of viral susceptibility or senescence occurs (Hayflick & Moorehead 1961, Hayflick 1965). Like primary cells, the cells in this type of culture maintain the normal diploid chromosome complement. Although semi-continuous cultures are easily established and provide an abundant source of cells, they may not be as susceptible to some viruses as true primary cultures; also at higher passage levels, the cells may vary in their ability to support virus replication. Examples of fibroblast strains are MRC5 and WI38.

Continuous cell cultures (cell lines). Characteristically, these cells may be serially subcultured indefinitely on glass or plastic surfaces. Some lines will also grow in suspension culture, unlike primary or semi-continuous cell cultures which require an anchorage on glass or plastic. Continuous cultures are produced either by transformation (spontaneous or engineered) of cell strains in vitro, or by the culture of cells taken from tumours. The number of cells required to initiate a culture on glass or plastic is low compared with that for primary cells or semi-continuous cell strains (i.e. high plating efficiency). Relative to the latter, requirements for serum or other nutrients are less, growth rate is faster and contact inhibition is lost. Consequently the cells have a tendency to overgrow, and often require more frequent attention than those in primary cultures. Although the cells of continuous lines are not necessarily tumorigenic in vivo, they are effectively immortal in vitro and their chromosome complement is heteroploid.

Patterns of respiratory metabolism are altered with increased production of acid from glucose. The ease of propagation of the continuous cell lines is to some extent offset by the need to maintain the pH of the culture around 7.0 by addition of buffer, or changing the medium, or both. Without this attention cells die or become detached ('metabolic degeneration'). Control of pH is partly effected by the addition of sodium bicarbonate to the medium, and incubation of the cells in a carbon dioxide-enriched atmosphere. Usually some phosphate buffer is also present. Recently the introduction of the zwitterionic buffer N-2-hydroxyethylpiperazine-N^1-3-ethanesulphonic acid (HEPES) (Good et al 1966; see Ch. 5) has simplified the growth of cell cultures since it overrides all other buffers present and does not require the presence of a CO_2-enriched atmosphere. This allows incubation of open cell cultures (e.g. in small Petri dishes) in a humidified incubator.

The following continuous cell lines are commonly used by diagnostic laboratories: HeLa (human cervical carcinoma), HEp2 (human epithelial), BHK 21 (baby hamster kidney), MDCK (dog kidney), RK 13 (rabbit kidney), Vero (African green monkey kidney) and a human rhabdomyosarcoma cell line (RD cells). HeLa and HEp2 cells are of use for the cultivation of herpes simplex virus, adenovirus, poliovirus and Coxsackie viruses. Some special clones of HeLa cells (e.g. HeLa 'Bristol' or 'Ohio') are susceptible to RSV and some rhinoviruses. Vero cells will also support growth of these viruses and are also used along with BHK 21 cells for growth of arboviruses. RK 13 cells and BHK 21 cells are of value for the isolation and propagation of rubella virus. RD cells are claimed to be of value for the isolation of Coxsackie A viruses.

This collection of continuous cell lines requires, however, to be supplemented with human diploid fibroblasts or epithelial cells for the culture of many enteroviruses and rhinoviruses. Ortho- and para-myxoviruses require combinations of human diploid fibroblasts, primary monkey kidney cells, MDCK cells and even on occasion (for some influenza A strains) inoculation of the chick embryo amniotic cavity (for chick embryo culture techniques, see 12th edn, Vol. 2, Ch. 10).

In the virological section of a microbiological

laboratory, the HeLa cell will be of the greatest utility. HeLa and HEp2 cells are malignant human epithelial cells. HeLa cells were derived from cervical cancer tissue taken from a negress. They contain a small number of copies of the genome of human papilloma virus type 18 and the racial origin of the donor of the cervical cancer cells is reflected in their possession of the fast isoenzyme of glucose-6-phosphate dehydrogenase. This marker, and other isoenzymes, are of central importance in establishing the identity of 'new' continuous lines of cells (Gartler 1967). The high plating efficiency and ease of growth of cells such as HeLa has led to numerous initially unrecognized episodes of cross-contamination of primary or semi-continuous cell cultures and consequently to claims of the establishment of 'new' stabilized continuous lines of, for example, human amnion and human hepatocytes. Inspection of the catalogue of the American Cell Culture Collection in which some cell strains or cell lines are categorized as having HeLa type isoenzymes rather than those of the tissue and animal from which they are said to be derived, will serve to illustrate the problem of cell to cell contamination. The problem is not confined to HeLa cells (e.g McCoy 'human synovial' cells are in fact mouse fibroblasts). However, some of the cell lines which have arisen as a result of contamination have altered characteristics, such as increased sensitivity to some viruses, compared with the presumptive parent line. Presumably the contamination represents an inadvertent cloning of a more sensitive subline.

The matter of fungal, bacterial, mycoplasma and cell contamination is discussed in greater detail below.

Tissue and organ cultures

It is unlikely that the microbiology laboratory will use these techniques but they are mentioned briefly for completeness.

Tissue cultures. The culture of small tissue fragments – rather than the cells dispersed from them by digestion – although not often used for routine diagnostic purposes, has in the past provided an alternative to monolayer cultures for viral culture. The technique has a particular application in the isolation of viruses in the 'latent' state. The culture of fragments of the tissue harbouring the virus (e.g. herpes simplex virus) may be successful when merely grinding the tissue and inoculating cell monolayers is not.

Small (1 mm³) pieces of tissue are attached to a glass or plastic surface in a tube or small Petri dish either by placing them in a drop of plasma and clotting this with thrombin, or more simply by warming (45°C) the glass or plastic in the vicinity of the fragments, before covering them with growth medium. On incubation, cells migrate from tissue fragments attached to the culture vessel surface. Migrating cells continue to multiply and eventually form primary monolayer cultures. Valuable primary cultures of fibroblasts (Green 1973) or epithelial cells (Stanley & Parkinson 1979) may be established from cultured tissue in this manner. Such cultures have the advantage that several cell types are available to support virus multiplication.

Organ cultures. Organ cultures are essentially cultured tissue pieces in which the architecture of the tissue is retained and the cells maintain their differentiated state. Migration of cells from the tissue fragments may be discouraged by culture manipulation (Paul 1970) or, in particular, by lowering the serum content of the growth medium. Organ cultures may be superior to cell monolayers, tissue cultures or other dedifferentiated cell preparations for the growth of some fastidious viruses. Thus, Tyrrell & Bynoe (1965) used organ cultures of ferret tracheas to isolate new rhinoviruses and coronaviruses.

Selection of culture media

A variety of media have been formulated for the growth of vertebrate cells in culture. These incorporate various concentrations of amino acids, vitamins, enzymes, growth factors and inorganic salts. Glucose, fructose or galactose are also added along with glutamine to provide a carbon source for cell metabolism. The more common of these media formulations are available in either single strength, concentrated or powdered forms from many commercial suppliers.

A variety of different media will usually provide adequate support for the growth of any one cell type. Selection of media for use in the diagnostic laboratory will often depend on the type of cells chosen for culture and on the commercial availability of different media formulations. Most laboratories are not equipped for the arduous task of media preparation from basic materials and the purchase of ready-to-use media is expensive. The use of commercially available media in powdered form, to be made up for use with ultra-pure water and sterile membrane filtration equipment, provides a convenient alternative.

There is a somewhat bewildering variety of medium formulations for cell culture; this is illustrated below in recommendations from Ham & McKeehan (1979), who should be consulted for details of media formulations and applications.

Cells in general	Parker 199, MEM, DME, F12K and MCDB 202
Human, monkey cells	Parker 199, BME, MEM, L15, RPMI 1640, CMRL 1969, MCDB 104 and MCDB 202
Rat, rabbit cells	MEM, 5A, F12, MCDB 104
Mouse cells	DME, CMRL 1415, MCDB 202 and MCDB 401
Chicken cells	Parker 199, DME, F12K and MCDB 202

In the particular circumstances of the virus section of the microbiology laboratory, it is probably simplest to use one of the variants of CMRL medium (named from *Connaught Medical Research Laboratories*). This complex medium contains all of the known cell nutrients; CMRL 1969 is optimal for use in the cell culture systems described below. It may be noted however, that when handling newly acquired cells, it is desirable to propagate them in the medium to which they are adapted before attempting innovations.

Conditions for growth of cell cultures

Optimum pH range for cellular growth is usually narrow and varies slightly with cell type. A pH of 7.1–7.5 is found to support growth of mammalian cells. Most culture media rely on bicarbonate buffer systems (CO_2/HCO_3^-) for pH maintenance. These media are formulated with $NaHCO_3$, and CO_2 is either provided by the cultured cells as a metabolic by-product (necessitating a tightly closed vessel) or by enrichment of the atmosphere using a CO_2 incubator. Media formulated with Hanks' balanced salt solution contain 0.33 g $NaHCO_3$/litre and are suitable for use in closed culture systems. Media containing Earle's salt solution have 2.20 g $NaHCO_3$/l and are more commonly used with open cultures incubated in a 5% CO_2 atmosphere (Paul 1970).

The synthetic buffer 4-(2-hydroxyethyl)-1-piperazine-ethanesulphonic acid (HEPES) may be used to control pH. Concentrations of between 10 mmol/l (2.38 g/l) and 25 mmol/l (5.95 g/l) effectively maintain pH and appear to be non-toxic to most cells (Shipman 1973) and viruses. HEPES buffered media are available from commercial suppliers or HEPES may be added to media preparations before filter sterilization. The pH is usually adjusted with sodium hydroxide.

Osmolality. The growth of cells in culture depends on an optimum range of osmotic pressures, usually between 280 and 320 mmol/kg (Ham & McKeehan 1979). Osmometers recording freezing point depression are conveniently used to measure the osmolality of culture media. Measurements should be taken after complete medium has been prepared and the pH adjusted with HEPES/NaOH, or after equilibration of bicarbonate buffered media with CO_2. Waymouth (1973) and McLimans (1979) should be consulted for further information concerning osmolality determinations.

Serum. Balanced salt solution, such as Hanks',* will support cell proliferation only when supplemented with serum, lactalbumin hydrolysate or other supplements. The serum

* Refer to *Methods* at end of this chapter.

has several functions. It provides essential amino acids, nucleic acid precursors and fatty acids and regulates the availability of the latter. It provides hormones and inhibits the proteases used for routine dissociation of cells for culture. Conventionally, fetal or new-born calf serum are used at concentrations of 5–15% (v/v) to promote cell growth and reduced to 0–2% (v/v) for maintenance of confluent monolayer cultures. Horse serum or human serum may be used; the former may be too stimulatory for continuous cell lines and the latter may contain antibody or be toxic. The proliferation of fastidious cells in culture often requires the use of fetal calf serum.

Sterile serum preparations are usually obtained from suppliers of biological reagents. As serum batches vary widely in their ability to support cell growth, it is usual to test samples from a batch before purchase. Satisfactory batches should then be acquired in substantial amounts and stored at −70°C. Repeated freezing and thawing should be avoided.

Antibiotics. Non-toxic antibiotic solutions may be incorporated into culture media for the prevention of bacterial and fungal infections. Antibiotics providing broad-spectrum protection from bacterial contaminants are: benzylpenicillin, 100 units/ml; gentamicin, 20–50 μg/ml; and tetracycline, 10 μg/ml. Amphotericin B, 3–4 μg/ml, or mystatin, 50 units/ml, are recommended for control of fungal infections. An extensive list of antibiotics and their concentrations for use in cell culture is given by Perlman (1979). Antibiotic powders are dissolved in sterile distilled water using aseptic precautions. The possibility of contamination of the antibiotic solution with microorganisms resistant to the antibiotics in the mixture must be borne in mind; if there is doubt about the adequacy of the aseptic techniques, the final solution should be filtered. Stock solutions should be stored frozen. Antibiotic solutions for addition to clinical specimens should be dispensed in convenient amounts in ampoules or bijou bottles which are used once and discarded, so as to avoid the cross-contamination between specimens that may arise from the use of a single bottle of antibiotic repeatedly opened and sampled.

Contamination of cell cultures

Cell cultures may be contaminated with bacteria, moulds, yeasts, mycoplasmas, viruses, or other eukaryotic cells and even amoebae (Fogh 1973). Contamination may originate from the environment, from the use of inadequately sterilized media or other solutions, from tissue specimens or from poor aseptic techniques.

Observation of the following measures will help to minimize contamination in the cell culture laboratory (Wolf 1979, Armstrong 1973):

1. Media and other solutions should be thoroughly tested for sterility* before use.
2. Serum purchased from supply houses should be certified as free from bacteria and mycoplasmas. Serum samples may be requested before purchase to confirm not only growth-promoting ability but also sterility.*
3. Cultures should be tested, at least twice a year, for mycoplasmas (Ch. 45) and other contaminants.*
4. Uncontaminated frozen cell stocks should be available for replacement of all cultures routinely handled by the laboratory.
5. Contaminated cultures should be immediately discarded and replaced with new stock cultures if possible. Contamination is usually considerable by the time it is detected and is therefore difficult, time-consuming or impossible to treat.
6. Treatment of contaminated cultures may be attempted if the organism is isolated and identified, and sensitivity tests are performed. Strict isolation procedures must be followed if the contaminant is to be confined to the original infected culture(s). Treatment of infected cultures with antibiotics may only suppress microbial growth and contaminating organisms may reappear when antibiotics are withdrawn.
7. The isolation and identification of contaminating organisms may help indicate the primary source of contamination.
8. It is not uncommon to find contaminants in cultures acquired from other laboratories. If possible, seed cultures should be purchased from the American (or other) Type Culture Collection or from supply houses which certify their cell stocks as being pure cultures not containing cellular or microbial contaminants.

9. Cultures imported from non-certified sources should be strictly isolated until sterility and verification tests can be completed.

10. Stock cultures should be handled infrequently and only by persons trained in aseptic techniques. Mouth pipetting should never be used in the cell culture (or any other) laboratory.

11. The use of laminar flow cabinets for culture manipulations will minimize contaminants from airborne sources.

Periodic checks of *cell identity* are required in order to detect cell-to-cell contamination and to establish the identity of cells acquired from other laboratories (see Nelson-Rees et al 1981; Stulberg 1973). Methods that may be employed are:

1. Chromosome counting.
2. Mixed haemagglutination test (Coombs et al 1961).
3. Analysis of isoenzyme pattern (Gartler 1967).
4. Immunofluorescence (Simpson & Stulberg 1963).
5. Cytotoxicity test (Greene et al 1964).

Of these techniques, isoenzyme analysis is effective (Peterson et al 1979). Kits for the determination of the isoenzymes of glucose-6-phosphate dehydrogenase are available (Corning Authentikit Systems, Innovative Chemistry Inc., PO Box 90, Marshfield, MA, 02050, USA).

LABORATORY PROCEDURES

Equipment for cell culture

Laminar flow cabinets. The danger of contaminating cultures with airborne organisms may be minimized by use of laminar flow cabinets. These cabinets are fitted with high efficiency particulate air (HEPA) filters which effectively sterilize the air flowing through the cabinet. Uninfected cultures may be manipulated in positive pressure laminar flow cabinets having either a horizontally or vertically directed air flow. Cultures containing potentially pathogenic organisms should be manipulated in biohazard cabinets which are designed both to protect the operator and to provide a working area with low numbers of microorganisms (Ch. 15).

Microscopes. An inverted microscope is necessary for the direct viewing of cells cultured in plastic or glass vessels. A microscope fitted with a phase contrast or a Nomanski differential interference illumination system will provide greater definition of cell structure and is particularly valuable when handling bottles or flasks of cells to be used to seed tubes. Tubes with cell monolayers inoculated with virus may be examined for viral cytopathic effect (CPE) at $\times$ 50 magnification with a simple binocular microscope with the substage condenser racked down and the iris diaphragm partly closed to provide contrast in the unstained cell sheet.

Incubators. Cultured mammalian cells achieve optimal growth when incubated at 35–37°C. If a Petri dish, microtitre plate or other open culture vessel is to be used, the loss of CO_2 and evaporation of culture medium can be prevented by the use of humidified incubators that maintain an atmosphere of 5% (v/v) CO_2 in air.

Water purification apparatus. A supply of highly purified water is mandatory for the preparation of cell culture media and all other solutions coming into contact with the cells and also for the final rinsing of all glass pipettes, culture and storage containers. Several approaches are available for water purification (Douglas & Dell'Orco 1979) including:

1. Treatment of tap water with a mixed-bed ion exchange unit followed by single or double glass distillation.

2. Preliminary filtration of tap water, reverse osmosis, mixed-bed deionization and submicron filtration.

3. If the laboratory has a supply of pre-treated water from a central purification system, it is advisable for this water to be further glass distilled or passed over activated charcoal, deionized and submicron filtered.

Conductivity meters are used to measure ionic contamination of water and for continuous monitoring of deionizer function; resistance readings at or in excess of 18 megohms have to be maintained. Although trace contamination of media with metallic ions may give rise to problems in growing and maintaining cells, contamination with organic products, some of which appear to be volatile and to distill over during attempted purification by double glass distillation, may be equally troublesome. It may also be noted that residual bacterial products, such as endotoxin, in solutions freed of bacteria by sterilization, may have untoward effects, e.g. activation of macrophages or lymphocytes in proliferation or other assays. Because of the central importance of highly purified water for virology, bacteriology, immunology and cell biology, investment in a water processing plant that will filter, deionize and remove organic trace contamination seems justified. Many systems are available; without prejudice, it may be mentioned that a machine such as the Millipore Super Q takes incoming water through a bed of activated charcoal, through a two stage reverse osmosis exchanger, through sequential deionizers and a submicron filter. The treated water – which otherwise would have to be stored in closed borosilicate carboys to prevent contamination from the air and container – is held in a vessel with a pump system which recirculates the water through the deionizers before dispensing.

Membrane filtration apparatus. Cellulose membrane filters are extensively used for filtration sterilization of culture media and other solutions in the cell culture laboratory. A wide range of vacuum, pressure or syringe operated membrane filtration systems is available. The autoclavable membrane filters used in such apparatus may be purchased with disk diameters of 13 mm to 293 mm and pore sizes varying from 8 μm to 0.025 μm (Millipore). Soluble wetting agents in some of the filters may effect cell growth. Such deleterious effects may be minimized by flushing the filter with glass-distilled water or by discarding the first 5–10% of the filtrate.

Glassware. Both high quality borosilicate glass and the less expensive soda glass are used routinely in the cell culture laboratory. Borosilicate glass is often preferred for medium storage bottles and cell culture vessels because it may be cleaned with strong solvents, is able to withstand repeated autoclaving and provides a neutral surface for cell attachment and growth. Soda

glass, although initially cheaper, cannot be autoclaved repeatedly, must be acid-washed (2% HCl) when new to remove excess soda, and may subsequently continue to impart traces of chemicals to stored solutions and chemicals.

Considerable care must be taken in the cleaning of glassware. Residual cell fragments from previous culture must be removed from cell culture tubes; used culture tubes should not be placed in discard buckets and allowed to dry out, but should be immersed in sodium hypochlorite or detergent and subsequently boiled or autoclaved to make them safe to handle and to give them a preliminary cleaning. This is followed by mechanical brushing and numerous rinses (8–10 with tap water and at least 2 rinses with purified water).

An important decision for the virus section of a microbiological laboratory is whether to route glassware through the central preparation facility of the laboratory. If glass preparation is centralized then all containers have to be washed to cell culture standard. Some selective media for bacteria utilize metallic salts such as potassium tellurite and thallium acetate; residual contamination with such compounds may be deleterious for cells.

Culture containers. Glass and disposable polystyrene plastic containers are routinely used for cell cultures. Laboratories culturing small quantities of cells or having inadequate staff or facilities for reprocessing glassware may find disposable plastics a useful alternative to glass. A number of companies produce plastic cell culture vessels sterilized by gamma irradiation, of high optical quality and with the internal surfaces coated or charged to facilitate cell anchorage and movement. There are also many brands of tubes and Petri dishes, including Sterilin, Falcon and Nunc.

Laboratories with adequate preparative facilities often use a combination of glass and plastic to meet their culture needs. Cell monolayers for routine use are cultured in glass bottles or tubes while plastic Petri dishes and flasks are used for establishing primary cultures. Plastic microtitre plates (e.g. Cooke or Linbro) are used for virus neutralization tests as they require less medium, antiserum and cells than tube cultures.

Roller drum apparatus. Once monolayer cultures have been established in tubes they are conveniently placed in rotating drums. The drums are tilted at an angle of 5° and mechanically rotated at 12–20 revolutions/h.

Roller bottle apparatus. Large volumes of cells may be obtained by growing monolayer cultures in cylindrical roller bottles. These bottles are inoculated with dispersed cells, placed horizontally in holders and rotated 5–12 times/h. Cells adhere to the cylindrical inner surface of the bottles and multiply to form monolayers.

Stoppers and rubber tubing. If stoppers are used rather than caps these should be either of white rubber or of silicone. Silicone has the advantage that it is non-toxic and does not become sticky on repeated sterilization but it is expensive and contracts at a different rate to glass so the stoppers are liable to fall out of the test-tubes at low temperatures. Black or red rubber stoppers should be avoided owing to their toxicity.

Instruments. These should be clean and sterile. Pre-packed disposable sterile scalpel blades are very useful because they do not have any coating of grease and so are not toxic to cells.

Subculture of semi-continuous or continuous cell cultures

1. Pour off culture medium and wash the cell sheet twice with phosphate buffered saline* (PBS; Dulbecco's Solution A, Ca and Mg free, pH 7.0) in order to remove serum.
2. Add a sufficient amount of trypsin-EDTA solution* to cover cells.
3. Incubate at room temperature until cell sheet appears opaque. At this stage cells will be rounded but not detached when observed with an inverted microscope. This process usually takes 1–3 min and must be determined for individual cell lines.
4. Remove excess trypsin solution. Cells will detach from culture vessel surface after approxi-

mately 2–3 min. The side of the flask may be tapped with the palm of the hand to dislodge any remaining cells.
5. Add a small amount of chilled growth medium and aspirate several times with a 10 ml pipette to suspend and separate the cells.
6. Dilute a small sample of the cell suspension with additional growth medium for cell counting or dispense directly into new growth vessels. Semi-continuous fibroblast cultures are generally passed from 1 culture container into 2 containers of the same surface area as the original vessel (or into 1 container having twice the surface area of the original). This is called a 1 to 2 split. A 1 to 6 up to a 1 to 10 split is common for continuous cultures. After counting*, cells may be seeded into tube cultures ($c.$ 1×10^5 cells/tube), microtitre plates ($c.$ 5×10^4 cells/well) or other culture vessels.

Preparation of primary human fibroblast monolayers

The following method may be used for the dissociation of neonatal foreskin or fetal skin tissue:

1. Collect fetus in a sterile covered container for transport to the laboratory. Place foreskin material in a collection bottle containing Dulbecco's phosphate buffered saline (PBS; Solution A) and antibiotics (penicillin 100 units/ml, gentamicin 50 μg/ml) for transport.
2. Aseptically excise fetal skin tissue and then treat in the same manner as foreskin tissue.
3. Chop tissues into small pieces using sterile fine curved scissors and wash a minimum of 3 times in fresh PBS containing antibiotics.
4. Mince tissues thoroughly using clean sterile curved scissors.
5. Transfer the minced tissue to a trypsinization flask containing $c.$ 50 ml of warmed (37°C) 0.25% (w/v) trypsin solution.*
6. Add a sterile Teflon-coated magnetic bar and place on a magnetic stirrer at 37°C. Stir moderately for $2\frac{1}{2}$–3 h.
7. Viability may be increased if dissociated cells are collected once or twice during the trypsinization process: the stirrer is stopped to allow the non-dispersed tissue to settle. Supernatant

fluids are collected and fresh trypsin solution is added to the flask for further stirring.

8. Centrifuge supernatant fluids after each collection for 5 min at 200 g and resuspend in 2–3 ml of chilled medium containing 15% (v/v) fetal calf serum.

9. Pool all cells obtained and count to determine cell yield and viability*.

10. Dilute the cell suspension to contain c. 2×10^5 cells/ml in growth medium containing 10% fetal calf serum and dispense into suitable culture vessels.

Preparation of human amnion cell cultures

(Duncan & Bell 1961) It is essential that any placenta that is to be used for tissue culture is not brought into contact with disinfectant; tissue from a Caesarian section is preferable. The placenta should be placed in a sterile beaker, covered and transported to the laboratory without chilling.

1. Suspend the placenta by the umbilical cord and free the amniotic membrane using scalpel, scissors and forceps.

2. Place the membrane in 100 ml Hanks' balanced salts solution (BSS)* with antibiotics (penicillin 100 units/ml, gentamicin 50 μg/ml).

3. Spread out the membrane in a large Petri dish and remove the mucus and blood clots by gentle scraping with the edge of a sterile microscope slide.

4. Wash 3 times in Hanks' BSS with antibiotics.

5. Put pieces of the membrane in a flask with 200 ml 0.25% (w/v) trypsin* in PBS (Ca and Mg free) and antibiotics and trypsinize for 30 min at 37°C, either shaking every 5 min or preferably using a magnetic stirrer.

6. Change the trypsin and leave for 4–4$\frac{1}{2}$ h at 37°C shaking every 30 min.

7. Filter through sterile gauze and wash filter with 100 ml Hanks' BSS with antibiotics.

8. Spin filtrate for 10 min at 1000 rev/min.

9. Discard supernatant.

10. Resuspend in 20 ml of propagating medium without serum.

11. Estimate the number of viable cells* and dilute to give 3.5×10^5 cells/ml.

12. Inoculate Roux bottles with 100 ml of cells and leave 3–4 days undisturbed.

13. Change medium.

Freezing of cells for storage

1. Harvest sub-confluent, logarithmically growing cells using subculture techniques.

2. Pool suspended cells (if replicate cultures are to be frozen) and determine the number of viable cells.*

3. Centrifuge cells at 500 g for 10 min.

4. Resuspend cells to desired concentration (2–8 $\times 10^6$ cells/ml) using chilled media containing 10% (v/v) dimethylsulphoxide (DMSO) and 20% (v/v) fetal calf serum.

5. Dispense 1–2 ml cell suspension into plastic cryopreservation ampoules (or Nunc screw-capped cryotubes) using a Pasteur pipette or syringe with an 18 gauge needle.

6. Place cryotubes or ampoules on suitable aluminium canes.

7. Cells should be cooled from room temperature to −70°C at approximately 1–2°C/min. This may be achieved by placing the tubes or ampoules in a polystyrene box in a −70°C freezer, or by using a controlled freezing rate apparatus in conjunction with a liquid nitrogen freezer.

8. Once at −70°C, the cells may be placed in the vapour phase of a liquid nitrogen freezer (−170°C) for long-term storage.

Recovery of frozen cells

1. Remove ampoule from liquid nitrogen and immediately thaw contents by agitation in a 37°C waterbath.

2. Swab ampoule with 70% ethanol and allow to dry.

3. Using heated, sterile scalpel blade, slice top off ampoule.

4. Withdraw contents with sterile Pasteur pipette and centrifuge 5 min at 200 g to remove DMSO solution. Resuspend in growth medium, place in culture vessel and incubate at 37°C. If DMSO solution is diluted at least 10-fold in growth media, cells may be placed directly from

ampoule into growth vessel. Replace media after the cells have attached, or after 24 h.

Specimens for virus culture

Collection and transport of specimens

The samples to be collected from the patient for virological tests have been considered in Chapters 47 and 48. Those taken for direct virus diagnosis often cover the requirements for virus culture. However, the maintenance of virus infectivity requires greater care in the handling and transport of the specimen than that needed to preserve virions or antigens for direct virus diagnosis.

Virus infectivity is generally better preserved in the cold than at room temperature. While it may be necessary to freeze specimens which are to travel long distances at high ambient temperatures, it should be borne in mind that some viruses, e.g. varicella-zoster virus and respiratory syncytial virus, suffer a greater loss of viability when the specimen is frozen than if it is maintained at 4°C on melting ice or in the refrigerator.

Most laboratories receive the majority of their specimens from nearby hospitals or clinics; under these conditions, the transport of specimens chilled but not frozen is preferable. Consideration should be given to sending ambulatory patients to the laboratory for collection of some types of specimen. Similarly, trained nursing or technical staff should be available to go, on request, into the wards of nearby hospitals and clinics to collect specimens. This arrangement not only ensures a higher and more consistent level of sample collection, but the documentation of the patient's condition on the request or application form is usually of a higher standard.

Tissue samples, body fluids or excreta should be forwarded to the laboratory in adequately sealed containers such as screw-capped Universal containers. Blood samples for virus culture are collected into heparinized containers, to allow separation of the leucocytes and erythrocytes, if required, from the plasma.

Swabs from lesions should not be allowed to dry out and the swab head should be broken off into a suitable virus transport medium (VTM)* immediately after collection. The composition of VTM tends to depend upon local laboratory preferences. There have been few controlled trials comparing viability of viruses in clinical specimens held in VTM (see Madeley 1977). In general, the transport medium combines a buffering system to maintain physiological pH with low concentrations of a protective protein and antibiotic to inhibit bacterial contaminants. Note that if virological specimens are also to be cultured for *Mycoplasma pneumoniae*, then streptomycin, gentamicin or other aminoglycosides should be omitted. VTM is conveniently dispensed into bijou bottles in 2–3 ml volumes. The protein seems to be of particular importance in preserving virus viability if the specimen is to be frozen.

Specimen preparation for virus culture

Protective gowns and gloves are worn. Procedures are performed in a safety cabinet.

Stock antibiotic solution for addition to samples for virus culture.

Benzylpenicillin	2000 units/ml
Gentamicin	1.6 mg/ml
Amphotericin B	50 μg/ml

Store in aliquots at −20°C.

Swabs (e.g. from possible herpes simplex). The specimen should have been received in VTM.* Vortex for 30 s, add 8 drops of antibiotic solution with a Pasteur pipette and inoculate 0.1 ml into suitable cell culture(s).

Nasopharyngeal aspirates (for RSV or enterovirus isolation). The specimen is centrifuged at 800 g for 10 min, to deposit cells for direct virus diagnosis (Ch. 48). The supernatant fluid is pipetted into a labelled bijou bottle, 8 drops of antibiotic solution are added with a Pasteur pipette, and 0.1 ml of sample inoculated into suitable cell culture(s).

Faeces. Prepare a 10–20% suspension of sample in PBS or maintenance medium (sugar cube size in 15 ml) in a sterile Universal container containing glass beads. Centrifuge the emulsion at 1000 *g*, 4°C for 20 min to deposit debris and most bacteria. Transfer 4 ml of supernatant (avoiding any fat floating on the surface) to a sterile bijou bottle and add 8 drops of stock antibiotic solution. As the preparation is frequently acid, the pH should be checked and adjusted to 7.0 with 8.0% (w/v) sodium bicarbonate solution.* Inoculate 0.1 ml into suitable cell culture(s).

Cerebrospinal fluid. Cerebrospinal fluid is inoculated directly (0.1 ml) into cell cultures, without any pre-treatment.

Other specimens. The above details cover most of the requirements of the general microbiology laboratory. For the preparation of other samples, such as post mortem and biopsy specimens, blood and urine, reference should be made to Chapter 48 and Schmidt (1972, 1979).

Inoculation and examination of cultures

Cell types suitable for the primary isolation of common human viruses have been discussed above. In summary, diploid human fibroblasts and a variety of continuous cell lines (e.g. HeLa) are suitable for HSV, Hep-2 cells are particularly suitable for RSV, and diploid fibroblasts plus HeLa or Hep-2 cells will cover many of the cultivable enteroviruses.

Duplicate tubes of each cell type are used for each specimen. The inoculum (0.1 ml) may be placed directly into the maintenance medium in the tubes. Alternatively, the virus in the inoculum may be allowed to adsorb on to cell monolayers devoid of medium; after 1 h the monolayers are rinsed and fresh-maintenance medium is added. The latter method has an advantage that any toxic material in the inoculum is removed from the cell culture tubes, but is obviously more laborious. The tubes are incubated, usually at 36°C (33°C for rhinoviruses),

either in stationary racks, or preferably in roller drums. The cell sheets are examined under the low power of the microscope on day 1 after inoculation and thereafter at 2 day intervals for appearance of cytopathic effects (CPE). Regular medium changes are necessary every 3–4 days to maintain a suitable pH and prevent the accumulation of toxic cell metabolites. It is possible to maintain cell culture monolayers in good condition for 14–28 days, depending upon cell type. Continuous (heteroploid) cell lines frequently show signs of overgrowth and 'metabolic degeneration' by 14 days; primary cell lines and fibroblast cell strains maintain good morphology for up to 28 days. In the absence of overt cytopathological effects in heteroploid cell lines by day 14, it is common practice to pass about 0.1 ml of cells and medium into fresh tubes of cells ('blind passage'); this increases the sensitivity of the isolation procedure and may facilitate the distinction between, for example, an adenovirus cytopathic effect and 'metabolic degeneration'.

Photographic illustrations of the cytopathic effects (CPE) produced by herpes simplex virus, adenovirus, respiratory syncytial virus and an enterovirus such as poliovirus or Coxsackie B have not been included here; reference may be made to the excellent illustrations given by White & Fenner (1986). However, the best way to gain familiarity with the CPE produced by these and other viruses, is to inoculate cell monolayers with prototype virus strains and to observe on a daily basis the process of degeneration of the cell monolayers.

Identification of presumptive isolates of viruses from clinical samples may be made, in the instance of herpes simplex virus and respiratory syncytial virus, by testing cell culture extracts in the direct virus diagnosis systems described in Chapter 48. Adenovirus antigen may be identified in a CF test with a known antiserum. Similarly, polioviruses and Coxsackie B viruses are identified by neutralization tests with known antisera as described below and in Chapter 49. The relevant chapters in Lennette & Schmidt (1979) may be consulted for further details of virus identification procedures.

Preparation of virus stocks

Virus stocks (for use in neutralization tests, etc.) are conveniently grown in 250 cm^2 disposable plastic culture flasks or roller bottles. Optimum conditions for the production of high titre stocks vary from virus to virus, but in general confluent monolayers should be inoculated at low multiplicity of infection (i.e. with dilute virus – low numbers of virus particles per cell in the culture) and harvested when 75–100% of the cell sheet shows CPE. High multiplicity infection gives faster results but tends to lead to the production of defective particles, and is therefore more suitable for antigen preparation rather than the production of infectious virus stocks. Cell-associated virus may be liberated by repeated freeze/thawing or sonication. Once produced, virus stocks should be stored in small samples at $-70°C$ or below.

Virus neutralization tests

Virus-specific neutralizing antibody in a patient's serum may be quantitated according to the ability of the serum to reduce the infectivity of a stock virus preparation. The test serum is diluted serially, incubated with a known amount of virus, and the mixture is then added to indicator cultures. The endpoint is arbitrarily defined; typically in the system described below, the highest dilution of serum ablating infectivity in 50% of the replicate virus-serum mixtures tested is taken as the titre. Neutralization tests are conveniently performed in flat-bottomed microtitre plates (cell culture grade, available from most manufacturers of laboratory plasticware). Depending on the virus involved, infection of the cultures may be judged by CPE, haemadsorption or metabolic inhibition.

The quantity of virus used in the test is important, and therefore the stock virus preparation must be accurately titrated before neutralization tests can be performed. The principles of virus titration are described in Chapter 49, and the method described here is for the determination of tissue culture infective doses (TCID50) in microtitre plates. In the test proper, an inoculum of 100 TCID50 per well is used; this reproducibly ensures infection of all cultures (unless inhibited by antibody) but retains a moderate degree of sensitivity to the presence of neutralizing antibody.

Sera to be tested for virus neutralizing ability should be promptly removed from the clot and stored frozen at or below $-20°C$. Neutralizing capacity diminishes during storage at 4°C.

Equipment required

Flat-bottomed microtitre plates suitable for cell culture.
Waterbath (56°C).
Multi-channel automatic pipette, 0.1 ml volumes.
CO_2 incubator.
Virus, cells and media as appropriate.

Titration of virus stock

The type of cell used will depend upon the virus to be cultured. For Coxsackie B virus neutralizing antibody tests, HeLa and Hep-2 cells are both suitable and easily maintained.

1. Harvest the cells to be used in the test and resuspend them to a concentration of 5×10^5/ml in growth medium (GM).

2. Dispense 0.1 ml of cell suspension into each of the wells of a flat-bottomed microtitre plate using a multi-channel pipette. Incubate overnight at 36–37°C, in a 5% CO_2 enriched atmosphere. The use of HEPES buffer (20 mmol/l) in the medium will obviate the need to seal the plates.

3. Next day, make 10-fold dilutions of virus stock in cell culture maintenance medium (MM; i.e. GM with less serum, see above). Ensure that a new pipette is used for each dilution step. Mix equal volumes of each dilution and MM, and incubate for 1 h at 37°C, to represent the neutralization step in the test proper. At least 0.5 ml of each mixture is required.

4. Using a multi-channel pipette, aspirate the GM from the wells of the microtitre plate, which should contain confluent cell monolayers. Replace by 0.1 ml of MM. Add 0.1 ml of each virus dilution to at least 4 wells of the plate.

5. Include 1 row of 4 or more 'cell' controls, containing 0.2 ml of MM only, to test for non-specific degeneration of the cell sheet during subsequent incubation.

6. Incubate the plate under the optimum conditions for virus growth (e.g. 36–37°C for Coxsackie B viruses) until clear CPE (or other effect, e.g. haemadsorption) develops at the lowest dilutions of virus.

7. Score the individual wells in the plate as infected or uninfected, and using the method of Reed & Muench described in Chapter 49, calculate the TCID50. The value obtained is the number of TCID50/0.1 ml of virus stock.

Micro-neutralization test for measurement of virus-specific antibody

1. Prepare microtitre plate(s) as for virus titration.

2. Next day, heat-inactivate test serum samples at 56°C for 30 min. Make serial two-fold dilutions of the inactivated serum in MM from, say, 1 in 10 to 1 in 320.

3. Next, dilute stock virus in MM to give 100 TCID50/0.1 ml. For example, if the virus titration gives a value of 10^7 TCID50/0.1 ml, then dilute the stock 1 in 10^5.

4. Mix an equal volume of diluted virus and each serum dilution. At least 0.5 ml of each mixture is required. Incubate at 37°C for 1 h (suitable conditions for most virus neutralizations).

5. It is necessary to include a back titration of virus to ensure that approximately 100 TCID50 was used in the test. Prepare several serial 10-fold dilutions of virus stock in MM. Mix each dilution with an equal volume of MM, and incubate as above.

6. Aspirate the medium from the wells of the microtitre plate(s). Replace by 0.1 ml of MM.

7. When incubation is complete, add 0.1 ml of virus-serum mixture to a minimum of 4 wells for each serum dilution. Also add 0.1 ml of each dilution of the virus control to a minimum of 4 wells.

8. High concentrations of serum alone may be toxic to the cell cultures. For serum controls, add 0.1 ml of a 1 in 10 dilution of each serum to 1 well on the plate.

9. Set up at least 4 cell control wells as for virus titration.

10. Incubate the plate under appropriate conditions until the virus controls show the desired pattern of CPE (indicating 100 TCID50). In the case of myxo- and paramyxoviruses, cultures are tested for haemadsorption after a suitable incubation period.

11. Determine the titre of the serum as the highest dilution eliminating infectivity in 50% of the 4 replicates of virus-serum mixtures. The method of Reed & Muench may be used to determine the 50% endpoint. Sera with a titre of 320 or greater will need to be retitrated at higher dilutions.

Cell culture tests for detection of bacterial toxins

Clostridium difficile cytotoxin

Post-antibiotic treatment diarrhoea may be associated with *C. difficile* infection (Ch. 38). To test for the presence of *C. difficile* cytotoxin in faeces, the following method may be used. (A quantitative procedure with microtitre plates is described in the *Methods* section of Ch. 38).

A faecal sample is prepared as for virus culture (see above).

1. Pipette 0.25 ml of sterile PBS into a 13 × 75 mm tube.

2. Pipette 0.25 ml of *C. sordelli* antitoxin (Wellcome) diluted 1 in 20 into another tube.

3. 0.25 ml of the 10–15% faecal suspension is added to each tube.

4. 0.25 ml from each tube is inoculated into one Hep-2 and one human foreskin fibroblast cell culture.

5. Working stocks of antitoxin are kept at 4°C and the concentrated antitoxin is stored at −20°C.

6. In the control (PBS) tubes, the presence of *C. difficile* toxin will produce a characteristic cytotoxic effect. This should be absent in the tubes containing antitoxin. Note that the CPE is usually evident within 24 h, but low levels of the toxin may not always be evident by then. It is therefore prudent to hold cultures for 48 h before reporting.

Escherichia coli enterotoxins

The detection of the toxins of *E. coli* strains that may be associated with diarrhoea makes use of various biological tests for toxins (Ch. 28). Other approaches include detection of the genes for enterotoxin production with nucleic acid probes, either excised inserts from plasmids labelled with ^{32}P (Moseley et al 1980) or synthetic oligonucleotide probes labelled with phosphatase (Peng Li et al 1987). ETEC kits based on oligonucleotide probes described by the latter authors are available from BRESA or Dupont. The biological tests include the ability of the heat-labile toxin of *E.coli* to alter the morphology of Chinese hamster ovary cells or Yl adrenal cells (Donta et al 1974, Guerrant et al 1974, Sack & Sack 1975). The latter authors should be consulted for details of media and propagation of the cells required for these tests.

Cell culture methods required for EBV antibody tests

For immunofluorescence (IF) tests to detect antibody to Epstein-Barr virus (EBV) use lymphoblastoid cells replicating virus (productive infection with presence of virion proteins) as targets. Commonly used lines are P₃HRl, derived from a patient with Burkitt's lymphoma, and B95–8, which are marmoset lymphocytes transformed in vitro with EBV. These cell types are suitable for the measurement of specific IgG, IgM or IgA antibodies to virus capsid antigens. Smears of the cells with the replicating virus are prepared on slides and examined by IF. For general notes on imunofluorescence methodology, refer to Chapters 10 and 49.

Propagation of lymphoblastoid cells

Growth medium is prepared as follows:

RPMI 1640	80 ml
Fetal calf serum	10 ml
NaHCO₃ (4.4% w/v)*	5 ml
Gentamicin	4 mg
Adjust pH to 7.4	

Method. Use 75 cm² cell culture flasks. Cells

require 'splitting' 1 to 5 every 4–7 days according to growth rate. To subculture, remove 10 ml of cell suspension and add to 40 ml of fresh growth medium in a 75 cm² flask. Record passage number and date.

Preparation of cell smears

Materials and reagents
10 ml conical centrifuge tubes.
Teflon-coated multiwell slides.
Cell counting chamber.
Fixative: cold acetone (−20°C) saturated with anhydrous $CaSO_4$ and filtered just before use (15 g $CaSO_4$/500 ml acetone).
Phosphate buffered saline (PBS) pH 7.4.

Method
1. Count* and adjust the lymphoblastoid cell suspension to contain 10^6 viable cells/ml.
2. Wash 10 ml of suspension twice in PBS.
3. Resuspend in 1 ml of PBS.
4. Add 1–2 μl of cell suspension to each well on slides. Dry under a fan and leave at room temperature for 1 h.
5. Immerse in fixative (−20°C) for 10 min. Dry under a fan.
6. Prepared slides may be stored for up to 6 months at −20°C provided they are kept dry. An airtight box containing silica gel is recommended for this purpose.

METHODS

Trypsin solution (0.25% w/v)

Trypsin (Difco 1:250)	2.5 g
Dulbecco's phosphate buffered saline (PBS) without calcium or magnesium (Solution A, see below)	1000 ml

Stir solution vigorously at room temperature for 4–5 h. Adjust pH to 7.4–7.5. Sterilize by membrane filtration.

To check the sterility of the trypsin preparation, pipette aseptically 0.1 ml from each 10 ml amount into 5 ml glucose broth. Incubate for 7 days at 37°C.

Tests for activity of trypsin

It is necessary from time to time to check the activity of the trypsin used in solutions to disaggregate the cells of tissues such as monkey kidney or human amnion. Two methods are given below.

Prepare a series of about 10 doubling dilutions, from 1 in 10 onwards, of the trypsin solution in Hanks' balanced salt solution (see below). Place 1 drop of each dilution on a strip of X-ray film together with 1 drop of Hanks' solution as a control. The strip is then placed on moist blotting paper in a Petri dish, covered and incubated for 30 min at 37°C. Remove the strip and allow to cool to room temperature, or run cold water over the reverse side (no film) until the gelatin has set firmly. Now flood the whole film gently with cold water. Wherever trypsin was present the gelatin will have been digested to water-soluble products and a punched out hole will appear in the film; the potency of the preparation is indicated by the endpoint. The control area (Hanks' solution) is not dissolved at all.

Alternatively, prepare a series of doubling dilutions of the trypsin solution in Hank's solution in 5 ml amounts. To each dilution, and a control tube containing Hanks' solution only, add a charcoal gelatin disc (Oxoid). Incubate for 90 min at 37°C. Examine every 30 min for trypsin activity, i.e. charcoal particles in suspension.

Trypsin-EDTA solution

EDTA (Disodium
  ethylenediaminetetra-acetic acid) 0.2 g
Trypsin (Difco 1:250) 1.0 g
Dulbecco's phosphate buffered
  saline (PBS) without
  magnesium or calcium 1000 ml

Stir solution vigorously at room temperature for 3–5 h. Adjust pH to 7.4–7.5. Sterilize by membrane filtration.

Sodium bicarbonate solution (1.4, 4.4 and 8.0%)

$NaHCO_3$ 14 g, or 44 g, or 80 g
Water 1000 ml

Dissolve $NaHCO_3$ in distilled water. Add a few drops 1% phenol red (see below) and pass CO_2 through the solution until colour is pale pink. Distribute in 1 oz bottles with as little air space as possible and screw caps on tightly. Autoclave for 20 min at 115°C. Store at 4°C.

Phenol red solution (1%)

Dissolve 10 g phenol red in 325 ml NaOH, 0.1 mol/l. Make up to 1000 ml with distilled water. Distribute in 20 ml amounts. Autoclave for 15 min at 121°C.

Hanks' balanced salt solution (BSS)

Stock solution A

1. NaCl 160 g
   KCl 8 g
   $MgSO_4.7H_2O$ 2 g
   $MgCl_2.6H_2O$ 2 g
   Distilled water 800 ml

2. $CaCl_2$ 2.8 g
   Distilled water 100 ml

Mix these two solutions slowly and make up volume to 1000 ml with distilled water. Add 2 ml chloroform and store at 4°C.

Stock solution B

$Na_2HPO_4.12H_2O$ 3.04 g
KH_2PO_4 1.2 g
Glucose 20 g
Distilled water 800 ml

When chemicals have dissolved add 100 ml of 0.4 % phenol red in NaOH (see below). Make up volume to 1000 ml with distilled water. Add 2 ml chloroform and store at 4°C.

Phenol red 0.4%

Dissolve 4 g phenol red in 325 ml NaOH 0.1 mol/litre. Make up to 1000 ml with distilled water. Distribute in 20 ml amounts. Autoclave for 15 min at 121°C.

Note. For some work, e.g. the fluorochrome detection of mycoplasmas with Hoechst 33258 stain, the phenol red solution is omitted.

For use

Stock solution A	100 ml
Stock solution B	100 ml
Distilled water	800 ml

Dispense in 100 ml amounts. Sterilize by auto-claving at 121°C for 20 min. Store at 4°C.

Dulbecco's phosphate buffered saline (PBS)

Solution A

NaCl	8 g
KCl	0.2 g
Na_2HPO_4	1.15 g
KH_2PO_4	0.2 g
Distilled water	1000 ml

Add a few drops of 1% aqueous phenol red (see above) until the solution is pale pink. The pH should be 7.3. Distribute in 100 ml amounts and autoclave for 20 min at 115°C. Store at 4°C.

Dulbecco's PBS solution B

$CaCl_2$	2.0 g
$MgCl_2.6H_2O$	2.0 g
Distilled water	100 ml

Dispense in 2.5 ml amounts in bijoux; sterilize for 20 min at 121°C. Store at 4°C.

Complete Dulbecco PBS

Add 0.5 ml solution B to 100 ml Dulbecco solution A to make the complete salt solution. The pH is 7.4.

Virus transport medium (VTM)

There are many formulations for VTM. For a laboratory using CMRL medium routinely, the following is recommended.

CMRL 1969 powder (Gibco, Flow)	10.8 g
HEPES	4.8 g
$NaHCO_3$	1.0 g
Benzylpenicillin	100 000 units
Gentamicin	40 mg
Sterile purified water	to 1 litre

Adjust pH to 7.2 with 10 mol/l NaOH (c. 0.5 ml), dispense aseptically into 4 ml amounts and store at 4°C.

Determination of cell numbers and viability

Dispersed cells are routinely counted using a Neubauer type haemocytometer chamber. When diluting cells for counting, a vital stain may be incorporated into the dilution media. Viable cells, which exclude the stain, can then be distinguished from stained non-viable cells. Trypan blue is commonly used for this purpose (see below).

1. Disperse cells and dilute 0.1 ml of cell suspension with 0.9 ml trypan blue solution in a separate container.

2. Moisten the supporting ridges of the haemocytometer chamber and apply coverslip.

3. After cells have sat for 4–5 min in trypan blue solution, resuspend and fill both sides of the chamber without overflowing.

4. Count the number of cells in the four corner squares and in the centre square of each side (10 squares).

5. Calculate the number of cells in the original suspension. Each square represents an area of $1 mm^2$ and has a depth of 0.1 mm. Therefore, the volume held by each square is $0.1 mm^3$ and the sample volume is 10×0.1 or $1 mm^3$. To determine the cell concentration of the original flask the following formula is used:

Number of cells counted × 10 (dilution factor) × 1000 (no. of mm^3 in $1 cm^3$) = number of cells/ml.

For example: when 250 cells are counted in 10 squares, the cell concentration in original solution = $250 \times 10 \times 1000 = 2.5 \times 10^6$ cells/ml.

6. To determine viability, count both stained and non-stained cell in a given area (at least 100 cells should be counted). The percentage number of viable cells is calculated as follows:

$$\frac{\text{Number of non-stained cells}}{\text{Number of stained and non-stained cells}} \times 100$$

Trypan blue solution

Trypan blue (vital stain, C.I. 23850)	0.40 g
NaCl	0.81 g

K_2HPO_4	0.06 g
Methyl *p*-hydroxybenzoate	0.05 g
Water	900 ml

Heat mixture to boiling, cool and adjust pH to 7.2–7.3 with 1 mol/l NaOH (approximately 8 drops). Adjust final volume to 1000/ml.

Sterility testing

The methods described by McGarrity (1979) for testing serum and media for bacterial and fungal contamination are presented.

Serum

1. Prepare duplicate sets of the following:
   a. Fluid thioglycollate broth, 5 ml/tube.
   b. Trypticase soy broth, 5 ml/tube.
   c. Sabouraud dextrose broth, 5 ml/tube.
   d. Sterile disposable tube.
   e. Blood agar plate.
2. Aseptically remove a 10 ml aliquot of serum for testing.
3. Add 3.0 ml serum to each disposable tube.
4. Add 0.5 ml serum to the remaining tubes.
5. Inoculate 0.1 ml on to each blood agar plate.
6. Incubate one rack of tubes and one agar plate at 37°C and the other set at 30°C.

7. Check the tubes daily for 2 weeks for evidence of contamination.

Medium

Culture medium is tested in the same manner as serum except that only one set of tubes and one agar plate are used (McGarrity 1979). These are incubated at 37°C and observed for 7–10 days. Medium should be sterility tested before antibiotics are added. If large batches of medium are filtered, samples for sterility testing are taken at the beginning, middle and end of the filtration process.

Cell cultures

Cell cultures are tested for contamination with *bacteria* or *fungi* as follows:

If cells are routinely grown in media containing antibiotics, establish some cultures without antibiotics when subdividing.

Examine cultures after several passages without antibiotics using the methods described for serum sterility test. Include both cells and culture fluid in the inoculum.

Tests for *Mycoplasma* in cell culture are described in Chapter 45.

REFERENCES

Armstrong D 1973 Contamination of tissue culture by bacteria and fungi. In: Fogh J (ed) Contamination in tissue culture. Academic Press, New York. p 51–64

Coombs R R A, Daniel M R, Gurner B W, Kelas A 1961 Recognition of the species of origin of cells in culture by mixed agglutination. 1. Use of antisera to red cells. Immunology 4:55

Donta S T, Moon H W, Whipp S C 1974 Detection of heat-labile *Escherichia coli* enterotoxin with the use of adrenal cells in tissue culture. Science 183: 334–336

Douglas W H J, Dell'Orco R T 1979 Physical aspects of a tissue culture laboratory. In: Jakoby W, Pastan I (eds) Methods in enzymology vol 58. Academic Press, New York. p 3–18

Duncan I B R, Bell E J 1961 Human amnion tissue culture in the routine virus laboratory. British Medical Journal 2:863

Fogh J (ed) 1973 Contamination in tissue culture. Academic Press, New York

Freshney R I 1983 Culture of animal cells: a manual of basic technique. Wiley, New York

Gartler S M 1967 Genetic markers as tracer in tissue cultures. National Cancer Institute Monograph USA 26:167

Good N E, Winget G D, Winder W, Connolly T N, Izawa S, Singh R M M 1966 Hydrogen ion buffers for virological research. Biochemistry 5:467

Green A 1973 Human biopsy material from genetic abnormalities. In: Kruse P F, Patterson M K (eds) Tissue culture methods and applications. Academic Press, New York. p 69–72

Greene A E, Coriell L L, Charney J 1964 A rapid cytotoxic antibody test to determine species of cell cultures. Journal of the National Cancer Institute 32:779

Guerrant R L, Brunton L L, Schnaitman T C, Rebhun L I, Gilman A G 1974 Cyclic adenosine monophosphate and alteration of chinese hamster ovary cell morphology: a rapid, sensitive in vitro assay for the enterotoxins of *Vibrio cholerae* and *Escherichia coli*. Infection and Immunity 10: 320–327

Ham R G, McKeehan W L 1979 Media and growth requirements. In: Jakoby W B, Pastan I H (eds) Methods in enzymology vol 58. Academic Press. p 44–93

Hayflick L 1965 The limited in vitro lifetime of human

diploid cell strains. Experimental Cell Research 37: 614–636

Hayflick L, Moorehead P S 1961 The serial cultivation of human diploid cell strains. Experimental Cell Research 25:585

Jakoby W B, Pastan I H (eds) 1979 Methods in enzymology vol 58. Academic Press, New York

Kruse P F, Patterson M K 1973 Tissue culture methods and applications. Academic Press, New York

Lennette E H, Schmidt N J 1979 Diagnostic procedures for viral, rickettsial and chlamydial infections, 5th edn. American Public Health Association, Washington

McGarrity G J 1979 Detection of contamination. In: Jakoby W B, Pastan I H (eds) Methods in enzymology vol 58. Academic Press, New York. p 18–29

McLimans W F 1979 Mass culture of mammalian cells. In: Jakoby W B, Pastan I H (eds) Methods in enzymology vol 58. Academic Press, New York. p. 194–211

Madeley C R 1977 Guide to the collection and transport of virological specimens. World Health Organization, Geneva

Moffat M A J 1973 Some cell culture procedures in diagnostic medical virology. In: Kruse P F, Patterson M K (eds) Tissue culture methods and applications. Academic Press, New York. p 611–617

Moseley S L, Huq I, Alim A R M A, So M, Samadpour-Motalebi M, Falkow S 1980 Detection of enterotoxigenic *Escherichia coli* by DNA colony hybridization. Journal of Infectious Diseases 142: 892–898

Nelson-Rees W A, Daniels D W, Flandermeyer R R 1981 Cross-contamination of cells in culture. Science 212: 446–452

Paul J 1970 Cell and tissue culture, 4th edn. Livingstone, Edinburgh

Peng Li, Medon P P, Skingle D C, Lanser J A, Symons R H 1987 Enzyme-linked synthetic oligonucleotide probes: non-radioactive detection of enterotoxigenic *Escherichia coli* in faecal specimens. Nucleic Acids Research 15: 5275–5287

Perlman D 1979 Use of antibiotics in cell culture media. In: Jakoby W B, Pastan I H (eds) Methods in

enzymology vol 58. Academic Press, New York. p 110–116

Peterson W D, Simpson W F, Hukku B 1979 Cell culture characterization: monitoring for cell identification. In: Jakoby W B, Pastan I H (eds) Methods in enzymology vol 58. Academic Press, New York. p 164–178

Sack D A, Sack R B 1975 Test for enterotoxigenic *Escherichia coli* using Y1 adrenal cells in miniculture. Infection and Immunity 11: 334–336

Schmidt N J 1972 Tissue culture in the laboratory diagnosis of viral infections. American Journal of Clinical Pathology 57:820

Schmidt N J 1979 Cell culture techniques for diagnostic virology. In: Lennette E H, Schmidt N J (eds) Diagnostic procedures for viral, rickettsial and chlamydial infections, 5th edn. American Public Health Association, Washington. p 65–139

Shipman C 1973 Control of culture pH with synthetic buffers. In: Kruse P F, Patterson M K (eds) Tissue culture methods and applications. Academic Press, New York. p 709–712

Simpson W F, Stulberg C S 1963 Species identification of animal cell strains by immunofluorescence. Nature (London) 199:616

Stanley M A, Parkinson E K 1979 Growth requirements of human cervical epithelial cells in culture. International Journal of Cancer 24: 407–414

Stulberg C S 1973 Extrinsic cell contamination of tissue culture. In: Fogh J (ed) Contamination in tissue culture. Academic Press, New York. p 2–27

Tyrrell D A J, Bynoe M L 1965 Cultivation of a novel type of common-cold virus in organ cultures. British Medical Journal 1:1467

Waymouth C 1973 Determination and survey of osmolality in culture media. In: Kruse P F, Patterson M K (eds) Tissue culture methods and applications. Academic Press, New York. p 703–709

White D O, Fenner F J 1986 Medical virology, 3rd edn. Academic Press, New York

Wolf K 1979 Laboratory management of cell cultures. In: Jakoby W B, Pastan I (eds) Methods in enzymology vol 58. Academic Press, New York. p 116–119

Appendix 1

Abbreviations and conversion factors

Mass

g = gram
kg = kilogram (1 kg = 1000 g)
mg = milligram (1 mg = 10^{-3} g)
μg = microgram (1 μg = 10^{-6} g)
ng = nanogram (1 ng = 10^{-9} g)
pg = picogram (1 pg = 10^{-12}g)
lb = pound weight avoirdupois (1 lb = 453.6 g)

Length and area

m = metre
cm = centimetre (1 cm = 10^{-2} m)
mm = millimetre (1 mm = 10^{-3} m)
μm = micrometre (1 μm = 10^{-6} m)
nm = nanometre(1 nm = 10^{-9} m)
in = inch (1 inch = 2.54 cm)
ft = foot (1 ft = 12 in)
in^2 = square inch (1 in^2 = 6.45 cm^2)

Volume

l = litre (1 litre = 1.76 pints)
ml = millilitre (1 ml = 10^{-3} litre)
μl = microlitre (1 μl = 10^{-6} litre)
oz = fluid ounce (1 oz = 28.41 ml)
ft^3 = cubic foot (1 ft^3 = 28.3 litre)
1 pint = 568 ml
1 gallon (British Imperial) = 8 pints
= 4.55 litres

Dilutions

Dilutions are stated as integers, not as fractions. Thus, a 'ten-fold dilution' denotes a dilution of one part of the original material in ten of the final solution. This is a dilution of 10, not 1:10, and not 10^{-1} or $\frac{1}{10}$. Similarly, titres (endpoint dilutions) are positive numbers, not fractions.

Pressure

1 normal atmosphere
= 1 bar
= 14.7 lb per in^2 (p.s.i.)
= 760 mm Hg
= 10^5 Newtons/m^2 (N/m^2)
= 100 kiloPascals (kPa)
1 mm Hg = 133 Pascals (Pa)
= 13.6 mm water

Temperature

C = Centigrade or Celcius; F = Fahrenheit
Conversion of °C to °F:
x°C = (1.8x + 32)°F

Other abbreviations

h = hour
min = minute
s = second
mol = mole (gram-molecular weight)
• mol/litre = molar (M)
rev/min = revolutions per minute (rpm)
mV = millivolt
LD50 = average lethal dose
MLD = minimum lethal dose
MHD = minimum haemolytic dose
% = per cent. The percentage concentration of a solution is stated as g of solute per 100 ml of solution, i.e. (w/v). Unless otherwise indicated the solvent is *water*. % (v/v) = ml of substance per 100 ml of mixture.
g = force of gravity
iu = international unit

Appendix 2

Postal regulations

Precautions to be observed by users of micro-biological services in the delivery of specimens to their local laboratories are outlined in Chapter 15 (see also Health and Safety Commission 1986). When pathological specimens have to be packaged and sent by post, special safety regulations apply at national and international levels. They must be rigorously observed.

National regulations for inland post

For users in the UK, the Post Office Guide (1986) gives details of requirements that apply in Britain. Deleterious liquids or substances, though otherwise prohibited from transmission by post, may be sent by authorized persons for medical examination or analysis to a recognized medical laboratory or institute, or to a qualified medical or dental practitioner, or a veterinary surgeon. Parcel post must not be used. Specimens should be sent by first class letter post or Datapost services under clearly specified conditions. Members of the public are not permitted to send pathological specimens by post, unless arrangements are made under the direction of an authorized laboratory. Pathological specimens known or suspected to contain Hazard Group 4 pathogens are not accepted for transmission by post in the UK. Users of laboratory services in other countries must observe the equivalent national. postal regulations.

In general, pathological material to be sent by post should have three layers of containment incorporating sufficient absorbent wrapping to prevent any possible leakage from the package if the primary container is damaged. The first component is usually a robust sealed container such as a sealed glass ampoule with lyophilized material, or a small screw-capped glass bottle with a watertight seal, or a swab or specimen securely sealed in a plastic or glass tube. The second component may be a protective cardboard or plastic tube with stoppered ends, or a sealable plastic bag or equivalent. This item is in turn immobilized by suitable absorbent packing. The third component is usually a stout fibreboard or cardboard box (or a wooden or metal case) and will normally also contain relevant correspondence and details of the specimen. The box, sealed and labelled, may be posted directly or may be sent in a padded envelope (e.g. Jiffy Bag). The packet must be conspicuously marked and bear the words PATHOLOGICAL SPECIMEN: FRAGILE WITH CARE.

If receptacles are supplied by a laboratory or institute, they should be submitted to Postal Headquarters, 33 Grosvenor Place, London SW1X 1PX, for confirmation that they comply with the conditions.

National regulations for overseas post

National regulations must be observed by those who wish to send pathological material for medical examination or analysis overseas. In the UK, pathological specimens for medical examination or analysis are classified as Perishable Biological Substances. These may be sent only in letter packets between officially recognized laboratories. Details of special packing conditions and the special labels required may be obtained from the address shown above.

International regulations

The World Health Organization Biosafety Manual (1983) gives information on safe shipment of specimens and infectious substances, with details of the packaging requirements. The Post Office Guide or other national equivalent should be consulted for advice on Customs Regulations and special safety requirements that might apply.

References

Health and Safety Commission Health Services Advisory Committee 1986 Safety in health service laboratories: the labelling, transport and reception of specimens. HM Stationery Office, London

Post Office Guide 1986 London (available from regional head post offices or from Postal Headquarters, 33 Grosvenor Place, London, SW1 1PX)

World Health Organization 1983 Laboratory biosafety manual. WHO, Geneva.

Appendix 3

Addresses of manufacturers and suppliers

Manufacturer/supplier	Address in UK	Address overseas
3M	3M Health Care Morley Street Loughborough Leicestershire LE11 1EP	3M Medical Products Div 3M Center Saint Paul Minnesota 55144 USA
ABBOTT	Abbott Laboratories Ltd Diagnostics Division The Business Centre Molly Millars Lane Wokingham Berkshire RG11 2QZ	Abott Laboratories Diagnostics Division Abbott Park North Chicago Illinois 60064 USA
AMERSHAM	Amersham International White Lion Road Amersham Buckinghamshire HP7 9LL	Amersham International 2636 S. Clearbrook Drive Arlington Heights Illinois 60005 USA
AMES	from MILES	
API	API Lab Products Ltd Grafton Way Basingstoke Hants RG22 6H	bioMerieux Laboratory Reagents Marcy I'Etoile 69260 Charbonnieres les Bains France Analytab Products Inc 200 Express Street Plainview New York USA
ARMOUR	Armour Pharmaceutical Co St Leonards House St Leonards Road Eastbourne Sussex BN21 3YG	Armour Pharmaceutical Co Suite 4000 1 Sentry Parkway Blue Bell Pennsylvania 19044. USA
ATCC		American Type Culture Collection 12301 Parklawn Drive Rockville Maryland 20852–1776 USA

Manufacturer/supplier	Address in UK	Address overseas
ATLAS	Atlas Chemicals Honeywell & Stein Ltd Mill Lane Carshalton Surrey	Atlas Chemicals Division ICI America Inc Hill Top Research Inc Miamiville Ohio USA
BAIRD & TATLOCK	Baird & Tatlock (London) PO Box 1 Romford Essex RM1 1HA	
BAYER	Bayer UK Ltd Bayer House Strawberry Hill Newbury Berkshire RG13 1JA	Miles Pharmaceuticals 400 Morgan Lane West Haven Connecticut USA
BBL	from BECTON DICKINSON	
BDH	BDH Chemicals Ltd Broom Road Poole Dorset BH12 4NN	E.M. Diagnostics Systems 480 Democrat Road Gibbstown New Jersey 08027 USA
BECTON DICKINSON	Becton Dickinson UK Ltd Between Towns Road Cowley Oxford OX4 3LY	BBL Microbiology Systems P O Box 243 Cockeysville Maryland 21030 USA
BEECHAM	Beecham Research Beecham House Great West Road Brentford Middlesex TW8 9BD	Beecham Laboratories Executive Offices 501 Fifth Street Bristol Tennessee 37620 USA
BEHRING	Behring Diagnostics Hoechst UK Ltd 50 Salisbury Road Hounslow Middlesex TW4 6JH	Behring Diagnostics 10933 N Torrey Pines Road La Jolla California 92037 USA
BIOGENEX		BioGenex Laboratories 6529 Sierra Lane Dublin California 94568 USA
BIO-RAD	Bio-Rad Laboratories Ltd Caxton Way Watford Business Park Watford Hertfordshire WD1 8RP	Bio-Rad Laboratories Chemical Division 1414 Harbour Way South Richmond California 94804 USA
BOEHRINGER	Boehringer Corp Ltd Bell Lane Lewes East Sussex BN7 1LG	Boehringer GmbH Mannheim West Germany

Manufacturer/supplier	Address in UK	Address overseas
BOOTS-CELLTECH	Boots-Celltech Diagnostics Ltd 240 Bath Road Slough Berkshire SL1 4ET	
BRESA		Biotechnology Research Enterprises SA Pty Ltd GPO Box 498 Adelaide South Australia Australia
BROWNE	Albert Browne Ltd Chancery House Abbey Gate Leicester LE4 OAA	SBW Medical Packaging Inc 9075 Knight Road Houston Texas 77054 USA
CALBIOCHEM	Calbiochem-Behring Cambridge BioScience 42 Devonshire Road Cambridge CB1 2BL	Calbiochem-Behring Inc PO Box 12087 San Diego California 92112 USA
CALTAG		Caltag Laboratories PO Box 86 Waverley New South Wales 2024 Australia
CAMLAB	Camlab Ltd Nuffield Road Cambridge CB4 1TH	
CAMPBELL BRUSHES	Campbell Brushes Ltd Cromwell Street Dudley West Midlands	
CAPPELL	from DYNATECH	Cappell Laboratories 237 Lacey Street PO Box 37 West Chester Pennsylvania 19380 USA
CARTER-WALLACE		Carter-Wallace Pty Ltd 6 Aquatic Drive French Forest New South Wales 2086 Australia
COMMONWEALTH SERUM LABS		Commonwealth Serum Laboratories 54 Poplar Road Parkville Victoria 3052 Australia
COOKE		Cooke Laboratory Products Cooke Engineering Co 900 Slaters Lane Alexandria Virginia 22314 USA

Manufacturer/supplier	Address in UK	Address overseas
CPHL	Central Public Health Laboratory 61 Colindale Avenue London NW9 5HT	
DAKOPATTS	from MERCIA	Dakopatts a/s Produktionsvej 42 PO Box 1359 DK-2600 Glostrup Denmark
DENLEY	Denley Instruments Ltd Natts Lane Billingshurst Sussex RH14 9EY	
DIAMED	from MAST	
DIFCO	Difco Laboratories PO Box 14B Central Avenue East Molesey Surrey KT8 OSE	Difco Laboratories Inc Box 1058A Detroit Michigan 48232 USA
DISPOSABLE PRODUCTS		Disposable Products PO Box 90 Ingle Farm 5095 South Australia Australia
DRG	DRG Hospital Supplies 1–3 Dixon Road Brislington Bristol BS4 5QY	DRG Medical Packaging Inc One University Plaza Hackensack New Jersey 07601 USA
DUPONT	DuPont (UK) Biotechnology Division Wedgewood Way Stevenage Hertfordshire SG1 4QN	Dupont Biotechnology Barley Mill Plaza Chandler Building Wilmington Delaware 19898 USA
DYNATECH	Dynatech Laboratories Ltd Daux Road Billingshurst West Sussex RH14 9SJ	Dynatech Laboratories Inc 14340 Sulleyfield Circle Chantilly Virginia 22021 USA
EDWARDS	Edwards High Vacuum Manor Royal Crawley West Sussex RH10 2LW	Edwards High Vacuum Inc 3279 Grand Island Bd Grand Island New York 14072 USA
ELECTRONUCLEONICS	American Hospital Supply Station Road Didcot Oxfordshire OX11 7NP	Electro-Nucleonics Inc 4809 Auburn Avenue Bethesda Maryland 20014 USA

Manufacturer/supplier	Address in UK	Address overseas
ELGA	Elga Ltd Lane End High Wycombe Buckinghamshire HP14 3JH	
ELKAY	Elkay Laboratories Ltd Unit 2 Crockford Lane Basingstoke Hampshire RG24 ONA	Elkay Products Inc 800 Boston Turnpike Shrewsbury Minnesota 01545 USA
ENZO BIOCHEM	from UNISCIENCE	Enzo-Biochemistry Inc 325 Hudson Street New York New York 10013 USA
ESSO	Esso Petroleum Co Ltd 106 London Road Kingston upon Thames Surrey KT2 6QX	
EVANS	Evans Medical Ltd 318 High Street North Dunstable Bedfordshire LU6 1BE	
EXOGEN	Exogen Clydebank Industrial Estate Beardmore Street Clydebank G81 4SA	
FALCON	from BECTON DICKINSON	
FLOW	Flow Laboratories Ltd Woodcock Hill Harefield Road Rickmansworth Hertfordshire WD3 1PQ	Flow Laboratories Inc 7655 Old Springhouse Road McLean Virginia 22102 USA
GALLENKAMP	Gallenkamp Belton Road West Loughborough Leicestershire LE11 0TR	Curtin Matheson Sci Inc 9999 Veterans Memorial Drive Houston Texas 77038 USA
GENETIC SYSTEMS		Genetic Systems 3005 First Avenue Seattle Washington 98121 USA
GEN PROBE		Gen Probe Inc 9620 Chesapeake Drive San Diego California 92123 USA

Manufacturer/supplier	Address in UK	Address overseas
GIBCO	Gibco Ltd PO Box 35 Trident House Renfrew Road Paisley PA3 4EF	Gibco Laboratory Life Technology Inc 3175 Staley Road Grand Island New York 14072 USA
GLAXO	Glaxo Laboratories Ltd Greenford Road Greenford Middlesex UB6 OHE	Glaxo Inc Five Moore Drive Box 13398 Research Triangle Park North Carolina 27709 USA
GULL LABS		Gull Laboratories 1011 East 4800 South Salt Lake City Utah 84117 USA
HARLECO		Harleco c/o Lab-Aids 1–3 Gondola Road Narrabeen 2102 New South Wales Australia
HENDLEY	C. A. Hendley Oakwood Hill Industrial Estate Loughton Essex IG10 3TZ	
HOECHST	Hoechst UK Ltd Hoechst House Salisbury Road Hounslow Middlesex TW4 6JH	Hoechst A. G. Postfach 800320 D-6230 Frankfurt Main 80 West Germany
HORWELL	Arnold Horwell Ltd 73 Maygrove Road West Hampstead London NW6 2PB	
ICN BIOMEDICALS	ICN Biomedicals Ltd Free Press House Castle Street High Wycombe Buckinghamshire HP13 6RN	ICN Biomedicals Inc ICN Plaza 3300 Hyland Avenue Costa Mesa California 92626 USA
INFRAKEM	Infrakem Ltd Unit 51D Bradley Hall Trading Estate Standish Wigan WN6 0XQ	
JANSSEN	Janssen Pharmaceuticals Grove Wantage Oxfordshire OX12 0DQ	Janssen Pharmaceutica N.V. Turnhoutsweg 30 B-2340 Beerse Belgium

Manufacturer/supplier	Address in UK	Address overseas
KIRKEGAARD & PERRY	from UNISCIENCE	Kirkegaard & Perry Inc 2 Cessna Court Gaithersburg Maryland 20879 USA
KOCH LIGHT	Koch Light Ltd Rookwood Way Haverhill Suffolk CB9 8PB	Genzyme Corporation 75 Kneeland Street Boston Massachusetts 02111 USA
KODAK	Kodak Ltd Kodak House Station Road Hemel Hempstead Hertfordshire HP1 1JU	Eastman Kodak Company 343 State Street Rochester New York 14650 USA
LAB M	Lab M Ltd Topley House PO Box 19 Bury Lancashire BL9 6AU	
LEEBROOK	Leebrook Scientific Ltd Claylands Cottage Works Claylands Road Bishop's Waltham Hampshire SO3 1BH	
LEITZ	E Leitz (Instruments) Ltd 48 Park Street Luton Bedfordshire LU1 3HP	Ernst Leitz D-6330 Wetzlar West Germany
LINBRO	from FLOW	
LINSCOTT	Linscott's Directory PO Box 55 East Grinstead Sussex RH19 3YL	
MA BIOPRODUCTS		Whittaker MA Bioproducts Inc PO Box 127 Biggs Ford Road Walkersville Maryland 21793 USA
MALLINCKRODT	from CAMLAB	Mallinckrodt Inc 675 McDonnell Boulevard Hazelwood St Louis Missouri 63134 USA
MARION	from MERCIA	Marion Scientific Corp Kansas City Missouri 64114 USA

Manufacturer/supplier	Address in UK	Address overseas
MAST	Mast Diagnostics Ltd Mast House Derby Road Bootle Merseyside L20 1EA	Mast Diagnostica GmbH Schubertstrasse D-2000 Hamburg 76 West Germany
MAY & BAKER	May & Baker Ltd Laboratory Products Liverpool Road Eccles Manchester M30 7RT	
MDH	Microflow Dent & Hellyer Walworth Road Andover Hampshire SP10 5AA	
MEDICAL WIRE	Medical Wire & Equipment Corsham Wiltshire SN13 9RT	Microdiagnostics 4090 Broadway New York New York 10032 USA
MERCIA	Mercia Diagnostics Ltd Brocades House West Byfleet Surrey KT14 6RA	
MILES	Miles Laboratories Ltd PO Box 37 Stoke Court Stoke Poges Slough SL2 4LY	Miles Laboratory Inc 30475 North Aurora Road Naperville Illinois 60566 USA
MILLIPORE	Millipore UK Ltd 11–15 Peterborough Road Harrow Middlesex HA1 2YH	Millipore Intertech PO Box 255 Bedford Massachusetts 01730 USA
MSD	Merck Sharp & Dohme Ltd Hertford Road Hoddesdon Road Hertfordshire EN11 9BU	Merck and Co Inc PO Box 2000 Rahway New Jersey USA
MSE	MSE Scientific Ltd Sussex Manor Park Gatwick Road Crawley Sussex RH10 2QQ	
NCTC	National Collection of Type Cultures Central Public Health Laboratories 61 Colindale Avenue London NW9 5HT	
NELSON	from MSE	

Manufacturer/supplier	Address in UK	Address overseas
NIAID		National Institute of Allergy & Infectious Diseases Bethesda Maryland 20014 USA
NORIT	Norit-Clydesdale Co Ltd 147 Millerstone Street Glasgow G31 1TG	
NORWICH–EATON	Norwich–Eaton Ltd Hedley House St Nicholas Avenue Gosforth Newcastle-upon-Tyne NE3 1LR	Norwich–Eaton Pharmaceuticals Inc PO Box 191 Norwich New York 13815 USA
NUNC	from GIBCO	
ORGANON	Organon-Teknika Ltd Science Park Milton Road Cambridge CB4 4BH	Organon-Teknika Corp 5300 SO Portland Avenue PO Box 19080 Oklahoma City Oklahoma 73144 USA
ORION	from GIBCO	Orion Diagnostica PO Box 83 SF-02101 Espoo Finland
ORTHO		Ortho Diagnostic Systems Raritan New Jersey 08869 USA
OXFORD	from BOEHRINGER	Oxford Laboratories Foster City California USA
OXOID	Oxoid Ltd Wade Road Basingstoke Hampshire RG24 OPW	Oxoid USA Inc 9017 Red Branch Road Columbia Maryland 21045 USA
PACIFIC		Pacific Diagnostics PO Box 309 Eastwood South Australia 5063 Australia
PAINES & BYRNE	Paines & Byrne Ltd Pabyrn Laboratories Bilton Road Greenford Middlesex UB6 7HG	
PENNSYLVANIA REFINING		Pennsylvania Refining Co Butler Pennsylvania USA

Manufacturer/supplier	Address in UK	Address overseas
PERMUTIT	The Permutit Company Ltd Permutit House 632/652 London Road Isleworth Middlesex TW7 4EZ	Portals Water Treatment 4328 N United Parkway Schiller Park Illinois 60176 USA
PFIZER	Pfizer Ltd Ramsgate Road Sandwich Kent CT13 9NJ	Pfizer Inc 235 East 42nd Street New York New York 10017 USA
PHARMACIA	Pharmacia Diagnostics Ltd Pharmacia House Midsummer Boulevard Milton Keynes Buckinghamshire MK9 3HP	Pharmacia Fine Chemicals Box 175 S-751 82 Uppsala Sweden Electro-Nucleonics Inc 350 Passaic Avenue Fairfield New Jersey 07006 USA
PHASE SEP	Phase Separations Ltd Deeside Industrial Park Queensferry Clwyd CH5 2NU	Phase Sep Inc 140 Water Street Norwalk Connecticut 06854 USA
RACAL	Racal Amplivox Beresford Avenue Wembley Middlesex HAO 1RU	
RADLEYS	Radleys London Road Sawbridgeworth Hertfordshire CM21 9JH	
RAVEN	Raven Scientific Ltd PO Box 2 Sturmer End Haverhill Suffolk CB9 7UU	
ROCHE	Roche Products Ltd Diagnostics Division PO Box 8 Welwyn Garden City Hertfordshire AL7 3AY	F. Hoffman-La Roche 4002 Basle Switzerland Roche Diagnostics Hoffman La Roche Inc 340 Kingsland Street Nutley New Jersey 07110 USA
SCANBUR		Scanbur Ltd Gl. Lellingegaard Bakkeleddet 9 DK 4600 Koge Denmark

Manufacturer/supplier	Address in UK	Address overseas
SERA-LAB	Sera-Lab Ltd Crawley Down Sussex RH10 4FF	
SEWARD	from OXOID	
SIGMA	Sigma Chemical Co Ltd Fancy Road Poole Dorset BH17 7NH	Sigma Chemical Co PO Box 14508 St Louis Missouri 63178 USA
SILENUS		Silenus Laboratories Pty 5 Guest Street Hawthorn Victoria 3122 Australia
SOUTHERN GROUP LABS	Southern Group Laboratories Hither Green Hospital Hither Green Lane London SE13 6RU	
STERILIN	Sterilin Ltd Sterilin House Clockhouse Lane Feltham Middlesex TW14 8QS	Bellco Glass PO Box 8 340 Edrudo Road Vineland New Jersey 08360 USA
STERISEAL	Steriseal Ltd Thornhill Road Redditch Worcestershire B98 9NL	
SUPELCO	from RADLEYS	Supelco Inc Supelco Park Bellefonte Pennsylvania 16823–0048 USA
SURGIKOS	Surgikos Ltd Kirkton Campus Livingston West Lothian EH54 7AT	
SYVA	Syva UK Syntex House St Ives Road Maidenhead Berkshire SL6 1RD	Syva Company 900 Arastradero Road Palo Alto California 94304 USA
TCS	Tissue Culture Services 2 Perth Estates Perth Avenue Slough SL1 4XX	

Manufacturer/supplier	Address in UK	Address overseas
TECHNICAL SERVICES	Technical Services Consultant PO Box 31 Bury Lancashire BL9 5RA	
THOMAS	from HORWELL	Thomas Scientific Arthur H Thomas Company 99 High Hill Road PO Box 99 Swedesboro New Jersey 08085–0099 USA
TURNER	James Turner Ltd Fleming Road Speke Liverpool L24 9LS	
UNISCIENCE	Uniscience Ltd 12–14 St Ann's Crescent Wandsworth London SW18 2LS	
UPJOHN	Upjohn Ltd Fleming Way Crawley Sussex RH10 2NJ	
VERNON–CARUS	Vernon–Carus Ltd Penwortham Mills Preston Lancashire PR1 9SN	
VIRION	Damon/IEC (UK) Ltd Lawrence Way Brewers Hill Road Dunstable Bedfordshire LU6 1BD	Virion GmbH Bron Bachergasse 18a D-8700 Wurzburg West Germany
WEBSTER		Arthur Webster Pty Ltd 226 Windsor Road Northmead New South Wales 2152 Australia
WELLCOME	Wellcome Diagnostics Temple Hill Dartford Kent DA1 5AH	Wellcome Diagnostics PO Box 100 Beaconsfield New South Wales 2014 Australia Burroughs Wellcome Corp Reagents Division 3030 Cornwallis Road Research Triangle Park North Carolina 27709 USA

Manufacturer/supplier	Address in UK	Address overseas
WHATMAN	Whatman LabSales Ltd Unit 1 Coldred Road Parkwood Maidstone Kent ME15 9XN	Whatman LabSales Inc 9 Bridewell Place Clifton New Jersey 07014 USA
WHITLEY	Don Whitley Scientific Ltd 14 Otley Road Shipley West Yorkshire BD17 7SE	Tekmar Company PO Box 371856 Cincinnati Ohio 45222-1856 USA
YOUNG	Archd Young & Son Ltd 37/39 Constitution Street Edinburgh EH6 7BG	
ZEISS	Carl Zeiss Ltd PO Box 78 Woodfield Road Welwyn Garden City Hertfordshire AL7 1LU	Carl Zeiss PO Box 1369–1380 D-7082 Oberkochen West Germany

Index